We dedicate this book to our wives (Ruti, Rosie, and Jane) and children,
whose patience, understanding, and support for this book,
and all our academic pursuits are taxed beyond measure.
You are our inspiration.

Contents

Contributors

Paul C. Adams, MD
Professor, Department of Medicine
University of Western Ontario
Division of Gastroenterology
Department of Medicine
London Health Sciences Centre, University Campus
London, Ontario, Canada
Iron Overload Diseases

Tracey D. Arnell, MD
Assistant Professor of Surgery
Harbor-UCLA Medical Center
Torrance, California
Diverticular Disease of the Colon

Nathan M. Bass, MD, PhD
Professor of Medicine
Medical Director, Liver Transplant Program
Division of Gastroenterology; Department of Medicine
University of California San Francisco
San Francisco, California
Drug-Induced Liver Disease

D. Montgomery Bissell, MD
Professor of Medicine
Director, Division of Gastroenterology & Liver Center
Department of Medicine
University of California, San Francisco
Attending Physician
University of California Hospitals & San Francisco
General Hospital Medical Center
San Francisco, California
Hepatic Porphyrias

Richard S. Bloomfeld, MD
Assistant Professor of Medicine
Section of Gastroenterology
Department of Medicine
Wake Forest University School of Medicine
Winston-Salem, North Carolina
Miscellaneous Disorders of the Esophagus

Henry C. Bodenheimer, Jr., MD
Chief, Division of Digestive Diseases
Beth Israel Medical Center
New York, New York
Complications of Chronic Liver Disease

Randall E. Brand, MD
Associate Professor of Medicine
Division of Gastroenterology
Department of Medicine
Evanston Northwestern Healthcare
Evanston, Illinois
Tumors of the Pancreas

Lawrence J. Brandt, MD
Professor of Medicine & Surgery
Albert Einstein College of Medicine
Chief of Gastroenterology
Montefiore Medical Center & Albert Einstein
    College of Medicine
Bronx, New York
Mesenteric Vascular Disease

Robert S. Bresalier, MD
Director, Gastrointestinal Oncology
Division of Gastroenterology
Henry Ford Health Hospital
Detroit, Michigan
Malignant & Premalignant Lesions of the Colon

Natalie H. Bzowej, MD, PhD
Assistant Clinical Professor
Division of Gastroenterology
Department of Medicine
University of California, San Francisco
Director, Clinical Hepatology Research
Division of Liver Transplantation
Department of Medicine
California Pacific Medical Center
San Francisco, California
Gastrointestinal Complications of Pregnancy

Michael Camilleri, MD
Atherton and Winifred W. Bean Professor
Professor of Medicine & Physiology
Mayo Medical School
Consultant in Gastroenterology & Hepatology
Mayo Clinic & Mayo Foundation
Rochester, Minnesota
Motility Disorders of the Stomach & Small Intestine

William D. Chey, MD
Associate Professor of Internal Medicine
Division of Gastroenterology
Department of Internal Medicine
University of Michigan
Ann Arbor, Michigan
Peptic Ulcer Disease

Heather J. Chial, MD
Instructor in Medicine
Mayo Medical School
Fellow in Gastroenterology & Hepatology
Mayo Clinic & Mayo Foundation
Rochester, Minnesota
Motility Disorders of the Stomach & Small Intestine

James C. Chou, MD
Associate Professor
School of Medicine
State University of New York at Stony Brook
Stony Brook, New York
Division of Gastroenterology, Hepatology, & Nutrition
Winthrop University Hospital
Mineola, New York
Esophageal Tumors

Albert J. Czaja, MD
Professor of Medicine
Division of Gastroenterology & Hepatology
Department of Medicine
Mayo Clinic & Mayo Medical School
Consultant, Gastroenterology & Hepatology
Division of Gastroenterology & Hepatology
Department of Medicine
Mayo Clinic
Rochester, Minnesota
Chronic Nonviral Hepatitis

Lorna Dove, MD, MPH
Assistant Professor of Medicine
Division of Digestive & Liver Diseases
Columbia-Presbyterian Medical Center
New York, New York
*Liver & Biliary Disease in Patients with Human
  Immunodeficiency Virus Infection*

J. Gregory Fitz, MD
Waterman Professor of Medicine and Head
Division of Gastroenterology & Hepatology
University of Colorado Health Sciences Center
Denver, Colorado
Approach to the Patient with Suspected Liver Disease

Chris E. Forsmark, MD
Associate Professor and Chief
Division of Gastroenterology, Hepatology, & Nutrition
Department of Medicine
University of Florida
Gainesville, Florida
Chronic Pancreatitis & Pancreatic Insufficiency

Rena Kramer Fox, MD
Assistant Clinical Professor of Medicine
Division of General Internal Medicine
Department of Medicine
University of California, San Francisco
San Francisco, California
Viral Hepatitis

Scott L. Friedman, MD
Chief
Division of Liver Diseases
Mount Sinai School of Medicine
New York, New York
*Liver & Biliary Disease in Patients with Human
  Immunodeficiency Virus Infection*

Ira S. Goldman, MD
Associate Professor of Clinical Medicine
Department of Medicine
New York University School of Medicine
New York, New York
Attending Physician
Division of Gastroenterology
Department of Medicine
North Shore University Hospital
Manhasset, New York
St. Francis Hospital
Roslyn, New York
Infections of the Liver

James H. Grendell, MD
Chief
Division of Gastroenterology, Hepatology, & Nutrition
Winthrop University Hospital
Mineola, New York
*Miscellaneous Disorders of the Stomach & Small Intestine
Acute Pancreatitis*

Frank G. Gress, MD
Associate Professor of Medicine
School of Medicine
State University of New York at Stony Brook
Stony Brook, New York
Chief of Endoscopy
Division of Gastroenterology, Hepatology, & Nutrition
Winthrop University Hospital
Mineola, New York
Esophageal Tumors

Adil Habib, MD
Assistant Professor of Medicine
Division of Gastroenterology
Medical College of Virginia
Virginia Commonwealth University
Associate Director, Liver Transplantation
McGuire Veterans Affairs Medical Center
Richmond, Virginia
The Liver in Systemic Disease

Samuel B. Ho, MD
Associate Professor of Medicine
Division of Gastroenterology
Department of Medicine
University of Minnesota
Staff Physician
Division of Gastroenterology
Department of Medicine
Veterans Affairs Medical Center
Minneapolis, Minnesota
Tumors of the Stomach & Small Intestine

Ira M. Jacobson, MD
Vincent Astor Professor of Clinical Medicine
Chief, Division of Gastroenterology & Hepatology
Weill Medical College of Cornell University
Attending Physician
Division of Gastroenterology & Hepatology
Department of Medicine
New York Presbyterian Hospital, Cornell Campus
New York, New York
Gallstones

William R. Jarnagin, MD
Assistant Professor of Surgery
Weill Medical College of Cornell University
Assistant Attending Surgeon
Division of Hepatobiliary Service
Department of Surgery
Memorial Sloan Kettering Cancer Center
New York, New York
Tumors of the Ampulla & Bile Ducts

Dennis M. Jensen, MD
Professor of Medicine
Division of Digestive Diseases
Department of Medicine
UCLA School of Medicine
Staff Physician
Division of Digestive Diseases
Department of Medicine
UCLA Center for the Health Sciences & VA Greater
Los Angeles Healthcare System
Los Angeles, California
Acute Upper Gastrointestinal Bleeding
Acute Lower Gastrointestinal Bleeding

Thomas A. Judge, MD
Assistant Professor of Medicine
Division of Gastroenterology
University of Pennsylvania School of Medicine
Philadelphia, Pennsylvania
Inflammatory Bowel Disease

Tya-Mae Y. Julien, MD
Clinical Fellow, Gastroenterology
Division of Gastroenterology
Department of Medicine
University of California—San Francisco
San Francisco, California
Miscellaneous Diseases of the Peritoneum & Mesentery

Rome Jutabha, MD
Associate Professor of Medicine
Division of Digestive Diseases
Department of Medicine
UCLA School of Medicine
Los Angeles, California
Acute Upper Gastrointestinal Bleeding

David J. Kearney, MD
Assistant Professor of Medicine
Division of Gastroenterology
Department of Medicine
University of Washington School of Medicine
Staff Physician
VA Puget Sound Health Care System
Seattle, Washington
Approach to the Patient with Gastrointestinal Disorders

Emmet B. Keeffe, MD
Professor of Medicine
Division of Gastroenterology & Hepatology
Department of Medicine
Stanford University School of Medicine
Chief of Hepatology
Co-Director, Liver Transplant Program
Stanford University School of Medicine
Stanford, California
Acute Liver Failure

Timothy P. Kinney, MD
Resident
Division of Internal Medicine
Department of Internal Medicine
Virginia Mason Medical Center
Seattle, Washington
Endoscopic Management of Biliary & Pancreatic Diseases

Lyn Knoblock, MD
Chief Resident
Division of General Surgery
Department of Surgery
University of Utah
Salt Lake City, Utah
Minimally Invasive Surgery for Gastrointestinal Diseases

Kavita Kongara, MD
Assistant Professor
School of Medicine
State University of New York at Stony Brook
Stony Brook, New York
Director, Gastrointestinal Diagnostic Motility Center
Director, Women's Center for Gastroenterology
Winthrop University Hospital
Mineola, New York
Esophageal Motility Disorders & Noncardiac Chest Pain

Richard A. Kozarek, MD
Clinical Professor of Medicine
Division of Gastroenterology
Department of Medicine
University of Washington
Chief
Division of Gastroenterology
Department of Medicine
Virginia Mason Medical Center
Seattle, Washington
Endoscopic Management of Biliary & Pancreatic Diseases

Douglas R. LaBrecque, MD
Professor of Internal Medicine
Director, Liver Service
University of Iowa College of Medicine
Iowa City, Iowa
Mass Lesions & Neoplasia of the Liver

John R. Lake, MD
Professor of Medicine and Surgery
Director, Division of Gastroenterology,
    Hepatology, & Nutrition
University of Minnesota Medical School
Director, Liver Transplantation Program
Fairview University Medical Center
Minneapolis, Minnesota
Liver Transplantation

Bret A. Lashner, MD, MPH
Director, Center for Inflammatory Bowel Disease
Department of Gastroenterology
Cleveland Clinic Foundation
Cleveland, Ohio
Miscellaneous Diseases of the Colon

Joel E. Lavine, MD, PhD
Professor of Pediatrics
Division of Gastroenterology & Nutrition
Department of Pediatrics
University of California, San Diego
Chief, Division of Gastroenterology & Nutrition
Department of Pediatrics
University of California, San Diego
    & Children's Hospital
San Diego, California
Pediatric Liver Disease

Gary R. Lichtenstein, MD
Associate Professor of Medicine
Division of Gastroenterology
Department of Medicine
Hospital of the University of Pennsylvania
Philadelphia, Pennsylvania
Inflammatory Bowel Disease

Keith D. Lindor, MD
Professor of Medicine
Division of Gastroenterology & Hepatology
Department of Internal Medicine
Mayo Clinic and Foundation
Chair; Consultant
Division of Gastroenterology & Hepatology
Mayo Clinic and Foundation
Rochester, Minnesota
Primary Disease of the Bile Ducts

Sarah A. Little, MB, ChB
Research Fellow, Division of Hepatobiliary Service
Department of Surgery
Memorial Sloan Kettering Cancer Center
New York, New York
Tumors of the Ampulla & Bile Ducts

Edward Lung, MD
Fellow, Division of Gastroenterology
Department of Medicine
University of California, San Francisco
San Francisco, California
Acute Diarrheal Diseases

Jacquelyn J. Maher, MD
Associate Professor of Medicine
Division of Gastroenterology
University of California—San Francisco
San Francisco, California
Alcoholic Liver Disease

George B. McDonald, MD
Professor, Division of Gastroenterology
Department of Medicine
University of Washington School of Medicine
Member and Head, Gastroenterology/Hepatology
    Section
Clinical Research Division
Fred Hutchinson Cancer Research Center
Seattle, Washington
*Hepatic Complications of Marrow & Stem
    Cell Transplantation*

Kenneth R. McQuaid, MD
Professor of Clinical Medicine
University of California—San Francisco
Director of Endoscopy
Section of Gastroenterology
San Francisco VA Medical Center
San Francisco, California
Dyspepsia & Nonulcer Dyspepsia

Sean J. Mulvihill, MD
Professor and Chair
Department of Surgery
University of Utah
University of Utah Health Sciences Center
Salt Lake City, Utah
Minimally Invasive Surgery for Gastrointestinal Diseases

Brent A. Neuschwander-Tetri, MD
Associate Professor of Internal Medicine
Division of Gastroenterology & Hepatology
Department of Internal Medicine
Saint Louis University
St. Louis, Missouri
The Liver in Systemic Disease

Don C. Rockey, MD
Associate Professor of Medicine
Director, Liver Center
Duke University Medical Center
Durham, North Carolina
Occult Gastrointestinal Bleeding

Thomas J. Savides, MD
Associate Professor of Clinical Medicine
Division of Gastroenterology
Department of Medicine
University of California, San Diego School
    of Medicine
San Diego, California
Acute Lower Gastrointestinal Bleeding

James M. Scheiman, MD
Associate Professor
Division of Gastroenterology
Department of Internal Medicine
University of Michigan Medical Center
Ann Arbor, Michigan
Peptic Ulcer Disease

Thomas D. Schiano, MD
Assistant Professor of Medicine
Division of Liver Diseases
Department of Medicine
The Mount Sinai Medical Center
New York, New York
Complications of Chronic Liver Disease

Lawrence R. Schiller, MD
Clinical Professor of Internal Medicine
University of Texas Southwestern Medical Center
Program Director, Gastroenterology Fellowship
Department of Internal Medicine
Baylor University Medical Center
Dallas, Texas
Malabsorption Disorders

Michael L. Schilsky, MD
Clinical Associate Professor of Medicine
Division of Liver Diseases
Department of Medicine
Recanati/Miller Transplantation Institute
The Mount Sinai School of Medicine
New York, New York
Copper Overload Diseases

James S. Scolapio, MD
Assistant Professor
Director of Nutrition
Division of Gastroenterology
Department of Medicine
Mayo Clinic Jacksonville
Jacksonville, Florida
*Nutritional Disorders & Their Treatment in Diseases
    of the Gastrointestinal Tract*

Edy Soffer, MD
Head
Center for Gastrointestinal Motility Disorders
Department of Gastroenterology
The Cleveland Clinic Foundation
Cleveland, Ohio
Esophageal Motility Disorders & Noncardiac Chest Pain

Stuart Jon Spechler, MD
Professor of Medicine
The University of Texas Southwestern Medical Center
    at Dallas
Chief, Division of Gastroenterology
Dallas Department of Veterans Affairs Medical Center
Dallas, Texas
Gastroesophageal Reflux Disease & Its Complications

Bruce E. Stabile, MD
Professor and Vice Chair, Department of Surgery
UCLA School of Medicine
Los Angeles, California
Chair, Department of Surgery
Harbor-UCLA Medical Center
Torrance, California
Diverticular Disease of the Colon

Nicholas J. Talley, MD, PhD
Professor of Medicine
University of Sydney
Nepean Hospital
Penrith, New South Wales, Australia
Functional Gastrointestinal Disorders

Raymond Thornton, MD
Department of Radiology
University of California, San Francisco
San Francisco, California
Imaging Studies in Gastrointestinal & Liver Diseases

Prashanthi N. Thota, MD
Fellow
Department of Gastroenterology & Hepatology
Cleveland Clinic Foundation
Cleveland, Ohio
Miscellaneous Diseases of the Colon

Rebecca W. Van Dyke, MD
Professor of Medicine
Division of Gastroenterology
University of Michigan School of Medicine
Attending Physician
University of Michigan Hospitals & Clinics
Staff Physician
Ann Arbor Veterans Administration
Ann Arbor, Michigan
Liver Disease in Pregnancy

Mark Lane Welton, MD
Associate Professor of Surgery
Chief, Colon & Rectal Surgery
Department of Surgery
Stanford University Medical Center
Stanford, California
Anorectal Diseases

C. Mel Wilcox, MD
Professor and Director
Division of Gastroenterology & Hepatology
Department of Medicine
University of Alabama Birmingham
Birmingham, Alabama
AIDS & the Gastrointestinal Tract

Teresa L. Wright, MD
Professor of Medicine
Division of Gastroenterology
Department of Medicine
University of California
Chief, Gastroenterology Section
Department of Veterans Affairs Medical Center
San Francisco, California
Viral Hepatitis

Wallace C. Wu, MBBS
Professor of Medicine
Section of Gastroenterology
Department of Medicine
Wake Forest University School of Medicine
Winston-Salem, North Carolina
Miscellaneous Disorders of the Esophagus

Judy Yee, MD
Associate Professor
Department of Radiology
University of California, San Francisco
Chief of Computed Tomography & Gastrointestinal
Radiology
Department of Radiology
VA Medical Center
San Francisco, California
Imaging Studies in Gastrointestinal & Liver Diseases

Rowen K. Zetterman, MD
Vice-Chair, Internal Medicine
University of Nebraska Medical Center
Interim Chief of Staff
Nebraska-Western Iowa HealthCare System
DVAMC
Omaha, Nebraska
Cystic Diseases of the Bile Duct & Liver

Preface

The second edition of *Current Diagnosis and Treatment in Gastroenterology* is a single-source reference for practitioners in both hospital and ambulatory settings, responding to a need for an up-to-date and accessible text covering all aspects of gastrointestinal and liver diseases with emphasis on practical features of diagnosis and patient management.

OUTSTANDING FEATURES

- Incorporation of up-to-date, cost-effective diagnostic approaches and therapeutic strategies.
- Comprehensive coverage of all major clinical aspects of gastrointestinal, hepatic, biliary, and pancreatic diseases.
- Authors are all experts who are currently directly involved in patient care and clinical teaching.
- Concise, readable format affording efficient use in various practice settings.
- Inexpensively priced.

INTENDED AUDIENCE

- Medical students and house officers will find the concise, clinically-oriented descriptions of diseases and their management, useful on a daily basis for both the care of patients and preparation for rounds and clinical conferences.
- Surgeons, family physicians, and internists who are not gastroenterologists will find this book helpful as an easy-to-use, ready reference and review.
- Nurses, nurse practitioners, physician's assistants, and other health care providers will appreciate the concise approach to clinical problems, combined with clear descriptions of the principles underlying the diagnosis and treatment of digestive diseases.

ORGANIZATION

The first chapter of *Current Diagnosis and Treatment in Gastroenterology* presents information on the general approach to the patient with symptoms and signs of gastrointestinal disease. Chapters 2–11 are symptom-oriented or relate to disease processes involving more than one organ such as gastrointestinal bleeding, acute diarrhea, functional disorders, and AIDS, as well as gastrointestinal problems related to pregnancy. Chapter 12 covers the evaluation and treatment of nutritional disorders. The rapidly evolving use of minimally invasive surgery for gastrointestinal diseases is summarized in Chapter 13. Chapter 14 describes the use of imaging studies for both gastrointestinal and liver diseases, and Chapter 15 covers the endoscopic management of biliary and pancreatic disease. Chapters 16–32 are organized by organ, providing information on diseases of the esophagus (Chapters 16–19), stomach and small intestine (Chapters 20–25), colon and rectum (Chapters 26–29), and pancreas (Chapters 30–32).

The final twenty-one chapters (33–54) consider diseases of the liver and bile ducts, beginning with a chapter on the approach to the patient with suspected liver disease. The subsequent chapters provide information on diseases of the liver and bile ducts both on the basis of etiology (eg, viral hepatitis, alcoholic liver disease) and on their impact on specific groups of patients (liver disease in children, during pregnancy, and following bone marrow transplantation). Individual chapters are also directed at liver failure, the liver in systemic disease, and liver transplantation.

ACKNOWLEDGMENTS

We would like to thank our chapter authors for their timely and practical contributions. We recognize that the time they spent in writing their manuscripts was at the expense of their families, to whom we extend our gratitude and apologies. We also would like to thank the editorial staff of McGraw-Hill for their expert assistance in working with the contributors and us to bring this second edition to publication. We particularly wish to acknowledge the support, guidance, and encouragement of Catherine Johnson, without whom this second edition would not have become a reality. To all of you we owe a debt of gratitude.

Scott L. Friedman, MD
Kenneth R. McQuaid, MD
James H. Grendell, MD
September 2002

SECTION I
General Approach to Gastrointestinal Diseases

Approach to the Patient with Gastrointestinal Disorders

David J. Kearney, MD

The primary functions of the gastrointestinal tract are the efficient processing of ingested nutrients and fluids and the elimination of undigested waste. The disruption of this process leads to a number of complaints. The cardinal symptoms that suggest gastrointestinal pathology are heartburn, dyspepsia, problems of swallowing (odynophagia and dysphagia), chest pain, hiccups, nausea and vomiting, gas, diarrhea, constipation, abdominal pain, weight loss, and occult or overt gastrointestinal bleeding. These symptoms may be attributable to problems intrinsic to the gastrointestinal tract or may be a manifestation of a systemic disorder. The complaints may represent minor problems that are easily corrected by a change in diet or lifestyle, or may be indicative of serious pathology. In this chapter, the approach to each of these symptoms will be addressed. For a discussion of the specific disease processes giving rise to these symptoms, the reader will be referred to the pertinent chapters.

SYMPTOMS OF ESOPHAGEAL DISEASE

The clinical history is extremely important in the diagnosis of esophageal disease. Complaints of heartburn, dysphagia, and odynophagia are highly specific and virtually always indicate an esophageal cause of symptoms. Less specific complaints that may be sometimes attributable to esophageal dysfunction include chest pain, belching, and hiccups. The approach to dysphagia and hiccups is discussed in subsequent sections.

Heartburn

Heartburn (pyrosis) is an extremely common symptom, occurring in 7% of Americans on a daily basis and in approximately one-third on a monthly basis. Pregnant women are commonly affected. Heartburn is usually defined as a feeling of substernal burning that radiates toward the neck from the epigastrium. Patients may use a number of other terms including "indigestion" and "acid regurgitation." Because heartburn is caused by the regurgitation of gastric acidic contents into the esophagus, it is generally improved, albeit transiently, by antacids. Heartburn occurs most commonly within 1 hour of meals or within 2 hours of reclining, especially if the patient has eaten a late meal or snack. Heartburn may be precipitated by foods that either decrease the lower esophageal sphincter pressure or cause direct mucosal irritation of the esophagus. It may also be precipitated by maneuvers that increase intraabdominal pressure (eg, lifting, bending, straining at stool, and exercise). Cigarettes potentiate heartburn by lowering the lower esophageal sphincter pressure and through relaxation of the sphincter during air swallowing. The clinical diagnosis of gastroesophageal reflux disease (GERD) based on the presence of a symptom of heartburn has a relatively high sensitivity of approximately 80% but a specificity of only 60%. In contrast, when heartburn clearly dominates the patient's complaints, the specificity increases to 90% with a positive predictive value for GERD of 80%. In other words, patients with a dominant complaint of heartburn are likely to have GERD. However, in patients who complain of a number of symptoms including heartburn and other associated dyspeptic symptoms (eg, pain, bloating, nausea), the diagnosis of GERD is less certain.

Regurgitation

Regurgitation describes the sudden, spontaneous reflux of small volumes of bitter tasting acidic material into the mouth. It most commonly occurs after meals, especially when bending over or at night. It is present in approximately two-thirds of patients with GERD but also occurs intermittently in up to one-half of healthy adults. It is distinguished from vomiting by the absence of nausea or retching. "**Water brash**" occurs when the mouth fills with clear, salty fluid. Water brash is not regurgitated fluid; rather, it occurs through salivary secretion stimulated through a vagally mediated reflex arc in response to acidic contents in the esophagus.

Regurgitation should be differentiated from **rumination,** which is the regurgitation of recently ingested food into the mouth with subsequent remastication and reswallowing or spitting out. Nausea and vomiting are absent. Rumination usually occurs in the immediate postprandial period. It occurs more commonly in males and in patients with severe psychiatric problems or the severely retarded. GERD and bulimia are often confused with rumination.

Odynophagia

Odynophagia is pain with swallowing. The discomfort may be a dull retrosternal pain or a severe, sharp sensation. Odynophagia usually reflects severe erosive disease. It is most commonly associated with infectious esophagitis resulting from *Candida,* herpes, and cytomegalovirus, especially in immunocompromised patients [eg, acquired immunodeficiency syndrome (AIDS), patients undergoing chemotherapy]. Dysphagia may also be present with these conditions. Odynophagia may also be caused by pill-induced ulcers (Table 1–1). Rarely, it may be caused by severe erosive esophagitis resulting from GERD or esophageal carcinoma.

Chest Pain

Recurrent chest pain resembling angina pectoris can originate from disorders of the esophagus. Cardiac disease (eg, coronary ischemia, coronary spasm, mitral valve prolapse, and microvascular angina) must first be definitively excluded in patients with typical or atypical angina. Approximately one-third of patients with chest pain who undergo cardiac catheterization have normal

Table 1–1. Causes of odynophagia.

Pill esophagitis
  Antibiotics
    Doxycycline
    Tetracycline
    Clindamycin
  Antivirals
    Zidovudine
    Zalcitabine
  Nonsteroidal antiinflammatory drugs
  Others
    Potassium chloride pills
    Quinidine
    Ferrous sulfate
    Ascorbic acid
    Phenytoin
    Theophylline
Infectious esophagitis
  Candida albicans
  Herpes simplex
  Cytomegalovirus
Corrosive esophagitis
Severe reflux esophagitis
Nonspecific ulcerations
  Primarily in AIDS

epicardial arteries and, therefore, are presumed to have a noncardiac source of pain. Causes of noncardiac chest pain include chest wall or thoracic spine pain, psychiatric problems (eg, depression and panic disorder), and esophageal dysfunction. Esophageal causes of chest pain include acid reflux (in up to 50% of patients), esophageal motility disorders, abnormal visceral nociception, and esophageal distention (see Chapter 17).

The clinical history is unreliable in distinguishing cardiac from esophageal causes of chest pain. Esophageal chest pain results in intermittent anterior chest discomfort. Esophageal chest pain may mimic coronary ischemia with substernal squeezing discomfort or may present as a burning sensation that radiates to the neck, jaw, or arm. Esophageal chest pain can be precipitated by exercise or emotional stress and is sometimes relieved by nitroglycerin. More commonly, however, esophageal chest pain presents with features that are not characteristic of cardiac ischemia, including pain that occurs during sleep, lasts for hours to days, or is precipitated by hot or cold liquids or meals. Symptoms may last from minutes to hours. The majority of patients with esophageal chest pain report other symptoms compatible with esophageal disease, such as heartburn, regurgitation, or dysphagia. However, chest pain is the only symptom in approximately 10% of patients. Also, up to one-half of patients with cardiac chest pain have associated esophageal symptoms.

Clinical Evaluation

A. SIGNS

The physical examination is almost always normal in patients with chest pain of esophageal origin. Weight loss and overt or occult gastrointestinal bleeding warrant further diagnostic tests to exclude complicated GERD, a gastric or esophageal malignancy, or other gastrointestinal pathology.

B. DIAGNOSTIC STUDIES

1. Upper endoscopy—Endoscopy is the study of choice for evaluating persistent heartburn, odynophagia, and structural abnormalities detected on barium esophagography. In addition to providing direct visualization of the mucosa, it allows the endoscopist to biopsy mucosal abnormalities such as Barrett's esophagus and to dilate esophageal strictures or rings.

2. Video esophagography—Oropharyngeal dysphagia is best evaluated with a rapid sequence videoesophagram. It is the initial diagnostic study of choice in most patients with oropharyngeal dysphagia (see section, "Dysphagia").

3. Barium esophagography—Patients with esophageal dysphagia usually are evaluated first with a radiographic barium study to differentiate between mechanical lesions and esophageal motility disorders. Although the information provided about esophageal motility is limited, it can provide strong clues to the diagnosis of certain motility disorders (eg, achalasia, diffuse esophageal spasm, and scleroderma esophagus). In patients in whom there is a high suspicion of a mechanical lesion (eg, patients with heartburn or weight loss and progressive dysphagia), many clinicians will proceed directly to an endoscopic evaluation without a barium study (see section, "Dysphagia").

4. Esophageal manometry—Motility of the esophageal body and lower esophageal sphincter is best studied using manometry. A small pressure-sensing catheter assembly is passed nasally into the esophagus, allowing manometric assessment of the lower and upper esophageal sphincters and esophageal body. Manometry provides information about the function of the lower esophageal sphincter and integrity of esophageal peristalsis. It is useful for documentation of impaired lower esophageal sphincter relaxation, weak or absent esophageal peristalsis, and disordered peristalsis. Esophageal manometry is indicated to establish the diagnosis in suspected cases of achalasia or diffuse esophageal spasm after more common causes of esophageal symptoms have been excluded by upper endoscopy or barium esophagography. This technique may be indicated rarely to document esophageal motor abnormalities in patients with suspected systemic diseases (eg, scleroderma) when this determination would help establish a definitive diagnosis. In patients undergoing fundoplication for gastroesophageal reflux, it should be performed preoperatively to document adequate peristaltic function. Finally, manometry is useful in determining the location of the lower esophageal sphincter before placing an esophageal probe for continuous ambulatory pH monitoring (usually located 5 cm above the lower esophageal sphincter).

Manometry is not useful in the diagnosis of GERD. Although it previously was employed in the evaluation of noncardiac chest pain, it is recognized now to be of limited usefulness because of the low likelihood of determining any clinically significant motility disorders.

5. Ambulatory esophageal pH monitoring—Esophageal pH can be monitored continuously by means of a small transnasal pH probe attached to a small, portable pH recording device. The probe and recorder are worn by the patient for up to 24 hours. The recording is then analyzed to determine a number of parameters. The most clinically useful information is the amount of gastroesophageal acid reflux (measured as the percentage of time below pH 4) in the upright and supine positions and for the total reporting period. Because a certain amount of acid reflux occurs in everyone, the definition of normal and abnormal values is somewhat arbitrary. Normal values are derived from studies of asymptomatic volunteers and vary between studies. In general, normal values of acid reflux (percentage time below pH 4) are less than 8.1% in the upright position, less than 3.0% in the supine position, and less than 5.5% for the total 24-hour period. The ambulatory pH study also is useful in determining whether a patient's symptoms correlate with documented episodes of acid reflux. A symptom index of greater than 50% (number of symptoms with pH<4/ total number of symptoms) × 100% is considered significant. Although ambulatory pH monitoring is the best method for diagnosing abnormal amounts of acid gastroesophageal reflux, it is seldom needed in the evaluation of patients with uncomplicated GERD who respond to acid suppression. For patients with typical symptoms who do not respond to standard therapies and do not have evidence of reflux esophagitis on endoscopy, ambulatory monitoring is useful in confirming or excluding GERD. Its principal value is in diagnosing GERD in patients with atypical symptoms (eg, including noncardiac chest pain, hoarseness, chronic cough, asthma, and aspiration pneumonia). Finally, ambulatory monitoring is useful in patients with GERD before performing antireflux surgery to document the severity of reflux, especially if symptoms are ambiguous or atypical.

DYSPHAGIA

General Considerations

Dysphagia refers to a sensation of impaired passage of food from the mouth to the stomach. Patients usually complain that the food "sticks," "hangs up," or "gets stuck" as it goes down the esophagus. Dysphagia should be distinguished from **odynophagia** (painful swallowing) and **globus** (a sensation of a lump in the throat), which involve different differential diagnoses. A carefully taken history will allow a correct diagnosis in approximately 80% of patients presenting with dysphagia.

Dysphagia can result from an abnormality at each stage of the swallowing process. The normal act of swallowing may be divided into oropharyngeal and esophageal stages. The oropharyngeal phase involves the process of chewing and mixing solid food with saliva so that individual food particles are sufficiently reduced in size and lubricated to allow easy passage through the pharynx and esophagus. With the voluntary initiation of swallowing, the food bolus is propelled posteriorly by the tongue into the pharynx. A rapid series of carefully orchestrated involuntary events follow in which the soft palate and larynx close (to prevent nasal regurgitation and aspiration), the upper esophageal sphincter opens, and a wave of pharyngeal peristalsis propels the food bolus into the upper esophagus. This involuntary process of food bolus transfer is controlled by the swallowing center located in the medulla oblongata. Respiration is inhibited centrally during the act of swallowing. Afferent input to the swallowing center is provided by cranial nerves V, X, and XI, and efferent motor function is provided by cranial nerves V, VII, IX, X, and XII. Once the food bolus has reached the upper esophagus, the esophageal phase of swallowing takes place. A primary peristaltic wave propels the food bolus down the esophagus. The lower esophageal sphincter relaxes in anticipation of the peristaltic wave, allowing passage of the food bolus into the stomach.

Dysphagia is usually classified as either *oropharyngeal* or *esophageal*. Oropharyngeal dysphagia (also termed transfer dysphagia) is produced by abnormal function of the pharynx or upper esophageal sphincter that impairs the preparation or transfer of food from the mouth to the upper esophagus. Esophageal dysphagia is caused by a mechanical or motor abnormality of the esophageal body that hinders movement of the food bolus through the esophagus into the stomach.

Clinical Findings

A. SYMPTOMS AND SIGNS

Oropharyngeal and esophageal dysphagia may be distinguished by a careful history and physical examination (Figure 1–1).

1. Oropharyngeal dysphagia—Patients with oropharyngeal dysphagia experience difficulty initiating swallowing. The problem is difficulty transferring a food bolus from the mouth to the esophagus. This may occur as a result of poor motor control of the tongue, jaw, or other oral structures or may be due to an abnormality of the swallowing reflex. Symptoms suggesting an oropharyngeal cause of dysphagia include nasal regurgitation, coughing during swallowing, or difficulty initiating a swallow. Repeated attempts by the patient to swallow are common. Dysphagia within 1 second after swallowing suggests oropharyngeal dysphagia. Oropharyngeal dysphagia is most commonly caused by neurologic or muscular disorders that are readily apparent at the time of physical examination. A speech disorder, cranial nerve deficits, abnormalities of motor function of the limbs, or a history of a recent cerebrovascular accident are frequently present. A small proportion of patients have symptoms produced by a structural abnormality of the pharyngeal region. A complaint of transfer dysphagia with regurgitation of undigested food contents, a gurgling noise after swallowing, halitosis, or nocturnal coughing suggests a Zenker's diverticulum. Table 1–2 lists the neurologic, motor, local/structural, and motility disorders that may cause oropharyngeal dysphagia.

Inspection of the oral cavity should be performed in patients complaining of oropharyngeal dysphagia paying particular attention to mucosal ulcerations, mass lesions, and dentition. Neurologic testing of the cranial nerves involved in swallowing (sensory: V, IX, X and motor: V, VII, X, XI, and XII) is important to rule out a neurologic deficit contributing to dysphagia. Examination of the neck is performed to exclude mass lesions or thyromegaly. Inspection of the limbs may show characteristic skin changes suggesting scleroderma or weakness suggesting a neuromuscular disorder. Patients with oropharyngeal dysphagia and hoarseness should be referred for otolaryngology consultation and direct laryngoscopy.

2. Esophageal dysphagia—Patients with esophageal dysphagia are able to transfer food from the mouth into the upper esophagus, but experience a sensation of food "hanging up" or "sticking" after it is swallowed. Esophageal dysphagia may be caused by two general categories of disease processes: (1) a structural or mechanical process impairing movement of a food bolus through the esophageal lumen (including structural ab-

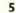

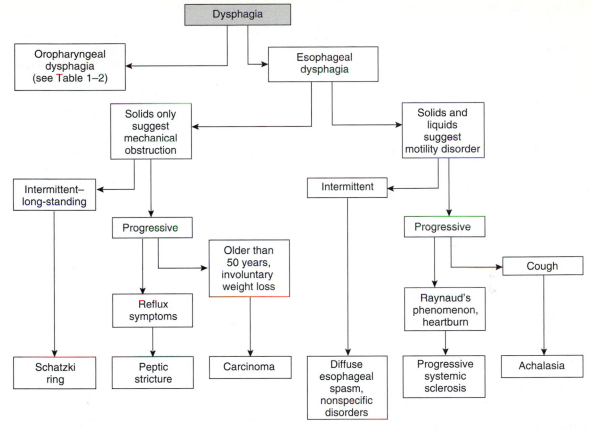

Figure 1–1. Algorithm illustrating the differential diagnosis for dysphagia. [Modified, with permission, from Castell DO: Esophagus: overview and symptom assessment. In: *The Esophagus*. Castell DO (editor). Little, Brown, & Company, 1992.]

normalities originating in the esophagus or extrinsically impinging upon the esophagus) and (2) motility disorders of the esophagus. Table 1–2 lists diseases that may cause esophageal dysphagia. These etiologies may be differentiated by several historical points.

a. Solid versus liquid dysphagia—Dysphagia to solids alone suggests a mechanical or structural abnormality, whereas dysphagia to both solids and liquids suggests a neuromuscular disturbance.

b. Intermittent versus progressive symptoms—A long history of intermittent dysphagia to solids (particularly steak or bread) suggests a fixed esophageal ring or web, which has not changed in size. In contrast, progressively worsening of solid food dysphagia suggests a peptic stricture, neoplasm, or achalasia.

c. Associated symptoms—An associated history of heartburn or acid regurgitation suggests scleroderma or a peptic stricture as the underlying abnormality. Suspicion of an esophageal neoplasm should be heightened

among older patients presenting with weight loss and a history of alcohol or tobacco use. Regurgitation of undigested food in association with coughing while in the recumbent position or recurrent pneumonia suggests achalasia. Associated symptoms of chest pain with intermittent dysphagia may indicate diffuse esophageal spasm or achalasia. Patients with AIDS may have dysphagia from opportunistic infections or mass lesions (eg, Kaposi's sarcoma and lymphoma) (see Chapter 2).

The physical examination usually is unremarkable in patients with esophageal dysphagia. Profound weight loss may be seen in patients with advanced esophageal malignancy or achalasia, but is uncommon in other benign conditions. The presence of a positive fecal occult blood test may be found in malignancy or reflux esophagitis.

B. DIAGNOSTIC STUDIES

Patients with dysphagia require a diagnostic evaluation to determine the cause. The available diagnostic tests

Table 1–2. Causes of dysphagia.

Oropharyngeal dysphagia
  Neurologic disorders
    Cerebrovascular accident (especially brainstem)
    Parkinson's disease
    Multiple sclerosis
    Brainstem tumors
    Bulbar poliomyelitis
    Peripheral neuropathies
    Huntington's disease
  Diseases of myoneural junction
    Myasthenia gravis
    Eaton-Lambert syndrome
    Botulism
  Muscular disorders
    Muscular dystrophies
    Dermatomyositis/polymyositis
    Sarcoidosis
    Metabolic myopathies (hypo- or hyperthyroidism)
    Amyloidosis
    Steroid-induced myopathy
  Structural abnormalities
    Oropharyngeal neoplasms
    Extrinsic compression (cervical osteophytes, thyromegaly)
    Esophageal web
    Zenker's diverticulum
  Upper esophageal sphincter (UES) dysfunction
    Cricopharyngeal achalasia
    Hypertensive UES
Esophageal dysphagia
  Intrinsic mechanical abnormalities
    Peptic (reflux-induced) stricture
    Esophageal carcinoma
    Esophageal webs/rings
    Schatzki ring
    Esophageal diverticula
  Extrinsic esophageal compression
    Mediastinal tumors
    Vascular compression
    Cervical osteophytes
  Esophageal motility disorders
    Achalasia
    Diffuse esophageal spasm
    Hypertensive lower esophageal sphincter
    Nonspecific motility disorders
    Chagas' disease
    Scleroderma/progressive systemic sclerosis
    Severe gastroesophageal reflux disease

include upper gastrointestinal endoscopy, barium esophagography (with or without videofluoroscopic assessment of swallowing), and esophageal manometry. Patients with oropharyngeal dysphagia should undergo a videofluoroscopic examination of deglutition. During this examination, barium of various consistencies is ingested by the patient and the swallowing sequence is recorded fluoroscopically. Anatomic and structural defects, as well as discoordination of muscular movements may be identified. This examination may also aid in nutritional management by determining the food consistency most easily swallowed by the patient as well as head and body positions that facilitate swallowing.

Patients with esophageal dysphagia may undergo either endoscopy or a barium swallow as the initial diagnostic evaluation. Under most circumstances, a barium swallow is favored as the initial study because it provides information about both structural lesions (strictures, tumors, rings or webs, cervical osteophytes) and esophageal motility. Endoscopy may overlook subtle mucosal rings or webs and is a poor means of assessing esophageal motility. However, for patients with persistent heartburn (suggesting a peptic stricture) or with significant weight loss (suggesting malignancy), endoscopy may be the study of first choice because it permits mucosal biopsy and dilation, as deemed necessary. Patients with suspected peptic strictures identified on barium swallow must undergo endoscopy in order to rule out esophageal carcinoma. Patients with lesions found on barium swallow that suggest carcinoma also must undergo endoscopy with biopsy for confirmation. Esophageal rings or webs identified on barium studies may benefit from endoscopic dilation and disruption, and thus should be referred for endoscopy as well. Findings suggesting achalasia on barium swallow (a dilated aperistaltic esophageal body and narrowed distal esophagus) warrant referral for esophageal manometry and endoscopy to exclude secondary causes of achalasia. Simultaneous nonperistaltic contractions seen on barium swallow suggest diffuse esophageal spasm, and manometry may be considered. The reader is referred to Chapters 16, 17, and 18 for a full discussion of the management of esophageal strictures, motility disorders, and malignant neoplasms.

DYSPEPSIA

Dyspepsia is a term used to describe upper abdominal symptoms. The term encompasses a variety of complaints including epigastric pain, bloating, fullness, belching, heartburn, nausea, or early satiety. Dyspepsia is synonymous with the term indigestion. **Nonulcer dyspepsia** (also termed **functional dyspepsia**) refers to dyspepsia of at least 3 months duration for which no biochemical or structural abnormality is found to explain the patient's symptoms. Patients with nonulcer dyspepsia have undergone appropriate investigations to rule out a structural abnormality as the cause of their symptoms. Nonulcer dyspepsia is the most common diagnosis following investigation of dyspeptic patients by endoscopy. **Uninvestigated dyspepsia** refers to patients with dyspepsia who have not undergone investigation to determine if a structural abnormality is present. Dyspeptic symptoms are very common and dyspepsia is one of the most common complaints evaluated by both general practitioners and gastroenterologists. Many persons with dyspepsia also have symptoms compatible with irritable bowel syndrome. Although dyspepsia is very common, most persons with dyspepsia never seek medical attention for their symptoms. A full discussion of dyspepsia and nonulcer dyspepsia is provided in Chapter 21.

Etiology

Approximately 50% of patients with uninvestigated dyspepsia who undergo endoscopy will have normal examinations and be classified as having **nonulcer dyspepsia**. **Peptic ulcer disease** is found in approximately 20% and **reflux esophagitis** in 15–20% of persons undergoing endoscopy for evaluation of dyspepsia. Although nonulcer dyspepsia has been used as a term to describe patients with dyspeptic symptoms and no obvious structural abnormality, it probably represents a heterogeneous group of disorders including nonerosive GERD, motility disturbances, abnormal visceral nociception, and pancreaticobiliary disease. Patients with nonulcer dyspepsia usually experience chronic symptoms. Other causes of dyspepsia include medication-induced dyspepsia (nonsteroidal antiinflammatory drugs, antibiotics, theophylline, digitalis, iron, niacin), dietary factors (alcohol, caffeine), endocrine/metabolic disturbances (diabetes mellitus, hyperthyroidism), and pancreaticobiliary disease (chronic pancreatitis, pancreatic cancer, sphincter of Oddi dysfunction, cholelithiasis). Gallstones usually cause severe pain that occurs in discrete episodes and lasts a few hours; this can usually be distinguished from functional dyspepsia. *Helicobacter pylori* gastritis in the absence of peptic ulcers has not been definitively shown to be a cause of dyspepsia. Gastric malignancy is found in 1–2% of patients with dyspepsia, nearly always among persons greater than 45 years of age with "alarm" symptoms (weight loss, dysphagia, bleeding, recurrent vomiting).

Clinical Findings

A. SYMPTOMS AND SIGNS

The clinical history is of limited usefulness in distinguishing among the causes of dyspepsia. The most important aspect of the clinical history is to determine whether "alarm symptoms" are present. Alarm symptoms include weight loss, persistent vomiting, dysphagia, anemia, or bleeding. The presence of any of these symptoms raises the suspicion of underlying malignancy or complicated ulcer disease and warrants prompt investigation by endoscopy. The type of dyspeptic symptoms (eg, whether the patient reports epigastric pain versus bloating) cannot be used to accurately differentiate between underlying peptic ulcer disease, nonulcer dyspepsia, or gastroesophageal reflux disease. Patients with underlying gastric ulcer, duodenal ulcer, GERD, or nonulcer dyspepsia often share similar symptoms; this makes the clinical history imprecise in directing therapy toward a specific disease state. However, predominant substernal burning (heartburn) and regurgitation are highly specific for GERD (see section, "Heartburn").

A thorough physical examination should be performed and may occasionally identify an abdominal mass lesion, evidence of gastrointestinal blood loss, or organomegaly. Routine laboratory studies including a complete blood count, electrolytes, serum calcium level, liver function tests, and fecal occult blood testing should be obtained, although the cost effectiveness of these studies remains unproven. Thyroid function testing, serum amylase, and a urine pregnancy test may also be performed when appropriate.

B. DIAGNOSTIC STUDIES

Because the history and physical examination are nonspecific, a diagnosis of dyspepsia in most cases requires special examinations. Upper endoscopy is highly accurate at diagnosing peptic ulcer disease, erosive GERD, and gastric neoplasms. However, at least one-half of patients with dyspepsia have normal or nonspecific findings on endoscopy. Although barium upper gastrointestinal series is less expensive, it is less accurate and is a suboptimal means of evaluating patients with dyspepsia. Abdominal ultrasonography should be obtained only when biliary or pancreatic disease is suspected. Computed tomography (CT) or magnetic resonance imaging (MRI) should be obtained only when there is a strong suspicion of intraabdominal diseases or to pursue abnormal findings on ultrasonography.

The decision as to when and how to investigate patients with dyspepsia depends on a number of factors. Patients who are age 50 years or older with new onset dyspepsia, alarm symptoms, physical or laboratory abnormalities, or are from regions endemic for gastric cancer should undergo a diagnostic endoscopy. In patients who are age 50 years or younger without alarm symptoms and normal physical and laboratory examinations (in whom the risk of malignancy is low), the optimal approach is controversial. With the recognition of the pivotal role of *H pylori* in peptic ulcer disease, a strategy of empiric testing and treatment for *H pylori* has been advocated as a cost-effective approach for patients with uninvestigated dyspepsia, since it decreases use of endoscopy. However, many patients test negative for *H pylori* infection or fail to respond to empiric *H pylori* treatment. These patients may benefit from an empiric trial of acid suppression, although the optimal management strategy remains unclear. A full discussion of these issues is discussed in Chapter 21.

HICCUPS

Hiccups (hiccoughs) is a complex reflex pattern characterized by a sudden contraction of the diaphragm inspiratory muscles that is terminated with an abrupt closure of the glottis, resulting in the characteristic "hiccup" sound. A brainstem "hiccup center" receives afferent activity from the central nervous system (CNS), vagus, or phrenic nerves and coordinates efferent activity via multiple nerves to the respiratory center and to the diaphragm (phrenic nerve), glottis (vagus nerve), scalenes (cervical plexus), and intercostals (thoracic nerves). Though usually a benign and self-limited annoyance, they may be persistent and occasionally reflect serious underlying illness. Persistent (intractable) hiccups appear to be without major consequences. Reports that hiccups lead to exhaustion, weight loss, or death are unsubstantiated. In patients on mechanical ventilation, hiccups can trigger a full respiratory cycle and result in respiratory alkalosis.

Causes of benign, self-limited hiccups include gastric distention (eg, carbonated beverages, air swallowing, overeating), sudden temperature changes (eg, hot or cold liquids, cold shower), alcohol ingestion, smoking, and emotional stress. Over 100 causes of recurrent or persistent hiccups have been identified. There are reports of hiccups lasting from 18 to 68 years. Causes of intractable hiccups can be related to any structure along the pathways of the phrenic and vagus nerves and may be grouped into the following categories:

- CNS—neoplasms, infections (meningitis, encephalitis), cerebrovascular accident, trauma, arteriovenous malformation, multiple sclerosis, surgery
- Metabolic—uremia, hypocapnia (hyperventilation), electrolyte imbalance, toxic (alcohol, medications), diabetes mellitus
- Irritation of vagus or phrenic nerve at any level: Head and neck: foreign body in ear, goiter, neoplasms
  Thorax: pneumonia, pleurisy, empyema, neoplasms, myocardial infarction, pericarditis, aneurysm, esophageal obstruction, reflux esophagitis
  Abdomen: subphrenic abscess, hepatomegaly, hepatitis, cholecystitis, gastric distention, gastric neoplasm, peritonitis, pancreatitis, pancreatic malignancy
- Surgical—general anesthesia, postoperative
- Psychogenic—excitement, stress, malingering, idiopathic

Clinical Findings

Patients with self-limited hiccups require no evaluation. Evaluation of the patient with persistent hiccups should include a history and physical examination (including neurologic examination), complete blood count (CBC), electrolytes, liver chemistry tests, and a chest radiograph. When the cause remains unclear, further testing may include CT of the chest and abdomen, echocardiography, bronchoscopy, and upper endoscopy.

Treatment

A number of simple remedies work by interrupting the reflex arc and may be helpful in patients with acute, benign hiccups:

1. Irritation of the nasopharynx—tongue traction, lifting uvula with spoon, catheter stimulation of the nasopharynx, eating 1 teaspoon of dry granulated sugar or a lemon wedge or vinegar.
2. Interruption of the respiratory cycle—breath holding, Valsalva, sneezing, gasping (frightful stimulus), rebreathing into a bag, compression of the thyroid cartilage.
3. Irritation of the vagus—supraorbital pressure, carotid massage.
4. Irritation of the diaphragm—holding the knees to chest, continuous positive airway pressure (CPAP) during mechanical ventilation.
5. Relief of gastric distention—belching, nasogastric aspiration.

In patients with persistent hiccups, therapy should be directed at relieving the predisposing cause. A number of drugs have been touted as being useful in the treatment of hiccups, but none has ever been tested in a controlled fashion. Chlorpromazine 25–50 mg orally or intramuscularly, or baclofen 5–20 mg orally every 6–12 hours are most commonly used. Other agents that have been reported to be effective in some cases include anticonvulsants (phenytoin, carbamazepine, valproic acid), metoclopramide, gabapentin, nifedipine, amitriptyline, nebulized lidocaine, and, occasionally, anesthesia. Unilateral phrenic nerve crushing may weaken the intensity but may not ablate hiccups, which have bilateral diaphragmatic involvement.

GASTROINTESTINAL GAS

Patients may complain of gaseousness as a descriptive term to describe many different gastrointestinal complaints, including bloating, borborygmi, abdominal pain, belching, cramping, and flatulence.

Belching

Belching or **burping** results when swallowed air is passed retrograde across the lower and upper esophageal sphincters and out of the oral cavity. Belching occurs frequently after meals, when gastric distention results in transient lower esophageal sphincter relaxation. It is more commonly seen in patients with GERD. Belching is restricted in the supine position because of the formation of a fluid "trap" at the gastroesophageal junction. Belching is also limited by surgical fundoplication; this may result in the "gas-bloat" syndrome.

Virtually all gas in the stomach comes from swallowed air. Each swallow draws 3–5 mL of air into the upper gastrointestinal tract, 80% of which is nitrogen. Swallowed oxygen is readily absorbed whereas there is minimal absorption of swallowed nitrogen. Swallowing excessive amounts of air may result in distention, belching, flatulence, and abdominal pain. Air swallowing is promoted by gum chewing, smoking, rapid eating, and drinking carbonated beverages. Also, some patients may consciously or unconsciously engage in forceful air swallowing (aerophagia). Conscious aerophagia occurs primarily in institutionalized or psychotic patients. (It is also a common parlor trick, usually performed by adolescent boys to generate loud, obnoxious eructations.) It may also occur subconsciously in anxious adults who relax the upper esophageal sphincter (UES) and draw air into the esophagus with negative intrathoracic pressure.

Belching is a normal physiologic reflex and does not denote gastrointestinal pathology per se. Chronic excessive belching is almost always caused by aerophagia. Evaluation of belching should be restricted to patients with other complaints (eg, dysphagia, distention, early satiety, or vomiting) that suggest more serious problems. Aerophagia and belching may be reduced by simple behavioral changes including chewing and eating food slowly, not drinking through a straw, and not chewing gum. In severe cases formal behavioral modification may be tried.

Flatus

The rate and volume of excretion of intestinal gas per rectum are highly variable. Normal volumes range from 500 to 1500 mL/d and the normal number of passages of gas per rectum ranges from 6 to 20 (mean 13.6) times/d. Intestinal flatus is derived from two sources: swallowed air and bacterial fermentation of undigested carbohydrates. Oxygen from swallowed air is readily absorbed, but no appreciable nitrogen absorption occurs because the partial pressure of nitrogen in the gut and

blood is similar. Swallowed air (nitrogen) that is not belched passes through the gut and leaves as flatus. Swallowed air may contribute up to 400 mL of flatus/d. Bacterial fermentation of undigested carbohydrates leads to the additional production of gas, particularly the odorless gases hydrogen, methane, and carbon dioxide. Except for situations in which there is bacterial overgrowth in the small intestine, the majority of fermentation takes place in the colon. Under normal circumstances, a small amount of fermentable substrates reaches the colon. These include lactose, fructose, bean starch, and complex carbohydrates derived from wheat, oats, corn, and potatoes. Gas production may be increased dramatically with diseases of malabsorption (eg, celiac sprue), or after ingestion of poorly absorbed carbohydrates (eg, lactose, lactulose, sorbitol). Lactase deficiency is a common cause of increased gas production. Gases derived from plant carbohydrates have little odor. In contrast, the digestion of meats and eggs may give rise to small quantities of odorous gases.

Determining normal from abnormal amounts of flatus can be difficult. In most cases no formal evaluation is needed. Asking patients how many times they pass flatus may provide a rough guide as to whether there is increased gas production. A work-up for malabsorption should be undertaken in patients who have diarrhea or signs or weight loss or anemia. The patient should be placed on a trial of a lactose-free diet as an initial step. Common gas-producing foods should be reviewed and the patient should be placed on an elimination trial. These include brown beans, cauliflower, brussel sprouts, broccoli, cabbage, onions, beer, red wine, and coffee. For patients with persistent complaints, fructose and complex carbohydrates may be eliminated, but such restrictive diets are unacceptable to most patients. The usefulness of activated charcoal or simethicone is dubious. The nonprescription agent "Beano" (α-galactosidase) reduces gas production after the ingestion of baked beans and other legumes. The complaints of chronic abdominal distention or bloating are common but do not correlate with increased intraabdominal gas or gas production. The majority of these patients have an underlying functional gastrointestinal disorder, eg, irritable bowel syndrome or nonulcer dyspepsia.

NAUSEA & VOMITING

Nausea is a vague, disagreeable sensation of "queasiness" or feeling sick to the stomach that may be followed by vomiting. **Vomiting** is the forceful expulsion of gastric contents through a relaxed upper esophageal sphincter and open mouth. Vomiting is brought on by coordinated gastric, abdominal, and thoracic contractions and is often preceded by nausea and by **retching**, spasmodic respiratory and abdominal movements (dry heaves). Vomiting should be distinguished from regurgitation and rumination (see section, "Symptoms of Esophageal Disease"). Rumination is not associated with nausea.

The act of vomiting is controlled by a center in the medulla that coordinates the respiratory, salivary, and vasomotor centers and the vagus nervous innervation of the gastrointestinal tract. The vomiting center may be stimulated by four different sources of afferent input:

1. Afferent vagal fibers [rich in serotonin 5-hydroxy-tryptamine ($5\text{-}HT_3$) receptors] and splanchnic fibers from the gastrointestinal viscera; these may be stimulated by biliary or gastrointestinal distention, mucosal or peritoneal irritation, or infections.

2. The vestibular system; this may be stimulated by motion or infections. These fibers have high concentrations of histamine H_1 and muscarinic cholinergic receptors.

3. Higher CNS centers; CNS disorders or certain sights, smells, or emotional experiences may result in vomiting. For example, patients receiving chemotherapy may develop vomiting in anticipation of the treatment.

4. The "chemoreceptor trigger zone" (CTZ) located outside the blood–brain barrier in the area postrema of the medulla; this area has chemoreceptors that sample both blood and cerebrospinal fluid that may be stimulated by drugs and chemotherapeutic agents, toxins, hypoxia, uremia, acidosis, and radiation therapy. This region is rich in serotonin $5\text{-}HT_3$ and dopamine D2 receptors. A list of the causes of vomiting are many; a simplified list is provided in Table 1–3.

Complications of vomiting include volume depletion, hypokalemia, metabolic alkalosis, pulmonary aspiration, rupture of the esophagus (Boerhaave's syndrome), and bleeding secondary to a mucosal tear at the gastroesophageal junction (Mallory-Weiss syndrome). Rarely, intraabdominal bleeding from splenic or hepatic laceration may occur as a complication of vomiting.

Clinical Findings

A. Symptoms and Signs

The history and physical examination are important in distinguishing among the causes of vomiting. Acute symptoms including chest or abdominal pain, CNS symptoms, fevers, or immunosuppression require a prompt diagnostic evaluation. Acute symptoms without abdominal pain are typically caused by food poisoning, infectious gastroenteritis, or drugs. Inquiry should be made into recent changes in medications, food ingestions, other viral symptoms of malaise or diarrhea, or

similar illness in family members. The acute onset of severe pain and vomiting suggests peritoneal irritation, acute intestinal obstruction, or pancreaticobiliary disease. Abdominal pain that precedes nausea and vomiting raises the suspicion of obstruction of the gut. Physical examination may reveal fever, focal tenderness, guarding, or rebound tenderness. Chronic vomiting suggests pregnancy, gastric outlet obstruction, gastroparesis, intestinal dysmotility, psychogenic disorders, CNS diseases, or systemic disorders.

If the patient is a female of child-bearing age, a pregnancy test should be performed, since pregnancy-related nausea and vomiting occur in up to 70–90% of pregnancies. Symptoms of nausea in pregnancy occur early in pregnancy and typically last all day, rather than being truly "morning sickness." If the patient has **vertigo** associated with nausea or vomiting, a thorough neurologic examination is required. Maneuvers involving a rapid change in head position can be used to diagnose benign positional vertigo. Associated symptoms including hearing loss, tinnitus, headache, visual changes, or loss of sensation should be sought. The goal is to distinguish peripheral causes of vertigo (benign positional vertigo, vestibular neuronitis, Meniere's disease, acoustic neuroma) from central causes of vertigo (multiple sclerosis, central nervous system tumor). The typical history for **vestibular neuronitis** is the rapid onset of vertigo, nausea, and vomiting that often follows a recent upper respiratory tract infection. **Acute labyrinthitis** usually has a history similar to vestibular neuronitis except that there is also hearing loss on the involved side. **Meniere's disease** (endolymphatic hydrops) typically presents as a sense of fullness in the ear, tinnitus, hearing loss, and vertigo. **Migraine headaches** are commonly associated with nausea and vomiting. **Cyclic vomiting syndrome** consists of self-limited attacks of nausea and vomiting often associated with a migraine headache or irritable bowel complaints; this syndrome is effectively treated with low-dose tricyclic antidepressants.

The timing of vomiting in relation to meals and the nature of the emesis may provide clues to the cause. Vomiting immediately after meals suggests bulimia or psychogenic causes but may also occur in pyloric stenosis from peptic ulcer disease. Vomiting undigested food 1 to several hours after meals suggests gastroparesis (eg, diabetes or postvagotomy) or a gastric outlet obstruction resulting from peptic ulcer disease or malignant neoplasm. Physical examination in these patients may reveal a succussion splash. Vomiting that occurs in the early morning may be seen in pregnancy, alcoholism, and uremia, and also with increased intracranial pressure. Patients with either acute or chronic symptoms should be asked about neurologic symptoms, such as headaches, stiff neck, vertigo, and focal paresthesias or weakness. Vomitus that contains truly undigested food

Table 1–3. Causes of nausea and vomiting.

Acute Nausea and Vomiting	

1. Infectious
    Viral gastroenteritis
        Norwalk agent
        Rotavirus
    Toxin-mediated (food poisoning)
        Staphylococcus aureus
        Bacillus cereus
        Clostridia perfringens
    Acute systemic infections
    Infections in immunocompromised hosts
2. Gastrointestinal mechanical obstruction
    Acute gastric outlet obstruction
        Pyloric channel ulcer
    Extrinsic small bowel obstruction
        Incarcerated hernia
            Inguinal, femoral, obturator, umbilical, incisional
        Volvulus
        Adhesions
        Malrotation
        Internal hernias
    Intrinsic small bowel obstruction
        Crohn's disease
        Small intestinal tumors
        Radiation stricture
        Foreign body (gallstone ileus)
        Intussusception
        Meckel's diverticulum
    Ileus
        Postoperative
        Medical illness
	3. Visceral pain
	    Appendicitis
	    Acute pancreatitis
	    Acute cholecystitis
	    Mesenteric ischemia
	    Peritonitis of any cause
	4. Central nervous system
	    Motion sickness
	    Labyrinthitis (Meniere's)
	    Migraine headaches
	    Increased intracranial pressure
	    CNS trauma
	    CNS tumors or pseudotumors
	    Meningitis, encephalitis
	5. Systemic conditions
	    Pregnancy
	    Myocardial infarction
	    Renal failure
	    Diabetic ketoacidosis
	    Radiation therapy
	    Reye's syndrome (children)
	6. Medications/topical irritation
	    Chemotherapeutic agents
	    Nonsteroidal antiinflammatory drugs
	    Antibiotics
	    Digoxin
	    Theophylline
	    Narcotics
	    Niacin
	    Heavy ethanol ingestion

Chronic Nausea and Vomiting	

1. Gastrointestinal mechanical obstruction
    Chronic gastric outlet obstruction
        Chronic peptic ulcer disease
        Gastric tumor
        Crohn's disease with duodenal stricture
        Pancreatic cancer with duodenal obstruction
    Small intestine obstruction
        Peritoneal carcinomatosis
2. Motility disorders
    Gastroparesis
        Diabetes mellitus
        Collagen vascular disorders (scleroderma)
        Postvagotomy
        Medication induced
        Idiopathic
	Small intestine motility disorders
	        Chronic intestinal pseudoobstruction
	        Familial visceral myoneuropathy
	        Paraneoplastic syndromes
	        Amyloidosis
	3. Psychogenic
	    Bulimia
	    Psychogenic
	4. Others
	    Increased intracranial pressure
	    Metabolic: hyperthyroidism, renal failure, Addison's
	    Medications

is seen in patients with achalasia. Otherwise, the presence of food contents suggests gastric outlet obstruction, proximal small intestine obstruction, or gastroparesis.

Evidence of dehydration should be sought, including orthostatic vital signs, skin turgor, and appearance of mucous membranes. Evidence of weight loss or a palpable abdominal mass raises the suspicion of malignant neoplasm. Abdominal distention raises the suspicion of small intestinal obstruction. A succussion splash may be present with gastric outlet obstruction or gastroparesis. Hernial orifices should be examined with careful attention to surgical scars. A careful neurologic and fundoscopic examination is required.

Many drugs can cause nausea and vomiting and it is important to obtain a complete medication history in order to exclude this as a cause. New onset symptoms that coincide with starting a new medication suggest a medication-induced side effect. Opiates, nonsteroidal antiinflammatory drugs (NSAIDs), theophylline, digitalis, antibiotics, and selective serotonin reuptake inhibitors are commonly prescribed agents that can cause nausea or vomiting. Other agents that cause nausea include misoprostol, colchicine, and chemotherapeutic agents. Carbon monoxide, arsenic, and fluoride poisoning are associated with nausea and vomiting. Other exposures that can lead to nausea and vomiting include spider bites (brown recluse, black widow), scorpion stings, and snake bites. In the latter conditions the exposure is usually evident from pain, erythema, and swelling at the site of puncture.

B. Laboratory Findings

Diabetes mellitus, adrenal insufficiency, and severe hypercalcemia may be causes of nausea and vomiting. Prolonged vomiting may in turn result in metabolic imbalances, the most common of which are metabolic alkalosis, hypokalemia, and either hyponatremia or hypernatremia. Prerenal azotemia may be present.

C. Special Examinations

In acute vomiting, a flat and upright abdominal radiograph may show evidence of obstruction, free intraperitoneal air, or dilated loops of small bowel. In patients with suspected mechanical small intestinal or gastric obstruction, a nasogastric tube should be placed for relief of symptoms. Aspiration of more than 200 mL of residual material in a fasting patient suggests obstruction or gastroparesis. This may be confirmed by a saline load test showing more than 400 mL of residual material on gastric aspiration performed 30 minutes after nasogastric instillation of 750 mL of normal saline. The cause of the gastric outlet obstruction is best demonstrated by upper endoscopy. Gastroparesis is confirmed by nuclear scintigraphic studies that show

delayed gastric emptying and either upper endoscopy or barium upper gastrointestinal series showing no evidence of mechanical gastric outlet obstruction. Abnormal liver function tests or amylase suggests pancreaticobiliary disease, which may be investigated with an abdominal sonogram or CT. CNS symptoms warrant CT or MRI of the brain. Cardiac ischemia may present with nausea and vomiting and an electrocardiogram should be obtained to evaluate this possibility.

Treatment

A. General Measures

The treatment of vomiting should be directed primarily at finding and correcting the underlying cause. Most causes of acute vomiting are mild, self-limited, and require no specific treatment. Patients should ingest clear liquids (broths, tea, soups, carbonated beverages) and small quantities of dry foods (soda crackers). For more severe acute vomiting, hospitalization is required. Because of the inability to eat and loss of gastric fluids, patients may become dehydrated and develop hypokalemia and metabolic alkalosis. Intravenous 0.45% saline with 20 mEq/L potassium is given in most cases to maintain hydration. A nasogastric suction tube for gastric decompression improves patient comfort and permits monitoring of fluid loss.

B. Antiemetic Medications

Medications may be given either to prevent or to control vomiting. Given the complexity of the various pathways that control and stimulate vomiting, it is not surprising that no single medication is effective in all patients. Combinations of drugs from different classes may provide better control of symptoms with less toxicity in some patients. The medications listed in Table 1–4 should be avoided in pregnancy.

1. Serotonin 5-HT$_3$ receptor antagonists—5-HT$_3$ receptors are found in both the central and peripheral nervous systems, with a high concentration in the gastrointestinal (GI) tract. Available 5-HT$_3$ antagonists include ondansetron, granisetron, and tropisetron. Efficacy appears to be similar among these agents. 5-HT$_3$ receptor antagonists are effective for chemotherapy-induced emesis, total body irradiation, GI motility disturbances, carcinoid syndrome, and nausea related to migraine headaches.

2. Dopamine antagonists—The phenothiazines, butyrophenones, and substituted benzamides have antiemetic properties that are due, at least in part, to dopaminergic blockade as well as sedative effects. Prochlorperazine (Compazine), promethazine (Phenergan), chlorpromazine (Thorazine), perphenazine (Trilafon), and thiethylperazine maleate (Torecan) are the

Table 1–4. Antiemetic dosing regimens.

	Dosage	Route[1]
Serotonin 5-HT$_3$ antagonist[2]		
Ondansetron	32 mg over 15 minutes beginning 15 minutes before chemotherapy; 4 mg over 2–5 minutes for postoperative vomiting	IV
	8 mg three times a day	PO
Granisetron	10 µg/kg over 5 minutes, 30 min before chemotherapy	IV
	1 mg twice a day	PO
Tropisetron	5–10 mg beginning 30 minutes before chemotherapy; 0.5–2 mg for postoperative nausea and vomiting	IV
	5 mg two to four times a day	PO
Dopamine antagonists		
Prochlorperazine	5–10 mg every 4–6 hours	PO, IM, IV
	25 mg suppository every 6 hours	PR
Promethazine	25 mg every 4–6 hours	IM, PR
Droperidol	2.5–5 mg	IV
Metoclopramide	10–20 mg every 6 hours	PO
	0.5–2 mg/kg every 6–8 hours	IV
Antihistamines/anticholinergics		
Diphenhydramine	25–50 mg every 4–6 hours	PO, IM, IV
Scopalamine patch	1.5 mg every 3 days	Patch
Dimenhydrinate	50 mg every 4 hours	PO
Meclizine	25–50 mg every 24 hours	PO
Sedatives/CNS altering agents		
Diazepam[3]	2–5 mg every 4–6 hours	PO, IV
Lorazepam[3]	1–2 mg every 4–6 hours	PO, IV
Dronabinol[4]	5 mg/m^2 1 hour before chemotherapy and every 2–4 hours prn	PO

[1]IV, intravenous; PO, oral; IM, intramuscular; PR, rectal.
[2]Approved for prevention of chemotherapy-induced nausea and vomiting and for treatment of postoperative nausea and vomiting. Use in other situations requires further study.
[3]Useful when given before chemotherapy in patients with anticipatory vomiting.
[4]Used primarily in the treatment of nausea and vomiting associated with chemotherapy; usefulness in other situations requires further study.

phenothiazines most commonly used. High doses of these agents are associated with antidopaminergic side effects, including dystonia, dyskinesia, and depression. These agents are commonly used antiemetics for a variety of situations. Phenothiazines are contraindicated if there is concomitant use of CNS depressants including alcohol.

3. Antihistamines—These have weak antiemetic properties, and are mainly used in the treatment of vomiting due to motion sickness and postoperative states. Commonly used agents include meclizine (Antivert) and diphenhydramine (Benadryl).

4. Sedatives—Benzodiazepines may be helpful in patients whose nausea and vomiting have a psychological component. These agents are useful in the treatment of the anticipatory nausea and vomiting associated with chemotherapy.

5. Corticosteroids—Dexamethasone is the agent most commonly used in the treatment of chemotherapy-induced nausea and vomiting. It has been shown to be useful alone or in combination with other antiemetic agents.

6. Dronabinol (tetrahydrocannabinol)—The major active substance in marijuana, this agent has been found empirically to have antiemetic properties. The mechanism is unknown. It is used for the control of nausea and vomiting related to chemotherapy. The dose is 5–15 mg/m^2, given 1–3 hours prechemotherapy and every 3–4 hours as needed after chemotherapy is given. Altered mood, motor, and cognitive function often limit its usefulness.

7. Acupressure—Pressure at the P6 point located on the wrist may be of benefit for motion sickness.

DIARRHEA

Diarrhea is a common symptom that can range in severity from an acute, self-limited annoyance to a severe, life-threatening illness. Diarrhea is defined as an increased liquidity or decreased consistency of stools. Many patients also complain of increased stool frequency. The use of the weight of stool per 24 hours (eg, >200 g) is less useful than a clinical definition of increased liquidity since some persons with formed stools have increased stool weight and some persons with normal stool weight have increased liquidity of stools. In clinical practice, quantification of stool weight is necessary only in some patients with chronic diarrhea. To properly evaluate the complaint of diarrhea, the physician must determine the patient's normal bowel pattern and the nature of the current symptoms.

In the normal state, approximately 10 L of fluid enter the duodenum daily, of which all but 1.0 L are absorbed by the small intestine. The colon resorbs most of the remaining fluid, with only 100 mL lost in the stool. The causes of diarrhea are myriad. In clinical practice it is helpful to distinguish acute from chronic diarrhea, as the evaluation and treatment is entirely different. A complete list of causes is given in the Table 1–5.

1. Acute Diarrhea

Etiology & Clinical Findings

Diarrhea that is acute in onset and present for less than 3–4 weeks is most commonly caused by infectious agents, bacterial toxins (either ingested preformed in food or produced in gut), or drugs. A careful clinical history may provide clues to the causative agent. Large volume watery diarrhea usually indicates a small bowel disorder whereas frequent small-volume stools suggest a colonic or rectal disorder. A similar recent illness in family members suggests an infectious origin. Recent ingestion of improperly stored or prepared food implicates food poisoning, especially if other people were similarly affected. Exposure to unpurified water (camping, swimming) may result in infection with *Giardia* or

Table 1–5. Causes of acute diarrhea.

Noninflammatory Diarrhea[1]	Inflammatory Diarrhea[2]
Viral	**Viral**
Norwalk virus	Cytomegalovirus[3]
Rotavirus	**Bacterial**
Protozoa	**1. Cytotoxin production**
Giardia lamblia	*E coli* O157:H7 (enterohemorrhagic)
Cryptosporidium	*Vibrio parahaemolyticus*
Bacterial	*Clostridium difficile*
1. Preformed enterotoxin	**2. Mucosal invasion**
Staphylococcus aureus	*Shigella*
Bacillus cereus	*Salmonella* sp.
Clostridium perfringens	Enteroinvasive *E coli*
2. Intraintestinal enterotoxin production	Aeromonal
E coli (enterotoxigenic)	*Yersinia enterocolitica*
Vibrio cholerae	Plesimonal
New medications	**3. Bacterial proctitis**
Fecal impaction	*Chlamydia*
	N gonorrhoeae
	Protozoal
	Entamoeba histolytica
	Intestinal ischemia
	Inflammatory bowel disease
	Radiation colitis

[1]Noninflammatory: Fever absent. Stool without evidence of blood or fecal leukocytes.
[2]Inflammatory diarrhea: Often with systemic features, including fever. Fecal leukocytes with or without gross blood usually present. (**Note:** Fecal leukocytes are variable in *Salmonella, Yersinia, V parahaemolytica, C difficile,* and *Aeromonas.*)
[3]Most commonly in immunocompromised patients, especially AIDS. Full causes of AIDS-associated diarrhea are discussed in Chapter 2.

Cryptosporidium. Recent foreign travel suggests "traveler's diarrhea." Antibiotic usage within the preceding several weeks increases the likelihood of *Clostridium difficile* colitis. Patients should be asked about any new medications. Finally, risk factors for human immuno-deficiency virus (HIV) infection or sexually transmitted diseases should be determined. Patients practicing unprotected anal intercourse are at risk for a variety of infections, including gonorrhea, syphilis, lymphogranuloma venereum, and herpes simplex. A variety of medications may cause diarrhea through various mechanisms and should not be overlooked. A full discussion of AIDS-associated diarrhea and acute diarrhea is provided in Chapters 2 and 8, respectively. The nature of the diarrhea helps distinguish among different infectious causes (see Table 1–5).

A. NONINFLAMMATORY DIARRHEA

Watery, nonbloody diarrhea associated with periumbilical cramps, bloating, nausea, or vomiting suggests a small bowel enteritis caused by either a toxin-producing bacterium [enterotoxigenic *Escherichia coli* (ETEC), *Staphylococcus aureus, Bacillus cereus, Clostridium perfringens*] or other agents (viruses, *Giardia*) that disrupt the normal absorption and secretory process in the small intestine. Prominent vomiting suggests viral enteritis or *S aureus* food poisoning. Though typically mild, the diarrhea (which originates in the small intestine) may be voluminous (ranging from 10 to 200 mL per kg/24 h) and result in dehydration with hypokalemia and metabolic acidosis due to loss of HCO_3^- in the stool (eg, cholera). Because tissue invasion does not occur, fecal leukocytes are not present.

B. INFLAMMATORY DIARRHEA

The presence of fever and bloody diarrhea (dysentery) indicates colonic tissue damage caused by invasion (shigellosis, salmonellosis, *Campylobacter, Yersinia,* amebiasis) or a toxin (*C difficile, E coli* 0157:H7). Because these different organisms involve predominantly the colon, the diarrhea is small in volume (<1 L/d) and is associated with left lower quadrant cramps, urgency, and tenesmus. Fecal leukocytes are present in infections with invasive organisms. *E coli* 0157:H7 is a toxigenic, noninvasive organism that may be acquired from contaminated meat and has resulted in several outbreaks of an acute, often severe, hemorrhagic colitis. Most of these outbreaks have been traced to contaminated ground beef (eg, hamburger, salami) that has been improperly prepared. It now is believed to be the most common cause of infectious bloody diarrhea in adults and the most common cause of hemolytic uremic syndrome in children. In immunocompromised and HIV-infected patients, cytomegalovirus (CMV) may result in intestinal ulceration with watery or bloody diarrhea. Infectious dysentery must be distinguished from acute ulcerative colitis, which may also present acutely with fever, abdominal pain, and bloody diarrhea.

C. ENTERIC FEVER

A severe systemic illness manifested initially by prolonged high fevers, prostration, confusion, respiratory symptoms followed by abdominal tenderness, diarrhea, and a rash is due to infection with *Salmonella typhi* or *paratyphi,* which causes bacteremia and multiorgan dysfunction.

Evaluation

In over 90% of patients with acute diarrhea, the illness is mild and self-limited and responds within 5 days to simple rehydration therapy or symptomatic antidiarrheal agents. In these cases a stool culture is unnecessary and has a low yield. Indeed, the isolation rate of bacterial pathogens from stool cultures in patients with acute diarrhea is less than 3%. Thus, the goal of initial evaluation is to distinguish these patients from those with more serious illness. In many outpatient clinics, an examination of the stool for fecal leukocytes is obtained in order to distinguish noninflammatory from inflammatory diarrhea. This test is easy to perform and is inexpensive. The presence of fecal leukocytes suggests an inflammatory diarrhea and warrants a stool bacterial culture.

Patients with signs of a severe infection require prompt medical attention. These signs include high fever [>38.5°C (101.3°F)], bloody diarrhea, abdominal pain, or diarrhea not improving after 4–5 days. Similarly, patients with symptoms of dehydration (excessive thirst, dry mouth, decreased urination, weakness, lethargy) and those with an immunocompromised state must be evaluated. Physical examination should note the patient's general appearance, mental status, volume status, and the presence of abdominal tenderness or peritonitis. Peritoneal findings may be present in *C difficile* and enterohemorrhagic *E coli.* Hospitalization is required in patients with severe dehydration, toxicity, or abdominal pain. Stool specimens should be collected from patients in order to examine for fecal leukocytes and bacterial cultures (see Table 1 –5). The rate of positive bacterial cultures in patients with dysentery symptoms is 60–75%. A wet mount examination of the stool for amebiasis also should be performed in patients with dysentery who have recently traveled to endemic areas or those who are homosexual. In patients with a history of antibiotic exposure, a stool sample should be sent for *C difficile* toxin testing. If *E coli* 0157:H7 is suspected, the laboratory must be alerted to do specific serotyping. In patients with diarrhea that persists for longer than 10 days, three stool examinations for ova and parasites also should be performed. Rectal swabs may be sent to a laboratory for *Chlamydia*, gonorrhea, and herpes simplex virus testing in sexually active patients with severe proctitis symptoms.

Sigmoidoscopy is warranted acutely in patients with symptoms of severe proctitis (tenesmus, discharge, rectal pain) and in patients with suspected *C difficile* colitis who appear ill. It may also be helpful in distinguishing infectious diarrhea from ulcerative colitis or ischemic colitis, especially in patients with bloody diarrhea.

Treatment

A. DIET

The overwhelming majority of adults have mild diarrhea that will not lead to dehydration provided the patient takes adequate oral fluids containing carbohydrates and electrolytes. Patients will find it more comfortable to rest the bowel by avoiding high fiber foods, fats, milk products, caffeine, and alcohol. Frequent feedings of fruit drinks, tea, defizzed carbonated beverages, and soft, easily digested foods (eg, soups, crackers) are encouraged.

B. REHYDRATION

In more severe diarrhea, dehydration can occur quickly, especially in children. Oral rehydration therapy containing glucose, Na$^+$, K$^+$, Cl$^-$, and bicarbonate or citrate is preferred in most cases to intravenous fluids because it is inexpensive, safe, and highly effective in almost all awake patients. An easy mixture is 1/2 teaspoon salt (3.5 g), 1 teaspoon baking soda (2.5 g NaHCO$_3$), 8 teaspoons sugar (40 g), and 8 ounces of orange juice (1.5 g KCl) may be diluted to 1 L with water. Alternatively, oral electrolyte solutions are readily available. Fluids should be given at rates of 50–200 mL/kg/24 h, depending on the hydration status. Intravenous fluids (lactated Ringer's solution) is preferred acutely in patients with severe dehydration.

C. SYMPTOMATIC AGENTS

Antidiarrheal agents may be used safely in patients with mild to moderate diarrheal illnesses to improve patient comfort. Opiate agents help decrease the stool number and liquidity and control fecal urgency. However, they should not be used in patients with bloody diarrhea, high fever, or systemic toxicity for fear of worsening the disease. Similarly, they should be discontinued in patients whose diarrhea is worsening despite therapy. With these provisos, these agents provide excellent symptomatic relief. Loperamide is the preferred agent; 4 mg is given initially, followed by 2 mg after each loose stool (maximum: 16 mg/24 h). Bismuth subsalicylate (PeptoBismol), two tablets or 30 mL four times daily reduces symptoms in patients with traveler's diarrhea because it stimulates sodium and water reabsorption, binds enterotoxins, and has a direct antibacterial effect; its role in other settings is poorly studied. Scores of other agents touted for their antidiarrheal action have undergone little or no controlled testing but appear to have minimal or no symptomatic benefit (lactobacilli, kaolin, pectin). Anticholinergic agents are contraindicated in acute diarrhea (eg, atropine).

D. ANTIBIOTIC THERAPY

1. Empiric treatment—The overwhelming majority of patients have mild, self-limited disease due to viruses or noninvasive bacteria, and empiric antibiotic treatment for these patients is not warranted. Even patients with inflammatory diarrhea caused by invasive pathogens most often have mild disease that will resolve within several days without specific treatment. However, for patients who appear to have signs of an invasive pathogen with moderate to severe symptoms of fever, tenesmus, severe abdominal pain, bloody stools, and positive fecal leukocytes, empiric treatment is recommended while awaiting the results of the stool culture. The drugs of choice are the quinolones (ciprofloxacin 500 mg twice daily) for 5–7 days. These agents have good antibiotic coverage against most invasive bacterial pathogens, including *Shigella, Salmonella, Campylobacter, Yersinia,* and *Aeromonas.* Treatment with antibiotics generally results in a shortened duration of illness by 1–2 days. Alternative agents are trimethoprim/sulfamethoxazole 160/800 mg twice daily or erythromycin 250–500 mg four times daily.

2. Specific antimicrobial treatment—Antibiotics are not generally recommended in patients with nontyphoid *Salmonella, Campylobacter,* or *Yersinia* except in severe or prolonged disease because they have not been shown to hasten recovery or reduce the period of fecal bacterial excretion. The infectious diarrheas for which treatment is clearly recommended are *Shigella,* cholera, extraintestinal salmonellosis, "traveler's diarrhea," *C difficile, Giardia, Entamoeba histolytica,* and the sexually transmitted infections (gonorrhea, syphilis, *Chlamydia,* and herpes simplex infection). Specific treatment of these organisms is discussed in Chapter 8.

2. Chronic Diarrhea

Etiology

The causes of chronic diarrhea may be grouped into six major pathophysiologic categories (Table 1–6).

A. OSMOTIC

As stool leaves the colon, the fecal osmolality is equal to the serum osmolality, ie, approximately 290 mOsm/kg. Osmotic diarrhea results when poorly absorbed osmoti-

Table 1–6. Causes of chronic diarrhea.

Osmotic diarrhea
  Lactose intolerance
  Medications: sorbitol, lactulose, antacids
  Factitious: magnesium laxatives or sodium sulfate laxatives
  Clues: Stool volume decreases with fasting; increased osmotic gap greater than 50 mOsm/L
Malabsorptive conditions
  Intestinal mucosal diseases: celiac sprue, Whipple's disease, eosinophilic gastroenteritis, Crohn's disease, small bowel resection
  Lymphatic obstruction
  Pancreatic disease: chronic pancreatitis, pancreatic carcinoma
  Small bowel bacterial overgrowth: motility disorders (vagotomy, scleroderma, diabetes), colonic-enteric fistulas, small intestinal diverticula
  Clues: Weight loss, fecal fat greater than 7–10 g/24 h stool collection, anemia, hypoalbuminemia
Secretory diarrhea
  Hormonal secretion: VIPoma, carcinoid, medullary carcinoma of thyroid, Zollinger-Ellison syndrome (gastrinoma)
  Bile salt malabsorption: ileal resection, Crohn's disease
  Medications
  Factitious: phenolphthalein, cascara, senna
  Villous adenoma
  Clues: Large volume (>1 L/d); little change with fasting (except with bile salt diarrhea); normal stool osmotic gap
Inflammatory conditions
  Ulcerative colitis
  Crohn's disease
  Microscopic colitis
  Radiation enteritis
  Malignancy: lymphoma, adenocarcinoma
  Clues: Fever, hematochezia or abdominal pain (absent in microscopic colitis)
Motility disorders
  Postsurgical: vagotomy, partial gastrectomy
  Systemic disorders: scleroderma, diabetes mellitus, hyperthyroidism
  Irritable bowel syndrome

---

cally active solutes are present in the gut lumen. These osmotically active solutes result in increased fecal water content and increased stool liquidity. Under normal circumstances, the major osmoles in stool are Na⁺, K⁺, Cl⁻, and bicarbonate. The stool osmolality may be estimated by multiplying the stool (Na⁺ + K⁺)/2 (multiplied by two to account for the anions). The osmotic gap is the difference between the *measured* osmolality of the stool electrolytes and the total osmolality of the

stool (which is approximately 290 mOsm/kg). The normal difference between the measured osmolality of stool (determined by stool electrolytes as shown above) and the total predicted osmolality of 290 mOsm/kg is less than 50 mOsm/kg. An increased osmotic gap implies the diarrhea is caused by ingestion or malabsorption of an osmotically active substance. The most common causes of osmotic diarrhea are disaccharidase deficiency (lactase deficiency), laxative abuse, ingestion of poorly absorbable carbohydrates (lactulose, sorbitol), and malabsorption syndromes (see the following section). A clinical hallmark of osmotic diarrhea is that it resolves during fasting. Osmotic diarrheas caused by malabsorbed carbohydrates are characterized by abdominal distention, bloating, and flatulence resulting from increased colonic gas production.

Disaccharidase deficiencies are extremely common and should always be considered in patients with chronic diarrhea. Lactase deficiency occurs in three-fourths of nonwhite adults and up to 25% of white adults. It may also be acquired after viral gastroenteritis, a medical illness, or gastrointestinal surgery. Sorbitol is a commonly used as a sweetener in "sugar-free" gums, candies, and some medications (elixirs); this may cause diarrhea in some patients. The diagnosis of sorbitol or lactose malabsorption may be established by an elimination trial for 2–3 weeks. The diagnosis may be confirmed by measuring a rise in breath hydrogen of more than 20 ppm after lactose or sorbitol ingestion, but this is seldom necessary.

Ingestion of magnesium or phosphate-containing compounds (laxatives, antacids) should be considered in enigmatic diarrhea. Surreptitious use should be considered, especially in young women with possible eating disorders and patients with psychiatric problems, a long history of vague or mysterious medical ailments, or employment in the medical field.

B. MALABSORPTIVE CONDITIONS

The major causes of malabsorption are mucosal diseases of the small intestine (eg, sprue), pancreatic insufficiency, intestinal resections (short-bowel syndrome), lymphatic obstruction, and small intestinal bacterial overgrowth. The hallmarks of malabsorption are weight loss, osmotic diarrhea, and nutrient deficiencies. Significant diarrhea in the absence of weight loss is unlikely to be malabsorption. The physical and laboratory abnormalities related to deficiencies of vitamins or minerals are discussed elsewhere. Briefly, they include anemia (micro- or macrocytic), hypoalbuminemia, low serum cholesterol, hypocalcemia, and an elevated prothrombin time.

In patients with suspected malabsorption, a quantification of the stool fecal fat should be performed. In patients with more than 10 g/24 h of fecal fat, further workup for malabsorption is indicated (see Chapter 23).

C. SECRETORY CONDITIONS

Diarrhea results from abnormal ion transport in enterocytes. Increased intestinal ion secretion or decreased ion absorption results in a watery diarrhea that is typically large volume (1–10 L/d). Secretory diarrhea has a normal osmotic gap and usually there is little change in stool output during the fasting state. In serious conditions, significant dehydration and electrolyte imbalance may develop. Major causes include endocrine tumors (stimulating intestinal or pancreatic secretion), bile salt or fatty acid malabsorption (stimulating colonic secretion), and laxative abuse (phenolphthalein).

D. INFLAMMATORY CONDITIONS

Diarrhea is present in the majority of patients with inflammatory bowel disease (eg, ulcerative colitis, Crohn's disease, microscopic colitis). A variety of other symptoms may be present including abdominal pain, fever, weight loss, and hematochezia (see Chapter 7).

E. MOTILITY DISORDERS

Abnormal intestinal motility secondary to systemic disorders or surgery may result in diarrhea due to rapid transit, or due to stasis of intestinal contents with bacterial overgrowth resulting in malabsorption. Patients with diarrhea due to rapid motility generally have <1 L stool/d and a normal osmotic gap. Mild steatorrhea may also be present. Perhaps the most common cause of chronic diarrhea is irritable bowel syndrome. In this idiopathic, chronic condition, patients have a variety of complaints including abdominal pain (often relieved by defecation), bloating, and disturbed defecation with fluctuating stool consistency and frequency (see Chapter 7). Although many of these patients complain of diarrhea, the majority, in fact, have a normal stool weight (see Chapter 6).

F. CHRONIC INFECTIONS

Chronic parasitic infections may cause diarrhea through a number of mechanisms. Although the list of parasitic organisms is lengthy, the most common organisms are *Giardia* and *E histolytica,* and the intestinal nematodes. Immunocompromised patients, especially those with AIDS, are susceptible to a number of infectious agents that can cause acute or chronic diarrhea (see Chapter 2). Chronic diarrhea in AIDS patients is commonly caused by *Microsporidia, Cryptosporidia,* cytomegalovirus, *Isospora belli,* and *Mycobacterium avium-intracellulare* (MAC).

Evaluation

The list of diagnostic tests available for the evaluation of chronic diarrhea is exhaustive. In most cases, however, a careful history and physical examination suggest the underlying pathophysiologic category that guides the subsequent diagnostic work-up (Figure 1–2). The following tests are commonly employed in the evaluation of chronic diarrhea.

A. STOOL ANALYSIS

1. Quantitative stool collection for weight and quantitative fecal fat—A 48–72 hour stool collection is useful to document the quantity of stool and whether steatorrhea is present. The patient should eat three moderately high-fat meals per day while collecting the stool specimen. Olestra should be avoided since it results in increased fecal fat measurements. A stool weight of more than 250 g/24 h confirms the presence of diarrhea, justifying further work-up. Patients with irritable bowel syndrome rarely have stool weight >500 g/24 h. A stool weight >1000–1500 g/24 h suggests a secretory process. Fecal fat in the range of 7–14 g/d can occur as a nonspecific phenomenon from any diarrheal illness, whereas fecal fat exceeding 14 g/d is more specific for disorders of fat digestion and absorption (eg, pancreatic insufficiency or small bowel mucosal disorders).

2. Stool osmolality—This can be performed on a spot stool specimen. Measurement of stool electrolytes allows calculation of the osmotic gap; if elevated the osmotic gap confirms the presence of osmotic diarrhea. The electrolytes should be used to calculate osmolality (see above) rather than performing direct measurement of fecal osmolality, since bacteria produce osmotically active substances that alter the measured osmolality. A stool osmolality less than the serum osmolality implies that water or urine has been added to the specimen (factitious diarrhea).

3. Stool laxative screen—In suspected laxative abuse, stool magnesium, phosphate, and sulfate levels may be ordered. Phenolphthalein is indicated by the presence of a bright red color after alkalinization of the stool. Bisacodyl can be detected in the urine.

4. Fecal leukocytes—The presence of leukocytes in a stool sample implies an underlying inflammatory diarrhea.

5. Stool for ova and parasites—In normal hosts, *Giardia* and *E histolytica* are considered.

B. LABORATORY TESTS

1. Routine tests—CBC, serum electrolytes, liver chemistry tests, calcium, phosphorus, albumin, thyroid-stimulating hormone (TSH), total thyoxine (T_4), β-carotene, and protime should be obtained. Anemia occurs in malabsorption (B_{12}, folate, iron) and inflammatory conditions. Hypoalbuminemia is present in malabsorption, protein losing enteropathies, and inflammatory diseases. Hyponatremia and nonanion gap metabolic acidosis may occur in profound secretory di-

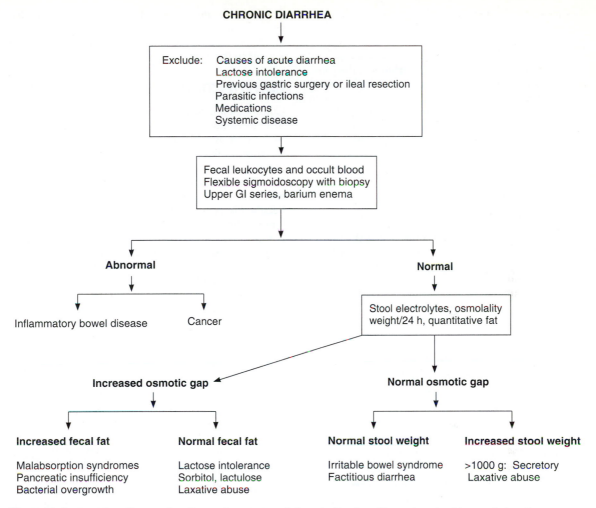

CHRONIC DIARRHEA

Exclude:
Causes of acute diarrhea
Lactose intolerance
Previous gastric surgery or ileal resection
Parasitic infections
Medications
Systemic disease

Fecal leukocytes and occult blood
Flexible sigmoidoscopy with biopsy
Upper GI series, barium enema

Abnormal

Inflammatory bowel disease   Cancer

Normal

Stool electrolytes, osmolality
weight/24 h, quantitative fat

Increased osmotic gap

Normal osmotic gap

Increased fecal fat

Malabsorption syndromes
Pancreatic insufficiency
Bacterial overgrowth

Normal fecal fat

Lactose intolerance
Sorbitol, lactulose
Laxative abuse

Normal stool weight

Irritable bowel syndrome
Factitious diarrhea

Increased stool weight

>1000 g: Secretory
Laxative abuse

Figure 1–2. Decision diagram for diagnosing causes of chronic diarrhea. [Reproduced, with permission, from McQuaid KR: Alimentary Tract. In: *Current Medical Diagnosis & Treatment 1996.* Tierney LM Jr, McPhee SJ, Papadakis MA (editors). Appleton & Lange, 1996.]

arrheas. Malabsorption of fat-soluble vitamins may result in an abnormal protime, low calcium, low carotene, or abnormal alkaline phosphatase.

2. Specific laboratory tests—In patients with suspected secretory diarrhea, serum vasoactive intestinal peptide (VIP) (VIPoma), gastrin (Zollinger-Ellison), calcitonin (medullary thyroid carcinoma), cortisol (Addison's), and urinary 5-hydroxyindoleacetic acid (5-HIAA) (carcinoid) levels should be obtained.

C. Colonoscopy or Flexible Sigmoidoscopy with Mucosal Biopsy

Examination may be helpful in detecting inflammatory bowel disease and melanosis coli, which indicates

chronic use of anthraquinone laxatives. Colonoscopy provides the advantage of inspecting the entire colon and terminal ileum, and may theoretically allow detection of Crohn's disease that may be missed by sigmoidoscopy alone. In cases in which the mucosa appears endoscopically normal, biopsies should be obtained to rule out the presence of microscopic colitis.

D. Upper Endoscopy

Upper endoscopy with small bowel biopsy is useful in suspected malabsorption due to mucosal diseases (eg, sprue, Whipple's disease, intestinal lymphoma). Upper endoscopy with a duodenal aspirate and small bowel biopsy is also useful in patients with AIDS and to document *Cryptosporidium, Microsporidia,* and MAC infection.

E. IMAGING STUDIES

After the above studies have been performed, the cause of the diarrhea will generally be clear and further imaging studies can be ordered as indicated. Calcification on a plain abdominal radiograph confirms chronic pancreatitis. An upper gastrointestinal series or enteroclysis study is helpful in evaluating Crohn's disease, lymphoma, or carcinoid. Abdominal CT is helpful in detecting chronic pancreatitis or pancreatic endocrine tumors.

Treatment

Treatment of chronic diarrhea is directed at the underlying condition. A number of antidiarrheal agents may be used in certain situations in patients with chronic diarrheal conditions.

A. NARCOTIC ANALOGUES

These may be used safely in most patients with chronic, stable symptoms.

1. Loperamide—4 mg initially; then 2 mg after each loose stool (maximum dose: 16 mg/d).

2. Diphenoxylate with atropine—One or two tablets to four times daily.

B. NARCOTICS

Because of their addictive potential these are generally avoided except in cases of chronic, intractable diarrhea.

1. Codeine—15–60 mg every 4 hours, as needed.

2. Paregoric—4–8 mL after liquid bowel movement.

3. Deodorized tincture of opium (10 mg morphine/mL)—5–20 drops four times per day.

C. OTHER AGENTS

1. Clonidine—α_2-Adrenergic agonists inhibit intestinal electrolyte secretion. Clonidine, available as a patch that administers 1 mg/d for 7 days or given as a tablet 0.1 mg two times a day initially and gradually increased to 0.4–0.6 mg/d, may be useful in some patients with secretory diarrheas, *Cryptosporidia,* and diabetes.

2. Octreotide—This somatostatin analogue stimulates intestinal fluid and electrolyte absorption and inhibits secretion. Furthermore, it inhibits the release of gastrointestinal peptides. It is very useful in treating secretory diarrheas due to VIPoma and carcinoid and in some cases of diarrhea associated with AIDS. Effective doses range from 50 to 250 μg subcutaneously three times daily.

3. Cholestyramine—This bile salt binding resin may be useful in patients with bile salt-induced diarrhea secondary to intestinal resection or ileal disease. A dose of 4 g one to three times daily is recommended.

CONSTIPATION

Constipation is best described as a perception of abnormal bowel movements that may include straining, hard stools, decreased frequency, and a feeling of incomplete evacuation. The frequency of "normal" bowel movements is broad, ranging from 3 to 12 per week; two or fewer bowel movements per week is considered abnormal. In many patients the complaint of constipation reflects a mistaken perception of what constitutes normal bowel habits. From a medical perspective, constipation is present when a patient has fewer than three bowel movements per week or when a patient has excessive straining at defecation. Constipation is extremely common and more often affects women than men. Surveys of the American population have shown a prevalence of constipation ranging from 2 to 20%, depending on the definition used. A marked increase in the complaint of constipation occurs with advancing age. Constipation is associated with a sedentary lifestyle, poor calorie intake, and the number of medications being taken (irrespective of their side-effect profile). Constipation is among the most common complaints encountered by primary care physicians and gastroenterologists, and the economic resources directed toward the evaluation and treatment of constipation are considerable.

The primary functions of the colon are the storage and conversion of liquid chyme to solid fecal bulk and the timely elimination of fecal contents. Approximately 1 L of liquid chyme passes daily through the ileocecal valve into the colon. Through a process of active colonic resorption of fluid and electrolytes and the activity of gut bacteria, this is converted to approximately 200 g of solid fecal waste. The colon may be divided into three functional regions: the proximal colon, the distal colon, and the rectum. In the proximal colon, which extends from the cecum to the hepatic flexure, fecal chyme is churned and mixed by rhythmic segmental and retrograde contractions that retard fecal passage and permit fluid resorption. Thus, this segment serves an important reservoir function. Intermittently, orthograde contractions occur that propel solid contents forward into the more distal colon. In the segment from the transverse colon to the rectosigmoid junction, orthograde rhythmic contractions occur that gradually move the more solid contents toward the rectum, allowing further fluid resorption. Two to three times daily there is a large propulsive movement that propels a larger amount of fecal contents distally. The rectum appears to fill slowly with solid contents from the sigmoid and serves as a storage area until elimination is convenient.

The process of defecation involves a complex array of autonomic and voluntary mechanisms. To permit defecation, the natural barriers to involuntary elimination must be overcome. Under normal circumstances, continence is assisted by the pelvic floor muscles (puborectalis and pubococcygeus), striated muscles that are innervated by the pudendal nerve and are under voluntary control. These muscles form a sling around the rectum to form an acute anorectal angle. In addition, the internal anal sphincter, which is under involuntary control, is tonically contracted. When the rectum becomes distended, the internal anal sphincter relaxes, due to spinal and intramural inhibitory reflexes. If elimination is not desired, voluntary contraction of the pelvic floor muscles and external sphincter prevents defecation until the internal anal sphincter tone returns. When defecation is desired, voluntary relaxation of the pelvic floor permits perineal descent and straightening of the anorectal angle. This is facilitated by assuming a squatting or sitting position. A Valsalva maneuver to increase intraabdominal pressure in conjunction with a mass rectal contraction permits evacuation.

Etiology

Given the complexity of colonic function and the defecatory process, constipation can occur for a variety of reasons. Constipation may occur as a result of abnormal motor function of the large intestine, which may be due to systemic disease, medications, or primary motor disorders of the bowel. Alternatively, abnormalities of the muscular structures of the anorectum (pelvic floor dysfunction) may lead to abnormal defecation and complaints of constipation.

The vast majority of constipated patients have mild symptoms that cannot be attributed to any structural abnormalities, intestinal motility disturbances, or systemic disease. Careful dietary review reveals that most of these patients do not consume adequate dietary fiber or fluids. Many patients ignore nature's "call to stool." In addition, immobility produced by chronic illness may lead to fecal retention and loss of rectal sensory cues to defecate, resulting in fecal impaction. The elderly in particular are predisposed to constipation because of a combination of poor eating habits, the use of medications that are constipating, decreased colonic motility, and physical limitations that may restrict ease of access to a bathroom or the ability to sit for defecation.

A. SYSTEMIC DISEASES

A variety of neurologic, endocrinologic, metabolic, and collagen vascular disorders may cause constipation (Table 1–7).

B. MEDICATIONS

A number of medications may produce constipation (see Table 1–7).

C. STRUCTURAL ABNORMALITIES

Colonic lesions that obstruct fecal passage (eg, malignancy) must be excluded in patients with constipation, particularly in patients over age 45 years with new-onset symptoms. The possibility of Hirschsprung's disease should be raised in younger patients with lifelong constipation.

E. IDIOPATHIC CONSTIPATION

The vast majority of patients with refractory constipation do not have an identifiable systemic disease or medication to which constipation may be attributed, and fall into the category of idiopathic constipation. These patients are categorized according to findings on colonic transit studies and studies of rectosphincteric function. These tests are described more fully in the section, "Diagnostic Studies."

1. Colonic inertia—The term "colonic inertia" describes an idiopathic delay in large bowel transit. The slow colonic transit is thought to be due to a decreased number of high-amplitude peristaltic contractions, or to uncoordinated motor activity in the distal colon that impairs the movement of fecal residues through the colon. Severe colonic inertia is more common in women, some of whom have a history of abuse or psychosocial problems. Colonic inertia may be part of a more generalized gastrointestinal dysmotility syndrome.

2. Pelvic floor dysfunction (also termed "outlet obstruction," "dyschezia," "anismus")—These patients have an inability to empty stool from the rectum. This may be due to the inability to relax the pelvic floor and external anal sphincter, or to muscular hypotonicity and excessive pelvic floor descent leading to an inability to expel stool. An abnormality in the relaxation of the puborectalis or sphincter mechanism results in impaired evacuation of the rectum and may occur with or without an abnormality of colonic transit. Pelvic floor dysfunction most commonly affects women. Difficulty evacuating stool can occur as a result of a variety of anatomic problems that impede or obstruct flow, some of which may benefit from surgery (eg, rectocele or intussusception). In other patients there is a failure to relax the pelvic floor during straining (anismus).

3. Constipation with normal colonic transit—Patients with a complaint of constipation often have normal colonic transit when evaluated by a radiopaque marker study. These patients' complaints are often due to irritable bowel syndrome. They should be treated with an aggressive bowel regimen without further investigatory studies.

Table 1–7. Causes of constipation in adults.

Lifestyle	**Systemic disease**
Low fiber	**Metabolic and endocrine**
Inadequate fluids	Hypothyroidism
Poor toilet habits	Hypercalcemia
Inability to sit on toilet	Chronic renal failure
Inadequate exercise	Diabetes mellitus
Medications	**Neurologic disorders**
Anticholinergics	Spinal cord lesions
Antidepressants	Multiple sclerosis
Neuroleptic agents	Parkinson's disease
Antihistamines	Hirschsprung's disease
Antiparkinsonian drugs	Autonomic neuropathy
Antihypertensives	Prior pelvic surgery with disruption of parasympathetics
Calcium channel blockers	**Others**
Clonidine	Amyloidosis
Cation-containing agents	Dermatomyositis
Iron supplements	Progressive systemic sclerosis
Calcium supplements	Depression
Aluminum-containing antacids, sucralfate	Dementia
Opiates	**Causes of refractory constipation**
Morphine	**Slow colonic transit**
Codeine	Idiopathic
Diphenoxylate	Chronic intestinal pseudoobstruction
Structural abnormalities	**Anorectal outlet disorders**
Perianal disease: fissure, thrombosed hemorrhoid	Rectocoele
Obstructing colonic carcinoma	Rectal intussusception
Colonic stricture: diverticular, radiation, ischemia	Rectal prolapse
Idiopathic megarectum	Perineal descent
	Anismus

Clinical Findings

A. SYMPTOMS AND SIGNS

The first step in the evaluation is to better define the nature of the symptoms. It is important to clarify whether the patient is complaining of decreased frequency of stools, painful evacuation, incomplete evacuation, or small hard stools. A history of excessive straining, the need to digitally extract stool, persistent rectal fullness, or pelvic floor descent suggest **pelvic floor dysfunction**. Patients may also report symptoms that occur between bowel movements (eg, pain or bloating) that suggest irritable bowel syndrome. The chronicity of the symptoms is perhaps the most important historical question. A recent change in bowel habits makes an identifiable cause more likely and requires investigation, whereas longstanding complaints suggest a functional origin. The patient should be questioned regarding toilet habits, including the time of day and duration of use. A history of exercise and dietary habits (with emphasis on fiber intake) should be obtained. Questioning the patient about whether he or she is depressed

is appropriate in the evaluation of constipation. There should be a thorough review of prescription and non-prescription medications, with special attention to use of laxative preparations.

In the majority of patients with constipation the physical examination is normal. Signs of systemic diseases, such as diabetes mellitus or hypothyroidism, should be sought. Distended bowel loops or a palpable abdominal mass suggest malignancy. The rectal examination may detect the presence of occult blood, rectal masses, anal fissures, fecal impaction, abnormal sphincter tone, or rectal prolapse. The sensation of the perineal area and the "anal wink" (a reflex contraction of the sphincter upon pinprick stimulation of the perianal area) reflex should be tested.

B. DIAGNOSTIC STUDIES

1. Routine studies—Initial laboratory studies include a screening blood count, chemistry panel, tests of thyroid function, and serum calcium. The selection of patients for further investigation depends on the patient's age, chronicity of symptoms, and the presence of occult or gross bleeding. Patients with a recent change in bowel habits, weight loss, or evidence of rectal bleeding require examination with flexible sigmoidoscopy and barium enema (or colonoscopy) to exclude mass lesions or stricture. Patients lacking these features who are 45 years of age or older should undergo a flexible sigmoidoscopy followed by an empiric trial of fiber supplementation and general measures (see the following section) if the flexible sigmoidoscopy is unrevealing. Patients who are 45 years of age or younger should initially be managed by a trial of fiber supplementation.

2. Specific studies—Studies of colonic motility and rectosphincteric function should be reserved for patients with severe symptoms who fail conservative measures of treatment, and who have had structural abnormalities ruled out with a colonoscopic or barium enema examination. This group of patients with intractable constipation constitutes a small proportion (estimated at <1%) of the total population of patients with constipation.

   a. Colonic transit study—The initial test of colonic motility performed should be a radiopaque marker intestinal transit study (Sitz-Mark, Konsyl Pharmaceutical, Fort Worth, TX). This is a simple technique that provides an assessment of overall colonic motor function. The test has been shown to be reproducible. This should be the first study performed for patients with persistent symptoms despite a trial of laxatives (and following a colonoscopy or barium enema to rule out structural lesions). Patients should be on a high fiber diet but should not use laxatives or enemas during the study. The simplest technique involves the ingestion of 24 radiopaque markers at time zero followed by a single abdominal radiograph 5 days later. In a normal study, 80% of the markers are evacuated by the fifth day. A modification of this protocol allows assessment of segmental colonic function by having patients ingest 24 markers on 3 consecutive days followed by radiographs on the fourth and seventh days. The total number of markers remaining on these radiographs are totalled, yielding an approximation of total colonic transit time. In addition, the markers in the right colon, left colon, and rectosigmoid can be tallied to give segmental transit times. Normal colonic transit time is approximately 35 hours; more than 72 hours is significantly abnormal. Patients with abnormal transit studies have what has been termed **colonic inertia.**

   The usefulness of a radiopaque marker transit study lies in its ability to identify patients who complain of constipation but have normal colonic motility. Some of these patients may have irritable bowel syndrome, and there appears to be a higher frequency of abnormalities on psychological testing in these patients as well. Patients with normal clearance of radiopaque markers do not require further colonic evaluation.

Radionuclide gamma scintigraphic techniques have also been developed to assess colonic function, and appear to correlate well with radiopaque marker transit studies. Although scintigraphic techniques are advantageous because of the ability to assess gastric and small bowel motor function in addition to colonic function, the use of this technique is likely to be limited by the higher cost and the need for nuclear medicine isotopes and equipment.

   b. Studies of pelvic floor function—Patients with symptoms suggesting an abnormality of the process of defecation (eg, digital extraction of stool, excessive straining) should undergo specialized studies to rule out pelvic floor dysfunction. The simplest way to test for pelvic floor dysfunction is to ask the patient to attempt to expel the examiner's finger during digital rectal examination. The puborectalis muscle should normally move posteriorly during this maneuver. Other specialized studies available to rule out pelvic floor dysfunction include the balloon expulsion test, anorectal manometry, and defecography. The **balloon expulsion test** involves inserting a urinary catheter into the patient's rectum and inflating it with approximately 50 mL of water. Although this test has not been formally validated, inability of the patient to expel the balloon is useful as a screening test for major dysfunctions of stool evacuation. **Defecography** can be performed with barium or scintigraphically. When performed with barium, it involves instillation of barium of stool consistency into the patient's rectum and fluoroscopically assessing rectal evacuation as the patient sits on a commode. Defecography allows determination of whether the anorectal angle opens (due to puborectalis relaxation) and the amount of pelvic floor descent. The presence of a rectocele or intussusception may also be detected, which may benefit from surgery. In addition, abnormal contraction of the pelvic muscles during attempts at defecation can be identified, a condition known as **anismus** or **pelvic floor dyssynergia.** This latter condition may benefit from biofeedback therapy. **Anorectal manometry** rarely may lead to the diagnosis of adult onset Hirschprung's disease (as evidenced by failure of rectal balloon distention to cause relaxation of the internal anal sphincter) and may also show evidence of abnormally high anal sphincter pressure suggesting anismus or evidence of decreased rectal sensation. An algorithm suggesting the appropriate use of these studies is shown in Figure 1–3.

Treatment of Chronic Constipation

A. GENERAL MEASURES

Attempts should be made to minimize use of any medications known to cause constipation, and to correct any metabolic abnormalities (eg, hypothyroidism). Regular exercise and an increase in fluid intake (at least

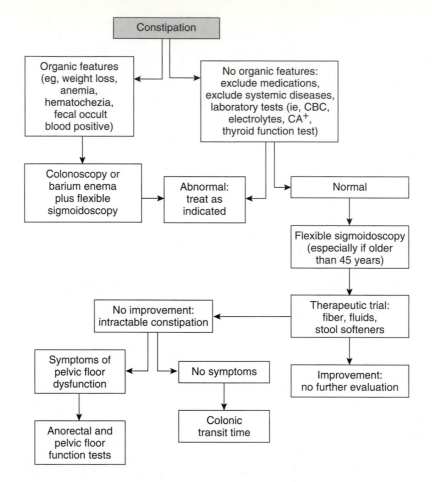

Figure 1–3. Algorithm suggesting appropriate diagnostic studies for constipation.

1500 mL/d) may also be beneficial. Patients should be encouraged to attempt defecation each day for 10–15 minutes approximately 30 minutes following breakfast.

B. DIETARY MODIFICATION

A gradual increase in dietary fiber to between 20 and 30 g daily is the mainstay of therapy. Fiber serves to increase stool bulk and water content. This may be partially accomplished through an increase in the intake of fruits, vegetables, or high-fiber breakfast cereals (All Bran and Fiber One each contains >10 g of fiber per serving), but for many patients a bulk-forming laxative is required. Patients should take fiber supplements in two daily doses, with meals. Increased bloating and gaseousness may occur with fiber supplementation, but this often subsides after several days of therapy. Although fiber benefits the majority of patients, it does not benefit those with severe colonic inertia or outlet disorders.

1. Bran powder—Between 1 and 2 tablespoons of bran powder twice daily mixed with fluids or sprinkled over foods is an inexpensive means of providing 10–20 g/d of fiber.

2. Fiber supplements—A variety of pharmaceutical supplements are available; they are, however, more expensive than bran powder. Preparations include psyllium and methylcellulose, 1 teaspoon to 1 tablespoon one to three times daily (both are natural fibers derived from vegetable matter). Polycarbophil, 1 g one to four times daily, is a synthetic fiber that may be less gas producing than natural fibers.

C. PHARMACOLOGIC THERAPY

With the exception of the bulk-forming laxatives (fiber), attempts should be made to minimize the regular use of laxative preparations. In patients with continued symptoms despite general measures and a bulk-forming laxative, addition of a small daily dose of a hyperosmotic laxative may be effective with minimal risk of long-term use.

1. Osmotic laxatives—These agents may be used to soften stools. They are commonly employed in elderly nonambulatory patients or institutionalized patients to prevent constipation and fecal impaction. They may be used safely long term and do not induce dependency. These agents cause osmotic retention of fluid in the bowel lumen. They are typically titrated to a dose that results in soft to semiliquid stools.

   a. Nonabsorbable sugars—Lactulose or sorbitol, 15–60 mL daily. Sorbitol is as effective as lactulose and is considerably less expensive. These sugars may result in significant bloating, cramps, and flatulence due to bacterial metabolism of unabsorbed carbohydrate.

   b. Saline laxatives—Magnesium hydroxide (milk of magnesia) is inexpensive and is dosed 15–30 mL daily. Patients may titrate the dose to obtain soft stools. Hypermagnesemia may result in patients with impaired renal function. Magnesium sulfate, sodium phosphate, and sodium sulfate are also osmotic/saline laxatives.

2. Emollient laxatives—Docusate sodium (50–200 mg per d) or mineral oil (1–2 tablespoons/d) may be given orally to promote stool softening. Mineral oil should be avoided in patients with decreased neurologic function owing to the risk of aspiration with pneumonitis.

3. Stimulant laxatives—Senna, bisacodyl, or cascara may be given if the above agents fail. In the past these agents have been thought to result in damage to the enteric nervous system ("cathartic colon"), although convincing evidence for this effect is lacking. Chronic use of anthraquinones (cascara, senna, casanthranol, danthron) may lead to melanosis coli, a condition without clinical consequence.

Treatment of Refractory Constipation

A. BIOFEEDBACK

In patients with pelvic floor dyssynergia (anismus) biofeedback appears to be effective in up to two-thirds of patients, particularly children. A visual feedback signal [most commonly the external anal sphincter electromyography (EMG) reading] is provided for the patient so that the relaxation of the pelvic floor structures may be achieved during attempts at defecation.

B. SURGERY

Selected patients with colonic inertia and severe symptoms who fail an aggressive trial of medical therapy have been shown to benefit from a subtotal colectomy with ileorectal anastomosis. Motility studies of the upper gastrointestinal tract must first be performed to rule out a generalized motility disturbance. Some anatomic problems (eg, rectal prolapse, vaginal rectocele) may benefit from surgical correction.

C. PSYCHIATRIC REFERRAL

Patients with depression or a history of sexual abuse may benefit from psychiatric therapy.

Treatment of Acute Constipation

Normal people and patients with chronic constipation can become acutely constipated in response to acute medical or surgical illness, dietary changes, medications, or travel. If several days pass since the last movement, the therapies previously described for chronic constipation will not be sufficient to induce a prompt evacuation and relief of discomfort. In such cases, cathartic or osmotic laxatives or enemas may be given. **Caution:** These agents should not be given to patients with a possible large bowel obstruction or fecal impaction.

A. CATHARTIC LAXATIVES (STIMULANT LAXATIVES)

These agents stimulate fluid secretion and colonic contraction resulting in a bowel movement within 6–12 hours after oral ingestion or 15–60 minutes of rectal administration. They may causes severe cramps and diarrhea. Agents used in the medical setting include cascara 4–8 mL orally, bisacodyl 5–15 mg orally or 10 mg suppository, and castor oil 15–45 mL orally. Castor oil is converted by intestinal lipases to products that stimulate intestinal secretion and motility and anthraquinones are converted to an active form by exposure to intestinal flora. Senna and phenolphthalein are common over-the-counter laxatives that are not generally prescribed. **Note:** Chronic use of any of these agents is discouraged and may in theory result in loss of normal colonic neuromuscular function.

B. OSMOTIC LAXATIVES

Osmotic laxatives produce a prompt evacuation in 0.5–3 hours, generally with less discomfort than cathartic laxatives. They are used in the medical setting as a bowel purgative before surgery or colonic examinations. Preparations include magnesium citrate 18 g/10 ounce, magnesium sulfate 10–30 g ("Epsom salts"), sodium phosphate 15–30 g (2–45 mL), and balanced polyethylene glycol lavage solution 1–4 L over 1 to 4 hours (GoLytely; Colyte).

C. ENEMAS

Enemas provide a simple and almost immediate means of relieving acute constipation. In some cases of severe constipation, it is best to treat with an enema first to promote comfortable fecal movement, before giving laxatives. Enemas vary in size and content: saline enemas 120–240 mL (nonirritating), tap water enemas 500–1000 mL (irritating), and oil retention enemas 120 mL (useful for hard or impacted stool).

Treatment of Fecal Impaction

Severe impaction of stool in the rectal vault may result in obstruction of further fecal flow leading to a partial or complete large bowel obstruction. A predisposition to fecal impaction occurs in situations in which the patient ignores the urge to defecate due to depression, dementia, inadequate access to toilet facilities, or prolonged bed rest or disability, and also in patients with neurogenic diseases of the colon or spinal cord disorders. When stool retention occurs from any cause, normal absorption of water continues and produces hard stool. Clinical presentation includes decreased appetite, nausea, vomiting, and abdominal pain and distention. There may be paradoxical "diarrhea" as liquid stool leaks around the impacted feces. Fever and leukocytosis may rarely occur. Firm feces is palpable on digital examination in the rectal vault. An abdominal plain film may show a large amount of stool in the colon, or rarely dilated loops of bowel and air–fluid levels. Initial treatment is directed at relieving the impaction with enemas or through digital removal of the impacted fecal material. Care should be taken not to injure the anal sphincter. Rarely, spinal or general anesthesia is required with manual disimpaction. If the hard stool cannot be reached manually, laxatives should be cautiously administered orally. Polyethylene glycol is a good choice in this setting. Long-term care is directed at maintaining soft stools and regular bowel movements (see section, "Treatment of Chronic Constipation").

WEIGHT LOSS

General Considerations

Body weight remains relatively constant over a lifetime and an involuntary decrease in body weight of at least 5% is a problem that requires clinical evaluation. In the clinical evaluation, the most important initial task is to document whether in fact weight loss has actually occurred. Approximately 50% of patients complaining of weight loss do not have a significant change in their body weight when previous clinic records are available for documentation. The amount of weight loss considered significant is usually defined as loss of 5% of total body weight within the past 6 months. When previously documented weights are not available for comparison, a change in clothing size, independent corroboration of weight loss by a family member, or clear recall of specific weights by the patient can serve as reliable indicators of significant weight loss. Once a history of weight loss is ascertained, it is important to determine if the weight loss is truly involuntary, or is due to dieting or increased exercise. Patients without a clinically apparent condition accounting for weight loss require investigation.

Weight loss of at least 5% of total body weight represents a significant caloric deficit. Rapid changes in weight are often due to a change in hydration with loss of water accounting for the decrease in weight. When water loss is excluded, approximately 3500 kcal must be expended in order to lose 1 lb of body weight. With this in mind, a 160-lb man must have a caloric deficit of approximately 28,000 kcal to lose 5% (8 lb) of his body weight. Such a caloric deficit may result from decreased intake of food, increased metabolic rate, malabsorption of nutrients, or a combination of these factors.

Etiology

There are numerous causes of weight loss. Table 1–8 lists diseases or conditions associated with weight loss through decreased intake of calories, increased basal metabolic rate, or malabsorption of calories. In the elderly, the causes of weight loss have been described as the 10 "D's" (see Table 1–8). Previous studies have shown that the most commonly identified causes of unexplained weight loss are malignant neoplasms, gastrointestinal disease, and psychiatric disorders. In these studies, approximately 10–25% of patients died within 1 year of initial evaluation. Approximately one-fourth of patients with weight loss will not have a definable cause for their symptoms following investigation. Patients without an identifiable cause of weight loss appear to have a better prognosis on long-term follow-up compared with patients with an identifiable cause. The most common malignant neoplasms identified in patients with weight loss are gastrointestinal, lung, genitourinary, hematologic, breast, and oral cancers. The gastrointestinal diseases include malabsorption, peptic ulcer disease, inflammatory bowel disease, diabetic enteropathy, motility disorders, GERD, pancreatitis, cholelithiasis, and Zenker's diverticulum. Benign gastric ulcers may result in weight loss due to anorexia. More recent case series suggest that between 40 and 60% of patients may have psychiatric diagnoses as the origin of weight loss, most commonly depression.

Clinical Findings

A. SYMPTOMS AND SIGNS

A careful history and physical examination along with a limited number of screening studies will lead to a diagnosis in the vast majority of cases. Most patients presenting with unexplained weight loss have symptoms or signs that will direct the work-up. The history should

Table 1–8. Causes of weight loss.

Decreased caloric intake
  Anorexia
    Malignant neoplasm
    Medications
    Psychiatric disorders
    Chronic renal disease
    AIDS
    Chronic alcoholism
    Eating disorders
  Swallowing disorders
    Oropharyngeal dysphagia
    Esophageal strictures
  Abnormal taste
    Medications
    Malignant neoplasms
    Psychiatric disorders
    Zinc deficiency
  Postprandial pain
    Chronic pancreatitis
    Chronic mesenteric ischemia
    Partial gastric outlet obstruction
    Partial intestinal obstruction
    Gastric bezoar
Increased metabolic rate
  Chronic obstructive pulmonary disease
  Congestive heart failure
  Hyperthyroidism
  Chronic infections (TB, fungal, endocarditis)
  Advanced malignant neoplasms
  Diabetes mellitus
  AIDS
Decreased caloric absorption
  Intestinal malabsorption (sprue, etc)
  Chronic pancreatitis
  Intestinal fistula
  Short bowel syndrome
  Bacterial overgrowth

include a careful review of systems. Pulmonary symptoms such as cough, shortness of breath, or hemoptysis should be sought. Complaints such as fever, anorexia, and weakness are nonspecific but should not be overlooked. Dyspnea on exertion, orthopnea, and chest pain may indicate significant underlying cardiovascular disease. Hematuria warrants an evaluation for urologic tumor. Polydipsia, polyuria, or polyphagia may lead to the diagnosis of poorly controlled diabetes. Uremia often leads to the diagnosis of anorexia. Gastrointestinal complaints such as dysphagia, odynophagia, nausea, vomiting, hematemesis, abdominal pain, hematochezia, change in stool caliber, and constipation should be sought. Diarrhea, especially with greasy, foul-smelling,

or difficult to flush stools, is suggestive of malabsorption of pancreatic insufficiency.

Behavioral disorders may account for weight loss and a history directed at diagnosis of these disorders is important. Depression is the most common psychological disorder associated with weight loss. Questions regarding sleep disturbances, anhedonia, or anorexia may unveil this diagnosis. Schizophrenia or other psychotic disorders may be associated with delusional thinking about food and eating. Eating disorders such as anorexia nervosa and bulimia are quite common; however, patients often deny these behaviors.

Careful documentation of medications used by the patient should be performed in order to rule out medication-induced dysgeusia, anorexia, or dyspepsia. A strong family history of cancer may also serve to direct the work-up. Smoking, alcohol, drug use, and risk factors for HIV infection should be recorded.

The physical examination should include a careful examination of the oral cavity to detect ulcerations, mass lesions, or poor dentition that may impair adequate oral intake. Poorly fitted dentures may produce pain with eating and subsequent weight loss. A search for lymphadenopathy should be performed as part of the evaluation for underlying disease. Evidence of obstructive lung disease, congestive heart failure, as well as abdominal, breast, or pelvic masses may also be present. Digital rectal examination with stool guaiac testing may also direct further evaluation.

B. Diagnostic Studies

Further studies should be directed according to abnormalities detected on history and physical examination. For example, patients with symptoms of dysphagia, abdominal pain, or guaiac positive stool should undergo appropriate endoscopic or radiographic evaluation aimed at detection of underlying gastrointestinal pathology. In patients in whom the history and physical examination are unrevealing, further diagnostic evaluation usually includes a limited number of radiographic and laboratory studies. Initial studies should include a sequential multiple analysis (SMA)-20, CBC, urinalysis, and chest x-ray. An erythrocyte sedimentation rate and thyroid function tests should also be performed. HIV testing should be performed if there are any risk factors present. If these studies are not helpful, an upper gastrointestinal series (or upper endoscopy) has been shown to be helpful. In a large prospective study in the United States, more than 80% of patients with an identifiable cause of weight loss have an abnormality on these screening laboratory or radiographic studies that suggests a diagnosis. If the above studies are unrevealing and there are no localizing symptoms or signs, screening measures for cancer are indicated including colonoscopy, cervical Pap smear in women, mammography (women aged 40 years or older) and prostate-specific antigen (men aged 50 years or older). CT of the abdomen or chest to detect occult malignant neoplasms, without symptoms or laboratory abnormalities suggestive of underlying disease, has a very low yield.

Prognosis

Patients who maintain their performance status despite weight loss and those without a significant smoking history are less likely to have a cause of weight loss identified on investigation. These patients generally have a good prognosis and are best managed by a period of observation. In contrast, patients who are heavy smokers, have a change in performance status, nausea or vomiting, a new or changed cough, or an abnormal physical examination are more likely to have significant underlying disease.

ABDOMINAL PAIN

Abdominal pain is one of the most common symptoms evaluated by primary care physicians and gastroenterologists. A wide variety of conditions can cause abdominal pain. The origin of the pain should be determined by a combination of clinical history, physical findings, laboratory values, and radiographic examination. A thorough, systematic evaluation is necessary in order to avoid overlooking potentially life-threatening conditions. The most important point is to first rule out life-threatening causes of abdominal pain, including dissecting aortic aneurysm, perforated viscus, or bowel obstruction. Before limiting the differential diagnosis to disease processes involving the abdomen, it is important to consider pulmonary processes and myocardial infarction as the underlying cause of symptoms. Abdominal pain can also be classified as acute or chronic. Patients with an acute onset of abdominal pain require an efficient and expeditious evaluation. Approximately one-third of patients admitted with abdominal pain will have no etiology identified following evaluation.

1. Acute Abdominal Pain

Clinical Findings

A. SYMPTOMS AND SIGNS

The history should include information about the location, time course, intensity, and character of the pain. Aggravating or alleviating factors should also be noted.

1. Location—Patients often have difficulty precisely describing the location of their abdominal pain. This is the result of several neuroanatomic factors. Sensation of the **abdominal viscera** is mediated by a network of af-

ferent C fibers that are stimulated primarily by stretching, inflammation, or ischemia. The abdominal viscera lack the dense network of somatic afferent fibers found in the skin; this limits precise localization of stimuli. A single splanchnic afferent nerve may provide sensory input from several organs and enter the spinal cord at more than one level, further contributing to imprecise localization. Embryologically, most abdominal organs are derived from midline structures, and retain bilateral innervation. As a result of this bilateral innervation, most abdominal pain is poorly lateralized and is instead reported in the midline. The exception occurs when organs assume a more lateral position, such as the kidneys, ureters, ovaries, and gallbladder. For these organs, pain produced by disease states usually is experienced on the corresponding side of the involved organ.

The superior to inferior location of pain in the abdomen is an imprecise indicator of the organ involved, but may suggest a foregut, midgut, or hindgut origin. Pain derived from foregut structures (eg, distal esophagus, stomach, proximal duodenum, liver, biliary system, and pancreas) most often presents with midline pain in the epigastrium. Pancreatic pain most often presents with pain in the midepigastrium or left side of the epigastrium with referred pain to the back. Pain derived from the midgut structures (eg, small intestine, appendix, ascending colon, and proximal two-thirds of the transverse colon) usually occurs in the periumbilical region, although pain derived from the ileum (such as Crohn's ileitis) can be localized to the right lower quadrant. Pain derived from hindgut organs (eg, distal transverse colon, descending colon, rectum, and sigmoid) most often presents in the midline lower abdomen between the umbilicus and symphysis pubis.

Pain originating from the **parietal peritoneum** is usually much better localized. Somatic afferent nerve fibers allow more precise localization of stimuli. The parietal peritoneum does not have the characteristic bilateral innervation found in the abdominal viscera, and the density of nerve fibers in the parietal peritoneum is significantly greater than in the abdominal viscera. This allows better identification of the origin of pain when the parietal peritoneum is irritated by bile, urine, pus, or luminal contents.

Referred pain is a term that describes pain localized to a site distant from the abdominal organ from which the pain originates. This occurs because of the common site of entry into the spinal cord of cutaneous sensory neurons and abdominal visceral afferents. Cutaneous and visceral afferents terminate on the same secondary neuron within the dorsal horn of the spinal cord, resulting in misinterpretation by the brain of the correct origin of the stimulus. For example, the biliary system is innervated by neurons terminating in segments T5–T9 of the spinal cord. Neurons derived from cutaneous dermatomes of the scapular area, back, and shoulder also enter the spinal cord at T5–T9. Biliary disease may thus stimulate the same secondary neurons commonly stimulated by cutaneous afferents of the shoulder and scapular region, resulting in complaints of shoulder and back pain. Complaints of shoulder pain may also be noted when processes that irritate the diaphragm (including subdiaphragmatic blood, pus, or masses, and pulmonary processes such as pneumonia) cause referred pain from the phrenic nerve (C3–C5). Associated findings in referred pain include skin hyperalgesia and increased tone of the abdominal wall muscles.

Visceral pain that is initially ill defined and midline in location may shift as the adjacent parietal peritoneum becomes inflamed or irritated. This is classically the case in acute appendicitis, which often presents initially with periumbilical pain that migrates to the right lower quadrant as the parietal peritoneum becomes irritated. Similar migration of pain can occur in acute cholecystitis, which initially presents with pain in the epigastrium but shifts to the right upper quadrant as the disease progresses. Perforated peptic ulcer may present as epigastric pain that moves to the right lower quadrant as spilled luminal contents cause inflammation in the area of the right paracolic gutter.

2. Time course—The onset of abdominal pain may be sudden (over seconds to minutes), rapidly progressive (over 1–2 hours), or gradual (over several hours) (Table 1–9). Sudden onset of abdominal pain suggests a catastrophic event such as a ruptured abdominal aneurysm, ruptured ectopic pregnancy, or perforated peptic ulcer. Pain that rapidly progresses over a few hours is seen typically in pancreatitis, cholecystitis, diverticulitis, bowel obstruction, renal or biliary colic, and mesenteric ischemia. Pain that progresses more slowly is more typical of peptic ulcer disease, distal small bowel obstruction, appendicitis, pyelonephritis, pelvic inflammatory disease, and malignant neoplasm, although it may be seen with many of the diagnoses in the more rapidly progressive categories as well. Pain occurring following the onset of vomiting often indicates a medical illness, whereas pain that precedes vomiting often indicates a surgical illness. Persistence of pain for over 6 hours after acute onset has a high likelihood of a surgical cause and requires admission for observation.

3. Intensity and description of pain—Certain characteristics of the type and severity of the pain may point toward a specific diagnosis. The pain of peptic ulcer disease is usually described as a dull, gnawing sensation of mild to moderate severity. Extremely intense pain of sudden onset suggests mesenteric ischemia or perforated peptic ulcer. "Colic" refers to episodic pain with intervening pain-free intervals. Whereas renal colic often presents in this fashion, biliary pain typically pre-

Table 1–9. Causes of acute abdominal pain.

Sudden onset (within seconds to minutes)
  Perforated peptic ulcer
  Ruptured aortic aneurysm
  Ruptured abscess or hematoma
  Esophageal rupture (Boerhaave's syndrome)
  Ruptured ectopic pregnancy
  Mesenteric infarction
  Myocardial infarction
Rapidly progressive (within 1–2 hours)
  Biliary colic
  Cholecystitis
  Renal colic
  Proximal small bowel obstruction
  Acute pancreatis
  Diverticulitis
  Appendicitis
  Mesenteric ischemia
Gradual onset (over number of hours)
  Appendicitis
  Cholecystitis
  Acute pancreatitis
  Diverticulitis
  Salpingitis
  Peptic ulcer disease
  Ectopic pregnancy (before rupture)
  Pyelonephritis
  Intraabdominal abscess
  Distal small bowel obstruction
  Incarcerated hernia
  Neoplasms with perforation
  Inflammatory bowel disease

sents with constant, steady pain without intervening pain-free intervals (the term biliary "colic" being somewhat of a misnomer). Pain that has a severe intensity and a "tearing" quality is commonly described in dissecting aneurysms. Patients with postprandial pain, food avoidance, weight loss, and known atherosclerotic disease should be evaluated for mesenteric angina.

4. Aggravating or alleviating factors—Actions that precipitate or improve the pain may help in determining the cause. Pain relieved by antacids suggests peptic ulcer disease or esophagitis. Pain worsened by movement suggests peritonitis, whereas constant movement by the patient in an attempt to find a comfortable position is commonly seen in bowel obstruction and renal colic. Patients with a retroperitoneal process (such as pancreatitis) commonly find partial relief by leaning forward, and aggravation by lying supine. Pain relieved by defecation may suggest a colonic source.

5. Physical examination—Examination of the abdomen is best performed before administration of narcotics or other medications that may affect the physical findings. The initial step is to observe the position and posture of the patient for clues that may suggest an underlying cause (as previously described). Vital signs may show tachycardia and hypotension indicative of intraabdominal hemorrhage or septic shock. The fever of appendicitis, diverticulitis, and cholecystitis is typically low grade, whereas high fevers are seen in cases of cholangitis, urinary tract infections, pelvic inflammatory disease, or perforation of a viscus with frank peritonitis.

Inspection of the abdomen may reveal a distended abdomen suggesting bowel obstruction or the presence of ascites, whereas a scaphoid, tense abdomen is seen in cases of peritonitis. Auscultation of the abdomen should be performed before palpation or percussion so as not to interfere with the interpretation of bowel sounds. Absence of bowel sounds is a sign of diffuse peritonitis. Intermittent hyperactive bowel sounds occurring concurrently with worsening of pain suggest a bowel obstruction. High-pitched hyperactive bowel sounds may also be seen in gastroenteritis. The presence of a succussion splash suggests gastric outlet obstruction.

Percussion of the abdomen allows assessment of the presence of peritonitis. Pain produced by light tapping indicates inflammation of the parietal peritoneum. This pain may also be elicited by asking the patient to cough or by gently agitating the gurney upon which the patient is lying. A distended abdomen with tympany upon percussion suggests a bowel obstruction.

Palpation of the abdomen is performed in order to assess the presence of rigidity or guarding, as well as to localize the site of maximal tenderness. Tightening (rigidity) of the abdominal wall musculature occurs as a reflexive response to peritoneal inflammation. This is assessed by gently compressing the abdominal wall musculature with both hands and assessing the relative softness or rigidity. Voluntary guarding refers to tightness or rigidity of the abdomen that relaxes when the patient takes a deep breath, whereas involuntary guarding refers to rigidity of the abdominal wall musculature that does not relax in response to deep inspiration. Involuntary guarding indicates peritoneal inflammation. Palpation of the abdomen should begin at the site most distant from where the patient localizes the pain, then gradually shift toward the site of pain. The presence of a focal site of pain produced by palpation is a useful finding that narrows the list of potentially involved organs. Tenderness over McBurney's point should be considered very strong evidence of appendicitis. Cholecystitis and salpingitis are often well localized as well, and salpingitis may be confused with appendicitis. Patients with an unimpressive abdominal examination

and complaints of severe, worsening pain should be suspected of having mesenteric infarction.

Murphy's sign refers to pain produced by deep inspiration during palpation of the right subcostal area and suggests acute cholecystitis. Pain produced by lightly punching the costovertebral angle ("punch tenderness") is often present in pyelonephritis. **Carnett's test** refers to the response of pain when the patient tenses the abdominal wall muscles by raising their head off the examination table. Worsening of pain during this maneuver suggests an abdominal wall source whereas improvement in the pain suggests a visceral origin. The **iliopsoas sign** refers to pain produced by passive extension of the leg and suggests a psoas abscess. The **obturator sign** refers to pain produced by rotation of the thigh in a flexed position. A rectal examination can reveal focal tenderness from an intraabdominal abscess or appendicitis. A pelvic examination is mandatory in female patients to look for evidence of salpingitis or adnexal masses. The inguinal and femoral canals, umbilicus, and surgical scars should be evaluated for the presence of incarcerating hernias.

B. LABORATORY TESTS

Although the majority of diagnoses can be made from a careful history and physical examination, laboratory studies help to confirm the diagnosis in many cases. Initial studies should include a CBC with differential count, electrolytes, renal function tests, liver function tests, amylase, and urinalysis. Pregnancy testing should be performed in women of child-bearing age. Typing and cross-matching of blood should also be performed in any patient potentially requiring surgery. An arterial blood gas specimen should be obtained in patients with peritonitis, pancreatitis, ischemic bowel, or hypotension to look for evidence of metabolic acidosis or hypoxemia.

A mildly elevated white blood cell (WBC) count is a nonspecific finding found in many inflammatory conditions. Likewise, a mild elevation of the serum amylase may be found in many conditions presenting with acute abdominal pain and is a nonspecific finding.

C. DIAGNOSTIC STUDIES

Plain radiographs can be very helpful in the initial evaluation of patients with acute abdominal pain. The films obtained should include an upright chest x-ray and supine and erect films of the abdomen. Plain films can identify cases of bowel obstruction, perforated viscus (free intraperitoneal air is often best seen on the upright chest film), air in the portal venous system or biliary system, calcifications (renal stones, chronic pancreatitis, gallstones), pneumatosis (air in the bowel wall), or bowel wall thickening. The abdominal films may also show loss of a normal psoas shadow, suggesting an intraabdominal inflammatory process. The chest x-ray can also show evidence of a pulmonary infiltrate, spontaneous pneumothorax, or sympathetic pleural effusion (due to subdiaphragmatic infection or irritation). To increase the detection rate of free air under the diaphragm on an upright chest x-ray, the patient should remain in the upright position for at least 5 minutes prior to obtaining the chest film.

Further x-ray studies may include angiography for patients suspected of having mesenteric ischemia, or contrast upper gastrointestinal studies for patients with possible perforated peptic ulcer (using a water-soluble contrast agent in order to avoid barium peritonitis). Lower gastrointestinal contrast studies are useful in evaluating cases of suspected colonic obstruction, and may be used diagnostically as well as therapeutically in patients with suspected colonic volvulus. Endoscopy is more sensitive and specific for mucosal abnormalities than contrast radiography.

Ultrasonography is a useful noninvasive test to show biliary abnormalities including cholelithiasis, ductal dilation, gallbladder wall thickening, and pericholecystic fluid. Abdominal ultrasound may also show evidence of acute appendicitis, abdominal masses, hydronephrosis, pelvic inflammatory disease, and other conditions that cause abdominal pain. CT may allow diagnosis of pancreatic disease, abdominal aortic aneurysms, intraabdominal fluid collections, diverticulitis, bowel obstruction, appendicitis, and malignancy. Magnetic resonance cholangiopancreatography allows noninvasive detection of biliary tract obstruction with sensitivity comparable to endoscopic retrograde cholangiopancreatography (ERCP). Other magnetic resonance imaging examinations are not commonly indicated in the evaluation of abdominal pain.

2. Chronic Abdominal Pain

Chronic abdominal pain is a very common complaint, and the origin of the discomfort is often difficult to determine. A wide variety of disease processes may cause intermittent or persistent abdominal symptoms. A useful method of categorizing abdominal pain is to distinguish between a history of discrete intermittent episodes of pain and nearly continuous discomfort. Separation of symptoms into these categories may help to narrow the differential diagnosis in many cases.

Chronic Intermittent Abdominal Pain

Pain that is intermittent (with intervening pain-free periods) can be caused by several categories of disease. Often, the disorders causing intermittent pain are correctable conditions. Clues suggesting the underlying cause may be found by evaluating the history, physical examination, and laboratory or radiographic studies.

A. CLINICAL FINDINGS

1. Symptoms and signs—Biliary tract disease (including cholelithiasis, choledocholithiasis, and sphincter of Oddi dysfunction) leads to intermittent discomfort usually localized to the right upper quadrant or epigastrium. The pain of chronic pancreatitis may be episodic and should be suspected in patients with chronic alcohol ingestion. Pain that occurs at approximately monthly intervals should raise the suspicion of endometriosis or mittelschmerz. Postprandial abdominal discomfort suggests chronic intestinal ischemia or intermittent intestinal obstruction (from internal or abdominal wall hernias, adhesions, or Crohn's disease). Abdominal pain relieved by bowel movements or associated with increased frequency or looseness of stools suggests irritable bowel syndrome. A radiculopathy in diabetic patients may cause abdominal pain. Similarly, spinal compression fractures may lead to nerve compression syndromes causing pain. Recent changes in medication should also be noted. Barbiturates may precipitate acute intermittent porphyria. Diuretics, tetracycline, sulfonamides, 6-mercaptopurine, and estrogen use may cause pancreatitis. Heavy metal poisoning can cause abdominal pain.

The physical examination can show jaundice, suggesting biliary tract disease. A distended, tympanitic abdomen suggests a bowel obstruction. The presence of hernias should also be assessed. Right lower quadrant fullness and pain or perianal disease may indicate Crohn's disease.

2. Laboratory and imaging studies—Routine laboratory tests may provide evidence of the underlying disease process. Anemia may be present in cases of inflammatory bowel disease or heavy metal poisoning. Liver transaminases, alkaline phosphatase, and bilirubin levels may be elevated in cases of symptomatic choledocholithiasis. An elevated alkaline phosphatase and bilirubin and a dilated bile duct suggest choledocholithiasis or sphincter of Oddi dysfunction. An elevated sedimentation rate (ESR) may indicate active inflammatory bowel disease or the presence of collagen vascular disease. A urine test for porphobilinogen should be done in cases of suspected acute intermittent porphyria.

Plain films of the abdomen may show evidence of bowel obstruction from an internal hernia or intussusception. Pancreatic calcification establishes a diagnosis of chronic pancreatitis. Abdominal ultrasonography may reveal gallstones or a dilated biliary tree. CT of the abdomen provides optimal imaging of the pancreas or intraabdominal malignancy. Colonoscopy is useful for ruling out cases of suspected colitis. ERCP is indicated in cases of sphincter of Oddi dysfunction, choledocholithiasis, and in some cases of suspected chronic pancreatitis. The appropriate use of these modalities for each of these disorders is provided in the chapters discussing each of these disease processes.

Persistent Abdominal Pain

Chronic persistent abdominal pain (present much or all of the time) may be related to underlying chronic disease or may be functional in origin. This complaint is an extremely common symptom among patients presenting to primary care physicians and gastroenterologists. A careful history is essential to guide the evaluation.

A. CLINICAL FINDINGS

1. Symptoms and signs—The history should define the location and character of the pain as well as aggravating or alleviating factors. Pain or discomfort present in the upper abdomen (between the xiphoid process and umbilicus) may be classified as dyspepsia. The clinical history is unable to reliably distinguish between peptic ulcer disease, GERD, gastric malignancy, or nonulcer dyspepsia as causes of dyspepsia (see section, "Dyspepsia"). Lower or mid-abdominal pain that is relieved by bowel movements or is associated with increased frequency or liquidity of stools suggests irritable bowel syndrome. Signs and symptoms of psychiatric disorders that may be associated with functional bowel complaints should also be sought (see Chapter 6). Weight loss and anorexia should raise the possibility of underlying malignancy (see section, "Weight Loss"). Chronic abdominal pain associated with steatorrhea, weight loss, or a history of alcoholism suggests chronic pancreatitis.

The physical examination is often unrevealing, but may show abnormalities that can direct the evaluation. Jaundice may suggest a pancreatic or biliary neoplasm. Palpation of abdominal mass lesions suggests a visceral neoplasm. The presence of ascites may be due to underlying liver disease, malignancy, or peritoneal disorders (see Chapter 10). A rectal examination may demonstrate occult blood, raising the question of peptic ulcer disease, inflammatory bowel disease, or an underlying neoplasm.

2. Laboratory and imaging studies—The appropriate use of laboratory and investigative studies in the evaluation of each disease category previously described is discussed in the respective chapters. The reader is directed to these chapters for a full discussion of the evaluation and management of each disorder.

REFERENCES

SYMPTOMS OF ESOPHAGEAL DISEASE

American Gastroenterological Association medical position statement: guidelines on the use of esophageal pH recording. Gastroenterology 1996;110:1981.

American Gastroenterological Association Technical Review on Management of Oropharyngeal Dysphagia. Gastroenterology 1999;116:455.

Browning TH: Diagnosis of chest pain of esophageal origin. A guideline of the Patient Care Committee of the American Gastroenterological Association. Dig Dis Sci 1990;35:289.

Kahrilas P, Clouse R, Hogan W: Policy and position statement: American Gastroenterological Association technical review on the clinical use of esophageal manometry. Gastroenterology 1994;107:1865.

Klauser AG et al: Symptoms in gastro-oesophageal reflux disease. Lancet 1990;335:205.

DYSPEPSIA

Bytzer P et al: Empirical H_2-blocker therapy or prompt endoscopy in management of dyspepsia. Lancet 1994;3443: 811.

Lassen AT et al: *Helicobacter pylori* test-and-eradicate versus prompt endoscopy for management of dyspeptic patients: a randomised trial. Lancet 2000;356(9228):455.

Loren L, Schoenfeld P, Fennerty MB: Therapy for *Helicobacter pylori* in patients with nonulcer dyspepsia. A meta-analysis of randomized, controlled trials 03-06-2001. Ann Intern Med 2001;134:361.

Talley NJ et al: Lack of discriminant value of dyspepsia subgroups in patients referred for upper endoscopy. Gastroenterology 1993;105:1378.

Talley NJ et al: Efficacy of omeprazole in functional dyspepsia: double-blind, randomized, placebo-controlled trials (the Bond and Opera studies). Aliment Pharmacol Ther 1998; 12:1055.

HICCUPS

Lewis JH: Hiccups: causes and cures. J Clin Gastroenterol 1985;7: 539.

GASTROINTESTINAL GAS

Kearney DJ, McQuaid KR: Gaseousness and indigestion. In: *Conn's Current Therapy.* Rakel RE (editor). W. B. Saunders, 1997.

Strocchi A, Levitt MD: Intestinal gas. In: *Gastrointestinal Disease,* 5th ed. Sleisenger MH, Fordtran JS (editors). W. B. Saunders, 1993.

NAUSEA & VOMITING

Allan GS: Antiemetics. Gastroenterol Clin North Am 1992;21: 597.

Grunberg SM, Hesketh PH: Control of chemotherapy-induced emesis. N Engl J Med 1993;329:1790.

Hanson JS, McCallum RW: The diagnosis and management of nausea and vomiting. Am J Gastroenterol 1985;80:210.

Kuver R, McDonald GB, Sheffield J: Nausea and vomiting. In: *Gastroenterology and Hepatology for the Primary Care Provider: Principles, Practice and Guidelines for Referral.* Kimmey MB, Lee SP (editors). University of Washington Division of Gastroenterology, 2001.

DIARRHEA

Aranda-Michel J, Giannella RA: Acute diarrhea: a practical review. Am J Med 1999;106:670.

Guerrant RL, Bobak DA: Bacterial and protozoal gastroenteritis. N Engl J Med 1991;325:327.

Park SI, Giannella RA: Approach to the adult patient with acute diarrhea. Gastroenterol Clin North Am 1993;22:483.

CONSTIPATION

AGA Technical Review on Constipation. Gastroenterology 2000; 119:1766.

Gattuso JM, Kamm MA: Review article: The management of constipation in adults. Aliment Pharmacol Ther 1993;7:487.

Prather CM, Ortiz-Camacho CP: Evaluation and treatment of constipation and fecal impaction in adults. Mayo Clinic Proc 1998;73:881.

Talley NJ et al: Functional constipation and outlet delay: a population based study. Gastroenterology 1993;105:781.

WEIGHT LOSS

Marton KI, Sox HC Jr, Krupp Jr: Involuntary weight loss: diagnostic and prognostic significance. Ann Intern Med 1981; 95: 568.

Rabinovitz M et al: Unintentional weight loss. A retrospective analysis of 154 cases. Arch Intern Med 1986;146:186.

Thompson MP, Morris LK: Unexplained weight loss in the ambulatory elderly. J Am Geriatr Soc 1991;39:497.

ABDOMINAL PAIN

Bender JS: Approach to the acute abdomen. Med Clin North Am 1989;73:1413.

Dominitz J, Sekijima J, Watts M: Abdominal pain. In: *Gastroenterology and Hepatology for the Primary Care Provider: Principles, Practice and Guidelines for Referral.* Kearney DJ (editor). University of Washington Division of Gastroenterology, 2000.

Silen W: *Cope's Early Diagnosis of the Acute Abdomen,* 18th ed. Oxford University Press, 1991.

AIDS & the Gastrointestinal Tract

2

C. Mel Wilcox, MD

Although the morbidity and mortality from acquired immunodeficiency syndrome (AIDS)-related complications have fallen dramatically because of highly active antiretroviral therapy (HAART), the gastrointestinal tract remains one of the most common organ systems in which complications occur during the course of human immunodeficiency virus (HIV) infection. This prevalence can be explained largely by the direct link of the gut to the external environment and the importance of the mucosal immune system in preventing infection. In general, most opportunistic disorders are not seen until the CD4 lymphocyte count falls below 200/μL. Thus, in the evaluation of patients with HIV infection, the CD4 lymphocyte count is very helpful in either narrowing or expanding the differential diagnosis.

In the evaluation of the symptomatic patient, both opportunistic and nonopportunistic diseases always deserve consideration. As with all opportunistic infections in AIDS, relapse is frequent in diseases of the gastrointestinal tract, since antimicrobial therapy does not truly eradicate opportunistic organisms in the immunosuppressed. In many patients, therefore, life-long therapy may be necessary. Many of these disorders result in significant morbidity, but rarely mortality. Therefore, therapy is directed toward improving the quality of life. The long-term prognosis for most disorders is dictated primarily by the degree of underlying immunodeficiency.

Monkemuller KE et al: Declining prevalence of opportunistic gastrointestinal disease in the era of combination antiretroviral therapy. Am J Gastroenterol 2000;95:457.

■ DISEASES OF THE OROPHARYNX

Clinical Findings

Oropharyngeal disease is a frequently recognized complication in HIV-infected patients. The most common disorder involving the oropharynx is candidiasis (thrush) and frequently is the first manifestation of HIV infection. Candidiasis appears as multiple white to yellow plaques that may be focal or may completely coat the pharynx. Occasionally, candidiasis may be manifested by erythema in the absence of recognizable plaques.

Herpes simplex virus (HSV) stomatitis may present at any point during the course of HIV disease, although it tends to be more severe with progression of immunodeficiency. Diffuse shallow oropharyngeal ulceration also involving the lips and nares is usually recognizable as HSV disease. Well-circumscribed focal ulcerations, which may be large and are typically painful, are usually of the aphthous type.

Other viruses occur less commonly. Epstein–Barr virus infection may produce oral hairy leukoplakia, which is manifested by whitish plaques on the lateral aspects of the tongue and is usually of no consequence. Cytomegalovirus (CMV) is a rare cause of oropharyngeal ulceration.

When oropharyngeal ulcers are very large, a fungal infection (histoplasmosis) or neoplasm (lymphoma) should be considered. Kaposi's sarcoma (KS) presents as a brownish-to-purple plaque or nodule on the hard or soft palate. Lymphoma appears as a mass-like lesion.

These entities can usually be distinguished by a thorough examination of the oropharynx. For oropharyngeal ulcers, biopsy may be required to exclude unusual infections or a neoplasm. The presence of these oropharyngeal lesions, especially when associated with esophageal symptoms (eg, odynophagia, dysphagia), should suggest coexisting esophageal disease. At many centers, oropharyngeal findings are used to guide empiric therapy for the patient with esophageal symptoms.

Treatment

Therapy will depend on the underlying etiology. Oropharyngeal candidiasis may be treated with short courses of antifungal agents, either local (clotrimazole troches) or oral systemic medications (ketoconazole, fluconazole, itraconazole). Corticosteroids are very efficacious for aphthous ulcers, however, long-term treatment is usually necessary due to recurrence.

Powderly WG, Mayer KH, Perfect JR: Diagnosis and treatment of oropharyngeal candidiasis in patients infected with HIV: a critical reassessment. AIDS Res Hum Retroviruses 1999;15: 1405.

■ DISEASES OF THE ESOPHAGUS

Esophageal disease is an important complication of AIDS. At least one-third of HIV-infected patients experience esophageal symptoms at some point during the course of the disease. Opportunistic infections are by far the most common cause of esophageal disease (Table 2–1). In fact, opportunistic esophageal disease may be the initial manifestations of HIV infection. In addition, prophylactic medications used to prevent opportunistic infections have shifted the incidence of other diseases, including esophageal disorders. Both opportunistic and nonopportunistic causes, therefore, should always be considered when evaluating these patients.

CANDIDA

 ESSENTIALS OF DIAGNOSIS

- *Most common cause of esophageal disease.*
- *Most common symptoms: dysphagia or odynophagia, or both; however, infection may be asymptomatic.*
- *Diagnosis established by barium esophagography, endoscopy, or presumptively by a symptomatic response to empiric antifungal therapy.*

General Considerations

Candida esophagitis is one of the most frequent opportunistic infections in patients with AIDS. Of HIV-infected patients with esophageal symptoms, *Candida* is the most common identifiable pathogen on endoscopy, occurring in up to 50% of patients. Oropharyngeal and esophageal candidiasis may be precipitated by the use of antibiotics or corticosteroids. In addition, *Candida* frequently coexists with other disease processes. Fungal cultures will usually yield *Candida albicans* and occasionally other *Candida* species or *Torulopsis glabrata.* Despite the vast numbers of yeasts involved in this infection, systemic dissemination does not occur, probably because the infection is limited to the superficial squamous epithelium.

Clinical Findings

A. Symptoms and Signs

The clinical presentation is broad, ranging from asymptomatic infection to severe symptoms with dehydration. Most commonly, **dysphagia** (difficulty in swallowing, described as the sensation of food sticking or slow transit of a food bolus) is the primary complaint (Table 2–2). Less frequently, **odynophagia** (painful swallowing in the substernal area), heartburn, or spontaneous substernal chest pain may be reported. The presence of fever, nausea, vomiting, and epigastric pain suggests some other cause.

The most important physical finding is the identification of oropharyngeal candidiasis. The prevalence of thrush is variable, ranging from 50 to 100% of symptomatic patients. The presence of thrush does not prove that *Candida* causes or contributes to the esophageal symptoms. Likewise, the absence of thrush does not exclude esophageal candidiasis.

B. Laboratory Findings

Candida esophagitis does not usually occur until the CD4 lymphocyte count falls to 300/μL or less. Additional laboratory abnormalities reflect the presence of other underlying processes.

C. Imaging

Barium esophagography is relatively insensitive for the detection of mild *Candida* esophagitis; however, most patients have severe disease at the time of diagnosis. The most common radiographic finding is diffuse mucosal irregularity resulting in a "shaggy" appearance mimicking diffuse ulceration (Figure 2–1). Focal disease or apparent mass lesions are unusual. A solitary ulceration in the absence of diffuse mucosal disease suggests a cause other than *Candida*.

D. Esophageal Brushings or Balloon Cytology

A cytology brush passed through a nasogastric tube, and a balloon cytology instrument used in a similar

Table 2–1. Causes of esophageal disease in AIDS.

Common	Infrequent	Rare
Candida albicans	Herpes simplex	Bacteria
Cytomegalovirus	virus	Mycobacteria
Idiopathic ulcer	Gastroesophageal	Noncandidal fungi
	reflux	Protozoa
	Kaposi's sarcoma	Lymphoma
	Pill-induced	
	esophagitis	

Table 2–2. Selected clinical features of common HIV related esophageal disorders.[1]

Feature	Etiology			
	Candida	**CMV**	**HSV**	**Idiopathic**
Oropharyngeal lesions				
Thrush	+++	+	+	+
Ulcer	——	+	++	+
Odynophagia	++	+++	+++	+++
Dysphagia	+++	+	+	+
Spontaneous chest pain	+	++	++	++
Fever	——	+	——	——
CD4 count (μL^3)	< 300	< 100	< 100	< 100
Radiography	Plaques	Ulcer	Ulcer	Ulcer
Endoscopy	Plaques	Ulcer	Ulcer	Ulcer
Diagnostic method	Empiric Rx Endoscopy	Endoscopy	Endoscopy	Endoscopy
Treatment	Fluconazole Ketoconazole Itraconazole	Ganciclovir Foscarnet Cidofovir Valganciclovir	Acyclovir	Prednisone

[1]+++, very common; ++, frequent; +, can occur; ——, not seen.

fashion, are reliable for the diagnosis and may abrogate the need for endoscopic or radiographic evaluation. Although sensitive and inexpensive, these diagnostic methods are rarely used, given the clinical practice of empiric oral systemic antifungal therapy for new-onset esophageal symptoms, and the fact that they will not reliably detect other causes, particularly in the patient with severe symptoms.

E. ENDOSCOPY

Endoscopic evaluation is the most sensitive diagnostic method. The endoscopic appearance is pathognomonic consisting of multiple yellow plaques, which may be isolated or confluent involving the entire esophagus. Esophageal brushings of these plaques will confirm yeast forms typical of *Candida*. Endoscopic mucosal biopsies will also substantiate the diagnosis as well as exclude coexisting causes.

Differential Diagnosis

In the patient with dysphagia and odynophagia, exclusion of other opportunistic infections is important. The patient with mild dysphagia and odynophagia associated with thrush is likely to have *Candida* esophagitis. In contrast, the patient with severe odynophagia without dysphagia resulting in an inability to eat is less likely to have *Candida* esophagitis, regardless of the presence or absence of thrush. In this setting, the most important causes to exclude are CMV esophagitis, idiopathic esophageal ulcer, and HSV esophagitis. Compli-

cating the approach to diagnosis is the fact that *Candida* may coexist with other esophageal disorders.

Complications

In contrast to other opportunistic infections in the immunocompromised host, *Candida* esophagitis is not truly invasive and thus does not result in disseminated infection. Because histopathologic ulcer is distinctly uncommon, perforation does not occur. Bleeding is rare and seen only in patients with an underlying coagulopathy or coexisting ulceration from some other cause.

Treatment

A number of oral systemic antifungal agents have established efficacy (see Table 2–2). Fluconazole is the most effective agent, and results in a clinical cure in over 90% of patients. This drug is an ideal agent given the high rate of renal excretion, long half-life of over 30 hours, and minimal toxicity. Ketoconazole appears somewhat less effective than fluconazole but is only one-third the cost; hepatotoxicity secondary to ketoconazole has been recognized. Itraconazole also appears efficacious. Antiacid therapy will significantly decrease the absorption of ketoconazole and itraconazole and should not be given concomitantly. Patients with refractory oropharyngeal or esophageal candidiasis due to drug resistance may require systemic therapy with amphotericin B. Both fluconazole and itraconazale are available as oral solutions.

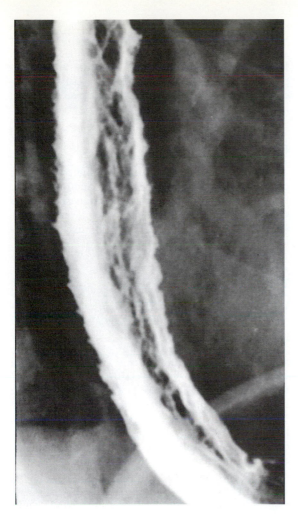

Figure 2–1. *Candida* esophagitis. There is diffuse mucosal irregularity.

Prognosis

Candida esophagitis is not a fatal disease but a marker of significant immunodeficiency. The long-term prognosis, therefore, is related to other underlying diseases and the absolute level of immunodeficiency. Relapse is very frequent, usually occurring within 2–4 months after clinical cure. Although indefinite suppressive therapy may be required if antiretroviral therapy is ineffective, fluconazole once weekly or intermittent treatment for recurrent symptoms may lessen the likelihood of resistance, minimize side effects, and be more cost effective.

Barbaro G et al: Fluconazole versus itraconazole for Candida esophagitis in acquired immunodeficiency syndrome. *Candida* esophagitis. Gastroenterology 1996;111:1169.

Bonacini M, Young T, Laine L: The causes of esophageal symptoms in human immunodeficiency virus infection. Arch Intern Med 1991;151:1567.

Levine MS et al: Opportunistic esophagitis in AIDS: radiographic diagnosis. Radiology 1987;165:815.

Lopez-Dupla M et al: Clinical, endoscopic, immunologic, and therapeutic aspects of oropharyngeal and esophageal candidiasis in HIV-infected patients: a survey of 114 cases. Am J Gastroenterol 1992;87:1771.

Wilcox CM, Monkemuller KI: Review article: the therapy of gastrointestinal infections associated with the acquired immunodeficiency syndrome. Aliment Pharmacol Ther 1997;11:425.

Wilcox CM, Monkemuller KI: Diagnosis and management of esophageal disease in the acquired immunodeficiency syndrome. South Med J 1998;91:1002.

CYTOMEGALOVIRUS

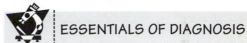 **ESSENTIALS OF DIAGNOSIS**

- *The most common viral cause of esophageal disease.*
- *Odynophagia almost uniformly present.*
- *Associated with concurrent extraintestinal disease.*
- *Histopathologic identification of viral cytopathic effect the most specific means of diagnosis.*

General Considerations

Prior exposure to CMV is almost uniform in HIV-infected patients. End-organ disease results from reactivation of latent infection. The reasons for reactivation in one organ as compared with other sites is unknown. Viremia can frequently be found, although its role in dissemination of disease is undefined. Concurrent disease of other gastrointestinal sites or the retina may be seen at the time of diagnosis, suggesting widespread reactivation or dissemination in some patients.

Clinical Findings

A. SYMPTOMS AND SIGNS

Odynophagia is the most consistent symptom. In contrast to *Candida* esophagitis, dysphagia is distinctly uncommon. The patient may disclose the presence of spontaneous (nonswallowing) substernal chest pain after close questioning. Heartburn is rare. Nausea, vomiting, and low-grade fever may be reported. Gastrointestinal bleeding can be the initial manifestation in the absence of significant esophageal symptoms. Concurrent intestinal and colonic disease may be suggested by the presence of diarrhea or abdominal pain. Altered vision may be an important clue to the presence of retinitis.

Physical findings are nonspecific. Concurrent oropharyngeal ulcerations are rare, however, thrush may be present.

B. LABORATORY FINDINGS

CMV gastrointestinal disease occurs in the setting of profound immunodeficiency; the CD4 lymphocyte count is almost always less than $100/\mu L$ and frequently less than $50/\mu L$. Serologic studies for CMV antibody are not helpful, given the uniform positivity in these patients.

C. IMAGING

Barium esophagography usually demonstrates one or more well-circumscribed ulcerations or a diffuse erosive pattern. Although characteristically large, ulcers may be variable in size and appearance, mimicking other disorders. Solitary or multiple large ulcers are not pathognomonic for CMV, but may be seen with the HIV-associated idiopathic esophageal ulcer (IEU) or pill-induced esophagitis. In contrast to *Candida* esophagitis, which has a more characteristic radiographic appearance, empiric antiviral therapy based on the radiographic findings alone is not appropriate, given the multiplicity of similar lesions. Computed tomography (CT), obtained for other reasons, may also reveal marked thickening of the esophagus.

D. ENDOSCOPY

Endoscopy is the diagnostic method of choice. Given the broad differential diagnosis of esophageal ulceration in these patients, endoscopy provides the opportunity for mucosal biopsy to establish a definitive diagnosis. As with esophagography, one or more well-circumscribed ulcers is the typical endoscopic finding. Multiple biopsies are required to reliably identify CMV cytopathic effect, as the inclusions may be few in number and atypical in appearance. Viral culture of biopsy specimens may be positive, but is less sensitive and specific than histopathologic examination.

Differential Diagnosis

CMV esophagitis must be distinguished from other causes of esophageal ulceration by endoscopic mucosal biopsy. An IEU is the most important lesion to exclude, given the similar clinical presentation, radiographic findings, and endoscopic features. Differentiation of these two disorders is important because they are managed differently. CMV is often missed when biopsy samples are inadequate or when viral cytopathic effect,

which may be infrequent or atypical, has not been identified. In this situation, *in situ* hybridization or antibody staining can help to confirm the diagnosis. Pill-induced esophagitis, HSV esophagitis, and gastroesophageal reflux disease (GERD) can usually be excluded based on history, endoscopic findings, and histopathologic results.

Complications

These lesions result in significant morbidity related to pain. Dehydration requiring hospitalization may result from severe odynophagia. Gastrointestinal bleeding is well recognized in the absence of a coagulopathy. Perforation has not been reported. Strictures may occur following antiviral therapy.

Treatment

Currently, only parenteral agents are available. Ganciclovir, foscarnet, and cidofovir yield a response rate of approximately 75% or greater. Choice of therapy should be based on the experience of the clinician with a particular agent and drug toxicity. The efficacy of oral valganciclovir has not been well studied for this indication. Ganciclovir is most frequently associated with bone marrow suppression and resultant leukopenia. In contrast, foscarnet may result in reduced renal function; hydration with drug administration reduces the frequency of renal insufficiency. Reductions in serum calcium and magnesium are also frequent with foscarnet and may be symptomatic, requiring supplementation. Therapy should be given for approximately 2–3 weeks, depending on the clinical response. Life-long therapy may not be required in all patients, as a long-term remission may occur after ulcers have healed completely.

If the patient becomes asymptomatic and shows no signs of retinal disease, close clinical monitoring without maintenance therapy is appropriate. If symptoms reappear, endoscopy should be performed to document recurrence. Long-term therapy after relapse should be individualized. Ophthalmologic examination at the time of diagnosis or recurrence is mandatory to exclude retinal disease, as the presence of CMV retinitis mandates life-long treatment. Ganciclovir is administered at a dose of 5 mg/kg twice daily, foscarnet at 90 mg/kg twice daily, and cidofovir at 5 mg/kg once weekly for 2–4 weeks. Elevation of serum creatinine during foscarnet therapy calls for a dose reduction. Myelosuppression with ganciclovir may be treated by giving bone marrow stimulators (granulucyte colony-stimulating factor) or switching to foscarnet. Similarly, if significant renal insufficiency occurs during foscarnet therapy, a change to ganciclovir may be appropriate.

Prognosis

Despite successful therapy, the median survival for patients with CMV esophagitis, in the absence of HAART, is less than 1 year. Although rarely the cause of death, esophageal disease is a marker of severe immunodeficiency, with death resulting from other AIDS-related illnesses.

Goodgame R: Gastrointestinal cytomegalovirus disease. Ann Intern Med 1993;119:924.

Wilcox CM et al: Cytomegalovirus esophagitis in patients with AIDS. A clinical, endoscopic, and pathologic correlation. Ann Intern Med 1990;113:589.

Wilcox CM, Schwartz DA, Clark WS: Esophageal ulceration in human immunodeficiency virus infection. Causes, response to therapy, and long-term outcome. Ann Intern Med 1995; 123:143.

HERPES SIMPLEX VIRUS ESOPHAGITIS

 ESSENTIALS OF DIAGNOSIS

- *Diagnosis confirmed by histopathologic or cytologic identification of viral cytopathic effect or by positive viral culture.*
- *Frequently associated with oropharyngeal ulceration.*
- *Relatively uncommon.*

General Considerations

In contrast to its occurrence in the immunocompromised host after transplantation or chemotherapy, HSV esophagitis is relatively uncommon in HIV infection. This infrequency may be explained only partially by the use of chronic acyclovir therapy in these patients.

Clinical Findings

A. Symptoms and Signs

As with other causes of ulcerative esophagitis, odynophagia and substernal chest pain are the most frequent complaints. Dysphagia, heartburn, nausea, vomiting, and fever are uncommon. HSV stomatitis has a characteristic appearance and its presence may provide an important clue to the diagnosis. However, as with other ulcerative esophageal disorders, thrush may be concurrently seen.

B. Laboratory Findings

The CD4 lymphocyte count is usually low (less than 200/µL).

C. Imaging

Barium esophagography most commonly demonstrates diffuse mucosal ulceration (Figure 2–2) or multiple well-circumscribed shallow ulcers with normal-appearing intervening mucosa. Large solitary ulcers are rare and more characteristic of CMV esophagitis or IEU.

D. Endoscopy

The most common endoscopic findings are a diffuse erosive esophagitis or multiple shallow ulcerations. Vesicles, which are the earliest manifestation, as well as large deep ulcers are rarely found. At endoscopy, cytologic brushings and mucosal biopsies may be used to

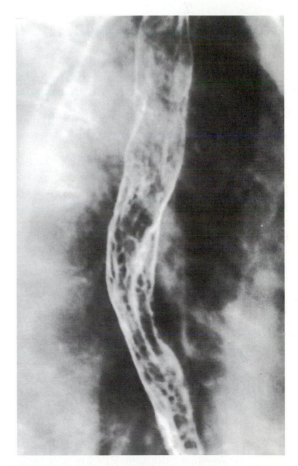

Figure 2–2. Herpes simplex virus esophagitis. There is diffuse superficial ulceration in the middle and distal esophagus.

identify characteristic viral cytopathic effect. In the presence of diffuse erosive disease, diagnosis becomes more difficult as HSV cytopathic effect is reliably identified only in squamous cells. In this situation, immunohistochemical stains to identify viral antigens may assist in the histopathologic diagnosis. Viral culture may also be performed, although as with CMV esophagitis, sensitivity and specificity may be greater with histologic examination of multiple biopsy specimens.

Differential Diagnosis

The most important causes to exclude are CMV esophagitis, IEU, and pill-induced esophagitis. As with other causes of ulcerative esophagitis, there are no truly pathognomonic radiographic or endoscopic features of HSV esophagitis; therefore, definitive diagnosis rests on the cytologic or histopathologic identification of viral cytopathic effect.

Treatment

Acyclovir is effective therapy, although resistance has been documented. Intravenous administration may be required when odynophagia is severe. The need for long-term therapy after diagnosis is not well established, although such treatment is common. The recommended dose is 5 mg/kg every 8 hours. Foscarnet may be used for treatment failures.

Genereau T et al: Herpes simplex esophagitis in patients with AIDS: report of 34 cases. The Cooperative Study Group on Herpetic Esophagitis in HIV Infection. Clin Infect Dis 1996;22:926.

Levine MS et al: Herpes esophagitis: sensitivity of double-contrast esophagography. AJR 1988;151:57.

IDIOPATHIC ESOPHAGEAL ULCERATION

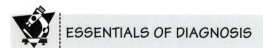

ESSENTIALS OF DIAGNOSIS

- *A common cause of esophageal ulceration.*
- *Diagnosis of exclusion.*

General Considerations

Idiopathic esophageal ulceration is a frequent cause of esophageal ulceration. Although HIV has been identified by immunohistochemical techniques in ulcer tissue from these patients, a similar prevalence of HIV has also been observed in other causes of esophageal disease,

such as CMV. HIV has not been found in squamous epithelial cells, but rather, in rare inflammatory cells in the ulcer base. Thus, it is unclear what role HIV mucosal infection plays, if any, in the genesis of these lesions. It has also been postulated that these lesions may be an autoimmune phenomenon, which is frequently seen in these patients, or the result of some as yet unidentified pathogen. A careful drug history must be obtained to exclude pill-induced disease.

Clinical Findings

A. SYMPTOMS AND SIGNS

The clinical presentation is similar to other causes of ulcerative esophagitis: commonly, odynophagia (which is usually severe), substernal chest pain, and occasionally dehydration and weight loss. Concurrent oropharyngeal ulcerations are infrequent.

B. LABORATORY FINDINGS

Idiopathic esophageal ulceration is seen in the setting of profound immunodeficiency with the CD4 lymphocyte count usually less than 100/μL. Self-limited esophageal ulcers have also been reported in patients with the HIV-associated seroconversion syndrome.

C. IMAGING

Typical findings on barium esophagography include one or multiple well-circumscribed ulcerations that may be shallow or deep (Figure 2–3).

D. ENDOSCOPY

The endoscopic appearance is one of single or multiple ulcerations of variable depth. As with CMV esophagitis, the intervening mucosa is normal. These findings are remarkably similar to CMV esophagitis. At the time of endoscopy, multiple biopsies of the ulcer base are necessary to exclude viral cytopathic effect.

Differential Diagnosis

The clinical, radiographic, and endoscopic findings are impossible to distinguish from CMV esophagitis. Multiple mid-esophageal ulcerations suggest a pill-induced esophagitis. Single or multiple distal ulcerations may mimic GERD; however, patients with GERD usually can be distinguished by a history of long-standing heartburn or regurgitation.

Complications

Sinus tract formation or fistulization to surrounding structures has been described, although frank perforation has not been reported. Bleeding may be seen.

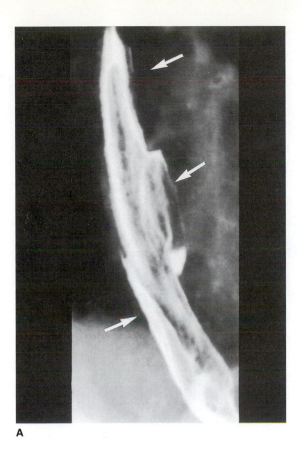

A

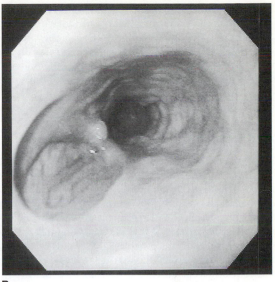

B

Figure 2–3. Idiopathic esophageal ulcer. **A:** There is a large deep ulcer in the mid-esophagus ***(arrow)***. The smaller ulcer seen proximally represents barium collecting in a healed ulcer ***(arrow)***. Barium is also seen in a large healed distal ulcer ***(arrow)***. **B:** Endoscopic photograph of the large esophageal ulcer. The mucosa surrounding the ulcer is normal. The endoscopic appearance is also compatible with CMV esophagitis.

Treatment

Corticosteroid therapy results in a dramatic response, with marked clinical improvement usually seen within the first few days of treatment. Prednisone administered at 40 mg/d orally, tapering 10 mg/wk for a 1-month course of treatment, results in a clinical and endoscopic cure rate of greater than 90%. Oral systemic antifungal therapy should be coadministered with prednisone to decrease the likelihood of symptomatic oropharyngeal or esophageal candidiasis, which may confuse assessment of the clinical response.

Prognosis

The long-term prognosis is related to the degree of immunodeficiency and the presence of other AIDS-defining illnesses. As with other opportunistic esophageal infections, IEU does not usually result in death. Relapse of IEU may be seen, usually occurring within the first several months after completion of therapy. Life-long low-dose corticosteroid therapy may be necessary for patients with frequent relapses to maintain a remission. Thalidomide has also shown efficacy in this disorder.

Alexander LN, Wilcox CM: A prospective trial of thalidomide for the treatment of HIV-associated idiopathic esophageal ulcers. AIDS Res Hum Retroviruses 1997;13:301.

Smith PD et al: Esophageal disease in AIDS is associated with pathologic processes rather than mucosal human immunodeficiency virus type I. J Infect Dis 1993;167:547.

Wilcox CM, Schwartz DA: Endoscopic characterization of idiopathic esophageal ulceration associated with human immunodeficiency virus infection. J Clin Gastroenterol 1993;16:251.

Wilcox CM, Schwartz DA: Comparison of two corticosteroid regimens for the treatment of HIV-associated idiopathic esophageal ulcer. Am J Gastroenterol 1994;89:2163.

MISCELLANEOUS DISORDERS

A variety of other opportunistic infections have been reported to involve the esophagus, including protozoa (*Cryptosporidia, Pneumocystis carinii*), bacteria (*Nocardia, Actinomyces*), *Mycobacterium* [*Mycobacterium avium* complex (MAC), *Mycobacterium tuberculosis* (TB)], as well as other fungi (*Histoplasma capsulatum*). These may be identified by appropriate histopathologic staining and culture of endoscopic biopsies. KS and non-Hodgkin's lymphoma (NHL) may also involve the esophagus.

Nonopportunistic processes, which always demand consideration in the appropriate setting, include GERD and pill-induced esophagitis. Reflux disease typically presents with symptomatic heartburn and distal esophageal disease radiographically and endoscopically. Pill-induced esophagitis has been documented from a number of drugs; in these patients, zidovudine (ZDV) and zalcitabine (ddC) have been reported.

APPROACH TO INITIAL MANAGEMENT

For patients without a prior AIDS-defining illness, the CD4 lymphocyte count provides considerable guidance in considering the plausibility of an opportunistic esophageal disorder. Given the prevalence of *Candida* esophagitis, the initial management of symptomatic patients usually consists of empiric oral systemic antifungal therapy, with fluconazole 100 mg daily after a 200-mg loading dose. This strategy may be employed in the presence or absence of thrush. In patients with severe esophageal symptoms associated with dehydration and weight loss, management should be individualized. For the patient without thrush, endoscopy may be appropriate to rapidly exclude ulcerative esophagitis.

Antifungal therapy with oral fluconazole usually results in rapid symptomatic improvement in the patient with *Candida* esophagitis and can be used as a diagnostic "test." In the absence of a prompt symptomatic improvement within 7–10 days of initiating treatment, endoscopy should be performed; barium esophagography or further empiric trials are not appropriate, given the high likelihood of ulcerative esophagitis requiring endoscopy with biopsy to exclude viral disease or IEU. Esophageal malignancy resulting from KS or NHL is uncommon, but may present with bleeding, or with dysphagia or odynophagia if the tumor is large and bulky. This suggested approach to management is summarized in Figure 2–4.

Connolly GM et al: Investigation of upper gastrointestinal symptoms in patients with AIDS. AIDS 1989;3:453.

Wilcox CM: Role of endoscopy in the investigation of upper gastrointestinal symptoms in HIV-infected patients. Can J Gastroenterol 1999;13:305.

Wilcox CM et al: Fluconazole compared with endoscopy for human immunodeficiency virus-infected patients with esophageal symptoms. Gastroenterology 1996;110:1803.

■ DISEASES OF THE STOMACH

In contrast to esophageal disease, symptomatic gastric disorders are uncommon in these patients. Diseases that affect the immunocompetent host, such as peptic ulcer, deserve consideration in the appropriate clinical setting, especially when the CD4 lymphocyte count is normal or has increased to >200/μL following HAART.

INFECTIONS & NEOPLASMS

Although a number of opportunistic pathogens have been documented to infect the stomach–including *Cryptosporidia, Toxoplasma,* fungi, *Leishmania,* and *Pneumocystis carinii,* the most common opportunistic pathogen is CMV. These infections may be asymptomatic and found incidentally, or result in nausea, vomiting, epigastric pain, or gastrointestinal bleeding. As in the normal host, asymptomatic *Helicobacter pylori* gastritis is common.

Hypochlorhydria occurs in 40–67% of patients with AIDS. Achlorhydria appears to be more common in those in the later stages of immunodeficiency. The pathophysiologic mechanisms underlying this reduced acid output are unknown, but may include antiparietal cell antibodies or the gastric secretory failure described

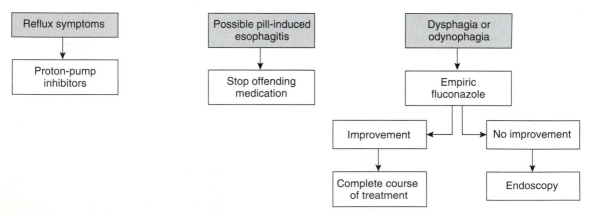

Figure 2–4. Suggested approach to the initial management of esophageal symptoms.

in other patients with severe systemic illnesses. Hypochlorhydria has important implications in relation to drug absorption and may predispose to gastrointestinal infections.

KS commonly involves the gastrointestinal tract, including the stomach; cutaneous disease is usually present. Although usually asymptomatic, KS may result in abdominal pain, obstruction, or bleeding when the lesions enlarge. NHL is usually symptomatic, presenting with obstruction or bleeding. Gastric adenocarcinoma is very rare.

Clinical Findings

A. SYMPTOMS AND SIGNS

Gastric infections usually cause nausea, vomiting, and epigastric pain. CMV may be associated with severe epigastric pain. Bleeding results from ulcerative lesions (acid-peptic, nonsteroidal antiinflammatory drug induced, CMV) or neoplasms.

B. LABORATORY FINDINGS

Opportunistic infections should be suspected when the CD4 lymphocyte count is less than 200/μL.

C. IMAGING

Upper gastrointestinal radiographic series may demonstrate thickened folds, indicative of gastritis. Gastric ulcers may have an acid-peptic etiology or be caused by CMV, neoplasms, or nonsteroidal antiinflammatory drugs (NSAIDs). Large-mass lesions resembling neoplasms have been described from CMV. KS usually appears as a large ulcerated mass or multiple well-circumscribed lesions. NHL results in a mass lesion. CT may identify wall thickening with CMV (Figure 2–5) or neoplasms (Figure 2–6).

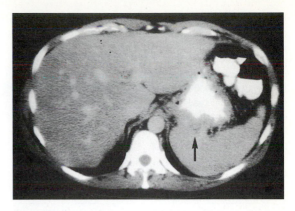

Figure 2–6. Gastric Kaposi's sarcoma. Nodularity and thickening, primarily of the posterior gastric wall *(arrow),* are seen.

D. ENDOSCOPY

In the patient with radiographic abnormalities and a low CD4 lymphocyte count, endoscopy with mucosal biopsy will often be required for diagnosis. The endoscopic appearance of KS is pathognomonic, and thus biopsy may not be required. Ulcerations should be biopsied to exclude an opportunistic infection or neoplasm.

Lake-Bakaar G et al: Gastric secretory failure in patients with the acquired immunodeficiency syndrome (AIDS). Ann Intern Med 1988;109:502.

Wilcox CM, Waites KB, Smith PD: No relationship between gastric pH, small bowel bacterial colonisation, and diarrhoea in HIV-1 infected patients. Gut 1999;44:101.

■ DISEASES OF THE PANCREAS

ESSENTIALS OF DIAGNOSIS

- *Epigastric pain, nausea, and vomiting are the most common manifestations.*
- *Exclude treatable causes.*

General Considerations

Elevation of the serum amylase concentration most commonly results from either increased levels of salivary amylase, macroamylasemia, or true pancreatic disease. De-

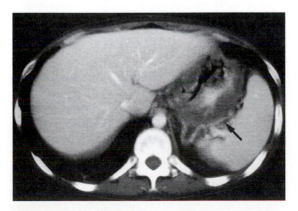

Figure 2–5. CMV gastritis. There is dramatic thickening of the gastric wall with "dirty fat" involving the gastrosplenic ligament *(arrow).*

spite the fact that a variety of opportunistic infections and neoplasms have been documented to involve the pancreas, pancreatic disorders are an infrequent clinical problem. As with the normal host, an inflammatory process is the most common expression of pancreatic disease. Pancreatitis may be caused by opportunistic infections (cryptospordia, CMV, MAC, TB), drugs [pentamidine, didanosine (ddI)], alcohol, choledocholithiasis, or, less frequently, neoplasms. The underlying cause may be suggested by the clinical setting.

Clinical Findings

A. Symptoms and Signs

Nausea, vomiting, and epigastric pain are highly suggestive of pancreatitis. The pain will frequently radiate to the back. The pattern of pain is constant and usually severe in intensity. Low-grade fever may be present.

B. Laboratory Findings

Pancreatic disease should be suspected when the amylase concentration exceeds two times the upper limits of normal. An elevation of serum lipase may help confirm a pancreatic origin of the amylase.

C. Imaging

Abdominal CT confirms the diagnosis of pancreatitis and identifies mass lesions or fluid collections. Pancreatic calcifications, retroperitoneal adenopathy, or other hepatic or splenic lesions may also be found by CT, further suggesting the underlying cause. CT-directed aspiration and biopsy of mass lesions or fluid collections with appropriate culture, staining, and pathologic evaluation may be necessary to exclude an infection or neoplasm. Ultrasound best excludes gallstones.

D. Endoscopy

Endoscopic retrograde cholangiopancreatography (ERCP) plays a valuable diagnostic and therapeutic role in the setting of suspected choledocholithiasis or in the jaundiced patient, as stones may be removed by endoscopic sphincterotomy and obstruction can be relieved by endoscopic stent placement, respectively.

Differential Diagnosis

The most likely cause depends on the clinical setting (eg, alcohol abuse or recent use of pentamidine). When the CD4 count is low, mass lesions or abscess may be related to opportunistic processes.

Complications

Complications of pancreatic disease in HIV infection are similar to those in the immunocompetent host. Chronic pancreatitis resulting from an opportunistic infection or neoplasm has not been described, probably as a result of short life expectancy.

Treatment

The treatment of pancreatitis depends on the cause. Reversible causes, such as alcohol and medications, should be excluded.

Prognosis

If a readily treatable process is found, the prognosis depends on the stage of immunodeficiency and the severity of the pancreatitis.

Dassopoulos T, Ehrenpreis ED: Acute pancreatitis in human immunodeficiency virus-infected patients: a review. Am J Med 1999;107:78.

Evrard S et al: Chronic pancreatic alterations in AIDS patients. Pancreas 1999;19:335.

■ DISEASES OF THE SMALL INTESTINE

 ESSENTIALS OF DIAGNOSIS

- *Most commonly manifested by diarrhea.*
- *Diarrhea usually of a large volume and can be associated with electrolyte disturbances and malabsorption.*

General Considerations

The small bowel is a frequent target of both opportunistic and nonopportunistic infections. Although small intestinal infection may be asymptomatic, symptoms eventually develop as immunodeficiency progresses and the infection worsens. Diarrhea and malabsorption are usually the direct result of intestinal infection. However, functional and morphologic abnormalities, such as reductions in enzyme activity (eg, lactase) and enterocyte hypoproliferation and dysmaturation, respectively, have been documented in patients with AIDS in the absence of any identifiable infection. This has been termed **AIDS enteropathy.** These functional and morphologic abnormalities do not appear to result from direct HIV infection of the enterocyte, as HIV has been found only in inflammatory cells in the lamina propria. On routine light microscopic examination of small bowel biopsies, increased inflammatory cells in the lamina propria and mild atrophy may be seen. Electron microscopic examination can be used to identify microsporidia, although routine light microscopic examination of appropriately stained specimens will usually be diagnostic. Additional small intestinal disorders potentially contributing to this enteropathy include bacterial overgrowth, neuropathic changes of the enteric nervous system, and alteration in release of enteric peptides.

Clinical Findings

A. Symptoms and Signs

Opportunistic infections of the small bowel typically cause intestinal secretion and diarrhea, with stool volumes greater than 1 L/d. For example, cryptosporidial diarrhea can be massive, with loss of over 10 L of stool per day, resulting in severe electrolyte disturbances, dehydration, and malabsorption. MAC is associated with a less severe diarrhea; however, malabsorption may be striking, given the disordered mucosal architecture caused by diffuse infiltration of macrophage-engulfed organisms in the lamina propria (termed the pseudo-Whipple's syndrome). Weight loss and fever are common with disseminated MAC infection in the absence of identifiable intestinal disease. Intestinal microsporidiosis is associated with mild to moderate diarrhea and malabsorption. In asymptomatic patients, this pathogen may be an incidental finding on small bowel biopsy. Tuberculosis may result in mass lesions of the distal small bowel, causing obstructive symptoms or frank perforation. Infections afflicting the immunocompetent host, such as giardiasis, will present similarly in the immunocompromised.

Both well-recognized viruses (rotavirus, Norwalk virus) and novel ones (picobirna, astra) have been documented and may be the cause of diarrhea when no diagnosis can be established by routine evaluation. CMV is infrequently isolated to the small bowel, but may present with abdominal pain (perforation has been reported) or diarrhea.

KS is usually asymptomatic; bleeding or obstruction may occur when the lesions becomes large. NHL may present with bleeding or signs of obstruction, since these neoplasms are usually large when clinically evident.

B. Laboratory Findings

Evidence of malabsorption and malnutrition, such as hypoalbuminemia and hypocholesterolemia, may be present, although these are nonspecific findings. Electrolyte disturbances such as hypokalemia and acidosis may reflect a secretory diarrhea. Blood cultures are important in providing indirect evidence for MAC or TB infection, and should be performed in the setting of persistent fever, weight loss, and diarrhea when the CD4 count is low (less than 100/μL).

C. Stool Analysis

Steatorrhea (positive qualitative fecal fat) may be found, although it is nonspecific. Fecal leukocytes do not result from small bowel mucosal infection. At least three sets of fresh stool should be examined to more reliably exclude an infectious cause. Specific stains for *Cryptosporidia, Isospora,* and MAC should be performed. Routine ova and parasite examination will identify *Giardia,* although multiple stool evaluations may be required to increase the diagnostic yield. Further development of immunofluorescent stains will help improve the diagnostic yield for *Cryptosporidia* and *Microsporidia.*

D. Imaging

Barium radiographic findings, such as bowel wall thickening, are often nonspecific; flocculation of barium results from failure of barium to adequately coat the mucosa as a result of excessive luminal fluid. Small bowel barium examination should not be routinely performed in the work-up of diarrhea as barium interferes with microscopic examination of the stool.

Abdominal CT may confirm the findings on the barium studies, such as small bowel thickening (Figure 2–7) or mass lesions (Figure 2–8); intraabdominal and retroperitoneal adenopathy suggest mycobacterial diseases, NHL, or less frequently KS. Mass lesions may result from KS or NHL and are rarely infectious in etiology (TB, MAC).

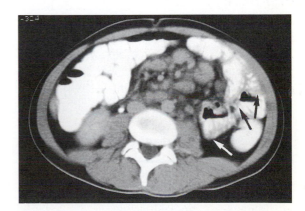

Figure 2–7. *Mycobacterium avium* complex enteritis. Thickening of the small bowel (***arrow***) is associated with diffuse mesenteric and retroperitoneal adenopathy.

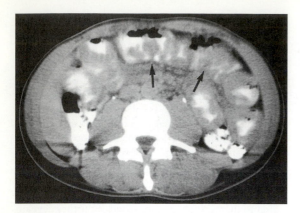

Figure 2–8. Non-Hodgkin's lymphoma involving the small intestine and colon. Loops of both small bowel ***(arrow)*** and colon are thickened. Multiple mass lesions are seen projecting into the colonic lumen ***(arrow).*** Adenopathy is also present.

E. ENDOSCOPY

Because most small intestinal pathogens causing diarrhea can be found by evaluation of multiple stool specimens, endoscopy with small bowel biopsy is infrequently required. Endoscopic evaluation is currently limited by the length of the endoscopes to the proximal small bowel (proximal jejunum). If multiple stool tests do not reveal a pathogen and small bowel infection is suspected clinically, endoscopically directed small bowel biopsy may be helpful to diagnose cryptosporidia, microsporidia, or MAC. Characteristic endoscopic abnormalities can be seen with MAC (yellow plaques, bowel wall thickening) and neoplasms (eg, KS and NHL).

Differential Diagnosis

Although a variety of both small bowel and colonic pathogens may result in diarrhea (Table 2–3), the clinician can distinguish the location of infection (small bowel versus colon) and thus site of diarrhea by history,

Table 2–3. Causes of diarrhea in AIDS.

Common	Infrequent	Rare
Cryptosporidiosis	Microsporidiosis	Tuberculosis
Cytomegalovirus	*Mycobacterium avium*	Histoplasmosis
Bacteria	complex	Amebiasis
Campylobacter		
C difficile		
Giardiasis		

physical examination, and routine laboratory tests (Table 2–4). *Giardia lamblia,* occurring in both the immunocompetent and immunodeficient individual, typically results in upper gastrointestinal symptoms such as nausea, bloating, flatulence, and periumbilical cramps. *Cryptosporidia* and *Microsporidia* may be difficult to differentiate clinically, although *Cryptosporidia* usually results in more significant diarrhea, and more commonly causes upper gastrointestinal symptoms (nausea). Significant epigastric and abdominal pain suggests CMV enteritis.

Regardless of the specific infectious causes, diarrhea tends to worsen with progression of immunodeficiency as the burden of pathogens increases. For example, *Cryptosporidia* may cause only mild diarrhea or be asymptomatic when the CD4 count is greater than 200/μL; however, diarrhea can be massive and life-threatening when the CD4 count is less than 50/μL.

Complications

Small bowel infections, particularly cryptosporidia, may be complicated by severe dehydration and life-threatening electrolyte disturbances. Weight loss is almost uniform with opportunistic small bowel infections. Bleeding can result from large neoplasms and infections causing mucosal ulceration (CMV, TB, and rarely MAC).

Treatment

Antimicrobial therapy should be directed toward the identified pathogen. Either chemotherapy, radiation

Table 2–4. Clinical features assisting in the differentiation of a small bowel from colonic diarrhea.[1]

Feature	Small Intestine	Colon
Stool frequency	Frequent	Frequent
Stool volume	Large	Small
Stool character	Watery	May be bloody
Electrolyte abnormalities	+++	——
Dehydration	++	——
Weight loss	+	+
Abdominal pain	+	++
Borborygmi	+	——
Upper gastrointestinal tract symptoms	+	——
Fecal leukocytes	Absent	Present with colitis

[1]+++, very common; ++, frequent; +, can occur; ——, not seen.

therapy, or both may be required for symptomatic neoplasms. No specific antimicrobial agent has shown consistent efficacy against cryptosporidia. Metronidazole has not been uniformly effective for microsporidiosis, although albendazole holds promise. Multidrug regimens may be efficacious in MAC. Overall, however, uniformly effective therapy for these pathogens is not available. HAART has been shown to be most effective against these small bowel infections, resulting in clinical and histologic remission. Treatment of opportunistic infections does not truly eradicate the infection; therefore, life-long therapy will be required for responders in the absence of HAART.

Prognosis

Long-term survival is primarily dependent on the degree of immunodeficiency. The lack of a response to treatment may result in progressive malabsorption and weight loss contributing to death. Severe diarrhea associated with cryptosporidiosis has a very poor prognosis.

Call SA et al: The changing etiology of chronic diarrhea in HIV-infected patients with CD4 cell counts less than 200 cells/mm[3]. Am J Gastroenterol 2000;95:3142.

Kotler DP, Orenstein JM: Clinical syndromes associated with microsporidiosis. Adv Parasitol 1998;40:321.

Schmidt W et al: Rapid increase of mucosal CD4 T cells followed by clearance of intestinal cryptosporidiosis in an AIDS patient receiving highly active antiretroviral therapy. Gastroenterology 2001;120:984.

Wilcox CM, Rabeneck L, Friedman S: AGA technical review: malnutrition and cachexia, chronic diarrhea, and hepatobiliary disease in patients with human immunodeficiency virus infection. Gastroenterology 1996;111:1724.

■ DISEASES OF THE COLON

Infections are the most common cause of colonic disease, including both nonopportunistic (bacteria, protozoa) and opportunistic (viruses, *Mycobacterium,* protozoa) causes. Abdominal pain, fever, bleeding, or perforation with peritonitis and an acute abdomen may be the initial manifestations of colonic disease.

BACTERIAL COLITIS

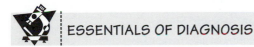 ESSENTIALS OF DIAGNOSIS

- *A frequent cause of acute diarrhea.*
- *Watery or bloody diarrhea.*

- *May be associated with relapse, requiring long-term antibiotics in those with severe immunodeficiency.*

General Considerations

The spectrum of bacterial pathogens causing colitis is similar to that in the normal host. The most frequently identified pathogen is *Campylobacter,* followed by *Salmonella* and *Shigella. Clostridium difficile* colitis is not infrequent and should always be considered in the appropriate setting. An increased risk for bacterial colitis may be seen in homosexual men engaging in oral–anal contact.

Clinical Findings

A. SYMPTOMS AND SIGNS

Bacterial colitis is associated with an acute diarrheal illness (less than 1 month in duration). The diarrhea is usually watery but may be bloody when colitis is severe. Lower abdominal pain and fever are frequent and may be prominent, suggesting peritonitis. Nausea and vomiting are uncommon.

Physical findings include fever and lower abdominal pain. Symptoms of proctitis (urgency, sense of incomplete evacuation, tenesmus, frequent low-volume stools) may be described. Digital rectal examination may demonstrate frank blood on the examining finger or a guaiac-positive stool.

B. LABORATORY FINDINGS

Bacterial colitis can occur at any stage of immunodeficiency. Electrolyte disturbances are infrequent, given that colitis does not typically cause a true secretory diarrhea. Blood cultures should be performed in the patient with fever and may be positive, especially with *Salmonella.*

C. STOOL ANALYSIS

Submitting fresh stool for bacterial culture is essential. Stool staining with Gram's stain or methylene blue to evaluate for fecal leukocytes is mandatory. Their presence documents colitis. They are almost uniformly found in the setting of bacterial colitis including *C difficile. Clostridium difficile* toxin should be excluded on fresh stool in the patient recently receiving antibiotics or the patient developing diarrhea while hospitalized, especially when associated with fecal leukocytes. Occasionally, bacteremia may be found when stool cultures are negative.

D. IMAGING

Routine abdominal radiographs are usually nonspecific, although in severe cases, thumbprinting or colonic dilation may be found. Barium enema examination plays no role in the evaluation of acute diarrhea, especially when bacterial colitis is suspected. As with small bowel disease, if barium enema is required for other reasons, all stool studies should be collected before the examination. In those with severe bacterial colitis, abdominal CT will often demonstrate colonic wall thickening.

E. ENDOSCOPY

Flexible sigmoidoscopic examination of the distal colorectum may be diagnostic for *C difficile* colitis when multiple or confluent yellow plaques are seen. The endoscopic appearance of bacterial colitis is nondiagnostic, resembling CMV colitis or idiopathic inflammatory bowel disease (ulcerative colitis, Crohn's disease). Sigmoidoscopic examination should be performed in the patient with suspected colitis when multiple (at least three) stool cultures and *C difficile* toxin titer are negative. In the hospitalized patient with diarrhea and fecal leukocytes, early sigmoidoscopy may expedite diagnosis and treatment.

Differential Diagnosis

In the patient with acute diarrhea, differentiation between small bowel (ie, giardiasis) and colonic causes may be difficult. Pathogens involving the small bowel typically cause upper gastrointestinal symptoms, such as nausea, vomiting, bloating and distention, borborygmi, and periumbilical abdominal cramps. Colonic disorders result in lower abdominal or left-lower quadrant pain and tenderness. Urgency, sensation of incomplete evacuation, tenesmus, and frequent low-volume stools are highly suggestive of proctitis or distal colitis. In general, *Cryptosporidia, Microsporidia,* and MAC cause small bowel disease and do not present acutely. Similarly, colonic processes such as CMV colitis or idiopathic inflammatory bowel disease are associated with chronic symptoms, however they may present acutely. These disorders can usually be differentiated by careful history, physical examination, and evaluation of multiple stool specimens, supplemented by sigmoidoscopic or colonoscopic evaluation where appropriate.

Treatment

The choice of definitive antimicrobial therapy depends on the culture and sensitivity results. Ciprofloxacin is the empiric therapy of choice for suspected bacterial colitis given the increasing bacterial resistance to trimethoprim-sulfamethoxazole. In contrast to the immunocompetent host with acute bacterial colitis, antibiotic therapy should be initiated in immunodeficient

patients with documented bacterial colitis. *Clostridium difficile* colitis can be treated with metronidazole, with oral vancomycin reserved for patients with severe life-threatening disease.

Prognosis

Antibiotic therapy is effective. Long-term suppressive therapy may be required to prevent relapse if severe immunodeficiency is present, particularly for patients with *Salmonella. Clostridium difficile* colitis does not appear to be associated with more severe disease, refractoriness to antibiotics, or a higher rate of relapse than in immunocompetent patients.

Cappell MS, Philogene C: *Clostridium difficile* infection is a treatable cause of diarrhea in patients with advanced human immunodeficiency virus infection. Am J Gastroenterol 1993;88:891.

Rene E et al: Intestinal infections in patients with acquired immunodeficiency syndrome. A prospective study in 132 patients. Dig Dis Sci 1989;34:773.

Smith DP et al: Gastrointestinal infections in AIDS. Ann Intern Med 1992;116:63.

CYTOMEGALOVIRUS COLITIS

 ESSENTIALS OF DIAGNOSIS

- *The most common opportunistic cause of colonic disease.*
- *Usually presents as chronic diarrhea.*
- *Associated with extraintestinal disease.*
- *Diagnosis most specific by histopathologic identification of viral cytopathic effect in mucosal biopsy specimens.*

General Considerations

As with the identification of CMV in other gastrointestinal sites, extraintestinal disease (ophthalmic disease) should be excluded at the time of diagnosis, given the implications for long-term management.

Clinical Findings

A. SYMPTOMS AND SIGNS

CMV colitis usually presents as a chronic (greater than 1 month) watery diarrhea in the setting of severe immunodeficiency. Fever, weight loss, and lower abdominal pain are common symptoms and signs. When the distal colorectum is involved, symptoms of proctitis may be reported. Gastrointestinal bleeding without diarrhea may be the initial manifestation of colitis. Other symptoms may be related to concurrent extraintestinal CMV disease, such as altered vision in CMV retinitis. Concurrent symptomatic upper gastrointestinal disease is rare.

Physical findings are nonspecific. Digital rectal examination is usually unremarkable, although tenderness may be elicited with associated anorectal disease.

B. Laboratory Findings

CMV colitis almost always occurs when the CD4 lymphocyte count is severely reduced (<100/µL). Serologic studies for CMV antibody are not helpful because they are uniformly positive in these patients.

C. Stool Analysis

The diagnosis should be suspected when multiple stool tests are negative in the setting of chronic diarrhea, weight loss, and severe immunodeficiency. Fecal leukocytes may be present with severe distal colitis.

D. Imaging

Routine abdominal radiographs are nonspecific. Barium enema examination should not be done for the routine evaluation of chronic diarrhea or if the diagnosis is suspected. Reported findings on barium enema, however, include a pancolitis, segmental colitis, or focal ulcerations that may be segmental or diffuse. Abdominal CT usually demonstrates focal or diffuse colonic wall thickening depending on the extent of involvement (Figure 2–9). As with bacterial colitis, these CT findings are highly suggestive of colitis, but not specific for any particular cause.

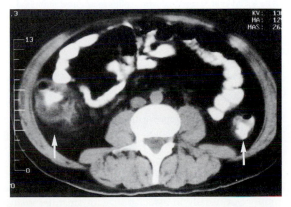

Figure 2–9. CMV colitis. The right colon and descending colon (**arrows**) are diffusely thickened. Similar findings may be seen with bacterial colitis.

E. Endoscopy

Endoscopic examination is necessary to establish the diagnosis. Viral cytopathic effect of CMV should be identified by histopathologic evaluation of biopsy specimens. Viral culture positivity of biopsy specimens is less sensitive and specific. In many patients, the region of disease will be continuous, beginning in the distal colorectum and extending proximally; thus, examination by sigmoidoscopy has a high yield. However, disease may be isolated to the right colon, thereby requiring full colonoscopy for diagnosis. Endoscopically, the most common appearance is a diffuse colitis mimicking bacterial colitis or idiopathic ulcerative colitis, or multiple ulcerations with normal-appearing intervening mucosa resembling Crohn's disease. Biopsies obtained throughout the colon may occasionally identify CMV in the absence of gross endoscopic abnormalities.

Differential Diagnosis

In the patient presenting with bloody diarrhea, lower abdominal pain, and fever, acute bacterial colitis should be excluded. Although CMV colitis may present with bloody diarrhea, it is more typically associated with a chronic watery diarrhea associated with weight loss and abdominal pain. *Clostridium difficile* colitis must be considered in those patients recently receiving antibiotics, or when the diarrhea develops during hospitalization. Patients presenting with acute diarrhea should have amebiasis excluded if they have traveled to an endemic area.

In the absence of colonic symptoms, differentiation from small bowel diarrhea may be difficult; these patients should have multiple stool specimens evaluated to exclude bacterial and parasitic diseases before undergoing endoscopy. Iatrogenic causes should always be excluded: eg, antibiotics (without associated *C difficile* colitis), medications that contain magnesium or phosphate, which may precipitate diarrhea, and enteral feedings. Antiretroviral agents are now recognized to be a frequent cause of mild diarrhea. A suggested approach for the evaluation of chronic diarrhea is provided in Figure 2–10.

Complications

Colonic perforation requires urgent surgical intervention. CMV colitis may also cause severe gastrointestinal hemorrhage. Dehydration and electrolyte disturbances are rare unless a concurrent small bowel disease is present.

Treatment

Intravenous treatment with either ganciclovir, foscarnet, or cidofovir is effective in approximately 75% of

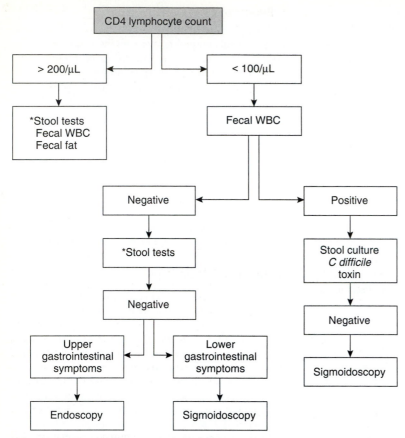

Figure 2–10. Suggested approach in the evaluation of chronic diarrhea.

*At least three sets of fresh stool for ova and parasites, bacterial culture, and C *difficile* toxin.

patients (see section, "Diseases of the Esophagus"). Drug selection should be based on toxicity as well as the clinician's level of comfort in administering the agent given the similar efficacies. In general, a longer course of treatment may be required for CMV colitis than for esophageal disease (usually 3–4 weeks), depending on the severity and extent of disease. As with esophageal disease, the need for life-long maintenance therapy is controversial. After a complete response, the patient should be followed clinically without maintenance antiviral therapy. If relapse occurs, reinduction therapy followed by maintenance therapy should be initiated. Documentation of retinal disease at diagnosis or during follow-up requires life-long maintenance therapy.

Prognosis

Despite a clinical response, CMV colitis is a marker of poor long-term survival, the mean survival being approximately 8 months.

Dieterich DT et al: Ganciclovir treatment of cytomegalovirus colitis in AIDS: a randomized double-blind, placebo-controlled multicenter study. J Infect Dis 1993;167:278.

Wilcox CM et al: Cytomegalovirus colitis in acquired immunodeficiency syndrome: a clinical and endoscopic study. Gastrointest Endosc 1998;48:39.

MISCELLANEOUS COLONIC DISORDERS

Infections

A variety of other opportunistic pathogens have been reported to infect the colon in these patients, including *Pneumocystis carinii* and *Histoplasma capsulatum. Mycobacterium avium* complex may involve the colon, although usually in association with small bowel disease. Similarly, *Cryptosporidia* may be identified on colonic biopsy but usually in association with small bowel infection. HSV infects squamous mucosa and therefore does not cause colitis; however, the distal colorectum may be involved in the setting of perianal disease.

Neoplasms

KS is the most common colonic neoplasm in HIV-infected patients. Colonic KS is usually associated with cutaneous disease as well as disease in the proximal gastrointestinal tract. Colonic KS, as with other gastrointestinal involvement, is most often clinically silent; however, bleeding, obstruction, or even perforation has been documented. NHL can involve the colon. These lesions are typically large, resulting in abdominal pain or obstruction; fever is often present (Figure 2–11). Barium enema examination or abdominal CT in the appropriate clinical setting may suggest the diagnosis. Colonic adenocarcinoma has also been reported in these patients. Colonoscopic biopsy will be required to make a definitive diagnosis of these neoplasms.

Idiopathic Inflammatory Bowel Disease

Given the prominent immunologic component of inflammatory bowel disease, the initial diagnosis of ulcerative colitis or Crohn's disease might be unexpected in these immunosuppressed patients. Interestingly, some HIV-infected patients with long-standing inflammatory bowel disease will have disease remission as the immunodeficiency progresses. Ulcerative colitis and Crohn's disease, therefore, are a diagnosis of exclusion in any HIV-infected patient with colitis. CMV colitis, bacterial colitis, and amebiasis should also always be excluded, especially if corticosteroid therapy is to be given.

Monkemuller KE, Wilcox CM: Diagnosis and treatment of colonic disease in AIDS. Gastrointest Endosc Clin North Am 1998;8:889.

■ DISEASES OF THE ANORECTUM

 ESSENTIALS OF DIAGNOSIS

- *Pain that worsens with defecation is a common complaint.*
- *Bleeding is seen with hemorrhoids, fissures, or, rarely, tumors.*

Clinical Findings

A. SYMPTOMS AND SIGNS

Anorectal disorders may cause significant morbidity, primarily as a result of pain. As with the general population, hemorrhoidal disease is the most common anorectal disorder and presents with anorectal pain or bleeding. Anal fissures cause anorectal pain, particularly with defecation, and may be associated with bleeding and rectal discharge. Fistulas, without any apparent underlying cause, may present with bleeding, pain, or discharge. Venereal diseases (syphilis, gonorrhea, *Chlamydia*) should be suspected in the patient with symptoms of proctitis who engages in unprotected receptive anal intercourse.

CMV may cause solitary anorectal ulceration with severe pain or bleeding. HSV is associated with perianal disease; rarely, a distal proctitis may be seen. Unex-

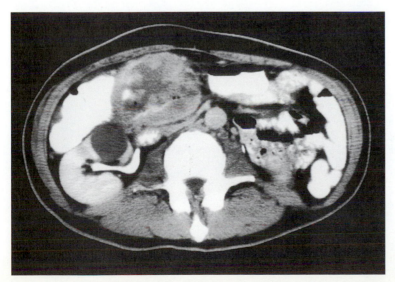

Figure 2–11. Colonic non-Hodgkin's lymphoma. A large mass lesion involving the proximal transverse colon is seen.

plained anorectal ulcerations have also been described in HIV-positive patients.

Neoplasms such as KS, NHL, cloacogenic carcinoma, and squamous cell carcinoma have been increasingly recognized. When these tumors ulcerate, pain and bleeding may occur; when they enlarge, obstruction results.

Physical examination plays an invaluable role in determining the underlying cause. Inspection of the perianal region may reveal ulcerations (neoplasms, infections such as HSV, CMV), mass lesions (KS, NHL, cloacogenic or squamous cell carcinoma), hemorrhoidal disease, or fissures. If digital rectal examination elicits exquisite tenderness, ulcerative disease of the anal canal is almost certainly present.

B. ENDOSCOPY

These patients may need to be sedated to obtain an adequate evaluation; surgical proctoscopic examination may be necessary to obtain adequate biopsy samples.

Sigmoidoscopic examination of the more proximal rectum may identify concurrent colitis or ulcers.

Treatment

Treatment depends on the underlying disorder. Local therapies and stool softeners are helpful for hemorrhoidal disease and fissures. When hemorrhoidal disease is precipitated by chronic diarrhea, antimotility agents to reduce stool frequency should be initiated. Medical therapy will be required for opportunistic infections. NHL responds to radiation therapy. Carcinomas respond poorly to therapy, although surgical excision has been used. Poor wound healing in the patient with severe immunodeficiency will limit the surgical options.

Brar HS, Gottesman L, Surawicz C: Anorectal pathology in AIDS. Gastrointest Endosc Clin North Am 1998;8:913.

Wilcox CM, Schwartz DA: Idiopathic anorectal ulceration in patients with human immunodeficiency virus infection. Am J Gastroenterol 1994;89:599.

Acute Upper Gastrointestinal Bleeding

Rome Jutabha, MD & Dennis M. Jensen, MD

This chapter discusses the diagnostic approach, acute and long-term management, and treatment options for acute upper gastrointestinal bleeding. **Acute upper gastrointestinal bleeding** refers to blood loss within the intraluminal gastrointestinal tract from any location between the upper esophagus to the duodenum at the ligament of Treitz. Specific causes of upper gastrointestinal bleeding will be reviewed and treatment modalities will be discussed (Tables 3–1 and 3–2).

The onset and severity of blood loss can range from intermittent and low-grade occult bleeding presenting as occult-blood-positive stools and iron deficiency anemia to very abrupt and massive blood loss presenting as hematemesis and hypovolemic shock. This discussion focuses on the medical and endoscopic management of severe, acute upper gastrointestinal bleeding that necessitates admission to an intensive care unit (ICU) and performance of emergency upper panendoscopy.

Acute upper gastrointestinal bleeding is responsible for significant morbidity and mortality. In addition, the costs to society in terms of hospital admission charges, lost work due to illness, and expense of maintenance therapy for prevention of rebleeding are staggering. Although there have been many advances in the past 50 years in critical care management, development of potent antisecretory medications, and new diagnostic and therapeutic technologies for acute upper gastrointestinal bleeding, the overall mortality rates have not changed significantly since 1945. More effective and safer endoscopic hemostasis modalities, such as thermal contact probes for control of nonvariceal hemorrhage and variceal band ligation for esophagogastric varices, have recently been developed and refined. Some of the randomized trials suggest improved morbidity and mortality rates for these new techniques as compared with traditional medical and surgical therapies.

By convention, upper gastrointestinal bleeding has been categorized as either variceal or nonvariceal in origin. **Gastroesophageal varices** are enlarged venous collateral channels that dilate as a consequence of portal hypertension. Varices gradually enlarge and eventually rupture, resulting in massive upper gastrointestinal hemorrhage. In contrast, **nonvariceal bleeding** results from disruption of esophageal or gastroduodenal mucosa with

ulceration or erosion into an underlying vessel. Some examples of nonvariceal lesions responsible for upper gastrointestinal bleeding include Mallory-Weiss tears, gastroduodenal ulcers or tumors, and Dieulafoy's lesions.

Before the development of diagnostic endoscopy and therapeutic endoscopic hemostasis, the distinction between variceal and nonvariceal bleeding was of great importance because they were diagnosed and managed differently. Furthermore, before liver transplantation was an option, the long-term prognosis for variceal bleeders was dismal because of end-stage liver disease. Now, the basic principles of resuscitation and the acute management of active upper gastrointestinal bleeding are the same for all patients, regardless of the origin of bleeding. The approach to acute upper gastrointestinal bleeding will be discussed in detail in the following section.

■ ACUTE MANAGEMENT OF SEVERE UPPER GASTROINTESTINAL BLEEDING

Patients experiencing severe upper gastrointestinal bleeding may present with dizziness, light-headedness, weakness, or pallor. They may also have palpitations, tachycardia, and hypotension. Patients may have anemia that is normochromic and normocytic. Blood loss is overt, demonstrated by vomiting or passing of blood in the stool.

The basic elements of the management of acute upper gastrointestinal bleeding include (1) prompt patient resuscitation and stabilization, (2) assessment of the onset and severity of bleeding, (3) regional localization of the bleeding site, (4) determination of the most likely cause of upper gastrointestinal bleeding, (5) preparation for emergent upper panendoscopy, (6) control of active bleeding or treatment of lesions at high risk of rebleeding with therapeutic endoscopy, (7) minimization of treatment-related complications, and (8) treatment of rebleeding episodes (Table 3–3).

Table 3-1. Causes of acute upper
gastrointestinal bleeding.

Ulcerative, erosive, or inflammatory diseases
  Peptic ulcer disease
    Gastric or duodenal ulcer disease
    Zollinger-Ellison syndrome
    Gastroesophageal reflux disease
  Stress ulcer
  Infectious causes
    Helicobacter pylori
    Cytomegalovirus
    Herpes simplex virus
  Drug-induced erosions, ulcers, or bleeding
    Aspirin
    Nonsteroidal antiinflammatory drugs (NSAIDs)
    Pill-induced ulcer (tetracycline, quinidine, potassium
      chloride tablets)
    Anticoagulation therapy
Trauma
  Mallory-Weiss tear
  Foreign body ingestion
Vascular lesions
  Varices
  Angiomas and Osler-Weber-Rendu syndrome
  Dieulafoy's lesion
  Watermelon stomach (gastric antral vascular ectasia)
  Portal hypertensive gastropathy
  Aortoenteric fistula
  Radiation-induced telangiectasia
Tumors
  Benign
    Leiomyoma
    Lipoma
    Polyp (hyperplastic, adenomatous, hamartomatous)
    Blue rubber bleb nevus syndrome
  Malignant
    Adenocarcinoma
    Leiomyosarcoma
    Lymphoma
    Kaposi's sarcoma
    Carcinoid
    Melanoma
    Metastatic tumor
  Miscellaneous
    Hemobilia
    Hemosuccus pancreaticus

Table 3-2. Therapeutic options for acute upper
gastrointestinal hemorrhage.

Medical therapy
  Peptic ulcer disease
    Antisecretory therapy (H_2-receptor antagonist, proton-
      pump inhibitors)
    Antacids
    Sucralfate
    Misoprostol
  Gastroesophageal varices
    Intravenous vasopressin with or without nitroglycerin
    Intravenous octreotide
    Balloon tamponade
Endoscopic therapy
  Peptic ulcer disease
    Thermal coagulation
      Multipolar electrocoagulation (bicap or gold probe)
      Heater probe
      Laser therapy
    Injection therapy
      Epinephrine
      Alcohol
    Combination therapy: thermal coagulation and injection
  Gastroesophageal varices
    Injection sclerotherapy
    Variceal band ligation
    Cyanoacrylate injection
    Combination therapy: sclerotherapy and band ligation
  Tumors
    Thermal probe (tumor, endoscopic bipolar, or heater
      probe)
    Laser ablation
    Thermal balloon catheter
Surgical therapy
  Nonvariceal (ulcer, tumor, or Mallory-Weiss tear)
  Variceal
    Portosystemic shunting
    Esophageal transection and devascularization
    Liver transplantation
Radiologic therapy
  Peptic ulcer disease
    Arterial embolization
    Intraarterial vasopressin infusion
  Gastroesophageal varices
    Embolization
    Transjugular intrahepatic portosystemic shunting

PATIENT RESUSCITATION & STABILIZATION

The fundamental principles of emergency medicine
apply to the patient presenting with acute upper gastrointestinal bleeding, namely, prompt assessment and
establishment of the ABCs (airway, breathing, circulation). Elective endotracheal or nasotracheal intubation
with or without mechanical ventilation is recommended before emergency endoscopy for patients with
shock secondary to massive bleeding, ongoing hematemesis, severe agitation or altered mental status, or
impaired respiratory status. This will facilitate both the
diagnostic and therapeutic endoscopies and minimize

Table 3–3. Management approach for acute upper gastrointestinal hemorrhage.[1]

Acute management
  Patient stabilization (ABCs)
    Respiratory stabilization (consider endotracheal
      intubation if altered respiratory status or ongoing
      hematemesis)
    Intravenous access
    Intravascular volume replacement
    Transfusions
      Packed red blood cells
      Fresh frozen plasma
      Platelets
  Focused history and physical examination
  Laboratory data
    CBC with platelet count
    Coagulation studies (PT/aPTT)
    Liver enzymes
    Chemistries
  Radiographic (if perforation suspected)
    Upright chest x-ray
    Abdominal x-ray
  Electrocardiogram
  Localization of bleeding site (upper GI vs lower GI vs
    small bowel)
  Surgery consultation
  Gastroenterology consultation for upper panendoscopy
    Diagnostic
      Localize source of bleeding
      Determine status of bleeding
      Risk stratification for further or recurrent bleeding
    Therapeutic
      Stop active bleeding
      Decrease the risk of recurrent bleeding
Long-term management
  Treatment of recurrent bleeding
    Repeat diagnostic and therapeutic endoscopy
    Angiography
    Surgery
  Preventive measures for peptic ulcer disease bleeding
    Maintenance antisecretory therapy
    Helicobacter pylori eradication
    Strict avoidance of ASA/NSAIDs
    Misoprostol
    Surgery
  Preventive measures for variceal bleeding
    β-blockers
    Obliterative endoscopic therapy
    Shunting
    Liver transplatation

[1]ABCs, airway, breathing, circulation; CBC, complete blood count; PT and aPTT, prothrombin time/activated partial thromboplastin time; GI, gastrointestinal; ASA, acetylsalicylic acid (aspirin); NSAIDs, nonsteroidal antiinflammatory drugs.

the risk of aspiration. The endotracheal tube can be removed after the effects of the premedication have worn off. In patients with hepatic encephalopathy, long-acting benzodiazepines should be avoided because they may exacerbate an already deteriorating mental status.

The importance of adequate resuscitation before diagnostic and therapeutic endoscopy cannot be overemphasized. Two large-caliber (18-gauge or larger) peripheral catheters should be inserted for intravenous access and volume replacement. High-risk patients (the elderly or those with known cirrhosis or coronary artery disease) should receive packed red blood cell transfusion to maintain the hematocrit above 30%. Young and otherwise healthy patients should be transfused to maintain their hematocrit above 20%. Patients with a coagulopathy (prolonged prothrombin time) or low platelet count should be transfused with fresh frozen plasma and platelets, respectively.

ASSESSMENT OF ONSET & SEVERITY OF BLEEDING

The onset of bleeding refers to acute versus chronic blood loss. Symptoms and signs suggestive of chronic bleeding include weakness, lethargy, occult gastrointestinal bleeding with occult-blood-positive stool, and iron deficiency anemia (hypochromic, microcytic). In contrast, acute upper gastrointestinal blood loss is usually overt, demonstrated by **hematemesis** (vomiting of fresh blood or clots), coffee ground emesis (vomiting of coffee-ground-like blood), **melena** (dark, tarry-appearing stool), or **hematochezia** (fresh blood or clot per rectum). Acute upper gastrointestinal bleeding causes tachycardia, orthostatic hypotension, or syncope. Massive bleeding may lead to hypotensive shock, myocardial infarction, and cardiopulmonary arrest.

DETERMINATION OF THE BLEEDING SITE

Once the patient has been adequately stabilized, the next step is to determine the site of bleeding (upper gastrointestinal versus lower gastrointestinal versus small bowel) to guide the diagnostic work-up. Emergent upper panendoscopy is indicated for patients with suspected acute upper gastrointestinal bleeding. Patient history, signs of upper gastrointestinal hemorrhage, and passage of a nasogastric tube will help distinguish upper gastrointestinal from lower gastrointestinal bleeding.

DETERMINATION OF THE CAUSE OF BLEEDING

The clinical history can yield useful information suggesting the site of gastrointestinal bleeding as well as the specific lesion. The medical history should include questions about prior episodes of upper gastrointestinal bleeding (ulcers or varices), liver disease, intestinal polyps or cancer, and blood transfusions. Pertinent symptoms include abdominal pain, nausea, vomiting, hematemesis, early satiety, anorexia, or weight loss. Medication history should include aspirin, nonsteroidal antiinflammatory drugs (NSAIDs), and anticoagulation therapy (warfarin or heparin). Social history should focus on intravenous drug use, alcohol abuse, and sexual partners.

Physical examination should include a rectal examination, a nasogastric tube aspiration, assessment of stigmata of chronic liver disease (jaundice, spider telangiectasias, ascites). Melena is suggestive of upper gastrointestinal bleeding, although it may be seen with small bowel bleeding or right-sided colonic lesions. Bright red blood per rectum or clot suggests a lower gastrointestinal bleeding source, although massive upper gastrointestinal bleeding may also present in this manner. A positive nasogastric aspirate yielding coffee ground material, clots, or bright red blood is highly suggestive of a recent upper gastrointestinal bleed. A negative nasogastric aspirate yielding clear fluid without bile will not exclude duodenal lesions, such as an ulcer.

Laboratory data can be useful for assessing the degree of bleeding, determining possible sources of bleeding, and guiding therapy. Laboratory studies should include a complete blood count (CBC), an automated chemistry panel that includes liver function studies [alanine aminotransferase (ALT), aspartate aminotransferase (AST), bilirubin, albumin, and total protein], and coagulation studies [prothrombin time (PT), partial thromboplastin time (PTT)]. It is important to keep in mind that the hematocrit may significantly underestimate the amount of blood loss during an acute bleed.

Serial hematocrits may be an indicator of ongoing bleeding or rebleeding and can help guide transfusions with packed red blood cells, fresh frozen plasma, and platelets. An electrocardiogram (ECG) should be obtained for all patients with significant cardiac risk factors. An upright chest and abdominal x-ray should be performed in patients with suspected intestinal perforation, obstruction, or pulmonary aspiration.

PREPARATION FOR EMERGENT UPPER PANENDOSCOPY

Both a gastroenterologist and a surgeon should be notified promptly of all patients with severe acute upper gastrointestinal bleeding. Patients with hemodynamic instability (shock, orthostatic hypotension, decrease in hematocrit of *at least* 6%, or transfusion requirement over two units of packed red blood cells) or active bleeding (manifested by hematemesis, bright red blood

per nasogastric tube, or hematochezia) should be admitted to an intensive care unit for resuscitation and close observation with automated blood pressure monitoring, ECG monitoring, and pulse oximetry.

Nasogastric tube or orogastric tube lavage should be performed to remove particulate matter, fresh blood, and clots. This will facilitate endoscopy and decrease the risk of massive aspiration.

CONTROL OF ACTIVE BLEEDING OR HIGH-RISK LESIONS

Diagnostic endoscopy can localize the site of acute upper gastrointestinal bleeding and stratify lesions at high risk versus low risk of bleeding. Stigmata of recent ulcer hemorrhage include active bleeding, visible vessel, or adherent clot (see Table 3–5). Endoscopic therapy should be limited to these high-risk lesions. Endoscopic treatments include thermal coagulation, injection therapy, and combination therapy. Specific modalities are discussed in further detail (see following section, "Treatment").

MINIMIZATION OF TREATMENT-RELATED COMPLICATIONS

Complications can arise prior to, during, or after endoscopy. Complications that can occur before endoscopy include aspiration (especially in a sedated, combative, or encephalopathic patient), hypoventilation (related to oversedation), and hypotension (due to inadequate volume replacement or transfusions in addition to sedation with narcotics). As previously mentioned, patients must be adequately resuscitated before endoscopy. Elective endotracheal intubation (with or without mechanical ventilation) may facilitate endoscopy and decrease the risk of aspiration.

Endoscopic complications are usually related to endoscopic hemostasis therapy and include precipitation or worsening of bleeding and perforation. Overly aggressive and repeated applications of thermal or injection therapy rarely increase the hemostasis rate but may increase the risk of treatment-induced complications. Therefore, a predetermined limit (amount of injection solution or total energy delivered) should be set and not exceeded.

TREATMENT OF PERSISTENT OR RECURRENT BLEEDING

For active bleeding that is not stopped or slowed down significantly with endoscopic therapy, alternative interventions such as surgery or radiographic modalities are indicated. For rebleeding lesions initially controlled by endoscopic therapy, endoscopy is repeated and the bleeding source is re-treated in the initial manner. If the bleeding persists or if rebleeding occurs after two therapeutic endoscopies, the patient is referred for surgery.

■ SPECIFIC CAUSES OF ACUTE UPPER GASTROINTESTINAL BLEEDING

This section discusses the diagnosis and management of specific causes of acute upper gastrointestinal bleeding, most common of which are peptic ulcer disease and gastroesophageal varices (Table 3–4).

ULCERATIVE OR EROSIVE DISEASES

Ulcerative or erosive diseases of the upper gastrointestinal tract that can cause acute upper gastrointestinal bleeding include peptic ulcer disease, Zollinger-Ellison syndrome, esophagitis, erosions of the stomach or duodenum, esophageal ulcers, stress-induced ulcers, infectious ulcers (herpes simplex virus, cytomegalovirus, or *Helicobacter pylori*), and medication-induced ulcers (aspirin, NSAIDs, pills).

1. *Peptic Ulcer Disease*

Pathophysiology

Mucosal erosions or ulcers develop from an imbalance between aggressive factors and the protective factors of the mucosa. Aggressive factors that can damage normal mucosal integrity include hyperacidity, pepsin, bile salts, ischemia, aspirin, and NSAIDs (which decrease

Table 3–4. Causes of severe upper gastrointestinal bleeding.[1]

Diagnosis	Number of Patients (%) (n = 948)
Peptic ulcers	524 (55)
Gastroesophageal varices	131 (14)
Angiomas	54 (6)
Mallory-Weiss tear	45 (5)
Tumors	42 (4)
Erosions	41 (4)
Dieulafoy's lesion	6 (1)
Other	105 (11)

[1]Data from the Center for Ulcer Research and Education (CURE) Hemostasis Research Group, UCLA School of Medicine and the West Los Angeles VA Medical Center.

the protective barrier by inhibition of mucosal prostaglandins), and *H pylori* (in duodenal and gastric ulcer, although the mechanism is not fully understood). Protective esophageal mechanisms include esophageal motility (clearance of refluxed acid), salivary secretions (bicarbonate), and the lower esophageal sphincter (prevents reflux). Gastric mucosal defenses include mucus, rapid epithelial renewal, and tissue mediators. Acute upper gastrointestinal bleeding occurs when an erosion or ulcer disrupts an underlying vein or artery.

 ESSENTIALS OF DIAGNOSIS

- *Abdominal pain, nausea, vomiting, and hematemesis or melena.*
- *Abdominal discomfort is improved with food or antacids.*
- *History of aspirin or NSAID use, history of peptic ulcer disease and upper gastrointestinal bleeding.*
- *Epigastric tenderness, succussion splash suggestive of outlet obstruction.*

General Considerations

Peptic ulcer disease is the most common cause of severe upper gastrointestinal bleeding, accounting for 30–50% of total cases. Bleeding peptic ulcers account for over 100,000 hospital admissions per year. Approximately 20–25% of ulcer patients with acute upper gastrointestinal bleeding have severe or recurrent bleeding. Their mortality rate is as high as 36%, due mainly to recurrent or persistent bleeding, surgical complications, or their underlying disease.

Clinical Findings

A. SYMPTOMS AND SIGNS

The symptoms of patients with bleeding ulcers are nonspecific and can range from silent disease to severe upper abdominal pain. Classically, ulcer pain is described as gnawing or cramping, lasting up to several hours, and relieved with food or antacids. Symptoms may recur episodically for a few weeks followed by asymptomatic periods for weeks or months. Other symptoms may include early satiety, abdominal distention, anorexia, nausea, or vomiting; these symptoms suggest a mechanical obstruction or altered gastroduodenal motility. Generally, however, only 30–40% of patients with severe ulcer hemorrhage have antecedent ulcer symptoms.

B. Laboratory Findings

Biochemical and hematologic abnormalities seen with upper gastrointestinal bleeding from peptic ulcer disease are nonspecific and may be seen with any cause of acute bleeding. These findings include acute anemia (normocytic, normochromic), elevated blood urea nitrogen (BUN) and creatinine (dehydration and prerenal azotemia), and prolonged bleeding time (due to aspirin or NSAID ingestion). An elevated serum gastrin level suggests Zollinger-Ellison syndrome.

C. Imaging

Endoscopy is the diagnostic method of choice because of high sensitivity and specificity. In addition, endoscopy can be used to collect biopsy specimens as well as to treat acute upper gastrointestinal bleeding (see following section, "Treatment"). Barium x-ray studies are less accurate and should not be performed during acute bleeding or when perforation is suspected. Angiography and radionuclide scans are rarely indicated in acute upper gastrointestinal bleeding, although angiography may be used to control acute bleeding with coil or Gelfoam embolization.

Differential Diagnosis

Benign peptic ulcer disease related to hyperacidity must be differentiated from ulcers caused by a malignant process (gastric or esophageal carcinoma), an infectious process, medications, or ischemia. The clinical history and endoscopic biopsies will help define the underlying cause. Other causes of upper abdominal discomfort include nonulcer dyspepsia, malignancy, cholelithiasis, and pancreatitis. However, most of these conditions are not associated with acute upper gastrointestinal bleeding.

Complications

Complications of bleeding peptic ulcer disease include pain, perforation, and obstruction. The latter are extremely rare in patients with bleeding ulcers. Other complications are related to endoscopy or therapeutic hemostasis. Complications associated with endoscopy include respiratory depression from premedication, aspiration, and perforation. Ulcers may enlarge or become deeper, or bleeding may worsen during or following endoscopic therapy because of tissue damage by the sclerosant or thermal coagulation.

Treatment

The immediate treatment of acute upper gastrointestinal bleeding secondary to peptic ulcer disease includes medical, endoscopic, and surgical interventions. Med-

ical treatments may decrease the risk of recurrent bleeding after hospital discharge but do not alter the hospital course. In the case of ulcer hemorrhage with no stigmata or minor stigmata of recent hemorrhage, there is a very low rebleeding rate on medical therapy (Table 3–5). Early refeeding of these ulcer patients may be beneficial and may decrease the hospital stay.

Medical treatments include antacids to neutralize gastric acidity, sucralfate, antisecretory therapy to decrease acid production, thereby accelerating ulcer healing and decreasing the long-term risk of ulcer recurrence and rebleeding, and prostaglandin analogs. Eradication of *H pylori* will decrease the risk of recurrent duodenal ulcer disease and may prevent recurrent bleeding.

In randomized prospective studies, patients with active bleeding or nonbleeding visible vessels have a better outcome with endoscopic therapy than with medical therapy (Table 3–6). Ulcers with a clean base or a flat pigmented spot are at low risk of rebleeding and should not be treated endoscopically. Adherent clots that are not easily removed endoscopically from the ulcer crater, ie, with irrigation or gentle suctioning, carry a 20–30% risk of rebleeding. These clots should not be routinely treated with endoscopic therapy because randomized studies have not demonstrated a benefit compared with medical therapy.

Endoscopic treatment of gastroduodenal ulcers with active bleeding or nonbleeding visible vessels include injection therapy with absolute alcohol (98%) (total volume less than 1.0 mL) or epinephrine (1:10,000 up to 10 mL); thermal coagulation with a heater probe,

Table 3–5. Endoscopic stigmata of recent hemorrhage in bleeding ulcers: prevalence and risk of rebleeding.

Stigmata	Prevalence (%)	Risk of Rebleeding (%)
Active arterial bleeding	10	90
Nonbleeding visible vessel	25	50
Adherent clot	10	25
Oozing without visible vessel	5	<20
Flat spot	15	<10
Clean ulcer base	35	<5

Adapted, with permission, from Freeman ML: The current endoscopic diagnosis and intensive care unit management of severe ulcer and other nonvariceal upper gastrointestinal hemorrhage. In: *Severe Nonvariceal Upper Gastrointestinal Hemorrhage.* Jensen DM (editor). Gastrointest Endosc Clin North Am 1991; 1:229.

Table 3–6. Rebleeding rates following medical versus endoscopic treatment.[1]

| | Rebleeding Rate (%) | | |
	Medical	Gold Probe	Heater Probe
Peptic ulcers			
Active arterial bleeding	90	35	22
Nonbleeding visible vessel	52	35	23
Nonbleeding adherent clot	30	35	35
Oozing bleeding without clot or visible vessel	10	N/A[2]	N/A
Flat Spots	7	N/A	N/A
Clean ulcer base	3	N/A	N/A
Dieulafoy's lesion			
Active arterial bleeding	100	40	40
Nonbleeding visible vessel	70	30	30
Mallory-Weiss tear without portal hypertension			
Active arterial bleeding	80	N/A	N/A
Nonbleeding visible vessel	<20	0	0

[1]Data from the Center for Ulcer Research and Education (CURE) Hemostasis Research Group, UCLA School of Medicine and the West Los Angeles VA Medical Center.
[2]N/A, not applicable.

multipolar probe, or bipolar probe; or laser therapy. Gastric ulcers along the lesser curvature and duodenal bulbar ulcers in the posterior wall are at high risk for massive upper gastrointestinal bleeding because of their proximity to large underlying arteries (left gastric and posterior duodenal arteries, respectively). If endoscopic hemostasis is unsuccessful, emergency surgery may be necessary.

Surgery is usually reserved for complicated peptic ulcer disease, such as persistent or recurrent upper gastrointestinal bleeding, nonhealing or giant ulcers, perforation, pyloric obstruction, or carcinoma. Emergency surgery for bleeding peptic ulcer disease is oversewing of the ulcer (to ligate the bleeding artery) plus truncal vagotomy (to decrease acid secretion) and pyloroplasty (drainage procedure). For nonemergency antiulcer surgery, more time-consuming procedures, such as highly selective vagotomy, can be performed laparoscopically.

Prognosis

The majority of patients with upper gastrointestinal bleeding from peptic ulcer disease will stop bleeding spontaneously and most will not rebleed during the hospitalization. However, a subgroup of patients is at high risk for recurrent bleeding. Clinical features suggestive of severe, recurrent upper gastrointestinal bleeding include hemodynamic instability, need for multiple transfusions, hematemesis of fresh blood or clots, hematochezia, the presence of a coagulopathy, and onset of bleeding during hospitalization. Endoscopic predictors of persistent or recurrent bleeding are active bleeding during endoscopy or a visible vessel. Endoscopic hemostasis should be reserved for these high-risk patients. Once patients are discharged from the hospital, the risk of recurrent ulcer bleeding is approximately 1% per month. This risk may be decreased significantly with maintenance H_2-receptor antagonist therapy. Eradication of *H pylori* in *H pylori*-positive patients with duodenal ulcer and prior upper gastrointestinal bleeding may significantly reduce both ulcer recurrence and rebleeding rates.

Chan FK et al: Preventing recurrent upper gastrointestinal bleeding in patients with *Helicobacter pylori* infection who are taking low-dose aspirin or naproxen. N Engl J Med 2001;344(13): 967.

Graham DY et al: Treatment of *Helicobacter pylori* reduces the rate of rebleeding in peptic ulcer disease. Scand J Gastroenterol 1993;28:939.

Hawkey CJ: Risk of ulcer bleeding in patients infected with *Helicobacter pylori* taking non-steroidal anti-inflammatory drugs. Gut 2000;46(3):310.

Jensen DM: Endoscopic control of nonvariceal upper gastrointestinal hemorrhage. In: *Textbook of Gastroenterology*. Yamada T et al (editors). Lippincott 1991:2618.

Jensen DM et al: A randomized controlled study of ranitidine for preventing recurrent duodenal ulcer hemorrhage. N Engl J Med 1994;330:382.

Jensen DM (editor): *Severe Nonvariceal Upper Gastrointestinal Hemorrhage.* Gastrointest Endosc Clin North Am 1991;1: 209.

Kovacs TOG, Jensen DM: Therapeutic endoscopy for upper gastrointestinal bleeding. In: *Gastrointestinal Emergencies.* Taylor MD et al (editors). Williams & Wilkins, 1992.

Lai KC et al: Treatment of *Helicobacter pylori* in patients with duodenal ulcer hemorrhage—a long-term randomized, controlled study. Am J Gastroenterol 2000;95(9):2225.

Ng TM et al: Non-steroidal anti-inflammatory drugs, *Helicobacter pylori* and bleeding gastric ulcer. Aliment Pharmacol Ther 2000;14(2):203.

NIH Consensus Conference: Therapeutic endoscopy and bleeding ulcers. JAMA 1989;262:1369.

Schoenfeld P et al: Review article: nonsteroidal anti-inflammatory drug-associated gastrointestinal complications—guidelines for prevention and treatment. Aliment Pharmacol Ther 1999; 13(10):1273.

Sung JJ: Management of nonsteroidal anti-inflammatory drug-related peptic ulcer bleeding. Am J Med 2001;110(1A):29S.

2. Stress Ulcers

Pathophysiology

There are relatively few data regarding critically ill patients hospitalized for a nongastrointestinal bleeding problem who subsequently develop upper gastrointestinal bleeding. Secondary upper gastrointestinal bleeding has been attributed to stress-related mucosal damage or stress ulceration. Despite its clinical importance, the pathogenesis of stress ulceration is not well understood. Some factors implicated in the pathogenesis of stress ulceration include acid hypersecretion in some patients, mucosal ischemia, and alteration in gastric mucus.

 ESSENTIALS OF DIAGNOSIS

- *Hematemesis or blood via a nasogastric tube in an ICU patient.*
- *Concomitant illness (multiorgan failure, sepsis, hypotension), trauma, major surgery, severe burn, prolonged mechanical ventilation.*

General Considerations

Stress ulceration implies that various physiologic stresses experienced by critically ill patients predispose them to developing ulcers. Risk factors for the development of stress ulcers include multiorgan failure, prolonged mechanical ventilation, hypotension (septic shock carries a higher risk for stress ulceration than hypovolemic shock), severe trauma, major surgery, severe central nervous system injury, and severe burn involving more than 35% of the body surface area **(Curling's ulcer).** Other factors that may play a role in secondary upper gastrointestinal bleeding include prior use of aspirin, NSAIDs, or steroids.

Clinical Findings

Patients with stress ulcer bleeding are often intubated and unable to report any symptoms. Signs of acute upper gastrointestinal bleeding in these patients include a falling hematocrit, a positive nasogastric aspirate of coffee ground material, bright red blood or clots, and melena. The diagnostic procedure of choice is upper panendoscopy.

Complications

The primary complication of stress ulceration is bleeding.

Treatment

Antacids, H_2-receptor antagonists, sucralfate, and omeprazole may be given prophylactically to high-risk patients to decrease acid production in hopes of decreasing the incidence of ulceration and upper gastrointestinal bleeding. However, these prophylactic therapies may not always be necessary, may not be uniformly effective, may increase the risk of nosocomial pneumonia, and can be both time consuming and expensive. Treatment of acute stress ulcer bleeding should include prompt resuscitation and urgent endoscopic hemostasis as outlined above for peptic ulcer disease. Although patients with stress ulcers may have oozing of blood from multiple foci, severe upper gastrointestinal hemorrhage occurring after admission to an ICU for an unrelated problem is most often due to a single large, deep ulcer with active bleeding or visible vessel. Endoscopic hemostasis is feasible but rebleeding and slow healing are common in this subgroup of patients.

Prognosis

Patients with upper gastrointestinal bleeding beginning or recurring in the hospital do more poorly than those with upper gastrointestinal bleeding prior to hospitalization. Patients with stress ulcer hemorrhage are at increased risk for recurrent bleeding and other complications, such as perforation and death, and are more likely to require emergency surgery. This may reflect the severity of their concomitant illnesses.

Bresalier RS: The clinical significance and pathophysiology of stress-related gastric mucosal hemorrhage. J Clin Gastroenterol 1991;13(Suppl 2):S35.

Cook D et al: Risk factors for clinically important upper gastrointestinal bleeding in patients requiring mechanical ventilation. Canadian Critical Care Trials Group. Crit Care Med 1999; 27(12):2812.

Fusamoto H et al: A clinical study of acute gastrointestinal hemorrhage associated with various shock states. Am J Gastroenterol 1991;86:429.

Tryba M: Prophylaxis of stress ulcer bleeding: a meta-analysis. J Clin Gastroenterol 1991;13(Suppl 2):S44.

Weber FH, Peura DA: Gastrointestinal bleeding in the critical care unit. In: *Gastrointestinal Bleeding.* Sugawa C, Lucas CE, Schuman BM (editors). Igaku-Shoin, 1992.

3. Medication-Induced Ulcers

Pathophysiology

Various medications play an important role in the development of peptic ulcer disease and acute upper gastrointestinal bleeding. Most notably, aspirin and NSAIDs can cause gastroduodenal erosions or ulcers, especially in elderly patients. A significant proportion of these patients develop bleeding ulcers. Steroids have also been implicated in ulcerogenesis, although this hypothesis has not been well established. Other medications that can cause pill-induced esophageal ulcers and bleeding include various antibiotics (doxycycline, tetracycline, clindamycin), potassium chloride, quinidine, and iron pills. Anticoagulation therapy with heparin or warfarin may exacerbate ongoing upper gastrointestinal bleeding or may precipitate bleeding from a previously nonbleeding lesion.

Clinical Findings

Patients with impaired esophageal motility (eg, scleroderma or esophageal strictures) are at increased risk for developing pill-induced ulcers. Patient history and medication history are essential in establishing the diagnosis. A history of dysphagia (difficulty with swallowing) or odynophagia (painful swallowing) after pill ingestion suggests a medication-induced ulcer.

Treatment

Medical treatment consists of discontinuation of the inciting medication. Patients on warfarin who are at risk of developing complications from active bleeding should be transfused with fresh frozen plasma and treated with vitamin K 10 mg subcutaneously daily for 3 days. Rebleeding is uncommon from medication-induced ulcers, thus, endoscopic therapy is rarely indicated except for control of active bleeding.

MALLORY-WEISS TEAR

Pathophysiology

Mallory-Weiss tears occur in the distal esophagus at the gastroesophageal junction, presumably after a bout of retching or vomiting, although often this antecedent is lacking. Bleeding occurs when the tear involves the underlying esophageal venous or arterial plexus. Patients with portal hypertension are at increased risk of massive bleeding from Mallory-Weiss tears compared with nonportal hypertensive patients.

ESSENTIALS OF DIAGNOSIS

- Antecedent nausea, retching, or vomiting followed by hematemesis.
- History of alcohol ingestion, chemotherapy, or medication ingestion.

General Considerations

In a series of about 1000 patients at UCLA admitted to the ICU with severe upper gastrointestinal bleeding, Mallory-Weiss tear was the fourth most common diagnosis, accounting for 5% (see Table 3–4) of all cases. Most tears heal uneventfully within 24–48 hours and will not be seen if endoscopy is delayed.

Clinical Findings

A. SYMPTOMS AND SIGNS

The classic patient with acute upper gastrointestinal bleeding from a Mallory-Weiss tear is a young or middle-aged man presenting with hematemesis following an episode of retching or vomiting after drinking alcohol. Other systemic symptoms and signs are usually lacking; if there is concomitant chest or abdominal pain, fever, or shortness of breath, then esophageal perforation must be ruled out.

B. IMAGING

Prompt endoscopy is the diagnostic procedure of choice. A Mallory-Weiss tear appears as an elliptical or longitudinal ulcer at the gastroesophageal junction, within a hiatal hernia, or on the gastric side just below the gastroesophageal junction. Upper gastrointestinal x-rays are usually nondiagnostic.

Differential Diagnosis

Mallory-Weiss tears must be distinguished from other ulcerative diseases of the esophagus, such as ulcerative reflux esophagitis, infectious esophagitis, or pill-induced esophageal ulcer. Mallory-Weiss tears are usually focal lesions with normal-appearing adjacent mucosa. In contrast, there is usually diffuse involvement of the distal esophagus with reflux or infectious esophagitis. Pill-induced ulcers are suspected by the history; usually these ulcers are more proximal in the esophagus.

Complications

Rebleeding may occur from the tear site. Perforation can occur spontaneously with repeated vomiting (Boerhaave's syndrome) or following endoscopic therapy.

Treatment

Because the majority of Mallory-Weiss tears stop bleeding spontaneously, endoscopic treatment is reserved for tears with active bleeding. Both injection therapy (epinephrine 1:10,000) and thermal coagulation have been used successfully to control active bleeding. The esophagus lacks a serosa and is very thin at the tear site. Therefore, injections or repeated coagulation should be avoided due to the risk of transmural injury and perforation. Thermal coagulation should not be performed in patients with portal hypertension and esophageal varices; sclerotherapy is preferable in such cases. Angiography can be performed to embolize a bleeding vessel. Surgical intervention, such as oversewing of the vessel, is rarely indicated. H_2 blockers, omeprazole, or sucralfate may be given to accelerate ulcer healing, although this is not of proven benefit.

Prognosis

The majority of Mallory-Weiss tears heal spontaneously within 24–48 hours. Bleeding usually stops spontaneously and rebleeding occurs rarely.

Bharucha AE, Gostout CJ, Balm RK: Clinical and endoscopic risk factors in the Mallory-Weiss syndrome. Am J Gastroenterol 1997;92(5):805.

Kovacs TOG: Endoscopic diagnosis and treatment of bleeding Mallory-Weiss tears. In: *Severe Nonvariceal Upper Gastrointestinal Hemorrhage.* Jensen DM (editor). Gastrointest Endosc Clin North Am 1991;1:387.

Younes Z, Johnson DA: The spectrum of spontaneous and iatrogenic esophageal injury: perforations, Mallory-Weiss tears, and hematomas. J Clin Gastroenterol 1999;29(4):306.

VASCULAR LESIONS

1. Gastroesophageal Varices

Pathophysiology

Esophageal and gastric varices are venous collaterals that develop as a result of systemic or segmental portal hypertension. The numerous causes of portal hypertension include prehepatic thrombosis (eg, portal or splenic vein), hepatic disease (eg, cirrhosis), and postsinusoidal disease (eg, schistosomiasis). Alcoholic liver disease and viral hepatitis (B and C) are the most common causes of intrahepatic portal hypertension in the United States. Isolated gastric varices can develop following splenic vein thrombosis (eg, acute or chronic pancreatitis or pancreatic tumor), causing segmental portal hypertension. Secondary gastric varices can develop after obliteration of esophageal varices with sclerotherapy.

ESSENTIALS OF DIAGNOSIS

- *Massive upper gastrointestinal bleeding (hematemesis, hematochezia, hypotension, tachycardia).*
- *History of chronic liver disease and cirrhosis.*
- *Prior episodes of variceal bleeding.*
- *Jaundice, spider telangiectasias, splenomegaly, ascites, encephalopathy, asterixis.*
- *Elevated liver enzymes, coagulopathy, thrombocytopenia.*

General Considerations

Nonbleeding esophageal varices that have never bled in the past may soon be treated prophylactically via endoscopy and variceal ligation. Active variceal bleeding can be acutely controlled by various endoscopic, radiologic, or surgical modalities. However, the risk of rebleeding remains high unless all distal esophageal varices are obliterated by serial endoscopic treatments or until portal hypertension is alleviated by portosystemic shunting or liver transplantation. Long-term survival is dependent on the severity of the underlying liver disease.

Clinical Findings

A. SYMPTOMS AND SIGNS

Nonspecific symptoms of variceal bleeding include hematemesis, melena, hematochezia, and dizziness. Mental confusion secondary to hepatic encephalopathy may be seen in patients with severe liver disease. Skin manifestations of cirrhosis include jaundice, spider telangiectasias, caput medusa, palmar erythema, and Dupuytren's contracture. Signs of portal hypertension include hemorrhoids, ascites, and splenomegaly. Patients with encephalopathy will have mental confusion and may develop asterixis and hepatic coma.

B. LABORATORY FINDINGS

Elevation of liver enzymes [ALT, AST, lactate dehydrogenase (LDH)] is seen with hepatocellular damage. Hyperbilirubinemia may be seen with decreased hepatic function. Poor liver synthetic function will result in hypoalbuminemia, hypocholesterolemia, and elevated PT. Pancytopenia may be secondary to hypersplenism or primary bone marrow suppression by alcohol. Progressive hypoglycemia and BUN and creatinine are seen with liver failure and hepatorenal syndrome.

C. IMAGING

Endoscopy is the diagnostic modality of choice. Endoscopic ultrasound may be useful for differentiating gastric varices from gastric folds. Barium x-rays may image large esophageal varices or large gastric folds suggestive of gastric varices, but the technique is not very sensitive. Portal vein angiography or abdominal CT may show venous collaterals and recanalization of the umbilical vein.

Differential Diagnosis

Nonvariceal causes must first be excluded before acute upper gastrointestinal bleeding can be attributed to varices. Peptic ulcer disease, esophagitis, and sclerotherapy-induced ulcers are often the source of upper gastrointestinal bleeding in patients with previous variceal hemorrhage.

Complications

Massive variceal bleeding may be uncontrollable, resulting in hemorrhage and death. Variceal bleeding may precipitate hepatic encephalopathy and hepatorenal syndrome. Local complications related to endoscopic therapy include secondary ulcers (ulcers induced by sclerotherapy or band ligation), chest pain, esophageal dysmotility, perforation, rebleeding from secondary ulcers, and strictures. Systemic complications of sclerotherapy include pulmonary or pericardial effusion, sepsis, fever, peritonitis, allergic reactions to the sclerosants, mediastinitis, and portal vein thrombosis.

Treatment

Various modalities are available for the acute hemostasis of bleeding esophagogastric varices. They include various medical, endoscopic, radiologic, and surgical treatments.

A. MEDICAL THERAPY

Because the most likely source of acute upper gastrointestinal bleeding is nonvariceal in origin (even in patients with prior variceal bleeding), diagnostic endoscopy should be performed prior to instituting empiric therapies. Medical therapies include intravenous vasopressin (bolus of 20 U over 20 minutes, then an infusion of 0.1–0.5 U/min) plus intravenous nitroglycerin (40 µg/min titrated upward to maintain systolic blood pressure above 90 mm Hg; maximum dose of 400 µg/min), intravenous octreotide (25–50 µg bolus, then 25–50 µg/h continuous infusion), and balloon tamponade (esophageal, gastric, or both). Tamponade balloons have been associated with many complications, such as aspiration and perforation; all patients must be intubated and adequately sedated and the balloon should not be inflated for over 24 hours. These therapies should not be instituted before endoscopic confirmation of variceal bleeding.

B. ENDOSCOPIC THERAPY

Endoscopic hemostasis is the treatment of choice for bleeding esophageal varices. The first objective of endoscopy is to identify a definitive source for the bleeding episode. Varices should be examined for stigmata of recent hemorrhage (active bleeding, adherent clot, red wale markings, hematocystic spots, veins on veins). If these stigmata are absent, nonvariceal sources of bleeding, such as ulcers or Mallory-Weiss tears, should be suspected and must be excluded. The vast majority of esophageal varices that bleed are located in the distal 5–10 cm of the esophagus, therefore, endoscopic treatments should be limited to this region. Endoscopic therapies include injection sclerotherapy, variceal band ligation, and combination therapy.

Gastric varices have been considered to be poorly responsive to endoscopic therapy because of high rebleeding rates from sclerotherapy-induced ulcers. Bleeding gastric varices can be technically difficult to treat endoscopically. Therefore, gastric varices should not be treated outside of randomized controlled trials. Recent studies report successful hemostasis and obliteration of gastric varices with intravariceal injections of absolute alcohol and cyanoacrylate, although the latter is not available in the United States.

1. Endoscopic injection sclerotherapy—Endoscopic injection sclerotherapy is the most well-established endoscopic treatment for bleeding esophageal varices. Endoscopic sclerotherapy has many advantages. It has proven safe and effective, it is low in cost and widely available, it is easy to learn and can be performed simply and rapidly, and it can be used in the outpatient setting for elective (obliteration) treatment. Numerous sclerotherapy techniques and various sclerosants have been used successfully for bleeding esophageal varices. A suggested sclerotherapy technique for bleeding esophageal varices is summarized in Table 3–7.

2. Variceal band ligation—Variceal band ligation is a new endoscopic modality for the treatment of bleeding and nonbleeding esophageal varices. The variceal banding technique is similar to hemorrhoid banding and involves placing small elastic bands around varices in the distal 5 cm of the esophagus. Varices are suctioned into the banding device and bands are released around the base of the varix by pulling a trip wire via the biopsy channel. The advantages of band ligation over sclerotherapy include fewer local complications (secondary bleeding from ulcers or strictures), no systemic side effects, and the need for fewer treatments for variceal obliteration. Some of the drawbacks of band ligation include a restricted endoscopic view (due to the banding device and blood pooling within the hood mechanism) and difficulty performing treatments in the retroflexed position in the fundus of the stomach.

Table 3–7. Endoscopic injection sclerotherapy technique for bleeding esophageal varices.[1]

Needle size	25 gauge
Needle length	4–5 mm
Sclerosant	
agent	Equal volume mixture of 3% sodium tetradecyl sulfate, 98% ethanol, 0.9 normal saline (TES)
Amount/injection	≤2–3 mL
Maximum volume	<50 mL[2]
Injection site	
Initial treatment	Bleeding site
Concomitant treatment	Each varix at GEJ[3] then 2.5 and 5.0 cm above GEJ
Follow-up treatment	Residual esophageal varices in the distal 5 cm
Adjuvant therapy	Ranitidine 150 mg twice daily
Treatment interval	1 week after initial treament, then once every 2–3 weeks until obliteration of distal esophageal varices

[1]Data from the Center for Ulcer Research and Education (CURE) Hemostasis Research Group, UCLA School of Medicine and the West Los Angeles VA Medical Center.
[2]Maximum volume of esophageal refers to volume to inject into all distal esophageal varices at GEJ, then 2.5 cm and 5 cm above the GEJ during first sclerotherapy session.
[3]GEJ, gastroesophageal junction.

3. Radiologic therapy—Radiologic therapies include venous embolization and transjugular intrahepatic portosystemic shunt (TIPS). TIPS is a new radiologic method of creating a portosystemic shunt via a transjugular approach to decrease portal pressure. It can control active variceal bleeding in patients who have failed endoscopic treatment and has been used for the treatment of refractory ascites. Some complications of TIPS include worsening of encephalopathy, shunt occlusion and rebleeding, and shunt migration. In addition, the procedure is expensive and is technically difficult to perform. Stenosis or TIPS occlusion occurs in at least 40% of patients followed for 6 months; repeat TIPS or other therapy is required to prevent recurrent variceal hemorrhage. This treatment should be reserved for patients with persistent variceal bleeding despite endoscopic treatments.

4. Surgical therapy—Surgical therapies include portosystemic shunting, esophageal transection and devascularization, and liver transplantation. Portosystemic shunting may decrease the risk of rebleeding; however, encephalopathy may worsen and overall survival is not improved. Esophageal transection and devascularization

have been utilized for acute hemostasis and prevention of rebleeding in Europe and Japan, but is not performed in the United States. Splenectomy is the treatment of choice for isolated gastric varices due to splenic vein thrombosis.

Prognosis

Variceal bleeding stops spontaneously in over 50% of patients. In those patients with continued bleeding, mortality approaches 70–80%. Medical treatments are only temporary measures and the patient is at high risk of rebleeding once these treatments are removed or discontinued. Each recurrent episode of bleeding carries a significant risk of mortality. The risk of rebleeding is high (60–70%) until gastroesophageal varices are obliterated by a subsequent endoscopic treatment of residual varices. Unfortunately, long-term survival is not improved following successful variceal obliteration. Propranolol therapy for patients undergoing elective sclerotherapy can further decrease the risk of rebleeding and may increase survival. The onset of massive upper gastrointestinal bleeding from gastroesophageal varices usually signifies advanced liver disease (Child class B or C). The majority of patients die within 6–12 months because of progressive hepatic decompensation, rebleeding, or other complications. Liver transplantation is the only treatment that significantly improves the long-term prognosis.

Gralnek IM et al: The economic impact of esophageal variceal hemorrhage: cost-effectiveness implications of endoscopic therapy. Hepatology 1999;29(1):44.

Imperiale TF, Chalasani N: A meta-analysis of endoscopic variceal ligation for primary prophylaxis of esophageal variceal bleeding. Hepatology 2001;33(4):802.

Jutabha R, Jensen DM: Endoscopic injection sclerotherapy for bleeding esophageal and gastric varices. In: *Advanced Therapeutic Endoscopy,* 2nd ed. Barkin JS, O'Phelan CA (editors). Raven Press, 1994.

Jutabha R, Jensen DM: Management of upper gastrointestinal bleeding in the patient with chronic liver disease. Med Clin North Am 1996;80(5):1035.

Laine L, Cook D: Endoscopic ligation compared with sclerotherapy for treatment of esophageal variceal bleeding. A meta-analysis. Ann Intern Med 1995;123(4):280.

Laine L et al: Endoscopic ligation compared with sclerotherapy for the treatment of bleeding esophageal varices. Ann Intern Med 1993;119:1.

Sarin SK et al: Prevalence, classification and natural history of gastric varices: a long-term follow-up study in 568 portal hypertension patients. Hepatology 1992;16:1343.

Stiegmann GV et al: Endoscopic sclerotherapy as compared with endoscopic ligation for bleeding esophageal varices. N Engl J Med 1992;326:1527.

Vinel J et al: Propranolol reduces the rebleeding rate during endoscopic sclerotherapy before variceal obliteration. Gastroenterology 1992;102:1760.

2. Angiodysplasia of the Upper Gastrointestinal Tract

Pathophysiology

In contrast to colonic angiomas, which are believed to develop from chronic low-grade venous obstruction associated with aging, the cause of upper gastrointestinal angiomas is unknown.

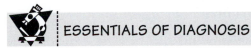 ESSENTIALS OF DIAGNOSIS

- *Chronic or acute recurrent episodes of bleeding.*
- *Long history of bleeding requiring multiple transfusions prior to diagnosis.*
- *Multiple nondiagnostic endoscopic procedures performed previously.*
- *Iron deficiency anemia and occult-blood-positive stools.*
- *Associated disorders—renal failure, von Willebrand's disease, aortic stenosis, cirrhosis, pulmonary disease.*

General Considerations

Other terms used synonymously with angioma include arteriovenous malformation, telangiectasia, vascular ectasia, and angiodysplasia. Upper gastrointestinal angiomas account for 1.2–8.0% of patients with occult-blood-positive stool and iron deficiency anemia. Infrequently, patients with upper gastrointestinal angiomas present with acute bleeding. Small bowel angiomas are the most common cause of gastrointestinal bleeding of obscure origin. Upper gastrointestinal angiomas may be suggestive of angiomas elsewhere in the gastrointestinal tract or may be part of the Osler-Weber-Rendu syndrome or hereditary hemorrhagic telangiectasia.

Clinical Findings

Bleeding from upper gastrointestinal angiomas is usually low-grade and intermittent, causing hemoccult-positive stools and iron deficiency anemia. Video endoscopy and enteroscopy are the diagnostic procedures of choice for evaluating upper gastrointestinal and small bowel angiomas. The classic angiographic features of intestinal angiomas include an early filling vein, a vascular tuft, and a late-draining vein.

Differential Diagnosis

Because upper gastrointestinal angiomas infrequently cause acute gastrointestinal bleeding, it is important to exclude other causes of upper gastrointestinal bleeding such as peptic ulcers, Mallory-Weiss tears, or varices. Incidental angiomas rarely bleed, therefore, treatment is not indicated.

Treatment

Hormonal therapy with combination estrogen and progesterone for bleeding angiomas has yielded conflicting results. Endoscopic therapy with thermal coagulation is the treatment of choice for bleeding upper gastrointestinal angiomas. Thermal coagulation may be performed with contact probes at a low power setting, eg, multipolar electrocoagulation (10–15 W × 1-second pulses) or heater probe (10–20 J/pulse). Nd:YAG laser may be used at a low power setting (40–100 W × 0.2–0.5 seconds). There is limited experience with injection therapy for upper gastrointestinal angiomas.

The endoscopic end point for thermal coagulation of angiomas is mucosal whitening and ablation of all visible angiomatous tissue. It is important to avoid excessive bowel distention, high-power generator settings, firm probe pressure, and repeated coagulation to the same area to minimize the risk of transmural injury and perforation. Surgical therapy such as intraoperative enteroscopy is reserved for failures of endoscopic and medical therapy.

Prognosis

Over one-half of patients stop bleeding spontaneously without any therapy. For patients with recurrent bleeding, endoscopic therapy can decrease the number of bleeding episodes as well as the transfusion requirement.

Chalasani N, Cotsonis G, Wilcox CM: Upper gastrointestinal bleeding in patients with chronic renal failure: role of vascular ectasia. Am J Gastroenterol 1996;91(11):2329.

Foutch PG: Angiodysplasia of the gastrointestinal tract. Am J Gastroenterol 1993;88:807.

Lewis BS et al: Does hormonal therapy have any benefit for bleeding angiodysplasia? J Clin Gastroenterol 1992;15(2):99.

Machicado GA, Jensen DM: Upper gastrointestinal angiomata. Diagnosis and treatment. In: *Severe Nonvariceal Upper Gastrointestinal Hemorrhage.* Jensen DM (editor). Gastrointest Endosc Clin North Am 1991;1:241.

Van Cutsem E, Rutgeerts P, Vantrappen G: Treatment of bleeding gastrointestinal vascular malformations with oestrogen-progesterone. Lancet 1990;335:953.

3. Dieulafoy's Lesion

Pathophysiology

Dieulafoy's lesion is a dilated aberrant submucosal vessel that erodes the overlying epithelium and is not associated with a primary ulcer. The cause of Dieulafoy's lesion is unknown, but it may be related to ischemia with thinning of the mucosa. Massive arterial bleeding occurs when the submucosal artery erodes through the gastric mucosa.

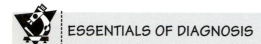

ESSENTIALS OF DIAGNOSIS

- Massive upper gastrointestinal bleeding with multiple nondiagnostic upper panendoscopies.
- Endoscopy reveals a visible vessel (actively bleeding or nonbleeding) without an associated ulcer.

Clinical Findings

Bleeding may be self-limited, although it is usually recurrent and can be massive. Diagnosis is best made with endoscopy during acute bleeding, which may reveal active arterial pumping from a point without an associated ulcer or mass lesion. In the absence of active bleeding, it may look like a raised nipple or visible vessel without an associated ulcer. The aberrant vessel is often not seen unless there is active bleeding from the site. Dieulafoy's lesions are usually located in the upper stomach along the high lesser curvature within 6 cm of the gastroesophageal junction.

Treatment

Endoscopic hemostasis with multipolar electrocoagulation or heater probe thermal coagulation is the treatment of choice for controlling acute bleeding. The risk of rebleeding after endoscopic therapy remains high because of the unusual size of the underlying artery. Surgical wedge resection, therefore, is recommended when endoscopic therapy fails. Endoscopic tattooing with India ink injections helps to locate the lesion intraoperatively. Recently, Doppler ultrasound has been used to confirm ablation of a Dieulafoy's lesion by documenting the absence of blood flow after injection therapy. There is no further risk of rebleeding from a Dieulafoy's lesion once it is surgically resected.

Ertan A: Image of the month. Recurrent painless, massive gastrointestinal (GI) bleeding obscure in origin. Dieulafoy's lesion. Gastroenterology 2000;118(5):820, 989.

Fockens P, Tytgat GN: Dieulafoy's disease. Gastrointest Endosc Clin North Am 1996;6(4):739.

Jaspersen D: Dieulafoy's disease controlled by Doppler ultrasound endoscopic treatment. Gut 1993;34:857.

McGrath K, Mergener K, Branch S: Endoscopic band ligation of Dieulafoy's lesion: report of two cases and review of the literature. Am J Gastroenterol 1999;94(4):1087.

Reilly HF, Al-Kawas FH: Dieulafoy's lesion. Diagnosis and management. Dig Dis Sci 1991;36:1702.

4. Watermelon Stomach (Gastric Antral Vascular Ectasia)

Clinical Findings

Watermelon stomach, or **gastric antral vascular ectasia,** has a characteristic endoscopic appearance of longitudinal rows of erythematous mucosa radiating from the pylorus into the antrum. The red stripes represent ectatic and sacculated mucosal vessels resembling the stripes on a watermelon. Diagnosis is based on the classic endoscopic appearance, but may be confirmed with endoscopic biopsy. Bleeding is most often chronic, with patients presenting with occult-blood-positive stools and iron deficiency anemia and requiring repeat transfusions. Occasionally, acute or massive upper gastrointestinal bleeding can occur.

Treatment

Acute bleeding may be controlled with endoscopic coagulation with heater probe, multipolar electrocoagulation, or laser therapy, which decreases the requirement for transfusion. Antrectomy will prevent recurrent bleeding.

Potamiano S, Carter CR, Anderson JR: Endoscopic laser treatment of diffuse gastric antral vascular ectasia. Gut 1994;35:461.

Tran A et al: Treatment of chronic bleeding from gastric antral vascular ectasia (GAVE) with estrogen-progesterone in cirrhotic patients: an open pilot study. Am J Gastroenterol 1999;94 (10):2909.

Yamada M et al: Gastric antral vascular ectasia successfully treated by endoscopic electrocoagulation. J Gastroenterol 1988;33 (4):546.

5. Portal Hypertensive Gastropathy

Clinical Findings

Portal hypertensive gastropathy or congestive gastropathy has a characteristic endoscopic appearance described as a fine, white reticular pattern separating areas of pinkish mucosa (snakeskin appearance). Histologically there is extensive edema and capillary and venous dilatation in the submucosa extending into the mucosa. The mucosa is friable and bleeding occurs presumably when the ectatic vessels rupture. It has been postulated but not proven that sclerotherapy increases the likelihood of developing portal hypertensive gastropathy by increasing back pressure; however, there is no correlation between the degree of portal hypertension and portal hypertensive gastropathy.

Bleeding gastroesophageal varices must be excluded before attributing acute upper gastrointestinal hemorrhaging to portal hypertensive gastropathy. Portal hypertensive gastropathy appears to be a rare cause of significant upper gastrointestinal bleeding in patients with cirrhosis.

Treatment

Treatments for bleeding from portal hypertensive gastropathy are directed at decreasing portal pressure, such as portocaval shunt surgery, TIPS, or low-dose propranolol (20–40 mg/d, then doubled each week until bleeding stops or diastolic blood pressure falls below 70 mm Hg or encephalopathy develops). Endoscopic thermal coagulation or injection therapy is ineffective for control of active bleeding. H_2 blockers, sucralfate, and surgical resection are also ineffective.

Hosking SW: Portal hypertensive gastropathy. Gastrointest Endosc Clin North Am 1992;2(1):111.

Primignani M et al: Natural history of portal hypertensive gastropathy in patients with liver cirrhosis. The New Italian Endoscopic Club for the study and treatment of esophageal varices (NIEC). Gastroenterology 2000;119(1):181.

Sarin SK et al: The natural history of portal hypertensive gastropathy: influence of variceal eradication. Am J Gastroenterol 2000;95(10):2888.

Toyonaga A, Iwao T: Portal-hypertensive gastropathy. J Gastroenterol Hepatol 1998;13(9):865.

Urata J et al: The effects of transjugular intrahepatic portosystemic shunt on portal hypertensive gastropathy. J Gastroenterol Hepatol 1998;13(10):1061.

Viggiano TR, Gostout CJ: Portal hypertensive intestinal vasculopathy: a review of the clinical, endoscopic, and histopathologic features. Am J Gastroenterol 1992;87(8):944.

6. Aortoenteric Fistula

Pathophysiology

Aortoenteric fistulas arise from a direct communication between the aorta and the gastrointestinal tract. Prior to 1960 the most common causes of abdominal aortoenteric fistulas were aortic aneurysm and infectious aortitis secondary to syphilis or tuberculosis. Now an infected prosthetic aortic graft eroding into the intestine is a more common cause. Other conditions that can result in an aortoenteric fistula include penetrating ulcer, tumor invasion, trauma, radiation therapy, and foreign body perforation. Pressure necrosis and graft infection have been implicated in the development of a fistula.

 ESSENTIALS OF DIAGNOSIS

- Massive upper gastrointestinal bleeding with a history of aortic prosthetic graft or abdominal aortic aneurysm.
- Endoscopy is often nondiagnostic in the absence of active bleeding or protruding prosthetic graft.
- Positive endoscopy may reveal a graft, adherent clot, or extrinsic pulsatile mass in the distal duodenum.

General Considerations

Aortoenteric fistula is a rare cause of acute upper gastrointestinal bleeding but is associated with a very high mortality rate if undiagnosed and left untreated. The third or fourth portion of the duodenum is the most common site for aortoenteric fistulas, followed by the jejunum and ileum.

Clinical Findings

A. SYMPTOMS AND SIGNS

Most patients have an initial herald bleed manifested by hematemesis or hematochezia, or both. This may be followed by a massive bleed resulting in hemorrhagic shock. Intermittent bleeding can be seen if a blood clot temporarily seals the fistula. About one-half of patients have abdominal or back pain, and fewer than 50% have fever or signs of sepsis. Infrequently an abdominal mass may be palpable or an abdominal bruit may be heard.

B. IMAGING

A high index of suspicion is needed to exclude this diagnosis. In a stable patient without active bleeding, endoscopy with a colonoscope (ie, enteroscopy) is the procedure of choice to rule out other causes of acute upper gastrointestinal bleeding, such as ulcers. Occasionally, endoscopy shows an aortic graft that has eroded into the bowel lumen. Abdominal computed tomography (CT) and aortography can be useful in confirming the diagnosis but may be unreliable. Exploratory laparotomy is indicated for patients with suspected aortoenteric fistula and severe, ongoing bleeding.

Treatment & Prognosis

The treatment for aortoenteric fistula resulting from an infected graft is emergent surgery for graft removal and intravenous antibiotics. The mortality rate of an untreated aortoenteric fistula is nearly 100%.

Abernathy W, Sekijima JH: Images in clinical medicine. Aortoenteric fistula. N Engl J Med 1997;336(1):27.

Antinori CH et al: The many faces of aortoenteric fistulas. Am Surg 1996;62(5):344.

Nagy SW, Marshall JB: Aortoenteric fistulas. Postgrad Med 1993; 93:211.

TUMORS

Pathophysiology

Acute bleeding from upper gastrointestinal tumors usually represents a late stage of disease in which the neoplasm has outgrown its blood supply, resulting in mucosal ulceration. Bleeding can occur from diffuse mucosal ulceration or from erosion into an underlying vessel.

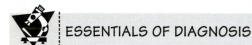

ESSENTIALS OF DIAGNOSIS

- *Anorexia, weight loss, early satiety, or dysphagia.*
- *Cachexia, hemoccult-positive stools, iron deficiency anemia.*
- *Upper endoscopy reveals an ulcerated mass with stigmata of recent hemorrhage (oozing, clot, or visible vessel).*

General Considerations

Neoplasms of the upper gastrointestinal tract account for less than 3% of cases of acute upper gastrointestinal bleeding. These tumors can be benign or malignant; malignant lesions may be either primary tumors or metastatic lesions. Benign lesions of the upper gastrointestinal tract include leiomyomas, lipomas, polyps, and blue rubber bleb nevus syndrome. Primary malignant tumors include adenocarcinoma, leiomyosarcoma, lymphoma, Kaposi's sarcoma, and carcinoid tumor; metastatic tumors to the upper gastrointestinal tract include melanoma, breast cancer, colon carcinoma, and lung cancer.

Clinical Findings

A. SYMPTOMS AND SIGNS

Esophageal tumors may produce luminal obstruction or ulceration causing **dysphagia** (difficulty swallowing) or **odynophagia** (painful swallowing). Bulky gastric tumors may cause anorexia and early satiety. Duodenal tumors can cause gastric outlet obstruction resulting in chronic nausea, vomiting, and bezoar formation. Ulcer-

ative tumors may cause perforation or fistulas, such as an esophageal-pulmonary fistula, which may present as recurrent aspiration pneumonia. Nonspecific signs of malignancy include cachexia and weight loss.

B. LABORATORY FINDINGS

Nonspecific laboratory findings include hypoalbuminemia and hypocholesterolemia (owing to malnutrition) and iron deficiency anemia (as a result of chronic bleeding). Metastatic colon carcinoma to the upper gastrointestinal tract may be associated with an elevated carcinoembryonic antigen (CEA) level.

C. DIAGNOSTIC TECHNIQUES

The diagnostic modality of choice is upper panendoscopy. Endoscopic findings suggestive of malignancy are irregular ulcer margins and an exophytic or fungating ulcerated mass. Endoscopic biopsy, brushing, or needle aspiration for histologic or cytologic examination is performed for definitive diagnosis. Endoscopic ultrasound is useful for staging local disease. Barium x-rays should be avoided if bleeding, obstruction, or fistulas are suspected because the barium will interfere with endoscopy and may result in barium peritonitis or aspiration. CT is helpful for staging and evaluating distant metastases.

Differential Diagnosis

Mucosal and submucosal upper gastrointestinal tumors must be differentiated from malignant extrinsic masses that erode through the upper gastrointestinal tract. Because such extrinsic masses involve the gut wall transmurally, endoscopic treatment should be conservative due to the high risk of perforation.

Complications

Complications of upper gastrointestinal tumors in addition to bleeding include cachexia, luminal obstruction (esophageal or duodenal tumors), perforation, and fistula formation.

Treatment

For potentially curable lesions, surgical resection is the treatment of choice. Large upper gastrointestinal tumors, either benign or malignant, that are symptomatic, ie, producing bleeding, obstruction, perforation, or fistulas, should be resected if the patient is a good surgical candidate. Endoscopic treatment for bleeding upper gastrointestinal tumors includes injection therapy, thermal contact probes (tumor probe, multipolar electrocoagulation, heater probe), and laser therapy. Rebleeding frequently occurs, thus, endoscopic hemostasis is a temporizing measure before staging and surgical resection. Medical therapy is most often palliative and consists of chemotherapy, radiation therapy, or both.

Prognosis

Patients with bleeding secondary to malignant upper gastrointestinal tumors have a very dismal prognosis, with the majority of patients dying within 1–3 months. Patients with benign upper gastrointestinal tumors that are successfully resected are cured.

Randall GM, Jensen DM: Diagnosis and management of bleeding from upper gastrointestinal neoplasms. In: *Severe Nonvariceal Upper Gastrointestinal Hemorrhage.* Jensen DM (editor). Gastrointest Endosc Clin North Am 1991;1:401.

MISCELLANEOUS CAUSES OF ACUTE UPPER GASTROINTESTINAL BLEEDING

1. Hemobilia

Hemobilia, or bleeding from the biliary system, is a rare cause of acute upper gastrointestinal bleeding. The classic triad of hemobilia includes biliary colic, obstructive jaundice, and occult or acute gastrointestinal bleeding. Some causes of hemobilia include hepatic trauma (eg, after liver biopsy), gallstones, hepatic or bile duct tumors, hepatic artery aneurysm, and hepatic abscess. The diagnosis is often overlooked, but the condition can be identified by endoscopy if there is active bleeding from the ampulla. A side-viewing duo-denoscope may be helpful in viewing the ampulla or for performing diagnostic endoscopic retrograde cholangiography. A technetium tagged red blood cell scan or selective hepatic arteriography may reveal the source of hemobilia. Hemobilia may be associated with obstructive jaundice and biliary sepsis. Treatment is directed at the primary cause of bleeding, utilizing surgical resection or arterial embolization.

2. Hemosuccus Pancreaticus

Bleeding from the pancreatic duct is also a rare cause of upper gastrointestinal bleeding. Pancreatic pseudocysts and pancreatic tumors are the most common causes of hemosuccus pancreaticus. Bleeding occurs when a pseudocyst or tumor erodes into a vessel, forming a direct communication between the pancreatic duct and blood vessel. The diagnosis may be made by endoscopy and a retrograde pancreaticogram, angiography, or abdominal CT. Complications related to the pseudocyst include infection and perforation. Surgical resection with ligation of the bleeding vessel provides definitive treatment. Mesenteric arteriography with coil embolization usually will control acute bleeding and may obviate the need for an operation.

Benz CA et al: Hemosuccus pancreaticus—a rare cause of gastrointestinal bleeding: diagnosis and interventional radiological therapy. Endoscopy 2000;32(5):428.

Kuganeswaran E et al: Hemosuccus pancreaticus: rare complication of chronic pancreatitis. Gastrointest Endosc 2000;51 (4 Pt 1):464.

Acute Lower Gastrointestinal Bleeding

4

Thomas J. Savides, MD & Dennis M. Jensen, MD

Lower gastrointestinal bleeding is generally defined as bleeding from below the ligament of Treitz. In this chapter, lower gastrointestinal bleeding will refer to **colonic bleeding,** while bleeding from between the ligament of Treitz and the ileocecal valve will be referred to as **small bowel bleeding.** Bleeding from the esophagus, stomach, or duodenum is **upper gastrointestinal bleeding.**

Patients with lower gastrointestinal bleeding usually present with bright red bleeding per rectum. The majority of patients (approximately 85%) have acute, self-limited, nonhemodynamically significant bleeds, such as occurs with hemorrhoids, colonic polyps, colon cancer, or colitis. Only 15% of patients will have severe, ongoing hematochezia, which is hemodynamically significant.

Severe bleeding that appears to be from a lower source may actually come from an area proximal to the terminal ileum, as 11% of patients with severe hematochezia actually have an upper gastrointestinal source (proximal to the ligament of Treitz) and 9% have a small bowel source (between the ligament of Treitz and the ileocecal valve) (Figure 4–1). Nearly all patients with severe hematochezia due to an upper gastrointestinal (GI) source will present with hypotension. Even with extensive diagnostic evaluation, the source of bleeding is not determined in 6% of patients with severe hematochezia. When severe bleeding is localized to the colon on the basis of colonoscopy or angiography, the bleeding lesion is located in the right colon 75% of the time.

The most common causes of severe lower gastrointestinal bleeding are shown in Table 4–1.

CLINICAL CHARACTERISTICS OF LOWER GASTROINTESTINAL BLEEDING

Hematochezia is defined as bright red blood passed per rectum; it is the most common presentation of lower gastrointestinal bleeding. Hematochezia usually suggests a left colon source of bleeding, although it may occur with brisk upper gastrointestinal or small bowel bleeding and rapid transit of blood.

Maroon stools are defined as maroon-colored blood mixed with melena, and are usually indicative of a lower gastrointestinal source (especially the right colon). However, upper gastrointestinal or small bowel bleeding with rapid transit of blood also can cause maroon stools.

Melena is defined as black, tarry, foul-smelling stools. Melena occurs when hemoglobin is converted to hematin or other hemochromes by bacterial degradation over a period of at least 14 hours. These degradation products cause the black color of melena. Melena usually indicates an upper gastrointestinal or small bowel site, although melena can occur from a right colon lesion if motility is slow. All black stools are not melena, as bismuth, charcoal, licorice, and iron preparations can turn the stool color black. For this reason it is important to do a guaiac test on all black stool for the presence of hemoglobin degradation products.

Occult bleeding occurs when there is no change in the color of the stool because only small quantities of blood pass into the gastrointestinal tract at any given time. This is detected by testing the stool with a guaiac card test.

INITIAL EVALUATION OF PATIENTS WITH RECTAL BLEEDING

The history should include direct questions, for example:

1. Does the blood coat the outside of formed, hard stool (suggesting internal hemorrhoidal bleeding), or is it mixed in with the stool (internal source)? Is there bloody diarrhea or tenesmus (eg, owing to colitis)?

2. Is this a chronic, intermittent problem, or an acute event?

3. Is there a history of gastrointestinal bleeding, previous gastrointestinal surgery, peptic ulcer, inflammatory bowel disease, vascular disease (suggesting the possibility of ischemic colitis), internal hemorrhoids, rectal trauma, change in bowel habits (cancer), weight loss (cancer), aspirin or nonsteroidal antiinflammatory drug (NSAID) use, alcohol abuse (upper gastrointestinal or rectal varices), abdominal pain (ischemia, inflammatory bowel disease), rectal pain (anal fissure, hemor-

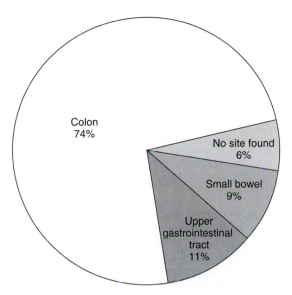

Figure 4–1. Actual bleeding sites in patients with hematochezia.

rhoids, rectal ulcer), constipation (hemorrhoids, mass), lack of pain (hemorrhoids, diverticula, angiodysplasia), recent antibiotics (antibiotic-associated colitis), or recent travel (infectious colitis)?

The following steps should be followed to ensure a complete physical examination:

1. Assess vital signs, particularly for the presence of shock or orthostatic hypotension.
2. Palpate the abdomen to assess for tenderness or masses.

Table 4–1. Frequency of colonic bleeding sites in patients with severe hematochezia.

Colonic diverticulosis	42%
Colorectal malignancy	9%
Ischemic colitis	9%
Acute colitis, unknown cause	5%
Hemorrhoids	5%
Postpolypectomy hemorrhage	4%
Colonic angiodysplasia	3%
Crohn's disease	2%
Other	10%
Unknown	11%

Data are from Longstreth GF: Epidemiology and outcome of patients hospitalized with acute lower gastrointestinal hemorrhage: a population-based study. Am J Gastroenterol 1997;92:419.

3. Evaluate stool color by rectal examination and perform guaiac card test to determine if blood is in the stool.
4. Perform anoscopy to look for active bleeding from internal hemorrhoids. The presence of a nonbleeding hemorrhoid implies that the bleeding site is probably not hemorrhoidal.
5. Perform nasogastric tube lavage (if bleeding is severe and patient is orthostatic). Even if no blood returns, there is still about a 15% chance that bleeding is from a site proximal to the ligament of Treitz. If bile returns, however, this virtually excludes an active upper gastrointestinal source of bleeding.
6. Measure hematocrit, mean cell volume, platelet count, prothrombin time, and partial thromboplastin time.

Figure 4–2 shows the algorithm for the initial assessment of rectal bleeding.

INITIAL ASSESSMENT & MANAGEMENT OF SUSPECTED LOWER GASTROINTESTINAL BLEEDING

Severe bleeding is defined as acute bleeding with either postural hypotension and/or a decrease in hematocrit of at least 8% from baseline after volume resuscitation.

Patients with **mild** lower gastrointestinal bleeding can be electively evaluated as outpatients. If the patient is younger than 50 years old, has a bleeding history characteristic of internal hemorrhoids, and has a normal hematocrit and mean cell volume, then flexible sigmoidoscopy should be performed to confirm the presence of hemorrhoids and exclude the possibility of a distal rectosigmoid polyp or cancer. Further evaluation with colonoscopy or an air-contrast barium enema may be indicated if a bleeding lesion is not found by flexible sigmoidoscopy. Patients 50 years of age or older should undergo a full colonoscopy if they present with new onset mild hematochezia, even if suggestive of hemorrhoids, because of the increased risk of colonic polyps and tumors (Figure 4–3).

Patients with **severe** lower gastrointestinal bleeding should be hospitalized for resuscitation, diagnosis, and treatment (Figure 4–4). Stabilization involves fluid resuscitation with saline and packed red blood cells and correction of any coagulopathy or thrombocytopenia. Patients with severe, acute gastrointestinal bleeding should be admitted to an intensive care unit and should be seen by both a gastroenterologist and a surgeon. Once a patient is medically stabilized, 4 L of a polyethylene glycol purge should be given over 3–4 hours, followed by semiurgent colonoscopy within the next

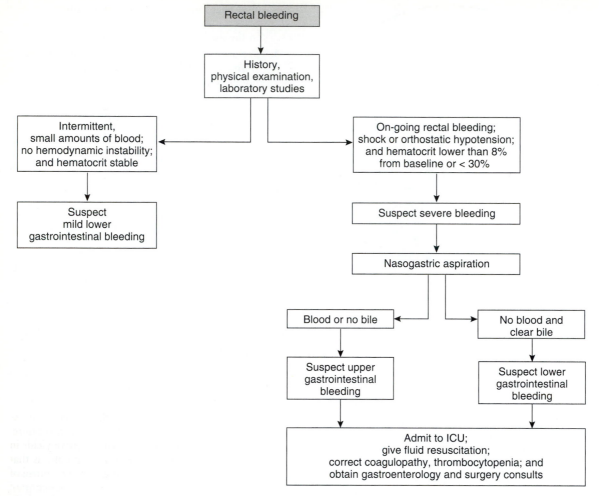

Figure 4–2. Initial assessment of rectal bleeding.

24 hours. The earlier the colonoscopy after the bowel purge, the more likely an actively bleeding lesion may be detected. Enough polyethylene glycol solution should be given such that the rectal effluent is relatively free of blood clots and debris. The polyethylene glycol may need to be given via a nasogastric tube. If a patient with profuse hematochezia cannot be medically resuscitated because of ongoing bleeding, then that patient should go immediately for surgical exploration and treatment.

DIAGNOSTIC & THERAPEUTIC OPTIONS

Anoscopy

Anoscopy is excellent for diagnosing bleeding lesions in the rectal canal, such as fissures, ulcers, or internal hem-orrhoids. Anoscopy may be used in conjunction with flexible sigmoidoscopy or colonoscopy in the evaluation of hematochezia.

Flexible Sigmoidoscopy

Flexible sigmoidoscopy uses a 65-cm instrument (as opposed to the colonoscope measuring 130–160 cm). It is mostly indicated for outpatient examination of patients younger than 50 years old who have mild lower gastrointestinal bleeding with an expected source located distal to the splenic flexure. Turn-around examination in the rectum is necessary to exclude isolated lesions that can be missed by rigid sigmoidoscopy. Sigmoidoscopy is not as reliable as anoscopy for diagnosing internal hemorrhoids.

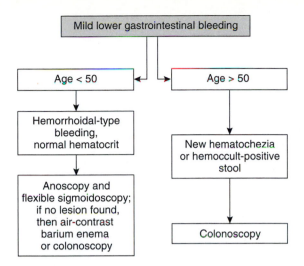

Figure 4–3. Diagnostic and therapeutic approach to mild lower gastrointestinal bleeding.

Colonoscopy

Colonoscopy should be the initial imaging procedure in patients with severe rectal bleeding after medical resuscitation. Four liters of an oral polyethylene glycol purge over 3–4 hours will clear the gastrointestinal tract of stool and blood. Colonoscopy can generally be performed safely, offering examination of the entire colon, including the cecum and possibly the terminal ileum. The bleeding site is determined by visualizing active bleeding from a lesion, stigmata of a recent bleed (such as a visible vessel or adherent clot), or blood in an area around a lesion without other lesions in that segment of bowel to explain the blood. Flat mucosal lesions, such as angiodysplasia, can be detected. Hemostasis can be performed through the colonoscope with bipolar probe coagulation, heater probes, epinephrine injection, hemoclips, or argon plasma coagulation. Complications from colonoscopy and colonoscopic hemostasis are rare and include perforation and induced bleeding.

Push Enteroscopy

When no source for the bleeding is seen with colonoscopy or esophagogastroduodenoscopy (standard endoscopy), then repeat upper endoscopy can be performed with a pediatric or adult colonoscope (130 cm long). Using the **push enteroscopy** technique, the endoscope can be passed 40–60 cm beyond the ligament of Treitz. Longer enteroscopes have been developed that measure 200–250 cm and can be advanced 80–120 cm beyond the ligament of Treitz. Forceps biopsies or therapeutic coagulation of bleeding lesions can be performed with these enteroscopes. Capsule endoscopy is currently being developed that may allow better visualization of bleeding lesions in the small intestine.

Barium Enema

There is no role for emergency barium enema in a patient with severe lower gastrointestinal bleeding. This test is rarely diagnostic because it cannot demonstrate vascular lesions and may be misleading if only diverticula are present. Subsequent colonoscopy will be necessary for obtaining biopsies if a suspicious lesion is seen on barium enema, and unlike colonoscopy or angiography, barium enema provides no opportunity for simultaneous therapy. Furthermore, barium enema will delay subsequent colonoscopy or angiography until the barium clears after several days. Nevertheless, air-contrast barium enema is indicated for complete evaluation of young adult outpatients (younger than 50 years old) with self-limited bright red blood per rectum when flexible sigmoidoscopy and anoscopy are negative.

Angiography

Angiography involves cannulating the femoral artery, then passing catheters into the superior mesenteric artery and inferior mesenteric artery and injecting contrast. Arterial bleeding can be detected only when the rate is 0.5 mL/min or greater. The diagnostic yield depends on patient selection, timing of the procedure, and the skill of the angiographer, with positive yields in 12–69% of cases. An advantage of angiography is that intravascular selective embolization can allow control of some bleeding lesions. The possible complications of angiography include bowel ischemia and infarction, hematomas, arterial embolization, and renal failure induced by contrast dye.

Nuclear Medicine Scintigraphy

Nuclear medicine scintigraphy involves injecting a radiolabeled substance into the patient's bloodstream, then performing serial scintigrams to detect focal collections of radiolabeled material. It has been reported to detect bleeding at a rate as low as 0.1 mL/min. Blood is removed from the patient, the red blood cells are labeled with ^{99m}Tc, and the labeled blood is reinjected into the patient. Scanning is typically performed early (1 and 4 hours after injection) and late (24 hours). An early scan that is positive is often more helpful than a delayed scan for localization of the bleeding site. The labeled red blood cells will circulate for at least 24 hours after injection, therefore, repeated scans can be performed in cases of intermittent bleeding.

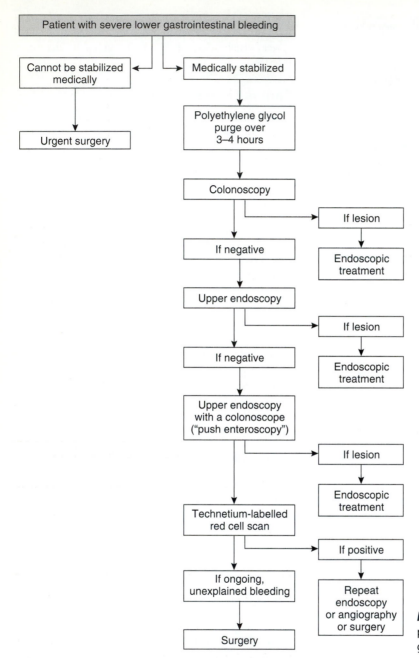

Figure 4–4. Diagnostic and therapeutic approach to severe lower gastrointestinal bleeding.

In patients with active bleeding, the red blood cell scan demonstrates a bleeding site in approximately 50% of patients; but the detection rate is lower with slower or intermittent bleeding. The most common false positive scan occurs when there is rapid transit of luminal blood, such that labeled blood is detected in the colon although it originated in the upper gastrointestinal tract. There is no therapeutic benefit from nuclear medicine scintigraphy.

Surgical Exploration

Surgical exploration is indicated for those patients with severe, ongoing hematochezia who cannot be medically resuscitated because of active blood loss. Patients with recurrent bleeding from a site previously localized by colonoscopy, angiography, or scintigraphy may also require surgical intervention. Preoperative localization of a lesion by endoscopy or angiography lowers the operative mortality risk.

Baum S: Angiography of the gastrointestinal bleeder. Radiology 1982;143:569.

Farrands PA, Taylor I: Management of acute lower gastrointestinal hemorrhage in a surgical unit over a 4-year period. J R Soc Med 1987;80:79.

Jensen DM, Machicado GA: Diagnosis and treatment of severe hematochezia. Gastroenterology 1988;95:1569.

Jensen DM, Machicado GA: Techniques of hemostasis for lower GI bleeding. In: *Medical Laser Endoscopy*. Jensen DM, Brunetaud JM (editors). Kluwer Academic Publishers, 1990;99.

Lewis BS, Waye JD: Chronic gastrointestinal bleeding of obscure origin: role of small bowel enteroscopy. Gastroenterology 1988;94:1117.

Nicholson ML et al: Localization of lower gastrointestinal bleeding using in vivo technetium-99m-labelled red blood cell scintigraphy. Br J Surg 1989;78:358.

Rex DK et al: Flexible sigmoidoscopy plus air contrast barium enema versus colonoscopy for suspected lower gastrointestinal bleeding. Gastroenterology 1990;98:855.

Ryan P, Styles CB, Chmiel R: Identification of the site of severe colon bleeding by technetium-labeled red-cell scan. Dis Colon Rectum 1992;35:219.

SPECIFIC DISORDERS CAUSING LOWER GASTROINTESTINAL BLEEDING

1. Colonic Diverticula

 ESSENTIALS OF DIAGNOSIS

- *Painless hematochezia.*
- *Most common cause of severe lower gastrointestinal bleeding in adults.*
- *Mostly located in the sigmoid colon.*

General Considerations

Diverticula are acquired lesions that occur with aging. Diverticula are herniations of colonic mucosa and submucosa through the muscular layers of the colon. What are called diverticula in the colon, are, in fact, pseudodiverticula, as true diverticula contain all layers of the intestinal wall. Colonic diverticula seem to form when colonic tissue is pushed out by intraluminal pressure. They vary in diameter from a few milliliters to several centimeters. The most common location is the left colon. Most colonic diverticula are asymptomatic and remain uncomplicated.

Diverticula are common in Western countries, with a prevalence of 50% in adults. In contrast, fewer than 1% of the African and Asian populations have diverticula. This has led to the hypothesis that regional differences in prevalence can be explained by the low amounts of dietary fiber in Western diets. Presumably, the low-fiber diet results in less stool content, longer fecal transit time, increased colonic muscle contraction, and, ultimately, increased intraluminal pressure that results in the formation of propulsion diverticula.

Diverticula occur at the point of entry of the small arteries that supply the colon, the **vasa recta.** The entry points of the vasa recta are areas of relative weakness through which the mucosa and submucosa can herniate when under increased intraluminal pressure. Bleeding usually occurs from vessels at the neck of the diverticula, but can occur from vessels at the base as well.

Clinical Findings

A. SYMPTOMS AND SIGNS

Patients generally present with painless hematochezia, although mild left lower quadrant discomfort may be present. Most patients have mild, self-limited bleeding, but occasionally severe bleeding occurs.

B. LABORATORY FINDINGS

Patients may have anemia with acute blood loss.

C. IMAGING

Colonoscopy after urgent bowel cleansing can identify diverticula as the source of bleeding based on active bleeding or fresh blood in a segment of colon with no other lesions but diverticula. Mesenteric angiography and radionuclide bleeding scans can also demonstrate diverticular bleeding if there is active bleeding and contrast extravasates into the colon lumen.

Differential Diagnosis

The main differential diagnosis in elderly patients is ischemic colitis and angiodysplasia, once internal hemorrhoids have been excluded. Other causes for painless hematochezia include polyps or tumors.

Complications

Patients with colonic diverticula can also develop diverticulitis (left lower quadrant pain, fever, elevated white blood cell count) or peridiverticular abscess, but these complications are extremely unusual in the presence of diverticular bleeding.

Treatment

Endoscopic treatment of bleeding diverticula has been reported with heater probe coagulation, bipolar probe coagulation, and epinephrine injection. Endoscopic treatment is best directed at the active bleeding site or visible vessel at the neck of the diverticulum, because this area is thicker than the base and therefore at less risk for perforation. Patients treated for bleeding diverticula have reportedly shown no recurrent bleeding during an average follow-up of 1 year.

Mesenteric angiography can demonstrate bleeding diverticula, and selective arterial infusion of vasopressin or selective embolization of mesenteric arterial branches can provide effective initial hemostasis. These patients often undergo subsequent elective surgical resection of the diseased area.

Surgical segmental colectomy is recommended for uncontrollable bleeding in patients who cannot be medically resuscitated or in whom bleeding cannot be stopped with endoscopic or angiographic means. Surgery may be considered in cases of recurrent diverticular bleeding in which the exact location of bleeding is fairly certain.

Prognosis

Diverticular bleeding will stop spontaneously in over 80% of patients but will recur in approximately 25% of these persons.

Most patients will have self-limited bleeding, which requires supportive care and accurate diagnosis. Those patients with profuse bleeding or recurrent bleeding can generally be managed successfully with surgical therapy.

Baum S et al: Selective mesenteric arterial infusions in the management of massive diverticular hemorrhage. N Engl J Med 1973;288:1269.

Goldberger LE, Bookstein JJ: Transcatheter embolization for treatment of diverticular hemorrhage. Radiology 1977;122:613.

Jensen DM et al: Urgent colonoscopy for the diagnosis and treatment of severe diverticular hemorrhage. N Engl J Med 2000;342:78.

Kim YI, Marcon NE: Injection therapy for colonic diverticular bleeding. A case study. J Clin Gastroenterol 1993;17:46.

McGuire HH, Haynes BW: Massive hemorrhage from diverticulosis of the colon: guidelines for therapy based on bleeding patterns observed in fifty cases. Ann Surg 1972;175:847.

Savides TJ, Jensen DM: Colonoscopic hemostasis for recurrent diverticular hemorrhage associated with a visible vessel: a report of three cases. Gastrointest Endosc 1994;40:70.

2. Internal Hemorrhoids

 ESSENTIALS OF DIAGNOSIS

- *Intermittent, self-limited bright red blood per rectum.*
- *Blood often coats outside of stool and is seen on tissue.*
- *Characteristic findings on anoscopy or sigmoidoscopy.*

General Considerations

Internal hemorrhoids are a plexus of veins just above the rectal squamocolumnar junction. Symptomatic hemorrhoids are common in adults, mostly associated with prolonged straining during bowel movements, chronic constipation, pregnancy, obesity, and low-fiber diet.

Clinical Findings

A. SYMPTOMS AND SIGNS

Bleeding is usually bright red blood per rectum that coats the outside of the stool. Fresh blood is often present on the tissue paper after wiping and in the toilet water. Bleeding from internal hemorrhoids is usually painless and may be associated with constipation, straining, or hard stool. Patients often have a life-long history of such intermittent bleeding. Patients may also note nonbleeding symptoms of hemorrhoids, such as prolapse, itching, or mucus discharge.

B. LABORATORY FINDINGS

The hematocrit is generally normal, although patients can occasionally lose large amounts of blood from hemorrhoidal bleeding.

C. IMAGING

Anoscopy is the best imaging modality for determining the presence of internal hemorrhoids, although they can also be detected with sigmoidoscopy. A slotted, metal anoscope is better than a clear plastic cylindrical anoscope in detecting hemorrhoids. Hemorrhoids should be suspected as the site of bleeding if active bleeding is seen, or if there is a fresh clot overlying a hemorrhoid. Otherwise, all other colonic sources of bleeding should be excluded.

D. GRADING

Internal hemorrhoids are graded for severity. Grade 1 are inside the rectal canal and do not prolapse. Grade 2 prolapse with bowel movements, but spontaneously go back into the rectal canal. Grade 3 are prolapsed (outside the rectal canal) but can be manually reduced. Grade 4 remain outside the rectal canal and cannot be reduced. Lower grades of internal hemorrhoids respond to medical therapy. Anoscopic therapy is effective for grades 1–3, and surgery is usually required for grade 4.

Differential Diagnosis

Bright red blood per rectum in a hemodynamically stable patient with a normal hematocrit implies a rectal source of bleeding. Besides internal hemorrhoids, the differential diagnosis includes external hemorrhoids, rectal varices, fissures, ulcers, polyps, tumors, and proctitis. External hemorrhoids that bleed may be acutely painful and are located outside the rectal canal.

Complications

Rarely, ongoing bleeding may occur that requires urgent treatment.

Treatment

A. MEDICAL THERAPY

Most patients will respond to warm sitz baths, lubricant rectal suppositories (with or without steroids), and increased dietary fiber.

B. ANOSCOPIC THERAPY

Injection sclerotherapy, rubber band ligation, cryosurgery, infrared photocoagulation, and bipolar and direct current electrocoagulation have all been successfully used to treat acute and chronic internal hemorrhoidal bleeding.

C. SURGICAL HEMORRHOIDECTOMY

Surgery is reserved for patients with chronic bleeding or other symptoms that cannot be controlled with medical or anoscopic treatment. Usually, such patients have grade 3 or 4 hemorrhoids, which require manual reduction or are not manually reducible.

Prognosis

Most patients will have resolution of bleeding with medical measures, whereas the patients who fail medical management will almost always respond to anoscopic treatment. Surgical treatment is reserved for patients who fail medical and anoscopic treatment.

Dennison AR, Wherry DC, Morris DL: Hemorrhoids: nonoperative management. Surg Clin North Am 1988;68:1401.

Jensen DM et al: Prospective randomized comparative study of bipolar electrocoagulation versus heater probe for treatment of chronically bleeding internal hemorrhoids. Gastrointest Endosc 1997;46:435.

Randall GM et al: Prospective randomized comparative study of bipolar versus direct current electrocoagulation for treatment of bleeding internal hemorrhoids. Gastrointest Endosc 1994;40:403.

3. Colonic Angiomas

 ESSENTIALS OF DIAGNOSIS

- Bleeding typically intermittent, mild, and painless, but can cause severe hematochezia.
- Mostly located in the right colon, but can be difficult to identify.

General Considerations

Colonic angiomas are also referred to as angiodysplasia, arteriovenous malformations, or vascular ectasias. These lesions, which are acquired with age, represent degeneration of previously normal blood vessels in the cecum and proximal ascending colon. They are not associated with systemic telangiectasias, which are contained and can occur at any age. Histopathology reveals a large, dilated, submucosal vein and, in advanced cases, dilated mucosal veins with small arteriovenous communications. Proposed explanations for angioma formation include the partial obstruction of submucosal veins passing through the colonic muscle layers, with eventual dilation of the submucosal and mucosal veins, and local mucosal ischemia.

By histopathologic injection studies, colonic vascular ectasias may be found in over 25% of asymptomatic persons over the age of 60. However, by colonoscopy, the frequency of incidental (asymptomatic) right colonic angiomata is less than 5%. An association between colonic angiomas and aortic stenosis has been reported, as has improvement of recurrent bleeding after aortic valve replacement, although the cause and effect of this relationship are unclear.

Clinical Findings

A. SYMPTOMS AND SIGNS

Elderly patients can present with occult bleeding manifested by iron deficiency anemia, or intermittent mild or severe episodes of hematochezia. There is no pain associated with angiomas.

B. LABORATORY FINDINGS

Acute bleeding causes an acute decrease in hematocrit; chronic bleeding causes microcytic anemia.

C. IMAGING

Colonoscopy reveals angiomas as red, spider-like subepithelial lesions in the right colon. The colonoscopic appearance of vascular lesions is influenced by blood pressure and intravascular volume, and lesions may not be evident until after a patient has had adequate fluid resuscitation. Sedation with meperidine hydrochloride during colonoscopy may make vascular lesions difficult to see because of splanchnic vasodilation, resulting in decreased mucosal blood flow; therefore, this drug should be used in minimal doses or reversed with naloxone during the procedure. Colonoscopic biopsy of suspected angiomas demonstrates histologic evidence of these lesions in fewer than 50% of biopsies. This may be related to tissue damage during processing or submucosal location of the lesions.

Angiography can identify the site of active bleeding if contrast material extravasates into the intestinal lumen. Bleeding is usually intermittent, and no active extravasation is found. Angiography can also demonstrate angiodysplasia even without active bleeding. The angiographic signs of angiodysplasia are (1) a densely opacified, slowly emptying dilated tortuous vein seen during the venous phase, (2) a vascular tuft seen during the arterial phase, which represents dilated mucosal venules, and (3) an early-filling vein in the arterial phase, which represents an arteriovenous communication.

Differential Diagnosis

Vascular lesions can also occur as part of systemic diseases. **Osler-Weber-Rendu** disease (hereditary hemorrhagic telangiectasias) is an autosomal dominant condition characterized by telangiectasias that affect mucocutaneous areas as well as internal organs. Patients may have telangiectasias involving the lips, mouth, face, hands, gastrointestinal tract, liver, lungs, and brain. Diffuse vascular lesions can also be seen in uremia, pseudoxanthoma elasticum, Ehlers-Danlos syndrome, and the CREST (calcinosis, Raynaud's phenomenon, esophageal dysmotility, sclerodactyly, and telangiectasia) variant of scleroderma.

Trauma during colonoscopy may cause artifacts that resemble colonic angiomata. Therefore, the colonoscopist must look closely for lesions before pressing the colonoscope against an area of mucosa.

Treatment

Endoscopic therapy allows colonic angiomata to be coagulated with either bipolar electrocoagulation, monopolar electrocoagulation, heater probe, or laser. Endoscopic coagulation can control acute bleeding from colonic angiomata in most patients, although at least 20% of patients will have recurrent bleeding and require additional colonoscopic treatment sessions. With long-term follow-up, patients who receive colonoscopic treatment of angiomata will have a significant decrease in frequency of bleeding episodes and number of units of packed red blood cells transfused per year, and an increase in mean hematocrit compared with pretreatment levels.

The main risks of colonoscopic coagulation of angiomata are perforation, postpolypectomy coagulation syndrome, and delayed bleeding. Perforation occurs in fewer than 1% of patients; **postpolypectomy coagulation syndrome,** defined by abdominal pain, focal rebound tenderness, fever, and leukocytosis without evidence of perforation, occurs in 2% and delayed bleeding occurs in 4% of patients.

Actively bleeding angiomata can be treated at the time of angiography with selective embolization of branches of the mesenteric artery using Gelfoam or metal coils. Surgery may also be useful in treating active bleeding and bleeding that recurs despite adequate endoscopic treatment.

Prognosis

Patients with bleeding angiodysplasia often have scattered or diffuse lesions in the colon and even other parts of the gastrointestinal tract. Although endoscopy, angiography, or surgery can stop acute bleeding, these patients are likely to have recurrent bleeding in the future. The goal of repeat endoscopic therapy is to reduce, if not totally eliminate, the number of bleeds, hospitalizations, and transfusions.

Boley SJ et al: On the nature and etiology of vascular ectasias of the colon. Degenerative lesions of aging. Gastroenterology 1977; 72:650.

Jensen DM, Machicado GA: Endoscopic diagnosis and treatment of bleeding colonic angiomas and radiation telangiectasia. In: *Prospectives in Colon and Rectal Surgery.* Schrock T (editor). Quality Medical Publishing, 1989.

Jensen DM: What to choose for diagnosis of bleeding colonic angiomas, colonoscopy, angiography, or helical computed tomography angiography? Gastroenterology 2000;119:581.

Reinus JF, Brandt LJ: Vascular ectasias and diverticulosis. Gastroenterol Clin North Am 1994;23:1.

4. Colon Cancer

 ESSENTIALS OF DIAGNOSIS

- *Weight loss.*
- *Change in bowel habits.*
- *Iron deficiency anemia.*

General Considerations

Colon cancer is one of the leading causes of cancer-related morbidity and mortality in the United States. Most patients with colon cancer present with occult gastrointestinal blood loss rather than hematochezia. For adult patients with hematochezia, determining the presence or absence of a colon cancer is imperative, because early diagnosis improves survival. Because a cancer must ulcerate for overt bleeding to occur, most bleeding cancers present at a relatively advanced tumor stage.

Clinical Findings

A. SYMPTOMS AND SIGNS

Patients with left-sided colonic cancers may note a recent change in bowel habits. This can be new constipation owing to an obstructing lesion, or can be diarrhea caused by only liquid stool passing around a distal colonic lesion. Some patients may have weight loss and a palpable mass, either on abdominal or rectal examination. Painless occult or overt rectal bleeding is the most common presentation.

B. LABORATORY FINDINGS

Patients often will have had chronic blood loss in addition to acute blood loss and will be found to have a microcytic and iron deficiency anemia. Patients with suspected colon cancer should not be screened with a carcinoembryonic antigen (CEA) test, as this is useful only after the diagnosis and primary treatment of the colon cancer.

C. IMAGING

Colonoscopy is the procedure of choice. Not only will the lesion be imaged, but biopsies can also be obtained at the same time. Flexible sigmoidoscopy combined with air-contrast barium enema has also been used for colorectal cancer screening of patients with hemoccult-positive stools.

Treatment

The most definitive therapy is surgical resection. Surgery is useful for both attempted cure and palliation by preventing colonic obstruction. If the patient is not able to undergo surgery because of other medical problems, then endoscopic therapy (especially in the rectum) can be attempted, using laser coagulation, bipolar probe coagulation, or injection of epinephrine or alcohol.

Eckhauser ML: The neodymium-YAG laser and gastrointestinal malignancy. World J Surg 1992;16:1054.

Randall GM, Jensen DM: Diagnosis and management of bleeding from upper gastrointestinal neoplasms. Gastrointest Endosc Clin North Am 1991;1:401.

5. Ischemic Colitis

 ESSENTIALS OF DIAGNOSIS

- *Sudden-onset, crampy, left lower abdominal pain followed by hematochezia.*
- *Radiographs show thick wall ("thumbprinting").*
- *Colonoscopy shows segmental submucosal hemorrhage.*

General Considerations

Ischemic colitis, which results from mucosal hypoxia, is caused by hypoperfusion of the intramural vessels of the intestinal wall, rather than by large vessel occlusion. Usually, this hypoperfusion is caused by vascular disorders, such as atherosclerosis or vasculitis, but it can also be caused by increased blood viscosity, such as occurs with polycythemia vera. Acute hypotension may also precipitate local ischemia in patients with vascular disease. Because of collateral circulation, the ischemic involvement is usually segmental and primarily affects the mucosal aspect of the intestine. The colon is mostly affected in the "watershed areas," such as the splenic flexure or rectosigmoid junction, in which there is reduced collateral circulation.

Clinical Findings

A. SYMPTOMS AND SIGNS

Patients usually present with sudden-onset, severe, crampy left lower quadrant abdominal pain with diarrhea and hematochezia. Physical examination should reveal bowel sounds and mild distention and tenderness. If there are peritoneal signs, transmural damage with perforation must be considered.

B. LABORATORY FINDINGS

Decreased hematocrit is noted, but transfusion is usually not required.

C. IMAGING

Abdominal radiographs typically demonstrate "thumbprinting", or thickening of the colon wall caused by intramural hemorrhage. Usually, there is segmental involvement, especially of the splenic flexure or rectosigmoid junction. Colonoscopy will reveal submucosal hemorrhage, ulceration, or necrosis. There is no role for angiography because large mesenteric vessels are not involved.

Differential Diagnosis

This includes acute infectious colitis, ulcerative colitis, Crohn's disease, and *Clostridium difficile*-induced pseudomembranous colitis.

Complications

Patients may develop severe intestinal ischemia or infarction with peritoneal signs, chronic segmental ulcerating colitis, colonic strictures, or fulminant pancolitis.

Treatment

Most patients' symptoms resolve within 24–48 hours, with radiographic or colonoscopic resolution by 2 weeks. Specific therapy is not needed for mild, self-limited disease. Treatment with 5-aminosalicylic acid or steroids may be useful, although effectiveness is not clearly proven. Attention should be paid to correcting any underlying medical conditions that may have contributed to the ischemia, such as cardiac disease, medications, vasculitis, or polycythemia vera. Patients with severe or ongoing bleeding should receive broad-spectrum antibiotics. If uncontrollable bleeding or peritoneal signs are present, surgical resection of the diseased bowel is indicated. Repeat colonoscopy several months after the bleeding episode can confirm healing and rule out other pathologies.

Boley SJ, Brandt LJ: Colonic ischemia. Surg Clin North Am 1992;72:203.

MacDonald PH, Beck IT: Mesenteric ischemia. In: *Current Therapy in Gastroenterology and Liver Disease,* 4th ed. Bayless TM (editor). Mosby 1994.

6. Radiation Colitis

 ESSENTIALS OF DIAGNOSIS

- *Symptoms begin weeks to months after radiation treatment.*
- *Recurrent hematochezia and rectal pain.*
- *Multiple telangiectasias seen on colonoscopy.*

General Considerations

Ionizing radiation can cause acute and chronic damage to the normal colon and rectum after radiation treatment for gynecologic, prostatic, bladder, or rectal tumors. Approximately 75% of patients who receive 4000 rads will develop acute, self-limited diarrhea, tenesmus, abdominal cramping, and rarely bleeding during the first few weeks. Chronic radiation affects occur 6–18 months after completion of treatment. Bowel injury resulting from chronic radiation is related to vascular damage, with subsequent mucosal ischemia, thickening, and ulceration.

Clinical Findings

A. SYMPTOMS AND SIGNS

Recurrent hematochezia and rectal pain are common.

B. LABORATORY FINDINGS

Hematocrit is decreased.

C. IMAGING

Endoscopy shows telangiectasias, strictures, ulcers, and inflammation. Barium studies reveal flattened mucosa with loss of haustral markings.

Treatment

Endoscopic bipolar coagulation, heater probe, argon plasma coagulation, or laser can coagulate the mucosal telangiectasias and result in decreased frequency of bleeding and transfusion requirements. Steroid or sucralfate enemas have been used with variable success. Patients with chronic blood loss require iron supplementation. Hyperbaric oxygen, topical formalin, and antioxidant therapy with vitamin C and E have also been reported to be useful in refractory cases. Rarely surgery is necessary for difficult to manage recurrent hematochezia.

Ahlquist D et al: Laser therapy for severe radiation-induced rectal bleeding. Mayo Clin Proc 1986;61:927.

Kochlar R et al: Radiation-induced proctosigmoiditis. Prospective, randomized, double-blind controlled trial of oral sulfasalazine plus rectal steroids versus rectal sucralfate. Dig Dis Sci 1991; 36:103.

Swaroop VS, Gostout CJ: Endoscopic treatment of chronic radiation proctopathy. J Clin Gastroenterol 1998;27:36.

Taylor JG, Disario JA, Buchi KN: Argon laser therapy for hemorrhagic radiation proctitis: long term results. Gastrointest Endosc 1993;39:641.

7. Inflammatory Bowel Disease

 ESSENTIALS OF DIAGNOSIS

- Painless, bloody diarrhea.
- Hematochezia more common in ulcerative colitis than Crohn's disease.
- Intermittent symptoms.

Clinical Findings

Patients may present with intermittent painless hematochezia. Laboratory findings include low hematocrit, low iron, and low albumin. Inflammatory bowel disease is diagnosed on the basis of friable, ulcerated, edematous mucosa seen during colonoscopy. Stool should be evaluated for ova and parasites, as well as *C difficile* to exclude infectious causes.

Treatment

Medical treatment consists of using 5-aminosalicylic acid products, steroids, or immunomodulatory agents. There is no role for endoscopic therapy. In cases of severe ulcerative colitis not responsive to intensive medical management, surgical colectomy may be necessary.

8. Infectious Colitis

 ESSENTIALS OF DIAGNOSIS

- Acute onset of bloody diarrhea.
- Abdominal pain, fever, or both are common.
- Stool cultures positive for organism.

Clinical Findings

Lower gastrointestinal bleeding can occur with infection by *Campylobacter jejuni, Salmonella, Shigella,* invasive *Escherichia coli, E coli* 0157, or *C difficile.* Rarely is there significant blood loss. Diagnosis is made by stool cultures and flexible sigmoidoscopy.

Treatment

Depending on the cause and severity, antibiotic treatment may be necessary. There is no role for endoscopic treatment. In severe cases of *C difficile* pseudomembranous colitis with impending perforation, surgical colectomy may be needed.

9. Rectal Varices

 ESSENTIALS OF DIAGNOSIS

- Hematochezia in patients with portal hypertension.
- Varices located proximal to internal hemorrhoids.

Clinical Findings

In response to portal hypertension, varices can develop in the rectal mucosa between the superior hemorrhoidal veins (portal circulation) and the middle and inferior hemorrhoidal veins (systemic circulation). With anoscopy or sigmoidoscopy, rectal varices are seen as vascular structures located several centimeters above the dentate line. The incidence of rectal varices increases with the degree of portal hypertension. About 60% of patients with a history of bleeding esophageal varices have rectal varices.

Treatment

Rectal varices can be treated similarly to esophageal varices, with either sclerotherapy or portosystemic shunts.

Hosking SW et al: Anorectal varices, haemorrhoids, and portal hypertension. Lancet 1989;8634:349.

10. Meckel's Diverticulum

 ESSENTIALS OF DIAGNOSIS

- Most common cause of gastrointestinal bleeding in children.

- *Painless melena or bright red blood per rectum ("currant jelly").*
- *Diagnosis with technetium scanning.*

Clinical Findings

Meckel's diverticula occur in 1–2% of the general population and are the most common cause of gastrointestinal bleeding in children. A **Meckel's diverticulum** is a congenital anomaly of the gastrointestinal tract in which there is incomplete obliteration of the vitelline duct, leaving an ileal diverticulum. It is located on the antimesenteric border of the ileum, within 100 cm of the ileocecal valve and is 1–10 cm long. Approximately one-half of Meckel's diverticula are lined with gastric mucosa. Most bleeding occurs in Meckel's diverticula that contain gastric mucosa because of acid-induced ulceration of adjacent ileal mucosa.

Preoperative diagnosis can be supported by a ^{99m}Tc sodium pertechnetate scan, which demonstrates ectopic gastric mucosa because it binds to parietal cells. This test has a sensitivity of about 75%, with 15% false-positive and 25% false-negative rates. The accuracy of the Meckel's scan may be improved with the use of pentagastrin or cimetidine, which increase the uptake of pertechnetate by parietal cells. In active bleeding, angiography may also be helpful.

Treatment

The condition is treated by surgical resection of the diverticulum.

11. Postpolypectomy Bleeding

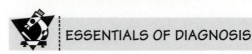

ESSENTIALS OF DIAGNOSIS

- *One percent risk after colonoscopic polypectomy.*
- *May occur up to 10 days after the procedure.*

Clinical Findings

Patients present with painless hematochezia hours to days after the colonoscopic polypectomy. Risk factors for postpolypectomy bleeding include polyp size greater than 2 cm, sessile polyp, elderly age, and use of aspirin, NSAIDs, or coumadin.

Treatment

The majority of postpolypectomy bleeding will usually stop spontaneously. Repeat colonoscopy with colonoscopic hemostasis (epinephrine injection, endoloop, hemoclips, or repeat snare coagulation) is usually successful in stopping active bleeding.

Waye et al: Complications of colonoscopy and flexible sigmoidoscopy. Gastrointest Clin North Am 1996;6:343.

Occult Gastrointestinal Bleeding[1]

5

Don C. Rockey, MD

OCCULT & OBSCURE BLEEDING

Occult gastrointestinal bleeding denotes chronic or intermittent loss of small amounts of blood of which the patient is unaware. That is, there is insufficient bleeding to cause obvious melena or hematochezia. Occult bleeding is by far the most common form of gastrointestinal bleeding, affecting at least 10% of the U.S. population. Instillation of 50 to 100 mL of blood into the stomach is required to produce melena. Thus, patients with gastroduodenal bleeding of up to 100 mL/d may have stools that appear normal. Occult bleeding therefore is most commonly identified in one of two ways. Occult blood may be detected directly by tests that assess the presence of fecal blood (the "fecal occult blood test"). Alternatively, chronic gastrointestinal bleeding with iron loss may manifest as iron deficiency anemia.

Obscure gastrointestinal bleeding refers to bleeding that persists or recurs and for which there is no obvious source found after routine endoscopic evaluation with upper endoscopy and colonoscopy. Obscure bleeding may be clinically evident, manifesting as recurrent melena or hematochezia. Alternatively, obscure bleeding may manifest as recurrent iron deficiency anemia or positive tests for fecal occult blood. Obscure bleeding is uncommon but poses a difficult diagnostic and management challenge.

FECAL OCCULT BLOOD

The most common form of occult gastrointestinal bleeding is that detected by fecal occult blood tests. When such tests have been applied to large populations, 2 to 16% of those tested are positive. Fecal blood loss in normal individuals varies from 0.5 to 1.5 mL/d; most fecal occult blood tests become positive at a level of around 2 mL of blood loss per day. However, fecal occult blood tests become consistent only at higher levels of fecal blood. A number of fecal occult blood tests are available and are commonly used as a screening test for colorectal cancer. When applied to large populations, these tests result in an 18–33% reduction in col-

orectal cancer mortality. The likelihood of detecting fecal blood depends on the fecal occult blood test used, the frequency with which the bleeding lesion bleeds, the intestinal transit time, and the anatomic level of bleeding (the latter feature influences intraluminal metabolism of hemoglobin, Figure 5–1). Thus, fecal occult blood tests are capable of detecting blood from lesions throughout the gastrointestinal tract.

Fecal Occult Blood Tests

The classic fecal occult blood tests are guaiac-based tests that take advantage of the fact that hemoglobin possesses pseudoperoxidase activity. Guaiac turns blue after oxidation by peroxidases in the presence of an oxygen donor such as hydrogen peroxide. Guaiac tests are more sensitive in detecting bleeding from the lower than from the upper gastrointestinal tract since hemoglobin is degraded in the gastrointestinal tract (see Figure 5–1). The characteristics of the different guaiac-based tests vary. Of the two most commonly used tests in the United States, Hemoccult II and Hemoccult II SENSA (both from SmithKline Diagnostics, Palo Alto, CA), the latter is substantially more sensitive in detecting fecal heme, however, this also results in reduced specificity.

The likelihood that a guaiac test will detect fecal blood (heme) is related to the quantity of heme present in the stool, which in turn is related to the size and location of the bleeding lesion. Blood from colonic lesions is more likely to be undegraded and therefore is easier to detect by guaiac-based tests than blood from upper intestinal sources. However, patient factors, such as stool transit time and mixing, as well as intraluminal degradation of heme may lead to variability in the content of fecal hemoglobin. Fecal hemoglobin levels must exceed 10 mg/g (10 mL daily blood loss) before Hemoccult II tests are positive at least 50% of the time, whereas stools with less than 1 mg/g hemoglobin still may be positive. Therefore guaiac tests are not sufficiently sensitive even for the detection of colonic lesions.

Dietary factors also affect the accuracy of guaiac test results (Table 5–1). Fecal rehydration improves their sensitivity, but reduces specificity. Although it is commonly believed that oral iron causes false-positive gua-

[1]This work was supported by the Burroughs Wellcome Fund (BWF Clinical Scientist Award).

Sites of gastrointestinal bleeding

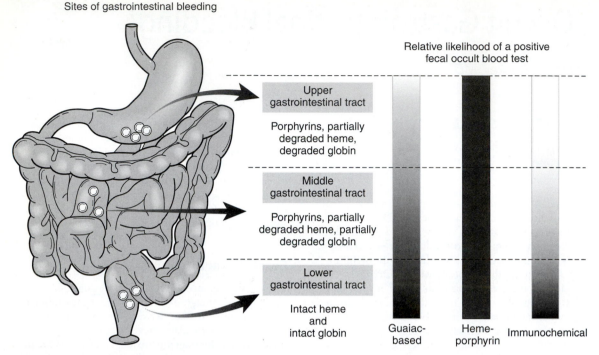

Figure 5–1. Sites of gastrointestinal bleeding, intraluminal metabolism of hemoglobin, and detection of intraluminal blood by fecal occult blood tests. Hemoglobin is cleaved to heme and globin by gastric pepsin and/or pancreatic proteases in the upper gastrointestinal tract. Heme that is not absorbed is converted to porphyrins and iron via poorly understood mechanisms. This fraction is not detected by guaiac tests but is detected by the heme-porphyrin assay (HemoQuant), which measures both heme and porphyrins, and is therefore a highly accurate indicator of bleeding, regardless of level. Globin in the upper gastrointestinal tract is digested by pepsin, pancreatic, and intestinal proteases and is thus not detected by immunochemical fecal occult blood tests. (Reprinted, with permission, from Rockey DC: Occult gastrointestinal bleeding. N Engl J Med 1999;341:38. Copyright © 1999 Massachusetts Medical Society. All rights reserved.)

iac tests, studies demonstrate that orally administered iron, even in large amounts, does not cause a positive guaiac reaction. The dark-green or black appearance of stool caused by iron should not be confused with a positive "blue" guaiac reaction. Bismuth-containing antacids and antidiarrheals also cause the stool to be dark and should not be confused with a positive guaiac reaction.

Immunochemical tests detect human hemoglobin epitopes and are highly sensitive—detecting as little as 0.3 mL of fecal blood. Further, they do not detect small quantities of blood arising from upper gastrointestinal sources (see Figure 5–1), and therefore have superior specificity to guaiac-based tests. However, they are limited by technical problems such as loss of hemoglobin antigenicity at room temperature and the requirement for laboratory processing. Newer slide immunochemical tests (ie, FlexSure OBT, SmithKline Diagnostics, Palo Alto, CA) may obviate these problems.

The heme-porphyrin test (HemoQuant, Mayo Medical Laboratories, Rochester, MN) uses a spectrofluorometric method to measure heme-derived porphyrin, and therefore allows precise determination of total stool hemoglobin. Substances that interfere with guaiac-based and immunochemical tests do not affect this test, however, nonhuman dietary heme (particularly myoglobin from meats) may confound the assay. The heme-porphyrin test is extremely sensitive in detecting occult blood loss, but the high number of false-positive tests has limited its usefulness as a screening tool.

Approach to Evaluation & Differential Diagnosis

The history and physical examination provide important diagnostic information in patients with occult bleeding. The history should be reviewed for medications that injure the gastrointestinal mucosa, including

Table 5–1. Characteristics of fecal occult blood tests.[1]

Variable	Guaiac	Heme-Porphyrin	Immunochemical
Detection characteristics			
Upper gastrointestinal	+	++++	0
Small bowel	++	++++	+
Right colonic	+++	++++	+++
Left colonic	++++	++++	++++
Test factors			
Bedside availability	++++	0	+
Time to develop	1 minute	1 hour	5 minutes to 24 hours
Cost	$3–5	$17	$10–20
False positives			
Animal hemoglobin	++++	++++	0
Dietary peroxidases	+++	0	0
False negatives			
Hemoglobin degredation	++	0	++
Storage	++	++++	++
Vitamin C	++	0	0

Derived from Rockey DC: Occult gastrointestinal bleeding. N Engl J Med 1999; 341:38.
[1]Relative comparisons are shown on a scale of 0 to ++++, with 0 being the negative and ++++ highly positive.

nonsteroidal antiinflammatory drugs (NSAIDs), alendronate, and potassium chloride and for the use of anticoagulants (see below). A family history of bleeding may suggest inherited disorders, such as hereditary hemorrhagic telangiectasia. A number of systemic disorders are important causes of occult bleeding, many of which have cutaneous manifestations. Patients with occult bleeding due to celiac sprue may have dermatitis herpetiformis. Neurofibromas, café au lait spots, and axillary freckles are found in patients with neurofibromatosis. The polyposis syndromes (Peutz-Jeghers syndrome, Gardner syndrome, Cronkite-Canada syndrome) have other cutaneous findings.

Virtually any gastrointestinal lesion can lead to occult bleeding, including lesions more often associated with acute bleeding. Lesions commonly responsible for occult bleeding are listed in Table 5–2. Although the colon has traditionally been considered to be the more common source of occult blood loss, the upper gastrointestinal tract is also an important site of occult bleeding. The most common causes of fecal occult blood include colon adenocarcinoma, large colonic adenomatous polyps (greater than 2 cm), gastroduodenal ulcers, colonic or small intestinal vascular ectasias, esophagitis, and erosive gastritis. Less common causes of occult bleeding include various small intestinal lesions (tumors, ulcers), upper gastrointestinal neoplasms (adenocarcinoma, adenomas), and Cameron lesions (erosions within hiatal hernias).

In asymptomatic patients found to have occult blood in the stool, investigation should initially be fo-

cused on the colon (Figure 5–2). Colonoscopy and air contrast barium enema are the most commonly used tests, although most experts recommend colonoscopy, where available. If air contrast barium enema is performed, a flexible sigmoidoscopy should also be performed to examine the rectosigmoid colon.

Colonoscopy is generally regarded as the more accurate test, although air contrast barium enema may accurately detect colonic malignancy and most large adenomas. However, there remains concern about the accuracy of air contrast barium enema, particularly for small adenomas. It is important to emphasize that any colon imaging modality—including colonoscopy—can miss important neoplastic lesions. Patients found to have a colonic polyp or suspicious mass on barium enema require a subsequent colonoscopic evaluation. Serious complications occur in less than 1/1000 diagnostic colonoscopies, however, serious complications with barium enema are extremely rare. Colonoscopy usually requires moderate sedation and therefore may pose increased risk in patients with multiple medical (especially cardiopulmonary) problems. Results with computed tomographic colonography with luminal views derived from three-dimensional computer reconstruction (virtual colonoscopy) suggest that this test may become an important test for colorectal cancer screening or evaluation of occult bleeding; however, this test is still not widely available. Ultimately, the provider's decision among colonoscopy, barium enema, and virtual colonoscopy will depend upon a variety of factors, including test availability and local expertise,

Table 5–2. Differential diagnosis of occult gastrointestinal bleeding.[1]

Mass lesions	Vascular
Carcinoma (any site)[2]	Vascular ectasia (any site)[2]
Large (> 1.5 cm) adenoma (any site)	Portal hypertensive gastropathy/colopathy
Inflammation	Watermelon stomach
Erosive esophagitis[2]	Hemangioma
Ulcer (any site)[2]	Dieulafoy's ulcer[4]
Cameron lesions[3]	Infectious
Erosive gastritis	Hookworm
Celiac sprue	Whipworm
Ulcerative colitis	Stronglyoidiasis
Crohn's disease	Ascariasis
Colitis (nonspecific)	Tuberculous enterocolitis
Idiopathic cecal ulcer	Amebiasis
Miscellaneous	Surreptitious
Long-distance running	Hemoptysis
Factitious	Oropharyngeal (including epistaxis)
	Pancreaticobiliary

Adapted, with permission, from Rockey DC: Occult gastrointestinal bleeding. N Engl J Med 1999;341:38. Copyright © 1999 Massachusetts Medical Society. All rights reserved.
[1]Potential lesions leading to all forms of occult gastrointestinal bleeding are shown. Some lesions that may lead to recurrent obscure bleeding are not listed (see text).
[2]Most common abnormalities.
[3]Linear erosions within a hiatus hernia.
[4]Large superficial artery underlying mucosal defect.

the patient's comorbid medical problems, and patient preference.

The upper gastrointestinal tract is also an important potential source of bleeding in patients with fecal occult blood. Indeed, in prospective clinical studies potential sources of occult bleeding are identified in the upper gastrointestinal tract more often than in the lower gastrointestinal tract (Figure 5–3). In all clinical studies, upper endoscopy led to the diagnosis of previously unrecognized upper gastrointestinal tract malignancies. In a high proportion of patients, upper endosocopy yielded findings that led to changes in patient management. Although guaiac-based fecal occult blood tests are believed to have a lower sensitivity for detecting blood from the upper gastrointestinal tract than from the colon, many of the lesions identified in the upper gastrointestinal tract nonetheless bleed enough to yield a positive test. Notwithstanding the results of these clinical studies, it is unknown whether it is cost effective to proceed with upper gastrointestinal (GI) tract investigation in patients with fecal occult blood and a normal colonic examination.

In patients with occult GI bleeding, the choice of initial investigation (ie, colonoscopy versus upper endoscopy) should be guided by the presence and location of GI symptoms (see Figure 5–2). Significant lesions in both the upper and lower GI tract are rare; hence, identification of an abnormality on either colonoscopy or

upper endoscopy that is felt to be consistent with occult bleeding (eg, a large mass, ulceration, or severe inflammation) usually precludes the need for endoscopic evaluation with the alternative study. Among patients without GI symptoms, it generally is recommended that a colonoscopy first be performed. If this study does not reveal a likely source of occult bleeding, upper endoscopy is recommended.

The appropriate evaluation for patients with occult blood found in stool obtained by digital rectal examination is controversial. Anorectal trauma and/or dietary factors in this setting may lead to false-positive tests. However, in both symptomatic and asymptomatic patients with fecal occult blood detected by digital rectal examination, the number of new lesions identified at endoscopic evaluation is substantial. In fact, the clinical significance of blood detected on digital rectal examination is similar if not greater than that detected in spontaneously passed stools. Thus, endoscopic evaluation of patients with a positive digital rectal examination probably is warranted.

A positive fecal occult blood test that occurs in patients receiving anticoagulants or low-dose aspirin should result in formal endoscopic evaluation. Although often ascribed to anticoagulant or aspirin therapy, fecal blood levels in patients therapeutically anticoagulated are normal. Low-dose aspirin alone results in minimally elevated fecal blood levels, whereas the com-

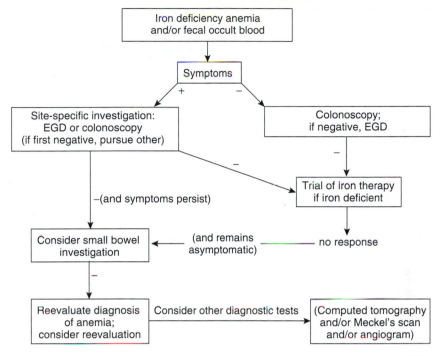

Figure 5–2. Algorithm for management of occult gastrointestinal bleeding (fecal occult blood and iron deficiency anemia). EGD, esophagogastroduodenoscopy.

bination of aspirin and warfarin caused higher elevations. Importantly, neither warfarin nor low-dose aspirin alone appears to cause positive guaiac-based fecal occult blood tests. In a prospective study evaluating the gastrointestinal tract in anticoagulated patients with positive guaiac-based fecal occult blood tests, 15 of 16 had significant lesions, 20% of which were malignant.

Treatment

Treatment of patients with fecal occult blood depends on the underlying disorder causing bleeding. Most mass lesions require surgical excision, whereas ulcerative processes can often be managed with medical therapy. Because NSAIDs cause gastrointestinal injury, these agents should be stopped, where possible, even in the absence of documented ulcer disease. Management of vascular ectasias may be problematic; these lesions often are multiple and may be difficult to locate. Hence, recurrent bleeding is common despite treatment of visible lesions.

The prognosis of patients with positive fecal occult blood tests but no significant identifiable gastrointestinal findings on upper and lower endoscopy appears to be favorable, but this has not been rigorously studied.

In most cases, no further evaluation is warranted. A very small proportion of patients will have continued or recurrent obscure bleeding manifested by hematochezia, melena, or the development of iron deficiency anemia and will require further diagnostic evaluation to try to localize a bleeding source.

IRON DEFICIENCY ANEMIA

Typical daily gastrointestinal blood loss is 0.5–1.5 mL/d, resulting in 0.25 to 0.75 mg of elemental iron loss. Additionally, a small amount of nonblood iron is lost in sloughed intestinal cells such that the usual daily iron loss is approximately 1 mg (Figure 5–4). Iron deficiency results when iron loss exceeds absorption, typically when blood loss exceeds 5–10 mL/d over long periods of time.

Iron deficiency anemia is the most cause of anemia. In the United States, 5–11% of adult women and 1–4% of adult men are iron deficient and 5% and 2% of adult women and men, respectively, have iron deficiency anemia. Iron deficiency anemia is most commonly identified in women during their reproductive years because of menstrual and pregnancy-associated iron losses. In other groups iron deficiency anemia is most commonly caused

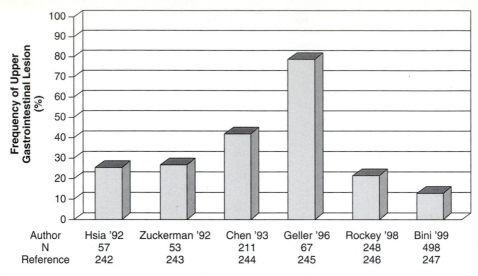

Figure 5–3. Frequency of upper gastrointestinal lesions in patients with fecal occult blood. Studies examining the frequency of upper gastrointestinal lesions in patients with fecal occult blood are depicted; these studies excluded patients with active bleeding. Some variation in the criteria used to ascribe a specific lesion to the positive fecal occult blood test exists.

by chronic occult gastrointestinal bleeding, although it may also be caused by poor nutrition or a malabsorptive disorder. Thus, the standard of care for men and postmenopausal women with iron deficiency anemia is to investigate the gastrointestinal tract for a possible source of chronic GI blood loss.

Approach to Evaluation & Differential Diagnosis

Although the diagnosis of iron deficiency is most accurately determined by a bone marrow biopsy, in routine clinical practice the diagnosis of iron deficiency and iron deficiency anemia is most often suggested by a low serum ferritin level. A ferritin value less than 30–40 µg/dL is a highly reliable indicator of iron deficiency. Unless another cause for iron deficiency is apparent, patients with iron deficiency anemia (with or without positive fecal occult blood tests) should be managed similar to those with fecal occult blood who do not have anemia (as described above). These two processes often are part of a continuum of disease. It is unclear whether patients with iron deficiency who do not have anemia also require endoscopic evaluation of the GI tract, however, recent data suggest this may be warranted.

Iron deficiency anemia due to occult GI blood loss can be caused by numerous gastrointestinal tract lesions (see Table 5–2). Historically, right-sided colonic can-

cers have been considered be the major cause of iron deficiency anemia. However, a number of studies have documented abnormalities in the upper gastrointestinal tract more commonly than in the colon (Table 5–3). Only 5% of patients had pathology identified in both upper and lower gastrointestinal sites. Although substantial available data emphasize that upper gastrointestinal tract evaluation is important in iron deficiency anemia, care must be taken when attributing iron deficiency anemia to lesions not expected to cause significant bleeding. Trivial lesions, such as mild inflammation and small adenomas, typically do not bleed enough to lead to iron deficiency.

Recently iron deficiency anemia due to *Helicobacter pylori*-associated gastritis and chronic blood loss was reported. Additionally, 20% of patients with iron deficiency anemia have gastric achlorhydria and atrophy (most commonly caused by *Helicobacter pylori*), implying that malabsorption of iron may be an important contributing factor to iron deficiency.

Gastrointestinal symptoms in patients with iron deficiency anemia may or may not guide gastrointestinal tract evaluation. Some investigators report that site-specific symptoms point to site-specific gastrointestinal lesions. Patients with symptoms (eg, change in stool caliber, epigastric pain, or heartburn) should have initial investigation directed toward the symptom location (see Figure 5–2). Because synchronous abnormalities in both the upper and lower gastrointestinal tract are un-

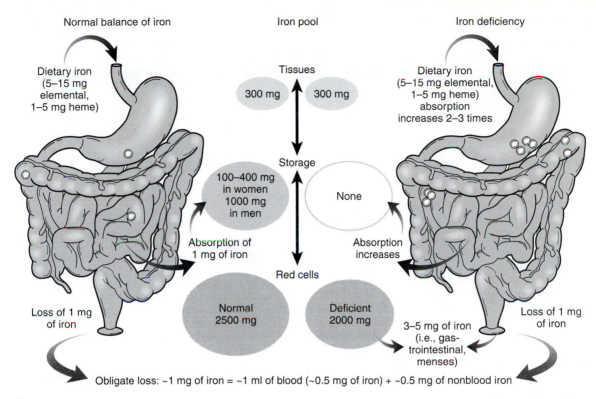

Figure 5–4. Gastrointestinal blood loss and iron balance. Normal obligate daily iron loss results from (1) blood loss in the gastrointestinal tract secondary to gastrointestinal mucosal microerosions or microulcerations and (2) iron in sloughed gut epithelial cells. Total daily iron loss is thus approximately 1 mg. The usual Western diet contains mostly elemental iron, of which about 10% is absorbed. Heme-iron, derived primarily from myoglobin in meats, is preferentially absorbed and accounts for 60–80% of the iron absorbed per day. Under normal circumstances, iron homeostasis is tightly regulated and daily iron loss is balanced by iron absorption. Iron deficiency results only when the dynamic, but limited, absorptive capacity of the small intestine is exceeded by iron loss. The time required to develop iron deficiency depends on the size of initial iron stores, the rate of bleeding, and intestinal iron absorption. Iron deficiency generally occurs only with increased loss of over 5 mL of blood daily. Importantly, anemia is a late manifestation of the iron-depleted state. (Reprinted, with permission, from Rockey DC: Occult gastrointestinal bleeding. N Engl J Med 1999;341:38. Copyright © 1999 Massachusetts Medical Society. All rights reserved.)

common, identification of an abnormality consistent with chronic bleeding (mass lesion, large ulceration, severe inflammation) usally makes evaluation of the remainder of the GI tract unnecessary. Patients who are asymptomatic usually undergo colonic evaluation first; when this is unrevealing, an upper gastrointestinal tract evaluation is also performed.

Iron deficiency in premenopausal women is common and the need for gastrointestinal tract evaluation to exclude occult GI blood loss is controversial. Iron deficiency anemia affects over 3 million women in the United States alone. As many as 12% of premenopausal women with iron deficiency anemia have been reported to have significant gastrointestinal tract

abnormalities, including a high proportion in the upper gastrointestinal tract, some of which are malignant. Therefore, the appropriate degree of evaluation in premenopausal women with iron deficiency anemia depends on the individual patient. For patients with gastrointestinal symptoms, weight loss, fecal occult blood, or severe anemia, gastrointestinal tract evaluation is clearly indicated. For asymptomatic women, gastrointestinal tract evaluation is appropriate if menstrual blood loss is disproportionate to the severity of iron deficiency anemia.

As for positive fecal occult blood tests, the tests used to evaluate patients with iron deficiency anemia include endoscopy (esophagogastroduodenoscopy and colon-

Table 5–3. Major gastrointestinal lesions identified in studies of patients with iron deficiency anemia.[1]

Lesion	Author (Total Number of Patients Evaluable)				
	Cook[2,6] (100)	McIntyre[2,7] (111)	Rockey[8] (100)	Kepczyk[9] (70)	Total (381)
Esophagus (%)					47
Esophagitis	14	15	6	10	
Cancer	1	NA	0	1	
Stomach					98
Ulcer	7	13	8	3	
Gastritis	14[3]	7	6	11	
Cancer	5	8	1	3	
Vascular ectasia	5	0	3	4	
Duodenal ulcer	1	10	11	3	25
Other upper	0	2	2	3	7
Small intestine					10
Celiac disease[4]	0	3	0	4	
Vascular ectasia	1	1	0	0	
Large intestine					85
Cancer	14	5	11	4	
Vascular ectasia	2	1	5	6	
Adenoma	6	4	5	6	
Colitis	1	2	2	1	
Other	0	3	3	4	
Upper lesion[5]	40 (47)	42 (51)	37	39 (43)	158 (41%)
Lower lesion	23	15	26	21	85 (22%)
Small intestine	2	4	0	4	10 (3%)
Upper + lower	7	0	1	12	20 (5%)
No GI lesion	35	50	37	6	128 (34%)

[1]Numbers shown are the reported lesions. Hiatal hernia alone, esophageal varices alone, hemorrhoids alone were not included as sources of chronic blood loss
[2]Barium enema was used to evaluate the colon in many patients.
[3]Duodenitis included.
[4]Duodenal biopsy was not performed to evaluate for celiac disease in all patients.
[5]Numbers shown represent those patients with abnormalities identified. The numbers in parentheses represent the number of reported lesions. For example, 47 lesions were identified in 40 patients by Cook et al.
[6]Cook IJ, et al: BMJ 1986;292:1380.
[7]McIntyre A, et al: Gut 1993;34:1102.
[8]Rockey D, Cello J: N Engl J Med 1993;329:1691.
[9]Kepczyk T, Kadakia S: Dig Dis Sci 1995;40:1283.

oscopy) and radiography (barium enema and upper gastrointestinal series). Radiographic studies are accurate in detecting masses and large ulcerating lesions, however, they are insensitive in detecting vascular ectasias and subtle mucosal lesions (ie, gastritis, esophagitis, colitis). Because patients with iron deficiency anemia have a high pretest probability of disease with the need for biopsy and/or endoscopic therapy, initial endoscopic investigation probably is more cost effective. Because sedation usually is given for endoscopic procedures, both the upper and lower endoscopy should be performed in the same visit to minimize overall risks.

In patients with iron deficiency anemia who have no apparent source of chronic blood loss found on examination of the colon and upper gastrointestinal tract, it is important to consider the small bowel as a potential site of chronic blood loss. Enteroscopy of the small intestine using a pediatric colonoscope or an enteroscope is useful for the evaluation of the distal duodenum and proximal jejunum, where it is sensitive for the detection of mucosal abnormalities (eg, vascular ectasias) and mass lesions. The distal jejunum and ileum can be radiographically evaluated for mass lesions with enteroclysis or small bowel follow through, however, chronic blood loss from a distal small bowel mass lesion is uncommon. The overall cost effectiveness of enteroscopy and small bowel radiography in the evaluation of patients with iron deficiency anemia is not established. Evaluation of the small bowel is not routinely performed in the initial evaluation of iron deficiency anemia, but is warranted in patients with persistent anemia and positive fecal occult blood tests.

A proportion of patients with iron deficiency anemia have no identifiable gastrointestinal tract abnormality after complete endoscopic evaluation. If iron deficiency anemia is refractory to iron supplementation, other tests should be considered to look for a source of chronic blood loss (eg, mesenteric angiography, computed tomography), especially if tests are positive for fecal occult blood. Celiac sprue causes malabsorption of iron as well as occult bleeding and should be considered in patients with iron deficiency, especially patients of northern European descent. Other explanations for iron deficiency anemia include nongastrointestinal blood loss, misdiagnosis of the type of anemia, or nutritional deficiency.

Treatment

The prognosis is excellent for patients with iron deficiency anemia found to have lesions amenable to medical therapy (ie, duodenal ulcer, esophagitis, large adenoma). Likewise, among patients who do not initially have identifiable gastrointestinal lesions, few are found to have significant gastrointestinal lesions at a later date. Iron therapy should be instituted once a diagnosis of iron deficiency anemia is established. Oral ferrous sulfate is inexpensive and effective (300 mg three times daily); ferrous gluconate or fumarate should be tried in patients who are intolerant of ferrous sulfate. Parenteral iron therapy is reserved for treatment of iron deficiency caused by severe malabsorption or in patients intolerant of iron supplements. In patients who do not respond to iron therapy, repeat gastrointestinal evaluation should be considered to be certain an important gastrointestinal lesion was not overlooked. Careful repeat examination of the stomach, duodenum (with small bowel biopsy), and colon may reveal previously overlooked lesions, especially "Cameron's ulcers" (erosions within a hiatal hernia), vascular ectasias, celiac sprue, and neoplasms. In patients with refractory iron deficiency anemia referred for enteroscopy of the small bowel, over one-third have a previously overlooked bleeding source identified within reach of the standard upper endoscope.

GASTROINTESTINAL HEMORRHAGE OF OBSCURE ORIGIN

Obscure bleeding manifests in two ways. Some patients have recurrent, clinically apparent gastrointestinal bleeding that is of unknown origin. In other patients, bleeding remains occult, evident as refractory or recurrent iron deficiency anemia or positive fecal occult blood tests. By definition, bleeding is labeled "obscure" only if readily identifiable causes of gastrointestinal

bleeding have been excluded, usually by esophagogastroduodenoscopy and colonoscopy. Determination of the source of obscure bleeding is important in order to target specific therapy. However, in some cases, localization can be exceedingly difficult.

Differential Diagnosis

Many different gastrointestinal lesions cause obscure bleeding but the more common abnormalities include vascular ectasias, neoplasms, Dieulafoy's ulcer, and Meckel's diverticulum. The lesions most commonly identified are in the small bowel, including tumors and vascular ectasias, which vary in frequency depending upon the patient's age. Tumors are more common in patients between 30 and 50 years of age, whereas vascular ectasias predominate in older patients. In patients less than 25 years of age, Meckel's diverticula are the most common source of small bowel bleeding. Additionally, varices and ulcers located in unusual locations should be considered. Several of the more important causes of obscure bleeding will be discussed subsequently.

Evaluation of Obscure Bleeding

Localization of the bleeding site should begin with history and physical examination. Although melena and hematochezia are usually associated with upper and lower gastrointestinal tract bleeding, respectively, it should be emphasized that patients with slow oozing from the distal small bowel or cecum may have melena and occasional patients with rapid upper gastrointestinal bleeding may present with hematochezia. Additionally, history and physical examination should focus on clinical features sometimes associated with "overlooked" lesions (Table 5–4).

In patients with obscure bleeding, repeat endoscopy directed at the most likely site of bleeding is warranted (Figure 5–5), and is especially helpful if performed during episodes of active bleeding. The endoscopist should

Table 5–4. Causes of obscure gastointestinal bleeding.

Vascular ectasias[1]
Small bowel neoplastic lesions
Hemosuccus panreaticus
Hemobilia
Aortoenteric fistula
Dieulafoy's ulcer (stomach > other sites)
Meckel's diverticulum
Extraesophageal varices (gastric, small bowel, colonic)
Diverticula (especially small intestine)

[1]Small intestinal lesions are particularly important.

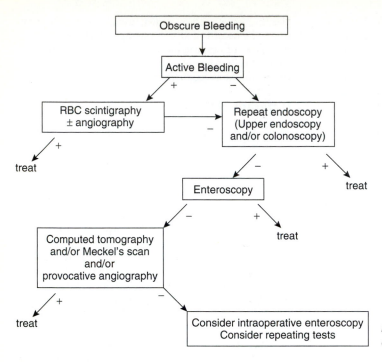

Figure 5–5. Algorithm for management of obscure gastrointestinal bleeding.

be familiar with the appearances of uncommon and/or subtle bleeding lesions. In patients with vigorous bleeding, a technetium-99 radionuclide scan or mesenteric angiogram should be performed. Although technetium scanning can suggest the location in the GI tract from which bleeding may arise, data assessing its impact on management in patients with obscure gastrointestinal bleeding are limited. Mesenteric angiography is less sensitive but more specific than technetium-99 radionuclide scanning for localization of a bleeding site. Other diagnostic tests (computed tomography, Meckel's scan) also may identify the site and/or cause of bleeding.

In patients with obscure bleeding in whom repeat upper and lower endoscopy is unrevealing, the investigation should be expanded to the small intestine with enteroscopy or radiography (see Figure 5–5). Enteroscopy, either "push" or "Sonde," is an important component of the initial evaluation for patients with obscure gastrointestinal bleeding.

Push enteroscopy denotes peroral insertion of a specialized long, flexible endoscope (or sometimes a standard pediatric colonoscope). Under moderate sedation, the enteroscope can be passed to the proximal jejunum, usually at least 50 to 60 cm beyond the ligament of Treitz. In clinical trials, push enteroscopy identifies a bleeding source in 24–75% of patients with obscure bleeding, although such high yield is not reported in clinical practice. Push enteroscopy is safe, widely avail-

able, and affords the opportunity for cauterization of vascular ectasias and biopsy of mucosal abnormalities.

Sonde enteroscopy involves placement of a long, small-caliber endoscope into the proximal small bowel. With time, subsequent peristalsis carries the endoscope to the distal small intestine. Subsequent withdrawal of the enteroscope permits visualization of much of the small bowel, leading to new diagnoses in a significant number of cases. Sonde enteroscopy requires a specialized instrument and operator expertise, and it is not widely available. Further, the instrument lacks a working channel; therefore, it does not afford biopsy or cautery therapy of bleeding lesions. Currently, its use is limited to centers of expertise and to patients with negative push enteroscopy.

Intraoperative enteroscopy permits visualization of most or all of the small intestine with an enteroscope (or standard colonoscope) that is manually advanced through the small bowel during laparotomy. This technique has been reported to detect abnormalities, which may be resected or cauterized, in up to 70–100% of patients. Unfortunately, this invasive technique does not always prevent recurrent bleeding.

A new, conceptually simple, approach to examine the small intestine is the use of a wireless imaging capsule. After demonstration of feasibility in animal models, wireless capsule endoscopy has been performed safely in humans. Its accuracy in the identication of small bowel bleeding sites is not established. An important limitation of capsule imaging is the inability to administer therapy of abnormal lesions.

An additional diagnostic approach in obscure bleeding is to provoke bleeding by administering vasodilators, anticoagulants, and/or thrombolytics and subsequently performing tagged RBC scintigraphy or visceral angiography. The diagnostic yield of this procedure is on the order of 20–40%. Although conceptually attractive, it must be emphasized that this is a highly specialized and potentially dangerous undertaking.

Small bowel radiography is of value in the identification of mass lesions of the small intestine beyond the reach of push enteroscopy. Standard small bowel radiography (or "barium meal" studies) are often inadequate to evaluate the distal small intestine. Enteroclysis effectively detects mass lesions of the small intestine but is inaccurate for the identification of mucosal lesions, particularly vascular ectasias. Because vascular ectasias are a major cause of obscure bleeding, enteroclysis is best reserved for those in whom the clinical suspicion of a mass lesion or small bowel diverticula is high and those who have negative push enteroscopy but persistent bleeding.

Diagnosis & Treatment of Specific Lesions

A. SMALL INTESTINAL VASCULAR ECTASIAS

Vascular ectasias, or angiodysplasias, are a common cause of obscure gastrointestinal bleeding that may be found in the upper gastrointestinal tract, small bowel, and colon. Patients with bleeding vascular ectasia may present with bright red blood, melena, or iron deficiency anemia, depending on the site of and rapidity of bleeding. The pathogenesis of vascular ectasias is unknown, but is probably linked to aging, as they are most commonly identified in elderly patients, over two-thirds of whom are over the age of 70. It is believed that repeated, partial, intermittent obstruction of the submucosal veins where they pierce the muscle layers of the colon leads to dilation and tortuosity of submucosal veins. Subsequently, the arteriolar-capillary-venular unit dilates, creating a small arteriovenous communication. Patients with bleeding vascular ectasias often have underlying chronic medical conditions, in particular renal failure. An association between vascular ectasias and aortic valve disease has been proposed (ie, "Williams syndrome"), but is dubious.

The role of therapeutic endoscopy in patients with vascular ectasias remains controversial. Endoscopic therapy may be successful for vascular ectasias localized to the stomach, duodenum, or colon, however, vascular ectasias often are multiple in number or outside the reach of endoscopy. These features significantly limit the efficacy of endoscopic intervention. Hence, demonstration and treatment of putative bleeding vascular ectasia do not always lead to improved outcomes. Cauterization of vascular ectasias leads to an improvement in hemoglobin and a reduction in blood transfusion requirements in some but not all cases.

Mesenteric angiography is useful in cases of active bleeding in order to diagnose and treat bleeding vascular ectasias. Angiography successfully identifies lesions in a high proportion of patients, and affords definitive treatment with intraarterial vasopression or embolization.

Some patients have chronic or recurrent clinically significant bleeding that is suspected to be caused by vascular ectasias that are outside the reach of the push enteroscope and colonoscopy but that cannot be identified by angiography. In some cases, intraoperative enteroscopy may be required. Intraoperative enteroscopy should be performed by an experienced endoscopist and surgeon. Although intraoperative endoscopy often identifes a "source of bleeding," surgical resection of these lesions does not always prevent recurrent bleeding. The reported rebleeding rates after intraoperative endoscopy vary from 20% to over 50%. Surgery is also required for patients with uncontrollable or hemodynamically significant bleeding. Surgical outcomes are best when resection is performed for a lesion that has been definitively localized to a specific portion of the gastrointestinal tract either by angiography or intraoperative endoscopy.

Medical therapy has been advocated for the treatment of obscure bleeding believed to be due to vascular ectasia. The pharmacologic compounds most widely utilized include estrogen/progesterone compounds. The mechanism by which these compounds prevent vascular ectasia bleeding is unknown, but may be related to enhanced clotting. The reported experience with estrogen/progesterone compounds has been conflicting. In a longitudinal study of 43 patients with proven or presumed vascular ectasias, treatment with Ortho-Novum 1/50 twice daily (1 mg of norethindrone and 0.05 mg of mestranol) for a mean of 535 days (range 25–1551) led to cessation of rebleeding in 38 patients receiving combination treatmen but in none of the five patients who received estrogen alone. Side effects of combination hormonal therapy include breast tenderness and vaginal bleeding in women and gynecomastia and loss of libido in men, leading to cessation of therapy in a significant proportion of patients. Notwithstanding the success reported in open treatment trials, small randomized controlled trials using estrogen/progesterone compounds have failed to demonstrate their effectiveness for prevention of bleeding from vascular ectasias.

Other pharmacologic agents, such as octreotide, aminocaproic acid, tranexamic acid, and danazol, have been reported to be effective for treatment of diffuse gastrointestinal and small bowel vascular ectasias. However, few controlled data support their use.

B. SMALL INTESTINAL MASS LESIONS

Neoplasms of the small intestine are an uncommon, but important potential cause of obscure gastrointestinal bleeding. A number of different benign and malignant tumors have been reported to cause bleeding. The most common benign tumors of the small intestine are leiomyomas. The most common malignant tumors are adenomas, adenocarcinomas, carcinoids, lymphomas, and sarcomas.

Evaluation of the small bowel with enteroscopy or radiography can identify mass lesions in most cases, however, exploratory laparotomy often is required to establish a specific histologic diagnosis. Management of small intestinal tumors depends on the primary diagnosis, but surgical resection is typically warranted.

C. AORTOENTERIC FISTULA

Aortoenteric fistulas are rare, but important, lesions responsible for upper and/or obscure gastrointestinal bleeding. They typically occur within 3 to 5 years after aortoiliac graft surgery in 0.5% of patients. Primary aortoenteric fistulas (ie, those arising in patients without prior vascular surgery) also have been reported. Aortoenteric fistulas typically involve the third portion of the duodenum as it crosses the abdominal aorta, but may involve other portions of the gastrointestinal tract. The fistula is believed to arise in most cases from subtle infection of the graft and perigraft area. Symptoms and signs of subacute infection (constitutional symptoms, low-grade fever, leukocytosis) in the appropriate clinical setting raise the likelihood of aortoenteric fistula.

The typical presentation is of upper gastrointestinal bleeding, which often occurs as a "herald" bleed that stops, but is followed within 1 or 2 weeks by massive, often fatal, bleeding. A high index of suspicion with the initial bleeding episode is required to make the diagnosis. All patients with previous aortic surgery and upper gastrointestinal bleeding should undergo esophagogastroduodenoscopy to examine the distal portion of the duodenum and to exclude other obvious causes of upper gastrointestinal bleeding. If the duodenum appears normal, abdominal computed tomography still may demonstrate periaortic inflammation and phlegmon, consistent with infection and suggestive of aortoenteric fistula. Angiography is rarely helpful.

Definitive therapy typically requires extensive vascular reconstructive surgery. The prognosis of patients with aortoenteric fistula has been historically poor (over 50% mortality rate), but because of increased recognition leading to earlier diagnosis, the prognosis appears to be improving.

D. HEMOBILIA

Hemobilia is due to hemorrhage into the biliary tract, most commonly caused by trauma, liver biopsy, gallstones, hepatic artery or portal venous aneurysms, liver abscess, and neoplasms. The most common cause of hemobilia is blunt or iatrogenic trauma. A high index of suspicion is necessary to make the diagnosis. The diagnosis is made either by visualizing blood emanating from the ampulla of Vater, and/or by angiography. Angiographic treatment with embolization may be effective, but surgical ligation of the hepatic feeding vessel is often required. Mortality from hemobilia is high, usually caused by other comorbid conditions.

D. HEMOSUCCUS PANCREATICUS

Hemosuccus pancreaticus is defined as bleeding from peripancreatic blood vessels into a pancreatic duct. Hemorrhage is most often caused by chronic pancreatitis with erosion of a pseudocyst into the splenic or a peripancreatic artery or formation of an arterial aneurysm that subsequently communicates with the pancreatic duct. The diagnosis may be made by endoscopic visualization of blood emanating from the papilla. A high index of suspicion, including a history of chronic pancreatitis, is required. Angiography is required to definitively identify the bleeding site, and may be used to administer therapeutic embolization. Surgery is often required to provide definitive control of bleeding.

SUMMARY

Occult gastrointestinal bleeding is the most common form of gastrointestinal bleeding. Its most common manifestation is occult blood in the stool, usually detected by guaiac-based fecal occult blood tests. Occult gastrointestinal bleeding may also present as iron deficiency anemia, which often results from chronic low-grade occult gastrointestinal bleeding. The approach to evaluation of patients with fecal occult blood and iron deficiency anemia is similar, and usually should begin with investigation of the colon. Colonoscopy is preferred, but flexible sigmoidoscopy plus air contrast barium enema may be an acceptable alternative. If evaluation of the colon does not reveal a bleeding site, evaluation of the upper gastrointestinal tract should be considered, and is required in patients with iron deficiency anemia. The role of small bowel investigation is controversial, and is best reserved for patients with iron deficiency anemia and persistent gastrointestinal symptoms or those who fail to respond to appropriate therapy. Celiac sprue should be considered as a potential cause of iron deficiency anemia in certain epidemiologic groups. The treatment and prognosis of patients with occult blood in the stool and/or iron deficiency anemia depend on the gastrointestinal tract abnormalities identified. Those without identifiable bleeding sites generally respond to conservative management and have a favorable prognosis. Patients with refractory iron deficiency anemia or clinically apparent but obscure bleeding make up a small fraction of all patients with gastrointestinal bleeding, but represent a considerable diagnostic and therapeutic challenge. These patients should undergo enteroscopic evaluation of the small bowel. In certain circumstances other diagnostic studies are indicated, including barium enteroclysis, mesenteric angiography, and abdominal computed tomography. Persistent or refractory occult or obscure bleeding is most commonly caused by multiple small intestinal vascular ectasias, the management of which is extremely difficult. Care for this group of patients requires a focused and experienced team approach.

REFERENCES

Allison JE et al: A comparison of fecal occult-blood tests for colorectal-cancer screening. N Engl J Med 1996;334:155.

Appleyard M et al: A randomized trial comparing wireless capsule endoscopy with push enteroscopy for the detection of small-bowel lesions. Gastroenterology 2000;119:1431.

Askin MP, Lewis BS: Push enteroscopic cauterization: long-term follow-up of 83 patients with bleeding small intestinal angiodysplasia [see comments]. Gastrointest Endosc 1996;43:580.

Barkin JS, Ross BS: Medical therapy for chronic gastrointestinal bleeding of obscure origin. Am J Gastroenterol 1998;93:1250.

Bergqvist D et al: Secondary aortoenteric fistulae—changes from 1973 to 1993. Eur J Vasc Endovasc Surg 1996;11:425.

Bini EJ, Micale PL, Weinshel EH: Evaluation of the gastrointestinal tract in premenopausal women with iron deficiency anemia [see comments]. Am J Med 1998;105:281.

Bini EJ et al: Is upper gastrointestinal endoscopy indicated in asymptomatic patients with a positive fecal occult blood test and negative colonoscopy? Am J Med 1999;106:613.

Bini EJ, Rajapaksa RC, Weinshel EH: The findings and impact of nonrehydrated guaiac examination of the rectum (FINGER) study: a comparison of 2 methods of screening for colorectal cancer in asymptomatic average-risk patients. Arch Intern Med 1999;159:2022.

Blackshear JL et al: Fecal hemoglobin excretion in elderly patients with atrial fibrillation: combined aspirin and low-dose warfarin vs conventional warfarin therapy. Arch Intern Med 1996;156:658.

Blanchard DK et al: Tumors of the small intestine. World J Surg 2000;24:421.

Bloomfeld RS et al: Provocative angiography in patients with gastrointestinal hemorrhage of obscure origin. Am J Gastroenterol 2000;95:2807.

Burt RW: Colon cancer screening [In Process Citation]. Gastroenterology 2000;119:837.

Chak A et al: Enteroscopy for the initial evaluation of iron deficiency. Gastrointest Endosc 1998;47:144.

Chak A et al: Diagnostic and therapeutic impact of push enteroscopy: analysis of factors associated with positive findings. Gastrointest Endosc 1998;47:18.

Eisner MS, Lewis JH: Diagnostic yield of a positive fecal occult blood test found on digital rectal examination. Does the finger count? [see comments]. Arch Intern Med 1991;151:2180.

Fenlon HM et al: A comparison of virtual and conventional colonoscopy for the detection of colorectal polyps. N Engl J Med 1999;341:1496.

Fine KD: The prevalence of occult gastrointestinal bleeding in celiac sprue [see comments]. N Engl J Med 1996;334:1163.

Geller AJ et al: The high frequency of upper gastrointestinal pathology in patients with fecal occult blood and colon polyps. Am J Gastroenterol 1993;88:1184.

Gordon RL et al: Selective arterial embolization for the control of lower gastrointestinal bleeding. Am J Surg 1997;174:24.

Gordon S, Bensen S, Smith R: Long-term follow-up of older patients with iron deficiency anemia after a negative GI evaluation. Am J Gastroenterol 1996;91:885.

Greenberg PD, Cello JP, Rockey DC: Asymptomatic chronic gastrointestinal blood loss in patients taking aspirin or warfarin for cardiovascular disease [see comments]. Am J Med 1996;100:598.

Hardcastle JD et al: Randomised controlled trial of faecal-occult-blood screening for colorectal cancer. Lancet 1996;348:1472.

Iddan G et al: Wireless capsule endoscopy. Nature 2000;405:417.

Kewenter J et al: The yield of flexible sigmoidoscopy and double-contrast barium enema in the diagnosis of neoplasms in the large bowel in patients with a positive Hemoccult test [see comments]. Endoscopy 1995;27:159.

Kronborg O et al: Randomised study of screening for colorectal cancer with faecal-occult-blood test. Lancet 1996;348:1467.

Landi B et al: Diagnostic yield of push-type enteroscopy in relation to indication. Gut 1998;42:421.

Lee JG et al: Serious gastrointestinal pathology found in patients with serum ferritin values <50 ng/ml. Am J Gastroenterol 1998;93:772.

Levin B, Hess K, Johnson C: Screening for colorectal cancer. A comparison of 3 fecal occult blood tests. Arch Intern Med 1997;157:970.

Lewis MP, Khoo DE, Spencer J: Value of laparotomy in the diagnosis of obscure gastrointestinal haemorrhage. Gut 1995;37:187.

Looker AC et al: Prevalence of iron deficiency in the United States. JAMA 1997;277:973.

Malden ES et al: Recurrent gastrointestinal bleeding: use of thrombolysis with anticoagulation in diagnosis. Radiology 1998;207:147.

Mandel JS et al: Reducing mortality from colorectal cancer by screening for fecal occult blood. Minnesota Colon Cancer Control Study [published erratum appears in N Engl J Med 1993;329(9):672] [see comments]. N Engl J Med 1993;328:1365.

Mandel JS et al: The effect of fecal occult-blood screening on the incidence of colorectal cancer. N Engl J Med 2000;343:1603.

Massey AC: Microcytic anemia. Differential diagnosis and management of iron deficiency anemia. Med Clin North Am 1992;76:549.

Nardone G et al: The efficacy of octreotide therapy in chronic bleeding due to vascular abnormalities of the gastrointestinal tract. Aliment Pharmacol Ther 1999;13:1429.

Ott DJ, Gelfand DW: The future of barium radiology. Br J Radiol 1997;70:S171.

Rex DK et al: Relative sensitivity of colonoscopy and barium enema for detection of colorectal cancer in clinical practice [see comments]. Gastroenterology 1997;112:17.

Rex DK et al: Colonoscopic miss rates of adenomas determined by back-to-back colonoscopies. Gastroenterology 1997;112:24.

Rex DK et al: Colorectal cancer prevention 2000: screening recommendations of the American College of Gastroenterology. Am J Gastroenterol 2000;95:868.

Risti B et al: Hemosuccus pancreaticus as a source of obscure upper gastrointestinal bleeding: three cases and literature review. Am J Gastroenterol 1995;90:1878.

Rockey DC: Occult gastrointestinal bleeding. N Engl J Med 1999; 341:38.

Rockey DC, Cello JP: Evaluation of the gastrointestinal tract in patients with iron-deficiency anemia. N Engl J Med 1993;329:1691.

Rockey DC et al: Relative frequency of upper gastrointestinal and colonic lesions in patients with positive fecal occult-blood tests. N Engl J Med 1998;339:153.

Rockey DC, Auslander A, Greenberg PD: Detection of upper gastrointestinal blood with fecal occult blood tests. Am J Gastroenterol 1999;94:344.

van Cutsem E, Rutgeerts P, Vantrappen G: Treatment of bleeding gastrointestinal vascular malformations with oestrogen-progesterone. Lancet 1990;335:953.

Vernava AM et al: Lower gastrointestinal bleeding. Dis Colon Rectum 1997;40:846.

Wilcox CM, Alexander LN, Clark WS: Prospective evaluation of the gastrointestinal tract in patients with iron deficiency and no systemic or gastrointestinal symptoms or signs. Am J Med 1997;103:405.

Winawer SJ et al: Colorectal cancer screening: clinical guidelines and rationale [published erratum appears in Gastroenterology 1997;112(3):1060] [see comments]. Gastroenterology 1997; 112:594.

Winawer SJ et al: A comparison of colonoscopy and double-contrast barium enema for surveillance after polypectomy. National Polyp Study Work Group. N Engl J Med 2000;342:1766.

Zaman A, Katon RM. Push enteroscopy for obscure gastrointestinal bleeding yields a high incidence of proximal lesions within reach of a standard endoscope. Gastrointest Endosc 1998;47:372.

Functional Gastrointestinal Disorders

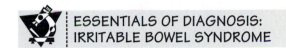

6

Nicholas J. Talley, MD, PhD

GENERAL CONSIDERATIONS

A large group of patients seen by primary care providers and gastroenterologists present with chronic or recurrent gastrointestinal symptoms that defy explanation despite structural (radiographic or endoscopic) and biochemical studies. These patients are generally labeled as having a *functional gastrointestinal disorder.* Up to 50% of outpatients referred to gastroenterologists ultimately are given this diagnosis.

A revised classification of functional gastrointestinal disorders (known as the *Rome II Criteria*) has been developed by an international group of clinical investigators. In this classification, symptoms attributable to disordered function in the oropharynx, esophagus, stomach, small or large bowel, anorectum, or biliary tree have been proposed to make up different functional disorders based upon clinical experience and epidemiologic data (Table 6–1).

The functional gastrointestinal disorders are important because they may be easily misdiagnosed and can cause considerable morbidity. Moreover, they are costly to society, not only in terms of medical expenditures but in time lost from work. Work absenteeism in persons with functional bowel complaints is double that of the general population; in one large survey, persons with functional symptoms missed an average of 9 days of work annually and those with irritable bowel syndrome missed over 13.

The best recognized functional gastrointestinal disorder is the irritable bowel syndrome (IBS), which is characterized by chronic or recurrent abdominal pain associated with disturbed defecation and, often, bloating. This chapter deals mainly with this prototypical functional disorder, however, much of the information is pertinent to all functional gastrointestinal disorders. Functional gastroduodenal disorders are addressed in another chapter.

ESSENTIALS OF DIAGNOSIS: IRRITABLE BOWEL SYNDROME

- *Abdominal pain associated with disturbed defecation.*
- *Abdominal pain relieved by defecation.*
- *Stools looser or more frequent at onset of pain.*
- *Stools harder or less frequent at onset of pain.*
- *Feelings of incomplete rectal evacuation.*
- *Mucus per rectum.*
- *Bloating or visible abdominal distention.*
- *Sigmoidoscopy and routine blood testing normal; further tests dependent upon clinical setting.*

Epidemiology

Functional gastrointestinal disorders are common even among otherwise healthy persons. At least one-third of adults have symptoms compatible with a functional gastrointestinal syndrome (Table 6–1). The worldwide prevalence of IBS is 10–20%, a rate that tends to be stable from year to year (Figure 6–1). The prevalence is higher in lower socioeconomic groups, which may reflect unknown environmental factors. Although most patients continue to have chronic, recurring gastrointestinal symptoms, up to 30% become asymptomatic over time.

For unknown reasons, the reporting of symptoms slightly declines with age, perhaps because older people are less likely to report minor symptoms or because there are changes in visceral sensory thresholds with advancing age. Functional bowel symptoms nonetheless are com-

Table 6–1. The Rome II classification of functional gastrointestinal disorders.

Disorder	Approximate Percentage Prevalence in United States[1]
Funtional esophageal disorders	
Globus	1
Rumination syndrome	1
Functional chest pain of presumed esophageal origin	5
Functional heartburn (no pathologic acid reflux)	5
Functional dysphagia	
Functional gastroduodenal disorders	
Functional (nonulcer or idiopathic) dyspepsia	4
Aerophagia	3
Functional vomiting	<1
Functional bowel disorders	
Irritable bowel syndrome	9
Two of three criteria:	
1. Discomfort or pain relieved by defecation	
2. Discomfort or pain associated with a change in stool frequency (increase or decrease)	
3. Discomfort or pain associated with a change in stool form (loose or hard)	
Functional abdominal bloating	4
Functional constipation	3
Functional diarrhea	2
Functional abdominal pain	1
Functional biliary pain (biliary dyskinesia)	<1
Functional anorectal disorders	
Functional incontinence	
Functional anorectal pain	8
Levator syndrome	1
Proctalgia fugax	7
Pelvic floor dyssynergia	2

[1]Twelve weeks or more of symptoms in the prior year.

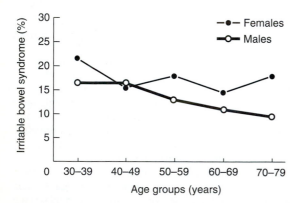

Figure 6–1. Prevalence of irritable bowel syndrome in a random sample of a representative county (Olmsted County, Minnesota) in the United States (*n* = 1163).

mon in the elderly, in whom they are more likely to be misdiagnosed or attributed to organic findings of uncertain significance, such as "symptomatic diverticulosis."

"Illness behavior" refers to the way people experience and cope with illness. Some ignore real symptoms while others misinterpret normal physiologic sensations as abnormal and seek medical care. Illness behavior may be learned. In one study, persons with IBS were more likely during childhood to have received gifts or remained home from school when they were sick than patients with peptic ulcer disease. Those with functional bowel symptoms are also more likely to see a physician for non-gastrointestinal complaints; this may reflect a general tendency to report symptoms (perhaps related to widespread abnormalities of visceral sensory thresholds or somatization), excessive health care seeking behavior (perhaps learned in childhood), or a combination of both.

Women tend to report more functional gut symptoms than men and are more likely to be diagnosed with

IBS in Western nations. It has been postulated that this gender difference is culturally related, since in some countries (eg, India) more men than women present with complaints consistent with IBS.

It is important to note that only a minority with functional gut symptoms—only 15–50% of adults with IBS—ever consult a physician. In evaluating the patient with chronic gastrointestinal symptoms, it is important for the provider to attempt to determine the reason the patient is seeking medical attention at this particular juncture.

Pathophysiology

Functional bowel disorders are characterized by symptoms that almost certainly arise from disparate causes. Several mechanisms may interact at any one time to induce symptoms (Figure 6–2). The evidence is clear that physiologic disturbances occur in the majority of patients, suggesting that symptoms are neither imagined nor the product of chronic somatization. However, a plausible disease model that takes into account all of the known abnormalities has yet to be derived, and none of the abnormalities is specific enough to be used as a diagnostic criterion. It is likely that both genetic and environmental factors contribute to symptom pathogenesis. The mechanisms identified to date that may be linked to specific symptoms in IBS are summarized in Table 6–2.

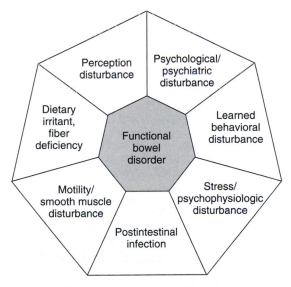

Figure 6–2. Potential mechanisms linked to functional bowel disease including irritable bowel syndrome. Therapy should ideally be targeted at reversing an individual's abnormal pathophysiology, but this remains largely impractical.

A. ABNORMAL VISCERAL PERCEPTION

Abnormal visceral perception may represent one of the key physiologic disturbances. Visceral sensory information is carried from the gut to the brain by vagal and spinal afferent nerves. In IBS, a subset of patients has a more "sensitive" bowel (rectum, colon, or small intestine) to distention compared with healthy control subjects. Increased rectal resistance and sensitivity to stretch or balloon distention has been found in the majority of patients with IBS. Furthermore, rectal hypersensitivity can be induced by repetitive high-pressure distentions of the sigmoid colon in patients with IBS (but not control subjects) who have normal baseline sensory thresholds. Whether increased gut sensitivity is due to an end-organ abnormality, increased relay of afferent inputs, or altered central processing is unclear.

Table 6–2. Pathophysiology of the irritable bowel syndrome.

Symptom	Putative Abnormalities
Abdominal pain	Increased responsiveness of colon and terminal ileum to meals
	Prolonged propagated contractions in terminal ileum
	Discrete clustered contractions in proximal small intestine
Constipation	Reduced high-amplitude colonic contractions
	Reduced whole gut transit
	Reduced ascending and transverse colon emptying
Diarrhea	Increased high-amplitude colonic contractions
	Increased feeding response
	Increased whole gut transit
	Increased colonic tone during fasting
	Increased ascending and transverse colon emptying
	Excess fluid secretin in ileum in response to bile acids
	Postinfection inflammation
Bloating/distention	Intestinal hypersensitivity (colon, small bowel)
	Inadequate gas expulsion
	Decreased ileocolonic transfer of chyme
	Not related to voluntary protrusion, lumbar lordosis, depression of diaphragm, failure of abdominal wall muscle activation
Feeling of incomplete evacuation/urgency	Rectal hypersensitivity

Visceral hypersensitivity in IBS is not explained by a generally low pain threshold. Studies show that functional bowel patients have normal thresholds for general somatic discomfort (eg, pain induced by immersion of the hand in ice water)—even those who have gut that is hypersensitive to balloon distention.

B. ALTERED GUT MOTOR FUNCTION

Although altered gut motor function previously was theorized to be of major significance in IBS, its importance presently is unclear. Abnormal colonic myoelectric activity (three cycles/min) was reported in the 1970s to be associated with IBS, but is now considered to represent either artifact or an epiphenomenon. Basal colonic motility is not altered in IBS, although the colon may be abnormally responsive to stress, cholinergic drugs, or hormonal factors (eg, cholecystokinin). Both small bowel and colonic transit may be disturbed and are correlated in some studies with the predominant symptom pattern in IBS (eg, fast transit in patients with diarrhea and slow transit with constipation).

Certain small intestinal motor patterns have been linked to the presence of abdominal pain in IBS. During periods of fasting, clusters of jejunal pressure waves occur in some patients with IBS that coincide with abdominal pain and disappear during sleep (Figure 6–3). Ileal propulsive waves associated with pain have also been documented in IBS (Figure 6–4). It has been postulated that abnormalities in sensory perception may induce alterations in local neural reflexes that in turn alter motor function in IBS.

C. EXTRAINTESTINAL MOTOR DYSFUNCTION

Extraintestinal motor dysfunction has been observed in the lung, urinary bladder, and gallbladder in IBS. These studies suggest that there may be a generalized abnormality either of smooth muscle or the nervous system. Extrinsic dysfunction could originate in the central nervous system or within the vagus nerve (which provides sensory and motor innervation of the stomach, small bowel, and proximal colon).

D. AUTONOMIC NERVOUS SYSTEM ABNORMALITIES

Vagal dysfunction and sympathetic adrenergic dysfunction have been documented in a minority of patients with IBS referred to specialist centers.

E. PSYCHOLOGICAL FACTORS

Gut function can be altered by acute stress or emotional factors. Coexistent psychiatric disease or a prior history of abuse or trauma may exacerbate acute psychological distress and, hence, bowel dysfunction in predisposed individuals.

It has been reported that 40–100% of patients with IBS have psychiatric disease, but this figure may be artificially high since these studies were based on patients seen at tertiary centers. A history of abuse (physical or sexual) is linked to chronic illness and multiple complaints. An

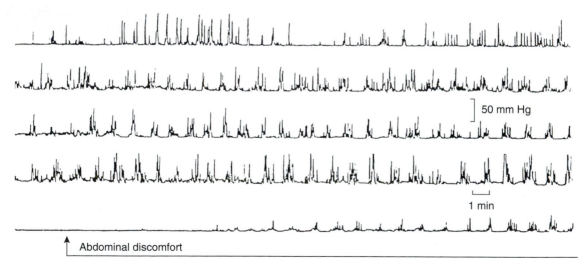

Figure 6–3. Fasting small bowel motility recordings in an irritable bowel patient. Note the clusters of contractions ("minute rhythm") associated with pain; this pattern is more frequently seen in irritable bowel patients than in control subjects. (Reprinted, with permission, from Kellow JE, Phillips SF: Altered small bowel motility in irritable bowel syndrome is correlated with symptoms. Gastroenterology 1987;92:1885.)

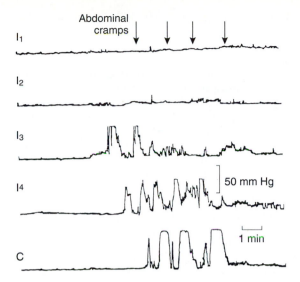

Figure 6–4. Motility recording from the terminal ileum (I_1–I_4) and cecum (C) in a patient with irritable bowel syndrome. Note the coincidence of abdominal pain with high pressure peristaltic waves propagated from ileum to colon. (Reprinted, with permission, from Kellow JE, Phillips SF: Altered small bowel motility in irritable bowel syndrome is correlated with symptoms. Gastroenterology 1987;92:1885.)

association between abuse and IBS has been found, both in medical patients and community subjects. In one study, 30% of female outpatients with IBS had a history of incest or rape. Those with a history of abuse are also more likely to suffer from psychiatric disease.

Persons with symptoms of IBS who consult for medical evaluation differ from subjects with similar symptoms who do not seek health care. Pain severity or the presence of other symptoms are poor predictors of consultation behavior. Studies have shown that those with symptoms of IBS who do not consult physicians have psychological profiles similar to asymptomatic persons; in contrast, those who seek care for their IBS tend to be more psychologically disturbed, or to have a history of a stressful life event or abuse. It is postulated that psychological factors infrequently cause functional symptoms, but when they coexist they probably enhance symptom severity and promote the seeking of health care. The excessive prevalence of psychiatric disease and psychological distress in patients with IBS likely is related to health care seeking and is not a cause per se of functional gut disease.

F. Diet

Environmental factors may potentiate or exacerbate functional symptoms. In susceptible patients, luminal contents such as sorbitol, fructose, and bile acids can induce symptoms, including diarrhea and bloating. Other dietary factors have been implicated in IBS, including deficient fiber intake and food intolerance, but convincing data are still lacking. In one trial, dietary exclusions followed by gradual, sequential reinstitution of foods induced symptomatic improvement in 50% of patients with functional diarrhea, providing some support for food sensitivity.

G. Infection

There is growing evidence that an acute, self-limited gastrointestinal infection may "prime" the gut, resulting in functional disturbances. A minority of IBS patients (10–25%) postdate the onset of their symptoms to a viral illness or travelers' diarrhea, and this association has been confirmed in prospective studies of acute bacterial gastroenteritis. A small but significant increase in rectal chronic inflammatory cells and enteroendocrine cells has been observed in postinfectious IBS. An excess of mast cells, which occur in close proximity to sensory nerves in the mucosa, has also been observed in the terminal ileum and colon of some patients with IBS, as has mast cell degranulation. It is likely that acute inflammation can permanently sensitize gut afferent receptors that sustain symptoms in predisposed individuals, even after the initial stimulus has disappeared and inflammation has healed.

Clinical Findings

A. Symptoms and Signs

A physician should strive to make a positive diagnosis of a functional disorder at the initial consultation. After taking a careful history and examining the patient, the experienced clinician can often correctly distinguish between a functional and organic disorder. The diagnostic tests should then be used to confirm the clinical impression. The physician should avoid the dangerous pitfall of pursuing a battery of expensive and invasive tests to exclude organic disease before applying a diagnosis of a functional gastrointestinal disorder.

Abdominal pain and disturbed defecation are characteristic of IBS, but these symptoms also occur transiently (Table 6–3) or chronically in a number of serious organic diseases (Table 6–4). The pain in IBS tends to be poorly localized, variable in nature, and may migrate around the abdomen. It is useful to remember that pain unrelated to defecation or pain induced by activity, menstruation, or urination is unlikely to be explained by IBS.

Bowel disturbance in IBS may be manifest by constipation or diarrhea, rectal urgency, feelings of incomplete emptying, or passage of mucus. Patients may use the term "constipation" to mean a variety of symptoms,

Table 6–3. Common causes of transient bowel symptoms.

Pregnancy, perimenstrual
Posthysterectomy
Dietary indiscretion
Travelers' diarrhea or constipation
Food poisoning, gastroenteritis
Bed rest or recent weight loss (constipation)
Nervous diarrhea (job interview, examinations, etc)

Adapted, with permission, from Heaton KW: Epidemiology of irritable bowel syndrome. Eur J Gastroenterol Hepatol 1994;6:465.

including infrequent defecation, straining with defecation, or incomplete evacuation. Similarly, patients may use the term "diarrhea" to refer to increased frequency of bowel movements (even hard or formed stools) rather than just to liquid or watery stools.

Specific symptoms help to discriminate IBS from organic disease. In a classic study from the United Kingdom, 15 symptoms were evaluated for their diagnostic value. It was found that four symptoms—relief of pain with bowel movements, more frequent stools with the onset of pain, looser stools at the onset of pain, and visible abdominal distention—were significantly more common in IBS, while two other symptoms—a feeling of incomplete rectal evacuation and mucus per rectum—tended also to occur more frequently (Table

Table 6–4. Differential diagnosis of chronic abdominal pain and bowel dysfunction.

Functional bowel disease
Drugs
    Constipation (eg, calcium channel blockers, antidepressants, aluminium-containing antacids)
    Diarrhea (eg, laxatives, antibiotics, magnesium-containing antacids)
Neoplasia (may be incidentally found in investigated patients)
Inflammatory bowel disease
Other types of colitis
    Infectious colitis
    Diverticulitis
    Ischemic colitis
    Radiation colitis
Psychiatric disease
    Depression
    Panic disorder
    Somatization
Intestinal parasites
    Giardia
    Stonglyloides

6–5). Of those with IBS, 94% had two or more of these six symptoms. These features, known as the "Manning criteria" (after the first author), have been confirmed to be of diagnostic value. The more symptoms that are present, the more likely is the diagnosis of IBS, especially in younger patients and in women. The Rome criteria, although more restrictive, have been shown to be highly specific for IBS.

Symptoms of gastroesophageal reflux are reported by one-third of patients with IBS. Other complaints frequently reported include headache, backache, fatigue, sexual dysfunction, and genitourinary symptoms. However, these features are not useful diagnostically.

"Alarm" (red flag) symptoms or abnormal findings on physical examination strongly point away from a diagnosis of IBS (Table 6–6). The physical examination in IBS and other functional disorders is usually normal, although there may be lower abdominal tenderness or abdominal scars. Localized abdominal tenderness that persists on tensing the abdominal wall muscles suggests abdominal wall pain (eg, from muscle strain, nerve entrapment, or myositis), which should not be misdiagnosed as functional pain. Local perianal disease or an abdominal mass argues against a diagnosis of IBS. Gynecologic examination can help to exclude pelvic inflammatory disease or endometriosis.

B. DIAGNOSTIC STUDIES

Selected investigations will help to exclude organic disease (Table 6–7). Laboratory tests are generally normal. Flexible sigmoidoscopy is not required for young patients with typical IBS symptoms who have no alarm features, but can be useful in some patients to confirm the clinical impression. In patients with diarrhea, sigmoid

Table 6–5. Discriminant value of symptoms identifying the irritable bowel syndrome (IBS) compared with organic bowel disease.

Manning Criteria	Organic (%)[1]	IBS (%)
Pain relief after defecation	30	81[2]
Looser stools at pain onset	27	81[2]
More frequent stools at pain onset	30	74[2]
Abdominal distention	21	53[2]
Mucus per rectum	21	47[3]
Feeling of incomplete rectal emptying	33	59[3]

[1]Percentage of patients with symptom.
[2]$P<0.05$.
[3]Trend toward significance at $0.05<P<0.1$.
Source: Manning AP et al: Towards possible diagnosis of irritable bowel. Br Med J 1978;2:653.

Table 6–6. Clinical features against a diagnosis of functional gastrointestinal disorder.

Weight loss[1]
Dysphagia[1]
Evidence of bleeding or dehydration[1]
Evidence of steatorrhea[1]
Recurrent vomiting[1]
Fever[1]
First onset in elderly patients
Symptoms wake the patient from sleep
New symptoms after a prolonged period
Progressive steady worsening of symptoms
Elevated erythrocyte sedimentation rate or C-reactive protein
Anemia or leukocytosis
Blood, pus, or excess fat in stool
Hypokalemia or persistent diarrhea during fasting
Stool weight > 350 g/d

[1]Alarm features (red flags).

biopsies may be obtained if the mucosa is normal to exclude collagenous or microscopic colitis, but the yield is very low. Colonoscopy should be performed to exclude colonic neoplasia in patients with IBS-like symptoms who are 50 years of age or older or have a family history of colon cancer; alternatively, flexible sigmoidoscopy and double-contrast barium enema may be performed. Lactase deficiency should be considered in patients with diarrhea and bloating or flatulence, especially Asians, blacks, Hispanics, Native Americans, and persons of Jewish descent. Either a 2-week trial of a lactose-free diet or lactose-hydrogen breath test may be performed. In patients with both IBS and lactase deficiency, withdrawal of lactose may not eliminate all symptoms.

C. DIFFERENTIAL DIAGNOSIS

In some cases, further testing is required to exclude organic disease. In patients with severe, refractory constipation who do not have a structural or metabolic cause evident from endoscopic, radiologic, and biochemical testing, it is important to consider two disorders: colonic inertia and outlet delay (pelvic floor dysfunction). Colonic inertia may be diagnosed using a radioopaque marker method. In this study, 24 radioopaque markers are ingested on three consecutive days. An abdominal radiographic flat plate is obtained on the fourth day; the total number of markers on Day 4 (multiplied by 1.2) represents the transit time in hours. Anorectal manometry, balloon expulsion, rectal sensation, and defecography are useful to detect pelvic floor dysfunction.

Severe diarrhea is not typical of IBS and also requires further consideration. A jejunal aspirate to examine for parasites and bacterial overgrowth may be worthwhile. Assessment of small bowel transit (eg, using breath hydrogen testing) or for bile acid malabsorption (eg, using ^{75}Se homocholic acid taurine) is of very limited value. A laxative abuser may present with apparent functional diarrhea but deny laxative use.

In patients with intractable pain or bloating, mechanical obstruction and intestinal pseudoobstruction need to be excluded by a radiographic barium small bowel study. Other diseases that should be considered in the differential diagnosis are presented in Table 6–4.

The presence of psychological distress is not helpful diagnostically. Many patients with organic disease also manifest psychological disturbances. However, it is important to screen for psychiatric disease, particularly depression (which may manifest by weight loss, sleep disturbances, and mood alterations), anxiety, and eating

Table 6–7. Laboratory investigations for suspected functional gastrointestinal disorders.

Representative Tests	Conditions Being Screened for
Recommended for all patients	
Hematology, ESR, and CRP[1]	Anemia, inflammation
Chemistry panel	Liver dysfunction, electrolyte disturbance
Thyroid function testing (optional)	Thyroid dysfunction
Recommended for suspected functional bowel and anorectal disorders	
Stool for blood	Bleeding
Flexible sigmoidoscopy (+/- biopsy)	Colitis, neoplasia
Stool/jejunal studies (microscopy, microbiology)	Infection (if diarrhea)
Colonoscopy or barium enema (> 50 years)	Colitis, neoplasia
Lactose tolerance test (optional)	Lactose intolerance
Colonic transit studies (optional)	Colonic inertia (if severe constipation)
Pelvic floor studies (optional)	Outlet obstruction (if severe constipation)
Stool/urine for laxatives (optional)	Surreptitious abuse

[1]ESR, erythrocyte sedimentation rate; CRP, C-reactive protein.

disorders. Panic attacks may accompany lower gastrointestinal symptoms; characteristically, these are discrete episodes of extreme fear or apprehension often accompanied by dyspnea, palpitations, chest pain, a choking or smothering sensation, dizziness, flushes, pins and needles sensation, sweating, or fainting.

Patients with somatoform disorder complain of a panoply of extraintestinal as well as gastrointestinal symptoms. Chronic pain syndrome patients have unexplained pain all of the time that is unrelated to defecation. Patients with these psychiatric diseases are extremely difficult to manage and should be referred when possible to a mental health program.

Principles of Management

The principles of management that apply to all functional gastrointestinal disorders are listed in Table 6–8. A step-wise approach to treatment is outlined in Table 6–9.

Patients seen in primary care practice often do not require drug or behavioral therapy. Patients referred to gastroenterologists tend to be more psychologically distressed and to be more difficult to manage.

A. Reassurance and Explanation

Reassurance and careful explanation of the epidemiology, pathophysiology, and natural history of symptoms in functional disorders are the most important aspect of therapy. The decision to seek health care may be influenced by the severity and type of symptoms, fear of serious disease, and psychosocial factors. The physician

should tell the patient that the symptoms are real, that they are common in the general population, and that will not lead to any life-threatening problems, such as cancer. The physician should explore the reasons the patient with chronic complaints has sought medical attention at this time. The patient may have fears of underlying disease (eg, the recent death of a relative with bowel or pancreatic cancer) that may explain the behavior and need specific attention from the physician. Changes in the patient's support system or recent life stresses may have led to symptom exacerbation or inability to cope with chronic symptoms.

It is important to avoid sending "mixed messages" to patients about the diagnosis of functional disorders. For example, a physician who states that serious disease is not a concern but who proceeds to order extensive and invasive diagnostic tests with little explanation may seriously undermine patient confidence. Providing an early positive diagnosis, spending time explaining the possible causes of the symptoms, and reassuring the patient about the benign prognosis represent a simple but effective form of supportive psychotherapy.

B. Precipitating Factors

Correction of precipitating factors, where present, can be therapeutic. Some patients may be helped by changing the diet (eg, eliminating lactose or known gas-producing foods in patients with diarrhea, flatulence, or bloating; increasing dietary fiber intake in patients with constipation), avoiding certain drugs (eg, excessive alcohol, caffeine, or sorbitol-containing gum), and reducing life stressors.

C. Diet

Dietary recommendations are particularly important in the treatment of patients with IBS. A high-fiber diet should be prescribed whatever the predominant bowel habit (although patients with constipation are more likely to benefit). A daily intake of 20–30 g of fiber is recommended, which is approximately double the amount in the normal American diet. The fiber content should be increased slowly to avoid increased bloating and flatulence. If patients are unwilling or unable to try such a diet, a commercially available fiber supplement (eg, methylcellulose, polycarbophil, or psyllium) should be started once daily and increased weekly by one dose per day until symptoms improve, or until a daily consumption of 5–10 g three times daily is achieved. Treatment with high fiber should not be abandoned unless it has failed to control symptoms over a 2- to 3-month period. If excessive flatus or bloating is a major symptom, an antigas diet should also be instituted. This involves avoidance of certain foods (eg, cabbages, beans, legumes, and lentils that are fermented in the colon), carbonated beverages, and foods containing sorbitol.

Table 6–8. Management principles in functional gastrointestinal disorders.

1. Make a positive clinical diagnosis based on the history and physical
2. Minimize invasive investigations and avoid giving "mixed messages," don't perform repeated testing without substantial indication
3. Determine the patient's agenda; ask why the patient with chronic symptoms has presented now
4. Provide education and firm reassurance
5. Try dietary modification
6. Set realistic treatment goals and center therapy around adjustment to illness and patient-based responsibility for care
7. Prescribe drugs sparingly, targeting the symptom(s) of most concern to the patient; remember the placebo response
8. Consider behavioral treatments or psychotherapy for moderate to severe cases
9. Organize a continuing care strategy

Table 6–9. Treatment of irritable bowel syndrome: A stepped-care approach.

Step	Severity	Clinical Picture	Management
1.	Mildly troubled/primary care	Fear of serious disease, anxious, worried, stress	Positive diagnosis Explanation Reassurance Dietary management Regular follow-up
2.	Complainer/secondary care	Uncertainty re: diagnosis; disturbed lifestyle	Reinforce above measures Stress management Target drugs to specific complaints
3.	Difficult/tertiary care	Coexistant psychiatric disease, possible secondary gain, disability, chronic pain	Avoid overtesting Low dose antidepressant Treat depression Treat anxiety Pain clinic

Adapted, with permission, from Drossman DA, Thompson WG: Irritable bowel syndrome: a graduated, multicomponent treatment approach. Ann Intern Med 1992;16:1009.

For constipation, adequate fluid intake and exercise may also be helpful.

D. Drug Therapy

Because the symptoms of functional gut disorders arise from a heterogeneous group of conditions, it is not surprising that drug therapy is often unsatisfactory. The placebo response is impressive in functional gastrointestinal disorders, ranging from 30% to 70% in controlled trials—even among patients who know that they are taking an inert pill. The large placebo effect may partly reflect the natural fluctuating course of functional symptoms that takes place in many patients. Patients tend to present when symptoms are worse, and may subsequently have spontaneous improvement. Patients may also be responding to the powerful influence of reassurance during the close follow-up that occurs in a clinical trial. Consequently, placebo-controlled trials are essential for determining whether a drug is truly efficacious in patients with functional disorders.

Unfortunately, most trials in this area have not been rigorously conducted. Systematic reviews of IBS studies have concluded that few trials provide convincing evidence of therapeutic efficacy over placebo. Drugs, therefore, should be used sparingly in most patients, and should be targeted at the major symptom or symptoms. It is useful to inquire whether a patient actually wants drug treatment; not all patients desire or need a drug after receiving firm reassurance, explanation, and general advice. It is also important to ask patients what they perceive as their dominant complaint; sometimes the answer is quite surprising. A bulking agent for constipation, imodium or cholestyramine for diarrhea, and an anticholinergic drug for postprandial IBS pain represent some examples of appropriately targeted drug treatment (Table 6–10). Although the risk of cathartic colon with stimulant laxatives appears to have been overemphasized, these drugs, although probably safe, often afford inadequate long-term symptom improvement in constipation-predominant IBS.

Experimental drugs that have been or are under evaluation for IBS include serotonin type 3-receptor antagonists (for diarrhea-predominant IBS), serotonin 4 agonists, and cholecystokinin antagonists (for constipation-predominant IBS), as well as selective antimus-

Table 6–10. Drugs for irritable bowel syndrome.

Predominant Symptom	Medication
Constipation	Bulking agent (eg, psyllium, methylcelluose, polycarbophil) Lactulose/milk of magnesia Polythylene glycol Enemas
Diarrhea	Loperamide Loperamide/simethicone Cholestyramine
Bloating	Simethicone Charcoal Lactobacillus
Flatus	α-D-Glactosidase enzyme with vegetable meals
Postprandial pain	Anticholinergic, eg, dicylomine, hyoscyamine (oral, sublingual)
Chronic pain	Antidepressant (see Table 6–11)

carinics, gonadotrophin-releasing hormone analogs, somatostatin agonists, and opioid agonists (for pain). However, their role is as yet uncertain.

Antidepressants may be particularly useful in patients with more persistent pain, resistant complaints, or impaired daily functioning (Table 6–11). Even those without associated depression may markedly improve. The mechanism of action is unknown, but central nervous system modulation of pain probably is important. Tricyclic antidepressants have been used most commonly for treatment of functional disorders. These agents should be started at a low dose and, if necessary, titrated upward; benefit is usually not apparent for 3–4 weeks. Side-effects are common and unpredictable, and a trial-and-error approach is required. If successful, treatment should be continued for 3–6 months before tapering the antidepressant and observing the clinical outcome. Although selective serotonin reuptake inhibitors have been used less commonly, they may also be considered. These agents should be used in full dose. Anxiolytics should generally be avoided, as they are potentially habituating, may interact with other drugs, and can induce a rebound effect on withdrawal.

E. Nonpharmacologic Treatments

Other approaches are of value in patients with persistent symptoms. Useful behavioral treatments include nonspecific relaxation therapy, hypnosis (which may reduce visceral gut perception and in controlled trials is beneficial in IBS), and biofeedback (most valuable in constipation with pelvic floor dysfunction). Psychotherapeutic approaches, such as cognitive-behavioral therapy (which usually includes anxiety management techniques and progressive muscular relaxation) and psychotherapy, are valuable, particularly in motivated patients whose complaints are exacerbated by environmental stressors or emotional difficulties. Patient support groups for IBS can be beneficial and patients should be made aware of their availability.

These approaches can all provide patients with a sense of greater control over their illness, promote healthy behavior patterns, and reduce anxiety. Least

Table 6–11. Commonly used antidepressant drugs in functional gastrointestinal disease.

Generic Name	Trade Name	Usual Daily Dose (mg)
Amitriptyline	Elavil	25–75
Doxepin	Sinequan	25–75
Imipramine	Tofranil	25–75
Nortriptyline	Pamelor	25–75
Trazodone	Desyrel	100 (divided doses)
Fluoxetine	Prozac	20–40 (morning)

Table 6–12. Reasons that patients with a documented functional gastrointestinal disorder seek health care.

1. New exacerbating factor (eg, side effect of treatment, dietary change, concurrent medical disorder)
2. New fear of serious disease (eg, death in the family)
3. Psychological or psychiatric comorbidity (eg, abuse, depression, anxiety)
4. Recent inability to socialize or work (eg, development of incontinence)
5. "Hidden agenda" (eg, laxative or narcotic abuse)

likely to respond are patients with unremitting pain and those who are resistant to the concept that psychological factors could be linked to their illness.

Prognosis

Prognostic studies have confirmed that once a diagnosis of IBS has been made, it is unlikely to be altered on follow-up. The physician should feel secure in making a diagnosis of functional gastrointestinal disease, which in addition, gives the patient the satisfaction of having a diagnostic label. The majority of patients continue to be symptomatic intermittently, but up to 30% will spontaneously become asymptomatic over time for unknown reasons. Follow-up of patients is therapeutic. Regular but brief visits are of particular help for those with unremitting symptoms. In such cases, it is essential to set realistic goals and help the patient to adjust to his or her illness; cure is not usually feasible but improved quality of life and better functional status can be achieved. If a patient with an established diagnosis returns unexpectedly, it is important to determine the reason (Table 6–12). Although the physician must be vigilant to a change in symptom status that may indicate the development of new organic disease, the physician should not yield to the patient's demand for testing in the absence of an objective change.

REFERENCES

Akehurst R, Kaltenhaler E: Treatment of irritable bowel syndrome: a review of randomised controlled trials. Gut. 2001;48:272.

Bennett G, Talley NJ: Irritable bowel syndrome in the elderly. Bailliere's Best Pract Res Clin Gastroenterol 2001;(in press).

Bytzer P et al: Low socioeconomic class is a risk factor for upper and lower gastrointestinal symptoms: a population based study in 15,000 Australian adults. Gut 2001;49:66.

Camilleri M: Management of irritable bowel syndrome. Gastroenterology 2001;120:652.

Creed F et al: Health-related quality of life and health care costs in severe, refractory irritable bowel syndrome. Ann Intern Med 2001;134:860.

Drossman DA, Thompson WG: The irritable bowel syndrome: review and a graduated multicomponent treatment approach. Ann Intern Med 1992;116:1009.

Drossman DA, Whitehead WE, Camilleri M: Irritable bowel syndrome: a technical review for practice guideline development. Gastroenterology 1997;112:2120.

Drossman DA et al (editors): *Rome II: The Functional Gastrointestinal Disorders.* Degnon, 2000.

Horwitz BJ, Fisher RS: Current concepts: the irritable bowel syndrome. N Engl J Med 2001;344:1846.

Jackson JL et al: Treatment of functional gastrointestinal disorders with antidepressant medications: a meta-analysis. Am J Med 2000;108:65.

Jailwala J, Imperiale TF, Kroenke K: Pharmacologic treatment of the irritable bowel syndrome: a systematic review of randomized, controlled trials. Ann Intern Med 2000;133:136.

Jones J et al: British Society of Gastroenterology guidelines for the management of the irritable bowel syndrome. Gut 2000;47(Suppl 2):1.

Koloski NA, Talley NJ, Boyce PM: Predictors of health care seeking for irritable bowel syndrome and nonulcer dyspepsia: a critical review of the literature on symptom and psychosocial factors. Am J Gastroenterol 2001;96:1240.

Levy RL et al: Irritable bowel syndrome in twins: hereditary and social learning both contribute to etiology. Gastroenterology 2001;121:799.

McKee DP, Quigley EMM: Intestinal motility in irritable bowel syndrome: is IBS a motility disorder? Dig Dig Sci 1993;38:1761.

O'Sullivan M et al: Increased mast cells in the irritable bowel syndrome. Neurogastroenterol Motil 2000;12:449.

Owens D, Nelson D, Talley NJ: The irritable bowel syndrome: Long-term prognosis and the physician-patient interaction. Ann Intern Med 1995;102:107.

Poynard T, Regimbeau C, Benhamou Y: Meta-analysis of smooth muscle relaxants in the treatment of irritable bowel syndrome. Aliment Pharmacol Ther 2001;15:355.

Ringel Y, Sperber AD, Drossman DA: Irritable bowel syndrome. Annu Rev Med 2001;52:319.

Schmulson M et al: Correlation of symptom criteria with perception thresholds during rectosigmoid distention in irritable bowel syndrome patients. Am J Gastroenterol 2000;95:2129.

Spiller RC et al: Increased rectal mucosal enteroendocrine cells, T lymphocytes, and increased gut permeability following acute *Campylobacter* enteritis and in post-dysenteric irritable bowel syndrome. Gut 2000;47:804.

Zighelboim J, Talley NJ: What are functional bowel disorders? Gastroenterology 1993;104:1196.

Inflammatory Bowel Disease

7

Thomas A. Judge, MD & Gary R. Lichtenstein, MD

Inflammatory bowel disease encompasses two distinct chronic, idiopathic inflammatory diseases of the gastrointestinal tract: Crohn's disease and ulcerative colitis. Although these two entities are frequently grouped together, it is important to appreciate the marked phenotypic differences between them, because these differences may have a profound impact on medical and surgical management. The incidence of Crohn's disease and ulcerative colitis in the United States is approximately 5 and 15 per 100,000 persons, respectively. There is evidence that the incidence of Crohn's disease has been increasing worldwide over the past several decades, although this rise appears to have plateaued over the past 10 years. The incidence of ulcerative colitis has remained fairly constant. The prevalence of these diseases, which is a more difficult parameter to measure, has been estimated at 90 per 100,000 persons for Crohn's disease and 200 per 100,000 persons for ulcerative colitis. The annual medical cost for the care of patients with inflammatory bowel disease in the United States is considerable and has been estimated to be $1.6 billion (1990 U.S. dollars) ($1.1 billion for Crohn's disease and $0.5 billion for ulcerative colitis). When adjusted for loss of productivity of patients, the total economic cost is estimated to be $2.2 billion. It is interesting to note, however, that approximately 2% of patients with inflammatory bowel disease account for 30–40% of the costs. These economic figures obviously do not address the personal and psychological toll of inflammatory bowel disease, particularly in patients with severe disease. Attention to the personal and psychological impact of this disease should be an important part of any treatment approach.

PATHOPHYSIOLOGY OF INFLAMMATORY BOWEL DISEASE

An in-depth discussion of the pathophysiology of inflammatory bowel disease is beyond the scope of this chapter. It is probably the result of the complex interaction of genetic susceptibility and numerous environmental influences. The pathophysiologic characteristics of Crohn's disease and ulcerative colitis are discussed together in this section for convenience only. The obvious phenotypic heterogeneity that is seen not only between Crohn's disease and ulcerative colitis but also

within subgroups of the two disorders (eg, pancolitis versus proctitis), underscores the theory that this is probably a clinically related but genetically diverse group of diseases. This genetic diversity most likely accounts not only for the variable clinical manifestations but also the variable clinical responses to standard medical treatments.

Immunologic Mechanisms of Tissue Injury

Inflammatory bowel disease is frequently referred to as an autoimmune disorder, but this appears to be a misnomer according to currently available information. In fact, there is little convincing evidence that there is an immune response directed against any specific self-antigen that would account for the inflammatory process observed in inflammatory bowel disease. There is, however, a large and growing body of evidence showing that there is an enhanced level of lamina propria T cell activation in patients with this disease (Figure 7–1). This notion is derived from a variety of observations, including increased expression of surface markers of T cell activation, increased production of T cell cytokines, and increased cytotoxic T cell function. This enhanced T cell activation leads to the recruitment of effector cells, such as neutrophils, and the subsequent elaboration of destructive substances, such as proteases and reactive oxygen metabolites. It appears that intestinal injury in inflammatory bowel disease is due to an "innocent bystander" mechanism as a consequence of enhanced nonspecific T cell activation rather than a directed attack against a self-antigen.

The trigger for T cell activation in inflammatory bowel disease is unknown. Animal models of colitis require the presence of enteric bacteria to initiate intestinal inflammation. There has been enthusiasm in the past for chronic mycobacterial infection as the underlying cause of Crohn's disease, but there has been no substantial support for this hypothesis. It is unlikely that a single trigger for T cell activation exists; it is more likely that mucosal T cells are activated by fairly ubiquitous antigens derived from enteric bacteria and their metabolic products. Underlying defects in mucosal immune function in patients with inflammatory bowel disease ultimately result in a state of perpetual T cell activation. The nature of these abnormalities in immune regulation is now the subject of

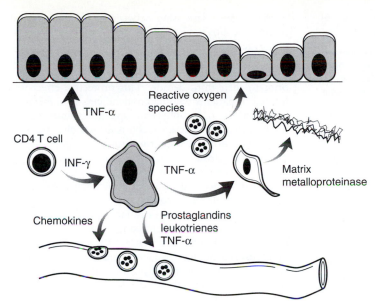

Figure 7–1. Pathogenesis of mucosal inflammation in inflammatory bowel disease. CD4+ T lymphocytes (activated by environmental antigens and enteric bacteria) stimulate macrophages within the lamina propria to release a variety of soluble proinflammatory mediators including prostaglandins, leukotrienes, chemotactic cytokines, and TNF-α. These bioactive agents enhance leukocyte recruitment and stimulate the release of potent tissue-injuring substances including reactive oxygen species and degradative enzymes from resident granulocytes, stromal cells, and activated macrophages that directly damage the epithelial cells and underlying mucosal tissues creating the ulcerations and edema that characterize these disorders.

considerable investigation. Potential sources of altered immune regulation include complex interactions among exogenous antigen, enhanced delivery of antigen (increased intestinal permeability), and a heritable propensity to mucosal immune dysregulation. The recent identification of NOD2 mutations in some families with hereditary Crohn's disease emphasizes the important relationship between mucosal responsiveness to enteric bacteria and the development of particular patterns of intestinal inflammation. It is plausible that additional variation in these factors and their interaction results in the variable expression of disease.

Other markers of immune dysregulation in inflammatory bowel disease appear to define particular disease phenotypes. Of special note is the description of antineutrophil cytoplasmic antibodies with a nongranular, perinuclear distribution (p-ANCA) in patients with ulcerative colitis. Their presence has been described in 60–70% of patients with ulcerative colitis and only occasionally in patients with Crohn's disease. Although p-ANCA does not appear to be involved in pathogenesis, its presence has been associated with the HLA-DR2 allele, whereas patients with ulcerative colitis negative for p-ANCA are more likely to be HLA-DR4 positive. This observation lends support to the notion of genetic heterogeneity within patients with ulcerative colitis.

Genetic Factors

Much of the evidence for genetic factors as a cause of inflammatory bowel disease is derived from family and twin studies. Although familial clustering of disease can frequently be explained by common environmental exposures, the finding of increased levels of concordance among monozygotic twins and discordance among spouses indicates a heritable predisposition. The age-corrected empiric risk of Crohn's disease for a first-degree relative of a patient with Crohn's disease is 5–8%, whereas that of a first-degree relative of a patient with ulcerative colitis is 2–5%. When rates of disease are compared in Jewish and non-Jewish families, the risk appears higher in Jewish families. An increased incidence of inflammatory bowel disease has long been reported in Jews, primarily in those of Ashkenazi origin. Given that Ashkenazi Jews living throughout the world have higher rates of inflammatory bowel disease than their geographically similar but non-Jewish counterparts, it is likely that Ashkenazi Jews represent a genetically predisposed segment of the population.

Twin studies further support the notion of an inherited susceptibility to inflammatory bowel disease. The concordance rates for monozygotic twins for Crohn's disease and ulcerative colitis are approximately 67% and 20%, respectively, whereas the rates for dizygotic twins are 8% and 0%, respectively. There have been no convincing reports that the risk of inflammatory bowel disease in the spouse of a patient varies from that in the general population.

Genetic analyses of families with high incidence of Crohn's disease or ulcerative colitis have identified several specific chromosomal regions with significant degrees of genetic linkage (Table 7–1). One such region, IBD1, contains the gene for NOD2, a protein that mediates recognition of bacterial products including

Table 7–1. Pathogenesis of inflammatory bowel disease: role of genetics.

Crohn's disease and ulcerative colitis are multigenic disorders; no single gene variant is sufficient to produce disease

Variations in genes from different pathways may generate a similar disease phenotype

Some disease-associated alleles may be specific for Crohn's disease or ulcerative colitis; others may be common to both disorders

Environmental trigger(s) are necessary for disease expression in susceptible individuals

---

lipopolysaccharide (LPS) by monocytes and macrophages. Point mutations in the 3′ LDD segment of NOD2 critical to bacterial recognition have been identified in over 10% of families with hereditary Crohn's disease (Figure 7–2). These mutations have also been described in normal control subjects who do not have Crohn's disease.

Environmental Factors

Higher rates of inflammatory bowel disease have been reported in urban areas than in rural areas. The disease also appears to be more common in higher socioeconomic status classes. It is possible, however, that living in a rural area and lower socioeconomic status are associated with more limited access to health care, and this leads to underreporting of incidence. It is interesting to note that this rural–urban disparity is observed in Sweden, where rural access to health care is excellent.

An increased risk of inflammatory bowel disease among users of oral contraceptives has been reported by several investigators in prospective and case–control studies. The relative risk of Crohn's disease and ulcerative colitis has usually been in the 2–3 range, although some studies have failed to show an increased risk. The mechanism by which oral contraceptive use may cause inflammatory bowel disease is not known.

An inverse relationship between appendectomy and ulcerative colitis has been suggested by several investigators. A recent large population-based analysis confirmed a significantly reduced incidence of ulcerative colitis in a cohort of patients who underwent appendectomy prior to their third decade. This protective effect was limited to patients who had appendicitis or mesenteric lympadenitis. As prophylactic appendectomies in patients with active ulcerative colitis do not alter the natural history of the disease, these findings would suggest distinct and possibly mutually exclusive patterns of intestinal inflammation in response to environmental stimuli in patients developing appendicitis and those who develop ulcerative colitis.

Another environmental risk factor that deserves special mention is cigarette smoking. There are now numerous studies that have consistently demonstrated a decreased risk of ulcerative colitis among smokers compared with nonsmokers. In addition, these studies usually show an increased risk of ulcerative colitis among former smokers compared with those who have never smoked. Meta-analyses have described a risk of ulcerative colitis among smokers as being 40% of that of nonsmokers. In contrast, cigarette smoking is associated with an increased risk of Crohn's disease. This risk applies to both current and former smokers, with a relative risk of 1.2–3.9 (current smokers) and 0.8–3.2 (former smokers). There is also some evidence that cigarette smoking may increase the likelihood of recurrence of Crohn's disease. The mechanism for the effects of smoking on inflammatory bowel disease is unknown. The increased risk of ulcerative colitis in former smokers is particularly interesting and unexpected.

Other potential environmental risk factors include diet and perinatal exposure to an inciting agent. Although food is the major source of nonbacterial antigen in the gut, no compelling dietary factor has been identified. The most consistent factor identified is increased consumption of refined sugars in patients with Crohn's disease, although the significance of this may be confounded by socioeconomic status. The occasional finding

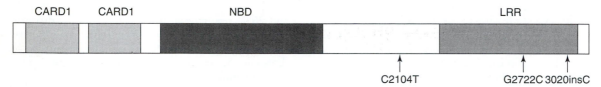

Figure 7–2. Crohn's disease-associated mutations of NOD2. Schematic depiction of the NOD2 gene product with putative functional domains. The allelic variants of NOD2 identified to date result in structural alterations of the 3′ portion of the NOD2 peptide, which includes a leucine-rich repeat (LRR) domain. The LRR physically interacts with bacterial lipopolysaccharide (LPS) to activate NF-κB. The frame shift mutation, 3020insC, results in a truncated peptide with marked hyporesponsiveness to LPS exposure *in vitro*.

of clustered birth dates among patients who have subsequently developed inflammatory bowel disease (primarily Crohn's disease) has led several investigators to hypothesize a common perinatal exposure to an inciting agent. There is some limited evidence of a greater than expected number of cases of Crohn's disease in individuals born at the time of a viral epidemic (eg, influenza, measles).

CROHN'S DISEASE

In the overwhelming majority of cases, the diagnosis of Crohn's disease is made on the basis of a constellation of characteristic radiologic, endoscopic, and histologic findings in the appropriate clinical setting. The combined radiologic and endoscopic appearances as well as the anatomic pattern of involvement form the basis of diagnosis. Histologic examination of biopsy specimens is useful in that it strengthens the diagnosis when the expected lesions are found and helps exclude other entities (see the following section, "Differential Diagnosis"). The diagnosis is rarely made solely on the basis of a biopsy.

The pattern of anatomic involvement in Crohn's disease is important and deserves special consideration. Crohn's disease may affect any portion of the gastrointestinal tract, but a few characteristic patterns of involvement account for most cases (Table 7–2). Approximately 40–50% of patients have involvement of both the terminal ileum and the cecum. About one-third have small bowel disease alone (usually of the terminal ileum), and approximately 20% have disease confined to the colon. Typically, the rectum is spared, and the pattern of involvement is often discontinuous, with intervening normal regions. The finding of discontinuous or "skip" lesions on colonoscopy or barium studies is characteristic. Overall, 75% of patients have small bowel involvement and about 90% of these have terminal ileal involvement. Crohn's disease may also involve the cryptoglandular structures of the anal canal (crypts of Morgagni) in up to one-third of patients, although this is especially common in patients with colonic involvement. Perineal disease alone is unusual. Involvement of the upper gastrointestinal tract (mouth, esophagus, stomach, and duodenum) is rare and almost always occurs in association with disease elsewhere.

Table 7–2. Patterns of involvement in Crohn's disease.

Pattern	Proportion at Presentation
Ileocecal disease	40–50%
Small bowel disease only	30–40%
Colon disease only	20%

Pathology

In patients with Crohn's disease, gross examination of the involved portion of bowel and its associated mesentery shows that they are thickened and edematous. Adipose tissue from the mesentery may be seen to spread over the serosal surface of the bowel, giving rise to the classic description of "creeping fat." Bowel loops are frequently adhered together or to adjacent structures. The gross mucosal lesion typically begins as an aphthous ulcer. As the disease process advances, these ulcers enlarge, deepen, and eventually coalesce to form transverse and longitudinal linear ulcers, giving rise to a cobblestone appearance. The base of these linear ulcerations may penetrate deeply, forming fissures in the underlying muscularis propria. This transmural penetration is the underlying mechanism leading to the abscess and fistula formation that frequently complicates Crohn's disease. Healing and fibrosis of these penetrating lesions may lead to stricture formation, another characteristic complication.

Histologically, transmural inflammation is the characteristic finding in Crohn's disease, as is a patchiness of the inflammatory infiltrate. Nonnecrotizing (noncaseating) granulomas are another characteristic but frequently absent lesion; thus, their absence is not helpful in excluding the disease. Although the presence of granulomas is probably a function of the diligence exercised in searching for them, they are present in only 60% of surgical specimens and 20% of endoscopic biopsy specimens. Even when granulomas are found on biopsy, their presence must be interpreted in the appropriate clinical context, as they may also be seen in association with gastrointestinal tuberculosis and sarcoidosis, *Yersinia* infection, and even disrupted crypts in severe crypt abscesses in ulcerative colitis. These granulomas in association with entities other than Crohn's disease frequently have a different appearance, and their specificity should be addressed by a gastrointestinal pathologist in cases in which the diagnosis of Crohn's disease is in doubt.

Clinical Findings

In most patients, Crohn's disease is characterized by intermittent exacerbations of disease separated by periods of complete or relative remission. A subset of patients has ongoing, persistent symptoms. As might be expected, the clinical presentation and findings are a function of not only the pattern of involvement but also the presence or absence of complications (see the following discussion). In addition, the clinical presentation can be divided into three general patterns that are independent of anatomic location: inflammatory, fibrostenotic (stricturing), and perforating (fistulizing) forms. Recognition of these patterns is valuable because flare-ups and postoperative recurrences of disease frequently tend to fit the same pattern for each individual patient, and the appreciation of these patterns provides a basis for a rational approach to treatment.

A variety of rating scales combining clinical and laboratory data are used to assess disease severity. These scales are cumbersome to use and serve primarily a research purpose. An overall assessment of severity is derived from the patient's complaints, impact of the disease on daily function, pertinent physical examination findings (eg, fever, mass), and the presence of abnormal laboratory parameters (eg, anemia, hypoalbuminemia). Attention to these parameters usually allows the clinician to categorize the patient as mildly, moderately, or severely ill.

A. Symptoms and Signs

The classic presentation of Crohn's disease is that of colicky right lower quadrant pain and diarrhea. Low-grade fever and weight loss are frequently present as well. High fever indicates a possible infectious complication (ie, abscess). Hematochezia occurs in a minority of patients, most often in those with colonic involvement. Patients with distal colonic involvement typically have more "colitic" symptoms, including frequent bowel movements, fecal urgency, and tenesmus.

Findings on physical examination may include signs of chronic illness and weight loss (eg, temporal wasting). The abdomen may be tender, most frequently in the right lower quadrant. A palpable right lower quadrant fullness or mass may be present; this typically corresponds to thickened and adherent loops of bowel, but may also be the manifestation of an intraabdominal abscess. A careful rectal examination may reveal evidence of a perirectal abscess, a fistula, or prominent skin tags representing healed perianal lesions.

The symptoms and signs of Crohn's disease are a function of the disease pattern. Patients with diffuse inflammatory disease of the small bowel may have an indolent presentation, with a prominent component of malabsorption and consequent weight loss and a less prominent complaint of abdominal pain. Patients with fibrostenotic disease may present primarily with complaints compatible with a partial small bowel obstruction, including diffuse abdominal pain, nausea, vomiting, and bloating. Physical examination may reveal distention and tympany. Patients with fistulizing disease may present with sudden onset of profuse diarrhea (due to an enteroenteric fistula), signs and symptoms of an intraabdominal abscess (eg, fever, localized tenderness), or cutaneous drainage (enterocutaneous fistula). Patients with enterovesicular fistulas may present with pneumaturia and recurrent urinary tract infections.

B. Laboratory Findings

In general, laboratory findings are nonspecific. Mild leukocytosis and thrombocytosis are frequently present. Anemia may be found. Marked leukocytosis suggests development of an abscess. The erythrocyte sedimentation rate (ESR) and C-reactive protein (CRP) are usually elevated. Hypoalbuminemia indicates disease severity and chronicity. Iron studies may reveal iron deficiency or an anemia of chronic disease. Serum vitamin B_{12} levels may be reduced secondary to ileal disease or resection. Stool studies may reveal leukocytes but no enteric pathogens. On occasion, bacterial overgrowth may also be present in individuals who have strictures or ileocolic resections, often resulting in vitamin B_{12} deficiency. Measurements of fecal fat may reveal steatorrhea if malabsorption is present.

C. Imaging Studies

Contrast radiography of the gastrointestinal tract provides valuable information in the diagnosis and management of Crohn's disease. Contrast studies of the small bowel allow documentation and delineation of the extent of small bowel disease. They are also useful in demonstrating and defining strictures and fistulas. Small bowel images can be obtained by a standard barium small bowel follow-through or by enteroclysis. Enteroclysis provides improved mucosal detail, but requires duodenal intubation for injection of contrast medium and air, which may be poorly tolerated by some patients. Characteristic findings of small bowel disease include "skip lesions," cobblestoning (owing to the intersection of transverse and longitudinal linear ulcers), and luminal narrowing ("string sign") and separation of bowel loops as a result of bowel wall thickening and edema. Computed tomography (CT) scan of the abdomen and pelvis is not a useful tool for establishing an initial diagnosis of Crohn's disease, but is crucial in the evaluation of complications related to the disease. It is the procedure of choice in determining whether an intraabdominal abscess is present. CT may also be useful in demonstrating enterovesicular fistulas or ureteral involvement by inflammatory masses.

Colonoscopy is the procedure of choice for evaluating the presence and extent of Crohn's disease involvement of the colon. Characteristic colonoscopic findings include aphthae (small shallow ulcers with a red halo), round or linear serpiginous ulcers juxtaposed to normal-appearing mucosa, "skip lesions," and rectal sparing. Biopsies of both affected and normal-appearing areas (particularly the rectum) confirm the variable and discontinuous nature of Crohn's disease. Colonoscopy also allows for intubation of the terminal ileum, allowing diagnosis of ileal disease, when present. For evaluation of colonic mucosal involvement, barium enema is inferior to colonoscopy, however it is superior for demonstrating colonic fistulas and strictures. Reflux of barium into the terminal ileum also may provide documentation of ileal disease. The presence of ileal disease is useful in differentiating Crohn's disease from ulcerative colitis.

Differential Diagnosis

The differential diagnosis of Crohn's disease is summarized in Table 7–3.

A. SMALL BOWEL AND ILEOCECAL DISEASE

Patients with ileocolonic Crohn's disease may have a relatively rapid onset of right lower quadrant pain, tenderness, and fever that is confused with acute appendicitis. The correct diagnosis may not be made except at laparotomy. Patients with ileocecal disease often report antecedent symptoms of pain and diarrhea preceding the acute worsening of symptoms. When the diagnosis of Crohn's disease versus appendicitis or periappendiceal abscess is in doubt, abdominal CT scanning may be useful. Other entities that must be

Table 7–3. Differential diagnosis of Crohn's disease.

Ileocecal small bowel disease
Infectious disease
  Acute appendicitis
  Cecal diverticulitis
  Pelvic inflammatory disease
  Ileocecal tuberculosis
  Yersinia enterocolitica infection
  Cytomegalovirus (immunosuppressed)
Noninfectious disease
  Celiac disease
  Ectopic pregnancy
  Cecal carcinoma
  Vasculitis (including Behçet's disease)
  Radiation enteritis
  Lymphoma or lymphosarcoma
  Eosinophilic gastroenteritis
  Chronic nongranulomatous ulcerative jejunoileitis
Colonic disease
Infectious disease
  Acute bacterial colitis (Salmonella, Shigella, Campylobacter)
  Amebic colitis
  Antibiotic-associated colitis (including Clostridium difficile toxin)
  Cytomegalovirus (immunosuppressed)
Noninfectious disease
  Ulcerative colitis
  Radiation colitis
  Ischemic colitis

considered in the acutely symptomatic patient include cecal diverticulitis, pelvic inflammatory disease (including tuboovarian abscess), and ectopic pregnancy. Menstrual and gynecologic symptoms, a pregnancy test, and pelvic ultrasound studies (using both the cutaneous and transvaginal views) aid in excluding gynecologic disorders.

Two infectious entities that may be confused with Crohn's disease are Yersinia enterocolitica and ileocecal tuberculosis. Yersinia may cause an acute self-limited ileitis. Diagnosis may be made by stool culture or serologic studies. Tuberculosis may cause ileocecal disease that is difficult to distinguish from Crohn's disease. In the United States, ileocecal tuberculosis is rare and frequently associated with active pulmonary disease. In immunosuppressed patients, particularly patients with acquired immunodeficiency syndrome (AIDS), cytomegalovirus may lead to ileocecal disease similar to that seen in Crohn's disease.

Other entities to consider include cecal carcinoma and gynecologic malignant tumors, particularly when there is a palpable mass. Celiac disease should be considered when diarrhea and weight loss are prominent symptoms.

Ischemic disease of the small bowel may resemble Crohn's disease and may be a result of use of oral contraceptives, radiation enteritis, or systemic vasculitis. A particularly interesting vasculitis is Behçet's disease, which may be associated with ileocecal disease that is virtually indistinguishable from Crohn's disease. Behçet's disease is usually differentiated by the presence of painful oral and genital ulcers.

Other rare entities included in the differential diagnosis of small bowel and ileocecal Crohn's disease include lymphoma, lymphosarcoma, eosinophilic gastroenteritis, and chronic nongranulomatous ulcerative jejunoileitis.

B. COLONIC DISEASE

In a small number of cases of Crohn's disease limited to the colon, differentiation from ulcerative colitis can be difficult (see the following section). Other entities included in the differential diagnosis of colonic Crohn's disease include acute colitis caused by bacterial infection with Salmonella, Shigella, or Campylobacter, colitis caused by cytomegalovirus or ameba, ischemic colitis, colitis associated with use of antibiotics (including Clostridium difficile colitis), or colitis resulting from radiation therapy.

Complications

A. PERFORATING DISEASE

A subgroup of patients has penetrating transmural disease that may lead to abscess or fistula formation. Free intraabdominal perforation is rare, due to the fact that the serosal surface of involved bowel usually adheres to adjacent structures.

Abscesses occur in up to 20% of patients with Crohn's disease and may be of an intraabdominal or extraabdominal type. The intraabdominal type is more common and may be located within the mesentery or between loops of bowel. Extraabdominal abscesses occur in the retroperitoneum and abdominal wall.

Fistulas result from the penetration of a sinus tract (presumably arising from a penetrating ulcer) into an adjacent structure, which may be a viscus or may extend externally to the skin. Fistulas complicate the course of Crohn's disease in approximately 40% of patients. They may be symptomatic or asymptomatic, depending on their course and physiologic consequences.

Enteroenteric fistulas are fairly common and may be asymptomatic or associated with high-output diarrhea, depending on the amount of gastrointestinal tract that is bypassed. Enterovesicular fistulas may present with pneumaturia and recurrent urinary tract infections. These fistulas may be well tolerated or associated with urinary sepsis. Enterocutaneous fistulas frequently arise from anastomotic sites after surgical resection or may occur *de novo*. Depending on size and location, enterocutaneous fistulas may have a low output or a high output associated with metabolic sequelae. Rectovaginal fistulas are usually the result of rectal or anal disease. Occasionally, enterovaginal fistulas occur, but these are seen most frequently in women who have had hysterectomies.

B. STRICTURES

Formation of recurrent strictures is the hallmark of the fibrostenotic variant of Crohn's disease and a common complication of Crohn's disease. Obstructive symptoms most often arise from fibrostenotic strictures of the ileum, but may be secondary to acute inflammation and edema, compression due to the mass effect of an abscess, or formation of adhesions. The typical clinical presentation of a stricture is caused by partial small bowel obstruction, which often resolves rapidly with conservative management. Patients complain of abdominal pain that occurs 1–2 hours after meals, loud borborygmi, and varying degrees of abdominal distention. More significant obstruction is manifested by severe pain, distention, and vomiting. Strictures are best demonstrated with barium studies, which usually reveal a narrowed segment of small bowel with dilatation of bowel proximal to the affected segment. Patients with strictures are at increased risk of developing bacterial overgrowth, which may lead to diarrhea and malabsorption. In patients with ulcerative colitis, the presence of a colonic stricture is worrisome for the development

of a colonic cancer. Alternatively, it may indicate that the patient actually has Crohn's colitis.

C. PERIRECTAL DISEASE

Perirectal Crohn's disease may result in anorectal fistulas and abscesses. Typically, the initial lesion is an abscess involving an anorectal gland located in the intersphincteric space. This abscess may extend along different tissue planes leading to cryptoglandular, perianal, ischiorectal, or supralevator abscesses or fistulas.

D. NUTRITIONAL DEFICIENCIES

Malnutrition from a variety of causes may complicate Crohn's disease. Patients may reduce caloric intake in an effort to minimize postprandial symptoms of abdominal pain, vomiting, or diarrhea. Extensive disease or resection of the ileum may lead to bile salt depletion with secondary B_{12} deficiency and fat malabsorption, which in turn may lead to deficiencies of fat-soluble vitamins. Unabsorbed colonic fatty acids compete for the calcium of dietary calcium oxalate. Dietary calcium oxalate is insoluble and excreted in the feces. However, as calcium–fatty acid complexes form, absorption of sodium oxalate is enhanced, potentiating the development of oxalate nephrolithiasis. In a small subgroup of patients, extensive jejunoileal disease results in a significant loss of absorptive surface and malabsorption of carbohydrates, proteins, and water-soluble vitamins. Multiple or extensive surgical resections may result in a short-gut syndrome.

E. OTHER CAUSES OF DIARRHEA

Diarrhea in Crohn's disease is not only caused by active intestinal inflammation but may also be the result of a structural consequence of Crohn's disease. Resection of the distal ileum (<100 cm) often results in moderate bile acid malabsorption and interruption of the normal bile salt enterohepatic circulation. Bile acids passing onto the colon cause electrolyte and water secretion. More extensive ileal resections (>100 cm) result in severe bile acid malabsorption that exceeds the hepatic synthetic capabilities of maintaining an adequate bile acid pool. This results in fatty acid malabsorption with diarrhea, which is further aggravated by bacterially hydroxylated long-chain fatty acids, which also induce water and electrolyte malabsorption. Patients with strictures and fistulas are predisposed to small bowel bacterial overgrowth, which also may cause diarrhea by disrupting bile acid enterohepatic circulation. Patients with fistulas may also have diarrhea if a significant portion of the gastrointestinal tract is bypassed.

F. CANCER

There is a clearly increased risk of small bowel adenocarcinoma in patients with Crohn's disease. Typically, these cancers arise in areas of long-term active disease. Segments of bypassed bowel may be particularly at risk. Although it has been estimated that the risk of small bowel cancer is 100-fold higher than in the general population, it should be noted that this type of cancer is rare in the general population, so the absolute risk is quite low. Among patients with Crohn's colitis, the risk of cancer is definitely increased. In patients with extensive colitis, the risk of developing cancer is as high as in patients with diffuse ulcerative colitis. Among patients with segmental disease, the risk is lower. Annual surveillance with colonoscopy is recommended in patients with Crohn's colitis.

Treatment

The goal of treatment in Crohn's disease is to restore well-being and an active life-style. A number of medications are available for the treatment of active Crohn's disease and for the maintenance of disease remission (Table 7–4). Although these agents may be beneficial, they also may have a number of serious side effects. Treatment of complications of this disease usually requires a joint effort by a gastroenterologist and a colorectal surgeon skilled in the management of inflammatory bowel disease.

Special attention should be given to the psychological impact of Crohn's disease. Although psychological factors have never been clearly shown to affect disease activity, they do have an impact on a patient's sense of well-being. Patients with inflammatory bowel disease may feel uncomfortable discussing their illness and symptoms even with close friends and family. Support groups and psychological therapies are an important adjunct to medical therapy (see the following discussion).

A. GENERAL APPROACH TO TREATMENT

1. 5-Aminosalicylic acid—Sulfasalazine has been the mainstay of treatment for both mild to moderately active Crohn's disease and ulcerative colitis for more than 50 years. 5-Aminosalicylic acid (5-ASA, or mesalamine) appears to account for most of the therapeutic effect of this agent. Sulfasalazine is 5-aminosalicylic acid that is linked to sulfapyridine by a diazo bond. When taken orally, 5-ASA is released primarily in the colon by the action of bacterial azoreductase (Figure 7–3). 5-ASA acts topically by a variety of mechanisms, including inhibition of synthesis of leukotriene B_4 (a potent chemotactic compound), impairment of phagocytosis, inhibition of interleukin-1 production, inhibition of NF-κB, inhibition of tumor necrosis factor-α (TNF-α), and scavenging of free oxygen radicals. At a dose of 3–5 g/d, sulfasalazine is moderately effective in the treatment of mild to moderate colonic and ileocecal Crohn's disease. Given its colonic release site, it is not surprising that this agent is no more effective than placebo in small bowel Crohn's disease. Side effects limit its use in a large proportion of patients (approximately 15–25%). Common side effects include nausea, vomiting, headache, rash, and fever. Some of these may be mitigated by a gradual escalation over 1–2 weeks to the full therapeutic dose of 1 g orally four times a day. Less common side effects include anemia, hemolysis, epidermolysis, pancreatitis, pulmonary fibrosis, and sperm motility disorders. Patients undergoing long-term

Table 7–4. Medical therapy for the induction and maintenance of clinical remission.[1]

	Induction of Remission		Maintenance of Remission		
	UC	CD	UC	CD (med)[2]	CD (surg)[2]
5-ASA	+++	+	+++	+/–	+/–
Antibiotics	+/–	+	–	–	+/–[3]
Corticosteroids	+++	+++	–	–	–
AZA/6-MP	+++[4]	+++[4]	+++	+++	+
MTX	+/–	++[4]	n.d.	++	n.d.
CSA	+++[5]	+/–	n.d.	+/–	n.d.
Infliximab	+[6]	+++[7]	+[6]	+++	n.d.

[1]UC, ulcerative colitis; CD, Crohn's disease; 5-ASA, 5-aminosalicylic acid; AZA, azathioprine; 6-MP, 6-mercaptopurine; CSA, cyclosporine A; n.d., no available data.
[2]Clinical remission induced by medical therapy (med) or surgical resection (surg) respectively.
[3]Short-term efficacy (~3 months) while antibiotics (metronidazole) are continued; effect absent at 1 year.
[4]Steroid-sparing effect also demonstrated.
[5]Small, uncontrolled series suggest efficacy in steroid-refractory ulcerative colitis.
[6]Data from preliminary studies (uncontrolled).
[7]Clinical trials performed in patients refractory to corticosteroids and AZA/6-MP.

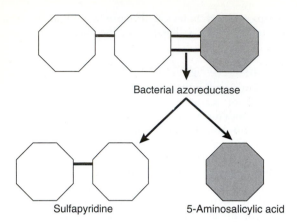

Figure 7–3. When taken orally, intact sulfasalazine is delivered to the colon, where bacterially derived azoreductase cleaves sulfasalazine's diazo bond, resulting in the release of the active 5-aminosalicylic acid moiety and the sulfapyridine carrier moiety.

Table 7–5. Oral mesalamine preparations.

Medication	Preparation	Release
Delayed release	Asacol	15–30% small bowel absorption
		Eudragit-S, coated Release at pH > 7
	Claversal Salofalk Rowasa	22–40% small bowel absorption
		Eudragit-L, coated Release at pH > 6
Sustained release	Pentasa	pH and time dependent
	Ethylcellulose microgranules	50% colonic delivery
Colonic release	Sulfasalazine 5-ASA bound via an azo bond to sulfapyridine	98% colonic delivery
	Balsalazide 5-ASA bound to an amino acid	>99% colonic delivery

sulfasalazine therapy should also be given folate, 1 mg/d orally, to prevent folate deficiency. Most side effects of sulfasalazine are attributable to the sulfapyridine moiety. This has led to the development of a variety of mesalamine (5-ASA) compounds that lack the sulfapyridine moiety.

Mesalamine in its native form is systemically absorbed in the proximal gastrointestinal tract and therefore is not topically available in the distal gastrointestinal tract. Delayed-release forms of mesalamine are coated in pH-sensitive methylacrylate (Eudragit). By adjusting the pH at which the methylacrylate dissolves, mesalamine may be released in the jejunum, ileum, or proximal colon. Mesalamine also is packaged in ethylcellulose microgranules, resulting in a time-dependent sustained release formulation that releases mesalmamine throughout the small and large intestine. Examples of delayed-release and sustained-release preparations are shown in Table 7–5. Asacol and Pentasa are available in the United States, whereas Claversal, Salofalk, and oral Rowasa are available in Europe. Two other compounds containing 5-ASA are olsalazine and balsalazide. Like sulfasalazine, both compounds have diazobonds that depend upon bacterial cleavage for colonic release of the active 5-ASA compound. Due to their release in the colon (not the small intestine), these agents are best suited for treatment of disease limited to the colon. Olsalazine is a 5-ASA dimer, and balsalazide has 5-ASA bonded to an inert peptide carrier (Figure 7–4). Olsalazine is approved for maintenance of remission only in ulcerative colitis. A side effect unique to

this agent is secretory diarrhea, which occurs in a significant minority of patients, limiting its usefulness in active Crohn's or ulcerative colitis.

Although Asacol and Pentasa are approved only for the acute and chronic treatment of acute ulcerative colitis, it can be seen from Figure 7–5 that their release characteristics have potential utility for the treatment of small and large bowel Crohn's disease. Although 5-ASA medications are effective in the induction of a clinical response of mildly to moderately active Crohn's disease, efficacy is less than for patients with acute ulcerative colitis. A variety of studies demonstrate that these mesalamine preparations have efficacy in both small bowel and ileocecal Crohn's disease, particularly when used at high dosages (4–4.8 g/d). The selection of a 5-ASA preparation is guided by the release characteristics of the drug and the distribution of disease in the patient. In general, these sulfasalazine analogs are well tolerated, with minimal side effects. Rare side effects include pancreatitis, nephrotoxicity, hair loss, and pericarditis.

Mesalamine is also available in enema and suppository preparations. Based upon largely uncontrolled clinical experience, these preparations may be efficacious for treatment of Crohn's disease involving the distal colon, rectum, or perirectal area.

Recent data suggest that mesalamine agents have limited efficacy for maintenance in patients who have

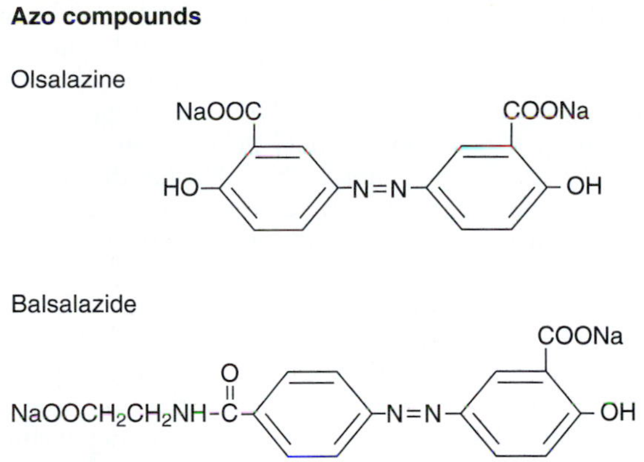

Azo compounds

Olsalazine

Balsalazide

Figure 7–4. Olsalazine and balsalazide are also diazo bonded and require degradation by bacterial azoreductase for the release of 5-aminosalicylic acid. Olsalazine is a 5-aminosalicylic acid dimer currently available in the United States. Balsalazide is 5-aminosalicylic acid diazo bonded to an inert carrier molecule recently approved for use in the United States.

achieved symptomatic remission from either medical or surgical treatment.

2. Corticosteroids—Corticosteroids have been the mainstay of medical treatment for patients with moderate to severe Crohn's disease. Their efficacy has been demonstrated in large cooperative trials performed in both the United States and Europe. Corticosteroids ap-

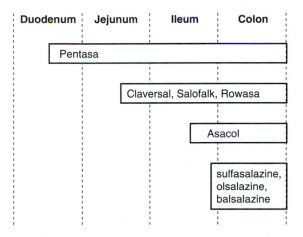

Figure 7–5. A schematic representation of approximate release and distribution sites in the gastrointestinal tract for a variety of 5-aminosalicylic acid agents that are either currently available or under development in the United States or Europe.

pear to act through a variety of mechanisms, including impairment of T cell function, impairment of chemotaxis and phagocytosis, and reduction of cytokine and eicosanoid synthesis. Most patients with moderate exacerbations of Crohn's disease achieve prompt remission with oral prednisone at doses of 40–60 mg/d for 1–2 weeks. Larger oral doses of prednisone are associated with significantly higher side effects without further improvement in clinical response. Severely ill patients with Crohn's disease should be hospitalized for exclusion of suppurative complications and treatment with intravenous methylprednisolone at a dose of 60 mg/d. Once remission is achieved, corticosteroids are converted to oral therapy and should be tapered at 5 mg/week increments over the next 8–12 weeks. Up to one-third of patients experience recurrent symptoms during the tapering period and require chronic corticosteroid therapy to maintain symptomatic remission. At doses less than 15–20 mg/d, slower tapering regimens (1–2.5 mg/week reduction) or gradual reduction of alternate day steroids may be required. Every effort should be made to avoid the long-term use of corticosteroids, however, because of their potentially devastating side effects. These include the typical cushingoid appearance ("moon faces"), cosmetic effects (such as acne), osteoporosis, hypertension, diabetes, psychosis, aseptic necrosis of bone, neuropathy, and myopathy. Patients should be treated with high dosages of 5-ASA compounds (eg, Pentasa 4 g/d or Asacol 4.8 g/d) in an effort to achieve some corticosteroid-sparing effect. The use of high-dose mesalamine has been shown to decrease the percentage of individuals who become steroid dependent but does not reduce the likelihood of having a future symptomatic flare-up. Crohn's patients with aggressive disease, disease that is refractory to corticosteroids, or disease requiring chronic corticosteroids to maintain symptom control should be given immunosuppressive medications. Use of immunosuppressants should be introduced early in the treatment course rather than after a prolonged course of high-dosage corticosteroids.

A potentially exciting class of corticosteroids introduced recently is topically active corticosteroids that have extensive first-pass hepatic metabolism resulting in diminished systemic effect. These agents include tixocortol pivalate, fluticasone propionate, beclomethasone dipropionate, and budesonide. These are available in Europe as enema preparations. An oral formulation of budesonide delivers the topical corticosteroid to the distal ileum via a delayed-release formulation, similar to that of delayed-release mesalamine preparations. Recent studies suggest that topical, oral budesonide may be as effective as systemic prednisolone in active Crohn's disease and may decrease the frequency of relapse. At recommended doses, budesonide is associated with minimal or no corticosteroid toxicity or suppression of the hypothalamic–pituitary axis. It has not been demonstrated to be effective for maintenance of medically or surgically induced remission. Recent preliminary data suggest that budesonide may promote corticosteroid withdrawal among patients who are dependent upon systemic corticosteroids. Further studies will be required to determine the role of budesonide versus systemic corticosteroids in patients with ileocolonic Crohn's disease.

3. Immunosuppressive drugs—The purine analogs 6-mercaptopurine and azathioprine play a vital role in the treatment of Crohn's disease. They are the drugs of choice for patients whose Crohn's disease is refractory to therapy with corticosteroids or requires chronic corticosteroid treatment to maintain symptom control. Purine analogs inhibit nucleotide synthesis. Their mechanism of action in inflammatory bowel disease is unclear, but may be related to inhibition of T cell clonal expansion. Azathioprine is nonenzymatically converted to 6-mercaptopurine following systemic absorption. Further metabolism in the liver results in the generation of 6-thioguanine nucleotide species, which are believed to be the agents responsible for clinical effectiveness. After absorption, azathioprine undergoes hepatic conversion to 6-mercaptopurine. These drugs therefore are used interchangeably, with the choice of agent largely dictated by physician preference and experience with drug dosing.

Although the effective dose of 6-mercaptopurine is frequently stated to be 1.0–1.5 mg/kg/d orally, recent studies suggest that optimal clinical response is achieved in those patients who achieve a 6-thioguanine level in excess of 235 pg/10^8 red blood cells (RBCs). The major limitation of therapy with purine analogs is their slow onset of action, resulting in a mean time to clinical response of 3 months, with full clinical response taking up to 6–9 months. Attempts to accelerate the time to clinical response through intravenous loading of azathioprine have not been demonstrated to be efficacious. However, recent studies from the Mayo Clinic suggest that nearly half of all patients receiving optimal oral dosing of either azathioprine (2.0–2.5 mg/kg/d) or 6-mercaptopurine (1.5–2.0 mg/kg/d) achieve a clinical response within 4 weeks. In practice, many patients initiate therapy at 50 mg/kg/d and the dose is escalated in 25 mg/d increments until either the recommended dose level is achieved, the desired clinical effect is observed, or significant leukopenia occurs. Data from a randomized, prospective trial have recently demonstrated that the induction of leukopenia in patients does not correlate with clinical efficacy, despite prior observations based upon retrospective data.

Patients should be fully informed of the toxicities of 6-mercaptopurine and azathioprine, which include marrow suppression, pancreatitis, hepatitis, and infections. Because of the potential for marrow suppression, complete blood counts should be monitored closely: weekly for the first month, biweekly for the next 2 months, and then monthly to every 3 months during long-term treatment. The risk of severe bone marrow suppression is particularly pronounced in 0.3% of individuals who are deficient in thiopurine methyltransferase (TPMT) activity. Measurement of TPMT activity or assessment of TPMT genotype identifies patients at high risk for toxicity from azathioprine and 6-mercaptopurine, however the role of TPMT testing in clinical practice is disputed. Pancreatitis occurs in 3–5% of patients, usually within the first month of therapy, and mandates discontinuation of the drug. Infections occur in 5–10% of patients, but severe infections occur in less than 2%. Of special concern is the theoretic risk of cancer in patients taking purine analogs. Lymphoma has been reported in renal transplantation patients taking azathioprine; however, there is little convincing evidence of an excessive risk of malignant tumors in patients with inflammatory bowel disease taking purine analogs. Patients should be made aware of this theoretic concern. Teratogenicity is also a theoretic concern, although no birth defects have been reported in children of patients with inflammatory bowel disease taking purine analogs. Although it may be prudent to avoid the use of these drugs in pregnant women and in women of child-bearing age who fail to use adequate birth control, the most significant risk during pregnancy is an active flare-up of Crohn's disease. These drugs therefore may be reasonable in pregnant women who require their use to maintain remission and in whom other less toxic medications, such as mesalamine, are ineffective. There are no controlled or uncontrolled trials assessing the efficacy and safety of these agents in pregnant patients.

Approximately 75% of patients treated with 6-mercaptopurine or azathioprine are able to eliminate or significantly reduce corticosteroid use. In addition, up to one-third of fistulas may close over a 2-year period of treatment. Because of their slow onset of action and the clinical setting in which they are used (for disease that is dependent on or resistant to corticosteroids), the purine analogs are usually used long term for chronic therapy or maintenance of remission. There is little rationale for using them for less than 4–5 years, as limited data suggest that the disease relapse rate associated with stopping the drug before this time is unacceptably high.

Other immunosuppressives have been investigated in the treatment of Crohn's disease, including cyclosporine and methotrexate. Randomized, placebo-controlled trials of cyclosporine have failed to demonstrate significant clinical benefit in active Crohn's disease. Furthermore, cyclosporine may result in severe neurologic and renal toxicity. Cyclosporine may be useful in the treatment of fistulas, although the relapse rate after discontinuation of the agent may be high.

Parenteral methotrexate (25 mg intramuscular injection once weekly) has been demonstrated to be effective both in the induction of clinical remission and in achieving a reduction or elimination of chronic corticosteroids. Unfortunately, there has been little study of the efficacy of oral methotrexate in either induction therapy or maintenance of clinical remission. The utility of methotrexate in the treatment of fistulizing Crohn's disease has not been evaluated to date in controlled trials.

4. Antibiotics—Metronidazole has been used extensively in the treatment of Crohn's disease. It appears to have efficacy in some subgroups of colonic and ileocolonic Crohn's disease, although there are few controlled supporting data. Metronidazole is widely used for treatment of perianal Crohn's disease, although controlled supporting data are lacking, efficacy appears to be limited, and recurrence is nearly universal once therapy is discontinued. Ciprofloxacin also has been demonstrated to be effective for induction of remission in mildly to moderately active Crohn's disease alone or in combination with metronidazole. Although other antibiotics, including clarithromycin, have been used in the treatment of Crohn's disease, there are few data to support their use.

5. Biologic agents—Research into the pathogenesis of Crohn's disease has demonstrated the importance of inflammatory mediators in the induction and maintenance of intestinal inflammation. One cytokine, TNF-α, is a critical factor in the mucosal inflammatory cascade associated with Crohn's disease. The introduction of anti-TNF-α therapies has dramatically affected the current treatment approach to patients afflicted with moderate to severe Crohn's disease.

Infliximab, a chimeric monoclonal antibody (75% human and 25% murine) directed against TNF-α, results in a rapid clinical response in 70–80% of patients with steroid-dependent or refractory Crohn's disease and leads to clinical remission in 48% of patients. The optimal dose of infliximab is 5 mg/kg administered as an intravenous infusion over 2 hours. Clinical response is maintained for 8–12 weeks in most patients. Side effects of infliximab therapy include infusion reactions, nausea, vomiting, fatigue, lupus-like reaction (anti-DNA antibodies), and the development of human antichimeric antibodies (HACA) against infliximab. The incidence of side effects is increased in patients with prolonged intervals between infusions. Concomitant use of immunosuppressive medications such as azathio-

prine or 6-mercaptopurine reduces the incidence of infusion reactions on repeat exposure to infliximab. Infliximab has also been demonstrated to be efficacious in the treatment of fistulizing Crohn's disease. Sequential infusions of infliximab (5 mg/kg) at 0, 2, and 6 weeks results in complete healing of perianal fistulas in 55% of patients. Repeated infusions of infliximab at 8-week intervals have been demonstrated to maintain clinical responses in both fistulizing and nonfistulizing Crohn's disease. The proper role of infliximab in the maintenance therapy of Crohn's disease has not been defined.

6. Nutrition—Aggressive nutritional support is an important adjunct in the treatment of Crohn's disease. Despite the fact that food is a major source of intraluminal antigen, there is no consistent evidence that elimination or highly restrictive diets have a role in the treatment of Crohn's disease. Lactose restriction may be helpful in some patients but is not mandatory in all patients. Patients with symptomatic fibrostenotic disease benefit from a low-residue diet. The use of growth hormone in conjunction with a high-protein diet for the induction and maintenance of clinical remission of Crohn's disease is under investigation.

Among patients with evidence of malnutrition, enteral nutritional therapy (rather than parenteral therapy) should be used. Of note, there is a large body of evidence in both the pediatric and adult literature that suggests that elemental enteral diets may be as effective as prednisone for the induction of remission, particularly in patients with small bowel disease. Because elemental solutions have an unpleasant taste, they usually require administration by enteral feeding tube, making them impractical for treatment in most cases. Elemental diets may be useful, however, in treating small bowel disease that is refractory to corticosteroids and in providing nutritional support for patients with short-gut syndrome.

Total parenteral nutrition should be reserved for patients in whom an enteral route is not feasible, as in high-output fistula or obstructive disease.

7. Education, group support, and psychological therapy—The psychological impact of a chronic intestinal disease upon patient quality of life should be considered. As with most chronic illness, fears surrounding the loss of well-being, risk of cancer, treatment, future complications, and possibility of death are common. Social support is an important factor leading to successful adjustment to a chronic disease. Patient education and concerns should be addressed by the physician and nurse, and through patient-based materials. The Crohn's and Colitis Foundation of America is an excellent source of educational material and provides an extensive network of peer support groups, which are invaluable to many patients. In a large proportion of patients, disease exacerbations impose limitations on personal and professional activities, resulting in significant psychological stress. In some patients, psychotherapy may aid in coping and may result in an enhanced sense of well-being.

B. Approach to Specific Problems and Complications

1. Perforating disease—Patients with abscesses usually require percutaneous or surgical drainage. When an abscess is suspected, broad-spectrum antibiotics should be instituted and the abscess should be localized by CT scanning. When possible, a catheter should be placed percutaneously under CT guidance and the abscess drained. After catheter drainage has slowed, the patient may be fed orally, with careful monitoring of catheter output. If the output is high, a course of total parenteral nutrition is required. Definitive surgery may be delayed for up to several weeks until the abscess is fully drained and the underlying Crohn's disease is brought under medical control with immunosuppressants and/or infliximab. This approach allows for a technically easier and more limited resection of the segment of involved bowel. Catheter drainage without subsequent surgery usually results in a persistent enterocutaneous fistula. If CT-guided drainage is not feasible or if there is evidence of peritonitis, immediate surgical intervention is required.

Fistulas associated with significant symptoms usually require surgery. Incidentally identified enteroenteric fistulas without significant metabolic consequences need no particular therapy. Fistulas causing severe symptoms and complex fistulas associated with abscesses require surgical management. In the case of moderately symptomatic enterovesicular, enterocutaneous, and enteroenteric fistulas, the options of medical versus surgical treatment must be considered.

Medical therapy requires a long treatment course (with azathioprine, 6-mercaptopurine, or infliximab) and at best is successful in only one-third of patients. Therefore, the ultimate decision between medical and surgical treatment is based on symptoms and patient preference. The introduction of infliximab has improved the success of medical therapy for enterocutaneous fistula; its effectiveness in the management of enterovesicular and symptomatic enteroenteric fistula remains under investigation. Before surgery is undertaken, bowel disease should be under good control.

2. Fibrostenotic disease—Patients with Crohn's disease presenting with obstructive symptoms due to stricture formation typically improve within 2–3 days with conservative therapy consisting of bowel rest, nasogastric suction, and intravenous hydration. It is reasonable to treat patients with evidence of active disease (on colonoscopy or contrast x-ray) with aggressive medical therapy, because inflammation may contribute to the partial obstruction. A low-residue diet may reduce the incidence of subsequent episodes of partial bowel obstruction. Patients with recurrent bouts of partial obstruction and patients who fail to respond to conservative therapy require surgery. Patients with complete bowel obstruction require urgent surgery. Surgery for stricturing disease may take the form of limited resection of the stenotic segment with primary anastomosis or stricturoplasty (technically similar to a pyloroplasty).

3. Perirectal disease—Treatment of perirectal disease requires a team approach with a gastroenterologist and an experienced colorectal surgeon. Draining fistulas may close with prolonged treatment with metronidazole, azathioprine, or 6-mercaptopurine. More severe disease should be treated with sequential infusions of infliximab and concurrent, prolonged immunosuppressive medication. Perirectal abscesses require surgical drainage. In patients with low-lying simple fistulas, simple fistulectomy in conjunction with medical therapy may be effective, resulting in 70–80% success in fistula elimination. Further surgery may be undertaken for persistent fistulas, but the successful repair is dependent on adequate control of the rectal or perianal disease. The use of noncutting seton catheters is effective in allowing the fistulas to drain adequately and should be used routinely in patients with complex fistulas. Severe perianal disease sometimes requires bowel rest, with total parenteral nutrition or fecal diversion. In truly refractory cases, especially when there is significant damage of the anal sphincters, proctectomy may be required. Rectovaginal fistulas commonly complicate perianal disease. They may close with intensive treatment with azathioprine, 6-mercaptopurine, or infliximab.

4. Other causes of diarrhea—As has been discussed previously, diarrhea may be the result of bacterial overgrowth, bile acid malabsorption, or bile acid depletion with secondary fat malabsorption. In patients with strictures or fistulas, bacterial overgrowth may contribute to the diarrhea. This should be considered, especially when there is little evidence of ongoing active Crohn's disease. A hydrogen breath test may be used to document bacterial overgrowth, but may be difficult to interpret in patients with fistulas. Often it is more practical to treat empirically with a course of broad-spectrum antibiotics (tetracycline, metronidazole, ampicillin/clavulanic acid, etc). Patients with ileal resections of less than 100 cm may have secretory diarrhea caused by the effects of unabsorbed bile salts on the colon. They may be treated empirically with bile acid-binding resins (eg, cholestyramine, 4 g orally two or three times daily). Diarrhea in patients with more extensive ileal resections may be due to bile salt depletion with secondary steatorrhea. Such patients will worsen following treatment with bile acid-binding resins because of further depletion of the bile acid pool. After documentation of steatorrhea, treatment requires a low-fat diet supplemented with medium-chain triglycerides, which are more readily absorbed without bile salt/micelle formation.

5. Prevention of relapse and postoperative recurrence—No drug has been proven effective in preventing relapse of Crohn's disease. This is particularly true of patients with quiescent disease who are receiving no current therapy. Patients with more aggressive disease requiring immunosuppressives are more likely to stay in remission if they continue to take the drugs. In many cases, it may be unclear whether therapy is suppressing ongoing active disease or preventing relapse in the setting of a true remission. Mucosal healing appears to determine the duration of clinical remission, as endoscopic and radiographic signs of recurrent inflammations precede the development of clinical symptoms. Immunosuppressive medications and infliximab have been shown to result in endoscopic healing in approximately 50% and 75% of patients, respectively. By contrast, corticosteroids result in endoscopic healing in less than 30% of patients and have not been demonstrated to maintain clinical remission. There does not appear to be any proven role for monitoring or treating patients who have endoscopic or radiologic evidence of active disease but who are in clinical remission.

Prognosis

The course of Crohn's disease is highly variable. The majority of patients lead productive, satisfying lives that are punctuated by intermittent episodes of disease relapse. It is important to remember that in placebo-controlled trials of active Crohn's disease, 30–40% of patients assigned to placebo nonetheless achieve a remission. In addition, 10–20% of patients with Crohn's disease have prolonged remissions after the initial episode of disease. Over the course of their disease, 60–70% of patients will require surgery, and of these, 50% will require subsequent surgery at some point. Mortality rates from Crohn's disease have declined over the past several decades because of improved management of suppurative and metabolic complications. Currently, mortality rates appear to be only slightly higher in patients with Crohn's disease compared with age-matched normal population control subjects; this may be due to cancer associated with Crohn's disease.

ULCERATIVE COLITIS

Ulcerative colitis is characterized by intermittent exacerbations and remissions of typical symptoms. For patients experiencing the first attack of ulcerative colitis,

the symptoms of cramping abdominal pain and diarrhea (often bloody) have a broad differential diagnosis. An initial attack of ulcerative colitis typically has a longer symptom prodrome than acute infectious diarrheal disorders. The diagnosis is made by exclusion of other causes of diarrhea (particularly infectious) and the typical findings seen on sigmoidoscopy or colonoscopy with biopsy. Supportive evidence of the diagnosis of ulcerative colitis is the absence of small bowel involvement or complications typical of Crohn's disease.

Pathology

The gross appearance of the colonic mucosa in ulcerative colitis varies with the extent and severity of disease. In mild disease, there is mucosal erythema, edema, and granularity with or without scattered, small erosions. The inflammation always begins in the distal rectum and spreads proximally in continuous fashion for variable distances. There is usually a sharp demarcation between the involved region of distal colon and the proximal uninvolved colon. In moderate to severe ulcerative colitis, colons exhibit large areas of ulceration and erosions with adherent mucopus, granularity, friability, and hemorrhage. In patients with long-standing ulcerative colitis, the colons lose the normal haustral folds and have a flat, featureless appearance. Inflammatory polyps or "pseudopolyps" may be present.

The characteristic histologic lesion of ulcerative colitis is the crypt abscess, which in its fully developed form is characterized by neutrophils within the crypt as well as in the crypt wall and the adjacent lamina propria. Although crypt abscesses are characteristic of ulcerative colitis, they may also be seen in acute self-limited infectious colitis as well as in Crohn's disease. The lamina propria in ulcerative colitis additionally is infiltrated with increased numbers of mononuclear cells, indicating chronicity. These chronic inflammatory cells are unusual in acute self-limited colitis but are common in Crohn's colitis. One of the helpful histologic findings in differentiating ulcerative colitis from acute self-limited colitis is the presence of crypt architectural distortion, characterized by gland branching, shortening (not reaching the muscularis mucosa), and loss of normal parallel distribution. Crypt architectural distortion is indicative of chronic, recurrent mucosal damage, consistent with chronic colitis. Another sign of disease chronicity is Paneth cell metaplasia, typically seen in the right colon. Many of these features of chronic mucosal damage may be seen in Crohn's colitis as well as ulcerative colitis. The inflammatory process in ulcerative colitis does not usually disrupt the muscularis mucosa. However, in patients with severe or fulminant disease, inflammation may extend into the submucosa or transmurally into the muscularis, resulting in the clinical picture of "toxic megacolon" (see below).

Clinical Findings

The clinical presentation of ulcerative colitis is dependent on both the extent of colonic involvement and the severity of the disease. Ulcerative colitis may involve anything from the rectum alone (ulcerative proctitis) to the entire colon (universal colitis or pancolitis). The hallmark of ulcerative colitis is that the rectum is always involved and disease extends proximally in a continuous fashion, without skip areas. In rare circumstances, there is rectal sparing, but this is most often due to prior topical treatments (enema or suppository) that have diminished the gross mucosal changes. Biopsies of the "spared" rectum usually reveal typical histologic changes of ulcerative colitis. Ulcerative colitis is categorized by the extent of involvement, however, there are no standard terms to describe this involvement. The terms most frequently used are ulcerative proctitis (usually limited to the distal 10–20 cm), left-sided colitis (which usually refers to disease limited to the colon distal to the splenic flexure), extensive colitis (which refers to colonic inflammation that extends proximal to the splenic flexure), and pancolitis (involvement of the entire colon, or proximal to the hepatic flexure). Because of the variability in definitions used to describe disease extent, it is difficult to quantify the percentage of patients who fall into each category at the time of presentation. Overall, about one-third of patients have pancolitis, 30–40% have disease limited to the rectosigmoid, and the remainder have some intermediate form.

For the purposes of this chapter, the extent of disease will be divided into two categories. Limited disease is defined as ulcerative colitis confined to the rectosigmoid and extensive disease extends beyond the rectosigmoid. The value of this classification is that this dichotomous distinction can be made by flexible sigmoidoscopy. Furthermore, distinguishing distal from extensive ulcerative colitis has implications for therapy and cancer screening. In contrast to extensive disease, distal disease may be expected to respond to topical therapies alone. In contrast to patients with distal disease, those with extensive disease have a substantially higher risk of developing colon cancer, warranting close surveillance.

As in Crohn's disease, there are a variety of ulcerative colitis disease activity scales that can be used to assess disease severity. An overall assessment of severity is derived from the patient's complaints (eg, number of bowel movements, the presence and amount of blood per rectum, and abdominal pain), the impact of the disease on daily function, pertinent physical examination findings (eg, fever, signs of intravascular volume depletion, tenderness), and the presence of abnormal labora-

tory parameters (eg, anemia, hypoalbuminemia). Attention to these parameters frequently permits the clinician to categorize the severity of illness as mild, moderate, or severe. Although there are numerous scales that grade the severity of colitis based upon endoscopic mucosal appearance, therapeutic decisions should be based primarily on clinical status, not endoscopic appearance.

A. SYMPTOMS AND SIGNS

Most patients with ulcerative colitis complain of bloody diarrhea, crampy abdominal pain, fecal urgency, and tenesmus. A small percentage of patients complain of bleeding or diarrhea alone. Fever and weight loss are present in approximately one-third of patients, and up to 15–25% have some extracolonic manifestation of ulcerative colitis (eg, eye, joint, and skin complaints). In general, patients with ulcerative colitis have had some symptoms for weeks to months prior to presentation, whereas patients with acute self-limited colitis typically have an abrupt onset of symptoms over a matter of hours or days.

The physical examination in patients with mild acute ulcerative colitis is usually normal except for mild left lower quadrant tenderness. In contrast, patients with severe ulcerative colitis have signs of volume depletion and systemic signs of toxicity, including fever >100°F, tachycardia, significant abdominal tenderness, and weight loss.

Patients with **toxic megacolon** (a rare, life-threatening form of ulcerative colitis) manifest signs of toxic colitis (fever >101°F, tachycardia, abdominal distention, and signs of localized or generalized peritonitis), with leukocytosis (white blood cell count usually >11,000/μL) and dilated colon (>6 cm) on plain abdominal x-ray.

B. LABORATORY FINDINGS

Abnormal laboratory parameters in patients with ulcerative colitis are not specific to ulcerative colitis but represent the degree of systemic impact. Patients with mild disease have a normal hematocrit, erythrocyte sedimentation rate (ESR), and albumin. Patients with more severe disease may exhibit anemia, leukocytosis, thrombocytosis, hypoalbuminemia, and elevated ESR. Stool studies for culture (enteric pathogens and, where indicated, *Escherichia coli* O157:H7), ova, and parasites and *Clostridium difficile* toxin should be negative.

C. IMAGING STUDIES

In the patient with acute colitis, endoscopy is useful to document the extent and severity of disease, to obtain biopsies that help distinguish inflammatory bowel disease from infectious or acute self-limited colitis, and to distinguish ulcerative colitis from Crohn's colitis. The endoscopic appearance of mild ulcerative colitis is characterized by erythema, granularity, loss of vascularity, and contact bleeding (friability). With increasing severity, there is pinpoint ulceration, spontaneous bleeding, and extensive frank ulceration. As previously stated, ulcerative colitis begins in the rectum and extends proximally in a continuous fashion. The most severe disease tends to be seen distally, unless there has been ongoing therapy per rectum. Random biopsies should be taken throughout the affected area. Separately labeled biopsies should always be taken in the rectum, particularly when there is some question of endoscopic sparing. In the setting of acute moderate to severe colitis, it is wise to limit inspection to the rectosigmoid with rectal biopsies (rather than perform pancolonoscopy) to reduce the risk of perforation of an acutely inflamed colon. A more complete endoscopic examination to assess the extent of involvement can be performed at a later date, after the disease has been adequately controlled.

With the widespread availability and superior accuracy of flexible endoscopy, contrast radiography of the colon has limited clinical usefulness in the diagnosis and management of acute ulcerative colitis. Double-contrast (air-contrast) barium enema in mild ulcerative colitis reveals a fine granular-appearing mucosa. With increased disease severity, discrete ulcers are seen. In more long-standing disease, there is loss of haustral markings, shortening of the colon, and, frequently, a tubular appearance of the colon. Typical filling defects representing pseudopolyps may be seen. Atypical masses or strictures raise concern for the presence of neoplasm.

Differential Diagnosis

The differential diagnosis of ulcerative colitis is summarized in Table 7–6.

There are a variety of infectious entities that must be considered. Acute self-limited colitis is most commonly caused by *Campylobacter, Salmonella, Shigella, Yersinia,* and *Escherichia coli* 0157:H7. Rectal biopsies frequently aid in differentiating acute self-limited colitis from ulcerative colitis. Amebiasis may cause a chronic colitis that can be confused with ulcerative colitis. Amebiasis should be excluded by mucosal biopsy and ova and parasite examination in patients who have traveled to endemic areas or are in contact with others from such areas. *Clostridium difficile* and antibiotic-associated diarrhea should be considered in patients who have taken antibiotics recently.

Of the noninfectious colitides, Crohn's colitis and ischemic colitis are usually able to be differentiated from ulcerative colitis by their pattern of distribution. Radiation-induced and diversion colitis are readily identified based on historic information. Collagenous and microscopic colitis are readily differentiated from

Table 7–6. Differential diagnosis of ulcerative colitis.

Infectious disease
  Acute bacterial colitis (acute self-limited colitis)
    Campylobacter
    Salmonella
    Shigella
    Yersinia
    Escherichia coli 0157:H7
  Antibiotic-associated diarrhea (including *Clostridium difficile*)
  Amebic colitis
  Immunocompromised host
    Cytomegalovirus
    Herpes simplex virus
    Neisseria gonorrhoeae
    Blastocystis hominis
    Chlamydia
Noninfectious disease
  Crohn's colitis
  Ischemic colitis
  Radiation colitis
  Collagenous or microscopic colitis

ulcerative colitis because they have a normal endoscopic appearance but evidence of chronic mucosal inflammation on histologic evaluation of mucosal biopsies.

In the immunocompromised patient, a variety of pathogens may cause proctitis or colitis, including cytomegalovirus, herpes simplex virus, gonorrhea, *Blastocystis hominis,* and *Chlamydia.* It is also noteworthy that there are reports of persistent ulcerative colitis activity in patients with ulcerative colitis who have subsequently developed AIDS.

Complications

A. TOXIC MEGACOLON

The true frequency of toxic megacolon in ulcerative colitis is unknown, but it is rare, appears to be decreasing in frequency, and now occurs in less than 2% of patients. Toxic megacolon usually occurs in patients with pancolitis, but has been reported in more limited disease. It may occur at any time during the disease course but is more likely early in the course. In some patients, the initial presentation of ulcerative colitis may be toxic megacolon. Reported mortality rates vary from 15% to 50%. Not unexpectedly, perforation at presentation is associated with a high mortality rate.

B. PERFORATION

Colonic perforation complicating severe colitis in the absence of toxic megacolon has been reported. Perforation of this type tends to occur during an initial episode of ulcerative colitis, and the sigmoid is the most common site of perforation. Free perforation is associated with a high mortality rate.

C. STRICTURE

Strictures are uncommon in ulcerative colitis, and the presence of a stricture should raise serious concern for an underlying malignant tumor. Colectomy should be strongly considered in a patient with long-standing ulcerative colitis and a stricture, even if mucosal biopsies are unrevealing. Dysplasia found in biopsies of a stricture is highly suspicious for the presence of underlying tumor and is an absolute indication for colectomy. When benign strictures occur in ulcerative colitis, they are usually seen in patients with extensive, chronically active disease.

D. MASSIVE HEMORRHAGE

Massive colonic hemorrhage requiring urgent colectomy is a rare complication of ulcerative colitis.

E. CANCER

Patients with chronic ulcerative colitis are at increased risk of developing colon cancer. The extent of colonic involvement and the duration of disease are strongly correlated with cancer risk. Although the estimates of the magnitude of risk vary, all studies report that the risk of colon cancer in patients with long-standing ulcerative colitis is significantly higher than in age-matched control subjects. Studies done at tertiary referral centers report a cancer risk of 13% after 20 years and 34% after 30 years of ulcerative colitis, whereas population-based studies report risks of 5.5% and 13% for 20 and 30 years, respectively. Patients with disease extending proximal to the splenic flexure carry the highest risk, whereas the risk in patients with ulcerative proctitis is similar to that of age-matched control subjects. Left-sided colitis is thought to have an intermediate risk. Because of the variability in the definition of left-sided colitis in available studies, it is difficult to determine whether the risk is significantly different than with pancolitis. For the purposes of risk assessment, it is probably more reasonable to categorize patients as having limited (low-risk) or extensive (high-risk) colitis.

In contrast to sporadic colon cancer, cancer arising in patients with ulcerative colitis does not necessarily develop from an adenomatous polyp but may arise from flat dysplastic epithelium, which cannot be distinguished at colonoscopy from adjacent nondysplastic mucosa. It is common practice to have patients with extensive ulcerative colitis for more than 7 to 8 years undergo yearly surveillance colonoscopic examination. At each examination, between two and four mucosal biopsies are taken at 10-cm intervals (at least 32 total biop-

sies) throughout the colon. These biopsies are taken randomly and from any raised mucosal abnormalities and evaluated for the presence of dysplasia. If dysplasia is present, it is categorized as either low grade or high grade. The finding of high-grade dysplasia (confirmed by a gastrointestinal pathologist) should prompt a recommendation for colectomy as an unrecognized carcinoma may be present in 30% of these patients. The management of patients with low-grade dysplasia is more problematic. Some investigators have recommended performing surveillance colonoscopy on patients with low-grade dysplasia at more frequent intervals. However, given the large sampling error associated with random biopsies, it may be prudent to recommend colectomy for confirmed low-grade dysplasia. The presence of low-grade or high-grade dysplasia in an endoscopically suspicious mass is called a **dysplasia-associated lesion or mass (DALM).** Because it is associated with a high rate of underlying neoplasm (approximately 50%), it is a clear indication for colectomy. Like patients without ulcerative colitis, older patients with ulcerative colitis may develop adenomatous polyps, which by their nature contain dysplastic cells. When adenomatous polyps are found, biopsies should be taken from the mucosa surrounding the polyp to look for evidence of dysplasia. In the absence of dysplasia in the surrounding mucosa, recent studies suggest that endoscopic resection of these polyps may be sufficient therapy. Given the high risk of colon cancer in patients with chronic, extensive ulcerative colitis, prophylactic colectomy should also be considered as an alternative to a program of routine colonoscopic surveillance (see the following section, "Surgical Treatment").

Treatment

The reader is directed to the treatment section on Crohn's disease for a more complete discussion of mechanism of action and side effects of the following classes of medications (Table 7–4). In this section, they are discussed primarily in the context of ulcerative colitis. The comments and section on group support, education, and psychological therapy appearing in the section on Crohn's disease are equally relevant to the treatment of ulcerative colitis.

A. GENERAL APPROACH TO TREATMENT

1. 5-Aminosalicylic acid—Sulfasalazine and mesalamine derivatives result in symptomatic improvement in 50–75% of patients with mild to moderate colitis within 4–8 weeks of therapy. Sulfasalazine has been the drug of choice for the treatment of mild to moderately active ulcerative colitis. There is little evidence to suggest that the newer preparations of this agent are any more efficacious than sulfasalazine in controlling inflammation when used in similar equivalent doses. One gram of sulfasalazine contains approximately 400 mg of mesalamine. Sulfasalazine is prescribed in doses of 3–6 g/d for active colitis (ie, 1.2–2.4 g/d of mesalamine). However, up to 25% of patients are intolerant of sulfasalazine or have a sulfa allergy.

Given this high rate of intolerance, other mesalamine (5aminosalicylate) derivatives are often used as first-line agents.

These newer 5-ASA preparations are capable of delivering higher concentrations of 5-ASA than sulfasalazine, with minimal side effects when used in high dosages. Patients can tolerate higher doses of mesalamine (2.4–4.8 g/d) with the newer formulations than with sulfasalazine. Two of the newer formulations (Asacol and Pentasa) have substantial release of mesalamine in the small bowel (15–30% for Asacol and 50% for Pentasa). Renal function and liver-associated enzymes should be monitored periodically in patients treated with high-dose 5-ASA compounds. Recently, balsalazide was approved for use in acute ulcerative colitis. This compound contains mesalamine (6.75 g balsalazide contains 2.4 g mesalamine) bound by an azo bond to an amino acid. In the colon, balsalazide is reduced by bacterial degradation, releasing mesalamine and the inert, unabsorbed amino acid. There is less than 1% absorption of mesalamine prior to entry into the colon. Balsalazide has been demonstrated to have efficacy comparable or superior to Asacol and sulfasalazine in several studies. Olsalazine is not used in treatment of acute colitis due to the moderate incidence of diarrhea.

Patients with disease limited to the rectum or rectosigmoid should be encouraged to use topical therapies applied per rectum once or twice daily. Patients with disease limited to the distal 10 cm of rectum may be treated with 5-ASA (mesalamine) suppositories. Patients with disease involving the proximal rectum or sigmoid colon should be treated with mesalamine enemas. It is important to consider that some patients with acute colitis will have difficulty retaining enemas and are better treated with oral medications until their disease is brought under control.

2. Corticosteroids—Patients with limited distal disease who fail to respond to topical or oral 5-ASA may be treated with hydrocortisone enemas (100 mg) once or twice daily. Corticosteroid foam and suppositories can be used for the treatment of ulcerative proctitis. There is significant systemic absorption of these preparations, particularly as the colonic mucosa heals, which may lead to full-blown Cushing's syndrome with long-term use. Topically active but rapidly metabolized corticosteroids may avoid many of these long-term toxicities.

Systemic steroids should be used for patients with mild to moderate ulcerative colitis unresponsive to oral 5-ASA and patients with severe colitis. Prednisone, at doses of 40–60 mg/d orally, induces remissions in 75–90% of patients with ulcerative colitis. As with Crohn's disease, long-term corticosteroid use should be avoided. Patients treated with corticosteroids should be treated concomitantly with 5-ASA preparations to take advantage of their potential "steroid-sparing" effects. After induction of remission within 1–2 weeks, corticosteroids are tapered slowly over a 6- to 8-week period.

3. Immunosuppressive drugs—There is substantial experiential but uncontrolled evidence supporting the efficacy of the purine analogs, 6-mercaptopurine and azathioprine, in the treatment of ulcerative colitis. As with Crohn's disease, they are indicated when a patient is refractory to or dependent on corticosteroids. The dosages, potential toxicities, and guidelines are the same as those described for Crohn's disease. Use of these agents in the treatment of ulcerative colitis has increased over the past several years because of their successful and largely safe use in Crohn's disease. It must be appreciated, however, that ulcerative colitis is a surgically curable disease. The risks and benefits of these drugs must be weighed against the risks and benefits of surgery. The decision in each case must be individualized and should be made only after the patient is fully informed. The process of educating the patient should include addressing any misconceptions about surgical treatment. It may be reasonable to use 6-mercaptopurine in selected patients who are early in the course of their disease or who have limited, distal colitis, but it is less reasonable to use these drugs to delay surgery in a patient with long-term, refractory extensive disease. Methotrexate is an alternative agent of use in the treatment of refractory or steroid-dependent ulcerative colitis. As with Crohn's disease, methotrexate appears to be efficacious when given by parenteral route (25 mg/week).

Cyclosporine A is efficacious in the treatment of severe ulcerative colitis refractory to intravenous corticosteroids. Typically, use of this drug has been confined to patients with severe disease despite at least 7–10 days of treatment with parenteral corticosteroids. In this patient group, intravenous cyclosporine (2–4 mg/kg/d) induces a rapid remission in approximately 80% of patients. However, up to 30–50% of these individuals ultimately require colectomy within the first 6 months for persistent symptoms or drug intolerance. If concomitant immunosuppressants are used, approximately 60–70% of patients who respond to cyclosporine may achieve remission and avoid colectomy. The toxicities associated with cyclosporine appear to be substantial in the population with inflammatory bowel disease, including seizures, hypertension, nephrotoxicity, and opportunistic infections. The use of cyclosporine may be considered in highly selected, fully informed patients as a bridge to therapy with the slower acting purine analogs. Recently, the use of infliximab in ulcerative colitis has been reported. Its role is evolving and being defined by clinical trials.

4. Surgical treatment—The indications for surgical treatment of ulcerative colitis include perforation, severe hemorrhage, disease refractory to medical therapy, or the development of dysplasia or cancer. The role of prophylactic proctocolectomy to prevent colon cancer in patients with long-standing, extensive, but medically controlled disease is controversial. It is usually held that the risk of cancer is too high to ignore but not high enough to warrant prophylactic proctocolectomy. However, it has not been definitively demonstrated that currently available colonoscopic surveillance techniques are adequate to prevent the risk of a cancer-related death. Patients should be informed of the limitations of colonoscopic surveillance and given the option of prophylactic proctocolectomy.

In the past, the standard ulcerative colitis operation was a proctocolectomy with either a standard (Brooke) ileostomy or a continent (Koch) ileostomy, which is technically more difficult to perform. In the past 15 years, major surgical advances have been made in restorative proctocolectomy. The operation most commonly performed is known as the ileoanal pull-through or ileal pouch–anal anastomosis. In this operation, an abdominal colectomy is performed, and a pouch is fashioned from the distal ileum and attached to the anus or distal rectum after rectal mucosectomy. Typically, a temporary diverting ileostomy is performed to allow the pouch and anastomosis to heal for several months, after which the ileostomy is taken down at a second operation. A more recent modification of this operation omits the rectal mucosectomy and instead anastomoses the ileal pouch to the distal rectum in close proximity to the dentate line (1–4 cm). This ileal pouch–distal rectal anastomosis is technically easier to perform. It is thought to have less risk for incontinence and in selected patients can be performed as a single-stage operation without a diverting ileostomy. The controversy around the ileal pouch–distal rectal anastomosis is related to the fact that some "transitional" epithelium is left intact that may be a source of future cancer risk as well as recurrent inflammation ("cuffitis"). In experienced hands, both operations have excellent outcomes. After 1 year, patients typically report an average of six bowel movements per day (one at night). Incontinence, impotence, and the need for pouch removal occur in less than 5% of patients. Pouchitis is the most common late postoperative complication. It is

characterized by increased stool frequency, urgency, cramps, and malaise. Pouchitis is believed to be related to bacterial stasis within the pouch and occurs more frequently in patients with ulcerative colitis than in patients with familial polyposis who have undergone prophylactic proctocolectomy and ileoanal pouch formation. Pouchitis occurs at least once in over 90% of patients with ulcerative colitis but usually responds well to a course of antibiotic treatment with metronidazole.

B. SPECIFIC TREATMENT RECOMMENDATIONS

1. Limited disease—In mild to moderate distal disease, mesalamine (5-ASA) suppositories (500 mg) or enemas (4 g) can be administered once or twice daily. If symptoms worsen or fail to improve over 2 weeks, hydrocortisone enemas (100 mg) may be substituted for or alternated with the 5-ASA preparation.

In patients who fail to respond to this regimen or who present with more severe disease, oral prednisone should be administered in doses of 40–60 mg/d. It is better to start at high doses in order to rapidly induce remission followed by drug tapering. Beginning with a low corticosteroid dose is more likely to result in treatment failure. In patients who relapse or fail to respond to a previously successful rectal regimen, it is important to consider the possibility of the proximal extension of disease. This can be evaluated with a flexible sigmoidoscopy or colonoscopy. Treatment with immunosuppressives may be considered in patients who are refractory to or dependent on corticosteroids (see the preceding section, "Immunosuppressive Drugs"). Severe disease is uncommon in patients with limited ulcerative colitis and is discussed below.

2. Extensive disease—In mild to moderate disease, sulfasalazine may be started at an oral dose of 500 mg twice per day and gradually increased over 1–2 weeks to a dose of 3–4 g/d. If the patient is allergic to or intolerant of sulfa, an alternative oral 5-ASA drug should be used (Asacol, 2.4–4.8 g/d, Pentasa, 4 g/d, or balsalazide 6.75 g daily). Patients taking sulfasalazine should be supplemented with folate, 1 mg/d orally.

In patients who fail to respond to this regimen or who present with more severe disease, oral prednisone should be administered in doses of 40–60 mg/d for 1–2 weeks to induce remission, followed by a gradual taper of 5 mg/week over 8–12 weeks. As discussed, it is best to start corticosteroids at high doses to induce remission, rather than starting at low doses followed by increasing doses for lack of efficacy. Severely ill patients should be hospitalized for bed rest, intravenous hydration, intravenous methylprednisolone (approximately 60 mg/d), and nutritional support (when indicated). Treatment with immunosuppressives may be considered in patients who are refractory to or dependent on corticosteroids (see the preceding section, "Immuno-suppressive Drugs").

3. Toxic megacolon—Toxic megacolon is a life-threatening complication of ulcerative colitis that requires an intensive team approach by a gastroenterologist and surgeon. Care is best provided in the intensive care unit setting. Management consists of aggressive fluid and electrolyte replacement, intravenous methylprednisolone (approximately 60 mg/d), broad-spectrum intravenous antibiotics, and placement of nasogastric and rectal tubes. Total parenteral nutrition should be considered, as enteral therapy may not be possible until later in the hospitalization. Frequent abdominal examination and daily or twice-daily abdominal and upright chest x-rays should be performed. Indications for surgical intervention include free intraabdominal air, colonic intramural pneumatosis, peritoneal signs on abdominal examination, and failure to improve within 24–48 hours. Patients who fail to improve within 48 hours are unlikely to improve and risk a poorer outcome if surgery is delayed.

4. Prevention of relapse—Patients who have achieved remission should be placed on maintenance therapy with 5-ASA, as these agents substantially reduce the incidence of relapse. For extensive disease, sulfasalazine 1 g twice daily, olsalazine 500 mg to 1 g twice daily, Asacol, 2.4 g/d, and Pentasa, 2 g/d, have been proven to reduce relapse rates. Patients with limited disease may be treated with rectal preparations on an every-other-day or every-third-day regimen. The optimal dosing regimen for all patients must be individualized.

Prognosis

There are few population-based studies that have examined the course of ulcerative colitis. A recent Danish study suggests that the likelihood of being in remission at any given time is 50%. The colectomy rate was 24% at 10 years and 30% at 25 years. The probability of colectomy was related to disease extent. At 5 years, the colectomy rate was 9% in proctosigmoiditis, 19% in "substantial" colitis, and 35% in pancolitis. The probability of maintaining capacity for work was 93% after 10 years of disease.

The severity of disease at presentation is somewhat predictive of the future disease course and probability of requiring a colectomy. Population studies suggest that for patients with limited disease at presentation, the risk of progression to extensive disease is 30–50% over 10 years.

Whether ulcerative colitis is associated with an increased mortality rate compared with that of the general population is controversial. Many previous reports of

poor outcome were derived from tertiary care centers, whose population included a large number of patients with severe or refractory disease and was not representative of most patients with ulcerative colitis. In the past, a high mortality rate was seen early in the course of patients presenting with severe disease. Given improved medical and surgical therapies, it is not clear whether this high rate still exists. Some recent population-based studies have failed to show increased mortality rates in patients with ulcerative colitis. Any higher rate of death in patients with chronic ulcerative colitis may be related to the increased incidence of colon cancer.

DIFFERENTIATING CROHN'S DISEASE FROM ULCERATIVE COLITIS

In approximately 75% of patients with Crohn's disease, there is characteristic involvement of the ileum seen on contrast x-ray. Crohn's disease limited to the colon may be difficult to differentiate from ulcerative colitis. In most cases, ulcerative colitis and Crohn's disease limited to the colon can be differentiated using the criteria summarized in Table 7–7. In 10–15% of cases of chronic colitis, a clear differentiation of ulcerative colitis and Crohn's disease cannot be made. This subgroup is usually referred to as "indeterminate" colitis.

EXTRAINTESTINAL MANIFESTATIONS OF INFLAMMATORY BOWEL DISEASE

Extraintestinal manifestations of inflammatory bowel disease are common, occurring in up to 25% of patients with inflammatory bowel disease. These manifestations can be divided into two types: those that occur during periods of active inflammatory bowel disease and those that occur at any time and are unrelated to the activity of bowel disease. Although these categories are conceptually useful, there are numerous examples of overlap between them.

Extraintestinal Manifestations Occurring during Active Inflammatory Bowel Disease

A. REACTIVE ARTHROPATHY

Acute synovitis is seen in up to 20% of patients with inflammatory bowel disease, primarily in patients with colitis (rather than small intestinal disease). Two forms of peripheral arthropathy have been described. Type 1 arthropathy is asymmetric and migratory, typically involving fewer than six large joints. The onset of arthritic symptoms corresponds to a flare-up in intestinal activity and usually resolves with treatment of the active bowel disease. Type 2 arthropathy, seen in 15% of patients, is a persistent nonerosive small-joint arth-

Table 7–7. Differentiating ulcerative and Crohn's colitis.

	Ulcerative Colitis	Crohn's Colitis
Clinical findings		
Perianal disease	Rare	Common (one-third of patients)
Fistulas	Rare	Common (up to 40% of patients)
Abscess	Rare	20% of patients
Stricture	Rare	Common
Colonoscopic findings		
Rectal involvement	Always	Usually spared
Pattern	Continuous, proximal extension from rectum	Usually skip lesions
Radiologic findings		
Ileal involvement	Rare, nonspecific "backwash ileitis"	75% of patients with Crohn's disease
Histologic findings		
Depth of inflammation	Usually limited to mucosa or submucosa, except in fulminant cases	Typically transmural
Granulomas	Only associated with crypts in severe colitis	20% of endoscopic biopsies

ritis. This subgroup is more likely to be HLA-B27 positive. Although this may be inaugurated by a flare-up of intestinal inflammation, the arthropathy may persist despite treatment of intestinal disease. The median duration of type 2 symptoms is 36 months, and a small subset develop a deforming arthritis. There is an overlap of this subgroup with other seronegative spondyloarthropathies such as postinfectious arthritis, Reiter's syndrome, and psoriasis-associated arthritis. Patients with either type 1 or type 2 reactive arthropathy may develop concurrent uveitis or erythema nodosum.

B. OCULAR MANIFESTATIONS

Episcleritis is the most common ocular manifestation of inflammatory bowel disease. It is more commonly seen in patients with Crohn's disease than ulcerative colitis. Characterized by a painless hyperemia of the conjunctiva and sclera, episcleritis occurs more commonly in patients with colitis or ileocolitis than ileitis, and its course closely follows the activity of the bowel disease. Episcleritis typically responds to topical antiinflammatory medications.

C. DERMATOLOGIC MANIFESTATIONS

Erythema nodosum is the most common dermatologic manifestation of inflammatory bowel disease. It is associated with both Crohn's disease and ulcerative colitis, but occurs more commonly in Crohn's disease. Erythema nodosum parallels the activity of the bowel disease in most, but not all, cases. It is frequently associated with reactive arthritis and uveitis.

Pyoderma gangrenosum is a serious dermatologic complication of inflammatory bowel disease. It is seen in equal frequency with ulcerative colitis and Crohn's disease. The relationship of pyoderma gangrenosum to the activity of bowel disease is not always clear. Patients with extensive and severe colonic involvement are more likely to develop pyoderma gangrenosum. In many patients, the pyoderma recedes with treatment of the underlying bowel disease, but there are many instances in which pyoderma develops or persists even after colectomy.

Extraintestinal Manifestations That May Occur at Any Time in a Patient with Inflammatory Bowel Disease

A. AXIAL ARTHROPATHY

Sacroiliitis is the most common axial abnormality associated with inflammatory bowel disease. It is seen in approximately 10% of patients with inflammatory bowel disease by plain x-ray but may be detected in most patients (two-thirds) by magnetic resonance imaging (MRI). Most cases are asymptomatic.

Ankylosing spondylitis has been estimated to be 30 times more common in patients with inflammatory bowel disease than in the general population and may complicate the course of disease in up to 5% of patients. There appear to be two subsets of patients who develop ankylosing spondylitis. Patients who are HLA-B27 positive have a high incidence of ankylosing spondylitis, typically with an accelerated course, whereas patients who develop ankylosing spondylitis and are HLA-B27 negative tend to have a benign course.

B. OCULAR MANIFESTATIONS

Scleritis and uveitis are two serious ocular complications associated with inflammatory bowel disease that may result in impairment or loss of vision. Neither entity appears to parallel the bowel disease activity. As stated previously, uveitis (particularly anterior uveitis) is seen in association with reactive arthritis and erythema nodosum. This clustering has a strong association with HLA-B27.

C. HEPATOBILIARY MANIFESTATIONS

Primary sclerosing cholangitis complicates the course of inflammatory bowel disease in 2–5% of patients. The overwhelming majority of cases are associated with ulcerative colitis. Primary sclerosing cholangitis is not associated with bowel disease activity, and its incidence is unaffected by colectomy. Many of the patients with primary sclerosing cholangitis have extensive colitis on colonoscopy but relatively mild or quiescent symptoms. Pericholangitis has been used to describe nonspecific elevations in alkaline phosphatase and transaminase levels, nonspecific portal inflammation, and chronic hepatitis in patients with inflammatory bowel disease with limited histologic lesions of primary sclerosing cholangitis. The majority of patients with evidence of pericholangitis do not progress to primary sclerosing cholangitis. Patients with primary sclerosing cholangitis are at markedly increased risk for developing cholangiocarcinoma. In addition, the incidence of colon cancer patients with ulcerative colitis and primary sclerosing cholangitis is significantly higher than in patients with ulcerative colitis alone.

Cholesterol gallstones occur with increased incidence in patients with ileal disease or resection, primarily due to a decrease in the bile salt pool.

INFLAMMATORY BOWEL DISEASE & PREGNANCY

Early reports suggested that women with inflammatory bowel disease were less fertile than an age-matched control population. More recent studies fail to show any difference in fertility for patients with ulcerative colitis, however, for women with Crohn's disease, the picture is unclear. Overall, the likelihood of having a successful pregnancy in women with inflammatory bowel disease is similar to the general population. For both ulcerative colitis and Crohn's disease, however, active disease at conception and during the course of pregnancy is associated with an increase in spontaneous abortions and premature delivery.

The effect of pregnancy on the course of inflammatory bowel disease appears to be similar for Crohn's disease and ulcerative colitis. Up to 75% of patients with inactive disease at conception remain inactive during pregnancy. Conversely, patients with active disease at conception are likely to remain active during the course of the pregnancy. Crohn's disease may flare up during the postpartum period, however ulcerative colitis is less likely to do so.

Treatment and management of inflammatory bowel disease during pregnancy are challenging. Gastrointestinal symptoms associated with a normal pregnancy can be confused with those associated with inflammatory bowel disease. Management is also made difficult by the limitation pregnancy imposes on the usual repertoire of diagnostic tests. Flexible sigmoidoscopy may be performed safely during pregnancy, but colonoscopy and x-rays should be avoided. Ultrasound (cutaneous and transvaginal) can be extremely helpful in some cases. Potentially life-threatening complications do require the use of radiologic and surgical interventions. Management in these situations is best accomplished by a team approach involving a gastroenterologist, colorectal surgeon, and high-risk obstetrician.

Drug treatment during pregnancy should follow the same approach as that in the nonpregnant patient. Untreated or undertreated inflammatory bowel disease poses a substantially greater risk to mother and fetus than appropriate drug therapies. There is a great deal of experience with sulfasalazine during pregnancy, and its use has not been shown to have any untoward effects on the fetus. It appears to be safe during breastfeeding as well. Folate supplements should be given when sulfasalazine is being used. A prospective randomized trial of oral 5-ASA demonstrates that these analogs also are safe during pregnancy, although many of these preparations are associated with measurable serum levels of 5-ASA, particularly when used at high doses. The safety of 5-ASA during breastfeeding has not been assessed in a prospective randomized fashion; however, the current opinion is that their use is safe.

Corticosteroids also are safe during pregnancy. Dosages are the same as for the nonpregnant patient. There are several reports of successful use of the purine analogs during pregnancy without apparent fetal toxicity. Nevertheless, these purine analogs should be avoided unless no other options exist, because the long-term effects on children born to these mothers still are unknown. It appears prudent to stop purine analogs in women who have accidentally become pregnant while taking them. Methotrexate is strongly contraindicated in pregnancy. Metronidazole previously was thought to be contraindicated during pregnancy, but recent information suggests this may be a safe drug during pregnancy, and current guidelines permit its use for short durations.

Both total parenteral nutrition and elemental diets have been used successfully to support the nutritional needs of pregnant women with inflammatory bowel disease. Elemental diets may be a reasonable first-line therapy in pregnant patients with small bowel Crohn's disease and may be especially useful in patients with small bowel disease that is refractory to or dependent on high-dosage steroids.

REFERENCES

Ekbom A et al: Ulcerative colitis and colorectal cancer: a population-based study. N Engl J Med 1990;323:1228.

Feagan B, Kumaranayake P: Methotrexate in inflammatory bowel disease. In: *Advanced Therapy of Inflammatory Bowel Disease.* Bayless T, Hanauer S (editors). Decker, 2000: 383–386.

Greenberg GR et al: Oral budesonide for active Crohn's disease: Canadian Inflammatory Bowel Disease Study Group [see comments]. N Engl J Med 1994;331:836.

Hay JW, Hay AR: Inflammatory bowel disease: costs-of-illness. J Clin Gastroenterol 1992;14:309.

Langholz E et al: Course of ulcerative colitis: analysis of changes in disease activity over years [see comments]. Gastroenterology 1994;107:3.

Lichtiger S et al: Cyclosporine in severe ulcerative colitis refractory to steroid therapy [see comments]. N Engl J Med 1994;330: 1841.

Rutgeerts P et al: A comparison of budesonide with prednisolone for active Crohn's disease [see comments]. N Engl J Med 1994;331:842.

Sandborn WJ: Pouchitis following ileal pouch-anal anastomosis: definition, pathogenesis, and treatment. Gastroenterology 1994;107:1856.

Sandborn W: A review of immune modifier therapy for inflammatory bowel disease: azathioprine, 6-mercaptopurine, cyclosporine, and methotrexate. Am J Gastroenterol 1996;91: 423.

Singleton JW et al: Mesalamine capsules for the treatment of active Crohn's disease: results of a 16-week trial. Pentasa Crohn's Disease Study Group. Gastroenterology 1993;104:1293.

Sutherland LR, May GR, Shaffer EA: Sulfasalazine revisited: a meta-analysis of 5-aminosalicylic acid in the treatment of ulcerative colitis. Ann Intern Med 1993;118:540.

Targan SR: The lamina propria: a dynamic, complex mucosal compartment: an overview. Ann N Y Acad Sci 1992;664:61.

Targan S et al: A short-term course study of chimeric monoclonal antibody cA2 to tumor necrosis factor-alpha for Crohn's disease. N Engl J Med 1997;337:1029.

Yang H et al: Familial empirical risks for inflammatory bowel disease: differences between Jews and non-Jews. Gut 1993;34: 517.

Acute Diarrheal Diseases

8

Edward Lung, MD

Acute diarrhea is a sudden alteration in normal bowel habits whereby normally formed stool (passed with a frequency ranging from daily to three times weekly) changes to frequent, multiple loose-to-watery stools. Diarrhea may be associated with increased frequency of defecation or increased liquidity of stools, or both, and often is accompanied by an abnormal increase in daily stool weight (>200 g/d). Therefore, acute diarrhea can be defined as the passage of a greater number of stools of decreased form from the norm lasting less than 14 days.

Pathophysiology of Diarrhea

A. NORMAL FLUID AND ELECTROLYTE ABSORPTION AND SECRETION

The small intestine and colon are normally involved in the absorption and secretion of fluid and ions. Absorption of nutrients and fluids far exceeds secretion, with most of the absorption occurring in the small bowel. Fluid absorption by the small intestine and colon is exceedingly efficient. The small intestine receives approximately 10 L/d of fluid consisting of oral intake and salivary, gastric, biliary, and pancreatic secretions. Of this, all but 1–1.5 L are absorbed in the small intestine. The colon resorbs most of the remaining fluid, with only 100 mL passed into the stool. The maximal absorptive capacity of the colon is 4–5 L every 24 hours, whereas that of the small intestine remains undefined.

B. MECHANISMS OF ACUTE DIARRHEA

Acute diarrhea may result from decreased absorption, increased secretion, increased osmolality of luminal contents, or a change in gut motility. Acute diarrhea may be classified clinically and pathophysiologically as either noninflammatory or inflammatory (Table 8–1).

1. Inflammatory diarrhea—Inflammatory diarrheas are caused by organisms or substances that disrupt the intestinal mucosal barrier through direct invasion or elaboration of cytotoxin. Disruption of the mucosa results in exudation of inflammatory cells, blood, and sera into the lumen. Clinical findings of inflammatory diarrheas are characterized by bloody, small-volume stools, often with associated lower abdominal cramping or urgency. Occasionally, symptoms including fever or shock may be present. The preferential intestinal site of involvement is the colon. Examination of a stool sample reveals numerous fecal leukocytes and red blood cells.

2. Noninflammatory diarrhea—Noninflammatory diarrheas are caused by organisms or substances that do not result in disruption or damage to the intestinal epithelium. Enterotoxins produced by infecting organisms stimulate excessive intestinal secretion of ions and water. Poorly absorbed substances, which are osmotically active, cause net fluid secretion into the intestinal lumen. The clinical hallmarks of infectious noninflammatory diarrhea are watery stools with minimal or no blood, and the absence of fecal leukocytes on stool examination. The small intestine is more likely to be affected.

Classification of Acute Diarrhea

Acute diarrhea may be classified according to clinical data obtained through the patient history, physical examination, and laboratory findings (Table 8–2). Once this has been done, any necessary diagnostic testing can be focused and reduced significantly.

Clinical Approach to the Evaluation of Acute Diarrhea

The objective in evaluating acute diarrhea is to identify patients with medically important diarrhea and provide appropriate triage. It is paramount to distinguish the patient with potentially life-threatening diarrhea from one with benign, self-limited disease to expedite delivery of specific therapy. This cannot be done on the basis of clinical findings alone and requires integration of data obtained from the patient history, physical examination, and laboratory tests (Figure 8–1).

A. PATIENT HISTORY

A careful, thorough history is the most important tool for uncovering the origin of diarrhea. The focus should be on the following areas.

1. Possible causative factors—The setting in which the diarrhea developed is useful in suggesting an origin. Questions should focus on the following factors:

- Travel history, including international, domestic, and wilderness travel.

Table 8–1. Inflammatory and noninflammatory diarrhea.

	Inflammatory Diarrhea	Noninflammatory Diarrhea
Clinical presentation	Small-volume, bloody diarrhea; lower abdominal cramping or pain; fecal urgency; tenesmus; sometimes, fever	Large-volume, watery diarrhea; upper or paraumbilical abdominal pain or cramping; possible nausea or vomiting
Presence of fecal leukocytes	Yes	No
Common causes	*Shigella, Campylobacter, Salmonella, E histolytica, Yersinia,* enteroinvasive *E coli, C difficile*	*Vibrio, Giardia, Cryptosporidia,* enterotoxigenic *E coli,* rotavirus, Norwalk virus, toxigenic food poisoning (*S aureus, C perfringens, B cereus*)

- Foods eaten, including types of foods or liquids ingested and locations at which food was eaten.
- Recent hospitalizations or closed community confinements, ie, nursing home, boot camp, dormitory.
- Recent use of antibiotics or new medication.
- Exposure to other similarly affected individuals.
- Sexual history, including receptive anal intercourse or oral–anal sexual contact.
- History of shellfish ingestion.
- Exposure to farm animals.
- Presence of systemic disease.
- Immune status [ie, human immunodeficiency virus (HIV), immunosuppressive therapy].

2. Severity of illness—The severity of the illness is determined through the interview and direct examination of the patient. It is important to elicit the following information: (1) appearance of stools, including the presence of blood; (2) frequency of bowel movements; and (3) the presence of other symptoms, including fever, abdominal pain, or volume depletion.

Physical examination may reveal signs consistent with systemic illness or volume depletion.

3. Duration of illness—Most infectious causes of diarrhea have a self-limited course. Prolonged diarrhea (more than 5 days duration) may indicate the presence of a more severe illness or a systemic illness with gastrointestinal manifestations.

B. PHYSICAL EXAMINATION

Examination of the patient may aid in determining the need for more aggressive therapy or hospitalization. Careful assessment should include the following:

- Overall appearance of the patient, including mental status (ie, toxic appearance).
- Vital signs, including high fever or hypotension.
- Postural changes in blood pressure and pulse.
- Skin turgor and mucous membrane examination.

- Abdominal examination for tenderness or peritoneal signs.
- Rectal examination for tenderness and for stool collection.

C. DIAGNOSTIC STUDIES

A variety of diagnostic tests are available, including stool cultures for enteric pathogens, tests for fecal parasitic or viral agents, and fecal leukocytes. Flexible sigmoidoscopy with biopsy may also be helpful. Tests should be used to help define a specific cause that has been suggested by the history and physical examination. They should not be considered the initial step but rather a supplemental step to support the clinician's suspicions of the cause. Despite the multitude of tests available, the cause cannot be determined in 20–40% of cases of acute diarrheal illness.

Diagnostic testing should not be performed routinely as most cases of acute diarrhea are self-limited. Diagnostic testing should be reserved for patients with severe illness, as suggested by one or more of the following:

- Profuse diarrhea with dehydration.
- Grossly bloody stools.
- Fever (oral temperature >38.5°C).
- Passage of more than six unformed stools per day or duration of illness >48 hours.
- Severe abdominal pain.
- Diarrhea in the immunocompromised or elderly.

The most frequently used tests are fecal leukocyte determination, stool culture for enteric pathogens, stool examination for parasites, *Clostridium difficile* toxin testing, and flexible sigmoidoscopy with biopsy.

1. Fecal leukocyte determination—Fecal leukocyte determination by microscopic examination of stool samples prepared by methylene blue staining is often recommended to screen for inflammatory diarrheas. Studies have suggested that stool cultures are unlikely to grow organisms in the absence of fecal leukocytes,

Table 8–2. Classification of acute diarrhea.

Noninflammatory diarrhea
  Viral disease
    Rotavirus
    Norwalk virus
    Cytomegalovirus
    Herpesvirus
  Bacterial disease (toxin-mediated)
    Nontyphoidal *Salmonella*
    S aureus
    B cereus
    C perfringens
    Listeria
  Protozoal disease
    G lamblia
    C parvum
  Medication-induced diarrhea
    Antacids (containing magnesium)
    Antibiotics
    Laxatives
    Miscellaneous drugs (colchicine, lactulose)
  Irritable bowel syndrome
  Dietary intolerance
    Disaccharidase deficiency (eg, lactase)
    Altered diet, with diarrhea induced by osmotic agent
      (eg, due to sorbitol ingestion)
Inflammatory diarrhea
  Bacterial disease
    Invasive disease
      Shigella
      Salmonella
      Campylobacter
      Yersinia
      Vibrio
      C difficile
      Enteropathogenic *E coli* (enteroinvasive)
    Toxin-mediated disease
      Enterohemorrhagic *E coli* (O157)
  Protozoal disease
    E histolytica
    Strongyloides stercoralis
  Mesenteric ischemia
  Radiation colitis
  Inflammatory bowel disease

therefore this test may be used to decide which stool samples should be sent for bacterial culture. However, this test has several limitations. The smear must be performed promptly on a fresh specimen, preferably collected in a cup rather than on a swab or a diaper. Furthermore, microscopy requires careful examination by a skilled microscopist. This examination is not specific for an infectious disorder, as other inflammatory conditions of the bowel (eg, inflammatory bowel disease, ra-

diation colitis) may also yield a positive result. The sensitivity of this examination is 60%. Because of these limitations, the role of testing for fecal leukocytes is unclear.

Nevertheless, the presence of fecal leukocytes supports the diagnosis of a bacterial cause of diarrhea in the context of the medical history. The Practice Parameters Committee of the American College of Gastroenterology recommends fecal leukocyte testing in patients with moderate to severe diarrhea. Furthermore, this committee recommends the use of empiric antibiotics in patients with fever who are positive for fecal leukocytes. Fecal leukocyte testing is probably not helpful in patients who develop diarrhea while hospitalized.

2. Fecal lactoferrin determination—The fecal lactoferrin latex agglutination assay was developed because of the limitations of fecal leukocyte testing. Stool lactoferrin is a byproduct of white blood cells, and its measurement is more precise and less vulnerable to variations in stool processing. Several studies have indicated that the lactoferrin assay is more sensitive than fecal leukocyte testing. As with fecal leukocyte testing, fecal lactoferrin will be elevated in any inflammatory process and it is not specific for infectious diarrhea. Disadvantages of lactoferrin testing include its cost and false-positive results in breast-fed infants. The role of fecal lactoferrin testing in the diagnosis of infectious diarrhea remains unclear.

3. Stool culture for enteric pathogens—Culturing the stool and determining a pathogen may aid in the management of diarrhea. However, results are often delayed and studies have shown that the yield from stool cultures is low. The indiscriminate use of stool cultures is expensive, with an estimated cost of between $900 and $1200 per positive result. Furthermore, the necessity of documenting a pathogen is not always clear as most infectious causes of diarrhea are self-limited. Fifty percent of cases of infectious diarrhea resolve in less than 3 days. In the patient with a high likelihood of an enteric pathogen as the cause of diarrhea, stool cultures may be useful to focus therapy. A stool culture should be obtained in a patient with fever, dysentery, severe diarrhea, or stools that contain leukocytes. Careful specimen collection is vital, because many enteric organisms are fastidious and stool specimens left at room temperature for a prolonged period may result in a false-negative culture. In most microbiology laboratories, a stool culture is routinely processed for the presence of only three enteric pathogens: *Shigella*, *Salmonella*, and *Campylobacter*. If high suspicion exists for the presence of other organisms (eg, *Yersinia*, *Vibrio*, and *Escherichia coli* O157:H7), the laboratory should be alerted, so that the appropriate tests can be arranged.

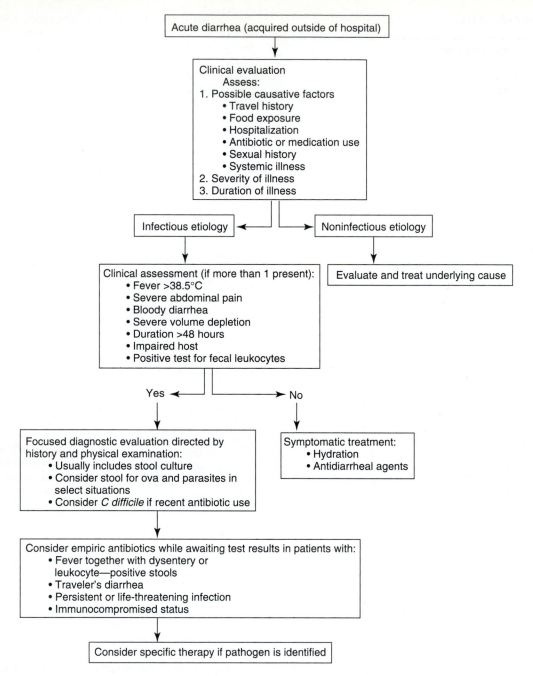

Figure 8–1. Clinical approach to the evaluation of acute diarrhea.

4. Stool examination for parasites—Routine examination of stool for ova and parasites is not cost effective in the work-up of acute diarrhea. Most parasitic infections have chronic presentations. If a patient has a high pretest likelihood of parasitic infestation, such as travel to an endemic region, exposure to infants, or diarrhea in a patient with acquired immunodeficiency syndrome (AIDS), stool should be obtained for ova and parasite examination. At least three stool specimens are needed to accommodate for the sporadic passage of parasites and ova in the stool.

5. *C difficile* toxin testing—In the patient with recent or remote antibiotic usage, hospitalization, closed-community living arrangement (eg, nursing home), or recent chemotherapy exposure, a stool sample should be obtained for *C difficile* toxin determination.

6. Endoscopy—Endoscopy is not usually needed in the diagnosis of acute diarrhea. Flexible sigmoidoscopy may be useful in the patient with signs and symptoms of proctitis (ie, tenesmus, rectal pain, and rectal discharge). Patients with moderate to severe illness suspected of *C difficile*-induced diarrhea may be considered for sigmoidoscopic examination, because the presence of pseudomembranes is highly suggestive of the diagnosis. In addition, flexible sigmoidoscopy may assist in distinguishing patients with other causes of bloody diarrhea (eg, inflammatory bowel disease, ischemic colitis) from those with infectious causes. Examination of the mucosa, including the distribution and endoscopic appearance of colitis, may be diagnostic, although infectious colitis may have an identical endoscopic appearance. Mucosal biopsies may be helpful in distinguishing inflammatory bowel disease from infectious colitis. Endoscopy may also be useful in the investigation of diarrhea in the setting of HIV infection.

D. THERAPY

1. Oral rehydration solutions—The most important risk with diarrheal illness is dehydration. Initial treatment must include rehydration. Patients with mild diarrhea can ingest extra fluids, such as fruit juices, with Saltine crackers. Patients with more severe diarrhea require oral rehydration solutions. These are effective because in small bowel diarrhea, intestinal glucose absorption via sodium–glucose cotransport remains intact. The World Health Organization (WHO) recommends that oral rehydration solutions (ORS) contain the following (per 1 L of water):

- 3.5 g sodium chloride;
- 2.9 g trisodium citrate or 2.5 g sodium bicarbonate;
- 1.5 g potassium chloride; and
- 20 g glucose or 40 g sucrose.

There are a number of oral rehydration solutions available over the counter, including WHO-ORS, Rehydralyte, Pedialyte, and Ceralyte. Solutions can be made by adding one-half teaspoon of baking soda, one-half teaspoon of salt, and four tablespoons of sugar to 1 L of water.

Although these glucose-based oral rehydration formulations correct dehydration, they do not reduce diarrhea. Conventional rehydration formulas focus on the enhancement of small bowel absorption of fluids. More recent strategies attempt to increase colonic absorption. Recent formulations incorporating amylase-resistant starch have shown benefit for cholera, in terms of a reduction in fecal fluid loss and a shorter duration of diarrhea. It is thought that the amylase-resistant starch is fermented in the colon to short-chain fatty acids, which may increase absorption of fluid in the colon. Future research in this field is anticipated.

2. Empiric antibiotic therapy—Empiric antibiotic therapy is rarely indicated for the treatment of acute infectious diarrhea. Most cases are effectively resolved by the host's cellular and humoral defense mechanisms. Fifty percent of cases of infectious diarrhea resolve in less than 3 days without antibiotics. Antibiotic therapy may result in prolonged duration of fecal excretion of the enteric pathogen, drug-related side effects (including *C difficile* diarrhea), and the development of bacteria resistant to multiple antibiotics. Antibiotic therapy may be considered, however, in these selected circumstances: (1) patients who present with signs and symptoms of bacterial diarrhea such as fever, bloody stools, and the presence of fecal leukocytes or occult blood in the stool; (2) to reduce fecal excretion and environmental contamination by a highly infectious agent (eg, *Shigella*); (3) for persistent or life-threatening diarrheal infections (eg, cholera); (4) for traveler's diarrhea, to accelerate resolution of symptoms in individuals who cannot afford to be indisposed by illness (eg, politician, concert pianist); or (5) for the immunocompromised host. Oral fluoroquinolones given twice a day for 3–5 days are suggested.

3. Specific antibiotic therapy—The treatment of specific intestinal pathogens is discussed below (Table 8–3).

4. Symptomatic therapy—Antimotility agents, including diphenoxylate (Lomotil) and loperamide (Imodium), may be used for the symptomatic treatment of acute diarrhea to reduce the number of bowel movements and diminish fluid and electrolyte losses. These agents should be avoided in the presence of fever or bloody stools. The dose of loperamide is 4 mg initially, then 2 mg after each unformed stool, not to exceed 16 mg/d for 2 days. The dose of diphenoxylate is 4 mg (two tablets) four times a day for not more than 2

Table 8–3. Indications for empiric and specific antimicrobial therapy in infectious diarrhea.[1]

Indication	Suggested Therapy
Fever (oral temperature >38.5°C) with one of the following: dysentery or those with leukocyte-, lactoferrin-, or hemoccult-positive stools	Quinolone[2]: NF 400 mg, CF 500 mg, OF 300 mg twice a day for 3–5 days
Shigellosis	TMP-SMZ[3] 160 mg/800 mg twice a day for 3 days or quinolone as above
Non-*typhi* species of *Salmonella*	Not routinely recommended, but if severe disease associated with fever and systemic toxicity or important underlying condition use TMP-SMZ 160 mg/800 mg or fluoroquinolone as above for 5–7 days
Campylobacter species	Erythromycin 500 mg twice a day for 5 days
Escherichia coli species	TMP-SMZ 160 mg/800 mg twice a day for 3 days or fluoroquinolone twice a day for 3 days
Enterotoxigenic (ETEC) Enteropathogenic (EPEC) Enteroadherent (EAEC) Enterohemorrhagic (EHEC)	Avoid antimotility agents; role of antibiotics is unclear and they should be avoided
Aeromonas/Plesiomonas	TMP-SMZ 160 mg/800 mg twice a day for 3 days
Vibrio cholerae	Tetracycline 500 mg four times a day for 3 days or doxycycline 300 mg as a single dose
Yersinia species	Antibiotics not usually required; for severe infections use combination therapy with aminoglycoside, doxycycline, TMP-SMZ, or quinolone
Parasites	
Giardia	Metronidazole 250 mg three times a day for 7 days
Cryptosporidium species	None; for severe cases consider paromomycin 500 mg three times a day for 7 days
Cyclospora species	TMP-SMZ 160 mg/800 mg twice a day for 7 days
Entamoeba histolytica	Metronidazole 750 mg three times a day for 10 days plus iodoquinol 650 mg three times a day for 20 days

[1]Adapted from DuPont HL: Guidelines on acute infectious diarrhea in adults. The Practice Parameters Committee of the American College of Gastroenterology. Am J Gastroenterol 1997;92:1962.
[2]Fluoroquinolones include norfloxacin (NF), ciprofloxacin (CF), and ofloxacin (OF).
[3]TMP-SMZ, trimethoprim-sulfamethoxazole.

days. Diphenoxylate has central opiate effects and may cause cholinergic side effects.

5. Probiotics—It is well established that maintainence of the normal intestinal microflora is essential in maintaining health. Colonization resistance refers to the ability of the microflora to resist proliferation of pathogens. The exact mechanism by which this occurs is poorly understood. Probiotics include bacteria that aid in recolonizing the intestine with normal bowel flora. Potential advantages of the use of probiotics include the following: they can reduce the use of antibiotics, they have multiple mechanisms of action making resistance less likely, and they are well tolerated. Probiotics may be useful in treating pediatric diarrhea, traveler's diarrhea, *C difficile* diarrhea, and antibiotic-associated diarrhea. The most extensively studied organisms include *Saccharomyces boulardii, Lactobacillus rhamnosus GG, Lactobacillus acidophilus,* and *Enterococcus faecium* strain SF68. They are usually administered as capsulated lyophilized powders or as fermented milk products. Proposed disadvantages of probiotic therapy include the risk of infection, quality control issues in the manufacturing of these agents, and a lack of placebo-controlled trials. Research in this area is needed before firm recommendations on the use of probiotics can be made.

■ INFECTIOUS CAUSES OF ACUTE DIARRHEA

VIRAL INFECTIONS

Although viral diarrhea is a major cause of gastroenteritis in the United States and the world (accounting for up to 40% of acute episodes), it accounts for few episodes of traveler's diarrhea. Rotavirus and Norwalk virus are the two most common agents in viral diarrhea in children and adults, respectively.

Rotavirus

The disease occurs primarily in children aged 3–15 months, with infections less common after 2 years of age. Adults can develop mild infection but rarely with the magnitude of diarrhea seen in the pediatric population. Typically, a child develops vomiting, followed by profuse, watery diarrhea. The average duration of illness is 5–7 days. Dehydration may develop rapidly in children and contributes significantly to the severity of the illness.

Rapid diagnosis can be achieved by detection of rotavirus antigen in feces by commercially available kits. In clinical practice, however, this usually is unnecessary.

RotaShield, a live oral vaccine initially approved for the prevention of rotavirus infection, was withdrawn from the market because of a possible increased risk of intussusception.

Symptomatic treatment is the mainstay of therapy. Rehydration is imperative and can be accomplished through oral rehydration solutions available commercially or through home preparation.

Norwalk Virus

Norwalk viruses have been implicated in up to 40% of nonbacterial diarrheal epidemics in the United States. Its role in traveler's diarrhea is not well defined.

The small intestine is the affected region during invasion by Norwalk virus. The exact mechanism of injury is unclear due to difficulty imaging the virus, even by electron microscopy. Morphologic and physiologic abnormalities appear to reverse within 1–2 weeks after infection.

The clinical spectrum of disease is varied, although all cases are mild. Diarrhea is the most prominent symptom, noted in up to 92% of patients. Abdominal pain, nausea, and vomiting are noted in up to 75% of patients. The duration of illness is usually 24–48 hours.

At this time, the virus cannot be cultured and stool viral antigen identification is not offered routinely. Diagnosis may be established by identification of viral antigen in the stool, when this is deemed necessary.

No specific treatment is available or required. Volume repletion for dehydrated patients is indicated.

Cytomegalovirus

Cytomegalovirus infection of the gastrointestinal tract can occur in the course of HIV infection when the CD4 lymphocyte count falls below 100/μL (see Chapter 2). Cytomegalovirus colitis accounts for up to 25% of cases of diarrhea in HIV patients.

The clinical spectrum of presentation is varied, ranging from abdominal pain, weight loss, fever, and watery diarrhea to hemorrhagic colitis with perforation. Cytomegalovirus colitis has been implicated in cases of appendicitis in AIDS patients.

Frequently, the CD4 lymphocyte count will be less than 100/μL. The demonstration of characteristic intranuclear cytomegalovirus inclusions on tissue biopsy is diagnostic. Immunohistochemical staining of tissue may be required to demonstrate the presence of the virus. Culture of cytomegalovirus from tissue biopsies is not helpful.

Colonoscopy with biopsy may be useful in determining the presence of cytomegalovirus colitis. Endoscopic appearances range from diffuse colitis to hemorrhagic colitis with deep, irregular ulcerations.

Ganciclovir, an acyclovir derivative, has been shown to be effective in most cases of cytomegalovirus colitis. For patients with neutropenia or ganciclovir resistance, foscarnet, a pyrophosphate analog, has been used for treatment.

BACTERIAL INFECTIONS

1. Noninvasive Infections

Food-Borne Gastroenteritis

Food poisoning is a frequently overlooked cause of diarrhea. Important clues to diagnosis can be found in the food history, the geographic location, the season of the year, and the order and timing of onset of symptoms. Of particular concern is the isolation of antibiotic-resistant pathogens from retail ground meats. The routine practice of administering antimicrobial agents to domestic livestock to prevent disease and promote growth is a factor in the emergence of these antibiotic-resistant bacteria. These organinsms can then be transferred to humans who ingest contaminated animal products.

Staphylococcus aureus

Staphylococcal food poisoning is caused by ingestion of preformed staphylococcal toxin, which accumulates in protein-rich foods that have been inadequately refrigerated. The most commonly implicated foods are cream-filled cakes, potato and macaroni salads, and ham. Staphylococcal enterotoxins are heat stable and cause symptoms through their effects on enteric autonomic sensory neurons and intestinal cell permeability.

Symptoms occur within 1–6 hours after ingestion of contaminated food. Approximately 75% of patients have nausea, vomiting, and abdominal pain, which are followed by diarrhea in 68%. Fever is exceedingly rare. The duration of illness is less than 24 hours.

Definitive diagnosis can be made by culturing *S aureus* from the contaminated food, or from the stools and vomitus of the patient. This may be considered in large outbreaks of presumptive food poisoning. Peripheral leukocytosis is rare, and white blood cells are absent on fecal smears.

Treatment is supportive, including adequate oral hydration and antiemetics. No role exists for antibiotics for eradication of ingested staphylococci.

Bacillus cereus

B cereus is a gram-positive, aerobic, spore-forming rod. Two separate enterotoxins are responsible for the distinct phases of illness, the emetic syndrome and the diarrheal syndrome, with the emetic syndrome being more common.

The onset of symptoms is 1–6 hours after ingestion of contaminated food, and the duration of illness is less than 24 hours. Acute symptoms include nausea, vomiting, and abdominal pain, which usually resolve within 10 hours. The emetic syndrome is more commonly associated with ingestion of fried rice, whereas the diarrheal syndrome is associated with ingestion of inadequately refrigerated prepared foods. The diarrheal syndrome occurs 8–16 hours after ingestion of contaminated food and produces a syndrome of profuse watery diarrhea and abdominal cramping. Nausea and vomiting are rare.

Treatment is supportive, with oral rehydration and antiemetics.

Clostridium perfringens

C perfringens is an anaerobic, spore-forming, gram-positive rod. It has been implicated in several distinct syndromes of food poisoning, with the most common type being a self-limited illness characterized by ingestion of organisms, with *in vivo* production of enterotoxin. Clostridial food poisoning is common in the setting of delayed serving of cooked meat and poultry products. When meat products are stored at room temperature, clostridial spores may germinate and be ingested, and elaboration of the enterotoxin may ensue.

The self-limited syndrome is characterized by onset of symptoms 8–24 hours after ingestion of the meat product. The onset of watery diarrhea and significant epigastric pain occurs, and this may be followed by nausea, vomiting, and fever, rarely. The symptoms resolve within 24 hours.

Microbiologic examination of the suspected food, with isolation of more than 10^5 organisms per gram of food, confirms the diagnosis of clostridial food poisoning. Fecal smears reveal no polymorphonuclear cells, and other laboratory testing is not indicated.

Treatment is supportive, with oral rehydration and antiemetics as needed.

Vibrio cholerae

V cholerae is a gram-negative, comma-shaped rod that produces a severe diarrheal disorder leading to profound dehydration; death may result within 3–4 hours in an untreated patient. Cholera toxin affects small intestinal fluid transport by increasing cyclic AMP, promoting secretion, and inhibiting absorption of fluid. The major vehicle of spread of cholera is contaminated food and water, particularly shellfish. *V cholerae* is endemic along the Gulf Coast of the United States.

The initial presentation is abdominal distention and vomiting, followed rapidly by diarrhea. The diarrhea is frequent, large in volume, and has the appearance of rice water. Patients may present with profound electrolyte abnormalities and volume depletion. Mild fever may be present.

Blood chemistries may be compatible with profound volume and electrolyte depletion and should be replaced accordingly. Bicarbonate and potassium are lost in significant quantities, and scrupulous replacement is warranted. Fecal cultures may be appropriate in the patient in whom a diagnosis of cholera is suspected and a lack of endemic exposure is demonstrated.

Treatment is primarily targeted at aggressive volume and electrolyte replacement. Most cases can be managed with oral rehydration solutions. Severe cases may require intravenous fluids. Antibiotics can reduce the volume and duration of diarrhea. Tetracycline, 500 mg three times a day for 3 days, or doxycycline, 300 mg as a single dose, are the drugs of choice. Aggressive management of volume status results in low mortality rates (usually <1%). Live and killed oral cholera vaccines are becoming available outside the United States. The new oral cholera vaccines appear to have higher protective efficacy compared with the older parenteral vaccines.

Pathogenic Escherichia coli

Pathogenic *E coli* is the major causative agent for traveler's diarrhea. The pathogenic mechanisms employed by this agent include elaboration of enterotoxin and diffuse mucosal adherence. There are several important agents:

1. Enterotoxigenic *E coli* (ETEC) accounts for approximately 50% of all *E coli* diarrhea cases and is the most common cause of traveler's diarrhea.

2. Enteropathogenic *E coli* (EPEC) causes a large proportion of the remaining cases of traveler's diarrhea.

3. Enteroadherent *E coli* (EAEC) appears to account for 15% of cases of traveler's diarrhea.

4. Enterohemorrhagic *E coli* (EHEC) is a rare cause of traveler's diarrhea but a major cause of sporadic

and epidemic cases of infectious bloody diarrhea (discussed separately).

Most patients with ETEC, EPEC, or EAEC have mild symptoms consisting of watery diarrhea, nausea, and abdominal cramping. The diarrhea is rarely severe, with most patients having five or fewer stools within 24 hours. The average length of illness is 5 days. Fever is present in fewer than a third of patients. Stools can be mucoid but rarely contain blood or white blood cells. Leukocytosis is uncommon. ETEC, EAEC, and EPEC are self-limited, with no significant sequelae.

Laboratory findings are nonspecific for *E coli* diarrhea, including rare fecal leukocytes, absence of other pathogens on stool culture, and occasional peripheral leukocytosis. EPEC and EHEC can be isolated in culture, and a latex agglutination assay specific for EHEC type O157 is available. However, other immunologic assays for ETEC are laborious and not widely available commercially.

Treatment is supportive, with the mainstay being adequate rehydration. Antimotility agents should be avoided in severe illness. ETEC will respond to trimethoprim-sulfamethoxazole or a quinolone given for 3 days. It is unknown if antimicrobial therapy will shorten the illness in EPEC diarrhea and EAEC diarrhea. As discussed below, antibiotics should be avoided in diarrhea due to EHEC.

2. Invasive Infections

Shigella

Shigella is the second most common food-borne disease in the United States. *Shigella* are typically food or water borne. *Shigella* organisms cause bacillary dysentery and produce an intense inflammatory response in the colon via elaborated enterotoxin and invasion.

Classically, shigellosis presents with crampy abdominal pain, fever, and multiple small-volume bloody, mucoid stools. Initial symptoms may consist of fever, abdominal pain, and watery diarrhea without gross blood, with a second stage with bloody stools occurring 3–5 days later. The average length of symptoms in adults is 7 days, with more severe cases persisting for 3–4 weeks. Chronic shigellosis can mimic ulcerative colitis, and a chronic carrier state is possible.

Extraintestinal manifestations of shigellosis may occur, including respiratory symptoms, neurologic symptoms such as meningismus, and hemolytic-uremic syndrome. An asymmetric oligoarticular arthritis may occur up to 3 weeks after onset of dysentery, mimicking Reiter's syndrome.

Fecal smears reveal multiple polymorphonuclear and red blood cells. Stool culture may be used for isolation and identification of antibiotic sensitivity.

The mainstay of treatment is adequate rehydration by oral or intravenous methods, depending on the severity of illness. Opiate derivatives should be avoided. Antimicrobial therapy is indicated to shorten the duration of illness and for public health issues. Trimethoprim-sulfamethoxazole or a fluoroquinolone twice a day for 3 days is the preferred antibiotic.

Nontyphoidal *Salmonella*

Nontyphoidal *Salmonella* is the leading cause of food poisoning in the United States. *Salmonella enteriditis* and *Salmonella typhimurium* are the causative agents. Infection is most common during the summer and fall months. Animals are a natural reservoir for nontyphoidal salmonellosis and, consequently, animal products derived from contaminated animals are the source of infection. Commonly implicated foods include eggs, poultry, milk, and beef.

The onset of illness is characterized by fever, chills, and diarrhea, followed by the variable presence of nausea, vomiting, and abdominal cramping. Grossly bloody diarrhea is uncommon. The duration of illness is usually less than 7 days.

Stool smears reveal moderate red and white blood cells. Blood cultures are positive in 5–10% of cases and are more common in HIV-infected patients.

The treatment in uncomplicated nontyphoidal salmonellosis is supportive care, with adequate hydration being paramount. Routine use of antibiotics is not recommended, because of increased incidence of resistant strains and prolongation of bacterial shedding. Indications for antibiotics include conditions that may complicate salmonellosis, including extremes of age (neonates and age >50), immunodeficiency, signs or symptoms of sepsis, or focal infections (osteomyelitis, abscesses). The antibiotic of choice is trimethoprim-sulfamethoxazole or a fluoroquinolone such as ciprofloxacin or norfloxacin by mouth twice a day for 5–7 days or a third-generation cephalosporin given intravenously in patients unable to tolerate oral medications.

Salmonella typhi

Salmonella typhi and *Salmonella paratyphi* are the causative agents of typhoid fever. Typhoid fever is characterized by a prolonged febrile illness with associated splenomegaly, delirium, abdominal pain, and other systemic manifestations. Typhoidal disease is a systemic disease and has few primary symptoms relating to the gastrointestinal tract. The source of the organism is usually contaminated water, poultry, or eggs.

After the initial bacteremia, the organism is sequestered in the reticuloendothelial system, resulting in hyperplasia of the system, including lymph nodes and

Peyer's patches within the small intestine. Progressive enlargement and ulceration of nodes may result in perforation of the small bowel or gastrointestinal hemorrhage.

The classic form of typhoid fever involves a 4-week cycle. The incubation period is 7–14 days. The first week is characterized by high fever, headaches, and abdominal pain. A pulse–temperature dissociation can be found. Approximately 50% of patients describe normal bowel habits. During the second week, splenomegaly and an evanescent rash are evident. The third week is characterized by decreasing mentation and increasing toxemia. Intestinal involvement, with greenish diarrhea and potential intestinal perforation, occurs during this period. The fourth week is characterized by defervescence and improved clinical status.

The diagnosis is established by isolation of the organism. Blood cultures are positive in up to 90% of patients within the first week of clinically apparent illness. Stool cultures become positive during the second and third weeks.

Intestinal perforation and gastrointestinal hemorrhage can occur during the course of the illness. Altered mental status and acute cholecystitis are less common; however, chronic infection of gallstones may attribute to a carrier state once the patient has recovered from the acute illness.

The traditional drug of choice is chloramphenicol, 500 mg orally four times a day for 2 weeks. However, due to problems with resistance, a high rate of relapse and chronic carriage, and potential bone marrow toxicity, third-generation cephalosporins and fluoroquinolones are preferred. Third-generation cephalosporins have demonstrated excellent efficacy against *S typhi* and should be administered intravenously for 7–10 days. Quinolones, such as ciprofloxacin, 500 mg twice a day by mouth for 14 days, have demonstrated high efficacy and a low resultant carrier state.

Oral (Ty21a) and parenteral (Vi) typhoid vaccines are recommended if travel to endemic areas is planned.

Campylobacter

Campylobacter species found in human infection include *Campylobacter jejuni* and *Campylobacter fetus,* more commonly found in immunocompromised hosts. Approximately 5–10% of all cases of bacterial diarrhea in the United States are caused by *C jejuni.* It accounts for up to 15% of cases of traveler's diarrhea from Asia. The most common route of transmission is from infected animals and their food products to humans, with chickens being the main source. Pathogenesis of disease is by toxin elaboration and mucosal invasion.

The clinical manifestations of *Campylobacter* infection vary widely, from asymptomatic disease to dysen-

tery. The incubation period is 24–72 hours after ingestion of organisms. Diarrhea and fever are present in 90% of patients, and abdominal pain and bloody stools in 50–70%. Other constitutional symptoms, such as fever, nausea, vomiting, and malaise, may also be present. The duration of illness is less than 7 days. Relapses can occur in as many as 25% of patients.

Fecal smears demonstrate numerous fecal leukocytes and the presence of red blood cells. Stool for culture will yield the presence of *Campylobacter.*

Campylobacter is sensitive to erythromycin and quinolones; however, debate has occurred regarding the need for antibiotic administration. Studies have revealed that inception of treatment after 4 days of onset of symptoms yielded no clinical benefit, except for decreased fecal excretion of organisms. Antibiotics are indicated in the severely ill patient or the patient with frank dysentery. If antibiotic therapy is initiated, erythromycin 500 mg twice a day orally for 5 days is effective. The most significant problem in the treatment of *Campylobacter* is the rise in resistance, most notably with the quinolones. As with all diarrheal illnesses, volume repletion and correction of electrolyte derangements are paramount.

Noncholera *Vibrio*

Noncholera *Vibrio* species have been associated with outbreaks of gastroenteritis. *Vibrio parahaemolyticus,* non-01 *V cholerae,* and *Vibrio mimicus* have been associated with the consumption of raw oysters. Diarrhea is usually self-limited, lasting less than 5 days. Diagnosis is made by stool culture and requires the use of selective media (ie, TCBS agar). Treatment is supportive with electrolyte and fluid repletion. Antibiotics have not been shown to shorten the duration of illness. However, for the patient with prolonged or severe diarrhea, some recommend the use of tetracycline.

Yersinia

Yersinia species are gram-negative, non-lactose fermenting coccobacilli. They are classified according to their somatic (O) and flagellar (H) antigens. The organism adheres to the epithelium with subsequent invasion. *Yersinia* produces a heat-labile enterotoxin that is elaborated at 25°C. The terminal ileum is the most common area of involvement, although the colon may also be invaded. *Yersinia* is found in streams and lakes, and has been isolated from many animals, which serve as reservoirs. Infections have been linked to contaminated dairy products and undercooked pork products.

Clinical presentation usually consists of diarrhea and abdominal pain, which can be followed by arthralgias and a rash (erythema nodosum or erythema multiforme). Fever and bloody stools are less frequent. Infected patients can present with mesenteric adenitis, with nausea, vomiting, and oral apthous ulcerations. Septicemia may occur with iron overload states, such as multiple blood transfusions, hemochromatosis, and deferoxamine therapy. Diagnosis is made by stool culture. Illness is usually self-limited, lasting from 1 to 3 weeks. Treatment is supportive with adequate hydration. Antibiotics are not usually required, however, they can be considered for severe infections or bacteremia. A combination of an aminoglycoside with a quinolone appears to be reasonable empiric therapy for sepsis. Deferoxamine therapy should be withheld.

Enterohemorrhagic *Escherichia coli* (Subtype O157)

Enterohemorrhagic *E coli* (EHEC) has become well recognized for its role in outbreaks of hemorrhagic colitis. Outbreaks have been attributed to contaminated undercooked ground beef, unpasteurized apple juice, milk, lettuce, and venison. Most cases occur within 7–10 days of ingestion of contaminated meat or water. Secondary infections may occur via a fecal–oral route among household contacts or children and personnel in daycare centers. EHEC may be the most common cause of infectious bloody diarrhea. Subtype O157:H7 may be associated with the development of hemolytic-uremic syndrome (HUS), especially in children. The Centers for Disease Control (CDC) has recommended that *E coli* O157 be considered for all persons with acute bloody diarrhea or hemolytic-uremic syndrome. EHEC is noninvasive but produces cytotoxin closely related to *Shigella* toxin, which produces endothelial damage, microangiopathic hemolysis, and renal damage. Shiga-like toxin may be produced by non-O157 strains of *E coli*. Testing for these organisms can be difficult, and toxin testing of stool or culture supernatants with Shiga toxin-based assays may be useful.

The onset of illness is characterized by moderate to severe diarrhea (up to 10–12 liquid stools per day). Initial diarrhea is nonbloody but frequently progresses to grossly bloody stools. Severe abdominal pain and cramping are common, and nausea and vomiting are present in about two-thirds of patients. Abdominal examination may reveal marked abdominal distention and diffuse abdominal or focal right lower quadrant tenderness. Fever occurs in fewer than one-third of patients and is of short duration. Up to one-third of patients require hospitalization.

Peripheral leukocytosis with a left shift is frequently present. Urinalysis may reveal hematuria or proteinuria or leukocyte casts. Evidence of microangiopathic hemolytic anemia (hematocrit <30%), thrombocytopenia ($<150 \times 10^9$/L), and renal insufficiency (blood urea nitrogen >20 mg/dL) is diagnostic of hemolytic-uremic syndrome.

Hemolytic-uremic syndrome may occur in 5–10% of patients and typically is diagnosed 6 days after the onset of diarrhea. Risk factors for developing hemolytic-uremic syndrome include extremes of age (especially children under 5 years) and prolonged use of antimotility agents.

Antibiotic use may also increase the risk. Approximately 60% of patients with hemolytic-uremic syndrome will have resolution of disease, 3–5% will die acutely, 5% will develop end-stage renal disease, and 30% will have long-term sequelae, such as proteinuria. Thrombotic thrombocytopenic purpura can occur but is less common than hemolytic-uremic syndrome. Central nervous system complications of thrombotic thrombocytopenic purpura, manifested by confusion, myoclonic jerking, and sensorimotor deficits, occur variably.

When EHEC is suspected, the laboratory must be alerted to culture stool specimens for *E coli* on sorbitol-McConkey agar. Specific serotyping usually is performed in special laboratories.

Treatment is supportive, with scrupulous attention to volume status and treatment of renal and vascular complications. Antibiotics have not been effective in reducing symptoms or the risk of complications of EHEC infection. In fact, several studies suggest antibiotic use may increase the risk of hemolytic-uremic syndrome. Antibiotics and antimotility drugs should be avoided. Fosfomycin may improve the clinical course, however, further studies are needed.

Aeromonas

Aeromonas species are gram-negative, facultative anaerobes. *Aeromonas* produces several toxins, including hemolysin, enterotoxin, and cytotoxin. Infections are associated with the ingestion of untreated water and appear to peak in the summer and fall.

Symptoms include watery diarrhea, vomiting, and mild fever. Occasionally, stools may be bloody. The illness is usually self-limited and usually resolves within 7 days. Diagnosis is made by stool culture.

Treatment is recommended for patients with prolonged diarrhea or conditions associated with an increased risk of septicemia, including malignancy, hepatobiliary disease, or immunocompromised states. Trimethoprim-sulfamethoxazole is the treatment of choice.

Plesiomonas

Plesiomonas shigelloides is a gram-negative, facultative anaerobe. Most cases are associated with ingestion of raw oysters or untreated water and travel to the tropics.

The most common symptoms are abdominal pain, fever, and vomiting. Patients can have bloody diarrhea. The illness is usually self-limited, lasting less than 14 days. Diagnosis is made by stool culture.

Antibiotics can shorten the duration of diarrhea. Trimethoprim-sulfamethoxazole is the treatment of choice.

PROTOZOAL INFECTIONS

Entamoeba histolytica

E histolytica is the causative agent of amebiasis, which is characterized as both an acute and a chronic illness. *E histolytica* has been reclassified into two species: *Entamoeba histolytica* and *Entamoeba dispar,* which is noninvasive. *E histolytica* causes amebic colitis and liver abscess. *E dispar* causes infection in sexually active homosexual males. Approximately 10% of the world's population are colonized with these organisms. Of these cases, 90% are due to nonpathogenic *E dispar*. Ten percent of infections with *E histolytica* will result in symptomatic disease. Amebiasis is transmitted by fecal–oral spread. A wide range of clinical states can be seen in amebiasis, from the asymptomatic carrier to the patient with frank dysentery or amebic hepatic abscess. Asymptomatic carriers have evidence of cysts in their stools but no clinical evidence of enteroinvasion. Patients with amebic dysentery demonstrate evidence of trophozoite and cyst passage into the stool.

E histolytica is directly invasive and is capable of mucosal invasion, with potential widespread distal dissemination. Histologically, colonic lesions demonstrate diffuse inflammation, with a dense cell infiltrate into the lamina propria. As the disease advances, ulceration occurs, eventually producing classic flask-shaped ulcers with undermined edges. Occasionally in severe cases, fulminant necrotizing colitis may occur.

The clinical spectrum of disease varies widely, from asymptomatic carrier to frank dysentery. In the patient with evidence of colitis, the presenting symptoms include diffuse lower abdominal pain, intermittent bloody, mucoid stools, anorexia, and malaise. The stool frequency may be 7–10 bowel movements within 24 hours. Physical examination may reveal diffuse or focal abdominal tenderness. In extremely ill patients, there may be signs of peritonitis and evidence of ileus suggested by abdominal distention.

Amebiasis may be associated with extraintestinal manifestations, including liver abscess, brain abscess, splenic abscess, pericarditis, and empyema. Most patients with liver abscess do not have a history of amebic colitis.

Stool samples for ova and parasites may reveal the presence of trophozoites and establish the diagnosis in

90% of patients. Serologic testing by indirect hemagglutination or enzyme-linked immunosorbent assay (ELISA) may detect elevated ameba serologies consistent with invasive disease. A warm saline wet mount of stool may reveal Charcot–Leyden crystals, which, although not specific for amebic colitis, raise suspicion for amebiasis.

Sigmoidoscopy may reveal discrete, small, flat, shallow-based ulcers, with overlying yellowish exudate. Frequently, the intervening mucosa is normal in appearance, in contradistinction to inflammatory bowel disease or other infectious colitides.

E histolytica should be treated and metronidazole is the drug of choice. Metronidazole, 750 mg three times a day for 10 days, should be followed by an intraluminally active agent such as iodoquinol, 650 mg three times a day for 20 days. In asymptomatic carriers, only a luminally active agent is required. In patients with amebic liver abscess, percutaneous drainage is not indicated for treatment as it does not shorten recovery time.

Giardia lamblia

G lamblia is an internationally distributed protozoan and accounts for 5% of traveler's diarrhea. Prevalence is highest in areas of poor sanitation and water treatment. It exists in both an encysted form and as a trophozoite. The parasite is common in freshwater streams and lakes in the Western United States, as well as in Eastern Europe. Animal vectors, particularly beavers, have been felt to be the source of contamination of waters in Rocky Mountain regions. Here, infection may occur in campers who drink contaminated lake or stream water or in international travelers. *Giardia* is also a common cause of diarrhea in daycare centers.

Giardia is transmitted by eating contaminated food, drinking contaminated water, or by fecal–oral contact.

The pathogenesis of diarrhea is unknown. Possible factors include inhibition of nutrient passage secondary to massive numbers of adherent parasites within the small bowel, epithelial damage, competition of the parasite and the host for nutrients, and mucosal invasion.

Patients with symptomatic giardiasis complain frequently of diarrhea, which may be acute in onset and loose to watery in consistency, with associated flatulence. Mucus may be present, but blood is absent from the stools. Steatorrheic stools may be described by patients, as well as symptoms of abdominal bloating, weight loss, and fatigue.

If steatorrhea is suspected, a Sudan stain may reveal the presence of fat in the stool. Laboratory evidence of malabsorption, with low carotene, vitamin B_{12}, or folate may be rarely present. Lactase deficiency occurs in 20–40% of cases.

There is no gold standard for the diagnosis of giardiasis. The first-line method of diagnosis is by demonstration of the trophozoite or cyst in the stool by microscopy. Due to a variable amount of organisms being shed at different times, three specimens on separate days should be obtained. The sensitivity of stool microscopy is 85% with three specimens. Another method for diagnosis is stool antigen detection by ELISA. The stool ELISA, which has a high sensitivity (95%) and specificity (98%), may be especially helpful for mass screening, as in the daycare setting. The final method of diagnosis is by examination of duodenal contents, by aspiration or biopsy with endoscopy. Although duodenal aspiration may reveal the presence of trophozoites, this is a cumbersome test that is done infrequently. The sensitivity of duodenal biopsy compared with duodenal aspiration has not been well determined. If stool studies are negative and the patient is having severe symptoms of diarrhea and malabsorption, endoscopy with biopsy may be helpful in examining for *Giardia* trophozoites in addition to ruling out other infectious or noninfectious causes.

Several excellent treatments exist for giardiasis. Metronidazole, 250 mg three times a day for 7 days, is the first-line treatment. If eradication of the organism is not successful at this dose, higher doses (500–800 mg orally three times a day for 7 days) are indicated. Albendazole, 400 mg a day orally for 3 days, may be useful if metronidazole therapy fails. Because *Giardia* may be difficult to identify from stool samples alone, empiric therapy may be given in patients with chronic watery diarrhea who have traveled to an endemic region.

Cryptosporidium parvum

C parvum is a coccidian protozoan that has been recognized as a common cause of bovine diarrhea. It has become more widely recognized as an important cause of chronic diarrhea in HIV-infected patients and in health care workers. In Latin America, *Cryptosporidium* causes up to 5% of cases of diarrhea in children and has occurred in daycare centers in the United States. Waterborne outbreaks have occurred in the Midwestern United States in normal hosts.

Cryptosporidia trophozoites attach firmly to intestinal epithelial cells, thereby destroying microvilli. Histologically, villi are blunted, with evidence of increased inflammatory cell infiltrate in the lamina propria.

Common presentation for acute cryptosporidial infection includes nausea, abdominal cramping, and low-grade fever, followed by a profuse, watery diarrhea. Nausea and vomiting may occur but are less common. Significant volume depletion may result from the profuse diarrhea. Physical examination may be remarkable for dehydration and mild diffuse abdominal tenderness.

A modified acid-fast stain of fecal smears may demonstrate cryptosporidial oocysts. This test lacks sensitivity, and immunofluorescent assays that are more sensitive are now available. Biopsy of the small intestine may reveal oocysts embedded in the microvillous border. Sigmoidoscopy may reveal hyperemic mucosa without frank ulceration or colitis.

Treatment is supportive, with volume repletion and correction of electrolyte derangements. In patients with intact immunologic status, the infection is self-limited and will resolve in approximately 14 days. To date, no effective antimicrobial agents have been identified for eradication of cryptosporidia. If symptoms are severe, consider paromomycin (a poorly absorbed aminoglycoside), 500 mg three times a day for 7 days.

Cyclospora cayetanensis

C cayetanensis causes gastrointestinal illness worldwide. The lifecycle of *Cyclospora* is unknown. Transmission is thought to be by the fecal–oral route and ingestion of contaminated water. Infection is common in patients with AIDS in Haiti and in travelers to Nepal. Several outbreaks have occurred in the United States. One outbreak, which occurred in the spring and summer of 1996 and 1997, was associated with ingestion of raspberries from Guatemala. More recently, this parasite has been linked to fresh basil.

Cyclospora causes pathologic changes in the small intestine, including villous atrophy and crypt hyperplasia by unknown mechanisms. The clinical presentation includes watery diarrhea, fatigue, abdominal pain, weight loss, fever, bloating, and nausea. The illness can be prolonged, lasting up to 12 weeks, if untreated. Diagnosis is by acid-fast microscopy of stool. Trimethoprim-sulfamethoxazole twice a day for 7 days is the treatment of choice.

SPECIAL CLINICAL SITUATIONS

1. Traveler's Diarrhea

Traveler's diarrhea is defined as the passage of three unformed stools within a 24-hour period, in conjunction with other gastrointestinal symptoms of nausea, vomiting, abdominal pain, tenesmus, or passage of blood or mucus with the stool. It typically occurs in a person who resides in an industrialized region and travels to a developing country. Traveler's diarrhea should also include diarrheal illness that is experienced 7–10 days after return to a developed area, as this period encompasses the incubation time of most enteropathogens. Up to 50% of travelers to developing countries are affected with diarrhea within the first 2 weeks of travel. After returning home, 10–20% of travelers will have the onset of diarrhea, which may last for longer than 1 week in 10% of patients and longer than 1 month in 2%.

Bacterial enteric pathogens are the causative agents in 80% of cases of traveler's diarrhea. The principal agents in most high-risk areas are, in decreasing order of importance, enterotoxigenic *E coli,* various species of *Shigella, C jejuni, Aeromonas* species, *Plesiomonas shigelloides, Salmonella* species, and noncholera *Vibrios.* Viral agents, such as rotavirus and Norwalk virus, are responsible for up to 10% of cases. Protozoa, such as *G lamblia* (in mountainous areas of North America and Russia) and *E histolytica,* are less common causes, despite their importance as pathogens within the developing country. *Cyclospora* (noteworthy for travelers to Nepal) and *Cryptosporidia* (Russia) may contribute to diarrhea in travelers. Parasites, such as *Strongyloides* and *Ascaris,* are not usually associated with diarrhea. The most important determinant of risk is the destination of the traveler. Low-risk regions (<10%) include Northern Europe, Canada, the United States, Australia, New Zealand, Japan, and Singapore. Moderate-risk regions (10–20%) include South Africa, countries bordering the Mediterranean Sea, and the Caribbean islands. High-risk regions (>30%) include Africa, Mexico, Central America, South America, and Asia (not including Singapore). Certain hosts appear to be at high risk, including patients with achlorhydria, postgastrectomy patients, persons with AIDS, and patients with secretory immunoglobulin A (IgA) deficiency.

Clinical Findings

Symptoms associated with traveler's diarrhea are variable. Most patients have a mild, self-limited clinical course consisting of 1–3 days of watery, nonbloody diarrhea, minimal other gastrointestinal complaints, and a lack of dehydration or fever. More severe illness may also be seen, with high fever, frequent bloody stools, abdominal pain, nausea and vomiting, and leukocytosis. Although clinical features on presentation may suggest the causative agent, severely ill patients warrant thorough assessment and close observation.

Prevention

A. FOOD AND WATER PRECAUTIONS

Because infectious agents of traveler's diarrhea are transmitted by the fecal–oral route, travelers should be advised about safe water and food practices. All travelers should be counseled to refrain from drinking tap water, iced drinks (including alcoholic beverages with ice), unpasteurized milk, and noncarbonated bottled water. Carbonated beverages and carbonated bottled water are bactericidal because of their low pH. Travelers should

be cautious when showering or brushing their teeth, as ingestion of pathogens can occur. If carbonated beverages are unavailable, travelers may achieve disinfection by boiling water at 100°C for 5–10 minutes, by halogenation using commercially available iodine or chlorine solutions, or by filtration via sediment filtration or resin contact devices.

Food may become contaminated at the source, as fertilization with human excreta is a common practice in developing countries. Additionally, food may become contaminated during preparation, or as a result of manipulation by a contaminated handler. Travelers should eat only foods that are served piping hot, and avoid raw vegetables and fruits that cannot be peeled. Foods requiring elaborate preparation or containing dairy products should be avoided. Only thoroughly cooked shellfish should be eaten.

B. PROPHYLACTIC MEDICATIONS

Despite the demonstrated efficacy of antibiotics and bismuth subsalicylate in preventing traveler's diarrhea, prophylactic antibiotics are not recommended uniformly for all travelers. Arguments against prophylaxis include the high cost of antibiotics, particularly the quinolones; potential adverse side effects, such as Stevens–Johnson syndrome and anaphylaxis (which occurs in 1 in 10,000 patients taking antibiotics); development of antibiotic resistance; and promotion of a false sense of security in the traveler, who may become less vigilant about what is eaten. The efficacy of antibiotics in reducing the duration of diarrhea if it develops raises the question of whether antibiotic prophylaxis or early self-treatment of diarrhea should be recommended.

Prophylaxis may be indicated in some travelers because of circumstances or inherent risk factors that would make a bout of diarrhea potentially dangerous. The following groups of travelers should be considered for chemoprophylaxis:

1. Travelers unable to tolerate any inactivity (eg, a professional athlete, performing artist, or politician).
2. Travelers with an underlying medical disorder in whom diarrhea may be poorly tolerated [eg, patients with diabetes mellitus, AIDS, inflammatory bowel disease, chronic renal failure, significant cardiac disease, or gastric pH that has been altered via surgical or medical means (eg, proton pump inhibitors)].
3. Travelers with a history of repeated bouts of traveler's diarrhea and known poor compliance with general food and water precautions.

The drug should be started on the day of arrival in the country and continued for 1–2 days after leaving the country. Prophylaxis should not be continued beyond 3 weeks, and if the traveler is to remain in the country for a longer time, prophylaxis should not be given because of its cost, potential side effects, and eventual acquisition of natural immunity over time. Recommended prophylactic regimens are outlined in Table 8–4.

Treatment

The treatment of traveler's diarrhea is outlined in Table 8–5.

A. FLUID REPLETION AND FOOD PRECAUTIONS

Assessment and treatment of dehydration are imperative in all patients with diarrhea. Because patients have a mild, self-limited disease, oral repletion of fluid is adequate. Flavored mineral water taken with Saltine crackers or a commercially available oral rehydration solution is frequently sufficient for replacement of ion and water losses. The repletion fluid should contain, at a minimum, glucose (which allows absorption via the small intestinal Na^+-glucose-amino acid cotransport mechanism), and should be caffeine free. Dairy products should be avoided because infectious diarrhea often results in transient lactase deficiency. Low-residue foods such as toast, rice, bananas, potatoes, boiled chicken, and applesauce may be added to the diet as diarrheal symptoms improve. High-fiber foods, raw fruits, and vegetables should be avoided, as they may exacerbate diarrhea.

B. ANTIBIOTICS

Antibiotics are indicated to treat diarrhea that is moderate to severe, characterized by three or more unformed stools daily, especially if associated with fever, blood, pus, or mucus in the stool. Antibiotics have been demonstrated to decrease the severity and duration of symptoms associated with traveler's diarrhea. Treatment with antibiotics decreases the duration of diarrhea from 59–93 hours to 16–30 hours. However, antibiotic

Table 8–4. Prophylactic regimens for traveler's diarrhea.

Agent	Dosage
Bismuth subsalicylate	Two tablets with meals and at bedtime (eight tablets/d)
Fluoroquinolones Ciprofloxacin 500 mg Norfloxacin 400 mg Ofloxacin 300 mg	One tablet once/d

Table 8–5. Management of traveler's diarrhea.[1]

Clinical Syndrome	Therapy
Vomiting	Bismuth subsalicylate two tablets every 30 minutes for eight doses (maximum of 2 days)
Mild diarrhea (no blood or fever)	Bismuth subsalicylate (as above) or loperamide 4 mg initially followed by 2 mg after each unformed stool (not to exceed 8 mg/d, use for < 48 hours)
Moderate to severe diarrhea (no blood or fever, but symptoms interfere with daily activities)	Fluoroquinolone (ciprofloxacin 500 mg twice a day, norfloxacin 400 mg twice a day, or levofloxacin 500 mg every day for 1–3 days plus loperamide (as above)
Dysentery with or without fever	Fluoroquinolone (as above) for 3–5 days

[1]Modified from De Las Casas C: Traveler's diarrhea. Aliment Pharmacol Ther 1999;13:1377.

use has been associated with prolonged fecal excretion of the pathogen, adverse side effects such as *C difficile* diarrhea, and development of multiply resistant bacteria. Specific antibiotic therapy is seldom indicated in traveler's diarrhea. Host immunity defenses are adequate to resolve most cases. Antibiotics are indicated for patients with severe, life-threatening illness, certain infectious agents to reduce environmental contamination (shigellosis), and prolonged diarrhea. When antibiotics are indicated, an oral quinolone is the first-line agent. The quinolones are active against most strains of enterotoxigenic *E coli*, *Campylobacter*, *Salmonella*, and *Vibrio*. In patients who cannot take quinolones (eg, pregnant women and children), trimethoprim-sulfamethoxazole is the drug of choice. It should be noted that widespread resistance has made this drug less effective.

C. ANTIDIARRHEAL AGENTS

Symptomatic treatment to reduce the frequency of unformed stool can be achieved with various antidiarrheal agents. Their mechanisms of action are as adsorbent, antimotility agent, or direct bactericidal. Adsorbents such as kaolin and pectin add bulk and thus decrease the liquidity of the stool without decreasing the stool quantity. Bismuth subsalicylate appears to have a variety of actions, including direct bactericidal effects via the bismuth moiety and antisecretory and antiinflammatory effects via the salicylate moiety. Given its safety, efficacy, and low cost, bismuth subsalicylate should be the first-line agent for treatment of acute infectious diarrhea. Opiate derivatives such as loperamide and diphenoxylate-atropine decrease intestinal motility, thus allowing increased intestinal contact time for absorption of salt and water. By inhibiting intestinal motility, these agents decrease the frequency of bowel movements and alleviate abdominal cramping. Opiate derivatives should be avoided in patients with clinical toxicity or significant bloody diarrhea because they may precipitate toxic megacolon or clinical deterioration.

NOSOCOMIAL DIARRHEA

Nosocomial diarrhea is defined as the onset of a change in normal bowel habits at least 72 hours after hospital admission for the purpose of clinical investigation. There must be at least two to three watery stools per day for more than 2 days. Patients over 70 years of age have the highest incidence (17–31 per 100 admission) and experience the highest mortality rates (21–83%). Possible etiologies of nosocomial diarrhea may be non-infectious or infectious. Noninfectious causes include fecal impaction, medications, and enteral feeding. *Clostridium difficile* infection is the most common infectious cause, whereas other enteropathogenic bacteria are unlikely. Increasing length of hospital stay has been identified as a significant risk factor for nosocomial infection in adult patients, with an incidence of almost 50% for hospital stays exceeding 21 days. The likelihood of nosocomial infections caused by enteropathogenic bacteria other than *C difficile* is rare and routine stool cultures and ova/parasite examinations are not cost effective if diarrhea begins 3 days after hospital admission ("3-day rule"). The yield of cultures in this setting is only 0.6% Patients with diarrhea developing in the hospital after 3 days should have specimens tested for *C difficile,* and noninfectious causes, such as antibiotic-associated or osmotic diarrhea, should be ruled out. As previously stated, the yield of stool cultures is low and this test should not be ordered routinely. A multicenter European trial has identified criteria for stool cultures in patients hospitalized more than 3 days that may reduce costs, yet provide rapid diagnosis for patients at increased risk for bacterial infection. These include patients over 65 years of age with preexisting comorbidity (cirrhosis, chronic renal failure, insulin-dependent diabetes mellitus, chronic obstructive pulmonary disease), neutropenia, and HIV infection.

1. Medication-Induced Diarrhea

Medication-induced diarrhea is a common cause of nosocomial diarrhea in the elderly patient. Medications implicated may include parasympathomimetic agents, cardiovascular medications, antimetabolites, antibiotics,

colchicine, antacids, or medications suspended in sorbitol. Enteral feeding preparations may also be a cause. A careful review of a patient's medication list is imperative before embarking on a costly, extensive diarrhea evaluation. A thorough history may implicate a temporal relationship to the inception of medication usage and the onset of diarrhea. A prolonged hospital stay with no change in medication usage may suggest a nosocomial pathogen as the source of diarrhea rather than a medication (Table 8–6).

Table 8–6. Agents implicated in drug-induced diarrhea, according to pathophysiologic mechanisms.[1]

Secretory
  Antineoplastics
  Auranofin (gold salt)
  Calcitonin
  Cardiac glycosides
  Colchicine
  Nonsteroidal antiinflammatory medications
  Prostaglandins (misoprostol)
  Stimulant laxatives (bisacodyl, phenolphthalein)
  Ticlodipine
Osmotic
  Laxatives and sugar-free products (lactulose, sorbitol, fructose, mannitol)
  Magnesium (laxatives, antacids)
  Secondary to maldigestion of carbohydrates
    Antibacterials (ampicillin)
    Acarbose (α-glucosidase inhibitor)
Motility
  Colchicine
  Macrolides (erythromycin)
  Thyroid hormones
  Ticlodipine
Exudative
  Antineoplastics
  Nonsteroidal antiinflammatory medications
  HMG-CoA reductase inhibitors (ie, simvastatin)
  Ticlodipine
Fat malabsorption
  Aminoglycosides
  Auranofin (gold salt)
  Biguanides
  Cholestyramine
  Colchicine
  Laxatives
  Methyldopa
  Octreotide
  Polymyxin, bacitracin
  Tetracyclines

[1]Modified from Chassany O, Michaux A, Bergmann JF: Drug-induced diarrhea. Drug Safety 2000;22:53.

2. Antibiotic-Associated Diarrhea

Diarrhea may occur during (more commonly) or after a course of antibiotics; there is usually no obvious pathogen. The disorder is dose related, and symptoms resolve promptly after discontinuation of the offending agent. The course is benign, with little evidence of systemic illness. Stool examination is negative for fecal leukocytes, and sigmoidoscopic examination is normal, with no evidence of inflammation on biopsy. The basis for diarrhea in these cases is unclear.

3. Clostridium Difficile Diarrhea & Enterocolitis

C difficile is a gram-positive, spore-forming anaerobic bacillus with a tendency to colonize the human intestinal tract when the normal enteric flora have been altered, particularly by antibiotic therapy. *C difficile* is able to survive for long periods of time in a hospital or chronic care facility setting in the form of heat-resistant spores. Asymptomatic carrier states are common in the elderly and serve as potential reservoirs for future outbreaks.

C difficile is the single most important infectious cause of nosocomial diarrhea. Outbreak clusters have occurred in hospitals and chronic care facilities. Current or prior use of antibiotics (within 3 months) is the most significant risk factor. It is unusual for *C difficile* colitis to develop in the absence of antibiotics, but this does occur. One such instance is after cancer chemotherapy. Increasing age and severity of underlying disease are important risk factors for *C difficile* infection. The most commonly implicated antibiotics include aminopenicillins (35% of cases), cephalosporins (30% of cases), and lincosamides, such as clindamycin (15% of cases).

C difficile colitis is a toxin-mediated disease. Toxin A, which is an enterotoxin, is capable of binding directly to the epithelium, eliciting a severe inflammatory reaction, which involves exudation of protein-rich materials that contain neutrophils, monocytes, and sloughed enterocytes and contributes to the formation of endoscopically apparent pseudomembranes.

Histologic studies show that pseudomembranes are made up of necrotic debri, mucus, and inflammatory cells that appear to well out over the surface epithelium in a "volcano" formation. Toxin B, a cytotoxin, is relatively inactive in animals, but can alter membrane function, inhibit protein synthesis, and inhibit cell division in cultured cells. Because of its lack of effect in animals, it was thought that toxin B played no role in the pathogenesis of *C difficile* diarrhea. It appears that all toxigenic strains of *C difficile* produce both toxin A and toxin B. Recent studies suggest that both toxins play a role in the pathogenesis of *C difficile*-associated enteric disease in humans. There have been reports of the isolation of toxin A-negative/toxin B-positive strains from patients with antibiotic-associated diarrhea.

Clinical Findings

A. SYMPTOMS AND SIGNS

A wide spectrum of clinical states is seen with *C difficile* infection, ranging from the asymptomatic carrier state to mild, self-limited diarrhea to fulminant pseudomembranous colitis with megacolon. In the patient with *C difficile* colitis, the onset of watery diarrhea and crampy lower abdominal pain may occur several days and up to 6 weeks after inception of antibiotic treatment. Approximately one-third of cases develop after discontinuation of antibiotics. The patient may pass up to 10–12 watery, occasionally blood-streaked stools per day. Grossly bloody stools are rarely seen. Patients may complain of abdominal distention, and fever may be present. The average duration of diarrhea is 1–2 weeks. Physical examination may reveal a distended abdomen with diffuse tenderness. In the extremely ill patient, evidence of peritoneal signs, including rebound tenderness and abdominal wall rigidity, may be present. In milder cases, patients may complain only of infrequent loose stools and mild, crampy lower abdominal pain. Fever is uncommon.

In the severely ill patient, megacolon with perforation may develop and is associated with a high mortality rate. Volume depletion and resultant electrolyte disturbances may contribute to the morbidity of the illness and should be monitored closely. Extensive ulceration may result in a protein-losing enteropathy with profound hypoalbuminemia, especially in patients who have had diarrhea for several weeks.

B. LABORATORY TESTING

In *C difficile* colitis, patients may have a mild peripheral leukocytosis. Fecal stool specimens may reveal leukocytes in up to 50% of patients. A positive *C difficile* tissue culture cytotoxicity assay is the most common method of diagnosis. It will detect toxin B. The advantages of the cytotoxin culture assay are its high sensitivity (94–100%) and specificity (99%). The major disadvantages of the cytotoxin assay are the expense and the turnaround time of 24–48 hours. A number of commercially available ELISAs are available. They are more rapid than the cytotoxin assay, however, they are less sensitive (70–90%). The tests are designed to detect toxin A, toxin B, or both. Due to its lower sensitivity, some favor the testing of three fecal specimens. Stool cultures for *C difficile* are difficult to perform, require several days to complete, and are not specific, because asymptomatic colonization occurs commonly in the hospital setting. Hence, they are not useful. As a general rule, if the initial stool samples are negative, repeat testing is not usually necessary or useful. Empiric therapy is often warranted if the clinical suspicion is high. Testing for cure of *C difficile* in patients with recent episodes that have been treated is not indicated, unless there are symptoms.

C. Endoscopy

Endoscopy is useful in a subset of patients with antibiotic-associated colitis. In patients with mild to moderate symptoms, the diagnosis of *C difficile* colitis is usually established by *C difficile* toxin assay alone. Endoscopy in such cases is unnecessary. When performed, it may show a spectrum of findings ranging from nonspecific colitis with edema, erythema, friability, and erosions, to the more classic pseudomembranous colitis.

In patients with more severe symptoms, it may be desirable to establish a diagnosis of *C difficile* colitis emergently, before the results of the toxin assay are available. Endoscopy can quickly establish the diagnosis of pseudomembranous colitis and helps to distinguish it from other clinical entities such as ischemic colitis or inflammatory bowel disease. The typical features of pseudomembranous colitis are colitis with white or yellow fluffy, loosely adherent plaques and copious mucopus. These changes are evident in the rectum and sigmoid in most patients.

D. Other Studies

Up to one-third of patients have exclusive right colonic involvement; hence, flexible sigmoidoscopy cannot reliably exclude the diagnosis. In the extremely ill patient, a roentgenogram of the abdomen may demonstrate ileus or megacolon, with edema of the colon. CT scanning may demonstrate a markedly thickened colon.

Treatment

The most important aspect in the management of *C difficile* diarrhea is to discontinue the offending agent. Diarrhea can resolve in 15–25% of patients without specific therapy. Antimotility agents, including loperamide and diphenoxylate, and narcotics should be avoided as they may delay clearance of the toxin. Two highly effective treatments exist for *C difficile* colitis: metronidazole and vancomycin. Both are effective when taken orally. Vancomycin has high luminal activity, with minimal absorption. Metronidazole is the drug of choice, however, because of lower cost and absence of metronidazole-resistant strains. Metronidazole, 250 mg orally four times a day for 10 days, is equally as effective as vancomycin, 500 mg four times a day for 10 days, with cure rates of >96%.

In the severely ill *C difficile* colitis patient, intravenous metronidazole, 250 mg every 6 hours, plus vancomycin, 500 mg every 6 hours by nasogastric tube or rectal tube,

should be administered. Approximately 10–20% of patients relapse and require a second course of antibiotics. Recurrence is rarely due to treatment failure or antibiotic resistance, and more likely results from germination of spores persisting in the colon or from reinfection with the same or a different strain from the environment. The most common therapy is a second course of the same antibiotic used to treat the initial episode. The response rate is excellent, nearly 92%. The optimal approach for patients with multiple relapses is unclear. Some authorities advocate prolonged treatment regimens with vancomycin, with gradual tapering of the dose to 125 mg every other day. Alternatively, combined regimens of vancomycin, 125 mg four times a day, and rifampin, 600 mg twice a day, for 7 days may be used. Use of lactobacilli, 1–2 g four times a day, or cholestyramine, 4 g twice a day, plus vancomycin is also expected to be effective. Reports have shown that serum antibody levels against *C difficile* toxins are low in patients with recurrent disease. Passive immunization with intravenous immunoglobulin has been used successfully to treat severe, recurrent *C difficile* colitis. Further studies are needed before firm recommendations regarding the use of γ-globulin can be made.

Probiotics, including *S boulardii*, appear to be promising in the treatment of *C difficile* diarrhea, however, further research is needed.

4. AIDS-Related Acute Diarrhea

Diarrhea is one of the most frequent symptoms in HIV-infected patients. As CD4 lymphocyte counts decrease below 200/μL, patients are at increased risk for opportunistic enteric infections, in addition to routine infectious agents. Although acute diarrhea may be seen with bacterial enteric pathogens, chronic diarrhea secondary to fungal, viral, and parasitic infections is much more prevalent (see Chapter 2).

5. Proctitis

Proctitis is defined as anorectal symptoms associated with sigmoidoscopic findings limited to the distal 15 cm of the rectum. It encompasses a broad group of clinical disorders with causative mechanisms, including infection, trauma, inflammatory bowel disease, and chemical injury.

Clinical Findings

A. Symptoms and Signs

Typically, patients complain of lower gastrointestinal symptoms, including tenesmus, fecal urgency, and frequent small-volume stools associated with mucoid or mucosanguineous discharge. Although rectal bleeding may be present, large-volume gastrointestinal bleeding is exceedingly rare. True diarrhea is uncommon, and symptoms of fever, weight loss, and malaise are usually absent.

A variety of disease processes may cause inflammation confined to the rectum (Table 8–7). A thorough, careful history should be taken, with close attention to the sexual history, concurrent medical illnesses, duration of illness, travel history, rectal trauma, and history of pelvic irradiation.

B. Diagnostic Studies

Stool culture for enteric pathogens may be useful. Rectal swabbing for specific bacterial and viral cultures may assist in determining the cause. Fecal leukocyte determination is usually positive, indicating active inflammation associated with proctitis.

Proctosigmoidoscopy is the examination of choice and may be accomplished with a rigid or flexible instrument. The endoscopic appearance of the rectal mucosa may aid in narrowing the cause; however, no findings are pathognomonic. Viral proctitis may be associated with discrete ulcerations or vesicles, with surrounding mucosal inflammatory changes. Characteristic endoscopic findings of inflammatory bowel disease may be seen within the distal rectum. Biopsies should be obtained for appropriate cultures and histologic examination.

Treatment

Therapy should be targeted toward the causative agent. For nonspecific ulcerative proctitis, topical cortico- steroids, 5-aminosalicylic acid suppositories, or enemas may be beneficial, with response rates of 70–90% after 4–8 weeks of treatment. Rarely, oral sulfasalazine may be required to ameliorate symptoms.

6. Diarrhea in Elderly Patients

Diarrheal illnesses may be particularly debilitating for elderly patients. In a report from the CDC, adults over age 74 years accounted for up to 51% of deaths due to diarrhea. Age per se is not a risk factor; however, it is a predictor of concomitant medical conditions that may predispose an elderly patient to development of diarrhea. Two important risk factors are nursing home residence and hospitalization. Individuals are at increased risk of fecal–oral contamination from other nursing home residents or supervising personnel. In addition, antibiotic administration during hospitalization is a significant risk factor for *C difficile* diarrhea in the elderly.

Elderly patients are at risk for routine bacterial, viral, and parasitic agents of diarrhea; however, noninfectious causes should be routinely considered. Iatrogenesis is an important cause of diarrhea in the elderly and should always be considered (Table 8–8).

Table 8–7. Differential diagnosis of proctitis.

Infectious causes	Traumatic proctitis
Bacteria	Foreign bodies
Aeromonas	Solitary rectal ulcer
Campylobacter	syndrome
Salmonella	Radiation proctitis
Shigella	Chemical- or drug-induced
Chlamydia	proctitis
Syphilis	Nonsteroidal antiinflam-
Gonorrhea	matory agents
Enteropathogenic *E coli*	Soap
C difficile	Hydrogen peroxide
Viruses	Fluorouracil
Herpesvirus	Gold and heavy metals
Cytomegalovirus	Miscellaneous causes
Parasites	Behçet's syndrome
Amebiasis	Amyloidosis
Schistosomiasis	Lymphoma
Inflammatory bowel disease	Fecal stream diversion
Crohn's disease	Connective tissue disorders
Ulcerative colitis	Vasculitis

Table 8–8. Noninfectious causes of diarrhea in elderly patients.

Iatrogenesis
 Antibiotics
 Antacids and acid-suppressing drugs
 Osmotically active laxatives (eg, milk of magnesia, lactulose)
 Enteral dietary supplements
 Miscellaneous drugs (eg, quinidine, digoxin, colchicine)
Systemic illness
 Diabetes mellitus
 Thyrotoxicosis
 Amyloidosis
 Scleroderma
 Uremia
Gastrointestinal disease
 Mesenteric ischemia
 Fecal impaction with overflow diarrhea
 Inflammatory bowel disease
 Obstructive lesions
 Malabsorption
 Chronic pancreatic insufficiency
Neoplasia
 Obstructive lesions
 Hormone-secreting tumors

REFERENCES

Bauer TM et al: Derivation and validation of guidelines for stool cultures for enteropathogenic bacteria other than *Clostridium difficile* in hospitalized adults. JAMA 2001;285:313.

Bennett RG, Greenough WB: Approach to acute diarrhea in the elderly. Gastroenterol Clin North Am 1993;22:517.

Bignardi GE: Risk factors for *Clostridium difficile* infection. J Hosp Infect 1998;40:1.

Chassany O, Michaux A, Bergmann JF: Drug-induced diarrhoea. Drug Safety 2000;22:53.

Chitkara YK, McCasland KA, Kenefic L: Development and implementation of cost-effective guidelines in the laboratory investigation of diarrhea in a community hospital. Arch Intern Med 1996;156:1445.

De Las Casas C, Adachi J, DuPont HL: Review article: travellers' diarrhoea. Aliment Pharmacol Ther 1999;13:1373.

DuPont HL: Guidelines on acute infectious diarrhea in adults. The Practice Parameters Committee of the American College of Gastroenterology. Am J Gastroenterol 1997;92:1962.

Elmer GW, McFarland LV: Biotherapeutic agents in the treatment of infectious diarrhea. Gastroenterol Clin North Am 2001; 30:837.

Fekety R: Guidelines for the diagnosis and management of *Clostridium difficile*-associated diarrhea and colitis. The Practice Parameters Committee of the American College of Gastroenterology. Am J Gastroenterol 1997;92:739.

Goodman L, Segreti J: Infectious diarrhea. Dis Mon 1999;45: 265.

Guerrant RL et al: Practice guidelines for the management of infectious diarrhea. Clin Infect Dis 2001;32:331.

Katz DE, Taylor DN: Parasitic infections of the gastrointestinal tract. Gastroenterol Clin North Am 2001;30:797.

Lopez AS et al: Outbreak of *Cyclosporiasis* associated with basil in Missouri. Clin Infect Dis 2001;32:1010.

Mead PS, Griffin PM: *Escherichia coli* 0157:H7. Lancet 1998;352: 1207.

Ramakrishna BS et al: Amylase-resistant starch plus oral rehydration solution for cholera. N Engl J Med 2000;342:308.

Savola KL et al: Fecal leukocyte stain has diagnostic value for outpatients but not inpatients. J Clin Microbiol 2001; 39:266.

Schiller LR: Diarrhea. Med Clin North Am 2000;84:1259.

Vesy CJ, Peterson WL: Review article: the management of giardiasis. Aliment Pharmacol Ther 1999;13:843.

Wong CS et al: The risk of the hemolytic-uremic syndrome after antibiotic treatment of *Escherichia coli* 0157:H7 infections. N Engl J Med 2000;342:1930.

Mesenteric Vascular Disease

9

Lawrence J. Brandt, MD

The gastrointestinal system performs a variety of energy-dependent processes, among which are motility, digestion, secretion, absorption, and cellular regeneration. Each of these vital functions relies on the adequate delivery of essential nutrients and oxygen, without which they cannot be performed properly. When the metabolic demands of the intestine outweigh its energy supply, ischemic injury may ensue. Intestinal ischemia produces a broad spectrum of disorders, the clinical presentation of which depends on many variables, including the onset and duration of the injury (acute or chronic), the distribution and the length of bowel affected (small bowel or colon), the type of vessel involved (artery or vein), the mechanism of ischemia (embolus, thrombus, or systemic hypoperfusion), and the degree of collateral flow.

The types of intestinal ischemia and their approximate incidences include colon ischemia (60%), acute mesenteric ischemia (30%), focal segmental ischemia (5%), and chronic mesenteric ischemia (5%). Acute mesenteric ischemia (AMI) involves that part of the intestinal tract supplied by the superior mesenteric artery and its branches, that is, the small intestine and ascending colon. Arterial causes of AMI are more common than venous, and emboli are more often responsible than thromboses.

Patients with AMI usually present during the ischemic episode, but because the amount of intestine involved is frequently extensive and the diagnosis is commonly made late (ie, after infarction has occurred), patients with AMI are more ill than those with colon ischemia (CI) and have higher morbidity and mortality rates. In contrast, patients with CI typically present after the ischemic episode when colonic blood flow has returned to normal, their complaints are relatively mild, their physical examination findings are usually minimally to moderately abnormal, and their risk of mortality is much lower than that of patients with AMI. Clinical presentations do overlap, however, and patients who present a diagnostic problem should be considered to have AMI until proven otherwise.

Angiography has a limited role in the evaluation of suspected CI because colonic blood flow usually has returned to normal on presentation. Colonoscopy or serial barium enemas are used to confirm the diagnosis of CI. On the other hand, angiography is an integral part of the diagnosis and management of suspected AMI as well as chronic mesenteric ischemia.

ANATOMY OF THE SPLANCHNIC CIRCULATION

The vascular supply to the abdominal viscera is via the three main branches of the abdominal aorta, namely, the celiac, the superior mesenteric artery, and the inferior mesenteric artery. Whereas some consistent patterns have been established, anatomic and angiographic studies have demonstrated a marked variability of these vessels. Anastomoses exist between branches of the major vessels, and as a result, if one artery is occluded, some flow may be maintained via the patent collateral. Furthermore, in certain areas a network of anastomosing arcades is present, which further reinforces this defense against ischemia; the anastomoses in the duodenum and rectum are quite rich, and ischemia is rare in these locations. In contrast, the vascular supply is less redundant in areas such as the splenic flexure and sigmoid colon where ischemic damage, therefore, is more commonly observed.

The celiac artery arises from the anterior aorta at the level of the twelfth thoracic vertebra or the first lumbar vertebra between the diaphragmatic crura. This vessel supplies the foregut structures from the distal esophagus to the second portion of the duodenum. The usual branches of the celiac artery are the hepatic, splenic, and left gastric arteries.

The common hepatic artery is quite variable in its origin and branches. It gives off the gastroduodenal artery, which branches into the right gastroepiploic artery and superior pancreaticoduodenal artery; the latter anastomoses with the inferior pancreaticoduodenal artery, a branch of the superior mesenteric artery (SMA). Anastomosis between these two vessels provides a rich blood supply to the duodenum and, as mentioned previously, safeguards it against ischemic insult.

Branches of the splenic artery, particularly the dorsal pancreatic artery, supply the pancreas while the left gastroepiploic artery and the short gastric arteries supply the greater curve, fundus, and cardia of the stomach.

The left gastric artery runs along the lesser curvature of the stomach toward the pylorus, supplying these areas as well as the anterior aspect of the stomach.

The SMA arises from the anterior aspect of the abdominal aorta at the level of the first lumbar vertebra and about 5–10 mm inferior to the celiac axis. The SMA originates behind the body of the pancreas and, as it travels inferiorly, crosses the third portion of the duodenum anteriorly. Under certain conditions, this part of the duodenum may become trapped between the SMA and the aorta, giving rise to the SMA syndrome. The SMA provides blood flow to the midgut structures, extending from the second portion of the duodenum to the mid or distal transverse colon. The major branches of the SMA include the inferior pancreaticoduodenal artery; the right colic, middle colic, and ileocolic arteries; and several separate jejunal and ileal branches. The jejunal and ileal vessels are connected through abundant primary, secondary, and tertiary anastomosing arcades that ultimately give rise to the vasa recta. As mentioned above, the inferior pancreaticoduodenal artery forms an important anastomosis with the celiac artery. The ileocolic artery divides into ileal and colic arteries, which supply the terminal ileum, cecum, and proximal ascending colon. The ileal artery eventually anastomoses with the distal-most SMA, forming a loop. The right and middle colic arteries usually arise from a common trunk; the right colic artery branches and supplies the ascending colon, while the middle colic artery travels in the transverse mesocolon and supplies the transverse colon. The marginal artery of Drummond, the arc of Riolan, and the central anatomic artery are collaterals that connect the SMA and inferior mesenteric artery (IMA).

The IMA originates at the level of the third lumbar vertebra, 3–5 cm above the aortic bifurcation. Its major branches are the left colic artery, the superior rectal artery, and a series of sigmoid arteries that form an anastomosing arcade around the sigmoid colon. The left colic artery supplies the distal transverse colon, the splenic flexure, and the descending colon and also forms an anastomosis with the middle colic artery. The superior rectal artery descends to provide blood to the rectum and forms anastomoses with the middle and inferior rectal arteries, each a branch of the internal iliac artery.

In regard to the microcirculation of the small intestine, the vasa recta enter from the mesentery, penetrate the wall of the intestine, and give off branches to the serosa, the external muscular plexus, and the submucosal vascular plexus. From the submucosa, arterioles ascend into each villus and arborize into a dense capillary network. Blood returns via subepithelial venules, which are in close proximity to the arterioles, creating a countercurrent system that has important implications during periods of ischemia. Specifically, an oxygen gradient exists from the base to the tip of the villus, and when oxygen delivery to the small intestine is compromised, the villus tip is the first area to sustain ischemic damage.

PATHOPHYSIOLOGY OF ACUTE MESENTERIC ISCHEMIA

Ischemic injury of the intestine occurs when there is inadequate delivery of oxygen and other nutrients to meet the intestine's various metabolic demands. Intestinal blood flow is controlled by a variety of factors—autonomic, humoral, and local—and relies on a rich anastomotic vascular network, both extraluminal and intraluminal. Each of these may influence and contribute to the generation of ischemic damage. Postischemic reperfusion also is important in this pathophysiologic process. Regardless of the cause, intestinal ischemia produces a spectrum of injury ranging from reversible function alterations to transmural necrosis of the bowel wall. Villus tips are the most sensitive to ischemia, and injury progresses from the intestinal luminal border toward the serosa.

Intestinal blood flow is controlled primarily by resistance arterioles and to a lesser degree by precapillary sphincters. A variety of vasoactive substances participate in the control of intestinal perfusion, either directly or indirectly; and specific substances may exert different effects in different regions of the intestine as well as in different layers of the bowel wall in the same segment.

The sympathetic nervous system, via stimulation of α-adrenergic receptors, causes arteriolar vasoconstriction that reduces mesenteric blood flow. However, blood flow ultimately returns to normal in the face of continued sympathetic stimulation, a process referred to as autoregulatory escape. The role of the sympathetic nervous system in the pathogenesis of AMI is unresolved at present. Angiotensin II also causes mesenteric vasoconstriction, an effect more pronounced in the colon than the small bowel and more pronounced in the muscularis than the mucosa. Vasopressin, released in states of volume depletion, results in a vasoconstrictive effect that is greater in the splanchnic circulation than it is in the systemic circulation. Arachidonic acid metabolites have been evaluated for their effects on mesenteric blood flow; several metabolites result in vasoconstriction, while others cause vasodilation. Several products of ischemia also exert vasodilatory effects, including hyperkalemia, acidosis, hyperosmolarity, and hypoxemia. Vasoactive intestinal peptide has been shown to cause vasodilation; the role of other gastrointestinal hormones in the regulation of intestinal blood flow is less certain. Recently, short-chain fatty acids have been demonstrated to result in dilation of colonic resistance arterioles.

Boley and colleagues demonstrated that when a major vessel is occluded, collateral pathways open immediately in response to a fall in arterial pressure distal to the obstruction. This compensatory mechanism augments blood flow to those areas beyond the obstruction, thereby ameliorating ischemic injury. If the obstruction is relieved early, blood flow returns to baseline values in the obstructed artery as well as in the collateral vessels. If, however, the obstruction persists, vasoconstriction develops in the distal vascular bed, resulting in elevated arterial pressure and diminished flow through the collateral pathways. Failure to relieve the obstruction promptly has been demonstrated to result in persistent vasoconstriction, which may continue even after the obstruction is corrected. If papaverine, a vasodilator, is given before or soon after the onset of vasoconstriction, this vasospasm can be reversed or even prevented. Persistent vasoconstriction helps explain the progression of ischemic injury despite relief of the obstruction in occlusive ischemia or correction of underperfusion in nonocclusive disease.

Relief of an arterial obstruction with subsequent reperfusion of ischemic tissue with oxygenated blood has been observed to aggravate tissue injury. Thus, the tissue damage produced by 3 hours of ischemia and 1 hour of reperfusion has been shown to be more severe than that of 4 hours of pure ischemia. There is evidence to suggest that reactive oxygen metabolites generated during ischemia with reperfusion mediate this enhanced injury. These metabolites are produced by xanthine oxidase. Molecular oxygen is sequentially reduced to hydrogen peroxide, superoxide, and hydroxyl radicals. The mechanism by which these metabolites cause injury involves damage to a variety of biomolecules, including nucleic acids, enzymes, and receptors. Hydroxyl radicals attack membrane-bound fatty acids resulting in lipid peroxidation, a process that alters membrane integrity and ultimately causes cellular swelling, lysis, and death. Free radical scavengers, xanthine oxidase inhibitors, and inhibitors of leukocyte chemoattractants, eg, platelet-activating factor (PAF), have been shown experimentally to protect the intestine from ischemia-induced reperfusion injury. Because most of these therapies require pretreatment to be effective, it is unlikely they will become clinically useful in their current formulations.

ACUTE MESENTERIC ISCHEMIA

 ESSENTIALS OF DIAGNOSIS

- *High index of clinical suspicion.*
- *Patient is usually older than 50 years with chronic cardiovascular disease.*
- *Early in course, abdominal pain is typically out of proportion to findings on physical examination.*
- *Angiography: diagnostic and potentially therapeutic.*

General Considerations

AMI is a medical and surgical emergency that demands prompt diagnosis and a coordinated and deliberate multidisciplinary approach, if death or the short bowel syndrome is to be avoided. AMI accounts for approximately one-third of episodes of intestinal ischemia but is responsible for most ischemia-related deaths. Mortality rates of 70–90%, once intestinal infarction has occurred, attest to the lethal nature of this disease if AMI is not recognized and treated promptly. Diagnosis before the occurrence of intestinal infarction is the single most important factor in improving survival for patients with AMI. A high index of clinical suspicion for AMI must be maintained; if combined with the early and liberal use of angiography in the correct clinical setting, this can improve the usual and excessive fatal outcome.

The various causes of AMI and their approximate incidences include SMA embolus (50%), nonocclusive mesenteric ischemia (NOMI) (25%), SMA thrombosis (10%), mesenteric venous thrombosis (MVT) (10%), and focal segmental ischemia (5%). The incidence of AMI has increased over the past 25 years owing to longer life expectancies and a heightened awareness of the various ischemic syndromes. The salvage of critically ill patients in intensive care units, who are subsequently prone to develop AMI, has also contributed to this increased incidence.

In the early part of this century, MVT was considered the most common cause of AMI, but it is likely that most cases of mesenteric ischemia believed to be MVT were actually caused by vasospasm secondary to NOMI. Today, SMA embolus is the most common cause of AMI, with the decreased incidence of NOMI reflecting improved ICU monitoring with rapid correction of volume deficits, shock, hemorrhage, congestive heart failure, and arrhythmias, each of which may result in reactive mesenteric vasoconstriction and NOMI if not treated promptly.

ARTERIAL FORMS OF ACUTE MESENTERIC ISCHEMIA

1. Superior mesenteric artery emboli (SMAE)— Emboli usually originate from a left atrial or ventricular mural thrombus, but can also arise from abnormal cardiac valves as well as from a left atrial myxoma. Many patients with SMAE have had previous peripheral emboli and approximately 20% have synchronous emboli to other arteries. Emboli tend to lodge at points of normal anatomic narrowing, usually just distal to the origin of a major branch.

2. Nonocclusive mesenteric ischemia (NOMI)— NOMI is caused by diffuse splanchnic vasoconstriction, which results from an extensive variety of conditions, each of which has in common splanchnic hypoperfusion. These conditions include a decrease in cardiac output with hypotension secondary to acute myocardial infarction, congestive heart failure, arrhythmias, and valvular heart disease; other shock states secondary to hemorrhage or sepsis; and renal failure, particularly in those requiring hemodialysis. Those undergoing major cardiac or intraabdominal operations are also susceptible. NOMI can attend SMAE, especially when diagnosis is delayed and the plan of management does not include intraarterial papaverine.

3. Superior mesenteric artery thrombosis (SMAT)— SMAT occurs at areas of severe atherosclerotic narrowing, most commonly at the origin of the SMA. The acute ischemic episode is commonly superimposed on chronic mesenteric ischemia, and 20–50% of these patients have a history suggesting intestinal angina in the weeks to months preceding the acute event. A history of coronary, cerebral, or peripheral artery ischemia is frequent.

Clinical Findings

A. Symptoms and Signs

AMI is associated with abdominal pain in 75–98% of cases. The pain usually develops suddenly and varies in character, intensity, and location. Classically, early in the course of AMI, the pain experienced by the patient is markedly out of proportion to objective physical findings; the patient may complain of severe abdominal pain, but the abdomen is soft, flat, and nontender. A history of postprandial pain in the weeks to months preceding the onset of severe pain is associated only with SMAT. Pain may be absent in up to 25% of patients with NOMI.

In patients in whom pain is absent, other signs and symptoms—such as unexplained abdominal distention or intestinal hemorrhage—may be the only manifestation of AMI. Bacteremia and diarrhea following cardiopulmonary resuscitation suggest NOMI; the bacteremia (and sepsis) is secondary to bacterial translocation across a segment of viable but ischemic bowel.

Occult blood may be found in the stool in up to 75% of patients with AMI. Right-sided abdominal pain associated with the passage of maroon or bright red blood in the stool, although characteristic of CI, also suggests the possibility of AMI, since the blood supply to the ascending and proximal transverse colon is provided by the SMA. Acute occlusion of the SMA initially results in increased bowel activity, and this heightened motor activity can result in rapid and forceful bowel evacuation early in AMI.

Whereas a paucity of physical findings is found early in the course of AMI, abdominal tenderness, rebound tenderness, and muscle guarding are all ominous signs, suggesting transmural necrosis and intestinal infarction. Nausea, vomiting, gastrointestinal bleeding, shock, and abdominal distention are also late features in AMI.

B. Laboratory Findings

Early in the course of AMI, there are no specific laboratory findings. On admission to the hospital, approximately 75% of patients with AMI have a leukocytosis above 15,000 cell/μL and about 50% have metabolic acidemia. Elevations of serum phosphate, amylase, lactate dehydrogenase, creatine phosphokinase, and intestinal alkaline phosphatase have been described, but these elevations occur late; the sensitivity and specificity of these and other markers of intestinal ischemia have not been established.

C. Imaging

Early in AMI, plain films of the abdomen are usually normal. Conversely, about 25% of patients with intestinal infarction also have normal plain films; plain films of the abdomen are not especially sensitive in detecting AMI and so a normal plain film does not exclude AMI. Nonspecific plain film findings may include a gasless abdomen, an adynamic ileus, or a small bowel pseudoobstruction pattern. Formless loops of small intestine and thumbprinting, the latter reflecting submucosal edema or hemorrhage, are more suggestive findings. Pneumatosis intestinalis, or portal vein gas, is a late finding, usually associated with transmural necrosis and infarction, and each portends a poor prognosis. The utility of plain films in AMI is not in diagnosis, but rather in its ability to rule out the presence of other entities that produce abdominal pain and mimic AMI.

Just as with plain films, findings on computed tomography (CT) may be normal or nonspecific in cases of ischemia or infarction. Nonspecific findings are seen in approximately two-thirds of cases of AMI on CT and include focal or diffuse bowel wall thickening, focally dilated fluid-filled loops of bowel, mesenteric edema, engorgement of mesenteric veins, and ascites. More suggestive but late findings include air in the bowel wall or mesenteric or portal venous gas. Intravenous contrast may demonstrate an arterial occlusion, which appears as a filling defect in the vessel lumen.

Angiography plays a critical role in both the diagnosis and management of patients with AMI. Angiography is performed only after a patient is adequately resuscitated, because the angiographic findings are similar in patients with NOMI and in those who are hypotensive or on pressors. In the latter two instances, mesenteric vasoconstriction is a normal and expected physiologic response, while in NOMI it is pathologic. The angiographic criteria for NOMI include narrowing of the origins of multiple branches of the SMA, irregularities in the intestinal branches, spasm of the arcades, and impaired filling of the intramural vessels. SMA emboli appear as well-delineated filling defects in the contrast column associated with obstruction to distal flow. Emboli tend to lodge in areas of vessel narrowing, usually just distal to the origins of major branches. SMA thrombosis usually occurs in a chronically atherosclerotic vessel. The diagnosis of SMAT is most often made on flush aortography, with the thrombosis located either at the origin of the SMA or within its proximal 2 cm. If angiographic criteria for NOMI, SMAE, or SMAT are met, intraarterial infusion of a vasodilator, specifically papaverine, may be indicated.

Treatment

The goals of treatment of AMI are early diagnosis by angiography, relief of persistent vasoconstriction by intraarterial administration of a vasodilator, and resection of any frankly necrotic bowel. Given the excessive mortality rate if ischemia is permitted to progress to infarction, broad selection criteria must be used in addition to early angiography if prompt diagnosis and successful treatment are to be achieved (Figure 9–1).

Initial treatment is directed toward correcting any precipitating causes of AMI. Treatment of acute congestive heart failure, stabilization of cardiac arrhythmias, and correction of blood volume or red cell deficits must precede any diagnostic studies. Given the physiologic redistribution of blood flow from the splanchnic to the systemic circulation in states of intravascular volume depletion, efforts at increasing intestinal blood flow will be futile if low cardiac output, hypotension, or hypovolemia persists. Shock is a contraindication to angiography because mesenteric vasoconstriction, as seen in NOMI, normally accompanies the shock state. Furthermore, intraarterial vasodilators should not be used to treat shock; they will increase the size of the mesenteric vascular bed and further reduce systemic blood pressure. If needed, placement of a pulmonary arterial catheter may be used to guide fluid management.

After volume resuscitation, patients are sent for plain films or CT scan of the abdomen, or both. These studies are obtained primarily to exclude other causes of abdominal pain such as perforated viscus or intestinal obstruction and not to establish the diagnosis of AMI. Both studies have a low sensitivity and specificity for mesenteric ischemia and infarction.

If the cause of the patient's abdominal pain cannot be elicited from the plain film or CT scan, visceral angiography is performed. Appropriate management depends on the angiographic findings (SMAT, SMAE, or NOMI) and the presence or absence of peritoneal findings.

Even when the decision to operate has been made based on clinical grounds, a preoperative angiogram should be obtained to help manage the patient before, during, and after laparotomy. Relief of mesenteric vasoconstriction, which may persist after the correction of the underlying cause, is essential in the treatment of emboli, thromboses, and the nonocclusive low flow states. For this purpose, papaverine should be infused at a rate of 30–60 mg/h through the SMA catheter. The complication rate of mesenteric angiography is usually acceptable and includes an approximately 6% incidence of transient acute tubular necrosis secondary to the contrast medium, an incidence of embolization of less than 1% (possibly resulting from the arterial catheter), and occasional catheter dislodgment with systemic infusion of papaverine and resultant hypotension.

Laparotomy is performed in AMI to restore arterial flow after an embolus or thrombus or to resect irreparably damaged bowel. Embolectomy, thrombectomy, or arterial bypass precedes the evaluation of intestinal viability, because bowel that initially appears infarcted may show surprising recovery after blood flow is restored. Short segments of bowel that are nonviable or of questionable viability after revascularization are resected and a primary anastomosis is performed. If extensive portions of bowel are of questionable viability, only the clearly necrotic bowel is resected and a planned reexploration, or "second look," is performed within 12–24 hours. The interval between the first and second operations is used to allow better demarcation of viable and nonviable bowel and to attempt to improve intestinal blood flow with intraarterial papaverine or by maximizing cardiac output.

Use of anticoagulants in the management of AMI is controversial. Heparin may cause intestinal or intraperitoneal hemorrhage, and except in the case of MVT, should not be given in the immediate postoperative period. Late thrombosis following embolectomy or arterial reconstruction occurs frequently enough that anticoagulation 48 hours postoperatively seems advisable. Given the high incidence of positive blood cultures in patients with AMI, broad-spectrum antibiotics are administered early and continued in the postoperative period.

Prognosis

If AMI is not diagnosed early and intestinal gangrene occurs, mortality rates are approximately 70–90%. Approached aggressively as outlined above, survival can be improved to about 55%. A decreased mortality rate has been demonstrated clearly in series in which routine angiography has been used to diagnose and treat patients with AMI. In those patients with angiographically proven AMI, but without peritonitis, survival rates approach 90%. Furthermore, if treated aggressively, the length of bowel requiring resection is diminished, allowing the patient a better chance of surviving with a functioning gastrointestinal tract.

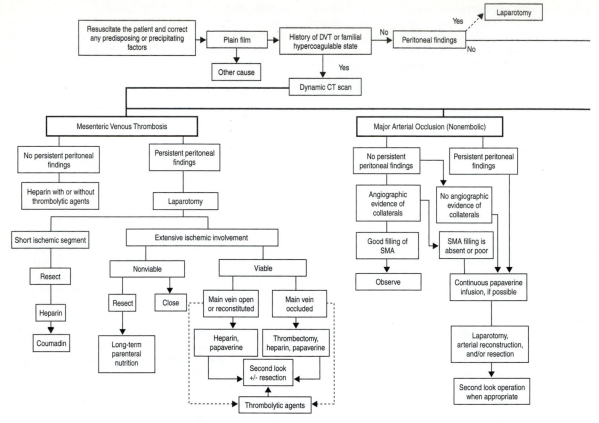

Figure 9–1. Algorithm for the diagnosis and treatment of acute intestinal ischemia. **Solid lines** indicate accepted management plans and **dashed lines** indicate alternate management plans. SMA, superior mesenteric artery; DVT, deep vein thrombosis. (Reproduced, with permission, from American Gastroenterological Association Medical Position Statement: guidelines on intestinal ischemia. Gastroenterology 2000;118:951.)

MESENTERIC VENOUS THROMBOSIS (MVT)

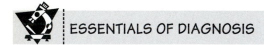

ESSENTIALS OF DIAGNOSIS

- Acute form: abdominal pain associated with a predisposing condition (eg, a hypercoagulable state).
- Chronic form: usually asymptomatic.
- Diagnosed by contrast CT or angiography.

General Considerations

Our understanding of the incidence, pathogenesis, and manifestations of MVT has evolved since its initial description in the late nineteenth century. Initially, MVT was believed to account for most cases of AMI. NOMI was described in the 1950s, and it is likely that patients felt to have MVT before that time in fact were suffering from NOMI; today MVT accounts for less than 5% of cases of AMI. Male-to-female ratios have been variable, ranging from 1.5:1 to 1:1, and the mean age of 48–60 years is lower than that of other forms of mesenteric ischemia.

Formerly an underlying cause of MVT was identified in less than 50% of patients. However, the condition responsible for the development of MVT today can be identified in over 80% of patients with the description of various hypercoagulable states (eg, factor V Leiden, deficiencies of antithrombin III, protein S, and protein C) and other prothrombotic conditions, including a variety of neoplasms and the myeloproliferative disorders. Other conditions associated with MVT

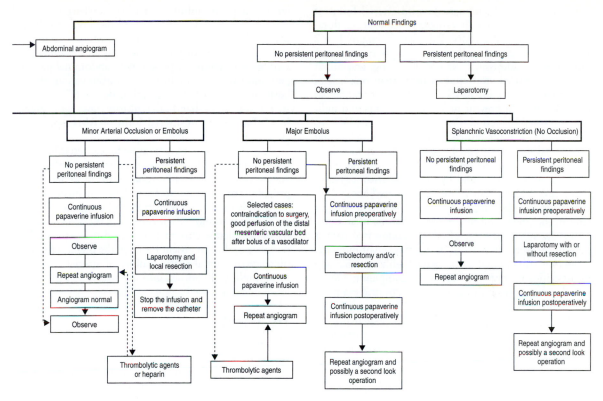

Figure 9–1. *(continued)*

include pregnancy, oral contraceptive use, portal hypertension, and a variety of intraabdominal processes, for example, pancreatitis, peritonitis, and inflammatory bowel disease. Rarely, nonthrombotic occlusion of the mesenteric veins secondary to venulitis or venous myointimal hyperplasia can simulate MVT.

With the advent of a variety of imaging modalities, the variability of clinical expressions of MVT became evident. MVT can be categorized into acute, subacute, and chronic forms, each of which will be further described in this section.

Pathophysiology

Ligation of the SMV in canines is associated with a variety of consequences, including dilation of the mesenteric vein, bleeding into the mesentery, cyanosis of the bowel with congestion and spasm, paralytic ileus, and the weeping of serosanguinous fluid from the bowel and mesentery into the peritoneal cavity. Hypovolemia, hemoconcentration, acidosis, and decreased flow in the SMA are also seen, resulting in death between 1 and 4 hours secondary to cardiovascular collapse. Release of the SMV ligature may be associated with residual arter-

ial spasm. In animals pretreated with heparin prior to SMV occlusion, death is prevented.

The propagation of the thrombus differs for different disease processes. For example, in MVT secondary to hypercoagulable states, the thrombus is believed to begin in small venous branches and extend toward the major trunks, whereas the opposite is felt to occur in MVT associated with portal hypertension or neoplasia. Intestinal infarction is rare unless the branches of the peripheral arcades and the vasa recta are involved. The extent of the venous collateral circulation also has a significant impact on the course of the disease after thrombus formation.

Clinical Findings

MVT can have an acute, subacute (weeks to months), or chronic onset. A previous history of deep venous thrombosis in the extremities may be elicited in up to 60% of patients.

A. SYMPTOMS AND SIGNS

The signs and symptoms of acute MVT are highly variable and nonspecific. Abdominal pain is present in more than 90% of patients and usually is out of proportion to physical findings. As with arterial forms of AMI, however, the pain is variable in its location, duration, character, and severity. Pain usually begins 1 to 2 weeks before admission, but may be present up to 1 month before admission. Nausea, vomiting, and occult blood in the stool are found in more than one-half of the patients with acute MVT. Hematemesis and hematochezia are each present in 15% of patients and indicate intestinal infarction. Physical findings of MVT include abdominal tenderness in almost all patients, and abdominal distention and hypoactive bowel sounds in about 80%. Temperature above 38°C is found in almost 50% of patients and hypotension with a systolic blood pressure less than 90 mm Hg is noted about 25% of the time. Guarding and rebound tenderness occur later in the course and may reflect intestinal infarction.

In the subacute form of MVT, abdominal pain is present for weeks to months in the absence of intestinal infarction. Abdominal pain, again highly variable and nonspecific, is the most common complaint; nausea and diarrhea occur only occasionally. Physical examination is usually normal.

Those patients with chronic MVT experience no symptoms at the time the thrombosis initially develops. They may either continue to remain asymptomatic or develop gastrointestinal hemorrhage secondary to esophageal or intestinal varices. Physical findings are those of portal hypertension, eg, splenomegaly if the portal vein is involved; however, there may be no abnormal findings with only SMV occlusion.

B. LABORATORY FINDINGS

In all forms of MVT, the laboratory findings are neither sensitive nor specific and therefore are not useful in confirming or excluding the diagnosis. The white blood cell count may be elevated above 12,000/μL in two-thirds of patients. Thrombocytopenia or pancytopenia secondary to hypersplenism may be seen in the chronic form.

C. IMAGING

Abdominal plain film findings of MVT are nonspecific. Whereas 75% of patients with acute MVT may have an abnormal abdominal film, 50% reveal a nonspecific ileus pattern. Portal venous air, air in the wall of the small bowel, and free intraperitoneal air are all ominous signs of intestinal infarction. Small bowel series typically reveals luminal narrowing from congested and edematous bowel wall, separation of loops due to mesenteric thickening, and thumbprinting secondary to submucosal edema and hemorrhage.

CT is capable of diagnosing MVT in more than 90% of patients. Specific findings using this modality include thickening and persistent enhancement of the bowel wall, an enlarged SMV with a central lucency

representing thrombus formation, a sharply defined vein wall with a rim of increased density, and dilated collateral vessels in a thickened mesentery. CT may be used as the initial diagnostic modality in certain clinical settings, for example, a patient with abdominal pain, no peritoneal signs, and a history of a deep venous thrombosis or an inherited coagulation defect (Figure 9–2). If, on the other hand, the history does not suggest MVT but rather an arterial form of AMI, splanchnic angiography is indicated.

Selective mesenteric angiography can establish a definitive diagnosis before bowel infarction, differentiate venous thrombosis from arterial forms of ischemia, and provide access for vasodilators if persistent arterial vasospasm is present. Angiographic findings in MVT include demonstration of a thrombus in the SMV with partial or complete occlusion; failure to visualize the SMV or portal vein; slow or absent filling of the mesenteric veins; presence of arterial spasm; failure of arterial arcades to empty; reflux of contrast into the artery; and prolonged blush in the involved segment of bowel.

Treatment

The treatment of acute MVT has changed over the years and now depends in part on whether the presence of intestinal infarction is suspected; several nonoperative approaches are proving to be successful in the subgroup of patients without bowel infarction (see Figure 9–1). In patients who have radiologic evidence of MVT and no signs of intestinal infarction, a trial of anticoagulation with heparin or thrombolysis with streptokinase

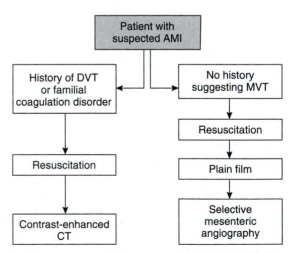

Figure 9–2. Evaluation of the patient with suspected acute mesenteric ischemia (AMI). DVT, deep vein thrombosis; MVT, mesenteric venous thrombosis.

has been successful. However, should signs of intestinal infarction develop, such as muscle guarding and rebound tenderness, laparotomy is mandated. Patients with peritoneal signs should undergo prompt laparotomy and resection of frankly necrotic bowel, followed by the administration of heparin. In patients who have received anticoagulation, the recurrence of the disease has decreased from about 25% to 13%, with a reduction in mortality rate. There are no studies to define how long patients with acute MVT should be maintained on anticoagulants. By convention, patients receive 7–10 days of heparin followed by an oral regimen of coumadin for 3–6 months. Of course, tendencies to coagulation, eg, thrombophilia and coagulation disturbances, may warrant lifelong anticoagulation.

In patients with long segments of bowel involved, the preoperative angiogram will help dictate whether thrombectomy is advisable. When blood flow is adequate through the major trunks or collaterals, only the portions of bowel believed to be irreversibly necrotic are removed; this is followed by the postoperative administration of heparin and transcatheter intraarterial papaverine to reduce the MVT-associated arterial vasospasm. A second-look operation is performed 12–18 hours later to assess bowel viability. Venous thrombectomy may be possible when there is complete thrombosis of the SMV at its junction with the portal vein.

In chronic MVT, treatment is directed at controlling symptoms, which usually consist of bleeding secondary to portal hypertension. Patients who are asymptomatic usually do not require treatment. The natural history of asymptomatic chronic MVT is not well known. The treatment of those patients with variceal bleeding is directed initially at control of the hemorrhage followed by treatment of the varices by endoscopy, portosystemic shunting, or surgical devascularization.

FOCAL SEGMENTAL ISCHEMIA (FSI)

 ESSENTIALS OF DIAGNOSIS

- In acute form it simulates appendicitis.
- In chronic form it may simulate Crohn's disease.
- Most commonly presents as small bowel obstruction with diarrhea or abdominal pain, distention, and vomiting.

Pathophysiology

Vascular insults to short segments of the bowel produce a broad spectrum of clinical features without the life-

threatening complications associated with more extensive ischemia. Some causes of FSI include atheromatous emboli, strangulated hernias, immune complex disorders, vasculitis, blunt abdominal trauma, radiation, and oral contraceptive use. With FSI there is usually adequate collateral circulation to prevent transmural infarction; perforation and peritonitis are uncommon. Limited necrosis may result in complete healing, a chronic enteritis simulating Crohn's disease, or a stricture. As a result, patients present with one of three clinical patterns: acute enteritis, chronic enteritis, or obstruction.

Clinical Findings

In the acute pattern, abdominal pain often simulates acute appendicitis. Physical findings are those of an acute abdomen, and an inflammatory mass may be palpated. Plain films of the abdomen early in the course are usually normal, but later may reveal a "sentinel loop" or a nonspecific ileus pattern. The chronic enteritis pattern may be indistinguishable from that of Crohn's disease, with symptoms including crampy abdominal pain, weight loss, fever, and diarrhea. Radiologically the diseases may be similar as well; however, Crohn's enteritis usually involves the terminal ileum, whereas FSI may occur anywhere in the small bowel. The most common presentation is of chronic small bowel obstruction with symptoms of abdominal pain, distention, and vomiting. Bacterial overgrowth in the dilated loop proximal to the obstruction may produce a blind loop syndrome and manifest with diarrhea. Radiologic studies reveal a smooth tapered stricture of varying length.

Treatment

Treatment of FSI is resection of the involved bowel.

COLON ISCHEMIA (CI)

 ESSENTIALS OF DIAGNOSIS

- Typically, left lower quadrant pain, followed by the passage of blood per rectum within 24 hours in an elderly patient.
- Diagnosed by serial colonoscopies or barium enemas.
- Prognosis usually is excellent.

General Considerations

Ischemic injury to the large intestine is a common disease in the elderly. The colon is the part of the gastrointestinal tract most susceptible to ischemia. A spectrum of ischemic injury to the colon is recognized, including reversible colonopathy (30–40%), transient colitis (15–20%), chronic ulcerating colitis (20–25%), stricture formation (10–15%), gangrene (15–20%), and fulminant universal colitis (< 5%). Regardless of the ultimate clinical expression of CI, the initial presentation of all forms may be identical and is not predictive of the disease course. Exceptions to this rule do exist, however, particularly when the right colon is affected as part of a more extensive process that also involves the small bowel; both are supplied by the SMA. This particular pattern of ischemia within the distribution of the SMA usually reflects an SMAE, SMAT, or NOMI; if not diagnosed and treated appropriately, it is associated with a mortality rate of 70–90%, as described earlier.

The true incidence of CI is difficult to determine for a variety of reasons. Many cases of transient or reversible ischemic damage are probably missed, either because the condition resolves before medical attention is sought, or barium enema or colonoscopy is not performed early enough to establish the diagnosis. Furthermore, the diagnosis of CI is not frequently considered, and many cases are misdiagnosed as infectious colitis or idiopathic inflammatory bowel disease. Rough estimates are that CI is seen in 1% of colonoscopies, 1 in 2000 admissions to a tertiary care hospital and 1 in 700 patient care visits among large office practices.

More than 90% of patients with noniatrogenic causes of CI are older than 60 years and have evidence of systemic atherosclerosis. There does not appear to be a significant gender predilection. CI in younger persons has been attributed to vasculitis (especially systemic lupus erythematosis), sickle cell disease, hypercoagulable states (especially factor V Leiden), medications (estrogens, danazol, vasopressin, gold, psychotropic drugs), cocaine abuse, and long-distance running.

Two special clinical situations associated with CI are its occurrence in patients with carcinoma of the colon and other potentially obstructing lesions and its association with aortic surgery. Less than 10% of patients may have an associated potentially obstructing lesion, especially colon carcinoma, diverticulitis, volvulus, fecal impaction, postoperative stricture, or radiation stricture. Typically, the associated lesion is distal and there is a segment of normal-appearing colon between the distal lesion and the proximal colitis. Radiologists and gastroenterologists must be careful not to overlook associated lesions in patients with CI. Surgeons must examine specimens of colon removed for carcinoma for evidence of ischemia near the anastomosis, because such involvement may lead to postoperative leaks or strictures. CI is a complication of elective aortic surgery in 1–7% of cases, but following surgery for ruptured abdominal aortic aneurysm its incidence may be as high as 60%. CI is responsible for approximately 10% of deaths after aortic grafting.

Pathophysiology

The precise etiology and pathogenesis of CI remains ill defined in most cases. In some instances, however, a cause can be identified, for example, ligation of the inferior mesenteric artery during repair of an abdominal aortic aneurysm. Indeed, ischemic injury to the colon may result from a variety of causes: iatrogenic and noniatrogenic, occlusive and nonocclusive, systemic and local. Most cases are considered to occur spontaneously and are believed to represent localized forms of nonocclusive ischemia, perhaps in conjunction with small vessel disease. Although a systemic low-flow state may be present, as in congestive heart failure or cardiac arrhythmias, in most instances no such condition exists to explain the ischemic episode.

Given that CI most often occurs in the elderly, age-related acquired abnormalities in the colonic vasculature have been sought. Postmortem angiographic studies of the mesenteric arteries have revealed an age-related tortuosity of the long colic arteries and pathologic specimens of the rectum of elderly patients have shown abnormalities of the musculature of the vessel wall. Neither of these two conditions, however, accounts for a significant percentage of causes of colon ischemia in aged subjects.

The ultimate process resulting in CI remains speculative. However, colonic blood flow is lower than that of any other intestinal segment, decreases with functional motor activity, and is greatly affected by autonomic stimulation. This unique combination may predispose the colon to ischemic injury.

Clinical Findings

A. SYMPTOMS AND SIGNS

Most instances of CI occur without explanation, in contrast to AMI, in which a major vascular occlusion or period of systemic hypoperfusion usually can be identified. Typically, CI presents with the sudden onset of mild, crampy, left-sided lower abdominal pain accompanied by an urgent desire to defecate. This is followed by the passage of either bright red or maroon blood mixed with stool over the ensuing 24 hours. The bleeding is not massive and blood loss requiring transfusion is so unusual as to suggest another diagnosis. Physical examination usually reveals only mild to moderate abdominal tenderness over the involved segment of bowel. The presence of peritoneal signs suggests colonic necrosis, gangrene, and perforation. Any part of the colon may be affected; however, the watershed areas, namely the splenic flexure and rectosigmoid, are the segments most commonly involved.

B. IMAGING

Plain films of the abdomen are usually nondiagnostic in patients with CI, but radiologic findings suggestive of CI include thumbprinting, transverse ridging, and a tubular appearance of the bowel. Thumbprinting of the colon may be seen in up to 20% of patients with CI and represents submucosal hemorrhage and edema. Although thumbprinting may be reflective of CI, especially in the correct clinical setting, other diseases—including inflammatory bowel disease, infectious colitis, pseudomembranous colitis, and certain malignant lesions—may produce this change as well. Gas in abnormal locations, such as the bowel wall, peritoneum, and portal vein, is indicative of colonic infarction.

If CI is suspected in a patient with no signs of peritonitis and an unremarkable abdominal plain film, colonoscopy or the combination of flexible sigmoidoscopy and a gentle barium enema should be performed within 48 hours of the onset of symptoms (Figure 9–3). Whichever test is selected, it should be performed early in the course, as the disease may evolve rapidly. If evaluation is delayed, initial characteristic lesions may be missed. If the patient is studied with serial examinations, which is sometimes the only way to suggest the correct diagnosis, the colon should show progression to a segmental colitis pattern within 1 week or reversion to normal within several weeks. Colonoscopy is preferable to barium studies because it is more sensitive in diagnosing mucosal abnormalities and biopsy specimens may be obtained at the time of examination. Hemorrhagic nodules may be seen on colonoscopy and correspond to the thumbprinting seen on radiologic evaluation. Other findings on colonoscopic inspection

may include an erythematous and congested mucosa, ischemic ulcerations, and mucosal gangrene. In cases in which the inflammatory response is excessive, lesions simulating strictures, polypoid neoplasms, or submucosal tumors may be seen. During colonoscopy, particular care must be taken to avoid overdistention with air, since pressures greater than 30 mm Hg, which may be attained on routine examinations, diminish colonic blood flow and cause a shunting of blood from the mucosa to the serosa, thereby producing or aggravating colon ischemia.

Although histologic evaluation of biopsy specimens obtained during colonoscopy often reveals a variety of nonspecific inflammatory changes also seen in other types of colitides, certain findings are more characteristic of ischemia. These include the preservation of cellular outlines referred to as "ghost" cells and hemosiderin-laden macrophages in the submucosa.

Stool studies are very important in excluding infectious causes of colitis that may mimic CI or agents that may even cause a hemorrhagic colitis. *E coli* O157:H7 is an organism that has been shown to elaborate toxins that may cause fibrin thrombi and produce hemorrhagic colitis in the elderly and in the young. This organism (which requires a special medium to be cultured) has been found by immunoperoxidase staining of archived colonoscopic biopsies and resected colon specimens in 10% of cases of CI. Cytomegalovirus (CMV) also may cause CI and many parasites may produce a segmental colitis that mimics CI.

Barium enema is also highly sensitive in the diagnosis of CI. The most characteristic early finding of CI is the presence of thumbprinting, seen in up to 75% of cases. Thumbprinting is not pathognomonic of CI, and if the diagnosis of CI is suspected, serial studies should be performed to demonstrate the evolution characteristic of this disease. Other findings may include transverse ridging, segmental ulcerations, and luminal nar-

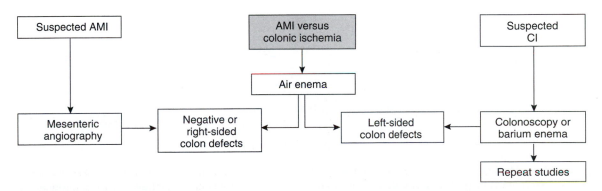

Figure 9–3. Management of suspected ischemic bowel disease. AMI, acute mesenteric ischemia; CI, colon ischemia.

rowing; ischemic inflammatory mass lesions may simulate colonic carcinoma. As mentioned previously, approximately 5% of patients with CI have a potentially obstructing lesion distal to the ischemic segment.

Mesenteric angiography is usually not indicated in the management of CI, as colonic blood flow has usually returned to normal by the time of presentation. Hence, angiography rarely shows any significant occlusions. Angiography may be indicated however, if AMI is a consideration, either because only the right side of the colon is affected or the clinical presentation does not allow a clear distinction between CI and AMI (see Figures 9–1 and 9–3). In the latter situation, if the plain films of the abdomen do not show the thumbprinting pattern characteristic of CI, an air enema is performed by gently insufflating air into the colon, either by using a hand bulb or during flexible sigmoidoscopy. On fluoroscopy, the submucosal edema and hemorrhage that produce the thumbprinting pattern of CI is accentuated by the column of air. If thumbprinting is not seen or is identified in the ascending colon only, mesenteric angiography is indicated. Because untreated AMI rapidly becomes irreversible, and optimal management requires angiography, AMI must be excluded before barium studies are performed.

Treatment

Because the outcome of CI usually cannot be predicted, serial examinations are necessary to determine the ultimate course of disease (Figure 9–4). When the physical examination does not suggest gangrene or perforation, the patient is treated expectantly. Parenteral fluids are administered, the bowel is placed at rest, and broad-spectrum antibiotics are given. There are no randomized controlled trials proving the use of antibiotics is effective to reduce morbidity and mortality, nor is it likely such studies will be forthcoming. Cardiac function is optimized and newly introduced or changed medications that cause mesenteric vasoconstriction, such as digitalis and vasopressors, are withdrawn if possible. Colonic distention is treated with rectal tube decompression and nasogastric aspiration. Serial evaluations of the colon and continuous monitoring of the hemoglobin, white blood cell count, and electrolytes are performed. Increasing abdominal tenderness, guarding, rising temperature, and paralytic ileus indicate colonic infarction and mandate laparotomy and colon resection.

If, as usual, CI resolves within several weeks, no further therapy is indicated. When segmental colitis develops, corticosteroid therapy does not appear to be beneficial and may predispose to perforation. Patients who

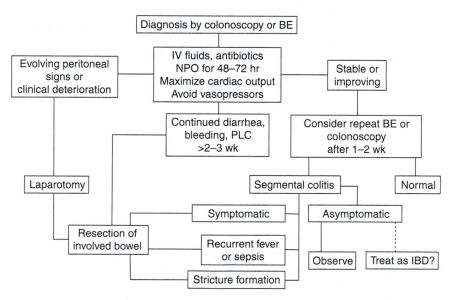

Figure 9–4. Management of colon ischemia. **Solid lines** indicate accepted management plans and **dashed lines** indicate alternate management plans. BE, barium enema; NPO, nothing by mouth; IV, intravenous; PLC, protein-losing colopathy; IBD, inflammatory bowel disease. (Reproduced, with permission, from American Gastroenterological Association Medical Position Statement: guidelines on intestinal ischemia. Gastroenterology 2000;118:951.)

are asymptomatic, but with roentgenographic or endoscopic evident of persistent disease, should have frequent follow-up examinations to determine whether the colon is healing, has persisting colitis, or is developing a stricture. Recurrent fevers, leukocytosis, and septicemia in otherwise asymptomatic patients with unhealed segmental colitis are usually caused by bacterial translocation across the damaged mucosa of the diseased bowel and are an indication for elective resection. In patients with diarrhea, rectal bleeding, or protein-losing colonopathy for more than 2 weeks, severe ischemic damage with colonic perforation is likely and early resection is suggested.

CI may not manifest symptoms during the acute insult but still may produce a chronic colitis frequently misdiagnosed as inflammatory bowel disease. Involvement is segmental, resection is not followed by recurrence, and the response to corticosteroid therapy is usually poor. Local steroid enemas may be helpful, but parenteral steroids should be avoided. In those whose symptoms cannot be controlled by medications, resection of the diseased segment is indicated.

If the ischemic process involves the muscularis propria with subsequent healing and fibrosis, an ischemic stricture may result. Strictures that produce no symptoms should be observed, as some of these will resolve over the next 12–24 months without specific therapy. Strictures that cause obstructive symptoms will require either dilation or resection.

A rare form of fulminating CI involving all or most of the colon and rectum has been identified. The clinical course is typically rapid and progressive and management is similar to other fulminant colitides, that is, total colectomy and ileostomy.

Prognosis

Usually symptoms of CI subside within 24–48 hours and healing is seen within 2 weeks. Two-thirds of patients with reversible disease exhibit intramural and submucosal hemorrhage or a reversible colonopathy, while one-third manifest a transient colitis. More severe reversible damage may take 1–6 months to resolve, but during this time, patients are usually asymptomatic. In less than 50% of patients with CI, irreversible damage results. Approximately two-thirds of these patients develop segmental colitis or stricture and one-third develop gangrene with or without perforation.

The prognosis of patients with CI-complicating shock, congestive heart failure, myocardial infarction, or severe dehydration is poor. One series reported these factors precipitating CI in 25% of patients, and 92% of patients who presented in shock died.

CHRONIC MESENTERIC ISCHEMIA (CMI)

ESSENTIALS OF DIAGNOSIS

- Postprandial abdominal pain, sitophobia, and weight loss.
- Diagnosed by angiography, which shows involvement of at least two of the three main splanchnic vessels.
- Treatment by surgical revascularization or percutaneous transluminal angioplasty.

General Considerations

CMI, or intestinal angina, is uncommon, accounting for less than 5% of all ischemic disease. The pathophysiology of this disease is most often related to atherosclerotic narrowing of the mesenteric vessels. These lesions are located proximally and at least two of the three major splanchnic vessels usually are involved before ischemia ensues. As these atherosclerotic narrowings develop over a period of time, usually an adequate collateral circulation has developed to prevent intestinal infarction, although this disastrous complication may occur if thrombosis suddenly develops in an involved artery. Similar to angina pectoris or intermittent claudication, in which blood flow is insufficient to meet the metabolic demands of exercise, the pain of CMI has been attributed to insufficient blood flow to satisfy the increased postprandial demands of motility, secretion, digestion, and absorption. The pain produced by intestinal angina typically occurs soon after eating, prior to food entering the small bowel, and is felt to be secondary to an increased demand for gastric blood flow as food enters the stomach. This requirement is satisfied by a "steal" of blood flow from the small intestine, depriving the intestine of its oxygen and nutrients.

Clinical Findings

A. SYMPTOMS AND SIGNS

The cardinal feature of CMI is abdominal discomfort or pain that usually occurs within 30 minutes after eating, gradually increases in severity, and then slowly abates over 1–3 hours. The pain is usually dull, gnawing, or cramping and is located in the periumbilical region or in the epigastrium. Pain is initially precipitated by large meals, however, as the disease progresses, the amount of food necessary to produce pain gradually diminishes until the patient ultimately becomes afraid to eat (sitophobia) and sustains weight loss. Malabsorption is seen in one-half of the patients, and gastroin-

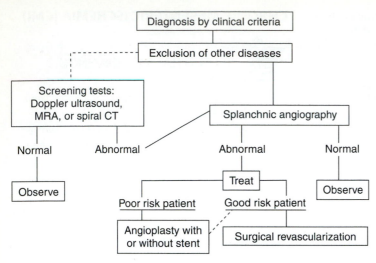

Figure 9–5. Management of chronic mesenteric ischemia. **Solid lines** indicate accepted management plans and **dashed lines** indicate alternate management plans. MRA, magnetic resonance angiography; CT, computed tomography. (Reproduced, with permission, from American Gastroenterological Association Medical Position Statement: guidelines on intestinal ischemia. Gastroenterology 2000;118:951.)

testinal dysmotility manifested by bloating, nausea, episodic diarrhea, or constipation also occurs.

Physical findings are usually limited and nonspecific, however, patients with advanced disease may appear cachectic with marked weight loss. The abdomen typically remains soft and nontender, even during painful episodes, although significant distention may be present. An abdominal bruit is common (especially with marked weight loss) but nonspecific.

Many patients have evidence of systemic atherosclerosis involving the heart, central nervous system, or peripheral vasculature.

B. DIAGNOSTIC STUDIES

Diagnosis is often difficult because of the vague nature of the complaints and the lack of a specific diagnostic test (Figure 9–5). Studies of malabsorption may reveal an elevated fecal fat excretion or decreased level of urinary D-xylose excretion, however, these are nonspecific tests and can be caused by a variety of diseases. Barium studies may be normal or reveal nonspecific evidence of either malabsorption or a motility disturbance. Doppler ultrasound, computed tomography, and magnetic resonance imaging are also limited by their lack of specificity, but are useful screening tests to identify patients who may or may not benefit from mesenteric angiography. Duplex ultrasound and magnetic resonance imaging may also be used to measure the effect of eating on splanchnic blood flow; intestinal blood flow normally increases after eating, whereas in patients with CMI, it does not.

Angiography in selected patients is quite helpful in the diagnosis of CMI, although all three major arterial vessels have been found occluded in asymptomatic patients. Single-vessel disease does not usually result in in-

testinal angina since the intestine within the distribution of the diseased vessel usually will be supplied by collateral vessels; at least two vessels usually need to be involved before the diagnosis of CMI can be considered. Angiographic views are taken anteroposteriorly to demonstrate the extent of the collateral circulation and laterally to show the proximal origins of the splanchnic vessels, especially the celiac axis, and SMA.

Treatment

Although CMI does not require urgent therapy, revascularization may be indicated if acute complete occlusion of the blood supply occurs, that is, if thrombosis is superimposed on preexisting arterial narrowing. Surgical revascularization should be performed on relatively healthy, "low-risk" patients with the typical pain of abdominal angina and unexplained weight loss, whose diagnostic evaluation has excluded other gastrointestinal diseases and whose angiogram shows occlusive involvement of at least two of the three major arteries. A variety of such surgical procedures exist, including aortovisceral bypass and transaortic visceral endarterectomy, each of which is associated with a reasonable operative risk and a good long-term prognosis. Success rates and recurrence rates range from 60 to 100% and 0 to 27%, respectively, with perioperative mortality rates of 0–16%. Success rates of percutaneous transluminal mesenteric angioplasty, alone or with stent insertion, are similar to those of surgical revascularization; rates of clinical success, that is, relief of symptoms, have varied from 63 to 100% with few mortalities. Angioplasty should, at present, be reserved for patients suspected or proven to have CMI who are too ill or who pose too great a risk for surgical revascularization.

REFERENCES

Allen RC et al: Mesenteric angioplasty in the treatment of chronic intestinal ischemia. J Vasc Surg 1996;24:415.

Bakal CW, Sprayregen S, Wolf EL: Radiology in intestinal ischemia: angiographic diagnosis and management. Surg Clin North Am 1992;72:125.

Boley SJ, Kaleya RN: Acute mesenteric ischemia: an aggressive diagnostic and therapeutic approach. Can J Surg 1992;35:613.

Brandt LJ, Boley SJ: Nonocclusive mesenteric ischemia. Annu Rev Med 1991;42:107.

Brandt LJ, Boley SJ: Colonic ischemia. Surg Clin North Am 1992;72:203.

Brandt LJ, Boley SJ: AGA technical review on intestinal ischemia. Gastroenterology 2000;118:954.

Cunningham CG, Reilly LM, Stoney R: Chronic visceral ischemia. Surg Clin North Am 1992;72:231.

Czerny M et al: Die akute mesenteriale ischamie. Zentralbl Chir 1997;122:538.

Genta RM, Haggitt RC: Idiopathic myointimal hyperplasia of mesenteric veins. Gastroenterology 1991;101:533.

Harward TR et al: Multiple organ dysfunction after mesenteric artery revascularization. J Vasc Surg 1993;18:459.

Inderbitzi R et al: Acute mesenteric ischemia. Eur J Surg 1992;158:123.

Kaleya RN, Boley SJ, Brandt LJ: Mesenteric venous thrombosis. Surg Clin North Am 1992;72:183.

Kaleya RN, Sammartano RJ, Boley SJ: Aggressive approach to acute mesenteric ischemia. Surg Clin North Am 1992;72:157.

Kornblith PL, Boley SJ, Whitehouse BS: Anatomy of the splanchnic circulation. Surg Clin North Am 1992;72:1.

Kubes P: Ischemia-reperfusion in feline small intestine: a role for nitric oxide. Am J Physiol 1993;264:G143.

MacDonald PH, Dinda PK, Beck IT: The role of angiotensin in the intestinal vascular response to hypotension in a canine model. Gastroenterology 1992;103:57.

Patel A, Kaleya RN, Sammartano RJ: Pathophysiology of mesenteric ischemia. Surg Clin North Am 1992;72:31.

Ritz JP et al: Prognosefactoren des mesenterialinfarktes. Zentralbl Chir 1997;122:332.

Su C, Brandt LJ: The immunological diagnosis of E. coli O157:H7 colitis: possible association with colon ischemia. Am J Gastroenterol 1998;93:1055.

Wolf EL, Sprayregen S, Bakal CW: Radiology in intestinal ischemia: plain film, contrast, and other imaging studies. Surg Clin North Am 1992;72:107.

Zimmerman BJ, Granger DN: Reperfusion injury. Surg Clin North Am 1992;72:65.

Miscellaneous Diseases of the Peritoneum & Mesentery

10

Tya-Mae Y. Julien, MD

The peritoneum is a serous membrane lining the peritoneal cavity that consists of a single layer of mesothelium and a thin basement membrane. The peritoneum lines the abdominopelvic walls and undersurface of the diaphragm (parietal peritoneum) and the intraabdominal organs (visceral peritoneum). Peritoneal folds support the viscera in the form of mesenteries, omenta, and ligaments. In men, the peritoneal cavity is a closed sac and only a small amount of intraperitoneal fluid is normally present. In women, the peritoneal cavity is in continuity with the female reproductive organs, and up to 20 mL of free fluid may be present depending on the menstrual phase. Acute peritoneal irritation (peritonitis) is associated with extrusion of inflammatory cells and serum which typically leads to ascites formation. Chronic injury may cause scarring with formation of adhesions. This chapter will discuss the less commonly encountered peritoneal diseases and will address the causes of nonportal hypertensive ascites. Ascites caused by chronic liver disease and portal hypertension will be discussed in Chapter 43.

GENERAL APPROACH TO ASCITES & PERITONEAL DISEASE

Patients with ascites typically present with increasing abdominal girth and nonspecific abdominal discomfort. Evaluation of the patient with ascites requires a careful history, physical examination, and peritoneal fluid analysis. A minimum of 1.5 L of fluid is felt to be necessary before ascites is detectable on physical examination. The physical diagnosis of ascites can be difficult in obese patients. Flank dullness is the most sensitive physical examination finding for the presence of ascites; the absence of flank dullness is strong evidence that little or no ascites is present. If flank dullness is detected, percussion should be repeated with the patient in the partial decubitus position to look for "shifting dullness." Looking for a "fluid wave" is seldom helpful as this is present principally in patients with massive ascites in whom the diagnosis is seldom in question. As the most common cause of ascites is portal hypertension, patients should be asked about risk factors for chronic liver disease (alcohol, hepatitis, blood transfu-

sions, intravenous drug use). The presence of spider angiomata, palmar erythema, gynecomastia, muscle wasting, splenomegaly, or abdominal wall collaterals suggests chronic liver disease and directs further studies.

Abdominal paracentesis is essential in the evaluation of the patient with ascites. The patient usually is placed in a semirecumbent position. The peritoneal cavity can be safely entered from either the midline suprapubic region or either lower quadrant provided there is dullness to percussion at the site. There should not be any scars or large vessels at the site. Using aseptic technique, the area should be disinfected and anesthetized with local anesthetic. To reduce the chance of postprocedure ascites leakage, the skin is pulled 1–2 inches to the side as the needle is passed slowly through the skin and peritoneum. For diagnostic paracentesis, a steel 1.5-inch 22-gauge needle is used; for therapeutic paracentesis a 16-gauge needle or multihole trochar needle is used.

The ascitic fluid should be visually inspected. Usual fluid is yellow-orange and transparent. Turbid fluid suggests the presence of white blood cells (>1000/µL). Milky fluid suggests the presence of triglycerides, as with chylous ascites. Bloody fluid may be caused by a traumatic tap, malignancy, or tuberculosis.

The initial paracentesis fluid should be sent for a cell count with differential, culture, and albumin (Table 10–1). Of these, the cell count is the most useful and requires only 10 µL for analysis. Fluid must be sent in a "purple top" ethylenediaminetetraacetic acid (EDTA)-containing tube to prevent clotting. Normal ascitic fluid contains less than 500 total white blood cells and 250 neutrophils/mL. Any inflammatory process can lead to an elevated ascitic fluid total white blood cell count (>500 cells/mL), however, a neutrophil count of >250 cells/mL usually is indicative of infection. Cultures are best performed by innoculation of blood culture bottles with 5–20 mL of ascitic fluid at the time of paracentesis. Positive culture results are obtained in up to 90% of cases when infection is present.

The serum-ascites albumin gradient (SAAG) has supplanted the transudate-exudate model for categorizing ascites. The serum and ascites albumin should be obtained on the same day. The gradient is calculated by subtracting the ascites albumin from the serum albu-

Table 10–1. Tests of ascitic fluid.

Routine	Secondary	Ancillary
Cell count	Gram's stain	AFB smear/culture[1]
Culture	Total protein	Amylase
Albumin	Cytology	Triglyceride
	Glucose, LDH[1]	Bilirubin

[1]AFB, acid-fast bacillus; LDH, lactate dehydrogenase.

min (eg, 3.5 g/dL − 2.5 g/dL = 1 g/dL). A calculated SAAG >1.1 g/dL suggests with 97% accuracy that portal hypertension is the cause of the ascites (for which there are multiple etiologies). A calculated SAAG <1.1 g/dL suggests that the pathophysiology of the ascites is not due to portal hypertension.

The clinical scenario directs further analysis (Table 10–2). In a patient with an elevated neutrophil count and suspected bacterial peritonitis, it is important to distinguish between spontaneous bacterial peritonitis and surgical ("secondary") peritonitis. The latter is suspected when a Gram's stain of the ascites demonstrates multiple different organisms or when ascites fluid analysis reveals an elevated total protein (>1 g/dL), low glucose (<50 mg/dL), and elevated lactate dehydrogenase (LDH). Tuberculous peritonitis may be suspected in patients with an elevated ascites white blood count, especially when there is a predominance of lymphocytes. Acid-fast bacillus (AFB) smear and culture should be sent in such patients, especially in immunocompromised hosts. Tuberculosis also should be suspected in cirrhotic patients with recurrent or poorly responding spontaneous bacterial peritonitis.

The ascites total protein measurement is of limited diagnostic value. Although most cases of malignancy-associated ascites (carcinomatosis, hepatocellular carcinoma) have a total protein >2.5 g/dL, malignancy is often associated with low protein ascites due to depressed serum albumin levels, especially in patients with concomitant liver disease and portal hypertension. Ascites total protein is of value in two situations. The first is in distinguishing among patients with suspected portal hypertension (ie, with an elevated SAAG). Almost all patients with portal hypertension caused by cardiac disease ("cardiac ascites") or hepatic venous thrombosis have an ascites total protein >2.5 g/dL. However, up to 20% of patients with uncomplicated cirrhotic ascites also have a value >2.5 g/dL. The second is to determine the risk of spontaneous bacterial peritonitis in patients with cirrhotic ascites; a total protein level <1.0 g/dL predicts an increased risk.

Cytologic studies should be ordered if lymphocytosis is evident in the ascitic fluid or if the patient has a

history of a solid organ tumor (eg, breast or colon carcinoma). Triglycerides may be sent when chylous ascites is suspected, and ascites amylase or bilirubin may be sent when pancreatic or biliary ascites are suspected.

"Mixed ascites" refers to the presence of portal hypertension in conjunction with another cause of ascites. Mixed ascites is characterized by a high SAAG (often due to cirrhosis) in conjunction with another process—such as peritoneal carcinomatosis or tuberculosis. Therefore, a high SAAG is diagnostic of portal hypertension but does not exclude the possibility of concomitant tumor or infection. Consideration of nonportal hypertensive causes is warranted in all patients presenting with ascites.

Abdominal imaging [ultrasound and computed tomography (CT)] aids in the detection of solid organ tumors, cystic lesions, lymphadenopathy, and infiltrative processes affecting the peritoneum. Ultrasonography is extremely sensitive for the detection of small amounts of ascites and can be used to guide paracentesis when ascitic fluid is modest or loculated. Radiologic-guided needle biopsy of masses discovered with these modalities is a useful minimally invasive technique that is safe in experienced hands.

Finally, laparoscopy is an important diagnostic modality in the evaluation of patients with ascites and a low SAAG. It is safe, well tolerated, and can be performed on an outpatient basis. Peritoneal diseases such as tuberculosis and carcinomatosis are best evaluated in this way.

Runyon BA: Care of patients with ascites. N Engl J Med 1994;330: 337.

Runyon BA et al: The serum-ascites albumin gradient is superior to the exudate-transudate concept in the differential diagnosis of ascites. Ann Intern Med 1992;117:215.

MALIGNANT ASCITES

Ascites in association with an advanced malignancy portends a poor prognosis. About two-thirds of such patients have peritoneal carcinomatosis, ie, direct or metastatic involvement of the peritoneum by cancer that results in alterations in the permeability of the peritoneum or obstruction of peritoneal lymphatics. The remainder have ascites due to massive liver metastases or hepatocellular carcinoma causing increases in portal pressures, or lymphatic obstruction resulting in chylous ascites (see below).

Patients usually present with nonspecific abdominal discomfort associated with increasing abdominal girth. Physical examination and imaging studies may show ascites and reveal the primary tumor. More than 75% of cases are adenocarcinomas arising within the abdomen. Ovarian, pancreatic, gastric, colonic, and uterine tumors

Table 10–2. Analysis of ascitic fluid.[1]

Condition	Fluid Inspection	Cell Count	SAAG[2] Total Protein	Gram's Stain and Culture	Other
Cirrhosis (uncomplicated)	Straw colored	WBC < 250/μL	SAAG > 1.1 g/dL, total protein < 2.5 g/dL	Negative	
Congestive heart failure	Straw colored	WBC < 1000/μL	SAAG > 1.1 g/dL, total protein > 2.5 g/dL	Negative	
Spontaneous bacterial peritonitis	Turbid or purulent	PMN > 250/μL (PMN=50–70% of WBC)	SAAG > 1.1 g/dL, total protein < 1 g/dL	Gram's stain 10% sensitive, culture 90% sensitive	
Secondary bacterial peritonitis	Turbid or purulent	PMN > 10,000/μL	SAAG < 1.1 g/dL, total protein > 2.5 g/dL	Gram's stain usually shows bacteria	Glucose < 50 mg/dL; ascitic LDH > serum LDH; plain films, CT to look for intraabdominal source of infection; increased ascitic amylase in pancreatic ascites or bowel perforation
Tuberculous peritonitis	Clear, turbid, hemorrhagic, chylous	Lymphocyte count 250–4000/μL	SAAG < 1.1 g/dL, total protein > 2.5 g/dL	AFB smear positive in < 5%, culture positive in 20%	Laparoscopy for dx—white nodules cover parietal surface + adhesions; biopsy—granulomas in 80%
Peritoneal carcinomatosis	Hemorrhagic	Positive cytology, WBC > 1000/μL (PMN+ lymphocytes)	SAAG < 1 g/dL, total protein > 2.5 g/dL	Negative	Laparoscopy to confirm dx

[1]WBC, white blood cells; PMN, polymorphonuclear cells; AFB, acid-fast bacillus; LDH, lactate dehydrogenase.
[2]SAAG (serum-ascites albumin gradient) = (serum albumin-ascites albumin). High gradient: SAAG > 1.1 g/dL suggests portal hypertension: cirrhosis, alcoholic hepatitis, portal vein thrombosis, Budd Chiari syndrome, massive liver metastases, or heart failure. Low gradient: SAAG < 1.1 g/dL suggests nonportal hypertensive etiology: nephrotic syndrome, tuberculosis, peritoneal carcinomatosis, pancreatic/biliary ascites, serositis.

are the most common abdominopelvic primary malignancies. Lymphoma lung and breast tumors are the most common extraabdominal primary malignancies.

The diagnostic evaluation should begin with paracentesis. The SAAG will usually be less than 1.1 mg/dL (indicating that the cause of ascites is not portal hypertension) and should prompt cytologic studies. At least a 1-L bottle of fluid should be sent for cellblock analysis, which has a diagnostic sensitivity of over 50% in patients with carcinomatosis. Of note, cytologic studies will typically be negative in patients with ascites sec-

ondary to hepatic metastases or hepatocellular carcinoma. The ascitic cholesterol level tends to be higher in malignant ascites, with a reported sensitivity exceeding 80%; however, a clear cut-off value has not been established. Ancillary tests of ascitic fluid such as fibronectin and α_1-antitrypsin are currently being evaluated for their use in differentiating malignant ascites from nonmalignant causes. Tumor markers, such as carcinoembryonic antigen, CA-125, and α-fetoprotein, may help to define the tumor of origin. Masses found on noninvasive imaging studies should be evaluated with radiologically guided percutaneous needle biopsy. Unexplained ascites with a low SAAG should be evaluated by laparoscopy if the diagnosis remains unclear after initial evaluation in order to exclude carcinomatosis. Tuberculous peritonitis and mesothelioma are alternative diagnostic considerations.

Therapy is directed toward relief of symptoms and improvement in the quality of life. Malignant ascites in the presence of hepatic metastases may respond to spironolactone. Large-volume therapeutic paracentesis is often useful, but palliation is of short duration. For patients with rapidly reaccumulating ascites, a peritoneovenous shunt will provide effective palliation in up to 70% of cases. However, complications occur in 25–50% of patients, most often due to shunt occlusion. In general, patients with primary gastrointestinal malignancy have a very poor short-term survival, and placement is not recommended in this group. At present, shunt insertion is recommended only for treatment of malignant ascites in nongastrointestinal malignancies after other nonsurgical therapies have failed. Overall survival rates for patients with nongastrointestinal malignancies are similar in patients treated with and without peritoneovenous shunts, but those treated with successful shunts may enjoy an improved quality of life.

The prognosis for most patients with peritoneal carcinomatosis is poor, with median survival rates of under 20 weeks. Patients with gastrointestinal primary malignancies do poorly compared with patients with gynecologic primary neoplasms (particularly ovarian carcinoma). However, maximum cytoreductive surgery combined with intraperitoneal chemotherapy, and advances in gene therapy may improve patient outcomes in future selected cases.

Bieligk SC, Calvo BF, Coit DG: Peritoneovenous shunting for nongynecologic malignant ascites. Cancer 2001;91(7):1247.

Elias D et al: Curative treatment of peritoneal carcinomatosis arising from colorectal cancer by complete resection and intraperitoneal chemotherapy. Cancer 2001;92(1):71.

Parsons SL, Watson SA, Steele RJ: Malignant ascites. Br J Surg 1996;83:6.

CHYLOUS ASCITES

Chylous ascites or chyloperitoneum refers to the presence of milky, lipid-containing thoracic or intestinal lymph within the peritoneal cavity. It is due to obstruction of lymphatic vessels (most often from tumor infiltration), or lymphatic injury secondary either to surgery in the retroperitoneum or trauma.

Patients may present with abdominal distention and malnutrition. Diarrhea may arise either from a protein-losing enteropathy or steatorrhea due to blocked small bowel lymphatics. Because peritoneal lymphatic vessels play a major role in the removal of particulate matter from the peritoneal cavity, impaired cellular immunity due to lymphocyte depletion predisposes to secondary infections.

Paracentesis reveals turbid milky fluid that separates into layers upon standing. Ether extraction clarifies the fluid if lipid is present. The triglyceride level in the fluid is often more than 1000 mg/dL and always exceeds the plasma level.

The possible causes of chylous ascites vary, depending on the patient's age and the acuity of onset of the illness. In children, up to 60% of cases are associated with a congenital lymphatic anomaly such as a lymphocele, lymphangiectasia, or lymphatic atresia. The most common cause in adults is cancer, which is present in over 80% of patients. Intraabdominal lymphoma that obstructs lymphatic outflow accounts for over half of cases. Inflammatory conditions and infections that involve the lymphatics such as mycobacteria [tuberculosis, *Mycobacterium avium* complex (MAC), especially in human immunodeficiency virus (HIV) disease], filariasis, pancreatitis, portal vein thrombosis, and mesenteric adenitis have been described. These entities lead to ascites by infiltrating lymph nodes, resulting in obstruction. Postoperative chylous ascites is uncommon and has been reported most often following extensive abdominal or retroperitoneal dissection.

Once chylous ascites has been documented, a CT scan of the abdomen should be obtained to evaluate for possible cancer. Lymphangiography is a useful study to document suspected leaks. Exploratory laparotomy may be necessary to exclude lymphoma with certainty.

Treatment is aimed at the underlying process. Although most chylous effusions heal spontaneously, early treatment is initiated to reduce the morbidity associated with lymphatic losses. Diuretics and salt restriction are ineffective and large-volume paracentesis gives only short-term relief. A low-fat diet supplemented with medium-chain triglycerides will decrease lymph flow and may be useful. Total parenteral nutrition and complete bowel rest decrease lymph flow and may allow small postsurgical leaks to heal. Large or persistent leaks may be repaired laparoscopically. Octreotide, the long-acting somatostatin analog, can reduce lymph flow, and its role in this setting is being examined. Placement of a peritoneovenous shunt has met with moderate success.

The prognosis of patients with chylous ascites depends on the underlying diagnosis. The 1-year survival rate in children is >80% but in adults is <30%.

Browse NL et al: Aetiology and treatment of chylous ascites. Br J Surg 1992;79:1145.

Keaveny AP, Karasik MS, Farber HW: Successful treatment of chylous ascites secondary to Mycobacterium avium complex in a patient with the acquired immune deficiency syndrome. Am J Gastroenterol 1999;94(6):1689.

TUBERCULOUS PERITONITIS

The incidence of tuberculosis in the United States has increased over the past decade due to HIV infection, immunosuppressive therapy following solid organ transplantation, and immigration. Abdominal involvement occurs in up to 5% of patients with tuberculosis but is more common in patients coinfected with HIV. The gastrointestinal (GI) tract is reported to be the sixth most common extrapulmonary site, and 15–50% of patients with GI involvement may have active pulmonary disease. Abdominal tuberculosis can involve the luminal gastrointestinal tract, liver, spleen, peritoneum, and female genital tract. The most common site of enteral tuberculosis is the ileocecal region. Tuberculous peritonitis occurs in less than 1% of cases of tuberculosis. The organisms may enter the peritoneal cavity through the bowel wall, by direct extension from the gynecologic tract, or by hematogenous spread from a primary pulmonary focus.

The diagnosis of tuberculous peritonitis is often difficult to make and requires a high index of clinical suspicion. Most patients will present with a triad of abdominal pain, fever, and weight loss, but anorexia, vomiting, and diarrhea are often reported. The pain may be diffuse or localized to the site of involvement. The onset usually is insidious, with symptoms present for many months before diagnosis. Abdominal distention caused by ascites or intestinal obstruction may be present. Abdominal tenderness is the most common physical examination finding, while hepatomegaly and clinically apparent ascites are variably present. In the United States, up to half of the patients with tuberculous peritonitis also have cirrhosis with portal hypertensive ascites. In such patients, the diagnosis of concomitant tuberculous peritonitis may be unsuspected and overlooked.

Routine laboratory and radiographic analyses are of limited diagnostic value. The total leukocyte count is usually normal and a mild anemia may be present. There may be evidence of malabsorption when the bowel is involved. Tuberculin skin tests are positive in over 70% of patients, but a negative test does not exclude the disease. Chest radiographs are abnormal in over two-thirds of patients, but active pulmonary tuberculosis is evident in only 14% of cases. Abdominal CT may reveal ascites or bowel wall thickening, nonspecific findings that mimic many other diseases including Crohn's disease.

When ascites is present, peritoneal fluid analysis may be informative and should be performed. The ascitic fluid protein exceeds 2.5 g/dL in more than 85%

of cases, and the glucose concentration usually is less than 30 mg/dL. The white blood cell count exceeds 250 cells/μL, with a predominance of lymphocytes. AFB smears on ascitic fluid are rarely positive. Cultures require weeks to mature and are positive in as few as 20% of diagnosed cases. Polymerase chain reaction (PCR) analysis for rapid detection of bacillus tubercles and ascitic adenosine deaminase levels are currently being evaluated as diagnostic tools.

Laparoscopy is the gold standard for the diagnosis of peritoneal tuberculosis. It allows a presumptive visual diagnosis in more than 85% of cases, and, with guided biopsy, allows a definitive diagnosis in over 97% of cases. The macroscopic findings include small (<5 mm) scattered yellowish-white nodules of fairly uniform size coating the visceral and parietal peritoneum, as well as adhesions between adjacent organs. Histologic analysis reveals caseating granulomas. In contrast, peritoneal carcinomatosis appears as larger whitish nodules of various sizes.

With proper therapy, tuberculous peritonitis is readily treated. Due to the emergence of multidrug-resistant tuberculosis, culture and sensitivity studies of biopsy specimens are imperative. Clinicians should maintain a high index of suspicion for tuberculosis so that antituberculin drug therapy, which is very effective in the absence of drug resistance, may be initiated early. Treatment delay is associated with significant mortality.

Bernhard JS, Bhatia G, Knauer CM: Gastrointestinal tuberculosis—an eighteen-patient experience and review. J Clin Gastroenterol 2000;30(4);397.

Karawi MA et al: Protean manifestations of gastrointestinal tuberculosis: report on 130 patients. J Clin Gastroenterol 1995;20 (3):225.

Marshall JB: Tuberculosis of the gastrointestinal tract and peritoneum. Am J Gastroenterol 1993;88(7):989.

Talwani R, Horvath JA: Tuberculous peritonitis in patients undergoing continuous ambulatory peritoneal dialysis: case report and review. Clin Infect Dis 2000;31:70.

PANCREATIC ASCITES

Pancreatic ascites is an uncommon complication of pancreatitis that is characterized by the presence of extravasated pancreatic enzymes into the peritoneal cavity. It is typically the result of disruption of the pancreatic duct or leakage from a pseudocyst, and may occur as a complication of either acute pancreatitis or chronic pancreatitis. Over 75% of cases occur in the setting of alcohol-related chronic pancreatitis—in which the cause of ascites may be inaccurately attributed to decompensated liver disease with portal hypertension. Less than 1% of patients with chronic pancreatitis develop pancreatic ascites. In approximately 80% of these cases, leakage arises from a pseudocyst communicating with a ductal disruption. The remainder of cases are due to ductal disruption in the absence of a pseudocyst. Blunt abdominal trauma with duct disruption is another important etiology.

In the setting of severe acute pancreatitis, peripancreatic fluid collections are common and most resolve spontaneously. Pancreatic ascites should be suspected when there is a gradual increase in abdominal girth and a persistently elevated serum amylase level. Patients with chronic pancreatitis typically present with increasing abdominal girth, weight loss, and pain due to distension. The intraabdominal pancreatic enzymes are inactive and do not cause painful ascites. Signs of chronic pancreatitis, such as steatorrhea or diabetes, or radiographic evidence of pancreatic calcifications may be present. Ultrasound or CT imaging demonstrates ascites. The majority of patients also have a pseudocyst, but the site of ductal disruption is seldom demonstrated by noninvasive imaging studies.

The diagnosis of pancreatic ascites is established by paracentesis. The ascitic fluid amylase is markedly elevated, often in excess of 10,000 units/mL. The ascitic fluid total protein level and albumin are also high due to leakage of enzyme-rich pancreatic fluid and exudate from the inflamed pancreas. The total protein is usually above 2.5 g/dL and the SAAG is less than 1.1 g/dL.

Effective management of pancreatic ascites requires collaboration among surgeons, biliary endoscopists, and interventional radiologists. Initial management involves bowel rest and parenteral nutrition in an effort to suppress pancreatic secretion, reduce fluid and protein loss, and improve nutritional status. Octreotide has been used to suppress pancreatic secretions, but its efficacy in pancreatic fistula closure and control of pancreatic ascites has not been consistently demonstrated in randomized controlled trials. Overall, response to conservative management may be successful in over 25% of patients. Definitive treatment depends on the degree and location of ductal disruption and the underlying cause of the pancreatic ascites. Endoscopic retrograde cholangiopancreatography (ERCP) guides therapy by delineating the site of ductal disruption and the presence of duct strictures. The majority of patients with persistent pancreatic ascites require surgical therapy with either partial pancreatic resection, cystgastrostomy, or cystjejunostomy. However, in specialized centers endoscopic transpapillary pancreatic duct stenting has resulted in complete resolution of pancreatic acites in selected cases, thus obviating the need for surgical intervention. Stents are placed across the pancreatic duct and either across the site of disruption into the proximal pancreatic duct, or across the disruption into the pseudocyst. Stenting may heal duct disruption by either occlusion of the leak or by bypassing the high-pressure pancreatic sphincter and allowing preferential flow through the low-pressure stent. In highly specialized centers, resolution of ascites is reported in >80% of cases with endoscopic treatment.

Bracher GA et al: Endoscopic pancreatic duct stenting to treat pancreatic ascites. Gastrointest Endosc 1999;49(6):710.

Kozarek RA et al: Endoscopic treatment of pancreatic ascites. Am J Surg 1994;168:223.

Li-Ling J, Irving M: Somatostatin and octreotide in the prevention of postoperative complications and the treatment of enterocutaneous pancreatic fistulas: a systematic review of randomized controlled trials. Br J Surg 2001;88(2):190.

BILIARY ASCITES

The most common causes of biliary ascites (bile extravasation into the peritoneal cavity) are complications of biliary tract surgery and trauma to the abdomen. Less common causes include percutaneous liver biopsy, transhepatic cholangiography, and rupture of the gallbladder due to gangrenous cholecystitis. The incidence of bile duct injuries worldwide has increased since the advent of laparoscopic cholecystectomy, and is associated with significant long-term morbidity (including recurrent stricture formation, cholangitis, and cirrhosis). An overall incidence of 0.3% (single center series) and 0.5% (multicenter series) has been reported with laparoscopic cholecystectomy compared with 0.5% with open cholecystectomy.

Patients with biliary ascites may remain asymptomatic or may present with severe abdominal pain due to peritoneal irritation. Uninfected biliary fluid does not usually cause peritoneal irritation. Patients may present with increased abdominal girth or vague upper abdominal discomfort. Laboratory testing may reveal elevation of serum bilirubin. Extravasation of infected bile will usually lead to suppurative peritonitis with fever, leukocytosis, and an acute abdomen. Ultrasound or CT imaging reveals intraabdominal fluid either around the liver, in the porta hepatis, or within the peritoneal cavity. Paracentesis reveals dark yellow fluid, with a bilirubin level greater than 6 mg/dL and exceeding that of serum.

Optimal management of biliary leaks requires close cooperation between hepatobiliary surgeons, biliary endoscopists, and interventional radiologists. Treatment depends on the etiology, anatomic location, and the duration of the leak. Major duct injuries generally require surgery. Localized collections of extravasated bile ("bilomas") often can be drained percutaneously with spontaneous resolution of a small bile duct leak. Persistent small bile duct leaks and cystic duct stump leaks are effectively treated with endoscopic sphincterotomy alone or endoscopically placed temporary biliary stents. These techniques facilitate leak closure by lowering intraductal pressure, allowing preferential bile drainage into the duodenum. Transhepatic biliary stents may be placed by interventional radiologists for isolated intrahepatic and proximal ductal injuries.

Branum G et al: Management of major biliary complications after laparoscopic cholecystectomy. Ann Surg 1993;217(5):532.

McMahon AJ et al: Bile duct injury and bile leakage in laparoscopic cholecystectomy. Br J Surg 1995;82:307.

Pencev D et al: The role of ERCP in patients after laparoscopic cholecystectomy. Am J Gastroenterol 1994;89(9):1523.

Ryan ME et al: Endoscopic intervention for biliary leaks after laparoscopic cholecystectomy: a multicenter review. Gastroint Endosc 1998;47(3):261.

MYXEDEMA ASCITES

Myxedema is a rare cause of ascites, complicating less than 4% of patients with clinically significant hypothyroidism. The mechanism of ascites formation is poorly understood, and may involve increased capillary permeability, impaired lymphatic drainage of extravasated albumin, or impaired free water clearance, due to low levels of circulating thyroid hormone. In addition, subtle heart failure may be present. Striking features of this condition include a high protein content of the ascitic fluid (>2.5 g/dL), a long duration of the ascites (typically months to years), and a dramatic response to thyroid replacement. Interestingly, the SAAG often is high—possibly due to cardiac failure with increased portal pressures. Diuretics are minimally beneficial. The diagnosis should be suspected in patients with high protein ascites and systemic evidence of hypothyroidism. Response is evident within a few weeks of initiation of thyroid replacement therapy.

de Castro F et al: Myxedema ascites. J Clin Gastroenterol 1991;13(4):411.

CHRONIC AMBULATORY PERITONEAL DIALYSIS-ASSOCIATED PERITONITIS

Chronic ambulatory peritoneal dialysis (CAPD) is utilized by 20–50% of all dialysis patients worldwide. Unfortunately, peritonitis remains a potentially life-threatening complication and is the leading single cause of treatment failure with this modality. Depletion of host immune defenses secondary to removal of opsonins with peritoneal fluid places this population at risk for infection. The main portal of entry of bacteria is the dialysis system, either at the catheter exit site or the tunnel through which the catheter crosses the abdominal wall. Strict aseptic technique and the use of new disconnect systems have led to a significant de-

crease in the incidence of peritonitis to 0.55 episodes per patient-year in 1998.

The clinical findings of CAPD-related peritonitis are generally mild compared with those of suppurative peritonitis. Fever, diffuse abdominal pain, and a cloudy dialysate are typical. The white blood cell count of the peritoneal fluid is more than 300/μL, with greater than 75% polymorphonuclear leukocytes. These changes may precede the development of cloudy fluid by 1 week. Although Gram-stained smears are positive in only 10% of samples, newer bacteria-concentrating techniques yield positive cultures in up to 90% of cases. Most cases are caused by a single organism, with *Staphylococcus epidermidis* and *Staphylococcus aureus* accounting for 50% of infections. Gram-negative organisms together account for an additional 25% (most commonly *Escherichia coli*, *Pseudomonas aeruginosa,* and *Klebsiella* sp.). Fungal peritonitis is uncommon but most serious.

Treatment consists of prompt administration of antibiotics (preferably intraperitoneally and on an outpatient basis) and elimination of the local infectious source. An increased frequency of exchanges also helps to resolve the infection. Heparin may be added to the dialysis bath to reduce the incidence of postinfection adhesions. Catheters should be removed in the setting of advanced cellulitis at the entry site, primary tunnel infection with persistent peritonitis beyond 5 days of therapy, fecal peritonitis, fungal peritonitis, and tuberculous peritonitis. As many as one-third of clinical episodes are sterile and may be due to a chemical constituent of the dialysate.

Monteon F et al: Prevention of peritonitis with disconnect systems in CAPD: a randomized controlled trial. Kidney Int 1998;54(6):2123.

Zelenitsky S et al: Analysis of microbial trends in peritoneal dialysis-related peritonitis from 1991 to 1998. Am J Kidney Dis 2000;36(5):1009.

CHEMICAL PERITONITIS

Chemical causes of peritonitis include spillage of sterile body fluids into the abdominal cavity (bile, chyle, and urine) as well as the introduction of irritant materials during surgery. Talc, cornstarch, cotton from sponges, and cellulose fibers from disposable gowns and drapes have all been associated with granulomatous peritonitis. Clinical symptoms typically manifest within 2–8 weeks of laparotomy and include fever, abdominal pain with tenderness, distention, and ascites. Peripheral eosinophilia may be present and birefringent crystals may be found in the ascitic fluid. Exploratory laparotomy reveals peritoneal nodules, adhesions, and ascites. Histologic analysis reveals granulomata and possible starch granules. The incidence of chemical peritonitis is rare since the inception of glove washing at the start of cases, and the prognosis is excellent.

Barium causes an intense peritoneal reaction when introduced through a perforated viscus and may cause a life-threatening suppurative peritonitis. For this reason, water-soluble contrast agents should be used when a perforated intraabdominal viscus is suspected. Treatment consists of antibiotics, prompt laparotomy with peritoneal lavage, and repair of the perforated viscus. Dense adhesions are a common long-term complication.

HIV-ASSOCIATED PERITONEAL DISEASES

The peritoneum in HIV patients may become involved in both acquired immunodeficiency syndrome (AIDS)-related and non-AIDS-related illnesses. Spontaneous bacterial peritonitis may occur in patients with cirrhotic ascites, while acute suppurative peritonitis may result from intestinal perforation. The most common cause of bowel perforation in AIDS patients is ileal or colonic cytomegalovirus infection. Peritonitis due to mycobacterial species, *Toxoplasma gondii, Cryptococcus neoformans, Pneumocystis carinii, Strongyloides, Ascaris, Leishmania,* and *Trypanosoma cruzi* has been reported. Kaposi's sarcoma may also cause peritoneal studding and ascites.

The evaluation of HIV-positive patients with peritonitis includes ascites fluid analysis, abdominal imaging, and often peritoneal biopsy. A high SAAG suggests portal hypertension and should prompt a search for chronic liver diseases due to hepatitis B or C, or alcohol. Routine bacterial cultures and special stains for AFB should be obtained.

In patients with a low SAAG, cytologic analysis is useful to evaluate for malignancy. Abdominal and pelvic CT may reveal lymphadenopathy, which may be present in patients with disseminated Kaposi's sarcoma or *Mycobacterium avium* complex. NonHodgkin's lymphoma often involves mesenteric, periportal, and retroperitoneal lymph nodes, and appropriate chemotherapy may improve morbidity and mortality.

Laparoscopy is an important diagnostic procedure in the HIV-postive patient with unexplained ascites or peritoneal disease. It allows inspection and directed biopsy of the liver and peritoneal surfaces, permitting detection of tuberculosis, other opportunistic infections and malignancy.

Chu CM et al: The role of laparoscopy in the evaluation of ascites of unknown origin. Gastrointest Endosc 1994;40:285.

Jeffers LJ et al: Laparoscopic and histologic findings in patients with the human immunodeficiency virus. Gastrointest Endosc 1994;40(2):160.

■ OTHER PERITONEAL DISEASES

FAMILIAL MEDITERRANEAN FEVER

Familial Mediterranean fever (FMF) is an autosomal recessive disorder characterized by recurrent febrile attacks, generalized peritonitis, pleuritis, pericarditis, and monoarthritis. The illness affects those of Mediterranean ancestry almost exclusively. Half of the affected individuals are of Sephardic Jewish descent, with Arabs, Turks, and Armenians comprising the majority of remaining cases. The pathogenesis is uncertain. Patients with FMF may lack one or more chemotactic factor-inactivating enzymes, thus precipitating inflammatory attacks.

Although a genetic test for FMF is now available (see below), the diagnosis in many patients is still made based upon clinical criteria and the exclusion of other causes of peritonitis. Patients usually present in the first or second decade of life. The major criteria for the diagnosis are recurrent fever alone or in combination with sudden attacks of serositis (involving the peritoneum, joints, or pleura), which are initial manifestations. Peritoneal attacks are marked by the sudden onset of fever, severe abdominal pain that may be diffuse or localized, and abdominal tenderness with guarding and rebound. The diagnosis should be suspected in young patients of appropriate ethnic origin or with a positive family history.

Most patients will have some leukocytosis and increased acute phase reactants [erythrocyte sedimentation rate (ESR), C-reactive protein]. Plain abdominal x-rays may show dilated loops of small bowel, with air–fluid levels consistent with ileus. If left untreated, the attack improves within 6–12 hours and ends with full recovery within 24–48 hours. In between attacks, patients feel entirely well. Attacks occur at unpredictable and irregular intervals. The associated arthritis may be prolonged, is usually oligoarticular, and may be associated with sacroiliitis.

Because patients have symptoms and signs that simulate an "acute abdomen," an exploratory laparotomy often is done at some point to exclude a surgical disease (appendicitis, salpingitis, perforated ulcer). Operative findings may show evidence of acute peritoneal inflammation with serous ascites that contains many polymorphonuclear leukocytes. Smears and cultures of the fluid are always sterile. To avoid confusion, an appendectomy is usually performed at the time of initial exploration. Other nonsurgical disorders that may be confused with FMF include acute intermittent porphyria, hereditary angioedema, abdominal epilepsy, polyarteritis nodosa, and systemic lupus erythematosis.

A major complication of FMF is the development of secondary amyloidosis, which occurs in up to 25% of patients. Renal amyloidosis (AA protein) is the leading cause of death in FMF patients.

The gene responsible for FMF, designated the MEFV gene, was recently cloned and is located on chromosome 16. A total of 19 mutations have been identified. Expressed in neutrophils, this gene codes for pyrin, a transcription factor that regulates the expression of target genes involved in immune suppression. PCR analysis of genomic DNA is now used to confirm the diagnosis in suspected cases. However, in about 40% of cases of FMF diagnosed by clinical criteria in the United States, no known mutation has been identified.

Colchicine is the only known effective treatment for the prevention and treatment of FMF. Its full mechanism is poorly understood, but it appears to alter leukocyte activity by interfering with microtubule function and neutrophil degranulation. Colchicine, 0.6 mg given two or three times a day, has been shown to decrease dramatically the frequency, severity, and duration of attacks. Over 85% of patients experience symptomatic improvement and a smaller number enjoy complete remission. This treatment has little long-term toxicity and should be prescribed to most patients as chronic, preventive therapy. Lack of improvement with colchicine is most commonly due to noncompliance or incorrect diagnosis. Colchicine has been documented to decrease the incidence of nephropathy by 67%, and it may even stablize renal disease once proteinuria has been detected.

In the absence of amyloid nephropathy, the prognosis for patients with FMF is excellent.

Babior BM, Matzner Y: The familial Mediterranean fever gene—cloned at last. N Engl J Med 1997;337(21):1548.

Livneh A et al: Criteria for the diagnosis of familial Mediterranean fever. Arthritis Rheum 1997;40(10):1879.

Scully RE et al: Case records of the Massachusetts General Hospital. Weekly clinicopathologic exercises, Case 25—1999. N Engl J Med 1999;341(8):593.

PSEUDOMYXOMA PERITONEI

Pseudomyxoma peritonei or "false mucinous tumor of the peritoneum" is a rare clinical condition characterized by copious amounts of gelatinous fluid and benign tumors that eventually fill the peritoneal cavity. It is believed to arise in most cases from a perforation of the appendix due to an adenoma, low-grade adenocarcinoma, or cyst. Although ascribed in older literature to ovarian disease, it is currently believed that the gynecologic tract is not a common source.

Patients present with increasing abdominal girth or subclinical appendicitis. A new-onset hernia and ab-dominal pain due to intermittent or chronic small bowel obstruction may be present. Ultrasound or CT scanning of the abdomen often shows ascites with multiple septations and semisolid masses along the peritoneal surfaces. However, the diagnosis is difficult to establish by imaging or percutaneous biopsy and is usually made at the time of laparotomy.

Reexploration for obstruction due to recurrent tumors was associated with significant morbidity in the past. However, cytoreductive surgery with complete peritonectomy combined with perioperative intraperitoneal chemotherapy has more recently resulted in an 86% 5-year disease-free survival rate.

Esquivel J, Sugarbaker PH: Clinical presentations of the pseudomyxoma peritonei syndrome. Br J Surg 2000;87:1414.

Witkamp AJ et al: Extensive surgical cytoreduction and intraoperative hyperthermic intraperitoneal chemotherapy in patients with pseudomyxoma peritonei. Br J Surg 2001;88:458.

PERITONEAL MESOTHELIOMA

Primary malignant peritoneal mesothelioma is a rare and highly aggressive tumor arising from the mesothelial surface lining the peritoneum. It accounts for approximately 30% of all mesothelial tumors. Approximately 25% of cases are associated with prior asbestos exposure, but the link between the two is less clear than with pleural mesothelioma. Mesothelioma incidence in industrialized nations has been steadily increasing, likely due to asbestos exposure after World War II, and is expected to reach its peak around 2020. Men are affected more often than women (2–4:1) and the median age at diagnosis is 55 years. The prognosis is extremely poor with a mean survival of under 12 months.

Patients present with increasing abdominal girth, ascites, abdominal pain, and weight loss. Abdominal CT often demonstrates ascites and sheetlike masses involving the omentum, mesentery, and peritoneum. Analysis of ascitic fluid reveals a SAAG <1.1 g/dL but the cytology is often negative. Laparoscopy usually is necessary and reveals extensive studding of all peritoneal surfaces with hard whitish nodules and plaques. On gross examination, the findings are indistinguishable from secondary carcinomatosis. Laparotomy may be required when findings on laparoscopy are inconclusive. Electron microscopy and immunohistochemical staining help distinguish mesothelioma from other peritoneal tumors.

Recent studies have identified female gender, lack of prior surgery, and completeness of tumor resection as favorable prognostic indicators. Treatment is evolving, and the use of cytoreductive surgery combined with anthracycline-based intraperitoneal chemotherapy is currently being explored in clinical trials. Nevertheless, prognosis remains dismal secondary to extensive disease at the time of presentation and ineffective curative therapy.

Sebbag G et al: Results of treatment of 33 patients with peritoneal mesothelioma. Br J Surg 2000;87(11):1587.

■ DISEASES OF THE MESENTERY

SCLEROSING MESENTERITIS

Sclerosing mesenteritis is a primary inflammatory process involving the mesenteric fat. It comprises a broad histologic spectrum from inflammatory to fibrotic lesions, and a multitude of terms have been ascribed to this clinical entity. Most lesions consist of chronic inflammatory cells, fat necrosis, and some degree of fibrosis. The cause is unknown, but trauma and infection may play a role in the initiation of damage to the mesenteric fat, with subsequent excessive lipid infiltration and fibrosis.

Patients generally present in the fifth or sixth decade with vague abdominal pain or a palpable abdominal mass. Retractile mesenteritis is a clinical variant associated with fibrotic thickening and shortening of the mesentery that can lead to intestinal obstruction.

Abdominal CT imaging may identify fat-filled mesenteric masses. The diagnosis is made during laparotomy or laparoscopy with biopsy, usually performed for the treatment of bowel obstruction or evaluation of an abdominal mass. The gross specimen reveals gray plaque-like masses at the root of the mesentery. Patients with retractile mesenteritis have a rubbery, thick mesentery resulting in retraction of the small bowel down to the mesenteric root. Adhesions and acute angulations of the small bowel are often seen and add to the propensity for intermittent bowel obstruction.

Sclerosing mesenteritis must be distinguished from neoplastic processes. Up to 30% of patients may have an associated neoplasm such as lymphoma. In the absence of associated tumor, the prognosis is good. Once the diagnosis of sclerosing mesenteritis is made, resection usually is not possible and should not be attempted. Bowel obstruction is best treated with surgical diversion or bypass. Recurrent symptoms are uncommon and most often are related to adhesions. Rare cases of disease progression have been noted, and a response to corticosteroids, colchicine, immunosuppressive therapy, and progesterone has been reported.

Emory TS et al: Sclerosing mesenteritis, mesenteric panniculitis and mesenteric lipodystropy: a single entity? Am J Surg Pathol 1997;21(4):392.

RETROPERITONEAL FIBROSIS

Retroperitoneal fibrosis (RPF) is an uncommon chronic inflammatory disorder characterized by slowly progressive fibrosis of fat and connective tissue in the retroperitoneum. The disease leads inexorably to compression of tubular structures within the retroperitoneum, including the ureters, lymphatics, nerves, and blood vessels. Approximately two-thirds of cases are idiopathic and the pathogenesis is poorly understood. Early pathologic findings include a mixture of macrophage, lymphocyte, and plasma cells, suggesting an immune-mediated process. Fibrosis subsequently develops, possibly in response to leakage of ceroid from retroperitoneal fat. RPF may be seen in conjunction with immune-mediated connective tissue disorders, other fibrotic processes such as mediastinal and mesenteric fibrosis, and various paraneoplastic syndromes.

The remaining one-third of cases of RPF are attributed to prior retroperitoneal infection, neoplasms (Hodgkins' lymphoma, sarcoma, carcinoid tumors), radiotherapy, hemorrhage, or medications (ie, secondary retroperitoneal fibrosis). An association between the serotonin-blocking agent methylsergide and RPF is well established. Cases of RPF have also been reported in patients taking other ergot derivatives, α-blocking agents, β-blocking agents, and some analgesics.

Patients are usually male and present in the fifth or sixth decade of life. The most common symptom is dull, poorly localized back and flank pain. This may be associated with fatigue, weight loss, and fevers. Laboratory findings include a leukocytosis and an elevated ESR. Encasement and compression of both ureters may lead to ureteral obstruction, azotemia, and eventual renal failure. Uncommonly, the fibrotic reaction may involve the aorta or iliac arteries leading to symptoms of arterial insufficiency, or may obstruct major veins resulting in deep venous thrombosis or lower extremity edema. A hydrocele is a relatively common finding due to increased pressure on the retroperitoneal structures. This diffuse fibrotic process may also extend anteriorly to obstruct the duodenum, common bile duct, or colon.

CT and magnetic resonance imaging (MRI) are the radiographic modalities of choice. RPF appears as a soft tissue mass that is isodense with muscle, obliterates fat planes, and encases the retroperitoneal structures. Pyelography will demonstrate the triad of medial deviation of the ureters, extrinisic ureteral compression, and delayed excretion of contrast with hydronephrosis—but these findings are nonspecific. Malignant RPF accounts for approximately 10% of all cases, and the presence of a retroperitoneal neoplasm must be excluded. Because definitive diagnosis is based on histologic analysis of adequate specimens, surgical biopsies are usually required.

Treatment goals include relief of ureteral obstruction with restoration of renal function, and control of inflammation. This can be accomplished by ureteral stent placement or lysis of ureteral adhesions. Corticosteroids have repeatedly been shown to be effective in reducing inflammation, particularly during the acute, early inflammatory stage. Other immunomodulators such as azathioprine and cyclophosphamide have also been used successfully. Tamoxifen has been used with some efficacy, possibly through the secretion of tumor growth inhibitor-β, an inhibitory growth factor.

Kottra JJ, Dunnick NR: Retroperitoneal fibrosis. Radiol Clin North Am 1996;34(6):1259.

Vivas I et al: Retroperitoneal fibrosis: typical and atypical manifestations. Br J Radiol 2000;73(866):214.

Gastrointestinal Complications of Pregnancy

11

Natalie H. Bzowej, MD, PhD

Disorders of the gastrointestinal tract during pregnancy are very common. This chapter is designed to provide the primary care physician, the obstetrician, and the gastroenterologist with an approach to the management of various gastrointestinal problems during pregnancy. For each disorder the pathophysiology, clinical findings, and treatment will be discussed.

Many gastrointestinal disorders are unique to pregnancy, but there are also those that occur coincidentally with pregnancy. In both instances many of the disorders are the result of hormonally induced alterations of gut motility that occur during pregnancy. This chapter will be divided into two main sections: (1) gastrointestinal disorders that are related to changes in motility and (2) nonmotility associated disorders. The indications, utility, and safety of endoscopic procedures as well as surgical problems during pregnancy will also be discussed.

Rational pharmacologic and nonpharmacologic approaches to the treatment of various problems during pregnancy, based on the best available information to date, will be described. In general, a minimalist approach to the use of medications in pregnancy is taken. Where applicable, the risks of treatment with a potentially harmful drug will be weighed against the risks of not being treated for the disorder.

If clinically appropriate, treatment with drugs should be initiated after the first trimester when organogenesis is completed. Because there are few data that address the safety of many commonly prescribed medicines, there are few category A drugs available for the treatment of gastrointestinal disorders. The current Food and Drug Administration (FDA) classification for drug therapy during pregnancy will be used when referring to medications:

Category A: Controlled studies in humans show no fetal risk.

Category B: Animal studies show no risk but poor human studies, or animal studies with some risk but no human risk.

Category C: Animal studies show risk but human studies are inadequate or lacking, or no studies in animals or humans.

Category D: Definite fetal abnormalities in human studies but benefits of drug may outweigh risk.

Category X: Contraindicated in pregnancy; fetal defects in animals or humans; risks outweigh benefits.

■ DISORDERS IN PREGNANCY ASSOCIATED WITH GASTROINTESTINAL DYSMOTILITY

Pregnancy has a major effect on gut motility, which results in many common problems such as gastrointestinal reflux, nausea and vomiting, hyperemesis gravidarum, constipation, diarrhea, and cholelithiasis. This occurs in large part due to the effect of high circulating levels of reproductive hormones, especially progesterone. Thus, most problems improve or resolve after delivery. In contrast, pregnancy has little if any effect on gastrointestinal secretion or absorption.

GASTROESOPHAGEAL REFLUX DISEASE (GERD)

Pathophysiology

Heartburn and other symptoms of reflux disease are very common during pregnancy and have been reported to occur in 30–80% of pregnant women. In many cases this represents a *de novo* problem that occurs during pregnancy. However, if a woman is symptomatic before pregnancy, this disease will likely be exacerbated during pregnancy. Symptoms worsen with increasing gestational age in part because of mechanical pressure from an increasing gravid uterus. Evidence for this exists from studies done in cirrhotic patients with ascites before and after aggressive diuresis. Considered a "pseudopregnancy" state, tense ascites has been shown to decrease lower esophageal sphincter pressures, which increase after ascites resolution. Studies indicate that symptoms parallel changes in circulating reproductive hormones, in particular progesterone and estrogen. These hormones result in a progressive relaxant effect on the lower esophageal sphincter. Hormonal levels peak by 36 weeks gestation, a time at which the lower esophageal sphincter pressure reaches a nadir. Sphincter pressure returns to normal after delivery when hormone levels normalize. No changes in basal or peak acid output are observed during pregnancy.

The factors that promote reflux also predispose patients to anesthesia-related aspiration of gastric contents, the most common cause of obstetric anesthesia morbidity and mortality.

Clinical Findings

Reflux symptoms are the same as in nonpregnant women and are most troublesome in the third trimester. It is usually mild with few patients developing complications such as erosive esophagitis or strictures. The diagnosis is almost always made from the clinical history and rarely requires the use of confirmatory tests. Radiologic imaging should be avoided in this setting. Although endoscopy can be done safely, it is rarely needed. It should be reserved for patients with worrisome symptoms such as dysphagia, bleeding, and weight loss. Ambulatory pH monitoring can be used for patients with symptoms that are atypical or fail to respond to empirical treatment.

Treatment

When choosing a treatment regimen, the potential adverse effects of medications on the fetus must be considered (Table 11–1). Whereas acid-reducing medications are prescribed liberally for nonpregnant women, life-style modifications should be initiated first in pregnant women. Life-style modifications include lifting the head of the bed, small frequent meals, and avoidance of foods that decrease lower esophageal sphincter pressure (fatty foods, caffeine, alcohol, and peppermint).

If nonpharmacologic methods fail, medications may be introduced in a stepwise fashion (see Figure 11–1). Whenever possible these medications should be prescribed after the first trimester. Sucralfate and/or antacids are considered safe because they are not systemically absorbed. H_2-receptor antagonists (H_2RA) can be introduced if these agents are inadequate. Although no controlled studies have been performed on the safety of H_2RA in pregnancy, there is anecdotal data for both cimetidine and ranitidine, suggesting they are safe even though they cross the placenta. Nevertheless, these agents should be used in the lowest effective doses. There are no controlled studies assessing the safety of prokinetic agents; hence, they should be used

cautiously. Few controlled or anecdotal data exist on the safety of proton-pump inhibitors during pregnancy. Therefore it is suggested that these agents should be reserved for patients with endoscopically confirmed evidence of severe reflux disease (erosive esophagitis or stricture).

The role in pregnancy of new endoscopic techniques for the treatment of reflux disease has yet to be elucidated. Surgery is rarely required and if deemed necessary should be performed in the second trimester. Women with a history of severe reflux disease who are planning a future pregnancy should consider surgical treatment before pregnancy.

NAUSEA & VOMITING

Nausea and vomiting are the most common gastrointestinal complaints in pregnancy and often are the first indication that someone is pregnant. Nausea occurs in 50–90% of pregnancies and is complicated by vomiting in 25–55%. These symptoms are on a continuum, varying from mild to severe. Mild to moderate symptoms that occur in the morning and resolve later in the day are often referred to as "morning sickness." Vomiting is most common during the first trimester, peaking around 10 to 15 weeks and subsiding by 20 weeks. More severe symptoms are known as hyperemesis gravidarum, which is characterized by intractable vomiting that results in dehydration, ketosis, electrolyte imbalance, weight loss, and, in some cases, the need for hospitalization. Hyperemesis gravidarum will be mentioned only briefly here, since it is discussed in more detail in Chapter 47.

Pathophysiology

The etiology of nausea and vomiting is unclear. Data suggest that high progesterone levels result in changes in gastric motility and tone. Premenopausal women have slower gastric emptying than men or postmenopausal women, suggesting that hormonal mechanisms affect gastric emptying. In animals, progesterone inhibits antral contractions. Studies also demonstrate delayed small bowel transit in pregnancy, which may also contribute to the symptoms.

The pathophysiology of hyperemesis gravidarum has been attributed to psychological factors, hormonal factors (eg, hyperthyroidism, hyperparathyroidism, effects of gestational hormones), liver abnormalities, abnormal gastric electrical activity, autonomic nervous system dysfunction, abnormal lipid metabolism, and nutritional deficiencies. None of these theories fully explains the pathophysiology. Hyperemesis gravidarum is more common in nulliparous patients, twin pregnancies, and women younger than 35 years of age (Table 11–2).

Table 11–1. Recommendations for use of gastrointestinal drugs in pregnancy.

Drug	Class	Comments
Antiulcer/dyspepsia		
Aluminum and magnesium hydroxide (Maalox, Mylanta)	B	Considered safe since nonsystemic; enters breastmilk, but breastfeeding not contraindicated
Bismuth subsalicylate (Pepto-Bismol)	C	Take with caution since salicylate absorption may occur in large doses
Calcium carbonate (Tums)	C	Considered safe since nonsystemic
H₂ blockers (nizatadine, famotidine, cimetidine, ranitidine)	B	Considered safe from clinical experience, although crosses placenta; largest experience with cimetidine more than ranitidine; secreted in breastmilk and breastfeeding not recommended
Misoprostol (Cytotec)	X	Use is contraindicated since it is an abortifacient; secreted in breastmilk and breastfeeding not recommended
Proton-pump inhibitors (omeprazole, esomeprazole, pantoprazole, rabeprazole)	B, C	Use with caution since it crosses placenta and minimal data in pregnant women; secreted in breastmilk and breastfeeding not recommended
Simethicone (Mylicon, Gas-X)	C	Considered safe; not known if it enters breastmilk, but no adverse neonatal effects expected
Sucrulfate (Carafate)	B	Considered safe since nonsystemic; not known if it enters breastmilk, but no adverse neonatal effects expected
Conscious sedation		
Meperidine (Demerol)	B	Considered safe; crosses placenta; peak cord concentration is 75% of maternal serum levels
Midazolam (Versed)	D	Avoid in pregnancy; crosses placenta; suggested increase in congenital malformations with the use of other benzodiazepines
Constipation		
Bisacodyl (Dulcolax)	B	Likely safe since not teratogenic in animals
Lactulose (Chronulac)	B	Likely safe since not teratogenic in animals
Magnesium hydroxide (Milk of Magnesia)	B	May promote sodium retention in the mother
Methylcellulose (Citrucel)	B	Considered an agent of choice since no systemic absorption
Mineral oil	C	Decreased maternal absorption of fat-soluble vitamins with neonatal hypoprothrombinemia and bleeding if used regularly
Phenolphthalein (Ex-Lax)		Excreted in breastmilk and may cause colic in breastfed infants
Polyethylene glycol (Golytely, Miralax)	C	Minimal data in pregnancy and no animal reproduction studies
Psyllium (Metamucil)	C	Considered an agent of choice since no systemic absorption
Senna (Senokot)	C	Minimal data in pregnancy
Sodium docusate (Colace)	C	Considered safe
Diarrhea		
Diphenoxylate hydrochloride plus atropine (Lomotil)	C	Use with caution since minimal data in pregnancy and breastfeeding; unknown if atropine and metabolite diphenoxylic acid are secreted in breastmilk
Loperamide (Imodium)	B	Likely safe since not teratogenic in animals
Octreotide (Sandostatin)	B	Likely safe since not teratogenic in animals
Inflammatory bowel disease		
Azathioprine, mercaptopurine	D	Clinical experience suggests it is safe; continue if required to prevent flare
Ciprofloxacin	C	Considered safe after first trimester; avoid in breastfeeding
Corticosteroids	C	Considered safe in pregnancy and breastfeeding (concern of adrenal insufficiency is theoretical)
Cyclosporine	C	Use only if deemed necessary in pregnancy; avoid in breastfeeding
Infliximab (Remicade)	C	Avoid in pregnancy
Mesalamine 5-ASA (Asacol, Pentasa, Rowasa suppository, and enema)	B	Considered safe in pregnancy and breastfeeding
Methotrexate	D	Avoid in pregnancy
Metronidazole (Flagyl)	D	Avoid in pregnancy

(continued)

Table 11–1. Recommendations for use of gastrointestinal drugs in pregnancy. (continued)

Drug	Class	Comments
Inflammatory bowel disease (*cont*)		
Olsalazine (Dipentum)	C	Minimal data in pregnancy
Sulfasalazine (Azulfidine)	B	Considered safe; does not cause significant displacement of bilirubin from albumin (do not stop during breastfeeding to prevent kernicterus)
Nausea and vomiting		
Cisapride (Propulsid)		Withdrawn from the market
Droperidol (Inapsine)	C	Clinical experience suggests it is safe
Dronabinol (Marinol)	B	Minimal data in pregnancy
5-HT3 receptor antagonists (dolasetron, ondansetron)	B	Minimal data in pregnancy
Metocolopramide (Reglan)	B	Considered safe from anecdotal data; crosses placenta
Prochlorperazine (Compazine)	C	Clinical experience suggests it is safe
Promethazine (Phenergan)	C	Clinical experience suggests it is safe

Clinical Findings

Symptoms typically start in the first trimester and resolve by the twentieth week of gestation. Vomiting that occurs or continues after the twentieth week of gestation should prompt a search for other causes (see Table 11–3). Symptoms are nonspecific, including nausea, vomiting, bloating, distention, anorexia, early satiety, and abdominal pain, but nausea and vomiting predominate. Hyperemesis gravidarum may complicate 0.3–1% of pregnancies and is generally a diagnosis of exclusion. Physical examination is unremarkable except in patients with severe vomiting who may have signs of dehydration. In general, the prognosis for mother and fetus is excellent. Fetal distress and demise can occur in severe cases.

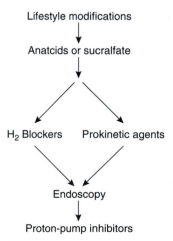

Figure 11–1. Algorithm for the stepwise treatment of gastroesophageal reflux in pregnancy.

Treatment

Most patients with pregnancy-associated nausea and vomiting are treated effectively with reassurance and dietary modifications. Patients should be instructed to eat frequent small meals (six small meals per day), to increase carbohydrate intake, and to decrease dietary fat intake. Ginger root recently has gained popularity for the treatment of nausea and vomiting and has been shown to be superior to placebo in controlled trials. Pyrodoxine (vitamin B_6) may be tried. For patients with refractory symptoms, the stepwise algorithm outlined in Figure 11–2 is recommended. As indicated, antiemetics are not used as a first line measure and should be reserved for patients who fail conservative therapy. Promethazine, a phenothiazine, or metoclopramide is recommended. It should be noted that doxylamine, a component of Bendectine, a previously used agent for nausea and vomiting, has been removed from the market due to suspected teratogenicity. As

Table 11–2. Factors associated with hyperemesis gravidarum.[1]

Factor	Odds Ratio
Maternal age > 35 years	0.6
High body weight	1.4
Nulliparity	1.4
Cigarette smoker	0.7
Twin gestation	1.5
Fetal loss	.07

[1]Reproduced, with permission, from Abell T, Riely CA: Hyperemesis gravidarum. Gastroenterol Clin North Am 1992;21:836. Klebanoff MA et al: Epidemiology of vomiting in early pregnancy. Obstet Gynecol 66;612:1985.

Table 11–3. Differential diagnosis of intractable nausea and vomiting in pregnancy.

Peptic ulcer disease
Severe gastrointestinal reflux
Cholelithiasis
Cholecystitis
Gastroparesis
Acute hepatitis
Pancreatitis
Urinary tract disease
Metabolic disorders
Central nervous system disorders

with all disorders of pregnancy, the benefits of drug therapy must outweigh the risks of treatment.

Patients with dehydration or ketosis require hospitalization and hydration with intravenous fluids. Rarely, hyperalimentation is required for patients with hyperemesis gravidarum who cannot tolerate enteral feedings. To exclude other causes of nausea and vomiting, screening laboratory tests should be obtained including thyroid studies, renal panel, liver chemistries, amylase, lipase, and calcium. Upper endoscopy may be performed if peptic ulcer disease is suspected. Ultrasonography is useful to detect twin or molar gestations.

As long as vomiting can be controlled and severe volume depletion prevented, the prognosis for hyperemesis gravidarum is good with no increased fetal or maternal complications.

CONSTIPATION

Pathophysiology

Constipation and altered bowel habits occur in 30–50% of pregnant patients. Constipation is attributed to progesterone-mediated slowing of intestinal motility. However, dietary changes, decreased fluid intake, reduction in exercise, ingestion of supplemental iron, and mechanical factors such as an enlarging uterus and weakening of the pelvic floor also may play a role.

Clinical Findings

Pregnant women may use the term "constipation" to refer to a decrease in the frequency of bowel move-

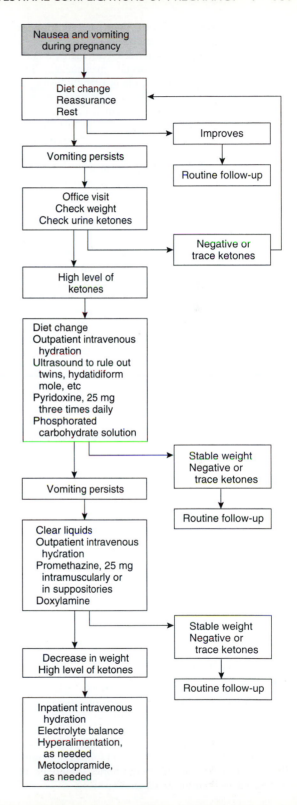

Figure 11–2. Algorithm for the management of nausea and vomiting in pregnancy. (Reproduced, with permission, from Kousen M: Treatment of nausea and vomiting in pregnancy. Am Fam Physician 1993;48:1279.)

ments or to hard stools. For the most part, constipation of pregnancy is an annoyance but seldom poses a serious threat to the mother or fetus. Occasionally, it is the presenting feature of colorectal malignancy. This should be considered when there is a family history of colon cancer or when worrisome symptoms such as hematochezia, iron deficiency anemia, or weight loss are noted. The differential diagnosis also includes obstruction, endocrine disorders, and other systemic illness (see Chapter 1). If serious organic disease is suspected, endoscopy should be performed; it should not be delayed until after pregnancy (see section, "Endoscopic Procedures").

Treatment

Constipation during pregnancy is initially treated with conservative measures, including increased fluids and dietary fiber to at least 25 g/d. Fiber supplements containing psyllium or methylcellulose are not systemically absorbed and they may be used without risk. If an initial trial of fluid and fiber is inefficacious, a trial of stool softeners is warranted (see Table 11–1).

Hemorrhoids occur commonly during pregnancy because of increased intraabdominal pressure and compromised venous return due to the gravid uterus. They can become symptomatic from straining due to constipation. In turn, they may exacerbate constipation due to perianal discomfort. Hemorrhoids also should be treated with fluid and fiber supplementation. Severe hemorrhoids may be treated with sitz baths and suppositories.

DIARRHEA

Pathophysiology

The etiology of diarrhea in the pregnant patient is similar to that in the nonpregnant patient. The incidence of infectious diarrhea is not increased during pregnancy, but infection is still the most common cause of acute diarrhea. Diarrhea also may be the first sign of preterm labor. Relaxin, secreted by the placenta during uterine contraction, may be the responsible agent.

Clinical Findings

Diarrhea that persists for longer than 48–72 hours, or diarrhea that is associated with signs of inflammation (eg, fever, hematochezia), warrants investigation with stool culture and testing for fecal leukocytes, ova, and parasites, and *Clostridium difficile* toxin. In patients with bloody diarrhea, *E coli* O157:H7 infection should also be considered. Empiric antibiotics should be restricted due to their potential teratogenicity.

Differential Diagnosis

Acute diarrhea in pregnancy may be caused by the usual infectious agents (ie, viral, bacterial, and protozoal), inflammatory bowel disease, or medications. Chronic diarrhea is unusual, but may be caused by irritable bowel syndrome, inflammatory bowel disease, malabsorption syndromes, or use of osmotic agents (see Chapter 1). Complications of severe diarrhea include dehydration with the threat of fetal demise. Patients with severe diarrhea warrant hospitalization.

Treatment

Treatment of diarrhea in pregnancy is directed at the underlying cause. Nonsystemic bulking agents are often of benefit (see Table 11–1). Systemic agents should be reserved for severe diarrhea complicated by dehydration, when the risk of dehydration outweighs the risk of the drugs (see Table 11–1). Antibiotics that appear to be safe during pregnancy are erythromycin and ampicillin. Metronidazole, sulfa drugs, and tetracycline should be avoided.

CHOLELITHIASIS & ITS COMPLICATIONS

Pathophysiology

Gallstones may be present before pregnancy or develop during pregnancy. Pregnancy promotes the formation of gallstones due to decreased gallbladder motility with stasis caused by high progesterone levels and decreased gallbladder responsiveness to cholecystokinin (CCK). In addition, bile is more lithogenic due to effects of estrogens and progesterone that lead to a decrease in bile acid enterohepatic circulation and a change in the ratio of chenodeoxycholic acid to cholic acid.

Clinical Findings

Although gallstone development is increased during pregnancy, most gallstones remain asymptomatic. Gallstones may lead to symptoms of biliary colic, acute cholecystitis, choledocholithiasis with jaundice or cholangitis, or acute pancreatitis.

Biliary colic during pregnancy is similar to the nonpregnant state: episodic epigastric or right upper quadrant pain with radiation to the back or shoulder that lasts up to several hours. Symptoms of cholecystitis and pancreatitis are also similar to those in the nonpregnant patient. Persistent epigastric or right upper quadrant pain, nausea, vomiting, fever, and leukocytosis suggest acute cholecystitis. Severe constant epigastric or periumbilical abdominal pain that is associated with increased amylase and lipase suggests acute pancreatitis. However, in pregnancy a broader differential diagnosis must be considered for these symptoms (Tables 11–4 and 11–5).

Table 11–4. Differential diagnosis of acute cholecystitis in pregnancy.[1]

Acute viral hepatitis
Acute alcoholic hepatitis
Duodenal ulcer
Acute pancreatitis
Pulmonary embolus
Right lower lobe pneumonia
Acute myocardial infarction
Acute appendicitis
Acute fatty liver of pregnancy
Preeclampsia
HELLP[2] syndrome

---

[1]Reproduced, with permission, from Scott LD: Gallstone disease and pancreatitis in pregnancy. Gastroenterol Clin North Am 1992;21:807.
[2]HELLP, hemolysis, elevated liver enzymes, and low platelet count.

The diagnosis of acute cholecystitis may be confirmed by abdominal ultrasonographic demonstration of gallstones or sludge within the gallbladder, a thickened gallbladder wall, and pericholecystic fluid. Ultrasonographic evidence of an echogenic focus within the common bile duct suggests choledocholithiasis. Ultrasound may be normal in patients with mild to moderate acute pancreatitis (see section, "Acute Pancreatitis").

Treatment

Because complications of asymptomatic gallstones are infrequent, there is no role for prophylactic cholecystectomy or oral dissolution therapy before or during preg-

Table 11–5. Differential diagnosis of pancreatitis in pregnancy.[1,2]

Acute cholecystitis
Penetrating duodenal ulcer
Ruptured spleen
Perinephric abscess
Acute cardiopulmonary events (embolus, infarction)
Acute appendicitis
Ruptured ectopic pregnancy
Hyperemesis gravidarum
Preeclampsia

---

[1]Reproduced, with permission, from Scott LD: Gallstone disease and pancreatitis in pregnancy. Gastroenterol Clin North Am 1992;21:811.
[2]This list also is expanded because of pregnancy-related conditions (preeclampsia, hyperemesis, ectopic pregnancy) and the effects of the enlarging uterus (appendicitis).

nancy. Chenodeoxycholic acid (Chenix) has teratogenic potential and is contraindicated. Ursodeoxycholic acid (Actigall) is safer, but the slow (and low) rate of gallstone dissolution makes this impractical for treatment during pregnancy.

For pregnant patients with symptomatic gallstones, surgical treatment (cholecystectomy) should be undertaken only when fetal and maternal survival are endangered. Surgery during pregnancy is not to be taken lightly. Whenever possible, most surgeons choose to perform a cholecystectomy electively in the postpartum period. Symptoms of biliary colic are managed expectantly unless they recur frequently, in which case surgery is indicated. Most cases of uncomplicated acute cholecystitis can be managed expectantly, however surgery is warranted when symptoms and signs fail to resolve, or when complications of cholecystitis intervene. Laparoscopic cholecystectomy during pregnancy can be performed safely and effectively during any trimester, but surgery in the second trimester is preferred, when the risk of spontaneous abortion is low and the uterus is not yet large enough to impinge upon the operating field.

Initial treatment of biliary ("gallstone") pancreatitis is supportive and includes hospitalization with intravenous fluids, bowel rest, and analgesia. Fetal loss rates with pancreatitis have been observed to be between 10 and 20%. Patients with an episode of biliary pancreatitis are at markedly increased risk of recurrent episodes of pancreatitis (>50%) due to further passage of gallbladder stones or sludge. In healthy nonpregnant patients, cholecystectomy usually is recommended to prevent further episodes of biliary pancreatitis and associated complications. During pregnancy, the risk of recurrent pancreatitis (with potential impact upon maternal or fetal survival) must be weighed against the risks of cholecystectomy. In patients in whom there is strong suspicion of retained common duct stones (protracted pancreatitis, persistent jaundice or abnormal liver chemistries, cholangitis) endoscopic retrograde cholangiopancreatography with sphincterotomy and stone extraction is indicated (see section, "Endoscopic Procedures").

■ DISORDERS IN PREGNANCY NOT ASSOCIATED WITH GASTROINTESTINAL DYSMOTILITY

DYSPEPSIA & PEPTIC ULCER DISEASE
Pathophysiology

Peptic ulcer disease is at least as common in pregnant women as it is in the general population. Similar to nonpregnant adults, the two major risk factors for peptic ulcer disease are the use of nonsteroidal antiinflammatory agents and infection with *Helicobacter pylori* (see Chapter 20).

There are conflicting data about acid secretion during pregnancy. Histaminase, an enzyme secreted by the placenta that inactivates histamine, may reduce acid production. In theory, a reduction in acid secretion may lessen the symptoms and severity of peptic ulcer disease during pregnancy. Some studies suggest that up to 90% of patients with a history of peptic ulcer disease are asymptomatic during pregnancy.

Clinical Findings

The symptoms of peptic ulcer disease are the same in pregnant and nonpregnant patients. Patients most commonly complain of dyspepsia, ie, intermittent epigastric pain or discomfort that may be relieved by eating meals or taking antacids. There may be associated complaints of heartburn, early satiety, nausea, and vomiting. The differential diagnosis of dyspepsia in pregnancy includes gastroesophageal reflux, nonulcer dyspepsia, biliary tract disease, and, in the first trimester, hyperemesis gravidarum. One-half to two-thirds of patients with dyspepsia have nonulcer dyspepsia or GERD—not peptic ulcer disease (see Chapter 21).

In uncomplicated peptic ulcer disease, the physical examination is unremarkable. Significant tenderness, a positive fecal occult blood test, or signs of ulcer complications warrant an in depth evaluation. There are no data to suggest that complications of peptic ulcer disease (bleeding, perforation, or obstruction) occur with increased frequency in pregnant women.

Diagnostic studies are reserved for patients with significant symptoms who fail to respond to conservative measures and initial medications (as below), or those with evidence of complications of peptic ulcer disease (bleeding, obstruction, penetration, or perforation). Upper endoscopy appears to be safe for both mother and fetus and is warranted when the findings of such a study may significantly alter therapy or in life-threatening situations (see section, "Endoscopic Procedures"). Upper gastrointestinal series should not be performed due to the risk of radiation to the fetus. Noninvasive testing for infection with *Helicobacter pylori* may be obtained using serologic tests, the nonradioactive [^{13}C]urea breath test, or fecal antigen testing. The radioactive [^{14}C]urea breath test is contraindicated in pregnancy.

Treatment

A stepwise approach to dyspepsia is recommended, similar to the approach mentioned in the treatment of

gastrointestinal reflux. First-line therapy is with conservative measures that include discontinuation of nonsteroidal antiinflammatory agents and eating small frequent meals. If dyspepsia continues, empiric medication therapy is begun without diagnostic studies. As mentioned earlier, antacids and sucrulfate are considered safe due to the lack of systemic absorption. H$_2$RAs, in particular cimetidine and ranitidine, may be used in patients with persistent dyspepsia.

There are minimal data on the safety of proton pump inhibitors in pregnancy. Omeprazole has demonstrated some fetal toxicity in animal studies (see Table 11–1). Therefore proton pump inhibitors should be initiated only after endoscopic evaluations have been performed that demonstrate significant pathology, such as a complicated ulcer. Misoprostol is an abortifacient and is therefore contraindicated. In pregnant patients with ulcers attributed to *H pylori*, antibiotic treatment should be deferred until after delivery, because many of the antibiotics used for treatment are considered toxic to the fetus.

ACUTE PANCREATITIS

Pathophysiology

The overall incidence of pancreatitis is not increased during pregnancy. When it occurs, pancreatitis is more common during the third trimester. The causes of acute pancreatitis during pregnancy are similar to those in the general population, however alcohol-induced pancreatitis is uncommon. Gallstones are the most common cause of pancreatitis during pregnancy. Drug-induced pancreatitis must be excluded. Diuretics, in particular thiazide diuretics, are commonly used during pregnancy and are known to cause pancreatitis. Hypertriglyceridemia-induced pancreatitis occurs, especially during the third trimester of pregnancy, because of a three-fold rise in serum triglyceride levels. This is thought to be due to estrogen-induced increases in triglyceride synthesis and very low-density lipoprotein secretion.

In a substantial number of pregnant patients with pancreatitis, the cause is undetermined—suggesting that pregnancy may alter pancreatic physiology. Limited data suggest that pregnancy may lead to increased enzyme and bicarbonate secretion and volume output, but the importance of this is unknown.

Clinical Findings

The symptoms of acute pancreatitis are similar to those in nonpregnant women. They include mid-epigastric or periumbilical pain that may radiate to the back, as well as nausea, vomiting, fever, and ileus. Because of the nonspecific nature of these symptoms, the diagnosis can be overlooked and the symptoms erroneously attributed to other diseases or pregnancy (see Table 11–5). Complications of pancreatitis result in a maternal mortality rate of 3.4% and fetal loss rate of 10–20%. Because acute pancreatitis is associated with a high risk to mother and fetus, it must be considered in every pregnant woman with abdominal pain.

The diagnosis of acute pancreatitis relies on the measurement of serum amylase and lipase levels. Serum amylase values tend to be lower during pregnancy due to increased renal amylase clearance, which may obscure the diagnosis. A rapid rise and fall in serum aspartate aminotransferase (AST) and alanine aminotransferase (ALT) levels and/or a rise in serum bilirubin level suggest gallstone-induced pancreatitis. A serum triglyceride level of more than 1000 mg/dL suggests hypertriglyceridemia as the causative factor.

Ultrasonography is a safe study in the pregnant patient with suspected pancreatitis. Unfortunately, the fetus or intestinal gas, or both, may obscure much of the pancreas. Features that are suspicious for pancreatitis are pancreatic edema and peripancreatic fluid collections. In addition, ultrasound provides useful information about the presence of cholelithiasis or biliary sludge. The presence of dilated intrahepatic or extrahepatic ducts suggests biliary obstruction, which is commonly due to choledocholithiasis. If possible, abdominal radiography or computed tomography (CT) imaging should be avoided due to the risks from radiation to the fetus. Magnetic resonance imaging (MRI) is without risk and may be useful to assess severe or complicated pancreatitis. Magnetic resonance cholangiopancreatography (MRCP) is a useful noninvasive method to look for retained common duct stones (choledocholithiasis).

Treatment

Treatment of pancreatitis in pregnant patients is the same as in nonpregnant patients. The mainstay of therapy is supportive, usually including hospitalization, intravenous fluids, analgesia, bowel rest, and nasogastric suction for significant nausea and vomiting.

Patients with gallstone-induced pancreatitis usually require elective cholecystectomy to reduce the risk of recurrent pancreatitis and its complications. Although laparoscopic cholecystectomy appears to be safe, surgery commonly is deferred until after delivery (see section, "Cholelithiasis & Its Complications"). ERCP with sphincterotomy and stone extraction may be necessary in patients with gallstone pancreatitis that is severe, worsening, or complicated by cholangitis. This procedure should be performed only by expert biliary endoscopists with the assistance of an anesthesiologist.

For patients with pancreatitis caused by hypertriglyceridemia, elimination of caloric intake during supportive therapy results in a fall in triglycerides and overall clinical improvement. Upon reinstitution of oral intake, nutritional needs can be met with dietary restrictions that generally maintain the triglyceride level less than 1000 mg/dL. If dietary measures alone are unsuccessful, total parenteral nutrition may be required. After delivery triglyceride levels usually fall. Thus, in patients who are near term, optimal management may be to induce labor early rather than initiate total parenteral nutrition. Such management should be determined on a case by case basis.

INFLAMMATORY BOWEL DISEASE (IBD)

Pathophysiology

The pathophysiology of IBD, which includes both Crohn's disease and ulcerative colitis (UC), is unknown in both pregnant and nonpregnant patients.

There are several interactions of this disease with pregnancy that warrant discussion: (1) the effect of the disease on fertility, (2) the effect of the disease on the course and outcome of pregnancy, and (3) the effect of pregnancy on the disease.

A. EFFECT OF IBD ON FERTILITY

Fertility appears to be normal in women with UC and in the majority of women with Crohn's disease. However, in some patients with Crohn's disease, pelvic inflammation, scarring of fallopian tubes or ovaries, poor nutrition, or dyspareunia may affect conception and reduce fertility. Some patients with IBD make a voluntary decision not to proceed with pregnancy.

There is no decrease in fertility in males due to IBD, except for drug-induced azospermia in men taking sulfasalazine. Sperm count normalizes within 2 months of discontinuing the medication.

B. EFFECTS OF INFLAMMATORY BOWEL DISEASE ON THE COURSE AND OUTCOME OF PREGNANCY

The activity of the disease is correlated with outcome of pregnancy. For patients with inactive UC or Crohn's disease, there is no increased risk of prematurity, spontaneous abortion, stillbirth, congenital anomalies, or maternal complications. For both UC and Crohn's disease, birth weights have been reported to be marginally lower.

In contrast, active Crohn's disease and, to a lesser extent, active UC cause a higher incidence of stillbirth. For this reason, every effort should be made to induce remission of IBD before undertaking pregnancy.

It remains unclear whether patients with UC who have undergone a previous ileoanal J-pouch can safely deliver vaginally. A cesarean section can be performed safely in these patients. A cesarean section should also be performed in patients with Crohn's disease who have active perineal disease.

C. EFFECTS OF PREGNANCY ON INFLAMMATORY BOWEL DISEASE

The effects of pregnancy on the course of IBD depend on the activity of the disease at the time of conception. In both UC and Crohn's disease, if the disease is quiescent at the beginning of pregnancy, it is likely to remain so throughout pregnancy (only one-third relapse, see Figure 11–3). However, if the disease is active at the time of conception, it is likely to remain so or even worsen during pregnancy (one-third remain active, one-third worsen, and one-third improve, see Figure 11–3).

Clinical Findings

The clinical features of IBD during pregnancy are similar to those in the nonpregnant patient. Signs and symptoms such as bleeding, pain, and diarrhea may occur. In patients known to have the disease before pregnancy, relapse of IBD is usually considered as part of the differential diagnosis for these symptoms. However, in patients without a prior history of IBD, the diagnosis may be obscured and the symptoms attributed to the effects of pregnancy.

Management is made difficult by limitations on the use of endoscopic or radiologic tests during pregnancy. In patients with known or suspected UC, flexible sigmoidoscopy can be safely performed during pregnancy to confirm disease activity before initiating therapy. In patients with known Crohn's disease, colonoscopy and barium radiography should be avoided, unless absolutely essential for management (see section, "En-

doscopic Procedures"). However, in patients with severe illness and no known history of IBD, these procedures sometimes are necessary to establish a definitive diagnosis. Complications of IBD are the same in pregnant and nonpregnant patients and are discussed in Chapter 7.

Treatment

Management of IBD during pregnancy is best approached by a team of physicians, including a gastroenterologist, a high-risk obstetrician, and a colorectal surgeon. Remission should be achieved before pregnancy and should be maintained during pregnancy. The consequences of a relapse are significant, and are thought to outweigh the risks of using medications to maintain a remission. Thus, the minimalist drug approach used in the majority of disorders of pregnancy is not advocated in IBD.

A number of drugs used for this disease have been given safely during pregnancy (see Table 11–1). Sulfasalazine readily crosses the placenta and is secreted in breastmilk. However, it has been used for many years without consequence, and is thus considered safe. Although it may displace bilirubin from fetal albumin during the third trimester, the risk of fetal kernicterus is considered negligible. Pregnant patients taking sulfasalazine should receive folate to prevent folate deficiency (1 mg twice a day). Mesalamine is also considered safe in pregnancy. There is only minimal excretion of aminosalicylic acid (5-ASA) and metabolites in breastmilk and breastfeeding is not contraindicated. Corticosteroids appear to be safe, but every effort should be made to maintain patients on the lowest dose possible. The risk of adrenal insufficiency in the fetus appears to be theoretical. With respect to antibiotics, ciprofloxacin is likely to be safe, but should be initiated after the first trimester and should not

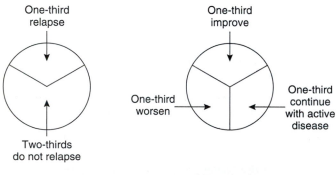

Figure 11–3. Effect of pregnancy on IBD.

be used in women who breastfeed. Metronidazole is best avoided throughout pregnancy. The use of immunosuppressant agents during pregnancy has been controversial. Azathioprine and mercaptopurine have been associated with some birth defects, although recent series report a low incidence. Recent data also suggest that the incidence of pregnancy-related complications was increased if the father was taking 6-mercaptopurine or azathioprine at the time of conception. Because these agents are often necessary to maintain remission, their use during pregnancy has grown in recent years with good outcomes. Thus, in clinical situations in which these drugs are considered necessary to maintain quiescence of disease activity, patients are being advised to conceive while on these medications and remain on these drugs during pregnancy. Methotrexate, on the other hand is contraindicated in both pregnancy and breastfeeding. There are very limited data on the use of cyclosporine and infliximab in this setting and these drugs are generally avoided.

Although surgery is associated with a significant risk of spontaneous abortion, it should be employed in cases of severe bleeding, perforation, and toxic megacolon unresponsive to medical therapy.

■ ENDOSCOPIC PROCEDURES

There is great reluctance to perform endoscopic procedures during pregnancy stemming from a scarcity of data documenting their safety and efficacy. Anecdotal reports and case–control studies suggest that endoscopy is generally safe. The approach used to decide whether a procedure should be performed is similar to the approach used to decide if a medication should be initiated during pregnancy: the risks and consequences to the mother of not doing the procedure must be weighed against the risks of the procedure to the fetus.

INTRAVENOUS SEDATION

A minimalist approach to the use of medications in pregnancy is generally applied and advocated for intravenous sedation. When it is feasible to perform endoscopic procedures without sedation, this approach should be taken first. In general, the pregnant patient is more willing and motivated to undergo an unsedated procedure. If sedation is required, meperidine is thought to be safe (see Table 11–1). Midazolam should be avoided since there is a suggested increase in the risk of congenital malformations with the use of other ben-

zodiazepines, including diazepam. Of note, no adverse events with midazolam itself have been reported.

UPPER ENDOSCOPY

Patients with symptoms suggestive of uncomplicated gastrointestinal reflux, peptic ulcer disease, or nausea and vomiting should be given an empiric course of treatment with conservative measures and medications before considering any endoscopic procedures. Endoscopy may be performed as needed for patients with severe symptoms that are unresponsive to empiric treatment or complicated disease. Case–control studies have shown no increase in endoscopic complications, premature labor, or congenital malformations with upper endoscopy (see Table 11–6). Endoscopic hemostasis reduces the risk of hypotension, hypoxia, and catecholamine release and is safer than performing surgery. Patients with known portal hypertension should have varices eradicated prior to pregnancy whenever possible. The 40–50% increase in plasma volume that occurs with pregnancy results in an increase in portal pressure and variceal size, which results in increased risk of hemorrhage. Sclerotherapy and banding have been performed without complications during pregnancy. The safety of propranolol and octreotide are unknown. Vasopressin should be avoided.

FLEXIBLE SIGMOIDOSCOPY & COLONOSCOPY

Gastrointestinal bleeding and diarrhea are the main indications for endoscopic evaluation of the lower gastrointestinal tract (see Table 11–6). Case–control studies have not shown an increase in endoscopic complications, premature labor, or congenital malformations when these procedures are performed. However, there is a theoretical concern that colonoscopy could cause spontaneous abortion. Given the younger age of most pregnant women, colonoscopy seldom provides more information than a flexible sigmoidoscopy. Fur-

Table 11–6. Indications for endoscopic procedures.

Gastrointestinal bleeding
Dysphagia
Odonyphagia
Weight loss
Iron deficiency anemia
Persistent nausea and vomiting
Diarrhea

thermore, flexible sigmoidoscopy requires no sedation. For these reasons flexible sigmoidoscopy is the prefererrd procedure for initial evaluation of the lower gastrointestinal (GI) tract in most instances. Colonoscopy should be restricted to patients in whom pathology of the right side of the colon is suspected.

ENDOSOCOPIC RETROGRADE CHOLANGIOPANCREATOGRAPHY (ERCP)

The most common indication for ERCP during pregnancy is for the evaluation and treatment of patients with suspected biliary tract disease, especially choledocholithiasis. When possible, it should be postponed until the postpartum period to avoid radiation exposure. However, it has been performed with increasing frequency during the past few years with few complications. Appropriate use of lead shielding of mother and fetus and minimization of fluoroscopy time are important measures that aid in the safe performance of this procedure.

In the nonpregnant patient, the acceptable radiation exposure levels for occupational and patient exposures is 5000 mrem to the whole body, 15,000 mrem to the eye, and 50,000 mrem to any single organ. The exposure limit for the fetus is 500 mrem, but most recommend limiting exposure to <100 mrem during the first trimester. Reports have estimated average fetal exposures with ERCP to be 59 mrem, well below these recommendations. These low levels are achieved in the hands of expert biliary endoscopists by limiting fluoroscopy to brief views, and avoiding hard copy x-rays. Cannulation of the common bile duct confirmed by aspiration of bile alone and stent placement without stone retrieval are techniques that further reduce the need for fluoroscopy. This often translates to less than 60 seconds of exposure. Sphincterotomy has been performed to prevent relapsing symptoms in an effort to postpone surgery until after delivery. It should be noted that randomized trials are needed to clarify whether this approach is truly safer than laparoscopic cholecystectomy.

PERCUTANEOUS ENDOSCOPIC GASTROSTOMY (PEG) TUBE PLACEMENT

This procedure is seldom performed in pregnant patients, because there rarely is a need and it is difficult to perform safely in the presence of the gravid uterus. However, when certain precautions are taken, the procedure is possible. The placement of this tube should be entertained only when the risk of parenteral nutrition is not acceptable and a nasogastric tube is not tolerated in the setting of persistent nausea and vomiting. In such cases, ultrasound marking of the dome of the uterus should be undertaken and transillumination should be unequivocal, since displacement of the colon and small bowel is common during pregnancy. In addition, care must be taken to anticipate the future growth of the uterus in an effort to prevent pressure necrosis as the abdomen enlarges.

■ SURGICAL DISORDERS

APPENDICITIS

The pathophysiology of appendicitis and other surgical disorders in pregnancy is the same as in nonpregnant patients.

Clinical Findings

Appendicitis is the most common surgical emergency in the pregnant woman, occuring more often in the second trimester. It may be confused with obstetric emergencies, including placental abruption, ectopic pregnancy, and ovarian torsion, as well as nonobstetric conditions such as acute cholecystitis, intestinal volvulus, and acute pancreatitis.

The disease tends to be more severe because there is increased vascularity in the intraabdominal tissues and a decreased ability of the omentum to wall off inflammation (it is displaced by the uterus). Furthermore, diagnosis often is delayed because the symptoms and physical findings of appendicitis are altered by pregnancy. The gravid uterus may shift the pain from the lower right to the upper right quadrant, confusing the diagnostic picture. Figure 11–4 shows the changes in location and direction of the appendix during pregnancy that account for the changes in the location of pain. Other clinical features including nausea, vomiting, fever, and leukocytosis are similar to those seen in the nonpregnant state.

Treatment

An ultrasound is often helpful in making the diagnosis. Appendectomy is the mainstay of treatment. Recently, laparoscopic appendectomy has been performed during pregnancy, resulting in less trauma than conventional surgery. Care must be taken to keep retractors away from the uterus, since they can trigger uterine contractions if placed against, or in close proximity to, the uterus.

Appendicitis results in 5% maternal and 15% fetal mortality. The diagnosis may be delayed in up to 35% of patients until perforation has occurred, resulting in even higher maternal and fetal mortality rates (19% and 43%, respectively).

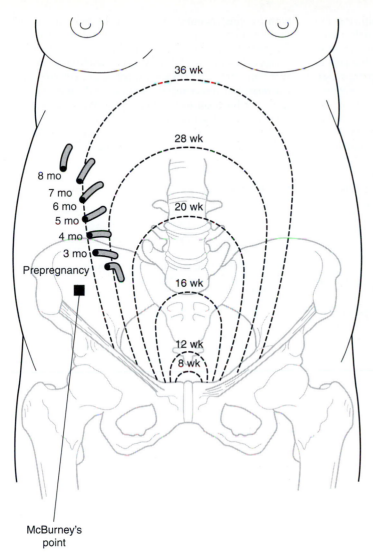

8 mo
7 mo
6 mo
5 mo
4 mo
3 mo
Prepregnancy

36 wk
28 wk
20 wk
16 wk
12 wk
8 wk

McBurney's
point

Figure 11–4. Changes in location and direction of the appendix during pregnancy in relationship to McBurney's point and the height of the fundus at various weeks of gestation. (Adapted, with permission, from Mahmoodian S: Appendicitis complicating pregnancy. South Med J 1992;85:19.)

VOLVULUS

Pathophysiology

Sigmoid volvulus may occur during the third trimester or the puerperium due to impact of the enlarged uterus on the sigmoid colon.

Clinical Findings

Patients report symptoms of abdominal pain, nausea, vomiting, and constipation, but these symptoms are nonspecific. Although the diagnosis is readily established by abdominal radiographic studies that demonstrate a torsed, dilated sigmoid colon and signs of a large bowel obstruction, the general reluctance to perform radiographic studies during pregnancy may delay diagnosis.

Treatment

Conservative treatment with sigmoidoscopic decompression should be attempted. Surgical intervention should be undertaken when endoscopic therapy is unsuccessful.

FECAL INCONTINENCE

Pathophysiology

It is now recognized that fecal incontinence may be a common complication of vaginal delivery. A third- or fourth-degree tear may complicate 0.7% of deliveries.

Significant damage to the external anal sphincter can result in gross fecal incontinence, unless the defect is repaired immediately. An even more common cause of fecal incontinence is damage during labor to the pudendal nerve as it passes through the sacrospinous ligament. This neurogenic trauma may lead to denervation of the pelvic floor muscles and external sphincter, resulting in fecal incontinence that may become apparent only years after delivery. The incidence of fecal incontinence due to pregnancy has been vastly underestimated, and many cases of "idiopathic" neurogenic fecal incontinence in elderly women are attributable to obstetric trauma. Recognition of fecal incontinence by primary care physicians, obstetricians, and gastroenterologists is important because it can be treated.

Clinical Findings

In patients with prior tears or episiotomies, physical examination may reveal evidence of external sphincter damage scarring, deformity, or a patulous appearance. Perineal sensation should be tested for sharp and dull sensation and the anal wink sign elicited. Absence of the anal wink may indicate the presence of pudendal neuropathy or a cauda equina lesion. Digital examination may reveal anatomic defects in the anomuscular ring. Strictures, scars, and gross resting and squeezing pressures can be assessed. Anal ultrasound, manometry, and electromyography detect defects in the external and internal sphincters, determining the presence or absence of nervous innervation, and localize the neurologic deficit.

Treatment

A bowel management program is the first element of therapy in most patients. A high-fiber diet is prescribed,

Table 11–7. Sample plan for doing Kegel exercises.[1]

Week	Repetitions
1	Three repetitions, 10 times a day
2	Three repetitions, 15 times a day
3	Three repetitions, 20 times a day, or six repetitions, 10 times a day
4	Three repetitions, 25 times a day, or six repetitions, 12 times a day
5	Three repetitions, 30 times a day, or six repetitions, 15 times a day
6	Three repetitions, 34 times a day, or six repetitions, 17 times a day

[1]Reproduced, with permission, from West L et al: Diagnosis and management of irritable bowel syndrome, constipation, and diarrhea in pregnancy. Gastroenterol Clin North Am 1992;21:802.

with patients encouraged to sit on the toilet for 20–30 minutes after eating, at the same time each day. Successful treatment is achieved in many mild cases with Kegel exercises (Table 11–7). Motivated patients with more severe symptoms who have some degree of neurologic impairment but intact rectal sensation and some external sphincter function may benefit from biofeedback therapy and pelvic floor retraining. Discrete muscular injury to the external sphincter with intact innervation may be amenable to surgical repair (see Chapter 28).

REFERENCES

Abell TL, Riely CA: Hyperemesis gravidarum. Gastroenterol Clin North Am 1992;21:835.

Amos JD et al: Laparoscopic surgery during pregnancy. Am J Surg 1996;171:435.

Axelrod AM et al: Performance of ERCP for symptomatic choledocholithiasis during pregnancy: techniques to increase safety and improve patient management. Am J Gastroenterol 1994; 89:109.

Borum ML: Hepatobiliary disease in women. Med Clin North Am 1998;82:51.

Brent RL: The effects of embryonic and fetal exposure to X-ray, microwaves and ultrasound. Clin Perinatol 1998;25:287.

Calhoun BC: Gastrointestinal disorders in pregnancy. Obstet Gynecol Clin North Am 1992;19:733.

Cappell MS: The safety and efficacy of gastrointestinal endoscopy during pregnancy. Gastroenterol Clin North Am 1998;27:37.

Chiloiro M et al: Gastric emptying and orocecal transit time in pregnancy. J Gastroenterol 2001;36:538.

Cosenza C et al: Surgical management of biliary gallstone disease during pregnancy. Am J Surg 1999;178:545.

DeLancey JOL: Childbirth, continence, and the pelvic floor. (Article review.) N Engl J Med 1993;329:1956.

Diav-Citrin O et al: The safety and efficacy of mesalamine in human pregnancy: a prospective controlled cohort study. Gastroenterology 1998;114:23.

Eliakim R, Abulafia O, Sherer D: Hyperemesis gravidarum: a current review. Am J Perinatol 2000;17:207.

Ghumman E et al: Management of gallstones in pregnancy. (Review) Br J Surg 1997;84:1646.

Gilat T, Konikoff F: Pregnancy and the biliary tract. Can J Gastroenterol 2000;14(Suppl D):55D.

Gouldman JW et al: Laparoscopic cholecystectomy in pregnancy. Am Surg 1998;64:93.

Hordnes K, Bergsjo P: Severe lacerations after childbirth. Acta Obstet Scand 1993;72:413.

Jamidar PA et al: Endoscopic retrograde cholangiopancreatography in pregnancy. Am J Gastroenterol 1995;90:1263.

Jewell DJ, Young G: Interventions for treating constipation in pregnancy. Cochrane Database Syst Rev 2001;2:CD001142.

Katz JA, Pore G: Inflammatory bowel disease and pregnancy. Inflamm Bowel Dis 2001;7:146.

Mabie WC: Obstetric management of gastroenterologic complications of pregnancy. Gastroenterol Clin North Am 1992;21: 923.

Meuwissen S et al: IOIBD questionnaire on the clinical use of aza-thioprine, 6-mercaptopurine, cyclosporin A, and methotrex-ate in the treatment of inflammatory bowel disease. Eur J Gastroenterol Hepatol 2000;12:13.

Moum B: Chronic inflammatory bowel disease and pregnancy. Scand J Gastroenterol 2000;35:673.

Nesbitt TH et al: Endoscopic management of biliary disease during pregnancy. Obstet Gynecol 1996;87:806.

Rajapakse RO et al: Outcome of pregnancies when fathers are treated with 6-mercaptopurine for inflammatory bowel dis-ease. Am J Gastroenterol 2000;95:684.

Ramin KD, Ramsey PS: Disease of the gallbladder and pancreas in pregnancy. Obstet Gynecol Clin North Am 2001;28:571.

Singer AJ, Brandt LJ: Pathophysiology of the gastrointestinal tract during pregnancy. Am J Gastroenterol 1991;86:1695.

Smoleniec JS, James DK: Gastrointestinal crises during pregnancy. Dig Dis Sci 1993;11:313.

Sultan AH et al: Anal-sphincter disruption during vaginal delivery. N Engl J Med 1993;329:1905.

Sungler P et al: Laparoscopic cholecystectomy and interventional endoscopy for gallstone complications. Surg Endosc 2000;14:267.

Swisher SG et al: Management of pancreatitis complicating preg-nancy. Am Surg 1994;60:759.

Vutyavanich T, Kraisarin T, Ruangsri R: Ginger for nausea and vo-miting in pregnancy: randomized, double-masked, placebo-controlled trial. Obstet Gynecol 2001;97:577.

Winbery SL, Blaho KE: Dyspepsia in pregnancy. Obstet Gynecol Clin North Am 2001;28:333.

Nutritional Disorders & Their Treatment in Diseases of the Gastrointestinal Tract

12

James S. Scolapio, MD

Gastrointestinal dysfunction can impair normal absorption and digestion of the food we consume. Such impairment can result in significant weight loss and malnutrition. Malnutrition may result from decreased intake, decreased absorption, or increased utilization. Examples of gastrointestinal dysfunction that can result in malnutrition include loss of intestinal absorptive surface area as occurs in large resections of the small intestine and stomach. Inflammation of the intestine from Crohn's disease and radiation therapy can both result in significant diarrhea and weight loss. Reduced digestive capability may also occur in patients with pancreatitis. Therefore, knowledge of gastrointestinal function and disease is important in the nutritional management of patients. Before intervening with nutritional support it is important to perform a careful nutritional assessment of the patient. The scope of nutritional support then focuses on three main points, which include *when, what,* and *how* to feed. This chapter will focus on the nutritional management of specific gastrointestinal illnesses.

NUTRITIONAL ASSESSMENT

When to Feed

Nutritional assessment is used to determine the nutritional reserve of the patient and help the clinician decide when to intervene with nutritional support. There is no gold standard for determining the nutritional status because there is no universally accepted marker of malnutrition. Albumin and prealbumin alone are not good markers of malnutrition since fluid redistribution and infection may reduce serum levels in the absence of malnutrition.

The clinical assessment of a patient's nutritional status involves a focused history and physical examination along with selected laboratory tests directed at detecting specific nutrient deficiencies. The history should include questions related to the amount of weight loss and food intake over the past 6 months and over the

most recent 2 weeks. Unintentional weight loss of greater than 10% within the previous 6 months is of concern and should be investigated. Usually, a careful history will aid the clinician in making a diagnosis and offering treatment. Following a focused history, the physical examination should begin by recording an accurate weight of the patient and comparing this weight with previously recorded weights.

The physical examination should also include a careful evaluation of the abdomen to determine bowel function. Physical signs of temporal muscle wasting and loss of subcutaneous fat are both signs of significant weight loss. The subjective global assessment (SGA) is a clinical method that encompasses the history and physical examination that are referred to above. The findings from the history and physical examination are subjectively scored as an A, B, or C, which rank patients as being well nourished (A), moderately malnourished (B), or severely malnourished (C) (Table 12–1). The use of SGA in evaluating hospitalized patients has been shown to give reproducible results with more than 80% agreement between two blinded observers assessing the same patient. Likewise, SGA was reported to be a better predictor of nutrition-related complications than traditional markers including creatinine-height index, delayed cutaneous hypersensitivity, and serum albumin.

Careful nutrition and disease assessment guides the clinician in determining *when* to intervene with nutritional support. If a patient is unable to take sufficient calories orally then administration of either enteral tube feeds or parenteral infusion is required. Patients should be fed by one of these methods within 7–10 days of being without oral intake. Within 7–10 days negative nitrogen balance occurs and the risk of infection and other morbidity substantially increases. Likewise, if a patient scores a C (severely malnourished) on the SGA, nutritional support should begin before Day 7 and usually within 48–72 hours of hospitalization. Likewise, a careful nutritional assessment should prevent starting nutritional support too early—the patient has not lost significant weight and has been without food for less

Table 12–1. Subjective global assessment score of nutritional status.

A. History

1. Weight change
   Overall loss in past 6 months: amount = # _____ kg
   Change in past 2 weeks: _____ increase
                                _____ no change
                                _____ decrease

2. Dietary intake change (relative to normal)
   _____ no change
   _____ Change: duration = # _____ weeks
                   type   _____ suboptimal solid diet _____ full liquid diet
                             _____ hypocaloric liquids   _____ starvation

3. Gastrointestinal symptoms that persisted > 2 weeks
   _____ None _____ Anorexia _____ Nausea _____ Vomiting _____ Diarrhea

4. Functional capacity
   _____ No dysfunction (eg, full capacity)
   _____ Dysfunction: duration = # _____ weeks
                                        _____ working suboptimally
                                        _____ ambulatory
                                        _____ bedridden

5. Disease and its relation to nutritional requirements
   Primary diagnosis (specify) _____
   Metabolic demand (stress) _____ None _____ Low _____ Moderate _____ High

B. Physical (for each trait specify 0 = normal, 1 + = mild, 2 + = moderate, 3 + = severe)
   # _____ Loss of subcutaneous fat (triceps, chest)
   # _____ Muscle wasting (quadriceps, deltoids, temporals)
   # _____ Ankle edema, sacral edema
   # _____ Ascites
   # _____ Tongue or skin lesions suggesting nutrient deficiency

C. SGA rating (select one)
   _____ A = Well nourished (minimal or no restriction of food intake or absorption, minimal change in function, weight
               stable or increasing)
   _____ B = Moderately malnourished (food restriction, some functional changes, little or no change in body masss)
   _____ C = Severely malnourished (definitely decreased intake, function, and body mass)

Reproduced, with permission, from Detsky AS et al: What is subjective global assessment of nutritional status? J Parenter Enteral Nutr 1987;11:8.

than 7–10 days. After the patient is assessed, calculation of energy and protein needs, or *what* to feed the patient, should be determined.

Caloric Requirements: What?

The energy and protein goals for most hospitalized patients are between 25 and 35 kcal/kg/d of total calories, which includes between 1.0 and 1.5 g/kg/d of protein. The aim is to achieve nitrogen balance without over-feeding, which can be detrimental by suppression of the immune system, predisposing the patient to infection. For most patients 100–120% of their actual total daily energy expenditure will keep them in nitrogen balance. The Harris-Benedict equation can be used to calculate basal energy needs:

$$\text{Woman (kcal/d)} = 655 + (9.6 \times \text{weight, kg})$$
$$+ (1.7 \times \text{height, cm}) - (4.7 \times \text{age})$$

$$\text{Men (kcal / d)} = 66 + (13.8 \times \text{weight, kg})$$
$$+ (5 \times \text{height, cm}) - (6.8 \times \text{age})$$

An activity factor of 20% is usually added to the basal needs of the patient. If weight gain is desired, an additional 500 kcal/d can be added, which should result in a gain of approximately 1 lb per week. In select cases such as morbid obesity and burn injuries, indirect calorimetry can be used to estimate basal caloric needs. Lipid or fat should supply approximately 30% or 1.0 g/kg/d of the total calories and protein should supply 1.0–1.5 g/kg/d. Carbohydrate should comprise the remaining calories. Most of the enteral formulas contain 1 kcal/mL (Table 12–2). They provide approximately 84% free water and 30–40% of the total calories as fat. Elemental diets contain very little fat and may be used in special circumstances. Disease-specific formulas including immune–enhancing formulas should be used only in very special circumstances.

When designing a parenteral formula it is important to have the help of an experienced pharmacist. Usually, a 1.5–2.0 L solution is given. In patients with congestive heart failure or renal disease total fluid volume may need to be restricted. As with enteral nutrition, lipids should make up approximately 30% of the total calories. Current lipid emulsions are polyunsaturated long-chain triglycerides from soybean or safflower oil. Crystalloid amino acids provide the protein source to total parenteral nutrition (TPN). Intravenous solutions with different amino acid compositions are available for different disease states such as high branch-chain amino acid formulas for hepatic encephalopathy. These formulas are much more expensive and data regarding their benefit are limited. Dextrose or glucose provides the remaining macronutrient once the amount of protein and lipid has been calculated. Hyperglycemia, which suppresses immune function, should be avoided to minimize the risk of infection. The goal in the hospital should be to maintain serum glucose between 110 and 200 mg/dL. Occasionally, insulin may be required to maintain blood glucose levels less than 200 mg/dL. Regular or short- acting insulin (0.05–0.2 units/g of dextrose) can be added to the TPN solution. The TPN infusion rate should be tapered over an hour before discontinuation to prevent hypoglycemia. The TPN solution also contains electrolytes, trace elements (zinc, copper, manganese, chromium, and selenium), and vitamins. Iron is not routinely included in the TPN because of the potential risk of anaphylaxis. Serum electrolytes should be checked at least twice weekly while a patient is receiving TPN in the hospital and adjusted accordingly with the help of a pharmacist. After the decision has been made to initiate nutrition support (*when*) and the goals for energy and protein have been calculated (*what*), the next step is the selection of access for feeding, or *how*.

Table 12–2. Enteral products.

Product[1]	kcal/mL	mL/can	Protein/L (g)	Osmolality (mOsm/kg water)	Fiber	Fat (%) (MCT + LCT; of Total Calories)[2]	MCT[2] (%) (from Total Fat)	Lactose
Osmolite (1)	1.06	237	37.1	300	No	29	20	No
Osmolite HN (1)	1.06	237	44.3	300	No	29	19	No
Osmolite HN Plus (1)	1.2	237	55.5	360	No	33	25	No
Nutren 1.0 (2)	1.4	240	40	300	No	33	25	No
Isosource HN (3)	1.2	250	53	330	No	30	50	No
Isocal (4)	1.06	240	34	270	No	37	20	No
Promote (1)	1.0	237	62.5	340	No	23	19	No
Jevity (1)	1.06	237	44.3	300	Yes	29	20	No
Peptamen (2)[3]	1.0	240	40	270	No	33	70	No
Vivonex TEN (3)[4]	1.0	Powder 300 mL mix/H$_2$O	38	630	No	3	0	No

[1]Product manufacturer: (1) Ross Laboratories Division/Abbott Laboratories; (2) Nestle Clinical Nutrition; (3) Novartis Nutrition; (4) Mead Johnson.
[2]MCT, medium-chain triglycerides; LCT, long-chain triglycerides.
[3]Semielemental.
[4]Elemental.

Nutrition Access: How?

Before starting nutritional support with either tube feeding or intravenous feeding, it is important to perform accurate calorie counts. Patients may be eating more than you think, and often with oral dietary supplements caloric goals can be met without a feeding tube or TPN. A trained dietician can be very helpful in this regard. If a patient cannot take sufficient nutrients orally, then the enteral route using a feeding tube should be considered. If a patient has gastrointestinal obstruction, feedings should first be attempted distal to the obstruction. Compared with TPN, enteral nutrition is less expensive, has been reported to have fewer infectious complications, and requires less laboratory monitoring. Nasogastric feeding is usually the most appropriate route. Delayed gastric emptying and regurgitation of gastric contents are indications for nasojejunal feeding.

With gastric feeding, gravity or continuous tube feeding can be used, whereas continuous infusion should be used for small bowel delivery. Gravity feeding into the small intestine can result in significant bloating and diarrhea. For most adults a soft 10 French nasogastric or nasojejunal tube is comfortable and clogging of the tube less of a problem than with smaller tubes. For most hospitalized patients, continuous infusion of the formula using a pump is recommended, because this method is generally better tolerated than gravity feeding. Feeding should be initiated with full strength product at 20–25 mL/h. Diluting formulas is not necessary. The rate may be increased every 12 hours in increments of 20–25 mL until the goal rate is reached.

Cyclic nighttime feeding permits some patients to eat more during the day. Gastric residuals should be checked in gastric-fed patients. A residual volume greater than 200 mL indicates delayed gastric emptying and increases the risk of aspiration. The infusion rate should be reduced or the tube advanced to the small intestine if there is a recurrent problem. Small bowel feedings do not require checking residuals. A gastrostomy or percutaneous endoscopic gastrostomy (PEG) tube is usually appropriate if feeding is anticipated to be more than 4 weeks. Nasal tubes for more than 4 weeks are uncomfortable for most patients and can cause significant nasal irritation. If a patient is having intraabdominal surgery, a gastric or jejunal feeding tube should be placed at surgery if adequate oral intake is expected to be delayed postoperatively. It is important to communicate with the surgeon prior to surgery regarding placement of a feeding tube.

In patients in whom enteral feeding is not possible, usually as a result of a mechanical bowel obstruction or an ileus, then TPN should be used. Parenteral nutrition can be given either through a peripheral vein (PPN) or through a central vein (CPN). Administration of nutrients into a peripheral vein is limited by the low rate of blood flow. The risk of phlebitis increases as the dextrose concentration increases above 5%. In some patients caloric needs of 25–35 kcal/kg/d can be met with PPN, avoiding the need of placing a central catheter. When a catheter is placed in a large central vein, the problem of phlebitis from a hypertonic solution is prevented. Direct subclavian placement of a central catheter has traditionally been the method of placement. However peripheral inserted central catheters (PICC) are now available and avoid the risk of a pneumothorax associated with the subclavian method and therefore should be used for purposes of nutritional support when possible. The following sections will focus on the management of specific diseases of the gastrointestinal tract.

ACUTE & CHRONIC PANCREATITIS

Severe acute pancreatitis is a hypermetabolic state characterized by increased energy expenditure, proteolysis, gluconeogenesis, and insulin resistance. Autodigestion by activation of pancreatic enzymes is the primary theory of the pathogenesis of acute pancreatitis. On the basis of this theory, nutritional management first focuses on avoiding pancreatic stimulation by withholding oral nutrients. Different compositions of diets are associated with different amounts of pancreatic secretion. Intraluminal fat is associated with more pancreatic amylase and lipase secretion compared with protein and carbohydrate. Intravenous fat, however, does not stimulate pancreatic secretion and therefore is safe to give in TPN. Serum triglyceride level should be monitored and kept below 500 mg/dL. Caution should be used in patients receiving the intravenous sedative propofol (Diprivan), which contains lipid (10% lipid emulsion). The amount of lipid in TPN should be reduced accordingly. Jejunal delivery (distal to the ligament of Treitz) of nutrients is also associated with less pancreatic stimulation than gastric or duodenal feeding. Defined elemental formulas also appear to cause less pancreatic stimulation than standard enteral formulas. There are limited data to suggest the benefit of antioxidants in acute pancreatitis.

Of patients presenting with acute pancreatitis, 80% have mild inflammation and usually have a self-limited hospital course returning to an oral diet within 7 days. Likewise, most patients admitted to the hospital with acute pancreatitis are not malnourished, that is, an SGA score of A. Therefore, because most are eating within this 7- to 10-day period, nutritional support with either tube feeding or TPN is not indicated. However, if a patient is thought to be malnourished, perhaps from coexisting alcohol-related liver disease, then nutritional support should be initiated before Day 7.

Despite improvement in specific nutritional parameters, studies have failed to show a direct effect of nutrition on morbidity or mortality of patients with mild pancreatitis. On the other hand, approximately 20% of patients admitted with pancreatitis have severe disease as determined by a variety of methods. In patients with severe pancreatitis, data would suggest the benefit of starting nutritional support within 48–72 hours of hospital admission. Patients with severe pancreatitis are unlikely to eat within 7–10 days. The optimal route, enteral versus parenteral, is not totally certain. More recent literature would indicate that the enteral route is more beneficial than TPN. A prospective, randomized study of 32 patients with severe pancreatitis suggests that jejunal feeding is as safe as TPN. Patients were fed within 48 hours of admission with either an elemental diet via a nasojejunal route or TPN. The enteral-fed patients normalized their elevated amylase and lipase levels just as well as the parenterally fed patients. The enteral group had significantly fewer problems with hyperglycemia and incurred less cost. In another study, nasojejunal feeding using a nonelemental formula improved disease severity and clinical outcome by modifying the acute phase response compared with TPN. Both studies would support the use of enteral nutrition in acute pancreatitis. Based on the current literature, this author's practice has been to feed enterally past the ligament of Treitz using an elemental or semielemental formula if patients will consent to a nasal tube. Often, patients refuse a nasal tube, in which case, TPN is used.

The question of when to begin oral *refeeding* is important since pain and pancreatic inflammation may relapse with feeding. A recent study suggests that the risk of relapse of pain increases if serum lipase is greater than three times normal, if patients have had a longer duration of pain (11 days versus 6 days), and if patients have a worse CT score (Balthazar score greater than D). The criteria this author uses to initiate oral feeding are (1) absence of abdominal pain, (2) return of appetite, (3) lipase less than three times normal, and (4) resolution of ileus with return of bowel sounds. Feeding is started with a clear liquid diet for the first 24 hours. The diet is then advanced as tolerated using a low-fat solid diet.

Protein–calorie malnutrition is common in patients with chronic pancreatitis. The cause of malnutrition is multifactorial, including fear of recurrent postprandial abdominal pain (sitophobia), steatorrhea, anorexia, and often coexistent alcoholism. Steatorrhea and azotorrhea (fecal protein loss) occur when lipase and trypsin secretion is reduced by 90%. Lipase secretion tends to decrease more rapidly than secretion of proteolytic enzymes; therefore steatorrhea occurs earlier in the disease course and is more severe than azotorrhea. Nutritional management first begins with appropriate management of a patient's abdominal pain. Analgesics should be given at least 30 minutes before meals to prevent postprandial exacerbation of pain. A meta-analysis failed to show a beneficial effect of exogenous pancreatic enzymes in relieving abdominal pain.

Treatment of exocrine insufficiency is centered on pancreatic enzyme replacement. The minimal dose of lipase required is 28,000 IU per meal. Standard pancreatic enzyme replacement consists of eight pancreatin tablets (eg, Viokase) with each meal. A newer preparation, Viokase 16, is available, which consists of 16,000 IU per pill. Therefore, two pills or 32,000 IU with each meal is recommended. It is important to administer the enzymes with meals and not before or after to ensure adequate mixing with each meal. Weight maintenance, symptomatic improvement of diarrhea, and a decrease in 72-hour fecal fat excretion are the goals of therapy. Dietary fat should not be restricted. If steatorrhea persists, the addition of a proton-pump inhibitor may be of benefit because low gastric and duodenal pH (pH < 4) can inactivate lipase. If this fails, the administration of an enteric-coated preparation may be effective (ie, Creon, Pancrease, Ultrase). Fat-soluble vitamins and vitamin B_{12} should be replaced if deficient.

SHORT BOWEL SYNDROME

Short bowel syndrome is a collection of signs and symptoms used to describe the nutritional and metabolic consequences following major resections of the small intestine. Diarrhea, fluid and electrolyte losses, and weight loss characterize the syndrome. The normal small intestine is approximately 600 cm in length. The length and health of the residual small bowel determine prognosis. Patients with less than 100–150 cm of remaining small bowel often require TPN for survival. Patients with part of their colon remaining and 50 cm or more of residual small bowel can usually survive without TPN. The terminal ileum is important in the specialized absorption of vitamin B_{12} and bile salts.

Following intestinal resection the remaining intestine undergoes a process of adaptation, which includes structural and functional changes to maximize nutrient and fluid absorption. Changes include villus cell hyperplasia and increased brush border enzyme activity. These changes can continue up to a year, but are usually noticeable within the first 3 months following resection. Various nutrient deficiencies can occur following resection. These include fat-soluble vitamin (A, D, E, and K), essential fatty acid, and trace element deficiencies. Parenteral supplementation is often required.

The dietary management of short bowel depends on whether a patient has a colon. The colon can convert complex carbohydrates to short-chain fatty acids (eg, acetate, propionate, and butyrate). The production of short-chain fatty acids stimulates sodium and water absorption and provides additional calories. Therefore patients with colonic continuity should receive a high complex carbohydrate diet (60% of total calories), whereas patients without colons do not require special diets. Patients should also be treated aggressively with antimotility agents to control stool losses.

Oral rehydration solutions are also beneficial for some patients with short bowel. Patients with colons and hyperoxaluria are at increased risk of calcium oxalate renal stones and should be placed on low-oxalate, low-fat diets. Foods such as chocolate, tea, cola, spinach, and rhubarb contain high concentrations of oxalate. Magnesium losses may also be problematic in the patient with short bowel and may require parenteral replacement since oral administration may worsen a patient's diarrhea. Other complications associated with short bowel include D-lactic acidosis, in which D-lactic acid is produced by fermentation of malabsorbed carbohydrate in the colon. Increased serum levels of D-lactic acid are associated with marked metabolic acidosis with an elevated ion gap. Carbohydrate-restricted diets may be needed. Various exogenous trophic factors, such as human recombinant growth hormone and glutamine, have been tried to enhance nutrient absorption in short bowel. The current literature would suggest no beneficial effect.

Studies with glucagon-like peptide 2 (GLP-2) and conjugated bile acid replacement look promising. Successful surgical treatment for short bowel includes intestinal tapering and lengthening and small bowel transplantation. Intestinal lengthening procedures have been reported exclusively in children, with long-term benefit reported at 10 years. Approximately 600 small bowel transplants have been preformed in the world with two-thirds in the pediatric population. Results of small bowel graft survival have improved with the introduction of tacrolimus (FK-506) immunosuppression. Current 1-year and 5-year small bowel graft survival is 64% and 40%, respectively. The 1- and 5-year survival with home parenteral nutrition (HPN) is 85% and 60%, respectively. Current indications for small bowel transplant include TPN-induced liver failure, recurrent catheter infection, and poor vascular access. As better immunosuppression therapy evolves, small bowel transplant will most likely become the treatment of choice for short bowel syndrome.

INFLAMMATORY BOWEL DISEASE

Whether the combination of complete bowel rest and TPN can be used successfully as primary therapy in patients with acute inflammatory bowel disease with or without the addition of other medical therapy including diet is controversial. The consensus of the literature would suggest that patients with acute Crohn's enteritis could be placed into clinical remission with the combination of bowel rest and TPN alone. Indirect evidence suggests that TPN is less effective than steroid therapy in active Crohn's disease. Results with TPN alone would suggest 3 to 6 weeks of TPN and bowel rest will achieve a clinical response rate of 64%. It is not well understood if it is the bowel rest or the nutrition that is responsible for the positive findings.

Perhaps correction of dehydration and replacement of various micronutrients are more important than bowel rest alone, since similar results have been observed in patients with Crohn's disease treated with oral (elemental and polymeric) formulas. Although enteral formulas are more effective than placebo, they appear less effective than corticosteroids. No consistent data support the clinical efficacy of any specific whole food. Although elemental diets were initially introduced as primary treatment for active Crohn's disease because of their presumed hypoallergenicity, a randomized study would suggest that both elemental and polymeric (standard) formulas are equally effective in Crohn's disease unresponsive to steroids. Administration of either an elemental, peptide-based or polymeric formula for 3 to 6 weeks is reported to achieve a remission rate of 68%, which is similar to the remission rate reported with bowel rest and TPN. Monounsaturated fatty acid (oleic acid), which is present in most enteral formulas, is not a precursor to arachidonic acid and eicosanoic synthesis, which may explain the beneficial effect observed.

On the other hand, the consensus of the literature would suggest that patients with Crohn's colitis and idiopathic chronic ulcerative colitis (CUC) do not respond any better to TPN and bowel rest than patients treated with prednisone and diet. A few studies would suggest that patients with Crohn's colitis might respond to bowel rest and TPN more so than CUC patients, but the numbers are too small to draw definitive conclusions. Elemental diets also have no benefit in Crohn's colitis and idiopathic CUC. Surgery should therefore not be delayed for an extended treatment period using TPN in patients with severe Crohn's colitis or CUC. Also reported in many of these studies is a 10% risk of complications associated with TPN, including pneumothorax from central catheter placement, catheter sepsis, and various metabolic complications. Therefore, before administering a therapy (TPN) with questionable benefit, the potential risks of therapy should be evaluated.

CHRONIC LIVER DISEASE & TRANSPLANTATION

Cirrhosis is perhaps one of the best examples of protein–calorie malnutrition. Following hepatic transplantation the reversal of protein–calorie malnutrition is clinically obvious. Poor dietary intake and altered substrate metabolism are the primary reasons for malnutrition in this group of patients. Substrate utilization in patients with cirrhosis resembles that of starvation marked by increased lipid oxidation and decreased carbohydrate utilization. In addition, insulin resistance is common. Some patients with cirrhosis may also have increased resting energy expenditures (REE). Malnutrition has a negative impact on survival. However, whether nutritional support with oral supplements, enteral feeding, or TPN improves survival is not entirely clear. A small bedtime snack of approximately 200 kcal has been reported to reduce the risk of malnutrition in patients with cirrhosis. Oral dietary therapy is the mainstay of nutritional treatment in this group of patients. Although nasogastric feeding tubes can be safely placed in most of these patients, use beyond 4 weeks is difficult because of nasal discomfort and risk of bleeding from thrombocytopenia and impaired coagulation.

Gastrostomy feeding tubes cannot be safely placed in most patients because of ascites and risk of peritonitis. Oral dietary treatment should not restrict protein and should limit sodium to less than 2.0 g/d. Protein should supply 1.5 g/kg/d of the total calories. Vegetable protein is better tolerated than animal protein because it produces less aromatic amino acids, which are thought to be responsible for hepatic encephalopathy. Branched-chain amino acids are helpful in the treatment of hepatic encephalopathy but should be used only in refractory cases. Fat-soluble vitamin levels should be checked and replaced if deficient. Serum vitamin A levels may not reflect hepatic vitamin A levels; therefore, replacement should be given with caution given the risk of vitamin A toxicity.

Orthotopic liver transplantation is the principal treatment for malnutrition in patients with cirrhosis. Within 4 months following transplantation, increased muscle mass is clinically obvious. Despite the increasing evidence of the prognostic importance of nutrition prior to transplantation, no randomized controlled studies have been published that evaluate the preoperative role of nutritional supplementation. Studies would support the benefit of early postoperative enteral feeding suggesting less infectious complications. In our experience most patients are eating within 48 hours posttransplant, therefore, we use enteral feeding and occasionally TPN only in select patients. Depending on the dose and duration of prednisone posttransplant, osteoporosis and hyperlipidemia may occur. In our experience, by using tacrolimus (FK 506) instead of cyclosporine immunosupression and by discontinuing prednisone at 4 months posttransplant, this has been less of a problem.

GASTROPARESIS & CHRONIC INTESTINAL PSEUDOOBSTRUCTION

The management of gastroparesis and chronic intestinal pseudoobstruction (CIP) centers on increasing propulsive function with pharmacologic agents and maintaining the nutritional well-being of the patient. In our experience, many of these patients also have functional complaints and are often taking narcotics, which should be minimized since they can significantly delay gastrointestinal motility. Patients with severe gastroparesis will often complain of early satiety and nausea shortly after a meal, whereas patients with CIP will complain of nausea and abdominal bloating 4 to 5 hours postprandial. The underling etiology of the CIP may also influence dietary therapy.

Patients with scleroderma may have reduced oral intake because of perioral skin sclerosis, which makes it difficult to chew food. In this case, a liquid diet through a straw may be helpful. Likewise, esophageal dysmotility and strictures from severe reflux may limit oral intake of both liquids and solids. Therefore, aggressive treatment of the reflux is often helpful in improving food intake. Bacterial overgrowth resulting in diarrhea and weight loss may also occur in patients with CIP and should be treated. Patients with systemic amyloidosis frequently complain of anorexia and bloating, usually the result of delayed gastric emptying and small bowel dysmotility. In addition, patients with amyloidosis may have macroglossia, which can impede the propulsion of food past the oropharynx. The primary dietary therapies in patients with delayed gastric emptying and CIP are similar.

Small frequent meals (six to eight) throughout the day are usually better tolerated than three large meals. A low-fiber, low-residue, lactose-free diet should be encouraged. A low-residue diet includes low fiber and omits foods such as whole grain, raw vegetables, and milk, which increase fecal residue. Because fat can delay gastrointestinal transit, a low-fat diet should be encouraged. Likewise, foods that produce intestinal gas should be avoided. Examples include dried beans and peas, cabbage, and dairy products. Avoiding use of straws and carbonated beverages and avoiding fast eating should minimize air swallowing. Sitting upright or walking after a meal should be encouraged. Blenderized pureed foods and commercial liquid formulas should be encouraged. Most commercial formulas are lactose and fiber free with less than 30% of the total calories as fat. An oral multivitamin should also be given. If a patient fails oral dietary therapy, the next step should be enteral feeding. Gastric tube feeding in most patients with gastroparesis will not work any better than oral feeding, and small bowel feeding is required. In our experience, a dual gastrojejunal tube works best. We find less leakage with the gastric entry site compared with direct percutaneous jejunal placement. Also, the gastric port can be used for venting and the jejunal port for feeding. If a patient can partially eat, tube feeds can be given nocturnally to allow for daytime eating. Elemental formulas are not needed since the intestinal mucosa is usually normal. TPN should be used only when patients have failed a trail of enteral feeding.

PERIOPERATIVE NUTRITION

Thirteen prospective studies evaluated the use of preoperative TPN in patients with gastrointestinal cancers who were considered at least moderately malnourished. Pooled analysis found that patients who received preoperative TPN for 7–10 days had 10% fewer postoperative complications. There was no difference in mortality between the TPN and the control group. There are insufficient data regarding preoperative tube feeding. The use of TPN in the immediate postoperative period has been evaluated in nine prospective studies in moderately malnourished patients. TPN had an approximate 10% increased risk of postoperative complications. No consistent difference in postoperative mortality was found. Four studies have evaluated postoperative tube feedings in similar patients and found no difference in morbidity or mortality. Postoperative nutritional support should, however, be given to those unable to eat 7–10 days postoperatively to prevent the adverse effects of negative nitrogen balance. Therefore, in most elective surgical cases, the data would suggest not delaying surgery for nutritional support.

HOME ENTERAL & PARENTERAL NUTRITION

With increased hospital costs there has been a shift to home treatment over recent years. Home health care companies have also emerged that have made home care more convenient for both the patient and clinician. The availability of home health care, however, should not encourage the premature hospital discharge of patients. Swallowing disorders are the most common indications for home enteral feeding. Poststroke and radiation therapy for head and neck cancer are the two most common indications for long-term gastrostomy feeding. Patients should be trained in the management of tube feeding before leaving the hospital. Portable pumps are available for those patients who are active and require continuous feeding. Home parenteral nutrition is used for those patients with intestinal failure, usually as the result of mechanical obstruction or inadequate surface area, ie, short bowel syndrome.

The most common complication of HPN is catheter infection. A patient on HPN with fever should be given close attention, often with empiric antibiotics started until blood cultures are final. Adequate sterile catheter training should be accomplished before a patient leaves the hospital. Other long-term complications of HPN include cholestatic liver disease and metabolic bone disease. Death in HPN-treated patients is primarily related to their underlying disease. Medicare remains the largest payer for home nutritional support reimbursement. Specific Medicare requirements must be met before a patient will qualify for reimbursement. Enteral nutrition is covered for patients who have a permanent (defined as greater than 3 months) disease that prevents food from reaching the small bowel. Calories must supply between 20 and 35 kcal/kg/d. Medicare will not cover a patient with a functioning gastrointestinal tract whose need is for reasons such as anorexia, nausea, associated mood disorder, or terminal illness. A certificate of medical necessity must be completed before leaving the hospital. Medicare qualifications for HPN likewise require a documented need of at least 3 months or longer. The patient must have a condition involving the small intestine that significantly impairs the absorption of nutrients or a motility disorder that impairs the ability of nutrients to be transported. Documentation of malabsorption and failure of tube feeding must be completed before qualification in most circumstances.

REFERENCES

Byrne TA et al: Growth hormone, glutamine and modified diet enhances nutrient absorption in patients with severe short bowel syndrome. J Parenter Enteral Nutr 1995;19:296.

Cabre E, Gassull MA: Nutrition in chronic liver disease and liver transplantation. Clin Nutr Metabolic Care 1998;1:423.

Detsky AS et al: What is subjective global assessment of nutritional status? J Parenter Enteral Nutr 1987;11:8.

Greenberg GR: Nutritional management of inflammatory bowel disease. Semin Gastrointest Dis 1993;4:69.

Kalfarentzos F et al: Enteral nutrition is superior to parenteral nutrition in severe acute pancreatitis: results of a randomized prospective trial. Br J Surg 1997;84:1655.

Klein S et al: Nutrition support in clinical practice: review of the published data and recommendations for future research directions. J Parenter Enteral Nutr 1997;21:133.

Levy P et al: Frequency and risk factors of recurrent pain during refeeding in patients with acute pancreatitis: a multivariate multicenter prospective study of 116 patients. Gut 1997;40:262.

Lipman TO: Grains and veins: is enteral nutrition really better than parenteral nutrition? A look at the evidence. J Parenter Enteral Nutr 1998;22:167.

Norgaard I, Hansen BS, Mortensen PB: Colon a digestive organ in patients with short bowel. Lancet 1994;343:373.

Scolapio JS et al: Effect of growth hormone, glutamine and diet on adaptation in short bowel syndrome. A randomized controlled study. Gastroenterology 1997;113:1074.

Scolapio JS, Malhi-Chowla N, Ukleja A: Nutrition supplementation in patients with acute and chronic pancreatitis. Gastroenterol Clin North Am 1999;28:695.

Scolapio JS et al: Nutritional management of chronic intestinal pseudo-obstruction. J Clin Gastrenterol 1999;28:306.

Scolapio JS et al: Survival of home parenteral nutrition-treated patients: 20 years of experience at the Mayo Clinic. Mayo Clin Proc 1999;74:217.

Szkudlarek J, Jeppesen PB, Mortensen PB: Effect of high dose growth hormone with glutamine and no change in diet on intestinal absorption in patient with short bowls: a randomized, double blind, cross over, placebo controlled study. Gut 2000; 47:199.

Windsor A et al: Compared with parenteral nutrition, enteral feeding attenuates the acute phase response and improves disease severity in acute pancreatitis. Gut 1998;42:431.

Minimally Invasive Surgery for Gastrointestinal Diseases

Lyn Knoblock, MD & Sean J. Mulvihill, MD

Beginning with the introduction of laparoscopic chole-cystectomy in 1987, gastrointestinal surgery has undergone revolutionary changes. New technology now allows many surgical procedures to be performed with "minimal access" to the thoracic or abdominal cavities, obviating the need for large, painful, and morbid incisions. In the minimal access approach, the operative visual field is provided by telescopes attached to miniaturized video cameras, with the image projected on television monitors. New instruments have been designed for use within the constraints of small incisions. General surgeons have been retrained to adapt to a new two-dimensional visual field. The technical limitations as compared with traditional surgery—including loss of tactile sensation and sensory feedback—are partially offset by improved resolution of anatomic detail through the magnification provided by the operating telescopes.

The initial driving force behind the rapid development of the minimally invasive approach was patient demand. The intuitive benefits of minimal access surgery, including minimal scarring, reduced pain, and quicker return to work, offer clear-cut advantages in many operations. In other operations, however, the advantages are less clear. The challenge for general surgeons today is to evaluate the outcome and costs of the minimally invasive approaches to gastrointestinal disorders, and compare these results with those obtained with traditional open surgical techniques.

DIAGNOSTIC LAPAROSCOPY

General Considerations

Diagnostic laparoscopy refers to the visual examination of the intraabdominal contents with a telescope. Diagnostic laparoscopy is useful in three general clinical scenarios: (1) evaluation of abdominal pain, (2) staging of abdominal tumors, and (3) evaluation of abdominal trauma.

Technical Considerations

Diagnostic laparoscopy is usually performed with the patient under general anesthesia, however, it is possible under local anesthesia. After adequate muscle relaxation, nasogastric and bladder catheters are placed to decompress the stomach and urinary bladder, respectively. The first goal is to create a working space (**pneumoperitoneum**) within the abdomen by insufflation of gas (usually CO_2) through a specially designed Verres needle. The **Verres needle** is a sharp hollow needle with a spring-loaded blunt tipped core designed to penetrate the abdominal wall with minimal risk of intraabdominal organ injury. If proper Verres needle placement is difficult or if the patient has had prior abdominal surgery, safe access to the abdominal cavity can be achieved through a small fascial and peritoneal incision for direct visual placement of a Hasson cannula. This method avoids the "blind" puncture of the Verres needle, reducing the risk of misplacement or accidental puncture of intraabdominal organs. Once the surgeon is confident of the Verres needle or Hasson cannula placement, CO_2 is insufflated to a maximum intraperitoneal pressure of 15 mm Hg.

After creation of the pneumoperitoneum, hollow ports or cannulas for telescope and instrument access are placed through the abdominal wall. These ports must be strategically situated for ideal surgical exposure and instrument access. The telescope, which has a fiberoptic light source for illumination, is connected to a camera with projection of the intraabdominal image on television monitors. If the diagnosis is not readily apparent after the initial inspection, a more thorough examination can be performed by placing additional ports to facilitate exposure. Satisfactory evaluation of the visceral and parietal peritoneal surfaces, liver, stomach, small bowel, colon, and pelvic organs can be achieved during routine diagnostic laparoscopy. If necessary, access to the retroperitoneum can be achieved to visualize the pancreas or retroperitoneal masses.

Prognosis

Refinements in video and instrument technology have helped make diagnostic laparoscopy an accepted procedure for the evaluation of abdominal pain, staging of malignant tumors, and evaluation of abdominal trauma. The overall accuracy of diagnostic laparoscopy in the evaluation of chronic or acute abdominal pain is reported to be 80–99%, reducing the need for exploratory laparotomy. When evaluating a patient for a malignant neoplasm, laparoscopy has proved useful in detecting small tumors (<2 cm) that are undetectable by conventional radiographic modalities (eg, computed tomography and ultrasound). Up to 40% of patients with pancreatic or gastric malignancies have unsuspected peritoneal or liver metastases discovered by diagnostic laparoscopy.

In trauma, diagnostic laparoscopy may be superior to peritoneal lavage in the evaluation of abdominal injury. Although both laparoscopy and peritoneal lavage have 100% sensitivity in detecting major intraabdominal injuries, the positive predictive value for therapeutic exploratory laparotomy has been reported to be 92% for laparoscopy compared with 72% for peritoneal lavage. Overall, the increased use of diagnostic laparoscopy has reduced the rate of unnecessary laparotomy, decreased morbidity, shortened hospital stays, decreased periods of disability, and lowered overall hospital costs.

MINIMALLY INVASIVE APPROACHES TO ESOPHAGEAL MOTILITY DISORDERS

General Considerations

Esophageal motility disorders represent a spectrum of disease states that range from absent peristalsis (**achalasia**) to hyperperistalsis (**diffuse esophageal spasm**). This array of disease processes can be further classified using a combination of clinical, radiographic, and manometric studies. Achalasia is the esophageal motility disorder most amenable to surgical treatment. It is a neuromuscular disorder of the esophagus associated with absence of the ganglion cells of the myenteric plexus and characterized by the classic triad of dysphagia, regurgitation, and weight loss.

The distinguishing radiographic feature of achalasia on barium esophagogram is a dilated esophagus with a "bird's beak" taper at the esophagogastric junction. Typically, esophageal manometry studies reveal (1) lack of progressive peristalsis throughout the body of the esophagus, (2) a high-pressure lower esophageal sphincter, and (3) failure of the lower esophageal sphincter to relax with swallowing. Endoscopy allows direct visualization of esophagitis and biopsy can be obtained to rule out the presence of cancer. Frequently a dilated body and narrowed lower esophageal sphincter (LES) can be observed. Treatment options for toxin achalasia include pharmacologic therapy, botulinum (BoTox) injections, pneumatic balloon dilation, and surgical myotomy. Pharmacologic therapy with smooth muscle relaxants, such as calcium channel blockers and nitrates,

usually fails to improve symptoms. They are reserved for patients with very mild symptoms or those who are not candidates for other therapies. BoTox injections are effective in the short term but frequently require repeated treatment. BoTox produces an inflammatory change in the distal esophagus, which may obliterate the plane of dissection between the mucosa and muscular layers. This places these patients at increased risk of esophageal perforation during a future surgical myotomy. Dilation is effective in 60–80% of patients. Repeat dilations are often necessary and approximately 50% have recurrent symptoms within 5 years. Dilation is associated with a risk of perforation and some patients have a new onset of heartburn. Laparoscopic Heller myotomy offers the best long-term results and is now the preferred initial approach in many patients with achalasia over other options, such as medical therapy, balloon dilation, or open surgery.

Laparoscopic Heller Myotomy

The patient is positioned supine and a general anesthetic is administered. After creation of the pneumoperitoneum, four or five operating ports are placed into the upper abdomen. The left lobe of the liver is retracted anteriorly. Division of the phrenoesophageal membrane exposes the esophagus. A longitudinal esophageal myotomy is created through the longitudinal and circular muscle layers over a distance of about 6 cm. The caudad extension of the myotomy is extended onto the anterior surface of the stomach for approximately 2 cm. The edges of the myotomy are separated by blunt dissection, so that approximately 50% of the circumference of the esophageal mucosa is visible. The vagus nerve trunks are identified and preserved. An antireflux procedure, such as a partial fundoplication, can be performed in conjunction with the myotomy to prevent reflux. Postoperatively, relief of dysphagia is usually immediate, and oral feedings are started the day after surgery. Patients are typically discharged from the hospital within 24–48 hours. In general, patients are pain free at the time of discharge and are able to return to work within 1 week.

Prognosis

After laparoscopic Heller myotomy, up to 95% of patients have symptomatic relief from dysphagia at 5 years follow-up. Persistent dysphagia is seen in 3–5% of patients and this is usually amenable to balloon dilation. The laparoscopic approach is as effective as the open technique and offers advantages of more rapid recovery and decreased postoperative pain. Experienced surgeons report conversion rates of less than 5%. A morbidity of 10–15% is similar to the open experience.

LAPAROSCOPIC TREATMENT FOR GASTROESOPHAGEAL REFLUX

General Considerations

Gastroesophageal reflux results from the abnormal entry of gastric contents into the esophagus, causing the classic symptoms of heartburn and regurgitation. This abnormal reflux is usually due to an abnormal transient relaxation of the lower esophageal sphincter, the presence of a hiatal hernia, or a combination of these factors. Other potentially important pathophysiologic factors include abnormal esophageal clearance, delayed gastric emptying, and increased intraabdominal pressure. Although symptoms of gastroesophageal reflux can be improved with H_2-receptor antagonists or proton-pump inhibitors the underlying pathophysiology is not corrected. Untreated gastroesophageal reflux can lead to serious complications, including esophagitis, stricture, bleeding, and aspiration. An important consideration is the pathophysiologic role of gastroesophageal reflux in the development of Barrett's metaplasia. This is now the most important risk factor for the development of esophageal cancer in the United States.

Diagnostic techniques, including fiberoptic endoscopy, esophageal manometry, and 24-hour esophageal pH monitoring, allow selection of patients most likely to benefit from surgery. Included are patients who have had a good previous response to proton-pump inhibitors, patients with complications of gastroesophageal reflux (eg, Barrett's and strictures), patients with pul-

monary symptoms (recurrent pulmonary infections and hoarse voice), and young patients. Antireflux surgery has been shown in large, controlled trials to be more effective than antacids and H_2-blocker therapy. A recent controlled trial comparing open antireflux surgery with standard omeprazole therapy found open surgery to be more effective. In this study if the dose of omeprazole was adjusted to either 40 or 60 mg/d when relapse occurred, the level of efficacy was not statistically different.

Laparoscopic Nissen Fundoplication

The primary goal of gastroesophageal reflux surgery is to reestablish the competency of the LES. The Nissen fundoplication is the most commonly performed antireflux operation, and the laparoscopic Nissen results in an anatomic equivalent to the open operation. After induction of general anesthesia and creation of the pneumoperitoneum, four or five abdominal ports are placed in the upper abdomen. The procedure begins with dissection of the phrenoesophageal membrane and diaphragmatic crura, which exposes the intraabdominal esophagus and hiatal hernia. The short gastric vessels are divided, mobilizing the upper stomach for the fundoplication. The crural defect of the hiatal hernia is repaired and a 2-cm-long, 360-degree wrap of the upper stomach is made around the intraabdominal segment of the esophagus (Figure 13–1). The wrap is loosely constructed over a 56-French bougie to avoid postoperative dysphagia or gas bloat syndrome. The vagus nerve trunks are identified and preserved.

Although this "floppy" Nissen fundoplication is the standard approach, the operation can be tailored to the

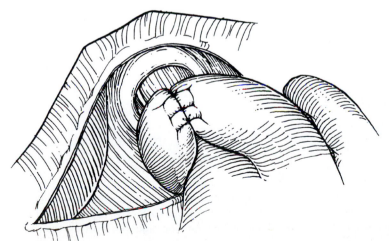

Figure 13–1. Laparoscopic Nissen fundoplication for gastroesophageal reflux. The hiatal hernia is repaired using crural sutures, and a 2-cm-long floppy, 360-degree wrap is constructed around the distal esophagus.

severity of reflux and the presence of associated pathology, such as defects in esophageal peristalsis or gastric emptying. In patients with defective peristalsis, a 270-degree wrap may be more appropriate to prevent dysphagia, although this view has been challenged. Patients with delayed gastric emptying benefit from concomitant pyloromyotomy or pyloroplasty.

Prognosis

Results of laparoscopic Nissen fundoplication, in terms of postoperative manometry and 24-hour pH monitoring, are equivalent to results achieved after traditional open Nissen fundoplication. Relief of heartburn is achieved in 80–90% of patients. Postoperative recovery of patients undergoing laparoscopic Nissen fundoplication is dramatically rapid compared with those undergoing open fundoplication, with typical hospital stays of 1–2 days and resumption of full physical activity within 1 week. Objective improvement in LES pressure and acid reflux, as measured by 24-hour pH monitoring, has been documented (Figure 13–2).

LAPAROSCOPIC TREATMENT OF PEPTIC ULCER DISEASE

General Considerations

Peptic ulcer disease traditionally was viewed as an imbalance between acid–pepsin secretion and mucosal defense. However, the management of patients with peptic ulcer disease has changed because of powerful evidence of the pathogenic role of the organism *Helicobacter pylori. Helicobacter* is present in the stomachs of 90% of patients with duodenal ulcers and 80% of patients with gastric ulcers. Treatment usually includes antibiotics, antisecretory medications, and bismuth preparations. Eradication is successful in 85–90% of patients with relapse rates of 6–14%. Today, surgery is reserved for the unusual patient refractory to antisecretory medications and eradication of *H pylori,* as well as those with complicated ulcer disease, including bleeding, perforation, and pyloric obstruction.

Laparoscopic Proximal Gastric Vagotomy

For the rare patient requiring elective surgery, laparoscopic proximal gastric vagotomy is the optimal procedure. This operation is anatomically equivalent to that performed during open surgery. The crucial elements include denervation of the distal 5 cm of the esophagus and proximal lesser curvature of the stomach, with preservation of the nerves to the pylorus and distal 6–7 cm of antrum (Figure 13–3). This procedure inhibits basal and vagally mediated acid and pepsin secretion but preserves normal gastric emptying.

Perforated duodenal ulcers are also amenable to laparoscopic treatment. The most common approach has been to combine simple closure of the perforation and

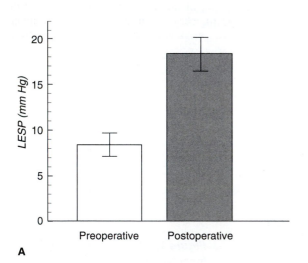
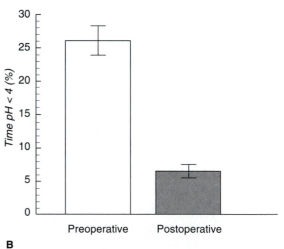

A   **B**

Figure 13–2. Results of laparoscopic Nissen fundoplication. **A:** Laparoscopic Nissen fundoplication results in a significant increase in lower esophageal sphincter pressure, compared with preoperative values. **B:** Laparoscopic Nissen fundoplication results in a significant decrease in the percentage of time the esophagus has a pH less than 4, compared with preoperative values.

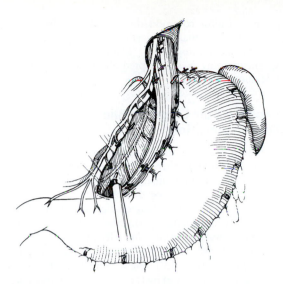

Figure 13–3. Laparoscopic proximal gastric vagotomy. The distal 5 cm of esophagus and the proximal stomach are denervated by dividing the anterior and posterior leaflets of the gastrohepatic ligament. The nerves of Laterjet innervating the antrum and pylorus are preserved.

placement of an omental patch. The laparoscopic approach allows a thorough lavage of the soiled peritoneal cavity. Simultaneous proximal gastric vagotomy is unnecessary unless the patient has had recurrent *Helicobacter* infection. Selected patients with gastric outlet obstruction due to peptic ulcer disease are candidates for laparoscopic truncal vagotomy and gastrojejunostomy. In this procedure, both vagal trunks are divided at the diaphragm and gastric drainage is achieved by a gastrojejunal anastomosis. The latter can be constructed with an endoscopic stapling device or by endoscopic suturing techniques.

Prognosis

Surgical treatment for peptic ulcer disease is less common with the widespread use of proton-pump inhibitors and treatment of *H pylori*. For patients refractory to medical therapy or those with complications such as bleeding, obstruction, or perforation, laparoscopic surgery is less invasive with shorter hospital stays and faster return to regular activity. Laparoscopic proximal gastric vagotomy resulted in appropriate reduction in basal and stimulated acid secretion, and low rates of recurrent ulceration in patients treated for chronic duodenal ulcers.

LAPAROSCOPIC APPROACH TO CHOLECYSTECTOMY

General Considerations

It was clear as early as 1989 that laparoscopic cholecystectomy offers clear benefits over open surgery. With decreased postoperative pain, shorter hospital stays, and earlier return to work, laparoscopic cholecystectomy quickly replaced open cholecystectomy as the gold standard operation. There are no absolute contraindications to laparoscopic cholecystectomy, but patients with severe abdominal adhesions or biliary anatomy that cannot be clearly defined often require an open procedure.

Laparoscopic Cholecystectomy

Laparoscopic cholecystectomy is performed under general anesthesia. The patient is laid in the supine position with sequential compression stocking in place. After induction of anesthesia, a Foley catheter and orogastric tube are placed to decompress the bladder and stomach. The abdomen is prepared and draped. A periumbilical incision is made and insufflation of the abdomen is performed using either a closed Verres needle or open Hasson technique. A 5- or 10-mm trocar is than placed through this incision and the telescope is introduced. After inspecting surrounding tissues to ensure injury secondary to trocar placement has not occurred, three additional ports are placed under direct vision. The second port, which is 5 or 10 mm in size, is placed in the mid-epigastric region and two 5-mm ports are placed in the right upper quadrant. Through the two right upper quadrant ports grasping instruments are used to retract the fundus of the gallbladder cranially and the infundibulum of the gallbladder laterally. This retraction exposes Calot's triangle and allows the surgeon to identify the cystic duct and artery, which can than be clipped and divided. Prior to division of the cystic duct a cholangiogram can be performed by placing a small catheter through a ductotomy and injecting radiopaque dye. Some surgeons perform a cholangiogram with every cholecystectomy, whereas others use a selective approach. A cholangiogram is absolutely required for patients with known common bile duct stones, for patients with recent pancreatitis or abnormal liver function tests, and when anatomy is unclear to the operating surgeon. After the cystic duct and artery have been divided the body of the gallbladder is dissected off the liver bed using electrocautery. The gallbladder is then removed via the mid-epigastric or periumbilical port site using a grasper or small bag. The 10-mm port site fascial edges are approximated and skin is closed. The Foley catheter and orogastric tubes are removed in the operating room. Patients are allowed to eat, drink, and ambulate immediately postoperatively. Pain is usually controlled with oral pain medications and most patients can be discharged the day of surgery.

Prognosis

Laparoscopic cholecystectomy is extremely effective at relieving symptoms related to gallstones. The major operative risk relates to the possibility of inadvertent bile duct injury. Initially, the risk of common bile duct injury with laparoscopic cholecystectomy was 10-fold higher than with open cholecystectomy. With improvement in laparoscopic techniques the rate of bile duct injury now approaches 0.2%, similar to that seen in the open technique (Table 13–1). Laparoscopic cholecystectomy is now the accepted gold standard operation for gallbladder disease.

LAPAROSCOPIC EXPLORATION OF THE COMMON BILE DUCT

General Considerations

Overall, choledocholithiasis is present in 10–15% of patients undergoing cholecystectomy. These stones usually have migrated from the gallbladder, but some form within the bile ducts. Common bile duct stones may cause biliary colic, obstructive jaundice, or cholangitis in patients with biliary tract disease; they may be asymptomatic and not be discovered until the time of operation for cholelithiasis; or they may become evident following cholecystectomy.

Diagnosis of common bile duct stones is suggested by liver function tests and ultrasound, but the most accurate method is cholangiography (intraoperative, endoscopic, or percutaneous).

The natural history of asymptomatic common bile duct stones is unknown, but because of their potentially serious sequelae, they should be treated when discovered. With technical improvements in laparoscopic in-

struments most common duct stones can be successfully removed laparoscopically. Endoscopic retrograde cholangiopancreatography (ERCP) and endoscopic sphincterotomy is an accepted alternative to common bile duct exploration.

Laparoscopic Common Bile Duct Exploration

Common bile duct stones may be approached laparoscopically through either the cystic duct (**transcystic access**) or the common bile duct (**choledochotomy**). The first step in transcystic access to the common bile duct is cystic duct dilation via a balloon-tipped catheter. Direct choledochoscopy is then performed with a miniaturized flexible telescope. Stones are entrapped with baskets under direct vision and extracted retrograde through the cystic duct. For proximal biliary stones and larger stones that cannot be removed by the transcystic route, a choledochotomy is made for insertion of a larger choledochoscope that can be directed anterograde or retrograde. After stone removal, the choledochotomy is closed over a rubber T-tube with absorbable, monofilament suture using intracorporeal suturing techniques.

Prognosis

Laparoscopic clearance of common bile duct stones can be accomplished, in expert hands, in up to 95% of patients. The postoperative convalescence of patients undergoing laparoscopic transcystic common bile duct exploration is no different from those undergoing laparoscopic cholecystectomy alone. When laparoscopic cholodochotomy and T-tube placement are performed, hospital stay is somewhat longer, and the T-tube must be removed at a later date. Decisions regarding approaches to common duct stones are best based on the clinical scenario, the patient's overall condition, and the expertise of the treating physicians (Figure 13–4).

Table 13–1. Comparison of laparoscopic and open cholecystectomy.

Group	Years Encompassed	Number of Patients	Mortality Rate (%)	Common Duct Injury rate (%)	Conversion Rate (%)	Postoperative Stay (Days)
Laparoscopic cholecystectomy						
Southern Surgeons	1990–1991	1,518	0.07	0.50	4.7	1.2
European	1989–1991	1,236	0	0.30	3.6	3.0
Louisville	1989–1991	1,983	0.10	0.25	4.5	2.1
Canadian	1990–1991	2,201	0	0.14	4.3	—
Open cholecystectomy						
Roslyn JJ et al	1989	42,474	0.17	0.20	NA	4
Morgenstern L et al	1982–1988	1,200	1.80	0.17	NA	5–7
Bredesen J et al	1977–1981	13,854	1.20	—	NA	—

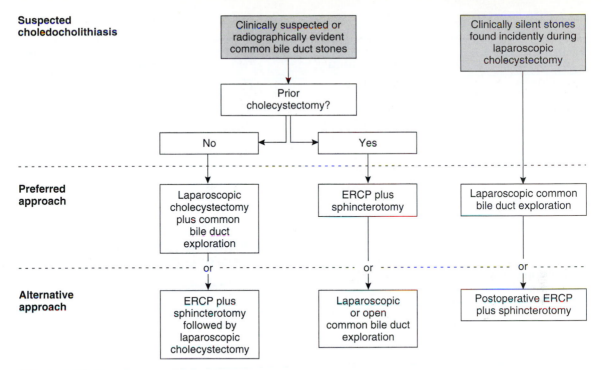

Figure 13–4. An approach to patients with choledocholithiasis.

LAPAROSCOPIC APPROACH TO APPENDICITIS

General Considerations

Although laparoscopic appendectomy was performed prior to laparoscopic cholecystectomy, it has not been accepted with the same enthusiasm. Unlike cholecystectomy, an open appendectomy can be performed through a small incision with minimal discomfort and a short hospital stay.

In several studies laparoscopic appendectomy has been shown to be associated with longer operative times and higher cost. Benefits of the laparoscopic approach have included improved diagnostic accuracy, lower wound infection rates, decreased pain, shorter recovery period, and faster return to work (Table 13–2). Controversy continues over the postoperative abscess rate with laparoscopic procedure. Several studies have indicated a higher abscess rate after the laparoscopic approach but six randomized study from 1993 to 1997 failed to show a significant increase after laparoscopy.

Laparoscopic Appendectomy

After creation of the pneumoperitoneum, a single port is placed below the umbilicus for insertion of the lap-

aroscope. Usually, the inflamed appendix is immediately evident in the normal anatomic position in the right lower quadrant. Rotational maneuvers and placement of accessory ports facilitate exposure of the difficult or retrocecal appendix. If the appendix is normal, a thorough laparoscopic exploration to identify other pathology is performed. Exposure and visualization of the abdominal cavity are usually superior to that achieved through a small right lower quadrant incision.

The technique for laparoscopic appendectomy is similar to that used in open surgery. The mesoappendix is dissected and the appendiceal artery is controlled with clips or a stapler. The appendix is ligated near the cecum with loops of absorbable suture material or stapled and then divided (Figure 13–5). The appendix is then placed into a plastic bag and withdrawn through a trocar site, thus preventing contact of the infected appendix with the skin incision. Postoperatively, patients generally do not require intravenous narcotic medication and are allowed oral feedings when hungry.

Prognosis

Laparoscopic appendectomy has been shown to be a safe acceptable alternative to open appendectomy. Although many reports indicate that the benefits are small

Table 13–2. Randomized controlled trials of laparoscopic versus open appendectomy.

Group (year)	Surgical Treatment	Number of Patients	Wound Infections (%)	Operating Time (min)	Postoperative (days)
Kum et al (1993)	Laparoscopic	52	0[1]	43	3.2
	Open	57	9	40	4.2
Pedersen et al (2001)	Laparoscopic	282	3[1]	60	2.0
	Open	301	7	40	2.0
Reiertsen et al (1977)	Laparoscopic	56	2	57	3.5
	Open	52	0	25	3.2
Attwood et al (1992)	Laparoscopic	30	0[1]	61	2.5[1]
	Open	32	12	51	3.8

[1]$P < .05$ compared with open appendectomy.

and do not justify the higher cost, there are some patients who may clearly benefit from this approach. The improved diagnostic accuracy seen with laparoscopic surgery is beneficial when the diagnosis is unclear. Obese patients who are at increased risk for postoperative wound infection benefit from the improved visualization and decreased wound infection rate associated with the laparoscopic approach. The typical hospital stay after laparoscopic appendectomy is less than 1 day.

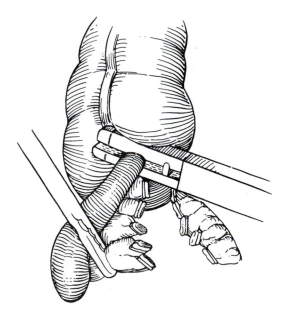

Figure 13–5. Laparoscopic appendectomy using a stapling device. Through a small suprapubic incision, a mechanical device divides the appendix between parallel rows of occluding staples.

LAPAROSCOPIC APPROACH TO COLON RESECTION

General Considerations

Large organs, such as the colon, are more difficult to resect laparoscopically than small organs, such as the gallbladder and appendix. The increased technical difficulty associated with laparoscopic colectomy results in longer operating times and increased operative cost. But like other laparoscopic procedures, it results in reduced postoperative pain, earlier return of bowel function, improved cosmetic results, and reduced hospital stay. Laparoscopic colectomy for benign disease is well accepted as a safe alternative to open colectomy. Indications for laparoscopic colectomy include diverticulitis, villous adenoma, polyposis, volvulus, inflammatory bowel disease, and rectal prolapse. Diverting procedures such as ileostomy or colostomy can also be performed through the laparoscopic approach. Concern has been raised, however, about the adequacy of laparoscopic colon resection for cancer. Two large randomized trials have recently been concluded and results should be reported in 2002.

Laparoscopic Colon Resection

The first technical issue related to laparoscopic colon resection is identification of the lesion. Because of the limited tactile sensation afforded by minimally invasive techniques, small lesions such as polyps may not be detectable with the laparoscope. Preoperative localization of these lesions by barium enema, or intraoperative confirmation of lesion position via colonoscopy, is required. Once the colonic segment of interest is identified, it is mobilized and suspended for access to its mesentery. Mesenteric transection is accomplished with hemostatic clips, a harmonic scalpel, or a stapling device.

Following mesenteric division, colonic resection and anastomosis are accomplished in one of two ways. Through a small incision, the colonic segment can be exteriorized, resected, and reanastomosed. This is termed **laparoscopic-assisted colectomy.** Alternatively, the colon can be divided and anastomosed intracorporeally, usually with the aid of mechanical stapling devices. With this technique, the specimen should be placed in a plastic bag to protect the wound edges during removal. After removal, the specimen must be immediately examined to ensure that adequate resection margins have been achieved. Finally, the anastomosis should be tested for integrity, either via direct inspection colonoscopically or via instillation of air or fluid intraluminally.

Prognosis

Laparoscopic colectomy for benign disease has been shown to be comparable to the open procedure with low morbidity and mortality. Conversion rates in several studies range from 5% to 40%. Laparoscopic colectomy is relatively difficult compared with other minimally invasive gastrointestinal operations. Virtually all colon resections, including right and left colectomy, low anterior resection, and abdominoperineal resection, can be performed with these techniques. It is not yet clear that an adequate cancer operation can be reliably performed laparoscopically. There have been several troubling reports of cancer recurrence at the trocar site. For now, laparoscopic colectomy is best performed in selected patients with benign disease or in the setting of prospective trials evaluating adequacy of a cancer operation.

LAPAROSCOPIC TREATMENT FOR HEMATOLOGIC SPLENIC DISEASE

General Considerations

Laparoscopic splenectomy has replaced the open procedure as the standard of care for nontraumatic splenic diseases. Many studies have shown that laparoscopic splenenctomy is safe and equally efficacious when compared with open splenectomy. The most common indication for laparoscopic splenectomy is immune thrombocytopenic purpura (ITP). Indications for surgery in patients with ITP include failure of medical therapy, a need for high-dose steroids to maintain remission, and relapse of symptomatic thrombocytopenia after initial response to therapy.

Laparoscopic Splenectomy

Laparoscopic splenectomy can be performed with the patient in a supine or right lateral decubitus position.

The lateral position can make visualization of hilar vessels difficult in patients with larger spleens. Four or five ports are placed for retraction, visualization, and dissection. The short gastric vessels are divided between clips or controlled with a harmonic scalpel. The lateral peritoneal attachments and splenic ligaments are dissected using electrocautery or a harmonic scalpel. The hilar vessels are isolated and clipped or stapled. The spleen is morcellized in a bag and removed by a suction device and forceps. The entire abdomen is then inspected for accessory spleens, with special attention paid to the splenic hilum, pancreatic tail, splenic ligaments, greater omentum, and small bowel mesentery.

Prognosis

Laparoscopic splenectomy is safe and efficacious for the treatment of nontraumatic splenic diseases. Studies comparing laparoscopic to open splenectomy have demonstrated decreased blood loss, decreased pain, faster return to normal diet, decreased pulmonary complications, shorter length of hospital stay, and faster return to normal activities. Although in the past large spleens were considered a contraindication to laparoscopic splenectomy, at many institutions these are now routinely removed laparoscopically without an increased complication rate. The conversion rate to an open procedure is less than 5% in most studies. The most common reason cited for conversion is bleeding. There are few absolute contraindications for laparoscopic splenectomy, but as with other laparoscopic procedures, severe cardiac or pulmonary disease may limit the patient's ability to tolerate a pneumoperitoneum. Because of the variceal dilation of the short gastric vessels seen in patients with portal hypertension and cirrhosis, these patients are not considered good candidates for the laparoscopic approach.

LAPAROSCOPIC APPROACH TO INGUINAL HERNIA REPAIR

Laparoscopic inguinal hernia repair is performed using one of two techniques. With the transabdominal preperitoneal (TAPP) approach, the abdominal cavity is entered and the peritoneum overlying the inguinal floor is incised and is elevated from the underlying structures. A large sheet of prosthetic mesh is placed over the entire myopectineal orifice and secured with sutures or staples. The peritoneum is then closed to reduce the frequency of postoperative adhesions to the mesh. Because the abdomen is entered there is an increased risk of injury to visceral or vascular structures. With the totally extraperitoneal (TEP) approach the insufflation and dissection are limited to the preperitoneal space.

With both techniques, the mesh is placed behind the fascial defect; the abdominal forces therefore work to stabilize the repair. Both techniques have a significant learning curve and require a general anesthetic. In a recent review of 34 studies overall recurrence rates were equivalent to the open technique and laparoscopic repair was associated with less postoperative pain and a more rapid return to normal activity.

LAPAROSCOPIC APPROACH TO PANCREATIC CANCER

An important advance in the management of patients with pancreatic cancer is the use of diagnostic laparoscopy for accurate staging of the extent of the disease. Diagnostic laparoscopy allows direct visualization and biopsy of capsular hepatic metastases and peritoneal implants. Diagnostic laparoscopy and computed tomography (CT) are complementary staging procedures. Up to 60% of patients thought to have resectable pancreatic cancer on radiographic grounds are found to have metastases at the time of laparotomy. Minimally invasive surgery plays an important role in accurately identifying patients who will not benefit from pancreatectomy, and to effectively palliate those with biliary or pancreatic obstruction.

Patients with pancreatic cancer can be broadly categorized into one of three groups. First, many patients are found, at radiographic staging, to have metastatic disease and are not candidates for curative pancreatectomy. These patients, however, may require palliation of bile duct obstruction and, in some cases, gastric outlet obstruction. A second group of patients has no radiographic evidence of metastases by CT, but is found at laparotomy to have small hepatic metastases or peritoneal implants. These patients are not suitable for pancreatectomy, but may benefit from palliative bypass procedures. The third group of patients has cancer limited to the pancreas and patients in this group are candidates for potentially curative resection. With the addition of laparoscopic staging, the morbidity and disability of nontherapeutic exploratory laparotomy are reduced.

Patients with bile duct obstruction from unresectable pancreatic cancer can be palliated in one of three ways. Patients with radiographic evidence of metastatic pancreatic cancer are best treated with endoscopic or percutaneous biliary stenting. A smaller number of patients found to have metastatic disease at the time of laparoscopy benefit from laparoscopic cholecystojejunostomy or choledochojejunostomy. In patients with concomitant duodenal obstruction, laparoscopic gastrojejunostomy is performed. This approach is summarized in Figure 13–6.

Recently, the results of open radical resection of pancreatic cancer have improved, both in terms of decreased operative morbidity and mortality and increased cure rates. Although laparoscopic pancreatectomy has been reported, at present this technique has limited applicability and open radical resection of the pancreas is still recommended for curative intent.

LAPAROSCOPIC APPROACHES TO OTHER GASTROINTESTINAL DISEASES

Laparoscopic Approach to Nonparasitic Liver Cysts

Nonparasitic liver cysts are largely asymptomatic and seldom produce functional abnormality of the liver. They can be solitary, multiple, or diffuse in the liver, as in polycystic liver disease. Asymptomatic liver cysts, whether solitary or diffuse, require no treatment. However, some become large, leading to palpable hepatomegaly and abdominal discomfort. These symptomatic patients are candidates for surgical treatment.

Today, laparoscopic fenestration of symptomatic liver cysts is the preferred approach for most patients. After induction of general anesthesia and creation of the pneumoperitoneum, diagnostic laparoscopy is performed and the liver cyst or cysts are identified. The roof of each cyst is widely excised by electrocautery and the excised cyst wall is sent for histologic examination. More than 90% of patients with solitary cysts have improved symptoms after this procedure. Patients with multiple, small cysts throughout the liver have a much higher rate of recurrence of symptoms after surgery. Laparoscopic treatment of liver cysts should be reserved for patients with symptomatic large or solitary cysts.

Laparoscopic Approach to Gastrostomy & Feeding Jejunostomy

For patients requiring access for enteral feeding, the preferred initial approach is percutaneous endoscopic gastrostomy (PEG). Some patients, however, do not tolerate gastrostomy feedings secondary to aspiration, and in others, because of technical reasons, the procedure cannot be performed safely. These patients are candidates for laparoscopic placement of gastrostomy or feeding jejunostomy catheters.

With minimally invasive techniques, feeding catheters are introduced into the gut lumen through the gastric or jejunal wall. Laparoscopic T-fasteners aid in the placement and security of the feeding catheters. These laparoscopic procedures are equivalent to their open surgical counterparts, except that the painful, disabling laparotomy incision is avoided. For patients with neurologic impairment and severe gastroesophageal reflux, a fundoplication procedure can be added to reduce the risk of aspiration.

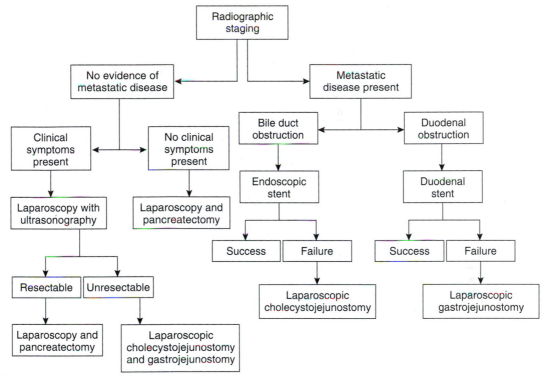

Figure 13–6. An approach to patients with pancreatic cancer.

Laparoscopic Approach to Pancreatic Pseudocysts

Patients who are candidates for internal drainage of pancreatic pseudocysts, particularly those in whom cystogastrostomy is considered, are candidates for a minimally invasive approach. In this operation, ports are placed percutaneously into the stomach, which is distended with gas, exposing the pseudocyst behind the posterior gastric wall. A cystogastrostomy is then created under direct vision with debridement of the pseudocyst cavity and, if necessary, biopsy of the cyst wall to exclude neoplasm. In small studies, this has been found to be a safe and effective approach for the treatment of large pseudocysts.

REFERENCES

ESOPHAGEAL MOTILITY DISORDERS

Annese V et al: Controlled trial of botulinum toxin injection versus placebo and pneumatic dilation in achalasia. Gastroenterlology 1996;111:1418.

Csendes A et al: Late results of a prospective randomized study comparing forceful dilation and esophagomyotomy in patients with achalasia. Gut 1989;30:299.

Hunter JG et al: Laparoscopic Heller myotomy and fundoplication for achalasia. Ann Surg 1997;225:665.

Vogt D et al: Successful treatment of esophageal achalasia with laparoscopic Heller myotomy and Toupet fundoplication. Am J Surg 1997;174:709.

GASTROESOPHAGEAL REFLUX

Bais JE et al: Laparoscopic or conventional Nissen fundoplication for gastro-esophageal reflux disease: randomized clinical trial. Lancet 2000;355:170.

Hunter JG et al: A physiologic approach to laparoscopic fundoplication for gastroesophageal reflux disease. Ann Surg 1996; 223:674.

Lundell L et al: Continued (5-year) followup of a randomized clinical study comparing antireflux surgery and omeprazole in gastroesophageal reflux disease. J Am Coll Surg 200l;192: 172.

Ortiz A et al: Conservative treatment versus antireflux surgery in Barrett's oesophagus: long-term results of a prospective study. Br J Surg 1992;79:1050.

PEPTIC ULCER DISEASE

Cadiere GB et al: Laparoscopic highly selective vagotomy. Hepatogastroenterology 1999;46:1500.

Donahue PE: Ulcer surgery and highly selective vagotomy: Y2K. Arch Surg 1999;134:1373.

Druart ML et al: Laparoscopic repair of perforated duodenal ulcer: a prospective multicenter clinical trial. Surg Endosc 1997; 11:1017.

Lee FYJ et al: Selection of patients for laparoscopic repair of perforated peptic ulcer. Br J Surg 2000;88:133.

CHOLECYSTECTOMY

Bredesen J et al: Early postoperative mortality following cholecystectomy in the entire female population of Denmark, 1977–1981. World J Surg 1992;16:530.

Larson GM et al: Multipractice analysis of laparoscopic cholecystectomy in 1983 patients. Am J Surg 1992;163:221.

Morgenstern L, Wong L, Berci G: Twelve hundred open cholecystectomies before the laparoscopic era. A standard for comparison. Arch Surg 1992;127:400.

Roslyn JJ et al: Open cholecystectomy. A contemporary analysis of 42,474 patients. Ann Surg 1993;218:129.

Savassi-Rocha PR et al: Laparoscopic cholecystectomy in Brazil: analysis of 33,563 cases. Int Surg 1997;82:208.

Z'Graggen K et al: Complications of laparoscopic cholecystectomy in Switzerland. A prospective 3-year study of 10,174 patients. Swiss Association of Laparoscopic and Thoracoscopic Surgery. Surg Endosc 1998;12:1303.

COMMON BILE DUCT EXPLORATION

Crawford DL, Phillips EH: Laparoscopic common bile duct exploration. World J Surg 1999;23:343.

Giurgiu DI et al: Laparoscopic common bile duct exploration: long-term outcome. Arch Surg 1999;134:839.

Liberman MA et al: Cost-effective management of complicated choledocholithiasis; laparoscopic trancystic duct exploration or endoscopic sphinterotomy. J Am Coll Surg 1996;182:488.

Lilly MC, Arregui ME: A balanced approach to choledocholithiasis. Surg Endosc 2001;15:467.

APPENDICITIS

Attwood SEA et al: A prospective randomized trial of laparoscopic versus open appendectomy. Surgery 1992;112:497.

Heikkinen TJ, Haukipuro K, Hulkko A: Cost-effective appendectomy. Open or laparoscopic? A prospective randomized study. Surg Endosc 1998;12:1204.

Kum CK et al: Randomized controlled trial comparing laparoscopic and open appendicectomy. Br J Surg 1993;80:1599.

Pedersen AG et al: Randomized clinical trial of laparoscopic versus open appendicectomy. Br J Surg 2001;88:200.

Reiertsen O et al: Randomized controlled trial with sequential design of laproscopic versus conventional appendicectomy. Br J Surg 1997;84:842.

COLON RESECTION

Gibson M et al: laparoscopic colon resections: a five-year retrospective review. Am Surg 2000;66:245.

Kockerling F et al: Laparoscopic resection of sigmoid diverticulitis: results of a multicenter study. Laparsocopic Colorectal Surgery Study Group. Surg Endosc 1999;13:567.

Metcalf AM: Laparoscopic colectomy. Surg Clin North Am 2000; 80:1321.

Schiedeck Th et al: Laparoscopic surgery for the cure of colorectal cancer: results of a German five-center study. Dis Colon Rectum 2000;43:1.

HEMATOLOGIC SPLENIC DISEASE

Baccarani U et al: Laparoscopic splenectomy for hematological diseases: review of current concepts and opinions. Eur J Surg 1999;165:917.

Glasgow RE, Mulvihill SJ: Laparoscopic splenectomy. World J Surg 1999;23:384.

Katkhouda N, Mavor E: Laparoscopic splenectomy. Surg Clin North Am 2000;80:1285.

Park A et al: Laparoscopic vs. open splenectomy. Arch Surg 1999; 134:1263.

INGUINAL HERNIA

Aeberhard P et al: Prospective audit of laparoscopic totally extraperitoneal inguinal hernia repair: a multicenter study of the Swiss Association for Laparoscopic and Thoracoscopic Surgery (SALTC). Surg Endosc 1999;13:1115.

Chung RS, Towland DY: Meta-analyses of randomized controlled trials of laparoscopic versus conventional inguinal hernia repairs. Surg Endosc 1999;13:689.

Grant A: EU Hernia Trialists' collaboration. Laparoscopic compared with open methods of groin hernia repair: systemic review of randomized controlled trials. Br J Surg 2000;87:860.

PANCREATIC CANCER

Conlon KC et al: The value of minimal access surgery in the staging of patients with potentially resectable peripancreatic malignancy. Ann Surg 1996;223:134.

Friess H et al: The role of diagnostic laparoscopy in pancreatic and periampullary malignancies. J Am Coll Surg 1998;186: 675.

Pisters PWT et al: Laparoscopy in the staging of pancreatic cancer. Br J Surg 2001;88:325.

Imaging Studies in Gastrointestinal & Liver Diseases

14

Judy Yee, MD & Raymond Thornton, MD

There have been important technological advances in the field of radiology in the past 5 years that have impacted significantly on imaging of gastrointestinal and liver diseases. This is a review of the various conventional and state-of-the-art imaging modalities available for gastroenterologic diagnosis. There is an initial presentation of the contrast media available for fluoroscopic gastrointestinal examinations along with their practical applications.

■ CONTRAST MEDIA FOR GASTROINTESTINAL EXAMINATIONS

Barium sulfate is the most commonly used contrast media for opacification of the gastrointestinal tract during fluoroscopy. The selected agent should allow for maximal diagnostic information while posing the least risk to the patient. The clinical history and condition of each patient will determine the appropriate selection of a contrast agent.

BARIUM SULFATE

Barium sulfate is an inert substance that is mixed with water to form a suspension. The weight-to-weight (w/w) and weight-to-volume (w/v) systems are used to describe the dilution. In general, high-density barium (85% w/w or 250% w/v) is used for double-contrast studies and low-density barium (50% w/w or 80% w/v) is used for single-contrast examinations. Barium sulfate provides the best contrast and anatomic detail during fluoroscopy and therefore yields the most diagnostic information.

Risks

If barium leaks into the peritoneal cavity, barium peritonitis occurs. Patients will exhibit signs of acute peritonitis; eventually, granulomas and scarring with adhesions will form. If barium leaks into the mediastinum, an inflammatory reaction occurs that may evolve into scarring and fibrosis; this process is less pronounced than in the peritoneal cavity.

Aspiration of barium into the lungs is usually of minimal clinical significance unless the quantity is large or the patient has significant lung disease. Barium itself is inert and nonirritating to the lungs. Barium has been used in the past for bronchography without complications.

Oral barium should never be given above a colonic obstruction because inspissation will occur. If colonic obstruction is a possibility, a single-contrast barium enema must be performed first.

IODINATED (WATER-SOLUBLE) CONTRAST AGENTS

Iodinated contrast agents used for opacification of the gastrointestinal tract—meglumine diatrizoate and diatrizoate sodium—are water soluble. These agents provide less contrast and reduced anatomic detail compared with barium and are therefore the second choice as contrast agents, based on diagnostic criteria. Iodinated contrast agents may be ionic (less expensive) or nonionic (more expensive).

Risks

There is no risk of chemical peritonitis if iodinated contrast material is spilled into the peritoneal cavity, because it will be absorbed. There may be risk of infection when there is contamination from the gastrointestinal tract.

The ionic iodinated contrast material that is most often used in clinical practice is hyperosmolar; its aspiration into the lungs causes a significant risk of chemical pneumonitis and pulmonary edema that may be intractable. Newer nonionic iodinated contrast agents are more isoosmolar and pose less of a risk when aspirated. However, these agents are more expensive than ionic iodinated contrast material and are not routinely used for opacification of the gastrointestinal tract.

Hyperosmolar iodinated contrast agents may also cause intraluminal movement of fluid, resulting in hypovolemia in children, debilitated patients, or patients with electrolyte imbalances.

PRACTICAL APPLICATIONS

- If a study is being obtained to evaluate for an esophageal perforation, then the study should be initially performed with a small amount of water-soluble contrast media. If no perforation is identified, the study is then repeated with barium.
- If a patient has signs, symptoms, or a history suggestive of an abdominal gastrointestinal tract perforation (eg, perforated duodenal ulcer, perforated colon, anastomotic leak in the immediate postoperative period), water-soluble contrast agents should be used.
- If a patient's condition or history suggests a risk of aspiration (aspiration risk may be assessed by initially giving a small sip of water to see if this induces coughing or choking) or esophagorespiratory fistula, barium should be used. Alternatively, at some institutions nonionic iodinated agents are administered. Examples include patients with depressed mental status who cannot reliably protect their airway, dysfunction of oropharyngeal swallowing mechanism, upper esophageal injury with edema, esophageal obstruction, or gastric outlet obstruction.
- In patients at risk for aspiration in whom a perforated ulcer is suspected, contrast should not be given unless exceptional circumstances exist. In select cases, water-soluble contrast may be carefully administered under fluoroscopic guidance into the stomach via a nasogastric tube. At the end of the study, the remaining contrast should be removed from the stomach via a nasogastric tube to prevent aspiration.
- Most radiologists prefer to wait at least 24 hours following endoscopic biopsy before performing a contrast study of the gastrointestinal tract.
- If there is clinical suspicion of bowel perforation following colonoscopy, computed tomography (CT) of the abdomen and pelvis with the administration of diluted water-soluble contrast per rectum may be more sensitive than conventional enema with diatrizoate sodium.

■ IMAGING MODALITIES

PLAIN FILM

Chest X-ray

An erect chest x-ray should be obtained in the setting of acute abdomen. This is the plain film study of choice for detection of pneumoperitoneum and can also be used to evaluate for chest pathology—such as basilar pneumonias—as the cause of abdominal pain.

Cost: $200–$250.

Plain Film of the Abdomen [Kidney, Ureter, Bladder (KUB)]

The symptom of abdominal pain does not mandate an abdominal film. Clinical judgment and suspected diagnoses in each case should determine if a patient will benefit from an abdominal film. Each film should be examined for abnormal air collections, calcifications, fluid, organomegaly, masses, and foreign bodies, and the bowel gas pattern should be evaluated. The most commonly obtained abdominal film is the supine view. An upright view of the abdomen may be helpful in cases of intestinal obstruction. The left lateral decubitus view may be used for suspected pneumoperitoneum in acutely ill patients when the upright view cannot be obtained.

Pneumoperitoneum is most commonly due to recent abdominal surgery. Persistent or increasing amounts of free air after 3–7 days suggests the possibility of a leaking surgical anastomosis. Perforated peptic ulcer is the second most common cause of pneumoperitoneum. Approximately 80% of perforated ulcers are located in the duodenum, and about 80% of perforated ulcers will result in sufficient free air that is detectable by plain film.

Other causes of pneumoperitoneum include perforation of an abdominal gastrointestinal tract neoplasm or diverticulum (Meckel's or sigmoid diverticulitis), perforated appendix, and traumatic or iatrogenic perforation following an endoscopy or enema. Extensions of air from the chest or retroperitoneum, or through the female genital tract, are other sources of free intraperitoneal air. Rarely, abscess rupture can result in pneumoperitoneum. In addition to the presence of air under the diaphragm, other radiographic evidence of pneumoperitoneum includes (1) **Rigler's sign** (outline of the inner and outer intestinal wall), (2) **football sign** (large ovoid air collection), (3) outline of the falciform ligament, (4) triangle of air seen between bowel loops, (5) perihepatic air, (6) **urachus sign** (outline of the middle umbilical ligament), and (7) **inverted V sign** (outline of the lateral umbilical ligaments).

Pneumoretroperitoneum may be seen as air outlining the kidneys or as streaks of air following the course of the psoas muscles. Causes include perforated duodenal ulcer or traumatic duodenal rupture, dissection of mediastinal air, or trauma or infection of the urinary tract.

Pneumatosis intestinalis, or gas within the bowel wall, may be primary or secondary. Primary or idiopathic pneumatosis is usually benign and most often involves the descending colon and sigmoid. About 85% of cases are secondary and may be due to intestinal ischemia (mesenteric arterial or venous thrombosis or decreased flow), bowel obstruction, trauma, infection, inflammatory bowel disease, connective tissue disorders, and chronic obstructive pulmonary disease. Primary pneumatosis appears radiographically as clusters of radiolucent cysts along the contour of the bowel wall. More linear collections of gas paralleling the wall of the bowel are seen with secondary pneumatosis. Small bowel involvement is more common with the secondary form.

Abnormal gas collections may also be contained within abscesses. Common locations of intraabdominal abscesses include the subphrenic space, lesser sac, Morison's pouch, and pouch of Douglas. Hepatic, splenic, and pancreatic abscesses may also contain air. Necrotic tumor containing air may suggest a fistulous tract to the bowel. Emphysematous cholecystitis can be diagnosed if gas is seen outlining the gallbladder wall or within the gallbladder lumen. It occurs more commonly in patients with diabetes and is thought to be due to ischemic changes of the gallbladder initiated by obstruction of the cystic duct by a stone.

Gas in the portal venous system is an ominous sign and is usually associated with mesenteric vascular thrombosis with associated intestinal ischemia and necrosis. This leads to the development of intramural gas and subsequent extension of gas through mesenteric veins to the portal vein. Gas in the portal venous system follows centrifugal portal venous flow and will appear as branching tubular lucencies extending into the liver periphery.

Gas in the biliary system may result from prior sphincterotomy or surgery, eg, choledochoenterostomy. It may also be seen with biliary-enteric fistula as a result of penetrating duodenal ulcer. Scarring of the ampulla owing to Crohn's disease, parasitic infection, or malignancy are other causes of pneumobilia. Rarely, biliary sepsis resulting from gas-producing bacteria can cause biliary tract gas. Biliary gas appears as centrally located tubular lucencies as it follows biliary drainage into the larger bile ducts.

Abnormal calcifications may also be detected on the abdominal film. Lamellated calcifications in the right upper quadrant are typical for gallstones. Only 10% of gallstones are radiopaque whereas 90% of urinary tract calculi are radiopaque. Porcelain gallbladder describes sheet-like wall calcifications of the gallbladder and is associated with a high incidence of gallbladder carcinoma, for which prophylactic cholecystectomy is recommended. A focal calcification in the right lower abdomen may represent an appendicolith, which is seen in 10–15% of patients with acute appendicitis. Mucocele of the appendix may appear as circular or rim calcification in the same location. Enteroliths may also be found in small or large bowel diverticula. Infections such as tuberculosis or *Pneumocystis carinii* can cause visceral or nodal calcifications. Alternatively, calcified

lymph nodes may represent metastatic tumoral involvement. Certain tumors more commonly calcify. Mucinous adenocarcinoma of the stomach, colon, and ovary can cause mottled or punctate calcifications in the primary tumor as well as in metastatic foci. Gastrointestinal tract leiomyomas and lipomas may also calcify. Pancreatic calcifications more commonly occur in association with chronic pancreatitis or pancreatic pseudocyst. Pancreatic tumors that calcify include the rare serous cystadenoma and mucinous cystic neoplasm.

Ascitic fluid initially accumulates in the pelvis, where symmetric bulges of increased density ("dog ears") may be seen on either side of the bladder. Thickening of the peritoneal flank stripe and increased distance (>3 mm) between the properitoneal fat and ascending colon are seen. With increased ascites, the right inferolateral margin of the liver becomes obscured and there is medial displacement of the liver and of the ascending and descending colon. With marked ascites there is diffuse haziness or a ground-glass appearance of the abdomen, and bowel loops may appear to separate or float centrally.

The **pattern of bowel dilatation** on the abdominal film can suggest adynamic ileus versus mechanical bowel obstruction. The radiographic pattern of **adynamic ileus** is uniform dilatation of both small and large bowel with gas present in the rectum. Clinically, the abdomen is distended and bowel sounds are decreased or absent. Adynamic ileus is common after abdominal surgery but may also be caused by peritonitis, hypokalemia, metabolic disorders, trauma, mesenteric ischemia, and various medications, such as morphine and barbiturates. Localized ileus in which there is an isolated loop of dilated bowel (**sentinel loop**) is due to an adjacent acute inflammatory process. Pancreatitis can cause dilatation of the proximal small bowel and transverse colon whereas appendicitis will cause dilatation of the cecum and distal ileum.

Mechanical small or large bowel obstruction will cause dilatation of bowel proximal to the level of obstruction. The contour of dilated bowel is also examined for evidence of thickening or of thumbprinting, which is suggestive of ischemia. Bowel obstruction at two different sites produces a closed loop obstruction. The appearance of air-fluid levels at the same height suggests an ileus, whereas the appearance of air–fluid levels at different heights is compatible with mechanical obstruction (Figure 14–1).

Adhesions, incarcerated hernia, tumor, and inflammatory bowel disease are common causes of small bowel obstruction. Colon carcinoma and diverticulitis are the most common causes of large bowel obstruction. Occasionally it may be unclear as to whether an obstruction is at the level of the distal small bowel or ascending colon. A barium enema should be the initial study before administering barium orally. Obstruction

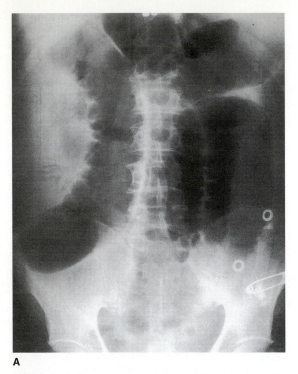

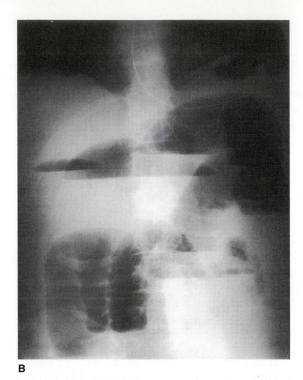

A   B

Figure 14–1. **A:** Supine plain film of the abdomen demonstrates multiple air-filled, markedly dilated small bowel loops with relative paucity of colonic air. **B:** Upright film of the abdomen in the same patient demonstrates air–fluid levels of different heights, consistent with mechanical small bowel obstruction. At surgery, adhesions were found in the distal ileum, causing obstruction.

from a sigmoid volvulus produces a distinctive inverted U-shaped dilated sigmoid, which is a type of closed loop obstruction (Figure 14–2). A contrast enema typically reveals a beak-like tapering of the contrast column at the site of mesenteric twist.

    Cost: $225–$350.

DEGLUTITION STUDY

The **deglutition study** is an assessment of swallowing function. The oropharyngeal phase of swallowing is a complex but organized series of events that transports a bolus from the oral cavity to the upper esophageal sphincter (cricopharyngeus). After relaxation of the cricopharyngeus, the bolus passes into the cervical esophagus and is propelled by peristalsis down the thoracic esophagus and into the stomach. Regulation of the swallowing mechanism is mediated by cranial nerves: (V) trigeminal, (VII) facial, (IX) glossopharyngeal, (X) vagus, and (XII) hypoglossal, all of which are involved with innervation of the intrinsic pharyngeal muscles. Support muscles are innervated by the accessory (XI) nerve and the first three cervical nerves.

The ingested bolus is transported from the mouth posteriorly into the oropharynx as swallowing starts. Pharyngeal peristalsis continues propulsion of the bolus through the hypopharynx. The larynx closes and elevates as the epiglottis deflects.

A. INDICATIONS

Impairment of the oropharyngeal swallowing mechanism can produce symptoms such as coughing, choking, dysphagia, regurgitation, and hoarseness. Aspiration pneumonia may be the initial sign of swallowing dysfunction. Symptoms often are nonspecific, and the patient may complain of a symptom distant from the actual location of a lesion. Patients with mid or distal esophageal mechanical obstruction may present with referred pharyngeal or cervical dysphagia.

    Oropharyngeal dysphagia may be caused by structural lesions (head and neck tumors, webs, diverticula), diseases of the central nervous system [cerebrovascular accident (CVA), neoplasms, poliomyelitis, extrapyramidal disease], muscle disorders (polymyositis, dermatomyositis), and myasthenia gravis.

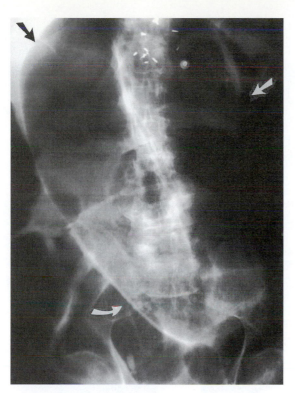

Figure 14–2. Large bowel obstruction due to a sigmoid volvulus. Air-filled dilated sigmoid has a distinctive inverted U-shaped appearance ***(arrows).*** This is a type of closed loop obstruction. Beak-like tapering is typically seen on contrast enema.

The deglutition study is a cooperative study performed by the radiologist and speech pathologist. During the study, patients are instructed to ingest barium liquids of various consistencies as well as barium-coated solids. If the patient demonstrates swallowing difficulty, various compensatory maneuvers may be attempted to relieve symptoms. The entire study is performed under fluoroscopy and is videotaped. This provides a dynamic recording of each phase of swallowing that can be reviewed frame by frame for complete evaluation.

B. Cost

$410–$550.

ESOPHAGRAM (BARIUM SWALLOW)

A complete esophagram consists of an evaluation of the oral cavity, pharynx, and esophagus. Although more extensive radiographic evaluation of oropharyngeal function is usually performed in a formal deglutition study, gross imaging of this area during the esophagram can

detect significant motility abnormalities. Mass lesions of the oral cavity, however, are not easily identified on barium study unless they are large.

Biphasic barium radiography of the esophagus using both single- and double-contrast techniques is the preferred method for evaluation of the esophagus. The advantages of each technique are discussed in the following sections.

Single Contrast

A. Indications

The single-contrast technique is used to study both the pharynx and the esophagus. Pharyngeal contour and distensibility are well demonstrated and webs, pharyngeal pouches, and Zenker's diverticulum can be detected. The single-contrast phase of the esophagram provides information on esophageal motility as well as esophageal contour and distension. Primary peristalsis is stimulated by the swallowing process and propels the bolus down the esophagus into the stomach. Secondary peristalsis is stimulated by focal distension, such as that due to residual bolus or reflux, and can start anywhere in the esophagus. Tertiary contractions are nonpropulsive segmental contractions that may occur in many asymptomatic patients and with increasing frequency in the elderly. Motility disorders of the esophagus, such as achalasia and diffuse esophageal spasm, are well demonstrated with the single-contrast technique. Esophageal motility disorders are optimally evaluated by videotape recording, although rapid filming by cine provides a more permanent hard copy of the examination.

Significant esophageal contour abnormalities, such as benign or malignant strictures, are evaluated with the single-contrast technique (Figure 14–3). More subtle strictures may be detected by the delayed passage of an administered barium pill. Extrinsic processes impressing on or displacing the esophagus are also well visualized on single-contrast images.

Varices will cause a scalloped or serpiginous contour of the esophagus with a changeable configuration depending on peristalsis, respiration, and the degree of distension. They are best seen on partially collapsed single-contrast views of the esophagus (Figure 14–4). Overdistension and peristalsis tend to obliterate these dilated submucosal veins. Traditionally, endoscopy has been more reliable than the esophagram in the detection of varices.

A single-contrast esophagram has limited usefulness in the diagnosis of gastroesophageal reflux. Spontaneous gastroesophageal reflux may occur during the single-contrast portion of the examination; however, this may not be clinically significant, since spontaneous reflux is observed fluoroscopically in 40% of asymptomatic individuals. On the other hand, fluoroscopic demonstration of reflux is found in only 40% of pa-

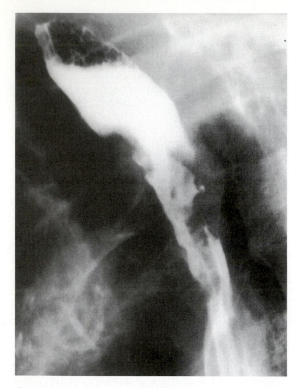

Figure 14–3. Single-contrast image of a typical malignant stricture due to squamous cell carcinoma located in the proximal esophagus with nodularity, fold thickening, and evidence of abrupt narrowing due to concentric mass. Contour abnormalities, such as benign or malignant esophageal strictures, are evaluated with the single-contrast technique.

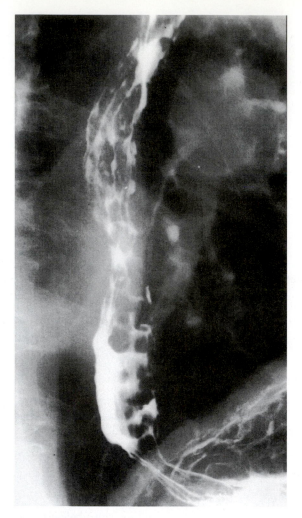

Figure 14–4. Multiple esophageal varices representing dilated submucosal veins. Varices are best visualized on partially collapsed single-contrast views. A scalloped contour of the esophagus with a changeable configuration is observed. Overdistension will obliterate the varices.

tients who have endoscopic evidence of reflux esophagitis. Although various provocative maneuvers, such as increasing intraabdominal pressure, have been used by radiologists to elicit reflux during the esophagram, the significance of the results obtained is controversial.

B. Contraindications

Single-contrast barium swallow is contraindicated in patients with esophageal perforation. In these patients, water-soluble contrast media may be administered. If no perforation is identified, a barium swallow may then be performed.

C. Patient Preparation

Patients should fast for at least 1 hour before the study.

D. Cost

$385–$410.

Double Contrast

A. Indications

Double-contrast imaging of the pharynx and esophagus is obtained as part of a standard biphasic esophagram. Mucosal lesions of the pharynx, such as lymphoid hyperplasia, ulcerations, and masses, are best seen with this technique. Most pharyngeal masses are malignant epithelial neoplasms (squamous cell carcinoma), although lymphomas, sarcomas, and benign tumors can occur in this location. An intraluminal mass or mucosal irregularity accompanied by asymmetric decreased distensibility is a suggestive finding.

Double-contrast views may also show extension of tumor into the valleculae, base of tongue, inferior hypopharynx, and pharyngoesophageal segment, which are areas that are difficult to evaluate by endoscopy. In addition, this technique can play a complementary role to endoscopy by allowing evaluation of areas distal to strictures or bulky masses. In patients in whom a pharyngeal carcinoma is detected, the esophagram may also demonstrate a second site of carcinoma in either the pharynx or esophagus. A second primary tumor develops in approximately 10% of patients with squamous cell carcinoma of the head and neck. About 1% of patients will develop synchronous or metachronous esophageal carcinoma.

Double-contrast esophagography allows significantly improved evaluation of the mucosa of the esophagus as compared with single-contrast images. The esophageal lumen is distended by administered effervescent granules and the esophagus is coated by high-density barium. This technique is best for identification of superficial esophageal carcinomas and for evaluation of malignant neoplasms in general (Figure 14–5). In cases of high-grade malignant esophageal strictures, double-contrast views may be difficult to obtain and the single-contrast technique is employed.

Double-contrast technique is the preferred method for demonstrating mucosal ulcerations, plaques, and nodular lesions associated with esophagitis. A granular or mildly nodular mucosal pattern with ulcerations involving the distal esophagus is typical for reflux esophagitis, especially if associated with a hiatal hernia or fluoroscopic evidence of gastroesophageal reflux.

More defined mucosal nodules with plaque formation, cobblestoning, or a shaggy-appearing esophagus are findings of *Candida* esophagitis. Recent studies have shown that the double-contrast technique is up to 90% sensitive in diagnosing esophageal candidiasis. Focal, shallow, mid-esophageal ulcerations may suggest herpes simplex, esophagitis, or drug-induced esophagitis. One or more giant superficial ulcers (>2 cm) is suggestive of cytomegalovirus (CMV) esophagitis, especially in patients with acquired immunodeficiency syndrome (AIDS).

The advantages of an esophagram are its low relative cost and low risk compared with endoscopy. Esophagoscopy, however, has the advantage of allowing biopsy samples or brushings to be taken for histology and culture.

B. CONTRAINDICATIONS

Double-contrast barium swallow is contraindicated in patients with esophageal perforation. In these patients water-soluble contrast media may be administered. If

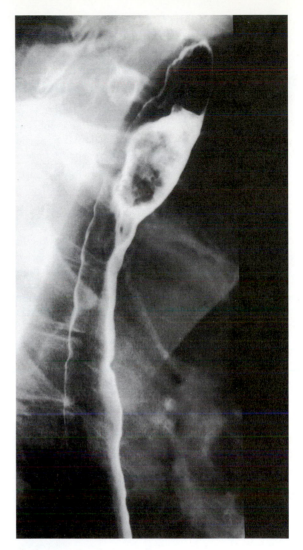

Figure 14–5. Double-contrast view from an esophagram demonstrating a large intraluminal mass of the proximal esophagus that represents squamous cell carcinoma. This technique is preferred for evaluating malignancy in general as well as for demonstrating mucosal lesions, such as those associated with esophagitis.

no perforation is identified, a barium swallow may then be performed.

C. PATIENT PREPARATION

Patients should fast for at least 1 hour before the study.

D. COST

$385–$410.

UPPER GASTROINTESTINAL STUDY

Biphasic barium evaluation is the radiologic study of choice for the stomach. This method takes advantage of the complementary information that can be obtained by the use of both the single- and double-contrast techniques.

The routine upper gastrointestinal study (UGI) series consists of double-contrast views of the esophagus, stomach, and proximal small bowel followed by single-contrast images of these areas in the prone or upright positions.

Single Contrast

A. INDICATIONS

Single-contrast images are obtained following the administration of low-density barium. Spot compression of portions of the lumen filled with barium will demonstrate filling defects due to thickened folds, large ulcerations, or masses (Figure 14–6). Abnormalities of motility and contour are well depicted, such as linitis plastica due to scirrhous adenocarcinoma of the stomach (Figure 14–7). Gastric varices are best seen on single-contrast or partially collapsed double-contrast images.

A single-contrast examination alone is performed in certain clinical settings. This includes patients who are

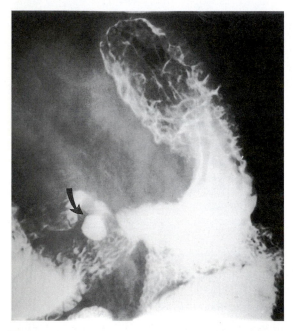

Figure 14–6. Large, rounded barium collection *(arrow)* representing a duodenal bulb ulcer crater seen with single-contrast technique on UGI series.

obtunded, debilitated, or have limited mobility, in whom a double-contrast study is not possible. Patients who have had recent abdominal surgery often cannot tolerate a double-contrast examination. In patients with suspected gastric outlet obstruction or gastric motility disorders, the single-contrast technique also is used. The primary cause of gastric outlet obstruction in adults is peptic ulcer disease involving the duodenal bulb or pyloric channel. These patients often have large amounts of residual fluid and debris in the stomach, making a double-contrast study impossible to perform.

B. CONTRAINDICATIONS

Suspected gastric or bowel perforation is a contraindication (in which case water-soluble contrast material is used).

C. PATIENT PREPARATION

An overnight fast is required prior to the study. Patients are asked to refrain from smoking on the day of the study to minimize gastric secretions.

D. COST

$600–$620.

Double Contrast

A. INDICATIONS

Double-contrast images are obtained following administration of an effervescent agent and high-density barium. This technique is best for demonstrating mucosal detail and is more sensitive for detecting erosions, ulcerations, and polyps. A double-contrast UGI series can define changes due to infectious gastritis, such as CMV or cryptosporidiosis, presenting as mucosal nodularity, ulceration, fold thickening, or antral narrowing. *Helicobacter pylori* gastritis may cause nonspecific fold thickening. However, endoscopy with biopsies and culture is required for the diagnosis of infectious gastritis.

Double-contrast study of mucosal abnormalities surrounding an ulcer is helpful in distinguishing benign versus malignant ulcers. Most gastric ulcers and almost all duodenal ulcers are benign. Features of a benign gastric ulcer include a round ulcer crater with a smooth mound of edema or regular mucosal folds that radiate to the rim of the crater. Benign ulcers tend to project outside the expected line of the gastric lumen when viewed in profile. Malignant gastric ulcers have an irregular eccentric ulcer crater with distortion of the surrounding mucosa. Radiating folds are nodular, thickened, and fused and do not extend to the crater edge. Malignant ulcers do not project beyond the gastric lumen when viewed in profile. Unequivocally benign gastric ulcers may be followed with a repeat radiographic study in 2–3 months until healing is com-

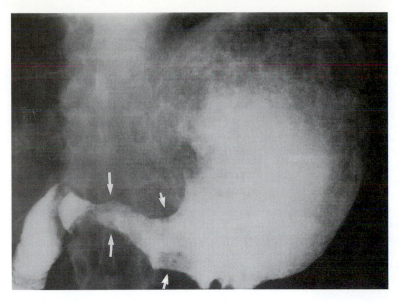

Figure 14–7. Single-contrast image from UGI series demonstrating markedly distended proximal stomach. Stomach shows retained fluid and debris with fixed rigid narrowing of the antrum *(arrows)* due to scirrhous adenocarcinoma (linitis plastica or leather bottle stomach). Double-contrast technique is not performed due to residual material in the stomach.

plete. However, equivocal or suspicious ulcers, or ulcers that do not heal after 2–3 months, require endoscopy with biopsy to exclude gastric malignancy. Mucosal lesions such as polyps or nodules (see Figure 14–8) and submucosal lesions such as leiomyomas are best imaged by double-contrast technique (see Figure 14–8).

B. CONTRAINDICATIONS

Double-contrast studies are contraindicated in patients who have complete gastric outlet obstruction, large amounts of retained gastric fluid, or suspected perfora-

tion, in which case water-soluble contrast material is used. They are unfeasible in patients who are unable to cooperate for the study or have limited mobility.

C. PATIENT PREPARATION

An overnight fast is required before the study. Patients are asked to refrain from smoking on the day of the study to minimize gastric secretions.

D. COST

$700–$750.

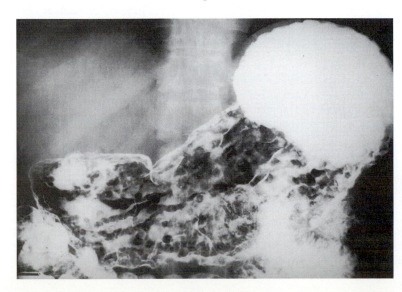

Figure 14–8. Multiple small nodular filling defects scattered diffusely throughout the stomach with central ulceration, causing bulls-eye appearance seen on this double-contrast UGI series. This is typical of hematogenous metastases to the stomach due to metastatic melanoma.

SMALL BOWEL FOLLOW-THROUGH EXAMINATION

The primary imaging modality for small bowel disease is the barium study. The small bowel follow-through (SBFT) is one of the most commonly employed techniques to evaluate diseases of the small bowel. A plain film of the abdomen is routinely obtained before contrast administration. SBFT is most often performed immediately following a double-contrast UGI series, for which the patient has already ingested an effervescent agent and high-density barium. Additional low-density barium is administered for the routine SBFT so as to completely fill the small bowel. Overhead radiographs and compression spot films of small bowel loops are obtained at sequential time intervals. Careful compression under fluoroscopy is essential to separate overlapping bowel loops. The terminal ileum and a portion of the cecum or ascending colon must be imaged before the study is complete. Normal transit of contrast through the small bowel into the colon is variable, most often spanning 1–2 hours. Accelerating agents such as metoclopromide or meglumine diatrizoate mixed with barium can be given in cases of slow transit.

The **dedicated SBFT** is a study performed independently of a UGI series. The patient ingests only low-density barium so that there is more uniform opacification of the small bowel. More accurate evaluation is possible, since artifacts from mixing of gas and barium suspensions of different density are avoided.

Over the past 5 years there has been increased use of a premixed suspension of barium and methylcellulose that is given to patients orally for a "see-through" SBFT. This allows for a translucent appearance of the small bowel resulting in improved evaluation of overlapping bowel loops and better delineation of bowel folds.

A. INDICATIONS

SBFT should be the initial study performed in patients with nonspecific symptoms (Figure 14–9) who elicit low clinical suspicion for small bowel pathology. These patients often have had negative findings on upper and lower endoscopy. Therefore, in most of these patients a "see-through" SBFT is preferred. SBFT is also indicated for further evaluation of high-grade small bowel obstruction located proximally within the first few feet of the jejunum (Figure 14–10). For these patients a dedicated SBFT using barium alone is preferred.

SBFT is technically less difficult and less expensive, and requires a smaller radiation dose than enteroclysis. It is the preferred study in female patients of child-bearing age with possible small bowel disease. A small percentage of patients who require enteroclysis but who refuse tube placement or who have unsuccessful tube placement will require SBFT.

B. CONTRAINDICATIONS

Small bowel follow-through is contraindicated in patients with bowel perforation.

C. PATIENT PREPARATION

An overnight fast is required before the study.

D. COST

$500–$530 (dedicated SBFT); $760–$800 (UGI with SBFT).

ENTEROCLYSIS (SMALL BOWEL ENEMA)

Enteroclysis is the optimal method for establishing small bowel as normal. After the administration of 10–20 mg of metaclopramide intravenously and topical anesthesia for the nostril and throat, a special balloon-tipped enteroclysis catheter containing a guidewire is inserted from the nose into the stomach and guided fluoroscopically into the proximal jejunum. Once the tip of the catheter is about 5 cm distal to the ligament of Treitz, the balloon is inflated. Barium followed by methylcellulose is infused at high rates via a pump into the jejunum. Careful compression spot films of each quadrant and overhead films are obtained. Difficulty in tube placement is encountered in patients with pyloric or duodenal scarring. Large sliding hiatal hernias or prior surgery, such as gastroduodenostomy and gastrojejunostomy, also may preclude tube placement.

Enteroclysis demonstrates excellent mucosal detail, fold pattern, and bowel distension (Figure 14–11). Through the adjustment of infusion rates, adequate distension of the entire small bowel can be achieved. This makes it easier to recognize areas of subtle narrowing that may not be detected on conventional SBFT. Enteroclysis is more invasive, requiring either nasal- or oral-jejunal catheter placement. Enteroclysis is also approximately twice as expensive as a dedicated SBFT, and delivers a higher radiation dose to the patient (one and one-half times greater than UGI with SBFT and three times greater than dedicated SBFT). However, enteroclysis has a shorter total examination completion time, approximately 30 minutes. Many studies demonstrate a high sensitivity (93–100%), specificity (89–99%), and accuracy (96–99%) of enteroclysis for evaluation of the small bowel.

A. INDICATIONS

Enteroclysis is particularly helpful in patients with partial small bowel obstruction, a history of radiation or pelvic surgery, suspected primary or secondary small bowel tumor, Meckel's diverticulum, malabsorption, and chronic unexplained gastrointestinal bleeding. (Arteriovenous malformations of the small bowel are a common cause of occult gastrointestinal bleeding but

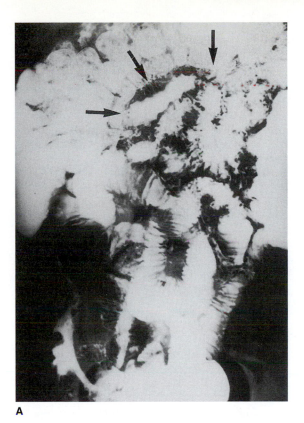
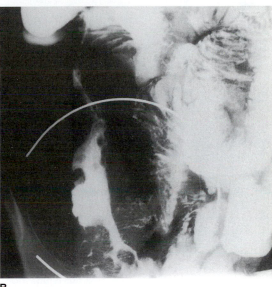

A

B

Figure 14–9. **A:** Overhead film from a small bowel follow-through examination with barium filling entire small bowel and proximal colon in a patient with nonspecific abdominal complaints. Fold thickening and nodularity are present, involving the jejunum *(arrow).* The terminal ileum is straightened, rigid, and narrowed. **B:** Spot compression view of the terminal ileum from the same patient showing "string sign," nodularity, and ulcerations typical of Crohn's disease.

cannot be demonstrated by enteroclysis.) Enteroclysis is the best examination for demonstrating the features of early Crohn's disease, such as a granular mucosal pattern, distorted folds, and small nodules. It is also the best study for evaluating the extent of involvement of Crohn's disease, especially if surgical management is being considered. This technique can help distinguish areas of fibrotic stricture due to Crohn's disease from spasm by demonstrating the degree of distensibility. Ulcerations, cobblestoning, and fistulas are particularly well demonstrated. Enteroclysis should also be performed if conventional SBFT is negative but there is high clinical suspicion of small bowel abnormality.

B. CONTRAINDICATIONS

Patients with complete small bowel obstruction or possible perforation should be excluded.

C. PATIENT PREPARATION

This is the same as for barium enema (to prevent artifacts and slow intestinal flow due to a filled ascending colon or ileum).

D. COST

$900–$1,000.

PERORAL PNEUMOCOLON

The peroral pneumocolon may be performed either as an individual examination or following SBFT. The patient ingests low-density barium, after which sequential films are obtained. When the oral contrast reaches the ascending colon to mid-transverse colon, air is insufflated through a rectal tube until the cecum is distended. This air then refluxes into the terminal ileum, providing a double-contrast appearance. Compression

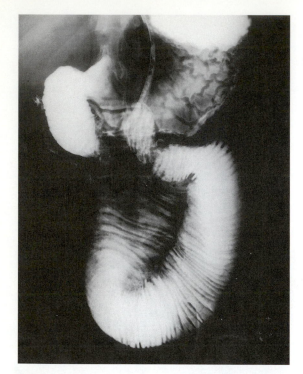

Figure 14–10. Small bowel follow-through examination in a patient with high-grade proximal jejunal obstruction due to an adhesion. The significantly dilated loop of proximal jejunum demonstrates a coiled appearance representing a closed loop construction.

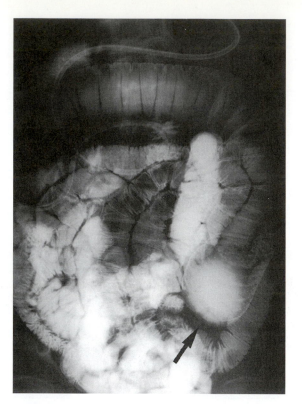

Figure 14–11. Enteroclysis or small bowel enema study that optimally demonstrates mucosal detail, fold pattern, and distension. This is the optimal study for evaluating partial small bowel obstruction. This patient has a dilated jejunal loop with a transition point to decompressed bowel, which is easily identified *(arrow)*. An adhesion found at surgery correlated exactly to this level in the jejunum.

spot films are obtained. Occasionally, glucagon is administered to relax the ileocecal valve and to facilitate reflux.

A. INDICATIONS

The peroral pneumocolon is used to specifically evaluate the terminal ileum. The peroral pneumocolon is more sensitive for disease of the terminal ileum than is the SBFT alone. The SBFT with peroral pneumocolon is often useful for patients with known terminal ileal disease, however, it is not as accurate as enteroclysis for proximal disease. It can also be used for evaluation of the ascending colon or cecum when a barium enema is unsuccessful or equivocal.

B. CONTRAINDICATIONS

It is contraindicated in cases of toxic megacolon.

C. PATIENT PREPARATION

This is the same as for barium enema (see the following section).

D. COST

$100–$125 added to cost of UGI series.

CONTRAST ENEMA

Thorough patient preparation for a barium enema, as described below, is essential for accurate interpretation of the study. In acute situations, such as obstruction or inflammatory bowel disease, colonic preparation may be unfeasible or limited. A plain film of the abdomen is obtained immediately before beginning a contrast enema. Residual contrast material from prior radiology study or retained fecal material may be detected, which may preclude the current examination. The bowel gas pattern is reviewed to evaluate for obstruction or pneumatosis. If toxic megacolon is suspected, contrast enema is contraindicated. Glucagon may be given intravenously to reduce colonic spasm during the study.

Single Contrast

About 15% of barium enemas are performed as single-contrast studies. Low-density barium is administered per rectum, and the leading edge of the contrast column is followed under fluoroscopy. Careful graded compression is applied as films are taken. The single-contrast examination is able to demonstrate bowel distensibility, contour deformities, larger filling defects, bowel obstruction, and fistulas or sinus tracts.

A. INDICATIONS

The single-contrast barium enema is performed in specific situations only. It is used for suspected large bowel obstruction and diverticulitis, in the very young or elderly, and in those who are debilitated or unable to cooperate for a double-contrast enema. Fistulas and sinus tracts involving the colon, such as in Crohn's disease, are particularly well demonstrated with the single-contrast technique. A good rule to remember is that a poor double-contrast enema is worse than a poor single-contrast enema.

B. CONTRAINDICATIONS

Single-contrast barium enema should not be performed in patients with toxic megacolon, suspected severe acute ulcerative colitis, or possible colonic perforation, or immediately after endoscopic biopsy (wait 24 hours). Also, it should not be used if a double-contrast examination is needed to evaluate the mucosa and to detect small lesions.

C. PATIENT PREPARATION

See the following section.

D. COST

$620–$660.

Double Contrast

The double-contrast barium enema involves the administration of high-density barium into the colon per rectum followed by air insufflation. It is also called **air-contrast barium enema (ACBE)** or **pneumocolon**.

A. INDICATIONS

ACBE is the recommended radiographic study for evaluation of mucosal detail. It is used for detecting polyps or tumors and for demonstrating early inflammatory disease of the colon, such as fine ulcerations and mucosal granularity (Figures 14–12 and 14–13).

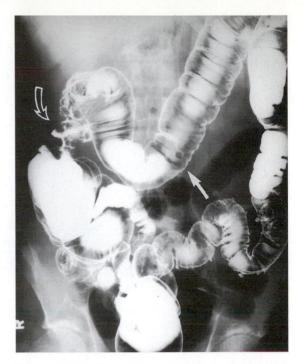

Figure 14–12. Typical "apple-core" annular carcinoma involving the ascending colon and hepatic flexure. Lesion is well demonstrated on this double-contrast barium enema **(open arrow)**. In addition, a small sessile polyp is present in the transverse colon **(arrow)** and there are small sigmoid diverticula.

The role of the double-contrast barium enema versus colonoscopy in the screening and detection of colorectal carcinoma remains controversial. Screening strategies are still evolving and being evaluated. CT colonography (virtual colonoscopy) is a new radiologic technique that combines helical CT and graphic software to create two- and three-dimensional views of the colon. It has been used successfully to detect colonic polyps and cancer in preliminary trials and will likely play a role in colorectal cancer screening. In the work-up of the individual patient, the clinician must consider a given method's cost effectiveness and proven efficacy in reducing mortality. Colonic lesions such as polyps or carcinomas greater than 1 cm are detected by barium enema with an accuracy of 90–95%, which is similar to the accuracy of colonoscopy. However, a recent study comparing double-contrast barium enema and colonoscopy in patients following polypectomy found that the barium enema examination had a sensitivity of 48% for polyps larger than 10 mm. Colonoscopy is more sensitive than barium enema for detecting polyps

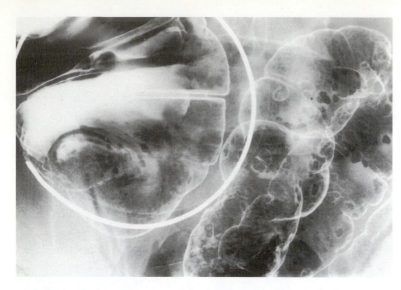

Figure 14–13. Spot view from a double-contrast barium enema revealing innumerable small polyps in a patient with familial adenomatous polyposis.

less than 7 mm, however, these diminutive polyps are rarely malignant, are often hyperplastic, and their clinical importance is unclear. In general, colonoscopy is about three times higher in cost than a barium enema and has up to a five times higher complication rate. Colonoscopy may be technically difficult in certain individuals and visualization of the whole colon may not be possible. In about 5% of patients, the cecum is not reached, and an estimated 10–20% of colonic lesions can be missed. Barium enema or CT colonography is the diagnostic tool for such situations and can offer evaluation of the right colon.

B. CONTRAINDICATIONS

These include the previously mentioned contraindications to single-contrast barium enema. Any patient with suspected colonic perforation requires a water-soluble contrast enema if the exact site of perforation needs to be demonstrated. Toxic megacolon is also a contraindication to barium enema. Colonic obstruction (eg, volvulus), diverticulitis, and colonic fistulas are better evaluated by the single-contrast technique.

C. PATIENT PREPARATION

A typical colonic cleansing preparation for contrast enema includes: (1) 24-hour clear liquid diet and no breakfast on the day of the study, (2) 350 mL magnesium citrate at lunch and four bisacodyl tablets in the evening before the study, and (3) one bisacodyl suppository in the morning of the study.

D. COST

$800–$900.

Water-Soluble Contrast Enema

A. INDICATIONS

The water-soluble contrast enema is primarily used in patients with suspected colonic perforation. This includes patients who have had recent instrumentation, surgery, or trauma. Water-soluble enemas can be used with caution in patients with the potential for perforation (such as those with colonic distension) when further anatomic delineation is necessary. Water-soluble contrast also is preferred for evaluation of possible colovesical fistula. Finally, the administration of water-soluble hyperosmolar contrast can also be used as a therapeutic maneuver to evacuate stool in cases of severe fecal impaction.

B. CONTRAINDICATIONS

Patients with toxic megacolon should be excluded.

C. PATIENT PREPARATION

Although a bowel preparation is preferred, water-soluble enemas are often obtained in situations in which colonic cleansing is not possible.

D. COST

$660–$750.

BILIARY IMAGING

Ultrasound

Real-time ultrasound is the imaging modality of choice for evaluation of the gallbladder and biliary ducts. The liver and pancreas are also routinely imaged when evaluating for biliary tract disease. Ultrasound is noninvasive and does not use ionizing radiation. Scanning units are portable and bedside examinations are possible. This modality can also be used to guide fine-needle biopsy, percutaneous transhepatic cholangiography, and biliary drainage procedures. **Intravenous cholangiography (IVC)**, which is associated with significant toxic reactions to the contrast material and poor opacification of the bile ducts in patients with a bilirubin greater than 2 mg/dL, has largely been replaced by sonography.

Relative limitations of ultrasound include the dependence of diagnostic accuracy on the skill of the operator performing the study, patient cooperation, and body habitus. Obese patients image poorly. Bowel gas or recently administered barium also will interfere with image quality.

A. INDICATIONS

Ultrasound has a 95% sensitivity for the detection of cholelithiasis. A gallstone can be diagnosed unequivocally when a mobile hyperechoic intraluminal mass is present with acoustic shadowing. Sonography has been demonstrated to be 15–20% more sensitive than oral cholecystography (OCG) and has a lower false-positive rate. Hence, it has largely supplanted OCG in most circumstances. Ultrasound is the initial examination of choice in cases of suspected acute cholecystitis because it is noninvasive, is readily available, and has excellent sensitivity for this entity. Sonographic findings supporting this diagnosis include the presence of gallstones, gallbladder wall thickening (greater than 3 mm), and pericholecystic fluid, and the detection of maximum tenderness directly over the gallbladder (sonographic **Murphy's sign**). When these findings are present there is a high (>90%) sensitivity in the diagnosis of acute cholecystitis (Figure 14–14). Ultrasound is less useful in the diagnosis of acalculous cholecystitis, demonstrating a 60–70% sensitivity for detection of this condition. The presence of gallbladder wall thickening is suggestive but not specific. Radionuclide imaging has a similar diagnostic sensitivity to ultrasound for acalculous cholecystitis.

Ultrasound is less capable of detecting choledocholithiasis than gallstones, with reported sensitivity ranging from as low as 13% to as high as 75%. The true sensitivity likely falls between these two figures. The difficulty arises in visualizing an intraductal stone, particularly if it is located in the distal common bile duct. These stones often do not demonstrate acoustic shadowing. Although dilated extrahepatic ducts are commonly seen in patients with choledocholithiasis, nondilated ducts are present in up to 30%, making sonographic diagnosis even more difficult. Therefore, a "negative" ultrasound does not reliably exclude chole-

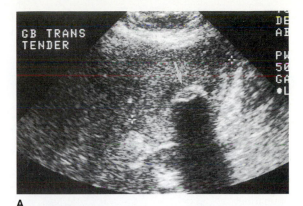

A

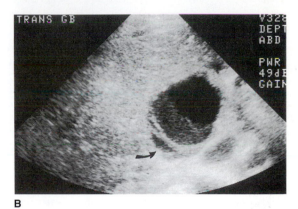

B

Figure 14–14. **A:** Ultrasound in a patient with acute cholecystitis, demonstrating a sludge-filled, thick-walled gallbladder containing a hyperechoic stone with acoustic shadowing *(arrow)*. A sonographic Murphy's sign was also present. Ultrasound has a high sensitivity for acute cholecystitis when these findings are present. **B:** Ultrasound of the gallbladder in another patient with acute cholecystitis demonstrating sludge and a small amount of pericholecystic fluid *(arrow)* but no stones. This patient had a sonographic Murphy's sign.

docholithiasis. Endoscopic retrograde cholangiopancreatography (ERCP) is the definitive diagnostic study.

Ultrasound is very valuable in the evaluation of the jaundiced patient with biliary obstruction. It is 95% accurate in the detection of biliary ductal dilatation although it may not be able to determine whether the obstruction is due to a stone, tumor, or stricture. Direct visualization of the bile ducts by ERCP or percutaneous transhepatic cholangiography is required to define the cause, at which time brushings and biopsies may also be obtained. CT has a sensitivity comparable to ultrasound for the diagnosis of bile duct obstruction and is more likely than sonography to demonstrate the cause.

A CT using thin sections through the pancreas and portal region should be obtained if tumor is suspected as the cause of biliary obstruction.

B. CONTRAINDICATIONS

There are none.

C. PATIENT PREPARATION

A fasting period of 6 hours is required to distend the gallbladder and decrease bowel gas.

D. COST

$350–$400; $600–$700 for complete abdominal examination.

Oral Cholecystogram

Contrast agents used for **oral cholecystography (OCG)** are absorbed through the intestinal mucosa into the bloodstream and are transported to the liver, where they are conjugated and excreted into the bile. If the cystic duct is patent, the conjugated contrast enters the gallbladder. The gallbladder mucosa resorbs water, thereby concentrating the contrast and opacifying the gallbladder. Iopanoic acid is the most commonly used OCG agent. It is the most lipid-soluble agent and requires bile salts and fat in the diet for absorption. Peak opacification occurs 17 hours after ingestion. Tyropanoate sodium is a newer agent that is more water soluble and produces gallbladder opacification in about 10 hours. It does not require bile salts for absorption and is not affected by lack of fat in the diet.

Nonvisualization of the gallbladder on OCG after administration of two consecutive doses of contrast agent is reliable evidence of gallbladder disease, if other causes can be excluded. Intrinsic gallbladder disease causing nonvisualization includes cystic duct obstruction, chronic cholecystitis, cholecystectomy, and anomalous gallbladder position. Extrabiliary causes of failure to view the gallbladder on OCG include fasting, failure to ingest contrast, vomiting, esophageal disorders (such as diverticula, obstruction, or hiatal hernia), gastric outlet obstruction, gastrocolic fistula, malabsorption states, diarrhea, ileus, acute pancreatitis or peritonitis, and deficiency of bile salts resulting from Crohn's disease or severe liver disease.

A. INDICATIONS

OCG is used as an adjunctive examination to ultrasound. It is obtained when the clinical symptoms are highly suggestive of cholelithiasis but the ultrasound either is normal or equivocal. OCG plays a role in helping to determine the eligibility of patients for nonsurgical treatment of gallstones. Chemical stone dissolution and biliary lithotripsy require knowledge of cystic duct patency as well as stone number, size, and composition: bile salt therapy requires small stones (<5 mm), whereas lithotripsy is most effective on a solitary stone less than 2 cm. Ultrasound can be used to measure stones smaller than 2 cm, but OCG is superior to ultrasound for sizing larger stones and for counting multiple stones. Noncalcified cholesterol stones are required for nonoperative therapy. Buoyancy is a sign of cholesterol stones on OCG (Figure 14–15). Gallbladder opacification on OCG establishes cystic duct patency.

Large doses of OCG contrast agent can cause renal failure. It will also cause the gallbladder to become very dense, which decreases the procedure's sensitivity for detecting small stones. Other side effects include diarrhea (25%), dysuria (14%), nausea (6%), and vomiting (0.5%).

B. CONTRAINDICATIONS

OCG cannot be performed in patients with bilirubin greater than 3 mg/dL or in pregnant patients.

C. PATIENT PREPARATION

The recommended dose of OCG agent is 3.0 g. For outpatients, a 2-day consecutive dosage schedule is used, with 3.0 g of iopanoic acid administered each day. The patient fasts overnight of the second day and radiographs are obtained the morning of the third day. For inpatients, a single dose of 3.0 g of iopanoic acid or other OCG agent is administered. If there is no image or a faint image of the gallbladder, a second dose of 3.0 g of contrast agent is given that evening and repeat radiographs are performed the next morning.

D. COST

$430–$480.

Percutaneous Transhepatic Cholangiogram

Percutaneous transhepatic cholangiography (PTC) is a technique that permits direct visualization of the biliary tree and may be extended during the same examination to include interventional biliary procedures. PTC is performed by percutaneous placement of a fine needle through the chest wall and the hepatic parenchyma and into a branch of either the right or left bile duct. A cholangiogram is then obtained by injection of water-soluble contrast directly into the biliary tree. Ultrasound, CT, or fluoroscopy may be used for guidance of the needle. The success of injecting a bile duct increases when the ducts are dilated. There is a 90–100% success rate for obtaining a diagnostic cholangiogram when intrahepatic

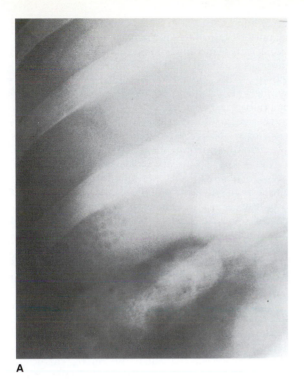
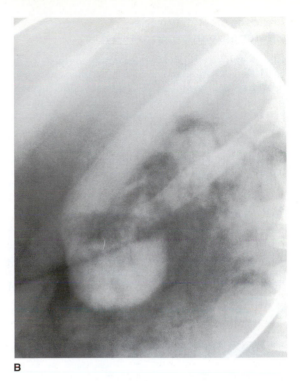

A
B

Figure 14–15. **A:** Supine view of an opacified gallbladder from an oral cholecystogram that contains multiple small noncalcified gallstones. **B:** Upright view of the same patient demonstrating buoyant stones that layer. Buoyancy on oral cholecystogram is a characteristic of cholesterol stones. These stones would be amenable to nonoperative therapy.

ducts are dilated. This drops to 70–85%, however, in patients with nondilated ducts.

Complications of PTC occur in about 5% of patients, including cholangitis, sepsis, hemorrhage, bile peritonitis, and pneumothorax.

A. INDICATIONS

Transhepatic cholangiography is obtained in the following situations:

- In patients with evidence of obstructive jaundice by noninvasive imaging in whom determination of the cause of obstruction is required for planning treatment. PTC is particularly helpful if there is a need to see the extent of a lesion located in the proximal biliary tree.
- For decompression of the biliary tree in patients with biliary obstruction. Drainage is achieved through the use of percutaneous catheter drainage or by the placement of stents in patients with unresectable malignant obstructions or benign strictures of the

bile duct. Retrieval of stones and dilatation of strictures can also be performed.

- Following a failed attempt at endoscopic retrograde cholangiography or for complications of endoscopic stent placement.

B. CONTRAINDICATIONS

Patients with abnormal clotting parameters, massive ascites, or diffuse hepatic metastases are excluded. Caution is advised in patients with renal insufficiency to avoid excessive intravascular administration of contrast medium.

C. PATIENT PREPARATION

All patients are premedicated with broad-spectrum antibiotics.

D. COST

$1,000–$1,100.

Endoscopic Retrograde Cholangiopancreatography

Endoscopic retrograde cholangiopancreatography (ERCP) is a procedure allowing for direct retrograde opacification of the biliary tree and pancreatic duct with a side-viewing duodenoscope. The patient is sedated and glucagon is given to induce atony of the duodenum. In the left lateral decubitus or prone position the endoscope is introduced orally and directed into the duodenum. Following cannulation of the papilla of Vater, water-soluble contrast is injected under fluoroscopy into either the pancreatic duct or common bile duct.

A. INDICATIONS

The most important indication for ERCP is obstructive jaundice. ERCP can demonstrate the cause as well as the extent of biliary obstruction. It is the preferred examination in patients with possible choledocholithiasis because stones can be extracted with balloons or gaskets after sphincterotomy. In patients with suspected periampullary tumor, ERCP permits direct visualization and biopsy of the papilla and duodenum (Figure 14–16). ERCP can identify intra- and extrahepatic strictures. It is the best modality for imaging primary sclerosing cholangitis and AIDS cholangiopathy. Alternate areas of narrowing and dilatation involving the intra- and extrahepatic biliary tree characterize sclerosing cholangitis. The intrahepatic tree may also appear pruned. AIDS cholangiopathy is due to opportunistic infection of the biliary system with *Cryptosporidium,* CMV, or *Microsporidium.* It can mimic sclerosing cholangitis radiographically. Shaggy irregularity of the common duct contour may also be seen. A distinguishing feature of AIDS-related cholangitis is the presence of papillary stenosis in many patients. Isolated papillary stenosis or a long common duct stricture may occasionally be seen without the intrahepatic findings in AIDS cholangiopathy.

Malignant stricture due to cholangiocarcinoma is well demonstrated by ERCP, typically appearing as an area of abrupt cutoff. Other causes of biliary ductal narrowing include postinflammatory or postsurgical strictures. Extrinsic compression of the biliary tree can occur secondary to hepatocellular carcinoma, portal adenopathy, or duodenal and pancreatic carcinoma. Decompression of the biliary system by endoscopic stent placement or balloon dilatation of benign or malignant biliary strictures involving the extrahepatic biliary tree can be achieved in more than 90% of cases. Intrahepatic strictures may be better approached by transhepatic cholangiography.

Opacification of the pancreatic duct is useful for diagnosing pancreatic carcinoma and pancreatitis, or for identifying a fistula extending from the pancreatic duct to a pseudocyst. Carcinoma of the pancreas head is often the cause of distal common bile duct stricture as well as stricture of the pancreatic duct in this region, producing the "double duct" sign (Figure 14–17). However, this appearance may also be seen with chronic pancreatitis due to stricturing within the pancreatic head. Findings of chronic pancreatitis also include dilatation of the pancreatic duct, often resulting in a tortuous, beaded, or "chain of lakes" appearance. Debris or calculi within the pancreatic duct may cause focal filling defects. Secondary branches of the pancreatic duct are enlarged and clubbed. Pancreatic parenchymal calcifications may be present and are diagnostic of chronic pancreatitis. Pseudocysts communicating with the duct may fill with contrast.

The success rate of ERCP is greater than 90% and is not dependent on the presence of ductal dilatation (unlike PTC). Failure to cannulate the papilla of Vater occurs in the following settings: papillary stenosis, severe duodenal inflammation or scarring, prior gastric surgery (particularly Billroth II), choledochocele, or juxtapapillary diverticulum.

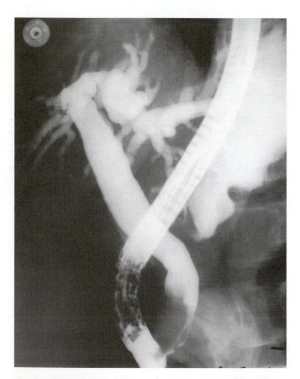

Figure 14–16. Film from an endoscopic retrograde cholangiopancreatogram (ERCP) of a jaundiced patient, showing dilatation of the intrahepatic and extrahepatic bile ducts. In the distal common bile duct there is a large irregular intraluminal filling defect due to a periampullary cholangiocarcinoma.

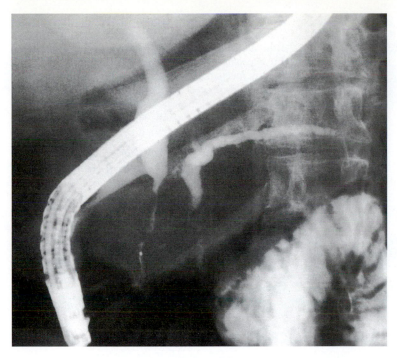

Figure 14–17. Film from an ERCP in a patient with pancreatic head carcinoma. Opacification of both the common bile duct and pancreatic duct reveals biductal strictures causing obstruction ("double duct" sign). This appearance is most commonly associated with pancreatic carcinoma but also may be seen with chronic pancreatitis.

The overall incidence of complications resulting from ERCP is about 2%. ERCP may cause injection-related pancreatitis, cholangitis, sepsis, duodenal perforation, and hemorrhage, particularly if a sphincterotomy is performed.

B. Contraindications

Caution is advised in patients with concurrent or recent acute pancreatitis, who are at a higher risk for developing procedure-related pancreatitis, and when pancreatic pseudocyst is present, since there is risk of developing abscess.

C. Cost

$1,300–$1,600.

Hepatobiliary Scan

The radiopharmaceutical used for the hepatobiliary scan is ^{99m}Tc N-substituted iminodiacetic acid (IDA). The most common analog is ^{99m}Tc diisopropyl-IDA (DISIDA) because it allows visualization of the hepatobiliary system at serum bilirubin levels up to 20 mg/dL. Following intravenous injection of DISIDA, there is rapid uptake by hepatocytes with subsequent conjugation and excretion into the biliary ducts. The liver is visualized within 5 minutes. The gallbladder, common bile duct, and duodenum are normally seen within 30–40 minutes. Diseases that affect liver perfusion,

cause hepatocyte dysfunction, or cause cystic or common duct obstruction will result in an abnormal scan.

A. Indications

Hepatobiliary scan is indicated in the following situations.

1. Cholecystitis—Cystic duct obstruction is present in the majority of patients with acute cholecystitis. In the correct clinical setting, acute cholecystitis can be diagnosed accurately if there is failure to see the gallbladder within 4 hours of injection and the patient demonstrates hepatic excretion into the common duct and small bowel (Figure 14–18). If there is delayed visualization of the gallbladder at 1 hour to 4 hours and cholecystokinin (CCK) or morphine has been administered, then the diagnosis is chronic cholecystitis. CCK stimulates gallbladder contraction and enhances biliary excretion, promoting gallbladder visualization in chronic cholecystitis. Intravenous morphine causes constriction of the sphincter of Oddi and increases the flow of radiopharmaceutical into the gallbladder.

The overall accuracy of hepatobiliary scintigraphy for acute cholecystitis is 95%. Normal visualization of the gallbladder reliably excludes acute cholecystitis. Nonvisualization or delayed visualization of the gallbladder (false-positive study) can be caused by nonfasting or prolonged fasting, hyperalimentation, acute pancreatitis, and hepatocellular dysfunction. False-negative

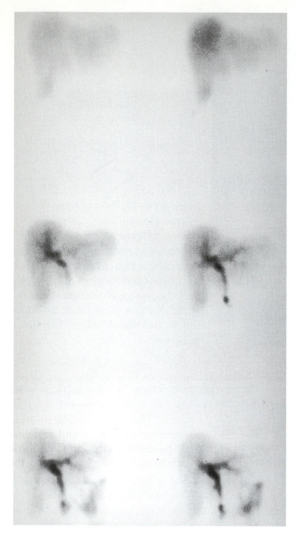

Figure 14–18. Acute cholecystitis. Activity is present in the common duct and small bowel within 30 minutes (images were taken at 5-minute intervals from 5 to 30 minutes). This study was continued for 4 hours and the gallbladder was not visualized.

studies may occur in patients with acalculous cholecystitis. Duodenal diverticulum, simulating the gallbladder or an accessory cystic duct, may also result in a false-negative study.

2. Cholestasis—If there is hepatic uptake but nonvisualization of the gallbladder, common duct, and small bowel, then common bile duct obstruction is suggested. Rarely, severe hepatocellular disease can produce a similar appearance. Findings on the hepatobiliary scan can help differentiate between intrahepatic cholestasis

owing to hepatocellular dysfunction and extrahepatic cholestasis resulting from common duct obstruction. Although both will cause a decrease in hepatic uptake, this is usually more impaired by hepatocellular disease than by mechanical obstruction. Hepatocellular disease is also characterized by normal or delayed visualization of bowel activity but lack of biliary dilatation. A partial common duct obstruction will cause delayed bowel visualization associated with a dilated bile duct.

3. Postsurgical complications—Complications of hepatobiliary surgery that result in abnormal biliary flow and biliary leakage can be easily identified with scintigraphy. Ductal obstruction resulting from retained stone or stricture is suggested by dilated ducts and delayed bowel visualization.

B. PATIENT PREPARATION

A fasting period of 6 hours is required before the study.

C. COST

$700–$800.

CROSS-SECTIONAL IMAGING

Modalities

A. COMPUTED TOMOGRAPHY

Recent advances in computed tomography (CT) include thinner slices, faster scan times, and higher spatial resolution, allowing for more accurate evaluation. The administration of intravenous contrast material with the rapid bolus technique permits improved detection and characterization of many lesions. CT is also used as guidance for percutaneous fine-needle aspiration biopsy and drainage catheter placement. Spiral CT eliminates respiratory motion artifacts and decreases the required amount of intravenous contrast. It requires a slip-ring scanner, which permits continuous imaging so that a large area of the body can be scanned quickly. The newest generation spiral CT scanner has multiple detectors and can scan the entire abdomen and pelvis in under 15 seconds.

1. Contraindications—CT is contraindicated in pregnancy. Renal insufficiency (creatinine >1.5–2.0 mg/dL) is a contraindication to the administration of intravenous contrast. The use of intravenous contrast also is associated with the risk of allergic reaction and, rarely, death.

2. Patient preparation—A fasting period of 4–6 hours is required before the study. Opacification of the gastrointestinal tract is necessary for abdominal-pelvic CT. Patients receive oral contrast approximately 1 hour before scanning. Some centers also administer rectal contrast before imaging the pelvis. A recent serum creatinine is necessary if intravenous contrast is to be given.

3. Cost—$1,700–$2,100; add $50–$70 for nonionic contrast.

B. ULTRASOUND

Ultrasound of the abdomen and pelvis is noninvasive, requires no ionizing radiation or iodinated contrast material, and is relatively inexpensive. In addition, units are portable so that bedside studies may be performed. Ultrasound is the best modality for determining the cystic versus solid nature of lesions, and it remains the primary modality for biliary imaging. Ultrasound is often used for following lesions such as pancreatic pseudocyst. Ultrasound guidance for percutaneous fine-needle biopsy or catheter placement is less expensive than CT. Endoscopic and intraoperative ultrasound are now more widely employed with the development of small high-resolution transducers and improved operator expertise.

1. Contraindications—There are none.

2. Patient preparation—A fasting period of 6 hours is required before the study.

3. Cost—$600–$700 for a complete abdomen examination.

C. MAGNETIC RESONANCE IMAGING

Magnetic resonance imaging (MRI) provides better tissue contrast than other radiographic modalities. It is noninvasive and does not require ionizing radiation or iodinated contrast material. Imaging can be performed in multiple planes (transaxial, coronal, sagittal, nonorthogonal). MRI can be used to clarify areas surrounding surgical clips that are not seen on CT because of induced artifacts. MRI is useful for evaluation of vascular

patency without the need for contrast material. Intravenous contrast material (gadopentetate dimeglumine) can be given to evaluate enhancement patterns and offer information complementary to that obtained by CT or ultrasound.

1. Contraindications—MRI is contraindicated in patients with pacemakers, intraocular metallic fragments, intracranial aneurysm clips, cochlear implants, some artificial heart valves, and some implanted metallic hardware.

2. Patient preparation—A fasting period of 6 hours is required. Glucagon is administered intramuscularly to inhibit peristalsis for abdominal-pelvic MRI.

3. Cost—$2,200–$2,400.

Esophagus

The most commonly used cross-sectional technique for evaluation of the esophagus is CT. It is useful for the evaluation of esophageal trauma, permitting detection of involvement of the mediastinum, lung, and pleural space. CT allows delineation of the extraluminal extent of disease.

CT is the best noninvasive method for staging esophageal carcinoma. It is limited in its ability to evaluate the actual depth of invasion in the layers of the esophageal wall. However, wall thickening or mass may suggest direct invasion of adjacent structures by causing a mass effect and loss of fat planes (Figure 14–19). Tumors demonstrating aortic or tracheobronchial invasion are considered unresectable. Pericardial and vertebral involvement may also be demonstrated on CT. Aortic invasion is suspected when there is obliteration of the

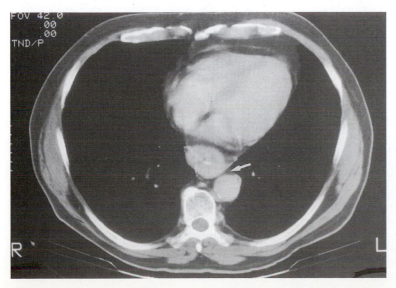

Figure 14–19. Circumferential distal esophageal mass due to squamous cell carcinoma. Note that the fat surrounding the mass is not infiltrated. There is a clear fat plane between the esophageal mass and the aorta *(arrow)*. This mass was subsequently resected.

triangular fat space between the esophagus, aorta, and spine or if there is contact of the esophagus involving more than 90 degrees of the aortic circumference.

The ability of CT to detect local tumor involvement is controversial. Published studies indicate that CT has a relatively high sensitivity and specificity for predicting mediastinal invasion with an accuracy of over 90% for staging esophageal carcinoma. However, most of these series consisted of patients with advanced disease. Local esophageal tumor involvement and mediastinal lymph nodes are more accurately assessed by endoscopic ultrasound (EUS). Thus, EUS is a superior technique for the preoperative evaluation of early esophageal cancer. Mediastinal lymph nodes are considered suspicious for malignancy when they are greater than 1 cm. However, the absence of enlarged nodes is not a reliable finding since CT cannot detect metastases in normal-sized nodes. Thus, CT has a low sensitivity but a high specificity for detection of malignant nodes.

MRI offers an alternative to CT for evaluating esophageal tumors although it has not been accepted widely for the staging of esophageal carcinoma. MRI of the esophagus may be limited by motion artifacts, long imaging times, cost, and availability. However, studies indicate that MRI is as accurate as CT for staging esophageal carcinoma.

EUS has played an increasing role for evaluation of the esophagus with greater availability. It plays a role complementary to CT and MRI in the staging of esophageal carcinoma. EUS allows visualization of the individual layers of the esophageal wall and can assess depth of invasion. Five alternating hyperechoic and hypoechoic layers are seen: mucosa (hyperechoic), deep mucosa (hypoechoic), submucosa (hyperechoic), muscularis propria (hypoechoic), and adventitia (hyperechoic). Esophageal carcinoma appears as a hypoechoic lesion with disruption of the normal layers.

EUS is 73–92% accurate in the T-staging of esophageal cancer. It has proven most useful for earlier stage tumors and gastroesophageal junction tumors, which are often difficult to evaluate by CT and MRI.

The accuracy of EUS for diagnosing periesophageal nodal metastasis ranges from 70 to 81%. Findings suggestive of malignant nodal involvement include well-circumscribed hypoechoic nodes with a rounded shape. Mediastinal and perigastric nodal involvement are considered regional disease whereas celiac axis nodal involvement, which can also be detected by EUS, is indicative of distant metastasis. A limitation of EUS is the poor depth of penetration of the high-frequency transducers (7.5 or 12 MHz) so that CT or MRI is still required to detect distant metastases, such as those to the liver. In addition, in about 25% of patients the transducer is unable to pass beyond a malignant stricture.

Stomach

The primary modalities for diagnosing gastric lesions are barium UGI series and endoscopy, both of which allow evaluation of the mucosa. CT allows evaluation of extraluminal malignancy, including distant metastases. Gastric carcinoma can appear as wall thickening or polypoid or ulcerative masses on CT. In addition to hematogenous and nodal metastases, direct tumor extension and peritoneal implants may also be detected. The role of CT in the preoperative staging of gastric carcinoma remains controversial. Earlier reports were favorable, but more recent series have better defined the limitations of CT. It has not proven reliable for detection of malignant adenopathy or pancreatic invasion. The overall accuracy of CT staging of gastric carcinoma is about 75%. At centers where all patients with gastric carcinoma undergo curative resection or palliative bypass, CT is not required preoperatively. However, if surgery is not always performed, preoperative CT may obviate laparotomy if diffuse metastatic disease is detected in patients who are asymptomatic or poor surgical candidates. Some surgeons request CT preoperatively to help in planning surgery. CT remains valuable in detecting distant metastases, particularly to the liver and lung. CT has proven more useful in the work-up of patients with gastric lymphoma and leimyosarcoma where it is able to show tumor extent, identify metastases, and localize for percutaneous biopsy. CT has also been used in planning radiation ports, evaluating response to therapy, and detecting recurrence.

MRI of the stomach and the gastrointestinal tract is still being developed. The advantages of MRI include multiplanar imaging (transaxial, coronal, sagittal), the lack of ionizing radiation or need for iodinated contrast, and fewer surgical clip artifacts. However, there are technical problems, such as motion artifact from respiration or peristalsis and the lack of an adequate oral contrast agent for luminal opacification. With the development of phased array surface coils with faster imaging sequences and echo-planar imaging, MRI may prove useful in the future for delineating gastric abnormalities, including staging of gastric carcinoma.

EUS is superior to CT in determining the depth of wall invasion by gastric carcinoma. It can also detect perigastric spread and local adenopathy that may not be apparent on CT. Gastric carcinoma appears as a hypoechoic, vertically oriented mass disrupting the five normal wall layers. EUS is 73–80% accurate in staging gastric carcinoma and 68–80% accurate in diagnosing nodal metastasis. Limitations include the poor depth of penetration and the inability to pass the EUS transducer beyond some obstructing lesions.

EUS can often distinguish lymphoma from carcinoma. Gastric lymphoma appears as an extensive horizontal infiltration of the wall involving predominantly the second and third layers with focal ulceration. Other indications for EUS include evaluation of submucosal lesions such as leiomyoma, leiomyosarcoma, lipoma, and gastric varices (Figure 14–20).

Bowel

CT is useful for evaluation of small and large bowel obstruction, tumor, ischemia, and inflammatory disease. Bowel dilatation, wall thickening, mesenteric involvement, and intramural air are easily demonstrated. CT can be used to characterize bowel disease as focal or diffuse, to determine the degree, symmetry, and contour of wall thickening, to demonstrate the pattern of enhancement, as well as to delineate extraluminal disease such as inflammatory changes, abscesses, ascites, adenopathy, and metastases.

Whereas benign diseases of the bowel cause circumferential and symmetric wall thickening, malignancy presents as an eccentric wall thickening or mass with luminal narrowing and an irregular outer contour. Bowel wall hemorrhage as a result of trauma, coagulopathy, or ischemia may be seen as high-density wall thickening. Findings of ischemic bowel are often nonspecific and include wall thickening and bowel dilatation. In addition, CT may identify thrombus within the mesenteric vessels or portal vein and is more accurate than plain films for identifying intramural air and portal venous gas owing to bowel infarction.

In the evaluation of Crohn's disease, CT can delineate the distribution of bowel wall thickening and is useful for identifying "creeping" mesenteric fat as well as complications of Crohn's, such as intraabdominal abscess, obstruction, and fistula. These findings are often helpful for differentiating between ulcerative colitis and Crohn's disease.

Infectious enteritis often produces nonspecific findings consisting of benign-appearing wall thickening with dilatation and increased intraluminal fluid. CT is slightly more sensitive than barium enema in detecting diverticulitis and is better able to demonstrate the extent of extraluminal disease. Thickened bowel wall, diverticula, and pericolonic involvement such as infiltration of the fat, abscess, and fistulas may be identified.

CT has been demonstrated to have a high sensitivity for diagnosing small bowel obstruction (SBO) as well as determining the location and cause. When clinical and plain film evaluation are equivocal, CT should be obtained. A barium SBFT should not be performed if there is the possibility that a CT scan will be obtained since the relative higher density barium given for SBFT will cause significant artifacts on CT making the CT nondiagnostic. CT can help to distinguish SBO from other conditions causing small bowel dilatation, such as ileus. In both small and large bowel obstruction, CT can demonstrate the level of obstruction by identifying a transition zone from dilated to decompressed bowel, and in some cases it can determine the cause of obstruction (Figure 14–21).

CT colonography (virtual colonoscopy) was first introduced in 1994 and since then has received widespread attention as a possible new tool for colorectal can-

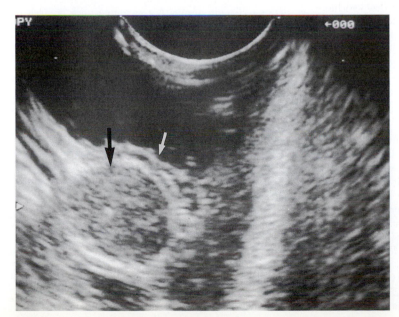

Figure 14–20. Endoscopic ultrasound (EUS) of a gastric leiomyoma **(black arrow)** arising in the submucosa. Note that the hyperechoic mucosa **(white arrow)** is intact and not thickened.

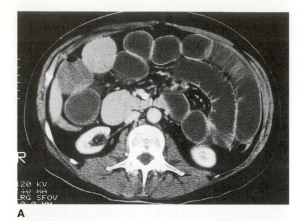

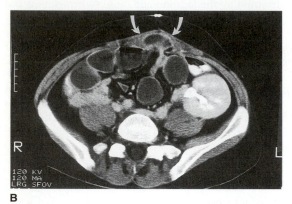

Figure 14–21. A: Patient with markedly dilated fluid-filled small bowel loops on CT who recently underwent pancreatic-renal transplant. Native kidneys are small. **B:** In same patient, note decompressed small bowel loop located anteriorly in the abdominal wall **(arrows)**, representing an incarcerated incisional hernia causing small bowel obstruction diagnosed by CT. Note the transplanted pancreas in the right pelvis and transplanted kidney in the left pelvis.

cer screening. CT colonography uses spiral CT data and a computer workstation to generate axial, reformatted, and three-dimensional endoluminal views of the colon. Interactive displays of the endoluminal view allow navigation through the colon similar to fiberoptic colonoscopy. Preliminary trials in larger patient groups have demonstrated excellent sensitivity of CT colonography for detection of clinically significant polyps (≥10 mm) of approximately 90% (Figure 14–22). However, confirmatory studies are needed in asymptomatic, screening patients. Excellent sensitivity has also been found for colorectal cancer (Figure 14–23). CT colonography has been found to have low sensitivity (26–59%)

for the detection of diminutive polyps smaller than 5 mm and also to have difficulty detecting flat lesions.

Patients must undergo a bowel cleansing regimen starting the day prior to the CT study. Colonic distention is achieved by retrograde insufflation of the colon with room air or carbon dioxide via a small rectal tube. The current CT colonography protocol requires scanning the abdomen and pelvis in supine and prone positions. CT colonography is a minimally invasive test and is very low risk. Other advantages of CT colonography include the relative fast examination time for the patient and no need for sedation. CT colonography can also evaluate the colon in patients with tight strictures or occlusive carcinomas. CT colonography lesion detection sensitivity is limited by inadequate bowel cleansing or poor colonic distention. Retained stool is the main cause of false-positive lesions on CT colonography. Current research includes the evaluation of fecal and fluid tagging with an ingested positive contrast agent that may then be combined with electronic subtraction of tagged material. In the future this may eliminate the need for bowel cleansing prior to CT colonography. Other research is targeted at computer-aided detection of colorectal lesions in attempting to decrease the radiologist's interpretation time, which has been found to range between 20 and 30 minutes.

MRI of the bowel is still under investigation and is not used widely except in evaluation of the rectosigmoid region. Colonic cleansing and rectal air insufflation aid in obtaining diagnostic images. In addition to the use of T1- and T2-weighted images, intravenous contrast (gadopentetate dimeglumine) may be used with T1 imaging to help stage rectal carcinoma and to detect recurrent tumor. A recurrent tumor is often of low signal (dark) on T1 images, but of mixed or high signal (brighter) on T2 images. Postsurgical fibrosis has a low signal (dark) on T1 and T2 images. Scar enhancement may normally occur for about 1–1.5 years following surgery.

CT and MRI are comparable in their ability to stage rectosigmoid tumors. Both modalities can also identify metastatic disease and adenopathy, although neither can distinguish malignant adenopathy from benign hyperplasia. MRI of the rectum using an endorectal coil is a newer technique that in initial studies appears promising in its ability to distinguish rectal wall layers and to detect perirectal adenopathy.

Transabdominal ultrasound is of limited use in the evaluation of bowel abnormalities. Ultrasound is able to detect distended fluid-filled bowel loops in cases of obstruction. However, air within the bowel will deflect the ultrasound beam and limit further evaluation of the abdomen. Ultrasound can also demonstrate bowel wall thickening resulting from tumor infiltration, inflammation, or hemorrhage.

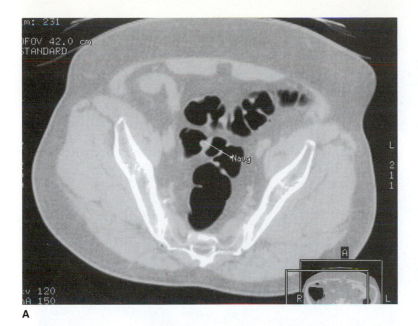

A

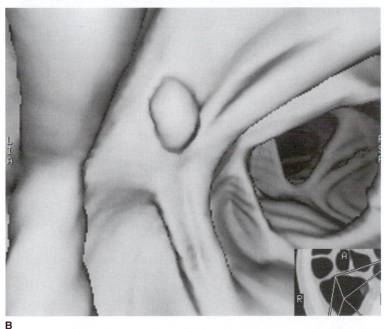

B

Figure 14–22. **A:** Axial image from a CT colonography examination shows a polyp located in the sigmoid colon. **B:** In the same patient, the polyp is easily identified on the three-dimensional endoluminal view.

Transrectal ultrasound (TRUS) permits excellent imaging of the lower two-thirds of the rectum and allows identification of the various layers of the wall. Studies performed so far indicate that TRUS is particularly useful in staging rectal tumors. Direct tumor extension and perirectal nodes that may be difficult to identify by CT and MRI are seen easily on TRUS.

Appendix

Plain film findings are often nonspecific in patients with appendicitis and may demonstrate an ileus pattern. Although seldom required to establish the diagnosis, single-contrast barium enema (SCBE) may reveal nonfilling of the appendix owing to extrinsic mass effect

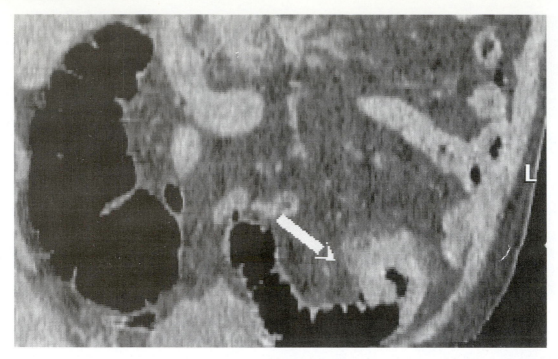

Figure 14–23. Coronal multiplanar reformatted view from a CT colonography examination demonstrates a large circumferential sigmoid carcinoma *(arrow)* with evidence of stranding and invasion into the pericolonic fat. L, patient's left.

on the cecum or terminal ileum. Although complete filling of the appendix on SCBE excludes the diagnosis of appendicitis, nonfilling or incomplete filling can occur in patients with a normal appendix and therefore is not specific for the diagnosis.

CT and ultrasound have been employed in diagnosing acute appendicitis. However, more recently CT is preferred over ultrasound because of its slightly higher diagnostic accuracy. CT has a high sensitivity (87– 89%), specificity (83–97%), and accuracy (93%) for the diagnosis of appendicitis. Findings include a thickened appendix (which may contain an appendicolith) and associated pericecal inflammation, fluid, or abscess (Figure 14–24).

CT has the ability to identify nonappendiceal disease that clinically may be confused for appendicitis. The extent of extraluminal disease is optimally demonstrated by CT, and it is particularly useful in patients with a suspected appendiceal perforation (eg, debilitated or immunosuppressed patients), severe clinical signs, or palpable right lower abdominal mass. CT is the best modality for distinguishing a periappendiceal phlegmonous (inflammatory) mass from an abscess. CT-guided percutaneous catheter drainage, when clini-

cally indicated, may be performed during the same examination if a periappendiceal abscess is identified.

Ultrasound has been shown to have a sensitivity of 77–89% and specificity and accuracy of over 90% for the diagnosis of acute appendicitis. The sonographic criteria used are an aperistaltic, noncompressible, thickened appendix (diameter >7 mm) (Figure 14–24).

The advantages of ultrasound include its lower cost compared with CT and the lack of ionizing radiation. Ultrasound should be the initial study performed in children as well as in young women of child-bearing age. Ultrasound (and transvaginal ultrasound) also has the ability to distinguish gynecologic disease from appendicitis. However, ultrasound is a more operator-dependent diagnostic modality and it may not be useful in obese or uncooperative patients. Ultrasound also is less useful than CT in identifying other intraabdominal causes of a patient's symptoms.

Liver

CT continues to be the preferred modality for the evaluation of focal hepatic abnormalities, including tumor, infection, and trauma. CT also can be used for identifi-

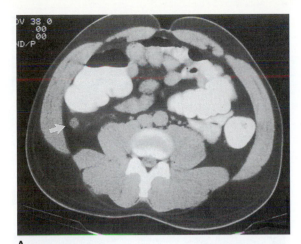

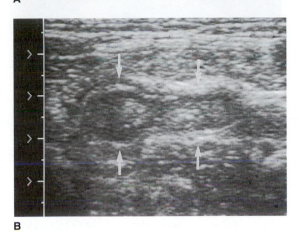

Figure 14–24. **A:** Patient with appendicitis found on CT to have a thickened appendix with mild periappendiceal stranding of the fat ***(arrow).*** **B:** Different patient who underwent ultrasound for abdominal pain, found to have a thickened appendix that was peristaltic and noncompressible, consistent with appendicitis ***(arrows).***

cation of diffuse liver diseases, such as fatty infiltration, cirrhosis, iron deposition (hemosiderosis, hemochromatosis), as well as infiltrative neoplasms. Technical advances have resulted in improved detection and characterization of mass lesions. Dynamic spiral CT scanning of the abdomen that takes place during a rapid power-injected intravenous contrast bolus is the established screening modality for liver lesions. With this technique, scanning of the liver occurs during arterial and venous phases of intravenous contrast administration, allowing optimal demonstration of mass lesions. De-

layed scanning at 4–6 hours can be performed to further increase sensitivity for lesions, due to iodine contrast uptake by normal tissue but not tumors.

CT arteriography (CTA) involves scanning of the liver during contrast injection directly into the hepatic or celiac artery via a catheter so that hepatic lesions are optimally enhanced and more easily detected. Most hepatic lesions derive their blood supply from the hepatic artery, whereas normal liver parenchyma receives 75–80% of its blood supply from the portal vein.

CT arterial portography (CTAP) is performed by scanning the liver during injection of contrast into the superior mesenteric artery. As contrast passes through the mesenteric artery and into the portal venous system, hepatic lesions may be seen as hypovascular compared with surrounding normal hepatic parenchyma, which enhances intensely. CTAP is the most sensitive technique (approximately 90%) for detecting hepatic metastases preoperatively and can accurately detail the precise hepatic segmental location of the metastatic deposits. Some studies indicate that CTAP can detect more than twice as many metastases as standard CT. However, because this technique is more invasive, it is used selectively for staging cancer or planning surgical resection. One drawback of CTAP is the high false-positive rate resulting from perfusion defects in up to 30% of cases.

Multidetector spiral CT is the newest modality for rapid scanning of the liver. The entire liver can be imaged within 20 seconds. Scanning occurs during arterial and venous phases of vascular enhancement. Dual-phase spiral CT, image reconstruction using thinner slices, and three-dimensional analysis can be performed to further enhance detection of smaller lesions.

Ultrasound is often the initial examination in the evaluation of nonspecific abdominal clinical signs and symptoms and in patients with suspected biliary disease. State-of-the-art equipment permits real-time scanning with duplex Doppler or color flow Doppler capabilities. This allows differentiation between blood vessels and bile ducts and can demonstrate vascular occlusion, flow in collateral vessels, and flow within liver tumors. Ultrasound is not employed as a screening modality if liver disease is suspected because small lesions (<1 cm) may not be detected. Hepatic sonography is useful for distinguishing cystic versus solid liver lesions, assessing the patient preoperatively or staging of tumors by evaluating lesion location and vascular invasion, evaluating for inferior vena cava, hepatic, and portal venous thrombosis, and evaluating liver transplant patients pre- and postoperatively.

The use of intraoperative ultrasound has increased with the improvement of small high-resolution transducers. Small linear array transducers can fit into small incision sites, and fingertip probes can be used to help locate small lesions. Intraoperative ultrasound is used to determine whether small lesions identified preoperatively are cystic or solid. It can demonstrate additional lesions that may be unsuspected preoperatively. This modality can be used to help plan surgical resection and to monitor hepatic cryotherapy. Intraoperative ultrasound has been shown to effectively detect liver nodules less than 1 cm that may not be visible or palpable during surgery. It is more sensitive than preoperative CT or ultrasound for detecting hepatic metastases and is as sensitive as CTAP.

MRI of the abdomen must include techniques to reduce motion artifacts due to respiration and peristalsis. Fast gradient-echo sequences have been developed in conjunction with the breath-holding technique and are performed in addition to standard T1 and T2 sequences. Dynamic MRI using gradient-echo imaging can be performed after intravenous contrast (gadopentetate dimeglumine) to evaluate the enhancement pattern of liver lesions (Figure 14–25).

The relative strength of MRI versus CT for liver tumor staging is controversial and related to differences in expertise as well as equipment and scanning protocols. At present, both CT and MRI are noninvasive and have high sensitivity and accuracy for lesion detection and characterization. MRI may be particularly helpful in cases of suspected focal fatty infiltration of the liver or for detecting hepatic iron deposition (hemosiderosis, hemochromatosis).

A. HEPATOCELLULAR CARCINOMA (HCC)

CT or ultrasound is usually the initial examination for hepatocellular carcinoma. These modalities may also be used as guidance for percutaneous fine-needle biopsy. CT findings of HCC include a heterogeneously enhancing necrotic mass that may be encapsulated. Vascular invasion can be seen, as can hemoperitoneum due to HCC rupture. HCC may also be identified using ultrasound. MRI can demonstrate fat-containing HCC, pseudocapsules, daughter nodules, and septations. Tumor thrombus in the portal and hepatic veins or inferior vena cava is as reliably demonstrated on both MRI and color flow Doppler. MRI should be performed in patients with severe cirrhosis when CT or ultrasound is equivocal, because MRI more easily detects and characterizes HCC against a background of abnormal parenchyma.

B. METASTASES

CT is the primary modality for the evaluation of hepatic metastatic disease because of its high sensitivity for liver lesions and because it can study the rest of the abdomen and pelvis for a primary malignant neoplasm or other metastatic lesions (Figure 14–26). Liver metastases typi-

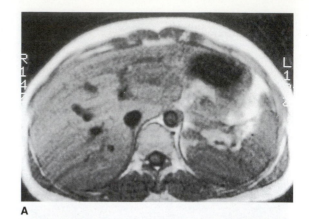

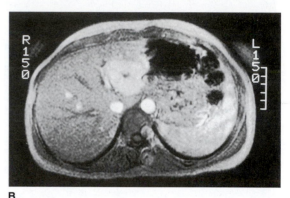

Figure 14–25. **A:** MRI of the liver using a T1-weighted sequence demonstrates a rounded lesion located in the left lobe. **B:** Fast gradient-echo image after administration of intravenous contrast (gadopentetate dimeglumine) showing immediate homogeneous enhancement of this lesion with a small central nonenhancing scar. This appearance and enhancement pattern is characteristic of focal nodular hyperplasia.

cally appear on CT as multiple rim-enhancing heterogeneous lesions that may have irregular margins. Although ultrasound can identify hepatic metastases, it provides less information about the rest of the abdomen and pelvis. MRI is preferred if a patient is allergic to iodinated contrast or if the CT findings are nonspecific. CTAP is the most sensitive modality for detection of hepatic metastases and should be performed if surgical resection of isolated hepatic metastases is being considered.

C. CAVERNOUS HEMANGIOMA

CT allows a reliable diagnosis of hemangioma when characteristic features are present. Lesions demonstrating early peripheral, nodular, or globular contrast en-

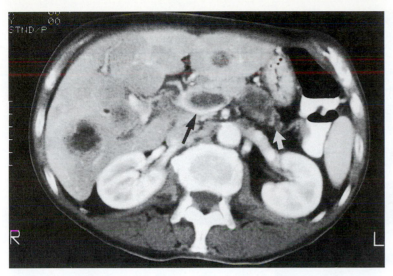

Figure 14–26. Low-density metastases are scattered throughout the liver, some with necrosis and some with rim enhancement. CT was able to demonstrate thrombosis of the main portal vein ***(black arrow)*** as well as the primary tumor, which was located in the pancreas ***(white arrow).***

hancement, which fills in centrally on delayed images, are typical of hemangiomas. However, these typical CT features are present in only 50–75% of cases. Incomplete fill-in may occur, especially in larger lesions that contain a central fibrous scar. If hemangioma cannot be confidently diagnosed by CT, other imaging studies may be helpful (Figure 14–27).

The typical ultrasound features of hemangiomas—well-defined hyperechoic lesions with increased through transmission —are seen in about 80% of cases. If such a lesion is identified incidentally during ultrasound imaging, the need for further evaluation is determined by clinical symptoms and liver function tests; follow-up sonogram in 3–6 months often is suggested to reevaluate the lesion. The patient with a known primary tumor, a hepatic tumor that has atypical sonographic features of hemangioma, or abnormal liver function tests should undergo additional imaging [CT, MRI, or ^{99m}Tc-labeled red blood cell (RBC) scan] to evaluate the hepatic lesion.

One of the major applications of abdominal MRI is in the evaluation of hemangiomas. Hemangiomas characteristically demonstrate a marked high signal (very bright) on heavily T2-weighted images and have an enhancement pattern similar to CT. MRI is about 90–95% accurate in the diagnosis of hepatic hemangiomas, but is much more costly than ^{99m}Tc RBC scintigraphy.

^{99m}Tc RBC scintigraphy identifies hepatic hemangioma as a focal area of increased activity on delayed imaging at 1–2 hours. This finding is present in 70– 90% of cases on planar imaging and in close to 95% of cases if single photon emission computed tomography (SPECT) is employed. ^{99m}Tc RBC scan with SPECT should be used for lesions greater than 1.5 cm,

whereas MRI is preferred for lesions less than 1.5 cm or for lesions adjacent to the heart or major vessels. This modality is safe and relatively inexpensive and is currently the modality of choice at many institutions for diagnosing hepatic hemangiomas.

Angiography was once considered the "gold standard" for diagnosing hemangiomas. It is only rarely performed now when all other noninvasive imaging modalities fail to establish the diagnosis. Fine-needle aspiration biopsies of hemangiomas with 20-gauge or smaller needles have been performed with a low incidence of complications. This may be warranted in some clinical situations to distinguish a lesion that has atypical features of hemangioma from a malignant lesion.

Pancreas

CT is the imaging technique of choice for the diagnosis of acute pancreatitis and for detecting related complications. Acute edematous pancreatitis appears as pancreatic enlargement with peripancreatic fluid and infiltration (Figure 14–28). CT can detect complications such as pseudocyst formation or pancreatic abscess, hemorrhage, and necrosis. Large areas of absence of pancreatic enhancement during dynamic contrast-enhanced CT correlates well with pancreatic necrosis and portends a worse prognosis. Associated biliary obstruction and gastrointestinal inflammatory changes may also be identified on CT. Features of chronic pancreatitis on CT include pancreatic atrophy with fatty replacement, calculi, pancreatic and bile duct dilatation, pseudocyst, venous obstruction, and pseudoaneurysm.

CT is considered the best screening and staging modality for pancreatic carcinoma. This tumor typically

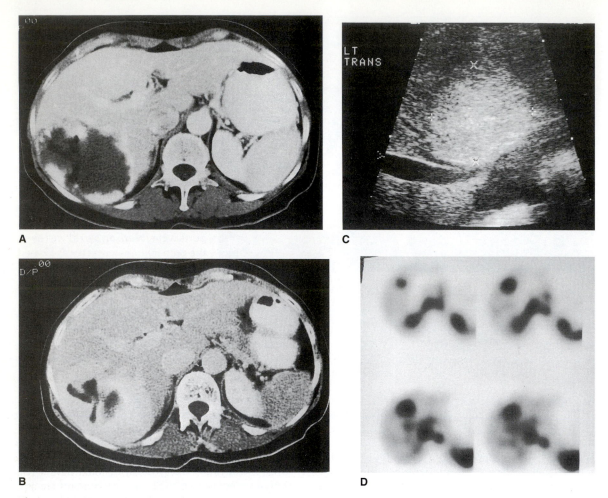

Figure 14–27. **A:** CT of a large cavernous hemangioma of the right lobe of the liver with initial peripheral nodular, globular enhancement. **B:** Delayed image demonstrating central fill-in of enhancement except for central fibrous scar. This appearance is typical of cavernous hemangioma of the liver. **C:** Ultrasound demonstrating a well-defined hyperechoic mass with increased through-transmission characteristic of hepatic hemangioma. **D:** ^{99m}Tc- labeled red blood cell scan with single photon emission computed tomography (SPECT), which should be used for lesions larger than 1.5 cm. These delayed images from a different patient show increased activity compatible with hepatic hemangioma. This modality is currently the modality of choice at many centers for diagnosing hepatic hemangiomas.

appears as a low-density mass with associated pancreatic duct obstruction. Rapid dynamic contrast-enhanced CT using thin ≤5-mm sections is recommended for maintaining a high detection rate. Less commonly a mass is not identified and only biductal (pancreatic and bile ducts) dilatation is present. CT can determine surgical resectability by evaluating for vascular involvement [loss of fat plane around the superior mesenteric artery (SMA)], infiltration of adjacent organs, and distant metastases. A CT-guided fine-needle biopsy of the pan-

creas is often helpful to confirm the diagnosis of pancreatic carcinoma. If CT or fine-needle biopsy does not confirm the diagnosis of pancreatic carcinoma, ERCP may be required. Spiral CT has been successfully applied to imaging the pancreas. Improved vascular enhancement and the ability to reconstruct images at overlapping intervals may improve detection of small pancreatic carcinomas as well as islet cell tumors.

With the widespread availability of CT, ultrasound is used infrequently for the diagnosis of pancreatic car-

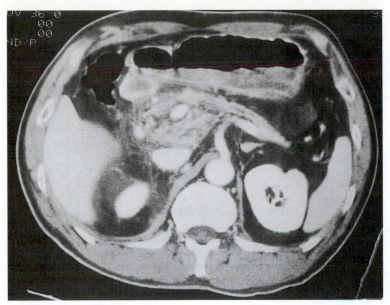

Figure 14–28. CT of the abdomen, demonstrating acute superimposed on chronic pancreatitis. CT is the technique of choice for imaging acute edematous pancreatitis. The pancreatic head is enlarged and there is infiltration of the peripancreatic fat with fluid present. The remainder of the pancreas is atrophied and the pancreatic duct is mildly dilated.

cinoma. Ultrasound has a reported sensitivity for pancreatic carcinoma of 80–95%. However, the sensitivity decreases when an adequate study is not obtained. Bowel gas may interfere with viewing the body and tail of the pancreas, and an incomplete examination occurs in up to 25% of cases. Sonographic findings include an irregular hypoechoic mass with dilatation of the pancreatic and bile ducts.

EUS has been demonstrated in preliminary studies to be highly accurate in the diagnosis and local staging of pancreatic carcinoma and is particularly useful for small tumors (<2 cm). CT or MRI for full staging is still necessary to detect distant metastases. The role of endosonography in clinical practice must be evaluated by further studies. Intraoperative ultrasound has proven useful in helping to distinguish between pancreatic carcinoma and inflammatory lesions. It can evaluate the pancreatic duct as well as identify pancreatic cystic lesions. Intraoperative ultrasound is an excellent modality for identifying small islet-cell tumors.

MRI of the pancreas is still being studied and has not gained wide acceptance because of its higher cost and decreased resolution compared with CT. MRI can identify pancreatic carcinomas and can delineate vascular involvement, biliary duct dilatation, and hepatic metastases. Fat suppression technique and contrast enhancement (gadopentetate dimeglumine) can improve detection of carcinoma, which appears as a low-signal (dark) mass with poor enhancement. MRI offers an alternative to CT in those patients who cannot receive intravenous iodinated contrast.

INTERVENTIONAL RADIOLOGY
Percutaneous Abscess Drainage

Percutaneous abscess drainage (PAD) has become the procedure of choice for treating many intraabdominal abscesses and fluid collections. The optimal therapeutic approach depends on the organism and on the cause, location, and appearance of the abscess. CT or ultrasound is used as guidance for percutaneous needle placement into an abscess, which should have a relatively well-defined wall. The abscess contents are aspirated and examined for leukocytes and bacteria. Once this is confirmed, the catheter can be placed. Follow-up care consists of a periodic sinogram or tube check every 3–5 days after tube insertion, until abscess resolution is confirmed.

A. LIVER

Most amebic abscesses of the liver are treated with antibiotics alone (metronidazole). Percutaneous drainage is performed in amebic abscesses with impending hepatic rupture, especially of left lobe abscesses, which can rupture into the thorax. PAD has also been performed successfully for large amebic abscesses (>8–10 cm) and in cases in which therapy is desired before serologic results are obtained.

Hydatid cyst was previously a contraindication to PAD because of the potential for anaphylaxis or peritoneal spread. However, PAD has been found to be safe in this situation, and transcatheter sclerosis has been performed. Surgical resection is still the preferred treatment modality for hydatid cyst of the liver in most centers.

Pyogenic abscesses are treated with a combination of PAD and antibiotic therapy, with cure rates of 70–90%. Pyogenic liver abscess can be due to biliary obstruction or to seeding from the gastrointestinal tract via the portal vein. Diverticulitis and inflammatory bowel disease are common causes that should be searched for and treated. The complication rate of PAD of the liver is low (<5%). Complications include pleural effusion, pneumothorax, hemorrhage, bacteremia, and peritonitis. Bile duct injury or biliary communication following drainage is uncommon.

B. SPLEEN

Splenic abscesses are uncommon, usually occurring in the setting of immunosuppression or bacterial endocarditis. Splenectomy has been the standard therapy although PAD has been successful in treating splenic abscesses with low morbidity (Figure 14–29). The most feared complication is hemorrhage. Multiple microabscesses due to hematogenous dissemination are not amenable to PAD.

C. PANCREAS

Pancreatic abscesses are optimally treated by surgical drainage and debridement. Percutaneous drainage is particularly difficult because pancreatic abscesses are often septated and poorly defined, and may be associated with necrotic tissue or fistulas. The material within pancreatic abscesses is often viscous and will not drain well through a catheter. In patients with severe necro-

tizing pancreatitis who are critically ill, PAD may be used as a temporizing therapy with surgery performed after improvement of the patient's clinical condition. PAD can be performed in patients who develop new pancreatic abscesses following surgery.

Percutaneous drainage of infected pancreatic pseudocysts remains controversial although it is now commonly performed as the initial therapy in many centers. Intravenous antibiotics are given and drainage is continued until the communication closes. If the distal pancreatic duct is obstructed, the fistulous communication may not close with percutaneous treatment and surgery may be required. The issue of surgical drainage versus PAD is still being debated, but PAD is used increasingly at many centers. Pseudocysts should be drained when they are enlarging, greater than 5 cm, painful, or are causing biliary, gastric, or duodenal obstruction. Complications occur in 5–10% of cases and include infection, fistula, rupture, and hemorrhage. Most noninfected pseudocysts do not require drainage.

D. BOWEL

Percutaneous drainage has been used successfully for enteric-related abscesses. This procedure is best performed under CT guidance so as to avoid traversing the adjacent intestine. PAD of periappendiceal abscesses allows drainage of infected inflammatory material, thereby permitting elective interval appendectomy at a later date. Peridiverticular abscesses treated by PAD also can facilitate subsequent surgical management by allowing bowel resection and primary anastomosis to be performed as a one-stage operation. Peridiverticular abscesses and periappendiceal abscesses treated by PAD

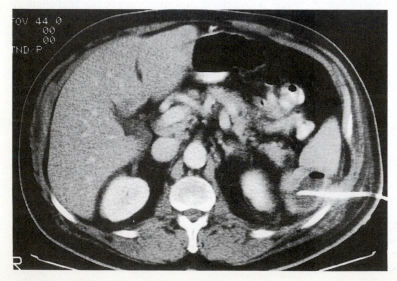

Figure 14–29. Successful CT-guided percutaneous catheter drainage of a splenic abscess in a patient with bacterial endocarditis. Multiple microabscesses of the spleen cannot be drained percutaneously.

have a success rate of over 90%. The need for interval appendectomy and subsequent bowel resection following PAD of appendiceal and diverticular abscesses is controversial. It is generally agreed that if surgery is not done, a barium enema should be performed to exclude an undiagnosed perforated tumor. Abscesses related to Crohn's disease may be treated successfully by PAD alone, without the need for surgery. Pelvic abscesses that cannot be drained by an anterior approach because of interfering bowel loops may be drained through transgluteal, transrectal, or transvaginal routes.

Angiography

A. GASTROINTESTINAL BLEEDING

Endoscopy is the primary diagnostic tool in patients with upper gastrointestinal hemorrhage. Endoscopy can identify the bleeding site or source as well as provide access for therapeutic intervention. If no source is identified and the patient has continued brisk bleeding, arteriography may be performed. Arteriography can identify and treat many causes of upper gastrointestinal bleeding, including varices, gastritis, ulcers, and Mallory-Weiss tears. Transcatheter treatment with intraarterial vasopressin (splanchnic vasoconstrictor) or embolotherapy often obviates surgery.

Colonoscopy is often not possible in patients with acute active lower gastrointestinal tract hemorrhage because blood obscures the endoscopic view. In this set-ting, nuclear scintigraphy or arteriography is performed. ^{99m}Tc sulfur colloid scan is a sensitive examination and is capable of detecting bleeding rates as low as 0.05–0.1 mL/min, which is one-fifth to one-tenth of the minimal rate seen by arteriography. However, sulfur colloid imaging will be positive only if bleeding is active within 10–15 minutes of injection. ^{99m}Tc-labeled red blood cell scan can detect rates of blood loss similar to sulfur colloid scans and has the advantage of allowing imaging up to 24 hours after injection. It is preferred in patients with intermittent bleeding. Causes of false-positive labeled RBC scan include gastric, kidney, and bladder uptake due to poor labeling efficiency. Neither of the scintigraphic studies will be helpful unless hemorrhage is ongoing, and neither can determine the origin of the bleeding.

If nuclear scintigraphy is positive, arteriography is performed. This study is useful for diagnosis as well as therapy (Figure 14–30). Lower gastrointestinal bleeding arteriography can locate the site of bleeding if bleeding exceeds 0.5 mL/min. Arteriography can diagnose angiodysplasia, arteriovenous malformation, vascular tumor, and bleeding diverticulum. In some situations subsequent transcatheter vasopressin or embolotherapy is performed in an attempt to arrest the bleeding. If nuclear scintigraphy or arteriography is negative, further work-up should include CT, colonoscopy, and barium studies. Barium studies should never be done in the initial work-up of gastroin-

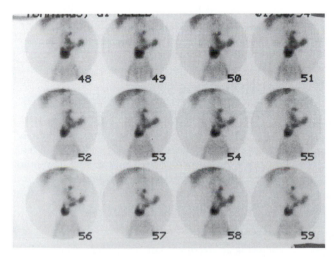

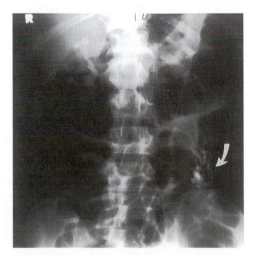

A

B

Figure 14–30. **A:** ^{99m}Tc-labeled red blood cell scan shows increased activity on delayed images in a patient with lower gastrointestinal hemorrhage. The configuration of the uptake is consistent with small bowel source. **B:** Superior mesenteric arteriogram shows extravasation of contrast in the region of the ileum with a tumor blush *(arrow)*. At surgery a bleeding carcinoid tumor was found.

testinal bleeding, since barium will interfere with subsequent angiography and endoscopy.

B. Mesenteric Ischemia

Early angiography is important in the diagnosis and treatment of mesenteric ischemia. Plain film findings often occur late in the course and include bowel wall thickening (thumbprinting), fixed bowel loops, a gasless abdomen, small bowel pseudoobstruction, and bowel distension to the level of the splenic flexure. Pneumatosis and portal vein gas are findings that indicate bowel necrosis and are associated with poor prognosis. CT and ultrasound can detect bowel abnormalities as well as vascular occlusions.

Mesenteric angiography is the diagnostic modality of choice for identification of occlusive disease [SMA embolus or thrombus, superior mesenteric vein (SMV) thrombus] versus nonocclusive disease (mesenteric vasoconstriction). SMA emboli usually occur in the setting of atrial fibrillation. The emboli appear as meniscoid filling defects at major branching points distal to the first 2 cm of the SMA. SMA thrombosis is usually seen in patients with preexisting atherosclerotic disease. Thrombus typically causes occlusion of the first 2 cm of the SMA.

SMV thrombosis may be idiopathic or occur in association with portal hypertension, hypercoagulable states, sepsis, or trauma. Angiographic findings include diffuse arterial spasm, slow arterial flow, and either absent visualization of the SMV or SMV thrombus. Nonocclusive ("low flow") mesenteric ischemia is due to arterial vasoconstriction commonly occurring in patients with underlying severe cardiac disease with low cardiac output or hypovolemic hypotension. During angiography, narrowing of the SMA branches is present with poor visualization of the SMV. In addition, focal or segmental spasm at branch points or diffuse spasm of the SMA system may be seen.

Mesenteric ischemia due to nonocclusive mesenteric ischemia is treated nonoperatively. In contrast, patients with SMA emboli or thrombus often require emergency surgery with embolectomy or thrombectomy with resection of infarcted bowel. A vasodilator such as papaverine may be infused into the SMA both before and after laparotomy and local resection. It may also be beneficial in patients with nonocclusive mesenteric ischemia. Patients with SMV thrombosis may be managed conservatively if collateral veins have formed. If peritoneal signs are present, laparotomy with bowel resection is often necessary.

C. Transjugular Intrahepatic Portosystemic Shunt

Placement of transjugular intrahepatic portosystemic shunt (TIPS) is a nonoperative treatment used for the management of acute variceal bleeding in patients with portal hypertension. In this procedure, the right or middle hepatic vein is accessed by passing a catheter through the right internal jugular vein and into the superior vena cava. A needle is advanced blindly from the hepatic vein out of the catheter and through the hepatic parenchyma into a branch of the portal vein. A wire is passed through the needle catheter into the portal vein system. An expandable metallic stent is then inserted across the tract, thereby creating a portal-systemic shunt.

TIPS is clinically indicated for patients with acute or recurrent variceal bleeding that is unresponsive to sclerotherapy and for patients with variceal bleeding who are awaiting liver transplantation. TIPS is also being evaluated as possible therapy for intractable portal hypertensive ascites. Contraindications for TIPS placement include severe right-sided heart failure, severe hepatic failure, polycystic liver disease, hypervascular hepatic masses, portal vein thrombosis, and sepsis.

Studies indicate that TIPS is an effective and safe method of decompressing portal pressure and controlling acute variceal bleeding (apparently as effective as surgical portocaval shunts and more effective than sclerotherapy, according to initial data). TIPS also avoids the need for surgery and general anesthesia and, due to its intrahepatic location, does not interfere with subsequent liver transplantation.

Reported complications of TIPS include intraperitoneal hemorrhage, hemobilia, bacteremia, and contrast-induced renal failure. Long-term complications include encephalopathy (in up to 20% of patients), recurrent variceal bleeding (18–26%), and shunt occlusion (in 10–20%). Shunt patency is usually maintained for up to 1–2 years, with occlusion related to the development of intimal hyperplasia.

RADIONUCLIDE SCANS

Gastroesophageal Reflux Study

The oral administration of ^{99m}Tc sulfur colloid rarely is used to evaluate patients presenting with atypical manifestations of gastroesophageal reflux, especially bilious vomiting or recurrent aspiration pneumonia. This technique is more sensitive than fluoroscopic barium esophagram or endoscopy for detecting reflux.

A. Technique

Following an overnight fast, the patient drinks 300 mL of acidic solution containing a radiotracer. With the patient in the supine position, images are obtained over the chest with an abdominal binder in place.

B. Cost

$690–$750.

Gastric Emptying Scan

This study is used for evaluation of gastric motility. It is most often employed in the evaluation of patients with suspected gastroparesis, especially diabetic gastroparesis or postvagotomy. The gastric emptying scan should not be the initial study for suspected mechanical gastric outlet obstruction. Although both liquid and solid phase emptying can be assessed, the solid portion of the study is more sensitive for detecting gastroparesis. For the liquid phase of the study, ^{111}In DTPA is used, and ^{99m}Tc sulfur colloid is used as the label for the solid phase (often tagged to egg whites). The normal time for one-half of the activity to leave the stomach is 90 minutes.

A. Technique

Following a fasting period of at least 4–6 hours, the patient consumes the labeled meal. Supine images are obtained every 15 minutes for 3 hours. The patient is required to sit up between each image.

B. Cost

$800–$900.

Liver-Spleen Scan

The liver and spleen both contain reticuloendothelial cells that readily take up ^{99m}Tc sulfur colloid from the blood. The pattern of uptake reflects the distribution of functioning reticuloendothelial cells as well as hepatic perfusion. The liver normally phagocytoses 80–90% of the tracer whereas the spleen sequesters 5–10% under normal circumstances. The bone marrow takes in a negligible amount of tracer. Lesions measuring 2–2.5 cm are readily identified. Smaller (1–1.5 cm) deep lesions may be detected by SPECT. Parenchymal defects demonstrated on this scan are nonspecific and cannot distinguish inflammatory from neoplastic lesions. However, the liver-spleen scan can detect some lesions that are missed by CT or ultrasound because of isodensity.

Causes of a solitary "cold" defect in the liver include hepatocellular carcinoma, metastasis, hemangioma, cyst, abscess, hematoma, and adenoma. Hepatic adenomas typically occur in young women with a history of oral contraceptive use. They usually do not contain a significant number of Kupffer cells and therefore will appear as an intrahepatic "cold" defect. In contrast, focal nodular hyperplasia (FNH) is a benign neoplasm that also occurs often in females. Because FNH contains Kupffer cells that are able to concentrate radiocolloid, it will appear indistinguishable (isodense) from the normal parenchyma or may occasionally appear as "hot" lesions with increased uptake. Multiple focal

"cold" intrahepatic defects are commonly due to metastatic disease, multiple cysts, or hemangiomas.

Diffuse liver disease may also be detected on liver-spleen scan. Cirrhosis is manifest by a small right hepatic lobe and an enlarged left lobe. Increased colloid uptake in the spleen and bone marrow typically is present. Causes of hepatomegaly with diffusely decreased colloid activity include infiltrative disorders, such as hepatitis or cirrhosis, fatty infiltration, passive congestion, lymphoma, and hemochromatosis.

Causes of splenic "cold" defects include cyst hemangioma, abscess, and malignancy. Splenic infarcts are typically identified by peripheral wedge-shaped defects. Splenomegaly may be due to portal hypertension, hemolytic anemia, lymphoma or leukemia, and infectious causes. The liver-spleen scan also may be used to localize accessory splenic tissue.

A. Technique

No patient preparation is necessary. Following the intravenous administration of ^{99m}Tc sulfur colloid, patients are imaged with multiple views, including anterior, posterior, lateral, and oblique positions.

B. Cost

$900–$950.

Meckel's Scan

Meckel's diverticulum represents the remnant of the omphalomesenteric duct and occurs in approximately 2% of the population. It is usually located within 100 cm of the ileocecal valve along the antimesenteric border of the ileum. There is a strong male preponderance, and the majority cause symptoms in children younger than 10 years. Most patients with Meckel's diverticula are asymptomatic; however, complications such as bleeding, obstruction, intussusception, and volvulus, can occur. Approximately 30% of Meckel's diverticula contain gastric mucosa, which increases the likelihood of complications. The frequency of ectopic gastric mucosa in symptomatic Meckel's diverticula is about 60%. In diverticula complicated by gastrointestinal hemorrhage, the incidence of ectopic gastric mucosa increases to over 95%.

Intravenous [^{99m}Tc]pertechnetate is secreted by gastric mucosa into the gastrointestinal tract. Radiopertechnetate also is secreted by the ectopic gastric mucosa located in a Meckel's diverticulum. It will be seen as a solitary focus of increased activity, usually located in the right lower quadrant of the abdomen. Activity in this focus should appear at the same time that activity appears in the stomach. Causes of false-positive results include inflammatory bowel disease, obstruction, urinary tract uptake (hydronephrosis), and intussusception. The accuracy of radiopertechnetate imaging for symptomatic Meckel's diverticulum is more than 95%.

A. PATIENT PREPARATION

Patients should fast for 6 hours to decrease gastric secretions and peristalsis. Patients should also empty the bladder and bowel before the imaging procedure.

B. TECHNIQUE

Following intravenous administration of radiopertechnetate, images are obtained in the supine position at 5-minute intervals up to 1 hour. Lateral views are also obtained. The administration of certain agents will improve localization: pentagastrin (increases pertechnetate uptake), glucagon (decreases peristalsis), or cimetidine (decreases pertechnetate secretion but not uptake).

C. COST

$800–$820.

Positron Emission Tomography (PET)

Positron emission tomography (PET) has become a useful tool in oncologic imaging because of its ability to image cellular metabolism. The most commonly used radiotracer, 2-[^{18}F]fluoro-2-deoxy-D-glucose (FDG), is a glucose analog. Images obtained reflect the uptake of glucose into cells. Because many tumors have rates of glycolysis higher than normal tissues, they exhibit increased uptake of FDG and appear as high intensity foci on PET-FDG images.

FDG is transported into cells by the glucose transporter. Once inside the cell, the molecule is phosphorylated by hexokinase. The phosphorylated molecule can neither advance down the glycolytic pathway nor exit the cell. Trapped within the cell, ^{18}F decays with a half-life of 110 minutes by emission of a positively charged electron called a positron. The positron, after exiting the nucleus, collides with an electron. This collision results in annihilation of the particles and emission of two photons at 180 degrees from each other. The detection of these annihilation photons by ring detectors is the basis for image production.

The sensitivity of PET is optimal for detection of lesions 1 cm or greater in size. Sensitivity for detection of lesions is compromised by hyperglycemia, and patients are routinely fasted prior to the examination. Image interpretation requires familiarity with the normal pattern of FDG uptake (most intense in brain, heart, kidneys, and urinary bladder) and appreciation for the heterogeneous pattern of activity common in normal livers. False-positive liver lesions have been reported in the setting of significant intrahepatic cholestasis. Against the background of normal biodistribution, foci of increased activity may represent a spectrum of

pathology spanning inflammatory and neoplastic etiologies.

A. COLORECTAL CARCINOMA

PET-FDG has been shown to be more sensitive than conventional modalities such as CT and MRI for detection of metastatic disease with high sensitivities in the range of 95–100%. Accuracy in the detection of hepatic metastases from colorectal carcinoma is essential when segmental hepatic resection is planned for cure (Figure 14–31). Sensitivity and specificity for detection of hepatic metastases were 95% and 100% by PET-FDG compared with 74% and 85% for CT in one series. Detection of otherwise occult metastatic disease has been shown to alter treatment planning in up to 60% of cases. PET-FDG can also assist in distinguishing tumor recurrence from postoperative scar. There is a limited but growing experience utilizing PET to document the response of metastatic lesions to chemotherapy. Uptake of ^{18}F-labeled flourouracil by tumor deposits has been shown to predict response to chemotherapy. After chemotherapy, decreased glucose utilization in lesions has been shown to correlate with a favorable response. If glucose utilization fails to decrease or if new lesions appear, alternative treatment therapies may be considered.

B. PRIMARY LIVER NEOPLASIA

Overall, PET-FDG has relatively low sensitivity for the detection of hepatocellular carcinoma, detecting 55% of tumors compared with a sensitivity of 90% by CT. Moderately to poorly differentiated tumors are more likely to show FDG uptake than are well-differentiated, low-grade tumors. Cholangiocarcinoma accumulates FDG avidly, making PET-FDG useful in differentiating benign from neoplastic strictures. Benign hepatic masses such as focal nodular hyperplasia and adenoma have been consistently reported to demonstrate little or no focal FDG uptake.

C. PANCREATIC NEOPLASIA

Sensitivity and specificity for the detection of pancreatic adenocarcinoma by PET-FDG have been shown to be 92% and 85%. PET-FDG is also useful for distinguishing chronic pancreatitis from tumor and for the detection of metastases. Positron emitters other than ^{18}F have been useful for imaging tumors of the endocrine pancreas.

D. ESOPHAGEAL CARCINOMA

The sensitivity of PET-FDG for detection of metastatic lymph nodes has been reported to range from 33 to 83% with optimum sensitivity for nodes 1 cm or larger. Metastatic deposits in lymph nodes as small as 4 mm have been identified using carbon-11, another positron

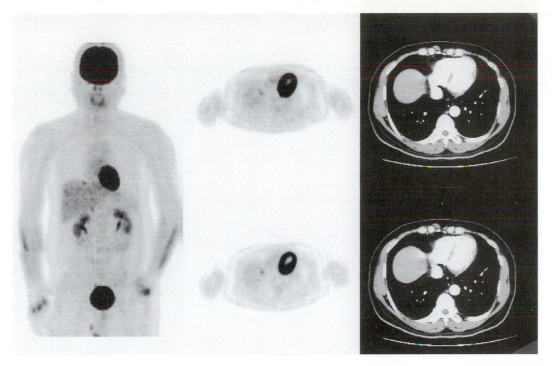

Figure 14–31. PET scan using FDG in a patient with metastatic colorectal carcinoma. A small focus of increased uptake is seen in the dome of the liver on both the whole body image and the axial image. Correlative CT scan shows a small enhancing mass high in the liver.

emitter, linked to choline. PET-FDG has been shown to be more sensitive than CT for the detection of distant metastases.

REFERENCES

Balthazar EJ et al: Acute appendicitis: CT and US correlation in 100 patients. Radiology 1994;190:31.

Bluemke DA, Fishman EK: Spiral CT of the liver. Am J Roentgenol 1993;160:787.

Botet JF et al: Preoperative staging of esophageal cancer: comparison of endoscopic US and dynamic CT. Radiology 1991;181: 419.

Botet JF et al: Preoperative staging of gastric cancer: comparison of endoscopic US and dynamic CT. Radiology 1991;181:426.

Choi JY et al: Improved detection of individual nodal involvement in squamous cell carcinoma of the esophagus by FDG PET. J Nucl Med 2000;41:808.

Delbeke D et al: Optimal interpretation of FDG PET in the diagnosis, staging and management of pancreatic carcinoma. J Nucl Med 1999;40:1784.

DelMaschio A et al: Pancreatic cancer versus chronic pancreatitis: diagnosis with CA 19-9 assessment, US, CT, and CT-guided fine-needle biopsy. Radiology 1991;178:95.

Dixon PM, Roulston ME, Nolan DJ: The small bowel enema: a ten-year review. Clin Radiol 1993;47:46.

Fenlon HM et al: A comparison of virtual and conventional colonoscopy for the detection of colorectal polyps. N Engl J Med 1999;341:1496.

Ferrucci JT: Liver tumor imaging. Am J Roentgenol 1990;155:473.

Ferrucci JT: Screening for colon cancer: programs of the American College of Radiology. Am J Roentgenol 1993;160:999.

Frazer D et al: CT of small bowel obstruction: value in establishing the diagnosis and determining the degree and cause. Am J Roentgenol 1994;162:37.

Frohlich A et al: Detection of liver metastases from pancreatic cancer using FDG PET. J Nucl Med 1999;40:250.

Gazelle GS et al: Efficacy of CT in distinguishing small bowel obstruction from other causes of small bowel dilatation. Am J Radiol 1994;162:43.

Hara AK et al: Detection of colorectal polyps with CT colography: initial assessment of sensitivity and specificity. Radiology 1997;205:59.

Khan MA et al: Positron emission tomography scanning in the evaluation of hepatocellular carcinoma. J Hepatol 2000;32: 792.

LaBerge JM et al: Creation of transjugular intrahepatic portosystemic shunts with the Wallstent endoprosthesis: results in 100 patients. Radiology 1993;187:413.

Levine MS, Laufer I: Perspective: the upper gastrointestinal series at a crossroads. Am J Roentgenol 1993;161:1131.

Levine MS, Rubesin SE, Ott DJ: Update on esophageal radiology. Am J Roentgenol 1990;155:933.

Maglinte DT, Torres WE, Laufer I: Oral cholecystography in contemporary gallstone imaging: a review. Radiology 1991;178: 49.

Niederau C, Grendell JH: Diagnosis of pancreatic carcinoma: imaging techniques and tumor markers. Pancreas 1992;7:66.

Ogunbiyi OA et al: Detection of recurrent and metastatic colorectal cancer: comparison of positron emission tomography and computed tomography. Ann Surg Oncol 1997;4:613.

Ott DJ, Pikna LA: Clinical and videofluoroscopic evaluation of swallowing disorders. Am J Roentgenol 1993;161:507.

Philpotts LE et al: Colitis: use of CT findings in differential diagnosis. Radiology 1994;190:445.

Rosh T et al: Staging of pancreatic and ampullary carcinoma by endoscopic ultrasonography—comparison with conventional sonography, computed tomography, and angiography. Gastroenterology 1992;102:188.

Soyer P et al: Detection of liver metastases from colorectal cancer: comparison of intraoperative US and CT during arterial portography. Radiology 1992;183:541.

Staib L et al: Is (18)F-fluorodeoxyglucose positron emission tomography in recurrent colorectal cancer a contribution to surgical decision making? Am J Surg 2000;180:1.

Takishima S et al: Carcinoma of the esophagus: CT versus MR imaging in determining resectability. Am J Roentgenol 1991; 156:297.

van Sonnenberg E et al: Percutaneous abscess drainage: current concepts. Radiology 1991;181:617.

Whitaker SC, Gregson RH: The role of angiography in the investigation of acute or chronic gastrointestinal haemorrhage. Clin Radiol 1993;47:382.

Yee J et al: Performance characteristics of CT colonography for the detection of colorectal neoplasia in 300 patients. Radiology 2001;219:685.

Zuckerman DA, Bocchini TP, Birnbaum EH: Massive hemorrhage in the lower gastrointestinal tract in adults: diagnostic imaging and intervention. Am J Roentgenol 1993;161:703.

Endoscopic Management of Biliary & Pancreatic Diseases

15

Timothy P. Kinney, MD & Richard A. Kozarek, MD

Endoscopic retrograde cholangiopancreatography (ERCP) was originally used to facilitate diagnosis in a variety of benign and malignant pancreaticobiliary disorders. In the past 25 years, however, since the original description of endoscopic sphincterotomy, it has evolved from a purely diagnostic modality to one that entails a therapeutic intervention 50–75% of the time. Thus, the majority of common bile duct calculi can be removed, most malignant biliary strictures can be stented, and a subset of biliary injuries is amenable to endotherapeutic procedures. Many of the questions that remain are technical: Is it safe to perform balloon dilation of the sphincter to remove stones? Should a dilating catheter or balloon catheter be used? In whom should we place an expandable metal prosthesis?

By way of contrast, endotherapy directed toward the pancreas is in its youth. Treatment of pancreatic calculi requires not only technical expertise but also a conviction that these calculi are more than epiphenomena, are not only the consequence of chronic pancreatitis, but also the cause of pain and relapsing attacks of clinical pancreatitis in a subset of patients. Treatment of benign and malignant pancreatic stenoses, in turn, requires a belief that impaired flow of pancreatic secretions causes clinical symptoms related to ductal obstruction. Finally, treatment of ductal disruptions presupposes that techniques used within the biliary tree can be readily adapted to the pancreatic duct with comparable results and an acceptable complication rate. Most of the above assumptions still await confirmatory studies before widespread application of these procedures can be recommended.

BILIARY DISEASE

Biliary tree processes amenable to therapeutic ERCP include calculi with or without concomitant jaundice, cholangitis, or pancreatitis; benign and malignant strictures; sphincter of Oddi stenosis or spasm; biliary fistulas; and miscellaneous conditions to include choledochocele, sump syndrome, biliary parasitosis, and acquired immunodeficiency syndrome (AIDS) cholangiopathy.

Calculus Disease

Endoscopic biliary sphincterotomy, developed simultaneously in Japan and Germany in the mid-1970s, is now widely applied for treating bile duct stones. Procedures require fluoroscopic monitoring, antibiotic precoverage, and access to a wide range of equipment. Using accessories that have evolved from free-hand to wire-guided, the endoscopist performs electrocautery incision of the distal bile duct to access the biliary tree. Balloon catheters or stone baskets are then used for subsequent calculus extraction (Figure 15–1). Most series and surveys suggest a success rate of approximately 85–95% for complete stone retrieval. This rate is contingent upon several factors, including stone size (large stones may require mechanical, extracorporeal, or electrohydraulic lithotripsy, dissolution therapy, or endoprosthesis placement). Other factors include concomitant biliary stricture, or the presence of variant anatomy such as juxtampullary diverticula, Billroth II gastric resection, and Roux-en-Y jejunal anastomoses. Complications, in turn, average 7–8% and the mortality rate is approximately 1% in the largest series. Complications include bleeding and pancreatitis, most frequently, but also acute cholecystitis in patients with intact gallbladders, bile duct or intestinal perforation (Figure 15–2), basket entrapment, and more mundane types of complications (drug reaction, aspiration, cardiopulmonary events) are all well described.

The above-mentioned success and complication rates have led practitioners to accept endoscopic sphincterotomy as the procedure of choice in postcholecystectomy patients who have common bile duct stones or the high surgical-risk patient who has an intact gallbladder. It is also the procedure of choice in most patients with acute cholangitis with or without a gallbladder. ERCP may be both diagnostic and therapeutic in a significant subset of patients with gallstone pancreatitis. Finally, the practice of laparoscopic cholecystectomy has radically altered the approach to choledocholithiasis in many centers. As such, open common bile duct exploration has been relegated to a small role in the treatment of choledocholithiasis.

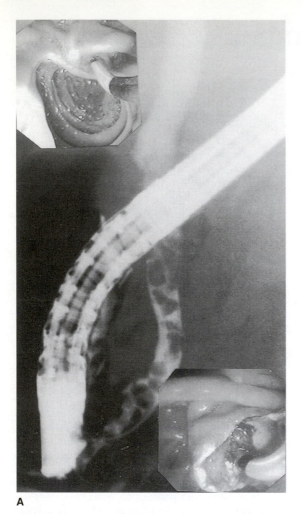

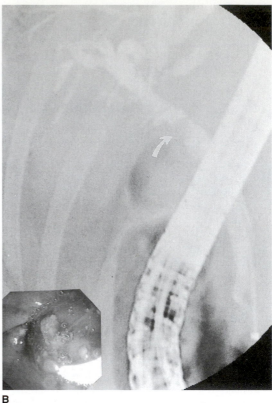

B

A

Figure 15–1. **A:** Cholangiogram demonstrating multiple calculi. Insets depict biliary sphincterotomy. **B:** Copious debris retrieved (inset) utilizing extraction balloon *(arrow).*

Cholangitis

Pus in the biliary tree occurs most commonly with impacted bile duct stones, but can also be a consequence of endoprosthesis occlusion. Presenting clinically with Charcot's triad (fever, jaundice, and hepatic pain) or Reynolds pentad (jaundice, pain, fever, change in mental status, and shock), bacterial cholangitis has a higher than 80% associated mortality rate when left undrained. Open surgical intervention carries mortality rates between 7% and 50%. Endoscopic drainage, in turn, is achieved by performing biliary sphincterotomy and placement of either a large-bore endoprosthesis or nasobiliary drain to effect ir-

rigation. Several studies document relative procedural safety and a mortality as low as 5% within 24 hours.

Pancreatitis

Gallstone pancreatitis may be mild when associated with calculus passage through the papilla of Vater. It can also be severe, recurrent, and associated with concomitant cholangitis, causing major morbidity (Figure 15–3). Given the known incidence of ERCP-induced pancreatitis, several studies have prospectively addressed whether urgent endoscopic intervention ameliorates or exacerbates presumptive biliary pancreatitis. In a classic

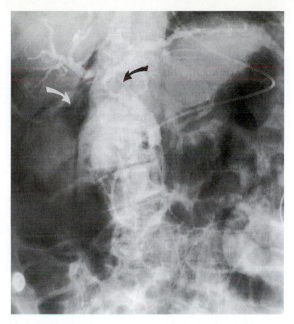

Figure 15–2. Nasobiliary drain ***(black arrow)*** in cholangitis patient who sustained perforation with sphincterotomy. Note para-psoas air ***(white arrow).*** Patient did well with conservative therapy.

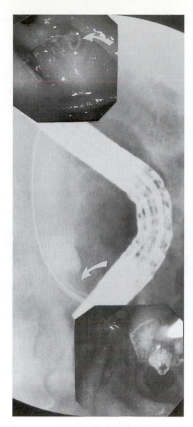

Figure 15–3. Arrows depict impacted calculus in patient with biliary pancreatitis. Lower inset shows stone retrieval following small sphincterotomy.

study by Neoptolemos et al, 121 patients were randomized to conventional medical therapy versus urgent ERCP and stone extraction, if indicated. Findings included the following: (1) ERCP did not appear to exacerbate the acute pancreatitis; (2) patients undergoing urgent ERCP/sphincterotomy had fewer complications (P = .03), particularly those with severe disease (P = .007) as defined by the Glasgow system for scoring severity; (3) hospitalization for the endoscopically treated group was approximately one-half that of the conservatively managed patients; and (4) there was no statistically significant difference in mortality between the two groups. Another study by Fan et al documented clinical improvement following sphincterotomy in patients with both mild and moderate biliary pancreatitis, suggesting that urgent ERCP should be considered in at least a subset of patients with gallstone pancreatitis. In particular, urgent ERCP resulted in a reduction in cholangitis with sepsis. A third study by Fölsch et al did not show the same benefit of urgent ERCP in acute biliary pancreatitis, however, patients with obvious obstructing stones or overt cholangitis were excluded, ie, those most likely to develop biliary sepsis. Current practice in the authors' institution is to use ERCP in patients with severe biliary pancreatitis, persistent liver function test abnormalities, recurrent biliary colic, or exacerbation of pancreatitis, and those who have evidence of cholangitis.

Interaction between ERCP & Laparoscopic Cholecystectomy for Stone Disease

Since the advent of laparoscopic cholecystectomy in 1989, practice patterns have varied widely with regard to the diagnosis and treatment of choledocholithiasis in patients undergoing cholecystectomy. Some recommend universal preoperative ERCP both to provide an anatomic "outline" for the surgeon and to remove stones when identified. However, such an approach exposes an excessive number of patients to the risk of ERCP—as 50–75% of preoperative ERCPs are normal. In some centers, magnetic resonance imaging of the bile duct (MRCP)—which is noninvasive—increasingly is used in such patients. Others recommend "selective" use of preoperative ERCP in patients in whom there is higher suspicion of common bile duct (CBD) stone (ie, elevated liver function tests, ultrasongraphic evidence of a dilated CBD, cholangitis, or pancreatitis). Other surgeons prefer to perform a routine cholangiogram at the time of laparoscopic cholecystectomy. Many small common duct stones can be retrieved through the cystic duct or pushed through the papilla. For common duct stones that cannot be removed laparoscopically, the surgeon must decide between open common duct exploration or postoperative ERCP with attempted stone extraction. At centers at which there is an experienced biliary endoscopist, postoperative ERCP is preferred to open exploration for most patients with retained common duct stones as well as patients who become symptomatic after laparoscopic cholecystectomy. Alternatively, intraoperative ERCP is used in a few centers to remove stones documented by operative cholangiography. Currently, approaches to choledocholithiasis are institutionally dependent, contingent on the relative skill and confidence levels of both the laparoscopic surgeon and biliary endoscopist. Institutions in which both the endoscopist and surgeon are uncomfortable with their ability to retrieve bile duct stones tend to do more preoperative MRCPs or ERCPs. If a stone is found at preoperative ERCP that cannot be removed, laparoscopic retrieval would be attempted, which, if unsuccessful, is followed by open exploration.

In the authors' institution, preoperative ERCP is restricted to patients with acute cholangitis, significant biliary pancreatitis, or obstructive jaundice. In all other cases undergoing laparoscopic cholecystectomy, intraoperative cholangiography is performed and if stones are found, attempts are made to remove them through the cystic duct. Postoperative ERCP is performed in patients in whom laparoscopic stone extraction is unsuccessful and in those who develop postoperartive biliary symptoms. This approach markedly limits the number of ERCPs performed to the subgroup of patients in whom the benefits outweigh the risks.

Stone Extraction without Sphincterotomy

Sphincterotomy is associated with a small but appreciable risk of severe acute complications (bleeding, pancreatitis, perforation) as well as the uncertain long-term consequences of sphincter ablation. Hence, a number of endoscopists perform balloon dilation of the sphincter rather than sphincterotomy prior to stone extraction. Although earlier studies suggested similar efficacy and complication rates, a U.S. multicenter trial revealed a 15% complication rate from balloon dilation compared with 4% with sphincterotomy. Most of the morbidity attributed to balloon dilation was due to moderate or severe pancreatitis, resulting in two deaths. For this reason, we perform balloon sphincter dilation only in the setting of severe coagulopathy, when the bleeding risk of sphincterotomy outweighs the risk of pancreatitis.

BILE DUCT STRICTURES

Benign Strictures

A. AMPULLARY SPASM–PAPILLARY STENOSIS

Sphincter of Oddi dysfunction may be caused by papillary stricture (stenosis) or disordered motility. Patients with sphincter of Oddi dysfunction from either subset typically present with postcholecystectomy biliary colic with fluctuating liver function test [increased aspartate aminotransferase (AST) and/or alkaline phosphatase] abnormalities. Papillary stricture may develop as a consequence of passage of small stones or "gravel," which leads to papillitis and scarring, resulting in biliary dilation. Over 90% of such patients derive relief of symptoms after biliary sphincterotomy. Alternatively, the "spastic" subset is caused by altered sphincter motility characterized by manometric abnormalities (hypertensive sphincter, tachyoddia) that usually does not lead to biliary dilation. A wide variety of diagnostic tests have been used to document sphincter dysfunction, including a morphine/neostigmine challenge ("Nardi test"), fatty meal ultrasound, nuclear medicine biliary scintigraphy, and conventional ERCP. Biliary manometry now is considered the gold standard for diagnosis of sphincter dysfunction by most endoscopists (Figure 15–4). A baseline biliary sphincter pressure of >35–40 mm Hg is abnormal. Endoscopic sphincterotomy in patients with a hypertensive sphincter has been associated with sustained relief in 60–90% of patients—being increased in patients with other demonstrated abnormalities (eg, elevated liver chemistries, ultrasonographic evidence of dilation of the biliary tract, or delayed drainage of the common bile duct demonstrated at ERCP). Balloon dilation of the sphincter is associated with a prohibitive risk of pancreatitis in such patients and has no sustained effect on sphincter pressure or patient symptoms.

Strictures Associated with Bile Duct Injury

Laparoscopic cholecystectomy is associated with a small but significant incidence of bile duct injuries. When discovered early, these injuries are frequently associated with a bile duct fistula. This problem will be discussed subsequently (see section, "Bile Duct Fistulas"). When discovered later, stenosis is often the result. Occurring

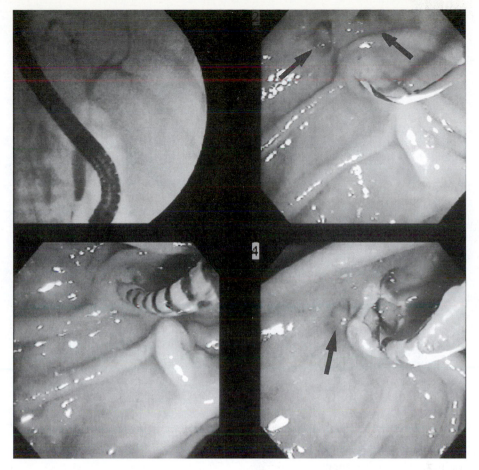

Figure 15–4. Manometry testing in a patient with periampulary diverticulae *(arrows)* followed by biliary sphincterotomy. Note normal cholangiogram.

as a consequence of a misdirected scalpel, scissors, clip, or cautery (Figure 15–5), or as a result of ischemic injury caused by devascularization, bile duct strictures traditionally have been treated surgically, most commonly with Roux-en-Y hepaticojejunostomy. However, results of endoscopic therapy for iatrogenic biliary injuries have been encouraging, with 70–80% of patients reported to be asymptomatic over follow-up periods of 3–6 1/2 years. The endoscopic approach requires sphincterotomy followed by balloon dilation of the stricture and subsequent placement of one or two endoprostheses (stents) across the stenosis. Stents are exchanged and the stricture redilated every 3–4 months for up to 1 year. Long-term follow-up is mandatory as restenosis may be subtle and may occur many years later—even after a "successful" surgical repair.

Miscellaneous Benign Strictures

Balloon dilation with or without endoprosthesis placement has been used for treatment of other benign biliary stenoses, including distal bile duct strictures associated with chronic pancreatitis, radiation stenoses, obstruction of the bile duct caused by an impacted stone in the cystic duct (Mirizzi's syndrome), and dominant strictures caused by sclerosing cholangitis. Biliary strictures caused by chronic pancreatitis usually are not treated effectively by the placement of endoprostheses. Most pancreatic strictures persist after stent placement. Long-term stent placement is often complicated by occlusion or migration. As such, many authorities recommend the placement of biliary stents for benign pancreatic disease only as a temporary measure or in patients

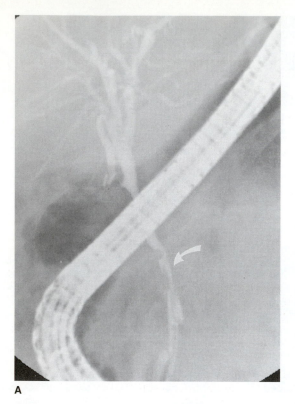

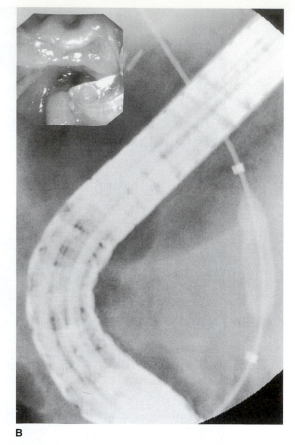

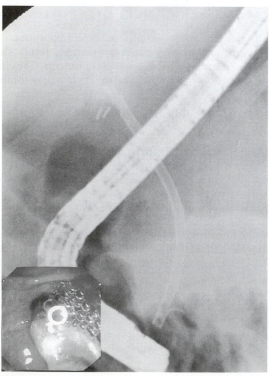

Figure 15–5. Asymmetric distal common bile duct stenosis as a consequence of cautery injury during laparoscopic cholecystectomy **(A)**. Stricture treated with balloon dilation **(B)** and stent insertion **(C)**.

who are poor operative candidates. In a subset of patients with sclerosing cholangitis, endotherapy of a dominant stenosis has been shown to improve liver function tests, decrease the incidence of secondary bacterial cholangitis, and delay or even obviate the need for liver transplant.

Malignant Biliary Strictures

The most common cause of malignant obstructive jaundice is carcinoma of the pancreatic head. Less common causes include carcinoma of the bile duct, gallbladder, ampulla, or duodenum, or nodal metastases to the porta hepatis. The vast majority of these neoplasms are unresectable for cure. For relief of biliary obstruction in patients with incurable malignancy, surgical resection or bypass, percutaneous stent or drain placement, or endoscopic drainage by dilation and endoprosthesis placement all are therapeutic options, depending upon the location of obstruction, expected survival, and other comorbid conditions.

Plastic Stents

Plastic (polyethylene) stents of different diameters (2.3–3.8 mm), lengths (3–15 cm), and configurations (straight, pig-tailed) are available for endoscopic placement. After placement of a wire across the area of stenosis, plastic prostheses are placed through the stenosis. Stent placement may be preceded by dilation and brush cytology, biopsy, or needle aspiration of suspected malignancy. Successful drainage is achieved in 85–90% of patients with malignant biliary obstruction with a median patient survival of approximately 5 months (Figure 15–6). About 15–30% of patients develop stent occlusion, necessitating stent replacement.

Randomized prospective studies of patients with malignant obstructive jaundice suggest that biliary enteric bypass surgery and endoscopic stent placement are equivalent with regard to adequacy of biliary decompression and long-term median survival. Endoscopic stenting caused significantly less procedure-related mortality, however, as well as fewer complications, lower costs, and shorter hospitalization compared with surgery.

Metallic Stents

Occlusion of polyethylene prostheses by bacterial biofilm is problematic. A number of metallic prostheses have been devised in the hopes that their large diameter (8–10 mm) will preclude or minimize plugging with biofilm. A variety of endoprostheses have been used including the conventional spiral Z stent, the Za stent, the Diamond, the Memotherm, and the biliary Endo-

coil, however most experience to date has accrued with the uncovered Wallstent (Figure 15–7). Prospective studies randomizing patients with malignant biliary obstruction to receive either the Wallstent or plastic stents have confirmed that the Wallstent affords longer stent patency, but no improvement in patient survival. The median stent patency of the Wallstent is 273 days compared with 126 days for a plastic stent. Placement of the Wallstent is associated with a 28% decrease in need for subsequent endoscopic procedures. Therefore, despite a 20-fold difference in cost between metallic and polyethylene prostheses, metal stents are more cost effective for treatment of malignant jaundice in patients with an expected survival of more than 3–4 months.

Bile Duct Fistulas

Bile duct fistulas may be caused by abdominal trauma, stone erosion, or liver transplantation, however, the majority occur after cholecystectomy. Fistulas may present with abdominal pain, nausea, distention, or fever. The diagnosis commonly is suggested by the presence of an intraabdominal fluid collection on abdominal ultrasound or computed tomography (CT). Biliary HIDA scintigraphy may document a biliary leak, but does not delineate the presence or extent of bile ascites, which may require percutaneous drainage.

Endotherapy has become the standard of care for treating most biliary fistulas and provides excellent results. By lowering intraductal pressures with either sphincterotomy alone or stent placement (in some cases supplemented by percutaneous drainage), fistula closure has been reported in 67–90% of patients. The efficacy of endotherapy for the treatment of biliary fistulas depends on the site of the leak (cystic duct, common duct, or intrahepatic duct), the presence of associated bile duct stricture, and the presence of biliary calculi or papillary stenosis (Figure 15–8). Most cystic duct or intrahepatic duct leaks close rapidly after placing a short 7–10 Fr plastic stent or after biliary sphincterotomy alone, if sphincter stenosis or a stone is present. Extrahepatic bile duct leaks also usually close, depending on the degree of ductal injury and whether the stent can be placed above an associated ductal stenosis.

Miscellaneous Conditions

ERCP has proven useful for the diagnosis and treatment of a number of other miscellaneous conditions. Sphincterotomy may be the definitive treatment for biliary ascariasis, choledochocele (Figure 15–9), and "sump syndrome" (ie, biliary colic or cholangitis caused by a narrowed side-to-side choledochoduodenostomy). Rarely, placement of a catheter across the papilla into the gallbladder has been used for decompression in

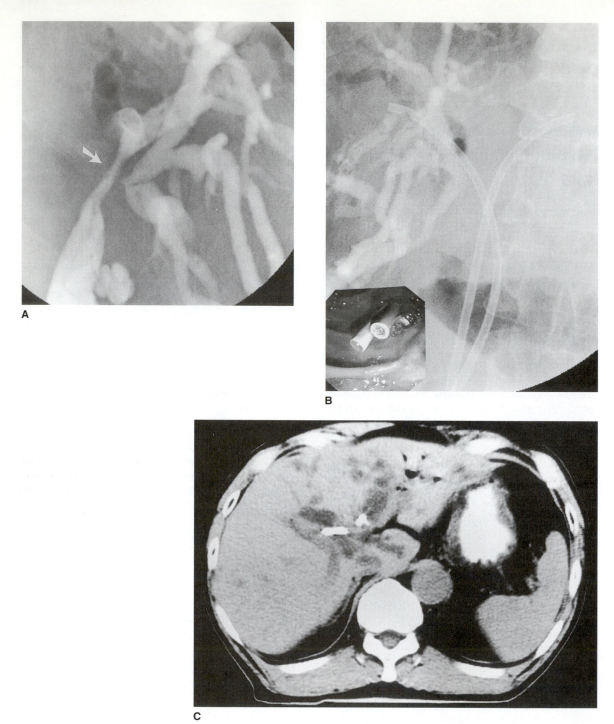

Figure 15–6. Tight bifurcation stenosis *(arrow)* in patient with cholangiocarcinoma **(A).** 10 Fr stents placed into right and left intrahepatic ducts **(B).** Note CT demonstrating adequate placement into dilated intrahepatic ducts **(C).**

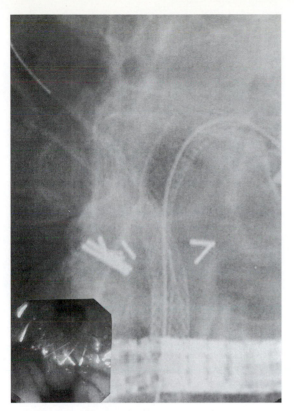

Figure 15–7. Bilateral Wallstents used in patient with bifurcation cholangiocarcinoma. Inset shows transpapillary stent in good position.

high-risk patients with acute cholecystitis and gallstone dissolution in poor surgical-risk patients with symptomatic cholelithiasis.

PANCREATIC DISEASE

Most commonly used for the diagnosis of pancreatitis or pancreatic malignancies, ERCP also has been widely applied therapeutically for the treatment of pancreatic disorders, although few controlled trials have been done to define efficacy. In patients with chronic pancreatitis, therapeutic interventions have included major or minor pancreatic duct sphincterotomy; calculus retrieval; transpapillary, transgastric, or transduodenal pseudocyst drainage; and dilation or stenting of pancreatic stenoses. Endoprostheses are also used to treat disrupted pancreatic ducts with fistulas. The use of endoprostheses to treat biliary chronic pancreatitis-induced bile duct stricture is discussed above (see section, "Miscellaneous Benign Strictures").

Sphincter Dysfunction/Sphincterotomy

Once considered high risk, endoscopic sphincterotomy of the major pancreatic duct can be undertaken fairly safely using either a conventional sphincterotome passed across the pancreatic orifice, or by cutting the sphincter with a needle-knife after placing a small stent into the pancreatic duct. Pancreatic sphincterotomy of either the major papilla or minor papilla may be used to treat presumed sphincter dysfunction or to facilitate passage of endoscopic accessories into the pancreatic duct (stents, stones, or dilators). Pancreatic endoprostheses have been placed in an attempt to relieve chronic pain or relapsing attacks of pancreatitis in some patients with presumed sphincter dysfunction, however they may induce focal pancreatitis and ductal stenoses. Accordingly, pancreatic duct sphincterotomy of either the major or minor papilla may be preferable to treat sphincter dysfunction.

Complications of pancreatic sphincterotomy include pancreatitis (9%) and bleeding (3.6%). In patients with chronic pancreatitis, long-term improvement in pain scores is reported in up to 60% of patients after pancreatic endotherapy with sphincterotomy, dilation, stent placement, and stone extraction.

Minor papilla sphincterotomy may be useful in patients with pancreas divisum and relapsing pancreatitis. Of 19 of 39 patients treated with minor duct sphincterotomy at the authors' institution for either pain or ductal disruption, approximately one-half were symptomatically improved and healing of ductal disruption occurred in 80%. Moreover, 11 of 15 patients had resolution of acute relapsing attacks. By contrast, patients with chronic pancreatitis caused by pancreas divisum are less likely to benefit from minor duct sphincterotomy. Procedure-related pancreatitis is noted in approximately 10% of patients.

Ductal Stenoses

Endoscopic therapy with dilation and stent placement generally is ineffective in the long-term treatment of pancreatic strictures, may cause pancreatic injury and stricture, and is associated with other complications (ie, pancreatic sepsis, stent migration into the duct, cholangitis, pseudocyst development, and hematobilia). Therefore, endotherapy is not an acceptable long-term treatment in most patients with pancreatic ductal strictures. Notwithstanding, placement of endoprostheses beyond pancreatic stenoses may be indicated for both diagnosis and therapy in high surgical-risk patient following catheter or balloon dilation (Figure 15–10). Cremer et al reported successful stenting of 75 of 76 patients with chronic pancreatitis and dominant duct strictures. Most also underwent major or minor duct

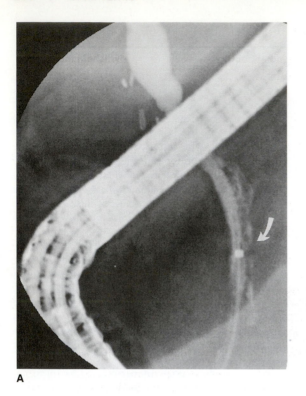
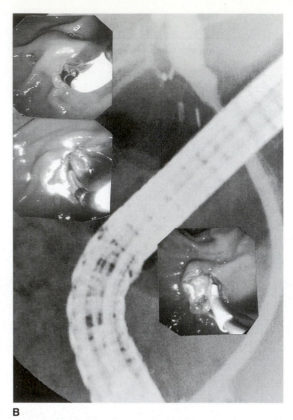

Figure 15–8. Irregular distal CBD leak as consequence of cautery injury **(A)** treated with sphincterotomy (insets) and **(B)** stent insertion.

sphincterotomy and some had extracorporeal shock wave lithotripsy for concomitant calculi. Ninety-four percent were symptomatically improved, although 11 ultimately underwent longitudinal pancreaticojejunostomy. Stent patency was estimated to be 1 year, with recurrent symptoms as a consequence of endoprosthesis occlusion. Less than 10% of patients had resolution of their stricture. Placement of double stents in proximal duct strictures may preclude the need for pancreatic head resection in a subset of patients. Even in the event of stent occlusion, drainage between the prostheses is often adequate to prevent recurrent obstructive pancreatitis and pancreatic sepsis.

Calculi

Pancreatic calculi are usually considered the consequence of chronic pancreatitis rather than the cause per se of pain or relapsing attacks of pancreatitis. However, in some patients pancreatic stones may obstruct the duct and cause symptoms. Kozarek et al achieved suc-

cessful stone retrieval in 10 of 11 patients utilizing conventional balloon or baskets following a pancreatic sphincterotomy (Figure 15–11). At a mean follow-up of 18 months, 8 of 9 patients with relapsing pancreatitis were symptom free. One of two chronic pain patients also was symptomatically improved. Similar data have been noted by Sherman et al, who reported partial or complete stone retrieval in 75% of 31 chronic pancreatitis patients, two-thirds of whom improved symptomatically.

Large, adherent, or impacted calculi must be fragmented prior to endoscopic retrieval. This has been done most commonly using extracorporeal shock wave lithotripsy (ESWL). Delhaye et al treated 123 patients with obstructing pancreatic calculi with ESWL after initial pancreatic duct sphincterotomy and nasopancreatic drain insertion. Virtually all stones could be fragmented and one-half of patients had subsequent complete stone retrieval. Complications included mild flare of pancreatitis in approximately one-third of patients. All patients were noted to have initial symptom relief

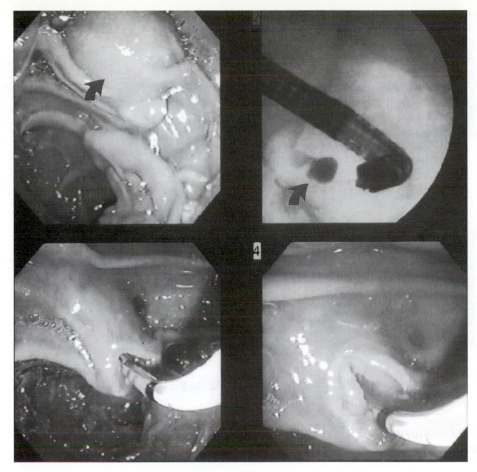

Figure 15–9. Choledochocele *(arrows)* causing recurrent obstruction and biliary colic is treated with sphinctero-tomy.

although one-half developed symptom recurrence as a consequence of stone migration or recurrence, ductal stenosis, or stent occlusion. Our group has documented statistically decreased pain, narcotic ingestion, and hospitalization rates in 40 patients treated with ERCP and ESWL. At a mean follow-up of 2 years, 80% of patients were able to avoid surgery.

Ductal Disruption

Ductal disruptions may present in the form of pseudo-cysts, pancreaticocutaneous fistula, pancreatic ascites, or chronic pleural effusion. Optimal treatment of these disruptions is contingent on both anatomic constraints and competing local expertise (surgical, interventional radiologic, and endoscopic). Kozarek et al have utilized transpapillary endoprosthesis to treat ductal disruptions associated with pancreatic ascites and with contained

fluid collections, including pseudocysts. Four patients rapidly resolved their ascites utilizing a combination of stent placement and a single large-volume paracentesis with no recurrence at a mean follow-up of 6 years. For contained fluid collections and pseudocysts, trans-papillary drains or stents were placed in 17 patients, 14 of whom had ultimate resolution of their fluid collections. Complications were noted in four patients, including mild pancreatitis in two, and stent occlusion with recurrent pseudocyst (1) and cyst infection (1). Both of the latter complications responded to stent exchange.

Pseudocysts can also be drained by endoscopic placement of a catheter across the duodenal wall or gastric wall into the pseudocyst. Transgastric or transduo-denal catheter drainage is facilitated by endoscopic ultrasonography to determine the distance between the mucosal surface and pseudocyst and to avoid vascular

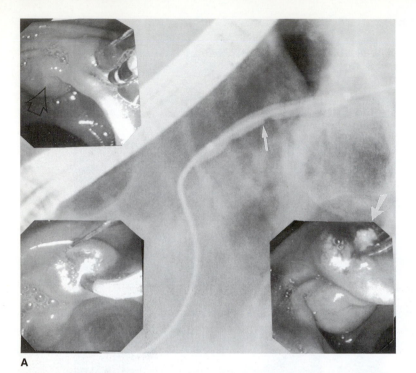

A

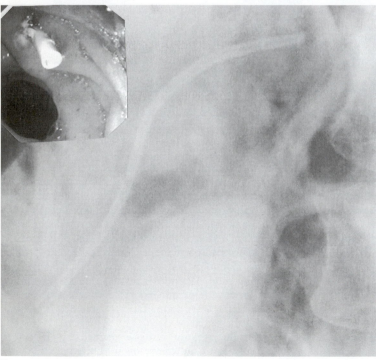

B

Figure 15–10. Pancreatic divisum patient with chronic pancreatitis, dorsal duct stricture treated with minor sphincterotomy (insets), balloon dilation *(arrow),* and stone extraction *(arrow)* **(A).** Open arrow depicts major papilla. Subsequent endoprosthesis insertion **(B).**

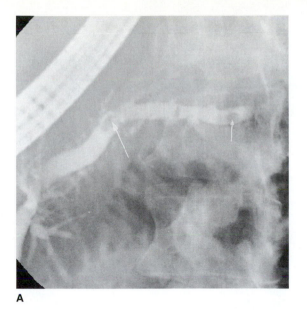

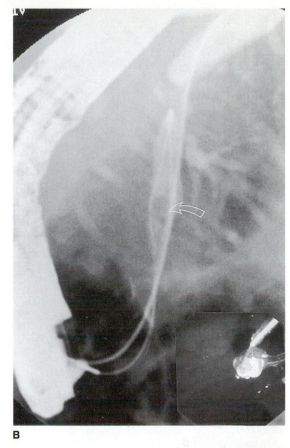

Figure 15–11. Arrows depict calculi **(A)** in patient with chronic pancreatitis. Basket retrieval of stones **(B:** *arrow,* inset)** following pancreatic duct sphincterotomy.

structures. A needle-knife sphincterotome is employed to enter the pseudocyst, followed by passage of a guidewire and drainage catheter(s) (Figure 15–12). Successful resolution of the pseudocyst is observed in about 75–80% of patients. Side effects include iatrogenic cyst infection, local hemorrhage, and retroperitonitis.

Miscellaneous

Pancreatitis or pancreatic neoplasms may result in splenic or portal vein thrombosis with the development of bleeding from gastric varices. Endoscopic sclerotherapy, injection of cyanoacrylate, or banding of gastric varices has been used to treat bleeding gastric varices. As discussed previously, distal bile duct strictures caused by chronic pancreatitis may result in cholestatis or cholangitis that may be treated acutely with endoscopic stent placement. Although endoprosthesis place-

ment is technically successful in most patients, stenosis resolution is unusual. Surgical bypass (choledochoduodenostomy or choledochojejunostomy) is the preferred long-term approach for good operative risk patients.

CONCLUSION

The endoscopic management of pancreaticobiliary disorders cannot be done in a vacuum. As such, the technical ability to apply a procedure does not imply that this procedure is superior to surgical or radiologic intervention, or even to comfort care in the functional Class IV (bed-ridden, moribund) patient. Clearly, well-controlled data demonstrate that patients with an unresectable pancreatic malignant growth causing obstructive jaundice fare equally well (or poorly) whether surgically bypassed or endoscopically stented. Moreover, data are ample suggesting that endoscopic sphinc-

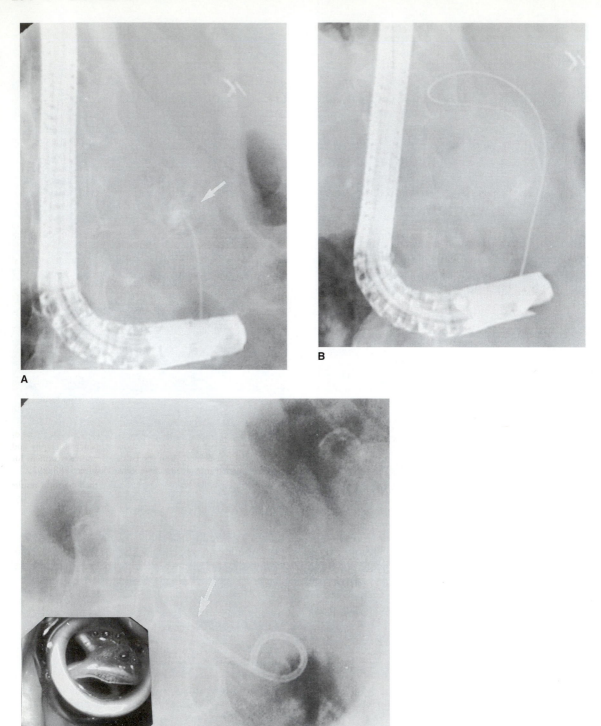

Figure 15–12. Transgastric puncture *(arrow)* into lesser sac pseudocyst **(A)** followed by guidewire insertion **(B)** and transgastric endoprosthesis placement **(C,** inset).

terotomy is the treatment of choice for most postcholecystectomy or high-risk patients with choledocholithiasis. A subset of patients with bile duct injury as well as those with diverse consequences of acute or chronic pancreatitis can also be managed endoscopically. Further experience in pancreatic endotherapy and controlled clinical trials are required before widespread application of this technology can be recommended.

REFERENCES

Adamek HE et al: Long term follow up of patients with chronic pancreatitis and pancreatic stones treated with extracorporeal shock wave lithotripsy. Gut 1999;45:402.

Baluyut AR et al: Impact of endoscopic therapy on the survival of patients with primary sclerosing choangitis. Gastrointest Endosc 2001;53:308.

Basso N et al: Laparoscopic cholecystectomy and intraoperative endoscopic sphincterotomy in the treatment of cholecystocholedocholithiasis. Gastrointest Endosc 1999;50:532.

Bourke MJ et al: Sphincterotomy-associated biliary strictures: features and endoscopic management. Gastrointest Endosc 2000;52:494.

Chang L: Preoperative versus postoperative endoscopic retrograde cholangiopancreatography in mild to moderate gallstone pancreatitis: a prospective randomized trial. Ann Surg 2000;231:82.

Cremer M et al: Stenting in severe chronic pancreatitis: results of medium-term follow-up in 76 patients. Endoscopy 1991;23:171.

Davids PHP et al: Randomized trial of self expanding metal stents versus polyethylene stents for distal malignant biliary obstruction. Lancet 1992;240:1488.

Delhaye H et al: Extracorporeal shock-wave lithotripsy of pancreatic calculi. Gastroenterology 1992;102:610.

DiSario JA et al: Endoscopic dilation of the sphincter for extraction of bile duct stones [abstract]. Gastrointest Endosc 2000;51:AB1.

Dumonceau JM et al: Endoscopic pancreatic drainage in chronic pancreatitis associated with ductal stones: long-term results. Gastrointest Endosc 1996;43:547.

Elton E et al: Endoscopic pancreatic sphincterotomy: indications, outcome, and a safe stentless technique. Gastrointest Endosc 1998;47:240.

Fan S-T et al: Early treatment of acute biliary pancreatitis by endoscopic papillotomy. N Engl J Med 1993;328:228.

Freeman ML: Mechanical lithotripsy of pancreatic duct stones. Gastrointest Endosc 1996;44:333.

Freeman ML: Complications of endoscopic sphincterotomy. Endoscopy 1998;30:A216.

Fölsch UR et al: Early ERCP and papillotomy compared with conservative treatment for acute biliary pancreatitis. N Engl J Med 1997;336:237.

Knyrim K et al: A prospective, randomized, controlled trial of metal stents for malignant obstruction of the common bile duct. Endoscopy 1993;25:207.

Kozarek RA: Endoscopy maneuvers for diagnosis and palliative treatment of pancreatic cancer. Problems Gen Surg 1997;14:13.

Kozarek RA: Endoscopic treatment of pancreatic pseudocysts. Gastrointest Endosc Clin North Am 1997;7:271.

Kozarek RA: Endoscopic therapy of complete and partial pancreatic duct disruptions. Gastrointest Endosc Clin North Am 1998;8:39.

Kozarek RA: Therapeutic pancreatic endoscopy. Endoscopy 2001;33:39.

Kozarek RA et al: Endoscopic approach to pancreas divisum. Dig Dis Sci 1995;40:1974.

Kozarek RA, Ball TJ, Patterson DJ: Pancreatic duct stone removal in the treatment of chronic pancreatitis. Am J Gastroenterol 1991;87:600.

Kozarek RA, Jiranek G, Traverso LW: Endoscopic management of pancreatic ascites. Am J Surg 1994;168:223.

Lai EC et al: Endoscopic biliary drainage for severe acute cholangitis. N Engl J Med 1992;326:1582.

Lau JY et al: Endoscopic drainage aborts endotoxemia in acute cholangitis. Br J Surg 1996;83:181.

Lehman GA et al: Pancreas divisum: results of minor papilla sphincterotomy. Gastrointest Endosc 1993;39:1.

Nelson DB et al: Technology status evaluation report: biliary stents. Gastrointest Endosc 1999;50:938.

Neoptolemos JR, London NJ, Carr-Locke DL: Controlled trial of urgent endoscopic retrograde cholangiopancreatography and endoscopic sphincterotomy versus conservative treatment for acute pancreatitis due to cholelithiasis. Lancet 1988;2:979.

Okolo PI, Pasricha PJ, Kalloo AN: What are the long-term results of endoscopic pancreatic sphincterotomy? Gastrointest Endosc 2000;52:15.

Ryan ME et al: Endoscopic intervention for biliary leaks after laparoscopic cholecystectomy: a multicenter review. Gastrointest Endosc 1998;47:261.

Saito M et al: Long-term outcome of endoscopic papillotomy for choledocholithiasis with cholecystolithiasis. Gastrointest Endosc 2000;51:540.

Sherman S, Lehman GA: Endoscopic pancreatic sphincterotomy: techniques and complications. Gastrointest Endosc Clin North Am 1998;8:115.

Smith AC, Dowsett JF, Russell RGG: Randomized trial of endoscopic stenting versus surgical bypass in malignant low bile duct obstruction. Lancet 1994;344:1655.

SECTION II
Esophageal Diseases

Gastroesophageal Reflux Disease & Its Complications

16

Stuart Jon Spechler, MD

The reflux of material from the stomach into the esophagus does not invariably result in disease. Indeed, normal individuals daily experience brief, asymptomatic episodes of gastroesophageal reflux that cause no esophageal injury. When the reflux of gastric material into the esophagus causes symptoms, tissue damage, or both, the resulting condition is called **gastroesophageal reflux disease (GERD).** Heartburn and regurgitation are the symptoms most frequently associated with GERD.

Reflux-induced esophageal injury **(reflux esophagitis)** is recognized endoscopically by the presence of erosions and ulcerations in the squamous epithelium of the esophagus. Reflux esophagitis can be complicated further by the development of esophageal strictures and columnar epithelial metaplasia **(Barrett's esophagus).**

Furthermore, the complications of GERD are not limited to the esophagus. In some patients, refluxed gastric material reaches the oropharynx and causes sore throat, burning tongue, and dental erosion. Aspiration of the refluxed material can cause laryngitis and pulmonary problems, including cough, bronchitis, and asthma. Thus, GERD can have protean clinical manifestations.

The development of GERD is a multifactorial process that involves dysfunction of mechanisms that normally prevent excessive gastroesophageal reflux and of mechanisms that normally clear the esophagus rapidly of noxious material.

Pathophysiology of Gastroesophageal Reflux Disease

A. ANTIREFLUX MECHANISMS

1. Lower esophageal sphincter (LES)—Normally, there is a positive pressure gradient between the abdomen and the thorax that tends to promote the reflux of material from the stomach into the esophagus. In the absence of effective antireflux mechanisms, this pressure differential would result in virtually continuous gastroesophageal reflux. One of the primary barriers to reflux is the LES, a 1.0- to 3.5-cm segment of specialized circular muscle in the wall of the distal esophagus that prevents reflux by maintaining a resting pressure some 10–45 mm Hg higher than that of the stomach (Figure 16–1).

Although the muscle of the LES cannot be distinguished morphologically from the muscle of the esophageal body, the LES exhibits a number of distinctive functional characteristics. Unlike muscle of the esophageal body, strips of LES muscle develop spontaneous tension on stretching and relax with transmural electrical stimulation. Gastroesophageal reflux can result from any of several types of LES dysfunction, including intrinsic weakness of the LES muscle that causes feeble resting LES pressure **(hypotonic LES),** inadequate LES response to increased abdominal pressure, and transient episodes of LES relaxation (Figure 16–2).

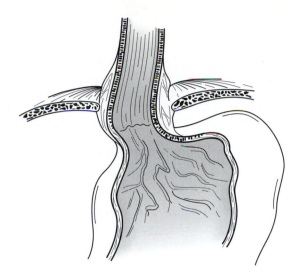

Figure 16–1. Lower esophageal sphincter anatomy. The esophagus passes into the abdomen through the esophageal hiatus, an opening in the right crus of the diaphragm. The distal few centimeters of circular muscle in the esophagus comprise the lower esophageal sphincter. (Reproduced, with permission, from the Clinical Teaching Project of the American Gastroenterological Association.)

When the resting pressure in the LES remains at or near zero **(feeble resting LES pressure),** the sphincter does not pose an effective barrier to reflux (Figure 16–2C). Normal individuals uncommonly exhibit such feeble resting LES pressures, and few episodes of gastroesophageal reflux in normal subjects are associated with this phenomenon. In patients who have severe GERD, however, approximately 25% of all episodes of acid reflux are associated with feeble resting LES pressure.

LES pressure rises rapidly with the sudden abdominal pressure elevations that occur during coughing, sneezing, or straining. Some patients, particularly those who exhibit feeble resting LES pressure, may have an inadequate LES response to increased abdominal pressure. If sudden increases in abdominal pressure are not accompanied by a commensurate rise in LES pressure, gastric material can be propelled into the esophagus (Figure 16–2B). The precise contribution of this mechanism to GERD is disputed, as is the contribution of the crural diaphragm to the observed increase in LES pressure.

Transient LES relaxation (TLESR) appears to be the most important LES mechanism for reflux (Figure

16–2A). During primary peristalsis **(peristalsis induced by swallowing),** the LES normally relaxes for 3–10 seconds to allow the swallowed bolus to enter the stomach. TLESRs, in contrast, are not preceded by a normal peristaltic sequence and last for up to 45 seconds. When LES pressure falls to zero during a TLESR, the sphincter does not function as an antireflux barrier. This phenomenon explains how patients with apparently normal resting LES pressures can experience frequent episodes of reflux.

The TLESR is part of the normal belch reflex that is triggered by gaseous distention of the stomach. In this situation, the TLESR allows gas to escape from the gastric fundus. The nucleus tractus solitarius in the medulla is involved in the reflex, both in integrating sensory information from the stomach and in controlling the neural circuits that trigger the TLESR. Medullary neurons with γ-aminobutyric acid B (GABA$_B$) receptors appear to inhibit TLESRs. Cholinergic blockade with atropine also inhibits TLESRs through a central mechanism. The sphincter relaxation that characterizes a TLESR is mediated by the activation of cholecystokinin-A receptors in LES muscle. Brief episodes of gastroesophageal reflux occur daily in normal individuals, and the vast majority of these episodes are the result of TLESRs. In patients with severe GERD, approximately 70% of reflux episodes are the result of TLESRs. TLESRs occur approximately two to six times per hour in normal subjects and three to eight times per hour in patients with GERD. Approximately 40–50% of TLESRs in normal subjects are accompanied by acid reflux, whereas acid reflux is observed in 60–70% of TLESRs in patients with GERD.

2. Crural diaphragm—The esophagus passes from the thorax into the abdomen through an opening in the right crus of the diaphragm called the **esophageal hiatus** (see Figure 16–1). When the crural diaphragm contracts, as occurs during inspiration, the crurae come together and pinch the distal esophagus. This pinching effect appears to function as an important barrier to reflux during inspiration and during other activities that increase intraabdominal pressure. In this fashion, the crural diaphragm serves as an external esophageal sphincter that buttresses the antireflux function of the LES. As evidence of the efficacy of this external sphincter mechanism, studies in dogs have shown that gastroesophageal reflux does not occur during transient LES relaxation unless the relaxation is attended by inhibition of the crural diaphragm. Furthermore, transient LES relaxation with inhibition of the crural diaphragm in dogs often is associated with contraction of the costal diaphragm that further promotes reflux. A similar se-

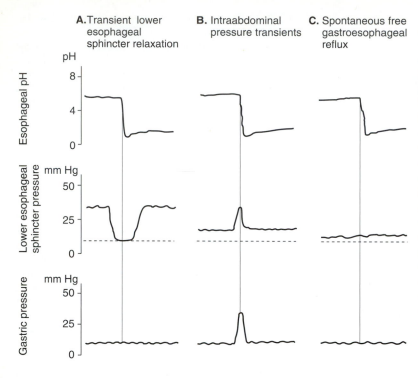

A. Transient lower esophageal sphincter relaxation

B. Intraabdominal pressure transients

C. Spontaneous free gastroesophageal reflux

Figure 16–2. Schematic representation of three different lower esophageal sphincter mechanisms for gastroesophageal reflux. Acid reflux (a drop in esophageal pH below 4) is represented by vertical lines. **A:** Acid reflux associated with a transient lower esophageal sphincter relaxation. **B:** Acid reflux during an inadequate lower esophageal sphincter response to increased intraabdominal pressure (note that the rise in lower esophageal sphincter pressure is not as great as the rise in gastric pressure). **C:** Acid reflux in a patient with feeble resting lower esophageal sphincter pressure. (Reproduced, with permission, from Dodds WJ et al: Mechanisms of gastroesophageal reflux in patients with reflux esophagitis. N Engl J Med 1982;307:1547. Copyright © 1982 Massachusetts Medical Society. All rights reserved.)

quence of events is seen in humans during belching, suggesting that gastroesophageal reflux during transient LES relaxation may occur through a variant of the belch reflex.

3. Anatomic features—In addition to the LES and the crural diaphragm, certain other anatomic features of the distal esophagus may contribute to the antireflux barrier (see Figure 16–1). For example, the acute angle formed by the junction of esophagus and stomach **(the angle of His)** may result in a one-way flap valve that prevents reflux. Also, a segment of the distal esophagus ordinarily is located within the abdomen where the segment is subject to external pressure that tends to force the walls together, thereby preventing reflux.

4. Effects of hiatal hernia on the antireflux barrier—Most patients with severe GERD have a sliding hiatal hernia in which both the esophagogastric junction and a portion of the gastric fundus protrude through the hiatus in the crural diaphragm into the chest. The susceptibility to gastroesophageal reflux induced by abrupt elevations of intraabdominal pressure has been found to correlate significantly with hiatal hernia size. It has been known for decades that large hiatal hernias are associated with low LES pressure, but only recently has the mechanism underlying this association been elucidated. During a standard esophageal

motility study, esophageal pressures are measured by transducers that are placed in the lumen of the esophagus. The LES pressure measured during such a study reflects pressure on the transducer that is generated by both the LES muscle (intrinsic sphincter) and the crural diaphragm (extrinsic sphincter). A better term for this value would be "gastroesophageal junction pressure," but the term "LES pressure" is conventional. With a large hiatal hernia, the LES muscle is displaced up into the chest, dissociated from the crural diaphragm. The intrinsic pressure generated by the sphincter muscle of the esophagus may be normal, but when separated from the crural diaphragm that ordinarily contributes to the pressure at the gastroesophageal junction, the measured LES pressure value appears to be low. With a large hiatal hernia that dissociates the internal and external sphincters of the distal esophagus, reflux may occur during the elevations in abdominal pressure caused by events such as inspiration, coughing, and straining. In this situation, the crurae can no longer buttress the LES by pinching the distal esophagus. Rather, contraction of the crurae creates an intrathoracic pouch of stomach whose contents are readily available for reflux. Compared with normal individuals, furthermore, patients with large hiatal hernias exhibit an increased frequency of TLESRs induced by gastric distention.

All of these mechanisms appear to contribute to GERD in patients who have large hiatal hernias, although it is difficult to quantitate that contribution. Clinicians should appreciate that hiatal hernia is not always associated with GERD, and vice versa. Finally, a study in opossums has shown that esophageal acid perfusion causes the long axis of the esophagus to shorten, an effect that could promote the development of a sliding hiatal hernia. This observation raises the possibility that hiatal hernia might be an effect rather than a cause of reflux esophagitis in some cases.

B. Gastric Contents

Gastroesophageal reflux causes esophageal injury only when the refluxed material is caustic to the esophageal mucosa. Potentially caustic agents that can be found in the stomach include acid, pepsin, bile, and pancreatic enzymes. The dramatic efficacy of potent inhibitors of gastric acid secretion (eg, proton-pump inhibitors) in the treatment of GERD emphasizes the importance of acid and pepsin in the pathogenesis of reflux esophagitis in most cases. However, refluxed bile or pancreatic secretions might contribute to esophageal damage for some patients.

Using sensitive radionuclide tests, some investigators have found delayed gastric emptying in more than 50% of patients with GERD. Delayed gastric emptying causes gastric distention that can stimulate gastric acid secretion and trigger transient relaxation of the LES. Both of these effects can be harmful for patients with GERD.

C. Esophageal Clearance Mechanisms

If caustic material is cleared quickly from the esophagus, no damage may result. Normally, the esophagus is cleared of acid by four important mechanisms: (1) gravity, (2) peristalsis, (3) salivation, and (4) intrinsic esophageal bicarbonate production. When a bolus of acid enters the esophagus, most of the material is cleared by the combined effects of gravity and peristalsis. The small quantity of residual acidic material that escapes clearance by gravity and peristalsis might cause mucosal damage if it were not neutralized by swallowed saliva, which is highly alkaline, and by bicarbonate produced by the esophageal mucosa itself.

GERD can be associated with conditions that impair esophageal clearance. For example, the severe reflux esophagitis that occurs in patients with scleroderma often is associated with disordered peristalsis that delays esophageal clearance. Reflux that occurs during sleep can be particularly damaging to the esophagus for several reasons relating to esophageal clearance. In recumbency during sleep, gravity retards the clearance of refluxed material. Swallowing and salivation virtually cease during sleep and, therefore, there is no primary peristalsis and little saliva available to clear acid from the esophagus. Cigarette smoking has been shown to increase esophageal acid exposure by increasing the frequency of acid reflux events and, perhaps, by decreasing salivary flow. Finally, hiatal hernia has been shown to interfere with esophageal clearance.

D. Esophageal Epithelial Resistance

Epithelial protective factors enable the esophagus to resist peptic injury (Figure 16–3). Ambulatory esophageal pH monitoring studies have shown that normal individuals experience brief episodes of acid reflux daily. Apparently, the normal epithelial defenses are sufficient to prevent these brief episodes from causing esophagitis. Most patients with reflux esophagitis have an abnormally prolonged duration of esophageal acid exposure that overwhelms the normal epithelial defenses (Figure 16–4). However, some patients have reflux esophagitis even though 24-hour pH monitoring studies demonstrate a normal daily duration of acid reflux. These patients may have yet uncharacterized defects in their epithelial protective factors.

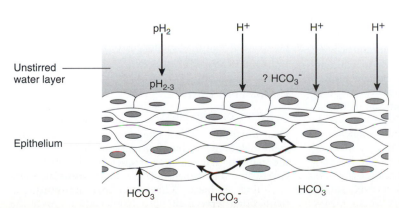

Figure 16–3. Preepithelial defenses. The esophageal preepithelial defenses against acid include the surface layer of mucus, unstirred water layer, and bicarbonate ions. [Reproduced, with permission, from Orlando RC: Esophageal epithelial defense against acid injury. J Clin Gastroenterol 1991;13(Suppl 2):S1.]

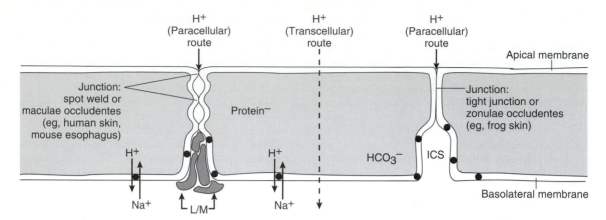

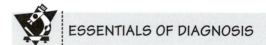

Figure 16–4. Epithelial defenses. The epithelial cell membranes, the intercellular junction complexes, and lipids and mucins (L/M) in the intercellular spaces all limit the penetration of H+ ions. Once within the cell, H+ ions are buffered by intracellular proteins and bicarbonate. The H+ ions also can be extruded by a Na+/H+ exchange mechanism. [Reproduced, with permission, from Orlando RC: *Gastroesophageal Reflux Disease: Pathogenesis, Diagnosis, Therapy.* Castell DO, Wu WC, Ott DJ (editors). Futura Publishing, 1985.]

E. NSAIDs AND GERD

Epidemiologic studies suggest that the ingestion of aspirin and other nonsteroidal antiinflammatory drugs (NSAIDs) can contribute to GERD. Patients with esophageal strictures appear to be especially susceptible to NSAID-induced esophageal injury. Many NSAID preparations are caustic to the mucosa, and severe local injury can result when a stricture impedes passage of the NSAID tablet into the stomach. Esophageal strictures themselves may be the result of NSAID-induced injury. For patients without strictures, the mechanisms whereby NSAIDs contribute to GERD are not clear.

F. *HELICOBACTER PYLORI* AND GERD

Helicobacter pylori are microaerophilic, gram-negative bacteria that are uniquely adapted for survival in the human stomach. More than 50% of the world's population is infected with *H pylori*. The infection causes a chronic gastritis that is associated with the development of intestinal metaplasia and cancer in the stomach. *H pylori* does not infect the esophagus. However, recent data suggest that gastric *H pylori* infection may protect the esophagus from GERD and its complications, perhaps by decreasing gastric acidity. There are reports of GERD developing after the eradication of *H pylori*. It has even been proposed that the declining frequency of *H pylori* infection in Western countries may underlie the rising frequency of adenocarcinoma in Barrett's esophagus (see below). Presently, the role of *H pylori* infection in the pathogenesis of GERD and its complications is controversial.

ESSENTIALS OF DIAGNOSIS

- *Heartburn and/or regurgitation.*
- *Esophagitis (eg, erosions, ulcerations).*

General Considerations

GERD can be defined as any symptomatic condition or anatomic alteration caused by the reflux of noxious material from the stomach into the esophagus. It is important to appreciate that by this definition, patients with GERD can have symptoms without objective evidence of esophagitis. The finding of reflux esophagitis on endoscopic examination confirms the diagnosis of GERD, but a normal esophagoscopy does not rule out GERD as a cause of symptoms.

Clinical Findings

A. SYMPTOMS AND SIGNS

Heartburn, the cardinal symptom of GERD, is an uncomfortable, hot or burning sensation located beneath the sternum. The sensation frequently originates in the epigastrium and radiates up the chest, sometimes into the throat or back. When describing heartburn, patients often wave their open hand vertically over the sternum, in contrast to patients with angina pectoris due to cardiac ischemia who typically hold their clenched fist stationary over the chest while describing their pain.

If refluxed gastric material reaches the oropharynx, the patient may experience the symptom of regurgitation wherein sour or bitter-tasting material appears in the mouth. Patients who have peptic strictures of the esophagus often complain of dysphagia. Even in the absence of a fixed stricture, however, dysphagia may be associated with the esophagitis and motility abnormalities that can accompany GERD. Odynophagia in patients with GERD suggests the presence of esophageal ulceration. Some patients describe the symptom of **water brash,** in which the mouth suddenly fills with saliva as a result of reflex salivary secretion stimulated by acid in the esophagus.

Heartburn associated with GERD can be aggravated by the ingestion of foods that predispose to reflux by decreasing pressure in the LES. These include chocolate, onions, peppermint, coffee, and foods that have a high content of fat and sugar. Certain foods have no affect on the LES but can cause the sensation of heartburn in patients with GERD by irritating the esophageal mucosa directly. These include spicy foods, citrus products, and tomato products. Certain practices that predispose to reflux by increasing intraabdominal pressure also can precipitate heartburn in susceptible patients. For example, many patients experience heartburn when they bend over, lift a heavy object, strain to defecate, or run.

Characteristically, heartburn caused by gastroesophageal reflux is relieved, if only temporarily, by antacids. For most patients with GERD, the symptom of heartburn can be eliminated by the administration of potent acid-suppressing agents.

B. DIAGNOSTIC TESTS

Table 16–1 lists the diagnostic tests that are commonly used to evaluate patients with GERD and the clinical questions for which these tests can supply answers.

Note that the barium swallow, endoscopic examination, and histologic examination of esophageal biopsy specimens are performed primarily to seek the anatomic alterations of reflux esophagitis. As previously noted, GERD is any symptomatic condition or anatomic alteration caused by the reflux of noxious material from the stomach into the esophagus. Based on this definition, patients can have GERD without anatomic alterations. For patients who have a characteristic history, for example, patients who complain of typical heartburn and regurgitation that respond readily to treatment with acid-suppression therapy, diagnostic tests are not necessary merely to establish the diagnosis of GERD. An **endoscopic examination** might be performed in such patients to seek evidence of esophagitis that could require more aggressive therapy or to look for complications, such as Barrett's esophagus, that cannot be diagnosed on the basis of history alone. However, a normal esophagoscopy would not eliminate acid reflux as the cause of symptoms.

Diagnostic tests may be required for patients with atypical signs or symptoms or for patients with typical signs and symptoms that do not respond well to acid suppression. A **barium swallow** can reveal signs of esophagitis including thickening of the esophageal folds, erosions, ulcerations, and strictures; it can also demonstrate the gastroesophageal reflux of barium. Radiography is considerably less sensitive than endoscopy for demonstrating esophagitis, however, and endoscopic examination has the added advantage that biopsy specimens can be obtained from any abnormal areas.

How often do patients with typical heartburn have endoscopic evidence of reflux esophagitis? Several studies suggest that esophagitis is present endoscopically in approximately 50–70% of patients with typical, frequent heartburn. **Histologic changes** of esophagitis are found more frequently, with over 90% of patients exhibiting histologic changes characteristic of GERD. The histologic changes of reflux esophagitis include lengthening of the papillae so that they occupy more than two-thirds of the thickness of the squamous mu-

Table 16–1. Clinical questions and diagnostic tests for GERD.[1]

	Is There Gastroesophageal Reflux?	Is There Esophagitis (Inflammation, Ulceration)?	Is There Barrett's Esophagus?	Is There an Esophageal Stricture?	Are Symptoms due to Acid Reflux?
Barium swallow	+	+	+	+++	–
Endoscopy	+	+++	+++	++	–
Esophageal biopsy	–	+++	+++	–	–
Bernstein test	–	–	–	–	++
Ambulatory pH monitoring	+++	–	–	–	+++

[1]Utility of diagnostic test for answering clinical question: –, not useful; +, somewhat useful; ++, useful; +++, very useful.

cosa, hyperplasia of cells in the basal zone so that this zone occupies more than 15% of the mucosal thickness, and infiltration of the epithelium with eosinophils and polymorphonuclear cells. The importance of the histologic changes of GERD are disputed, however, and most authorities hold that the endoscopic findings have more clinical relevance.

Several studies suggest that severity of heartburn is not a reliable index of esophagitis. There appears to be no significant correlation between the severity of heartburn reported by the patient and the severity of reflux esophagitis on endoscopic examination. In fact, patients can have severe esophagitis with no heartburn. The precise frequency of this situation is not clear, as asymptomatic patients seldom have endoscopic examinations, but a number of reports have described patients who had severe ulcerative esophagitis with no complaints of heartburn. It appears that less than two-thirds of patients with esophagitis complain of frequent heartburn.

Diagnostic tests may be needed for patients who have atypical chest pains with features that are suggestive, but not entirely characteristic, of reflux-induced heartburn. For example, occasionally patients are encountered who complain of a burning sensation in the lower chest that does not radiate, that is unaffected by activities, and that is only partially or unreliably relieved by antacids and antisecretory drugs. This is not typical heartburn, and it is not clear that the symptom is triggered by acid reflux even if endoscopic examination demonstrates esophagitis.

The **acid perfusion (Bernstein) test** has been used in this situation to support acid reflux as the cause of symptoms. During this test, the esophagus is perfused with 0.1 N hydrochloric acid. Reproduction of the patient's chest pain with acid perfusion implicates GERD as a cause of the chest pain and suggests a role for antireflux therapy. This test has limited sensitivity and specificity, however, and has largely been replaced by ambulatory esophageal pH monitoring.

Ambulatory monitoring of esophageal pH can be used to document the pattern, frequency, and duration of acid reflux, and to seek a correlation between reflux episodes and symptoms. In most ambulatory systems, an episode of acid reflux is defined (somewhat arbitrarily) as a drop in esophageal pH below 4. Standard 24-hour pH monitoring records a number of different variables, such as the total number of reflux episodes, the number of episodes longer than 5 minutes in duration, and the duration of the longest episode.

The single most clinically applicable variable appears to be the total percentage of the monitoring period that esophageal pH remains below 4. In normal individuals, esophageal pH remains below 4 for less than 4.5% of the 24-hour monitoring period. Most patients who have both endoscopic signs and symptoms of GERD also have abnormal 24-hour esophageal pH monitoring studies, whereas subjects with no such signs and symptoms usually have normal studies. It is difficult to determine the precise sensitivity and specificity of the test, however, because there is no universally accepted "gold standard" for the diagnosis of GERD.

In theory, protracted esophageal pH monitoring should be very useful in establishing that acid reflux is the cause of heartburn in individual patients. In practice, however, the correlation between discrete episodes of acid reflux and heartburn is poor. For example, although normal individuals often experience brief episodes of acid reflux during the day (particularly after meals), these episodes usually are not associated with heartburn. Even in patients with heartburn who have endoscopic evidence of reflux esophagitis, 24-hour esophageal monitoring reveals that fewer than 20% of episodes of acid reflux (defined as a drop in pH of less than 4) are accompanied by heartburn. These observations indicate that most episodes of acid reflux do not trigger the sensation of heartburn.

It is not clear why only a minority of episodes of acid reflux cause heartburn. It appears, however, from experimental studies that provocation of pain is dependent on the pH of the refluxate and the length of time of acid exposure. The duration of acid perfusion required to produce pain is a function of the pH of the perfusion solution, ie, the lower the pH, the shorter the duration of acid perfusion necessary to produce heartburn. The frequency with which acid perfusion induces pain also is related to the pH. In one study all patients experienced heartburn during perfusion with solutions of pH 1, whereas only 50% of patients experienced pain during esophageal perfusion with solutions of pH 2.5–6. Once a subject had experienced pain with an acid solution, subsequent perfusions of the same solution caused pain more rapidly than the first perfusion. During 24-hour pH monitoring, reflux episodes associated with pain were significantly longer than those without pain, and often were preceded by another episode of heartburn. These findings suggest that the reflux of strongly acidic material is more likely to cause heartburn than weakly acidic material. Furthermore, once an episode of reflux has caused pain, the esophagus may become sensitized so that subsequent reflux episodes are more likely to be painful.

Treatment

When planning a management strategy for patients with GERD, it is important to appreciate that the efficacy of any antireflux therapy is inversely related to the severity of the underlying reflux esophagitis, ie, the worse the esophagitis, the poorer the healing rate. A

Table 16–2. Official indications, dosage, and duration of treatment for commonly prescribed antireflux medications.[1]

Drug	Official Indication	Recommended Dosage	Recommended Duration
Cimetidine	Erosive esophagitis diagnosed by endoscopy	800 mg twice a day or 400 mg four times a day	12 weeks
Famotidine	Short-term treatment of symptoms or esophagitis due to GERD including erosive or ulcerative disease diagnosed by endoscopy	20 mg twice a day symptoms / 20 mg or 40 mg twice a day for esophagitis	6 weeks / 12 weeks
Nizatidine	Endoscopically diagnosed esophagitis including erosive and ulcerative esophagitis and associated heartburn due to GERD	150 mg twice a day	12 weeks
Ranitidine	Treatment of symptoms and endoscopically diagnosed erosive esophagitis	150 mg twice a day symptoms / 150 mg four times a day esophagitis	No limit specified
Metoclopramide	Short-term treatment for adults with symptomatic documented gastroesophageal reflux who fail to respond to conventional therapy	10–15 mg four times a day	12 weeks
Cisapride	Symptomatic treatment of patients with nocturnal heartburn due to GERD	10–20 mg four times a day	No limit specified
Omeprazole	Short-term treatment of erosive esophagitis that has been diagnosed by endoscopy; short-term treatment of symptomatic GERD poorly responsive to customary medical therapy usually including a histamine H_2-receptor antagonist	20 mg four times a day	4–8 weeks

[1]Recommendations as specified in the *Physician's Desk Reference* 1995; Medical Economics Data Production Co., Montvale, NJ.

treatment that is highly effective for patients with mild esophagitis may be virtually useless for patients with severe disease. This section outlines a stepwise approach to the therapy of GERD. For patients who are found to have severe, ulcerative, reflux esophagitis, it may be appropriate to begin therapy immediately with potent acid suppression (eg, by administering a proton-pump inhibitor) rather than proceeding stepwise through trials of agents less likely to effect healing. Conversely, it may not be appropriate to begin the treatment of very mild GERD with a proton-pump inhibitor. The official indications, dosage, and duration of treatment for commonly prescribed antireflux medications are listed in Table 16–2.

A. LIFE-STYLE MODIFICATIONS

The management of GERD traditionally begins with life-style modifications (Table 16–3) aimed at reducing acid reflux and minimizing the duration of contact between refluxed material and the esophageal mucosa. The head of the bed is elevated on 4- to 6-inch blocks to exploit the effect of gravity in clearing the esophagus of noxious material.

Obese patients are advised to lose weight, with the rationale that obesity may contribute to reflux by in-

creasing abdominal pressure; dieting also helps patients avoid fatty foods that promote reflux. Bedtime snacks can stimulate gastric acid production and trigger transient LES relaxation. Both of these effects promote the reflux of gastric acid during sleep, a time when swallowing and salivation decrease dramatically. With no swallowing to initiate peristalsis and no saliva to buffer retained acid, reflux during sleep can be especially damaging.

Tobacco and alcohol consumption should be avoided because these agents may decrease LES pressure and

Table 16–3. Life-style modifications for GERD.

Elevate the head of the bed
Weight loss for obese patients
Avoid
 Bedtime snacks
 Chocolate, fatty foods, and carminatives
 Cigarettes and alcohol
 Drugs that decrease lower esophageal sphincter pressure and delay gastric emptying
Nonsteroidal antiinflammatory drugs

because cigarette smoking also decreases salivation. Fatty foods, chocolate, and carminatives (spearmint, peppermint) contribute to GERD by decreasing LES pressure and by delaying gastric emptying. Drugs that have anticholinergic effects (eg, phenothiazines, tricyclic antidepressants), theophylline preparations, and calcium channel blocking agents can decrease LES pressure and delay gastric emptying; these medications should be avoided if possible. NSAIDs can be caustic to the esophageal mucosa, and these agents also should be avoided.

B. H₂-RECEPTOR BLOCKING AGENTS

In some patients who have mild GERD, life-style modifications alone can be very effective therapy and medications may not be necessary. For these patients, antacids with or without alginic acid can be used as necessary for occasional episodes of heartburn. For patients who remain symptomatic despite the implementation of life-style modifications, a histamine H₂-receptor blocking agent (cimetidine, famotidine, nizatidine, or ranitidine) often is the next step. When administered in conventional doses, H₂ blockers relieve symptoms of GERD and heal esophagitis within 12 weeks in approximately one-half to two-thirds of patients. If relief is not complete, the dose of the agent can be increased, although many physicians will proceed to a proton-pump inhibitor if conventional-dose histamine H₂-receptor blocker therapy fails.

C. PROKINETIC AGENTS

Prokinetic agents can decrease gastroesophageal reflux by increasing LES pressure, and by enhancing gastric and esophageal emptying. Presently, the only prokinetic agent available for use in the United States for GERD is metoclopramide, a dopamine antagonist that can be effective in treating patients who have relatively mild disease. Metoclopramide increases pressure in the LES, and enhances gastric emptying by coordinating motor activity in the stomach, pylorus, and duodenum. The use of this agent often is limited by its frequent side effects, including agitation, restlessness, somnolence, and extrapyramidal symptoms, that occur in up to 30% of patients.

D. SUCRALFATE

Sucralfate is an exceptionally safe medication that has been found to be effective in the treatment of mild reflux esophagitis. In several studies performed outside of the United States, the efficacy of sucralfate in relieving symptoms and healing esophagitis appeared to be similar to that of the H₂-receptor blockers. Sucralfate can be administered either in tablet form or as a suspension.

E. PROTON-PUMP INHIBITORS

The proton-pump inhibitors (PPIs) omeprazole, lansoprazole, rabeprazole, pantoprazole, and esomeprazole are the most effective of the available agents for the treatment of GERD. In patients with mild to moderately severe reflux esophagitis treated with PPIs in conventional dosages, healing rates of 80–100% can be expected within 8–12 weeks. Very severe (grade 4) reflux esophagitis may persist despite conventional-dose PPI therapy in up to 40% of cases, however. In most such resistant cases, the esophagitis usually can be healed by increasing the dose of the PPI. Recent studies also have shown that aggressive acid suppression with PPIs improves dysphagia and decreases the need for esophageal dilation in patients who have peptic esophageal strictures.

For patients with severe GERD who respond to PPIs, GERD returns shortly after stopping the drug in the majority of cases, and maintenance therapy is required. For most patients, the dose of PPI necessary to maintain remission is at least the dose required to heal the acute esophagitis. For patients with severe GERD, furthermore, the PPI maintenance dose requirement often increases with time. One long-term study of patients who had severe GERD treated with a maintenance dose of omeprazole (20 mg/d) found that relapses occurred frequently (at the rate of 1 per 9.4 treatment-years), and that patients often required increasing doses of omeprazole (up to 120 mg/d) to maintain GERD in remission.

The profound acid suppression that can be achieved with the use of PPIs has raised theoretical concerns regarding their long-term safety. Protracted acid suppression can elevate the serum level of gastrin, a hormone that has trophic effects on the stomach and colon, and might result in colonization of the stomach with bacteria that can convert dietary nitrates to carcinogenic nitrosamines. These effects conceivably might contribute to the development of gastric and colonic neoplasms. Furthermore, some data suggest that sustained acid suppression with PPIs might hasten the development of gastric atrophy in patients who are infected with *H pylori*, and that chronic PPI therapy might interfere with vitamin B₁₂ absorption. Despite these theoretical concerns, there are no reports of tumors or nutritional deficiencies clearly attributable to the use of PPIs after more than a decade of extensive clinical experience with these agents.

F. COMBINATION THERAPY

Most patients treated with PPIs in conventional dosages do not exhibit complete suppression of gastric acid secretion. Approximately 70% of individuals who take a PPI twice a day experience nocturnal gastric acid breakthrough (defined as a gastric pH <4 for more than 1 hour at night). Brief episodes of acid reflux occur frequently during these breakthrough periods in patients with GERD. For some patients taking a PPI twice daily, nocturnal acid breakthrough can be abolished by adding a histamine H_2-receptor blocker at bedtime. It is not clear that this approach is desirable, however. Complete elimination of acid reflux usually is not necessary to effect the healing of reflux esophagitis. Indeed, most patients who are treated with a PPI in conventional dosage exhibit complete healing of their symptoms and signs of GERD. No clear clinical benefit yet has been demonstrated for the practice of adding a histamine H_2-receptor blocker at bedtime to PPI therapy.

A few older investigations have explored the value of combination drug therapy for the healing of GERD. The great efficacy of the PPIs used as single agents in this condition has discouraged investigators from undertaking new studies on combination therapy. Drug combinations that have been studied have included an H_2 blocker plus either sucralfate or a prokinetic agent. Cimetidine (1200 mg/d) combined with sucralfate (5 g/d) was found to be superior to cimetidine alone for relieving daytime heartburn and for improving the endoscopic signs of esophagitis. For patients unresponsive to treatment with cimetidine alone, the addition of metoclopramide resulted in symptomatic improvement significantly more often than the addition of placebo, but side effects of metoclopramide were frequent. A combination of ranitidine (300 mg/d) plus metoclopramide (40 mg/d) was not found to be as effective as omeprazole alone (20 mg/d) in healing the signs and symptoms of esophagitis. Some studies explored combination therapy with the prokinetic agent cisapride, but these studies are of historical interest only because cisapride has been withdrawn from general use due to serious side effects (lethal arryhythmias). For patients with moderately severe reflux esophagitis, the use of combination therapy may eliminate the need for treatment with a PPI. However, the addition of a second medication increases the cost of therapy and the potential for side effects. Furthermore, the long-term benefit of combination therapy has not been demonstrated. For patients who are refractory to single-agent therapy (with an H_2 blocker, sucralfate, or a prokinetic), a change to a PPI generally is more likely to effect healing than the addition of a second drug.

G. ANTIREFLUX SURGERY

There are a number of different antireflux operations (eg, Nissen, Belsey, Toupet fundoplication), but all share some fundamental features. In all of these procedures, the surgeon creates an intraabdominal segment of esophagus, reduces the hiatal hernia, approximates the diaphragmatic crurae, and wraps a portion of the gastric fundus around the distal esophagus (fundoplica-

tion). The mechanisms whereby these maneuvers create a barrier to gastroesophageal reflux are not clear, but several have been proposed. For example, the surgery narrows the angle of His, which may create an antireflux flap-valve effect. Restoration of the distal esophagus to the positive pressure environment of the abdomen also may prevent reflux. Reduction of the hiatal hernia and approximation of the diaphragmatic crurae may restore the antireflux effects of the crural diaphragm. The fundoplication itself may act as a one-way valve, and also may prevent the distention of the gastric fundus that can trigger TLESRs.

Surgical reports generally have described excellent results for fundoplication, with more than 85% of patients experiencing relief of their signs and symptoms of GERD. However, few studies on this issue have been prospective and randomized, and the duration of follow-up generally has been short. A large Department of Veterans Affairs cooperative study conducted in the late 1980s prospectively compared the efficacy of available medical and surgical therapies for GERD. The 247 study subjects all had GERD complicated by Barrett's esophagus, esophageal ulceration, esophageal stricture, or severe erosive esophagitis. Antireflux life-style modifications were prescribed for all patients regardless of treatment group. Patients were randomly assigned to receive one of three types of treatment: continuous medical therapy, symptomatic medical therapy, or surgical therapy. Continuous medical therapy included antacid tablets and ranitidine taken on a daily basis regardless of symptoms; metoclopramide and sucralfate were added in a stepwise fashion for patients who remained symptomatic. For patients in the symptomatic medical therapy group, drug therapy was used only for control of symptoms. Therapy in these patients began with antacid tablets; ranitidine, metoclopramide, and sucralfate were added in a stepwise fashion for symptoms that could not be controlled with antacids alone. Patients in the surgical therapy group had Nissen fundoplications. All three therapies resulted in significant improvements in the symptoms and endoscopic signs of GERD for up to 2 years (Figure 16–5). However, surgical therapy was significantly better than both medical therapies administered for the 2-year duration of the study. Overall satisfaction with therapy also was better for patients in the surgical group. This prospective, randomized study clearly demonstrated that surgical therapy was superior to medical therapy (without PPIs) for the short-term treatment of GERD.

Antireflux surgery now can be performed laparoscopically, and a number of reports have described the short-term results of laparoscopic fundoplication. The technique of laparoscopic Nissen fundoplication is virtually identical to that of the open procedure, and the mortality rate is between 0.2% and 0.4%. The

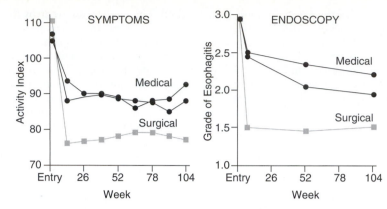

Figure 16–5. Results of the Veterans Affairs cooperative study on GERD (Spechler SJ: Comparison of medical and surgical therapy for complicated gastroesophageal reflux disease in veterans. The Department of Veterans Affairs Gastroesophageal Reflux Disease Study Group. N Engl J Med 1992;326:786). Patients were randomly assigned to receive one of three types of treatment: continuous medical therapy, symptomatic medical therapy, or surgical therapy. The left panel shows the effects of therapy on the activity index score, an index of GERD symptom severity [range of scores: 74 (no symptoms) to 172 (worst symptoms)]. The right panel shows the effects of therapy on the endoscopic signs of esophagitis [range of scores: 1.0 (no esophagitis) to 4.0 (esophageal ulceration)]. The points on the graphs represent mean values ± SE. The two medical groups are represented by black lines and the surgical group by gray lines. (Reproduced, with permission, from the Clinical Teaching Project of the American Gastroenterological Association.)

laparoscopic approach has become popular, not because it is safer or because it produces a better functional result than the open procedure, but because of proposed advantages in the degree of postoperative discomfort, duration of hospital stay, and cosmetic outcome. Two recent randomized trials of laparoscopic and open Nissen fundoplication found no significant differences in the functional results of the two procedures (ie, relief of symptoms of GERD, reduction in esophageal acid exposure). However, one of those studies was terminated prematurely because an interim analysis showed an excess of adverse outcomes in the group treated laparoscopically. Furthermore, at least one study has shown that the primary factor involved in overall patient satisfaction with antireflux surgery is the relief of symptoms of GERD, not the operative approach. These observations suggest that the availability of laparoscopic surgery should not be a major factor in the physician's decision regarding the advisability of fundoplication. The primary decision for the clinician is whether the patient should have an antireflux operation, not how the operation should be performed.

A recent report has described the results of a follow-up study on the patients who participated in the Veterans Affairs cooperative study on reflux disease previously described. Using a professional search agency, the investigators determined the whereabouts of 239 (97%) of the original 247 study patients. Of the 160 known survivors, 129 agreed to participate in the follow-up study that included a GERD history, GERD symptom scoring, endoscopic examination, and completion of the SF-36 general health and well-being form. There were 79 deaths involving 33 (40%) of the 82 surgical patients and 46 (28%) of the 165 medical patients. Survival over a period of 140 months was significantly shorter in the surgical group ($p = 0.047$, RR 1.57, 95% CI 1.01–2.46). During the follow-up period of 10–13 years, surgical patients were significantly less likely to take antireflux medications regularly, and when antireflux medications were discontinued, their symptoms of GERD were significantly less severe than those of the medical patients. However, 62% of the surgical patients took antireflux medications on a regular basis, and there were no significant differences between the groups in the rates of neoplastic and peptic complications of GERD, overall physical and mental well-being scores, and overall satisfaction with antireflux therapy. For reasons that are not clear, antireflux surgery was associated with a significant decrease in long-term survival. The investigators concluded that antireflux surgery should not be advised with the expectation that patients with GERD will no longer need to take antisecretory medications or that the procedure will prevent esophageal cancer for those with GERD and Barrett's esophagus.

H. Endoscopic Antireflux Procedures

Two endoscopic therapies for GERD recently have been approved by the Food and Drug Administration—the Bard endoscopic suturing system and the Stretta radiofrequency energy system. The Bard endoscopic suturing system uses an endoscopic sewing machine device to plicate the gastroesophageal junction from the mucosal side. The Stretta system delivers radiofrequency (microwave) energy that creates thermal lesions in the LES muscle. Presently, there are no controlled trials demonstrating the efficacy of the procedures, but small clinical studies have described promising results. It is not clear how the procedures create an antireflux barrier (if in fact they do), and the safety of the techniques is questionable even though no serious complications were observed in the small clinical studies. The role of these procedures in the treatment of GERD is not yet clear.

Complications

A. Esophageal Stricture

Peptic strictures form when reflux-induced ulceration stimulates fibrous tissue production and collagen deposition in the esophagus. These strictures typically cause slowly progressive dysphagia for solid foods, such as meats and breads. Liquids alone do not cause dysphagia unless the stricture is associated with an esophageal motility disorder such as scleroderma. Patients with peptic strictures often modify their diets to avoid the foods that produce dysphagia but, unlike patients with malignant strictures, profound weight loss is uncommon.

The length of peptic strictures varies from fine, focal narrowings to long constrictions that involve virtually the entire esophagus. On barium swallow, peptic esophageal strictures characteristically have a smooth, tapered appearance. Radiography is more sensitive than endoscopy for demonstrating subtle esophageal narrowing, particularly when the radiographic examination includes swallowing of a solid bolus, such as a barium tablet or a barium-soaked marshmallow. Radiography does not reliably distinguish benign and malignant esophageal strictures, however, and endoscopic examination with biopsy and brush cytology of the esophagus is necessary to exclude cancer. Other conditions that can mimic peptic esophageal stricture include esophageal narrowing due to radiation, infectious esophagitis, or the ingestion of caustic substances, such as lye. Also, a variety of medications taken in pill form (eg, tetracycline, NSAIDs) can cause caustic injury with stricture formation if the pills linger in the esophagus. Unlike peptic strictures that usually involve the distal esophagus, pill-induced stricture often involves the proximal esophagus at the level of the aortic arch.

Peptic strictures usually are treated by the peroral passage of devices that dilate the esophagus. These devices include fixed-size dilators (eg, mercury-filled rubber bougies, Savary-Gilliard dilators) and balloons that can be inflated within the stricture. For strictures that are neither very tight nor tortuous, the passage of mercury-filled rubber bougies often is effective. Tight or tortuous strictures can be treated with dilators that are passed over a guidewire that is positioned within the stricture using either fluoroscopic or endoscopic guidance. As previously mentioned, aggressive acid suppression with PPIs both improves dysphagia and decreases the need for esophageal dilation in patients who have peptic esophageal strictures. Strictures can also be dilated surgically, and this procedure can be combined with an antireflux operation. Rarely, intractable strictures require resection. In such cases, the esophagus is reconstructed with a segment of bowel.

B. Barrett's Esophagus

Barrett's esophagus is a condition in which a metaplastic columnar epithelium replaces squamous epithelium in the distal esophagus. The condition is a sequela of reflux esophagitis in most cases, and is a strong risk factor for adenocarcinoma of the esophagus and gastroesophageal junction.

1. Histology—Histologic examination of biopsy specimens obtained from patients with Barrett's esophagus can reveal any of three types of columnar epithelia: (1) gastric fundic-type epithelium that has a pitted surface lined by mucus-secreting cells, and a deeper glandular layer that contains chief and parietal cells; (2) junctional-type epithelium that has a foveolar surface and glands lined almost exclusively by mucus-secreting cells; and (3) specialized intestinal metaplasia (also called specialized columnar epithelium) that has a villiform surface and intestinal-type crypts lined by mucus-secreting columnar cells and goblet cells (Figure 16–6). The former two epithelial types can be morphologically indistinguishable from epithelia normally found in the stomach. Specialized intestinal metaplasia, in contrast, is readily distinguished from normal gastric epithelia. Specialized intestinal metaplasia also is the most common and important of the three epithelial types found in Barrett's esophagus. Dysplasia and carcinoma in this condition invariably are associated with intestinal metaplasia.

2. Diagnosis—On endoscopic examination, columnar epithelium in the esophagus can be recognized by its characteristic red color and velvet-like texture that contrast sharply with the pale, glossy appearance of the adjacent squamous epithelium. Consequently, endo-

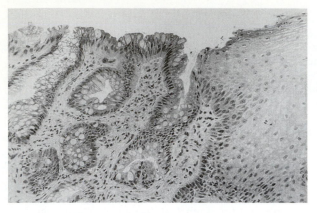

Figure 16–6. This photomicrograph of a biopsy specimen obtained at the squamocolumnar junction in the distal esophagus shows an abrupt transition from stratified squamous epithelium to specialized intestinal metaplasia. Both the surface and the intestinal-type glands of the specialized columnar epithelium are lined by mucus-secreting cells and goblet cells (H&E; original magnification ×200). (Reproduced, with permission, from Spechler SJ: Prevalence of metaplasia at the gastroesophageal junction. Lancet 1994; 344:1533. © by The Lancet Ltd., 1994.)

scopists recognize Barrett's esophagus easily when they see long segments of columnar epithelium extending up the esophagus, well above the junction with the stomach (Figure 16–7). The diagnosis of Barrett's esophagus is clear when long segments of columnar epithelium extend to the mid-esophagus and beyond. Substantial diagnostic difficulties can arise, however, when patients are found to have short segments of columnar lining in the distal esophagus. Several factors contribute to the diagnostic problems in these cases. One major confounding factor lies in identifying the precise point at which the esophagus joins the stomach (the esophagogastric junction). Anatomists, radiologists, and physiologists all have used different landmarks to identify the junction, most of which are not applicable by endoscopists. Endoscopic criteria that have been used to recognize the esophagogastric junction include the point at which the tubular esophagus flares to become the sack-like stomach, and the proximal margin of the gastric folds. The distal esophagus *in vivo* is a dynamic structure whose appearance changes constantly, however. The location of the point of flare varies with respiratory and peristaltic activity and with the degree of esophageal and gastric distention. With no "gold standard" for localizing the esophagogastric junction, it can be difficult to ascertain whether columnar epithelium found in this area lines the distal esophagus or the proximal stomach (the gastric cardia). Adding to the diagnostic confusion, some investigators have claimed that gastric mucosa normally can extend at least 2 cm into the distal esophagus. Therefore, the finding of gastric-type epithelia in this distal esophageal segment does not establish a diagnosis of Barrett's esophagus.

Confronted with these diagnostic difficulties, investigators who designed studies on Barrett's esophagus often attempted to avoid making false-positive diagnoses by including only those patients whose esophageal columnar lining extended some specified distance (eg, >3 cm) above the esophagogastric junction. Although many gastroenterologists have adopted those investigative criteria into their clinical practices, diagnostic standards for Barrett's esophagus that are based on a specified extent of columnar lining clearly are arbitrary. For example, if 3 cm is selected as the diagnostic criterion for Barrett's esophagus, then patients who have 2.5 cm of metaplastic columnar lining (with potential for neoplastic change) will be ignored. Furthermore, criteria based on the extent of esophageal columnar lining are subject to the considerable imprecision of endoscopic measurement.

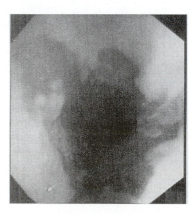

Figure 16–7. This endoscopic photograph of the distal esophagus shows long segments of red, columnar epithelium extending well above the esophagogastric junction. This is the characteristic endoscopic appearance of Barrett's esophagus.

In an attempt to avoid the diagnostic difficulties described, some investigators have chosen to define Barrett's esophagus by the presence of specialized intestinal metaplasia anywhere in the esophagus, regardless of extent. Even this approach does not eliminate diagnostic problems. Intestinal metaplasia in the stomach can be histologically indistinguishable from esophageal intestinal metaplasia, and inadvertent biopsy of an intestinalized gastric cardia could result in a false-positive diagnosis of Barrett's esophagus. Although intestinal metaplasia in the gastric cardia, like its counterpart in the esophagus, may well predispose to cancer of the esophagogastric junction, there is an obvious conceptual problem inherent in calling intestinal metaplasia of the stomach "Barrett's esophagus."

Perhaps the major problem in defining Barrett's esophagus solely by the presence of specialized intestinal metaplasia relates to the frequency with which short segments of this epithelium can be found in the region of the esophagogastric junction. In one recent study, all patients scheduled for elective endoscopic examinations in a general endoscopy unit, regardless of the indication for the procedure, had biopsy specimens obtained at the squamocolumnar junction (the Z-line) in the distal esophagus irrespective of its appearance and location. Among 142 patients who had columnar epithelium involving <3 cm of the distal esophagus, 26 (18%) were found to have specialized intestinal metaplasia in hematoxylin and eosin (H&E) stains of biopsy specimens from the squamocolumnar junction. Signs and symptoms of esophagitis were not reliable markers for the presence of intestinal metaplasia, and the metaplastic epithelium found in the study patients would have gone unrecognized if the protocol had not mandated the acquisition of biopsy specimens from a normal-appearing squamocolumnar junction. A number of studies have confirmed these findings that short, inconspicuous segments of specialized intestinal metaplasia can frequently be found at the squamocolumnar junction. The role of GERD in the pathogenesis of these short metaplastic segments is not clear. Some authorities refer to this condition in which intestinal metaplasia lines <3 cm of the distal esophagus as "short-segment Barrett's esophagus."

Barrett's esophagus of the endoscopically obvious variety ("long-segment Barrett's esophagus") traditionally has been associated with severe GERD and with a high risk for developing adenocarcinoma. The risks for GERD complications and cancer development have not yet been established for patients with short segments of intestinal metaplasia at the esophagogastric junction. Some data suggest that these risks are substantially different for patients with short segment disease. Therefore, it may not be appropriate to include patients with long segments of esophageal intestinal metaplasia and those with short segments both under the rubric "Barrett's esophagus."

There remains substantial controversy regarding the diagnostic criteria for Barrett's esophagus. An alternative diagnostic system that does not rely on arbitrary and imprecise endoscopic measurements has been proposed. Whenever columnar epithelium is seen in the esophagus, regardless of extent, the condition is called "columnar-lined esophagus." In these cases, biopsy specimens are obtained from the esophageal columnar lining to seek specialized intestinal metaplasia. The condition can then be classified as either "columnar-lined esophagus with specialized intestinal metaplasia" or "columnar-lined esophagus without specialized intestinal metaplasia." If desired, the term "Barrett's esophagus" can be applied to the subset of patients with columnar-lined esophagus who have long, endoscopically obvious segments of columnar epithelium extending well above the esophagogastric junction. Most of the latter patients are found to have specialized intestinal metaplasia. Regardless of the diagnostic system used, the clinician should recognize that most studies on Barrett's esophagus have included only patients with endoscopically obvious disease. It is not clear that the conclusions of these studies are applicable to patients who have short segments of specialized intestinal metaplasia in the region of the esophagogastric junction. Barrett's esophagus traditionally has been associated with severe GERD and with a high risk for adenocarcinoma. Many patients with short segments of specialized intestinal metaplasia have no apparent GERD, and their risk for developing adenocarcinoma may be far less than that for patients with long segments of intestinal metaplasia.

Further studies are needed to define the epidemiology and natural history of this condition. The remainder of this chapter deals primarily with studies of patients who had endoscopically obvious disease. Unless otherwise specified, the term "Barrett's esophagus" refers only to such patients.

3. Clinical features—Columnar-lined esophagus with intestinal metaplasia has been described in children as young as age 5, but Barrett's esophagus usually is discovered in middle-aged and older adults. The average age at diagnosis is approximately 55 years. White males predominate in most series and, for unknown reasons, Barrett's esophagus appears to be uncommon in blacks and Asians.

Most patients are seen initially for symptoms of underlying GERD, such as heartburn, regurgitation, and dysphagia. The Barrett's epithelium causes no symptoms, and even may be more resistant to acid-peptic injury than the native squamous mucosa. Many patients with endoscopically apparent Barrett's esophagus have no symptoms of GERD, however, and recent data suggest that the large majority of patients with Barrett's esophagus do not seek medical attention for esophageal symptoms. Among patients identified by physicians, the GERD associated with Barrett's esophagus often is severe and associated with esophageal ulceration, stricture, and hemorrhage.

A variety of physiologic abnormalities have been described that might contribute to the severity of GERD in patients with Barrett's esophagus (see Table 16–1). For patients with these abnormalities, the gastric contents available for reflux are exceptionally caustic because they contain high concentrations of acid, bile, and pancreatic secretions. Patients who have extreme hypotension of the LES are exceptionally predisposed to the reflux of their caustic gastric contents. Poor esophageal contractility interferes with clearance of the refluxed material, allowing protracted contact with the esophageal epithelium. With diminished sensitivity to esophageal pain, reflux may not induce the symptoms that lead patients to seek medical attention to prevent further damage to the esophagus. Finally, decreased secretion of epidermal growth factor might delay the healing of the reflux-induced injury. With all these abnormalities, it is not surprising that GERD frequently is severe in patients with Barrett's esophagus.

Given the propensity for severe GERD in patients with Barrett's esophagus, it has been assumed that the metaplasia should progress in extent over the years as more and more columnar epithelium replaced reflux-damaged squamous epithelium. Surprisingly, however, recent studies suggest that in most cases Barrett's esophagus develops to its full extent relatively quickly, neither progressing nor regressing substantially with time. The length of esophagus lined by Barrett's epithelium does not differ significantly among various age groups. Furthermore, no significant change in the extent of Barrett's epithelium is found among patients who have had follow-up endoscopic examinations performed after a mean interval of 3 years. It is not clear why Barrett's esophagus usually does not progress in extent, despite ongoing GERD.

4. Cancer risk—Barrett's esophagus is a risk factor for adenocarcinoma of the gastroesophageal junction. Adenocarcinomas develop in Barrett's esophagus at the rate of approximately 0.5% per year. The frequency of adenocarcinoma of the gastroesophageal junction has been increasing in the United States at a rate exceeding that for any other cancer to the point that adenocarcinomas comprise approximately 50% of all esophageal malignancies in this country.

Carcinogenesis in Barrett's esophagus appears to begin with genetic alterations that activate protooncogenes (eg, c-*erb*-B) and disable tumor suppressor genes (eg, *p53*). These DNA abnormalities endow the cells with certain growth advantages. The advantaged cells hyperproliferate, and in so doing acquire more genetic changes that result in neoplasia with autonomous cell growth. When enough DNA abnormalities accumulate, clones of malignant cells emerge that have the ability to invade adjacent tissues and to proliferate in unnatural locations. Before the cells acquire enough DNA damage to become frankly malignant, the earlier genetic alterations often cause histologic changes that can be recognized by the pathologist as dysplasia.

Dysplasia in Barrett's epithelium is defined as a neoplastic alteration of columnar cells that remains confined within the basement membranes of the glands from which the cells arose. Dysplasia is the precursor of invasive malignancy, and the finding of dysplasia can provide an opportunity to initiate therapy to interrupt the progression to invasive cancer. Endoscopic surveillance for cancer in Barrett's esophagus is performed primarily to seek high-grade dysplasia, with the rationale that resection of the dysplastic epithelium may prevent the progression to invasive malignancy.

The usefulness of dysplasia as a biomarker for a malignant neoplasm is limited by the problem of biopsy sampling error. For example, patients who have esophageal resections performed for high-grade dysplasia in Barrett's esophagus often are found to have an inapparent malignant neoplasm in the resected specimen. These cancers were missed by the endoscopist preoperatively because of biopsy sampling error, a problem that can be reduced by increasing the number of biopsy specimens obtained during endoscopic examinations. Although it has been reported that clinicians can differentiate high-grade dysplasia from early adenocarcinoma in Barrett's esophagus by rigorously sampling the esophagus extensively, the extensive biopsy protocol required may be too rigorous to be clinically applicable.

Another problem with dysplasia as a biomarker for malignancy is the fact that the natural history of dysplasia is not well defined. Available data suggest, however, that high-grade dysplasia progresses to malignancy often and rapidly. Up to 25% of patients with high-grade dysplasia may progress to invasive cancer during a follow-up period of 2–46 months. This appears to be an alarming rate of progression to malignancy. In some cases, however, high-grade dysplasia has persisted for years with no apparent progression to carcinoma.

Noting the shortcomings of dysplasia as a biomarker for malignancy, investigators have studied alternative biomarkers, such as flow cytometry, ornithine decarboxylase activity, mucus abnormalities, chromosomal abnormalities, oncogenes, tumor suppressor genes, growth regulatory factors, and endosonographic findings. None of these biomarkers has been shown to be superior to the histologic finding of dysplasia for predicting the development of malignancy in Barrett's esophagus, however. Despite the problems, the finding of dysplasia remains the best biomarker for the clinical evaluation of patients with Barrett's esophagus.

5. Treatment—There is no specific treatment for Barrett's esophagus other than treatment of the underlying reflux esophagitis. Furthermore, neither medical nor surgical therapy for GERD reliably results in the regression of the columnar epithelium. In recent studies, regression has been achieved by ablation of Barrett's epithelium using thermal or photochemical energy combined with the administration of a PPI. The rationale for this approach is the hypothesis that in the absence of acid reflux, damaged esophageal tissue should heal normally by regeneration of squamous mucosa.

A number of reports document the feasibility of endoscopic ablation of Barrett's epithelium, but none of them has established the benefit of the technique. The procedures entail some risk, and have not been shown to reduce the risk of esophageal cancer. Also, it is not clear whether life-long, intensive acid suppression will be necessary to prevent return of the columnar epithelium. Further studies addressing these issues are necessary before endoscopic ablation of Barrett's epithelium can be recommended for general clinical application.

6. Management recommendations—The management of patients with Barrett's esophagus is disputed, and will remain so until studies demonstrate the cost-effectiveness of endoscopic surveillance and clarify the natural history of high-grade dysplasia. Clinicians reviewing the available data on these issues might reasonably arrive at different conclusions regarding management. With minor modifications, the following management approach is recommended by the American College of Gastroenterology:

1. Patients with Barrett's esophagus should undergo surveillance endoscopy and biopsy at an interval determined by the presence and grade of dysplasia. GERD should be treated aggressively prior to surveillance endoscopy to minimize confusion caused by inflammation in the interpretation of biopsy specimens. The technique of random, four-quadrant biopsies taken every 2 cm in the columnar-lined esophagus for standard histologic evaluation is recommended.

2. For patients with no dysplasia, surveillance endoscopy is recommended at an interval of every 2–3 years. For patients with low-grade dysplasia, surveillance endoscopy every 6 months for the first year is recommended, followed by yearly endoscopy if the dysplasia has not progressed in severity. For patients with high-grade dysplasia, two alternatives are proposed after the diagnosis has been confirmed by an expert gastrointestinal pathologist:

   a. One alternative is intensive endoscopic surveillance until intramucosal cancer is detected.

The guideline does not recommend a specific interval for such surveillance, but some investigators have studied such patients at an interval of every 3 months.

   b. The other alternative is to recommend esophageal resection.

Although not specifically recommended in the practice guidelines, clinicians can consider the use of experimental ablative therapies such as photodynamic therapy for their patients with high-grade dysplasia in Barrett's esophagus, *provided the therapy is administered as part of an established, approved research protocol.* The use of ablative therapies outside of research protocols cannot be encouraged at this time.

REFERENCES

Baldi F et al: Acid gastroesophageal reflux and symptom occurrence. Analysis of some factors influencing their association. Dig Dis Sci 1989;34:1890.

Berenson MM et al: Restoration of squamous mucosa after ablation of Barrett's esophageal epithelium. Gastroenterology 1993;104:1686.

Cameron AJ, Lomboy CT: Barrett's esophagus: age, prevalence, and extent of columnar epithelium. Gastroenterology 1992;103:1241.

Cameron AJ et al: Prevalence of columnar-lined (Barrett's) esophagus. Comparison of population-based clinical and autopsy findings. Gastroenterology 1990;99:918.

Dent J et al: Mechanisms of lower oesophageal sphincter incompetence in patients with symptomatic gastro-oesophageal reflux. Gut 1988;29:1020.

DeVault KR, Castell DO, and The Practice Parameters Committee of the American College of Gastroenterology: updated guidelines for the diagnosis and treatment of gastroesophageal reflux disease. Am J Gastroenterol 1999;94:1434.

Devesa SS, Blot WJ, Fraumeni JF Jr: Changing patterns in the incidence of esophageal and gastric carcinoma in the United States. Cancer 1998;83:2049.

Dodds WJ et al: Pathogenesis of reflux esophagitis. Gastroenterology 1981;81:376.

Frierson HF Jr: Histological criteria for the diagnosis of reflux esophagitis. Pathol Annu (Part 1) 1992;27:87.

Haggitt RC, Dean PJ: Adenocarcinoma in Barrett's epithelium. In: *Barrett's Esophagus: Pathophysiology, Diagnosis, and Management.* Spechler SJ, Goyal RK (editors). Elsevier, 1985.

Hameeteman W et al: Barrett's esophagus: development of dysplasia and adenocarcinoma. Gastroenterology 1989;96:1249.

Hassall E: Barrett's esophagus: new definitions and approaches in children. J Pediatr Gastroenterol Nutr 1993;16:345.

Helm JF et al: Effect of esophageal emptying and saliva on clearance of acid from the esophagus. N Engl J Med 1984;310:284.

Herrera JL et al: Sucralfate used as adjunctive therapy in patients with severe erosive esophagitis resulting from gastroesophageal reflux. Am J Gastroenterol 1990;85:1335.

Hetzel DJ et al: Healing and relapse of severe peptic esophagitis after treatment with omeprazole. Gastroenterology 1988;95: 903.

Hewson EG, et al: Acid perfusion test: does it have a role in the assessment of noncardiac chest pain? Gut 1989;30:305.

Holloway RH, Dent J: Pathophysiology of gastroesophageal reflux. LES dysfunction in gastroesophageal reflux disease. Gastroenterol Clin North Am 1990;19:517.

Inauen W et al: Effects of ranitidine and cisapride on acid reflux and oesophageal motility in patients with reflux oesophagitis: a 24-hour ambulatory combined pH and manometry study. Gut 1993;34:1025.

Jamieson GG: Anti-reflux operations: how do they work? Br J Surg 1987;74:155.

Johnson DA et al: Esophageal acid sensitivity in Barrett's esophagus. J Clin Gastroenterol 1987;9:23.

Kahrilas PJ: Cigarette smoking and gastroesophageal reflux disease. Dig Dis 1992;10:61.

Kahrilas PJ, Clouse RE, Hogan WJ: American Gastroenterological Association technical review on the clinical use of esophageal manometry. Gastroenterology 1994;107:1865.

Klinkenberg-Knol EC, et al: Long-term treatment with omeprazole for refractory reflux esophagitis: efficacy and safety. Ann Intern Med 1994;121:161.

Koufman JA: The otolaryngologic manifestations of gastroesophageal reflux disease (GERD): a clinical investigation of 225 patients using ambulatory 24-hour pH monitoring and an experimental investigation of the role of acid and pepsin in the development of laryngeal injury. Laryngoscope 1991; 101:1.

Lagergren J et al: Symptomatic gastroesophageal reflux as a risk factor for esophageal adenocarcinoma. N Engl J Med 1999; 340:825.

Lanas A, Hirschowitz BI: Significant role of aspirin use in patients with esophagitis. J Clin Gastroenterol 1991;13:622.

Levine DS et al: An endoscopic biopsy protocol can differentiate high-grade dysplasia from early adenocarcinoma in Barrett's esophagus. Gastroenterology 1993;105:40.

Lieberman DA, Keeffe EB: Treatment of severe reflux esophagitis with cimetidine and metoclopramide. Ann Intern Med 1986; 104:21.

Mansfield LE: Gastroesophageal reflux and respiratory disorders: a review. Ann Allergy 1989;62:158.

Marks RD et al: Omeprazole versus H_2-receptor antagonists in treating patients with peptic stricture and esophagitis. Gastroenterology 1994;106:907.

Mattox HE III, Richter JE: Prolonged ambulatory esophageal pH monitoring in the evaluation of gastroesophageal reflux disease. Am J Med 1990;89:345.

McCallum RW: Gastric emptying in gastroesophageal reflux and the therapeutic role of prokinetic agents. Gastroenterol Clin North Am 1990;19:551.

Mittal RK: Current concepts of the antireflux barrier. Gastroenterol Clin North Am 1990;19:501.

Mittal RK, Rochester DF, McCallum RW: Electrical and mechanical activity in the human LES during diaphragmatic contraction. J Clin Invest 1988;81:1182.

O'Connor HJ: Helicobacter pylori and gastro-oesophageal reflux disease—clinical implications and management. Aliment Pharmacol Ther 1999;13:117.

Orlando RC: Esophageal epithelial defenses against acid injury. Am J Gastroenterol 1994;89:S48.

O'Sullivan GC et al: Interaction of LES pressure and length of sphincter in the abdomen as determinants of gastroesophageal competence. Am J Surg 1982;143:40.

Peghini PL, Katz PO, Castell DO: Ranitidine controls nocturnal gastric acid breakthrough on omeprazole: a controlled study in normal subjects. Gastroenterology 1998;115:1335.

Reid BJ: Barrett's esophagus and esophageal adenocarcinoma. Gastroenterol Clin North Am 1991;20:817.

Robinson M et al: Omeprazole is superior to ranitidine plus metoclopramide in the short-term treatment of erosive oesophagitis. Aliment Pharmacol Ther 1993;7:67.

Sampliner RE and The Practice Parameters Committee of the American College of Gastroenterology: updated guidelines for the diagnosis and treatment of gastroesophageal reflux disease. Am J Gastroenterol 1999;94:1434.

Shaheen NJ et al: Is there publication bias in the reporting of cancer risk in Barrett's esophagus? Gastroenterology 2000;119: 333.

Sloan S, Rademaker AW, Kahrilas PJ: Determinants of gastroesophageal junction incompetence: hiatal hernia, LES, or both? Ann Intern Med 1992;117:977.

Smith JL et al: Sensitivity of the esophageal mucosa to pH in gastroesophageal reflux disease. Gastroenterology 1989;96:683.

Smith PM et al: A comparison of omeprazole and ranitidine in the prevention of recurrence of benign esophageal stricture. Gastroenterology 1994;107:1312.

Sontag SJ: The medical management of reflux esophagitis. Role of antacids and acid inhibition. Gastroenterol Clin North Am 1990;19:683.

Spechler SJ: Barrett's esophagus. Curr Opin Gastroenterol 1994; 10:448.

Spechler SJ: Comparison of medical and surgical therapy for complicated gastroesophageal reflux disease in veterans. The Department of Veterans Affairs Gastroesophageal Reflux Disease Study Group. N Engl J Med 1992;326:786.

Spechler SJ: Complications of gastroesophageal reflux disease. In: The Esophagus. Castell DO (editor). Little, Brown and Company, 1992.

Spechler SJ: Epidemiology and natural history of gastroesophageal reflux disease. Digestion 1992;51(Suppl 1):24.

Spechler SJ: Laser photoablation of Barrett's epithelium: burning issues about burning tissues. Gastroenterology 1993;104: 1855.

Spechler SJ: Barrett's esophagus: an overrated cancer risk factor. Gastroenterology 2000;119:587.

Spechler SJ et al: Prevalence of metaplasia at the gastroesophageal junction. Lancet 1994;344:1533.

Spechler SJ et al: Long-term outcome of medical and surgical treatments for gastroesophageal reflux disease. Follow-up of a randomized controlled trial. JAMA 2001;285:2331.

Tytgat GNJ: Dilation therapy of benign esophageal stenoses. World J Surg 1989;13:142.

Esophageal Motility Disorders & Noncardiac Chest Pain

17

Kavita Kongara, MD & Edy Soffer, MD

The esophagus is a 20- to 22-cm muscular conduit between the oropharynx and the stomach. Functionally, it can be divided into three zones: the upper esophageal sphincter (UES), the esophageal body, and the lower esophageal sphincter (LES), which, in the healthy state, serve a dual function: to propel food from the pharynx to the stomach and to prevent/minimize esophageal exposure to gastric contents. The pharynx, UES, and proximal one-third of the esophagus are composed primarily of striated (skeletal) muscle; the distal two-thirds of the esophagus and LES are composed of smooth muscle. The esophageal muscle consists of an outer longitudinal layer, an inner circular layer, and the myenteric plexus, which lies between these two layers.

Voluntary and involuntary mechanisms act together in the esophagus to coordinate function. Primary peristalsis is initiated by the act of swallowing and results in the passage of a food bolus past the UES, through the esophageal body, and into the stomach via the relaxed LES. Secondary peristalsis is a progressive contraction that occurs only in the esophagus and is induced not by a swallow, but rather by stimulation of sensory receptors in the esophageal body. This is usually secondary to distention by a bolus (such as that not entirely cleared by primary peristalsis) or to reflux of gastric contents.

Disruption of central nervous system (CNS) function (medullary swallowing center) or any of the esophageal components (including the sphincters or body) can result in various esophageal motor abnormalities. It is, therefore, important for the clinician to recognize these disorders and offer therapy, which can be very effective in some instances.

UPPER ESOPHAGEAL SPHINCTER & HYPOPHARYNGEAL DISORDERS

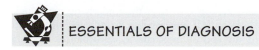

ESSENTIALS OF DIAGNOSIS

- *Oropharyngeal dysphagia (difficulty in transferring material from the mouth or pharynx into the esophagus); usually most severe with liquids.*
- *Nasal or oral regurgitation, aspiration, and coughing with swallowing.*
- *Documentation with cine-esophagogram.*

General Considerations

The oropharyngeal phase of swallowing is quite complex, because the nasal cavity and airway must close during a swallow to convert the oropharynx from an air conduit to a food conduit. There are four phases of oropharyngeal swallowing:

1. Oral-preparatory phase
2. Reflex initiation phase
3. Pharyngeal phase
4. Pharyngeal-esophageal phase

Any condition that affects the muscle or its innervation is capable of affecting the integrity of the muscular response and therefore coordination of the oropharynx. Oropharyngeal dysphagia results from the uncoordinated, feeble, or absent contractions of the tongue, pharynx, or hypopharynx. In general, neurologic disorders tend to result in oropharyngeal incoordination, while muscular disorders can cause weak pharyngeal contractions. Dysphagia is usually the most prominent esophageal symptom, but is often only one of a constellation of symptoms of a neuromuscular disorder.

Table 17–1 lists the various disorders that may cause oropharyngeal dysfunction, including disorders of the CNS, peripheral nervous system, and muscle. Cerebrovascular accidents are the most common CNS cause.

Diseases affecting the UES and cervical esophagus lead to oropharyngeal dysphagia, which involves difficulty in transferring the food from the mouth to the esophagus. Patients with this disorder have true difficulty with the act of swallowing and cannot propel the food bolus into the esophageal body. Various neuromuscular, skeletal, or structural lesions have been described to cause oropharyngeal dysphagia.

Table 17–1. Causes of oropharyngeal dysphagia.

Neurologic Causes	Muscular Causes	Structural Causes
Cerebrovascular accident	Muscular dystrophies	Zenker's and other diverticula
Parkinson's disease	Polymyositis	Neoplasms
Wilson's disease	Amyloidosis	Postoperative changes
Amyotrophic lateral sclerosis		Postradiation changes
Myasthenia gravis		Extrinsic compression (eg, cervical osteophytes)
Multiple sclerosis		
Brainstem tumors		
Tabes dorsalis		
Poliomyelitis		
Diphtheria		
Botulism		
Rabies		

Swallow-induced opening of the UES is the result of both relaxation of the sphincter and pulling by the suprahyoid muscles. Inadequate opening is commonly the result of fibrosis, which can cause increased intra-bolus pressure in the pharynx, which in turn can lead to the formation of a Zenker's diverticulum, which is formed by a herniation of hypopharyngeal mucosa through an area of weakness in the posterior wall between the pharyngeal constrictor muscle and the cricopharyngeal sphincter (Killian's triangle). Another entity, cricopharyngeal bar, is also thought to represent reduced muscle compliance rather than decreased relaxation.

Clinical Findings

A. SYMPTOMS AND SIGNS

Oropharyngeal motility disorders result primarily in oropharyngeal dysphagia despite repeated efforts at swallowing. Liquids can be more of a problem than solids and patients are often observed to cough, choke, or have nasal regurgitation during a meal. Because this type of dysphagia often has a neurologic basis, patients often have dysarthria (impaired articulation of speech) and dysphonia (impaired quality of the voice). Patients with a Zenker's diverticulum have retention of food and secretions that classically leads to halitosis, delayed regurgitation, recurrent aspiration, and, in some cases, pneumonia. Interestingly, patients with oropharyngeal dysphagia are often able to point to, or localize the site

of dysfunction, which correlates well with findings on radiologic studies. Noteworthy is the extremely common complaint of globus, which refers to a nonpainful sensation of a lump or fullness in the throat. With globus, bolus transfer into the esophagus is normal and swallowing may actually improve the feeling of fullness. Some believe it to be due to a dysfunction of the UES, but its etiology remains unclear in most cases.

B. IMAGING STUDIES

The study of choice for the evaluation of oropharyngeal dysphagia is the videofluoroscopic study of the "modified barium swallow." This test allows slow-motion replay of a swallow, which is done with boluses of different texture to define the mechanisms and severity of dysfunction. In specialized centers it can be interpreted with the aid of a speech therapist who can help to make therapeutic recommendations. Rare structural causes of oropharyngeal dysfunction, such as tumors, require further evaluation with plain x-ray or computed axial tomography (CAT) scan of the neck.

C. MANOMETRY

Standard manometry has a very limited role in the evaluation of the oropharyngeal region and is no longer utilized in the clinical evaluation of oropharyngeal dysfunction.

D. ENDOSCOPY

Upper endoscopy is not helpful in the evaluation of oropharyngeal dysfunction and, in a case of suspected Zenker's diverticulum, should be avoided or approached with extreme caution.

Differential Diagnosis

The differential diagnosis of oropharyngeal dysphagia is listed in Table 17–1.

Complications

Complications of the various disorders that cause oropharyngeal dysphagia include weight loss, malnutrition [in some cases requiring the placement of a percutaneous endoscopic gastrostomy (PEG) tube] and aspiration pneumonia.

Treatment

The ideal therapy is to treat the underlying neurologic impairment and, if not possible, to proceed with treatment of the specific mechanical disturbances seen on fluoroscopic examination. In addition to the overall neurologic rehabilitation therapy, speech therapists are often able to help by working with patients in developing new swallowing techniques with the goal of resuming a modified oral diet. In some instances this is not possible and a patient will require the placement of a PEG tube to avoid becoming malnourished. If a structural lesion is present, surgical therapy can be effective, as in the case of a patient with a Zenker's diverticulum that undergoes diverticulectomy and UES myotomy.

Prognosis

Much like therapy, the prognosis of the patient depends directly on the self-limited or progressive nature of the underlying neuromuscular process. Many patients who develop oropharyngeal dysphagia as a result of a confined cerebrovascular accident are able to reclaim their swallowing mechanism with time and are able to resume adequate oral intake. Others with more progressive disorders, such as Parkinson's disease, muscular dystrophy, or multiple sclerosis, might develop recurrent aspiration pneumonia, malnutrition, and may even die.

MOTILITY DISORDERS OF THE BODY OF THE ESOPHAGUS

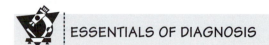

ESSENTIALS OF DIAGNOSIS

- *Dysphagia to solid foods and liquids.*
- *Chest pain (see the section, "Noncardiac Chest Pain").*
- *Confirmation of abnormal motility by barium study/esophageal manometry.*

General Considerations

Esophageal dysphagia is characterized by motor dysfunction, typically of the smooth muscle portion and/or the LES, which leads to a failure in the transport of a food bolus to the stomach. There are a number of structural and neuromuscular defects that can cause symptoms in patients. Some are better defined, as in the case of achalasia, and others cause nonspecific motility abnormalities whose clinical significance remains unknown.

Esophageal peristalsis consists of a sequential contractile wave, which advances the contents from the proximal to the distal end as seen in Figure 17–1. Neural control of the esophagus is by way of the vagus and neurons within the myenteric plexus. The LES is controlled by both excitatory cholinergic neurons and inhibitory neurons releasing nitric oxide (NO) and vasoactive intestinal polypeptide (VIP).

Motility disorders of the esophagus include the well-described achalasia, which results in aperistalsis and failure or incomplete relaxation of the LES upon deglutition. The cause of achalasia is unknown, but suggested theories include infectious, autoimmune, or environmental etiologies. Neuropathologic features of achalasia include loss of ganglion cells within the myenteric plexus of the distal esophagus, degenerative changes of the vagus nerve and in the dorsal motor nucleus of the vagus, as well as a decrease in inhibitory neurotransmitters in the myenteric neurons, such as VIP and NO. Other described motility disorders include the nutcracker esophagus, diffuse esophageal spasm, and hypertensive LES. Diffuse esophageal spasm (DES), or incoordinated motility, is a disorder seen in approximately 3–10% of patients with unexplained chest pain and dysphagia and is associated with simultaneous distal esophageal contractions intermixed with normal peristalsis. A barium esophagram can demonstrate the characteristic "corkscrew" appearance of DES. Although 3–5% of patients with DES are thought to progress to achalasia, the overall prognosis is excellent and symptoms tend to be stable and may spontaneously improve. Nutcracker esophagus is a manometric abnormality with high-amplitude peristaltic contractions (HAPCs) greater than 180 mm Hg, commonly seen in patients with chest pain. It is unclear if it represents a true disorder because no direct correlation exists between HAPC and chest pain and reduction in HAPC correlates poorly with improvement in symptoms. Treatment of both DES and nutcracker esophagus remains limited and is often best done with frequent physician–patient interactions, reassurance, and, in some cases, low-dose antidepressants. Hypertensive lower esophageal sphincter (HLES) is an uncommon manometric abnormality defined as an increased resting LES pressure >45 mm Hg with normal residual pressure following swallows and normal peristalsis. It is seen in patients with chest pain, dysphagia, nutcracker esophagus, or even gastroesophageal reflux disease (GERD). Nonspecific esophageal motility disorders or ineffective esophageal motility (Table 17–2) are a group of manometric abnormalities including mostly low-amplitude contractions or nontransmitted contractions and have been referred to as ineffective esophageal motility. These abnormalities can be seen in patients with GERD, but their relation to symptoms or to the pathophysiology of GERD remains to be determined.

Clinical Findings

Healthy asymptomatic individuals can have nonspecific manometric abnormalities, hence symptoms cannot al-

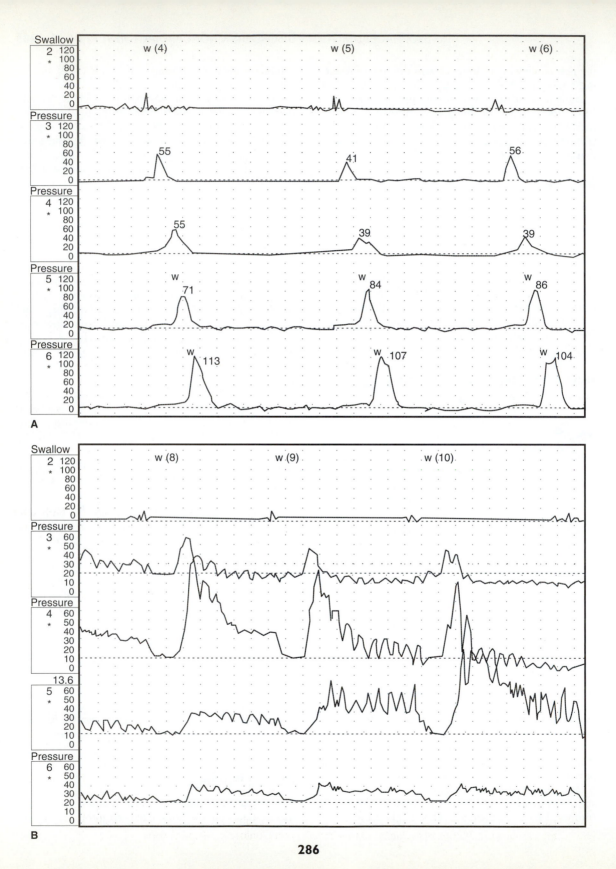

Table 17–2. Classification of primary esophageal motility abnormalities.

Functional Defect	Descriptive Term	Manometric Findings
Aperistalsis	Achalasia (a true disorder)	Absent distal peristalsis[1]
		Elevated resting LES[2] pressure (>45 mm Hg)[3]
		Incomplete LES relaxation (residual pressure >8 mm Hg)[3]
		Elevated baseline esophageal pressure[3]
Incoordinated motility	Diffuse esophageal spasm	Simultaneous contractions ≥20% wet swallows, with intermittent peristalsis[1]
		Repetitive contractions (≥3 peaks)[3]
		Prolonged-duration contractions (>6 seconds)[3]
		Retrograde contractions[3]
		Isolated incomplete LES relaxations[3]
Hypercontractile	Nutcracker esophagus	Increased distal peristaltic amplitude (≥180 mm Hg)[1]
		Increased distal peristaltic duration (>6 seconds)[3]
	Hypertensive LES	Resting LES pressure >45 mm Hg[1]
		Incomplete LES relaxation (residual pressure >8 mm Hg)[3]
Hypocontractile	Ineffective esophageal motility	Increased nontransmitted peristalsis (≥30 %)[4]
		Distal peristaltic amplitude,[4] <30 mm Hg in ≥30 swallows
	Hypotensive LES	Resting LES pressure <10 mm Hg[1]

[1]Required for diagnosis.
[2]LES, lower esophageal sphincter.
[3]May be seen, not required.
[4]Either or both may be seen.
Reproduced, with permission, from Katz PO et al: Non-achalasia motility disorders. In: *The Esophagus,* 3rd ed. Castell D, Richter JE (editors). Lippincott Williams & Wilkins, 1999.

ways be clearly attributed to the presence of a manometric abnormality. Up to 33% of patients seen for chest pain, or dysphagia, will be found to have a motility abnormality upon evaluation. It is the role of the gastroenterologist to determine which of the abnormal findings are relevant, knowing the particular history of the patient, and then to individualize treatment. Diagnosis of an esophageal motility disorder is usually based on (1) the combination of symptoms—chest pain, dysphagia, regurgitation, or weight loss—and (2) abnormal motility by barium x-ray studies or esophageal manometry.

The history is often extremely helpful in determining the correct diagnosis in patients with esophageal dysphagia, and a few basic questions can narrow the etiology:

1. Does the dysphagia occur with solids only, or solids and liquids?
2. Is the dysphagia intermittent or progressive?
3. Are there associated clues: heartburn, pulmonary symptoms, chest pain, weight loss, or heartburn? (Figure 17–2).

Patients who complain of dysphagia to both solid foods and liquids are likely to have an esophageal motility disorder. Patients with intermittent solid and liquid dysphagia may have diffuse esophageal spasm; those with progressive solid and liquid dysphagia may have achalasia; and those with progressive solid and liquid dysphagia with prominent symptoms of heartburn may have scleroderma. Patients with achalasia may also have pulmonary symptoms (nocturnal cough, recurrent pneumonia) or weight loss. Progressive dysphagia to solids (especially meat and bread) suggests mechanical obstruction by tumor or a peptic stricture. Intermittent dysphagia to solids is suggestive of a Schatzki's ring. Patients with GERD may present with either dysphagia resulting from peptic stricture or gross esophagitis, or a

Figure 17–1. **A:** Manometry of the esophageal body in a normal subject. All leads are spaced 5 cm apart. Leads 6, 5, 4, and 3 are positioned in the body of the esophagus, 3, 8, 13, and 18 cm above the lower esophageal sphincter. Lead 2 is in the pharynx. Note that after each wet swallow (w), a peristaltic wave passes through the esophageal body. **B:** Manometry of the lower esophageal sphincter in a normal subject. Leads 3, 4, 5, and 6 are spaced 1 cm apart. Lead 2 is in the pharynx. With a wet swallow (w), the lower esophageal sphincter pressure falls to the level of the gastric baseline pressure **(dotted line),** and then returns to its tonic level of contraction.

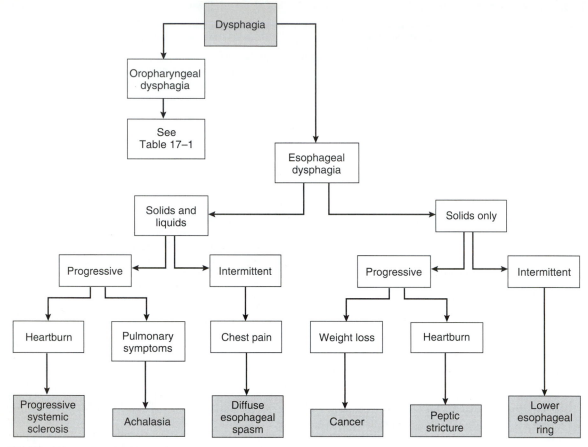

Figure 17–2. Dysphagia algorithm. The cause of dysphagia in most patients can be determined by the history.

combination. Infectious or radiation-induced esophagitis may cause dysphagia or odynophagia (pain during swallowing). Finally, neoplasms of the esophageal body and gastric cardia may present with dysphagia, which is usually progressive and accompanied by weight loss.

A. SYMPTOMS AND SIGNS

Dysphagia resulting from dysfunction of the esophageal body is described as a feeling that the bolus gets "stuck" or "hung up" on the way down. This may be accompanied by pain or discomfort. The patient typically describes difficulty in swallowing both solid foods and liquids. Notably, although most patients feel as though the bolus stops at the level of the suprasternal notch, the area of obstruction may be well below that. Patients with esophageal motility disorders may also present with chest pain, which may mimic angina pectoris. The pain is often substernal, burning, or pressure-like and may radiate into the neck or down the left arm. Pain may or may not be related to eating or swallowing; it may

occur at rest or may awaken the patient from sleep; and it is frequently made worse by stress. The pain may resolve spontaneously, or antacids or nitrates may be required for relief. In most cases, the clinical history will not differentiate between cardiac and esophageal chest pain. Patients with esophageal chest pain often report other esophageal symptoms, such as heartburn, regurgitation, or dysphagia, which also may be reported by patients with coronary disease.

B. MANOMETRY

Esophageal manometry can be used to measure the strength (amplitude) and duration and sequential nature of the contractions of the esophageal body as well as the resting pressure and relaxation of the upper and lower esophageal sphincters. This technique involves passage of a small, flexible catheter with pressure sensors through the nose and into the esophagus. The catheter may be water perfused or house miniature solid-state pressure transducers. Normal esophageal motility consists of orderly, sequential peristaltic contractions of normal amplitude and duration down the body of the esophagus. Normal values for esophageal manometry (amplitude and duration of contractions, percentage of peristaltic contractions, and percentage of abnormal contractions) have been derived from the study of healthy volunteers. Normal lower sphincter function consists of resting pressure within the normal range and complete or near complete relaxation following a wet swallow. In achalasia, there are two characteristic manometric findings: aperistalsis of the esophageal body and partial or absent relaxation of the lower sphincter (Figure 17–3). In the past, the terms "classic" and "vigorous" achalasia were used to distinguish patients with low-amplitude isobaric waveforms (classic) from those with relatively higher amplitude simultaneous contractions (vigorous). These distinctions, however, are of little clinical usefulness. The most common motility disorder in patients with chest pain is nutcracker esophagus. Other such disorders include diffuse esophageal spasm, hypertensive lower esophageal sphincter, and nonspecific esophageal motility disorder (see Table 17–2).

C. IMAGING STUDIES

Radiographic examination of the esophagus should include double-contrast esophagram and videoesophagram. The advantage of the double-contrast technique is visualization of the extended esophagus and its mucosal surface; this is helpful in identifying small neoplasms and esophagitis. The video portion of the examination is done with the patient in different positions with ingestion of barium, barium tablets, or food mixed with barium for the purpose of assessment of esophageal motility disorders as well as Schatzki's rings and peptic strictures.

D. ENDOSCOPY

Endoscopy is required in all patients with achalasia to rule out **pseudoachalasia,** a syndrome that occurs in certain malignant tumors. This syndrome typically involves tumors of the gastric cardia and causes symptoms by compressing the gastroesophageal junction or infiltrating the myenteric plexus, or may be produced as a paraneoplastic phenomenon, by distant tumors. Pseudoachalasia may also be seen in patients with amyloidosis, sarcoidosis, or Chagas' disease.

Differential Diagnosis

The differential diagnosis for esophageal dysphagia is shown in Figure 17–2.

Complications

Complications of achalasia include weight loss, nocturnal regurgitation, airway obstruction, the development of squamous cell carcinoma, esophageal diverticula, and pulmonary infections. The frequency of squamous cell carcinoma developing in achalasia varies greatly, reflecting major differences between studies. Currently no clear guidelines exist regarding surveillance. Complications of scleroderma include peptic stricture and food impaction. Serious complications from other esophageal motility disorders are rare.

Treatment

A. ACHALASIA

The current therapies for achalasia can be divided into medical and surgical categories. There is no curative therapy in either category that can reestablish normal esophageal peristalsis and allow the LES to relax completely. However, therapies have been shown to be effective in reducing LES pressure and, more importantly, in improving patient symptoms. Recommended treatments include drug therapy, botulinum toxin injection, pneumatic dilation, and esophagomyotomy. Of these, only pneumatic dilation and surgical myotomy can significantly decrease the resting pressure of the LES and can thus be considered definitive and not palliative therapy.

1. Drug therapy—Pharmacotherapy may be used as a temporary measure in selected patients prior to definitive therapy. These patients include those who are awaiting definitive therapy, are completing their evaluation, or wish to delay their decision about definitive therapy. In addition, pharmacotherapy may be appropriate for patients who refuse definitive therapy, are uncooperative, or are not candidates for definitive therapy because of advanced age or other illnesses.

Calcium channel blockers have been studied the most in a clinical setting. Nifedipine, 10–20 mg sublingually 30 minutes before meals, may be used. Despite initial interest in pharmacologic therapies, recent data from the literature and long-term experience indicate that they may best be used as palliative measures prior to more definitive treatment.

2. Botulinum toxin injection—Botulinum toxin prevents acetylcholine release from nerve terminals. As a result, the toxin decreases lower esophageal sphincter pressure when injected into the sphincter muscle. Although botulinum toxin injection is safe and well tolerated, its effects are transient. The efficacy of botulinum toxin injection for achalasia at 1 month is approximately 70%. However, this drops in most studies to 36–50% at 1 year. Therefore patients would require further injections at 6 months to maintain effectiveness. However, it is useful therapy for the short term with minimal side effects, therefore, it should, be considered the treatment of choice for the older, debili-

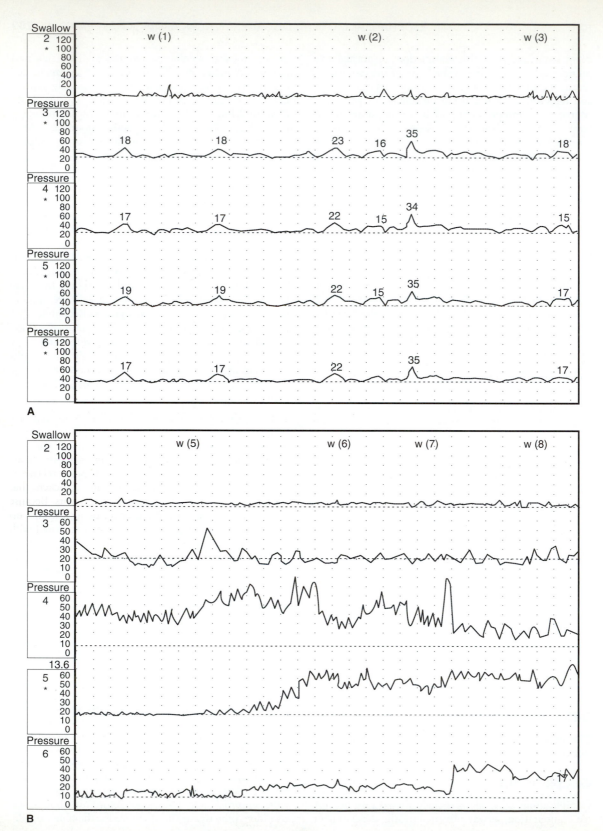

tated patient in whom complications of pneumatic dilation or the morbidity of surgery cannot be tolerated.

3. Pneumatic dilation—In pneumatic dilation, a balloon is used to forcefully disrupt the lower esophageal sphincter muscle. The procedure is often done on an outpatient basis. The most widely available balloon is the Microvasive Rigiflex Achalasia Dilator (Microvasive, Watertown, MA). In recent studies, pneumatic dilation was up to 85% effective after a mean follow-up of 6.5 years. However, LES pressures increase over time leading to repeat dilation rates between 7 and 38% in the literature. Early complications include perforation (3.3%), aspiration pneumonia (0.8%), and death (0.2%). The late complication of gastroesophageal reflux occurs in only 2% of patients treated with pneumatic dilation. Older patients respond more favorably to pneumatic dilation when compared with younger patients. This fact, and the recent advent of successful laparoscopic repair, should be considered in the treatment of young and otherwise healthy individual with achalasia. Ultimately the choice depends on patient preference and the surgical/medical expertise available.

4. Esophagomyotomy—Surgical esophagomyotomy is more efficacious than pneumatic dilation in relieving dysphagia. A modified Heller procedure is usually employed in which a myotomy of the circular muscle layers is performed down to the level of the mucosa. The myotomy extends 1–2 cm onto the stomach and up to several centimeters above the lower sphincter. Csendes and coworkers randomly treated 81 patients with achalasia (11 with Chagas' disease) with surgical myotomy or forceful pneumatic dilation. At a mean follow-up time of 5 years, 95% of patients who had undergone myotomy had a good or excellent result, compared with only 65% of those treated with pneumatic dilation. The myotomy is usually performed by extending the incision 1- to 2-cm distal to the gastroesophageal junction, in addition to including an antireflux procedure. With the advent of laparoscopic techniques, the morbidity of achalasia surgery has decreased significantly and the majority of achalasia surgery today is being performed laparoscopically.

Laparoscopic modified Heller myotomy in most series has an efficacy rate of >70%, with a conversion rate to open myotomy of 2.1% and a complication rate with tear or perforation of 4.5%. The procedure usually takes between 120 and 160 minutes with an average hospital stay of 2–5 days. The most common medical complications include GERD and dysphagia, but the rates are no different with open versus laparoscopic technique. Most surgeons currently opt for a Dor or Toupet wrap following the myotomy (anterior or posterior partial wrap, respectively) because proton-pump inhibitor therapy is highly effective in the treatment of mild GERD, and it is more problematic to treat dysphagia.

The respective skills of the local surgeon and gastroenterologist should be considered in formulating a plan for the therapy of each individual achalasia patient, including consideration of the patient's quality of life, health status, preferences, and costs. Now that laparoscopic Heller myotomies can be performed with markedly less morbidity and cost, surgery has become a more attractive alternative for the treatment of achalasia, especially in the young and otherwise healthy patient.

OTHER ESOPHAGEAL MOTILITY DISORDERS

Treatment of the remaining esophageal motility disorders is less straightforward with mixed success rates reported for a variety of measures that have been attempted. The use of smooth muscle relaxants, including nitrates and calcium channel blockers, has been shown to provide relief for some patients. Because of the concomitant relaxation effect of such agents on the lower sphincter, however, problems associated with GERD may be increased. Psychotropic drugs, bougienage, behavioral therapies, and surgical myotomies have been used with success in selected patients (Table 17–3).

PROGNOSIS

The prognosis for patients with esophageal motility disorders is generally good. The life expectancy of patients with achalasia is no different from that of patients without the disorder. Surveillance for squamous cell carci-

---

Figure 17–3. **A:** Manometry of the esophageal body in achalasia. The leads are placed in the same manner as in Figure 17–1A. With a wet swallow (w), simultaneous, low-amplitude, nonperistaltic waves are seen in all leads in the esophageal body. These contractions are virtually identical in all four leads. Note that the baseline esophageal pressure (normally 0 cm H_2O) is elevated to 20 cm H_2O, because the esophagus is filled with fluid. **B:** Manometry of the lower esophageal sphincter in achalasia. The leads are placed in the same manner as in Figure 17–1B. The baseline lower esophageal pressure is elevated. With wet swallows, little relaxation in the lower esophageal sphincter pressure occurs, and it remains well above the gastric baseline (**dotted line**).

Table 17–3. Potential therapies for esophageal motility abnormalities.

Treatment Modality	Dose	Mode of Administration
Reassurance		
Nitrates		
Nitroglycerin	0.4 mg sublingually	Usually before meals and as needed to prevent attacks
Isosorbide	10–30 mg orally	30 minutes before meals
Visceral analgesic		
Imipramine	50 mg orally	Bedtime
Sedatives, antidepressants		
Alprazolam	2–5 mg orally	Four times daily
Trazodone	50 mg orally	Three or four times daily
Calcium channel blockers[1]		
Nifedipine	10–30 mg	Four times daily
Diltiazem	60–90 mg	Four times daily
Smooth muscle relaxant[1]		
Hydralazine	25–50 mg orally	Three times daily
Botulinum toxin[2]	80 U	Injection into LES[3] via endoscopy
Static dilatation	56–60 French bougie	Repeat as needed
Pneumatic dilatation[4]		
Esophagomyotomy[5]		

[1]Orthostatic hypotension is a common complication of this class of drugs.
[2]Single uncontrolled study.
[3]LES, lower esophageal sphincter.
[4]May be indicated if dysphagia is a prominent symptom.
[5]Rarely indicated (intractability).
Reproduced, with permission, from Katz PO et al: Non-achalasia motility disorders. In: *The Esophagus,* 3rd ed. Castell D, Richter JE (editors). Lippincott Williams & Wilkins, 1999.

noma may be advisable in these patients, but this issue remains controversial.

NONCARDIAC CHEST PAIN

Pathophysiology

Chest pain may occur in patients with cardiac, gastrointestinal, psychiatric, or musculoskeletal disorders. Determining which disorder is truly the cause of the chest pain is difficult, as many purported disorders do not meet strict criteria for causation and may be epiphenomena. Pain has been thought to result from reflux, esophageal motility disorders, or visceral hypersensitivity. Several studies have demonstrated that multiple disorders may affect a single patient, and it is often difficult to establish which disorder is responsible for the pain.

The mechanism and cause of pain in most patients remain speculative. Abnormal esophageal contractions and distention may cause chest pain in patients with achalasia by stimulating mechanical nociceptors or inducing esophageal ischemia. Stimulation of acid-sensitive esophageal chemoreceptors may cause pain in patients with gastroesophageal reflux. Cardiac ischemia can be demonstrated in patients with microvascular angina when sophisticated tests are performed, although the degree of chest pain seems disproportionate to the severity of ischemia. Provocative testing (see the section, "Clinical Findings") induces pain in patients with chest pain of undetermined etiology but not in subjects without the disorder.

Increased visceral sensitivity to normal physiologic or minor noxious stimuli, commonly referred to as **heightened visceral nociception,** or visceral hyperalgesia, may be the underlying abnormality in many patients with chest pain of undetermined etiology and the common thread linking several disorders in a single patient. This theory is supported by the fact that these patients frequently exhibit an increased sensitivity to visceral stimuli such as distention or acid reflux. The mechanism responsible for this heightened sensitivity is not known, but may involve malfunction of the nociceptor itself, the ascending nociceptive pathway, the CNS, the descending antinociceptive pathway, or neurotransmitter release. Several neurotransmitters have been identified that play a role in pain perception and transmission including substance P, calcitonin gene-related peptide, and serotonin. Specific antagonists of the 5-HT$_3$ receptor may block visceral pain perception and may be an effective therapy in the future for patients with chest pain of undetermined etiology.

ESSENTIALS OF DIAGNOSIS

- *Exclusion of life-threatening conditions, usually coronary artery disease (ideally with an angiogram).*
- *Search for the two common and treatable conditions that may present with chest pain: GERD and panic disorder.*
- *Suspicion for unusual causes of chest pain (eg, biliary colic, costochondritis, aortic aneurysms, or peptic ulcer disease).*

General Considerations

Noncardiac chest pain, more aptly termed unexplained chest pain (UCP), is alarming for both patient and physician because it may herald a potentially life-threatening condition. The first step in the evaluation of all patients with chest pain is to diagnose and treat such conditions, most commonly ischemic heart disease. However, as many as 30% of cardiac catheterizations in patients with chest pain will reveal normal or insignificantly diseased coronary arteries. Although this subset of patients has a low mortality rate (cardiac survival exceeds 98% at 10 years), their quality of life is poor and the yearly cost of their medical care is estimated to be $3500. Once life-threatening conditions have been excluded, the two most important conditions to recognize are gastroesophageal reflux and panic disorder, both of which are common and treatable.

Gastroesophageal reflux is found in 25–50% of all patients with chest pain of undetermined etiology studied with ambulatory pH monitoring. Such monitoring quantifies esophageal acid exposure and also establishes the temporal correlation of spontaneous chest pain with reflux episodes (positive symptom index)(Figure 17–4). A diagnosis of GERD can lead to relief of chest pain with effective treatment.

Patients with psychiatric disorders (eg, panic disorder, anxiety, and depression) commonly have abnormal esophageal motility. Panic disorder is present in 30–50% of patients with chest pain of undetermined etiology who undergo psychiatric evaluation and is the most common psychiatric illness in these patients. This disorder must be excluded in all patients with disabling chest pain and a history of depression or social phobias. The diagnosis may be suggested by the history or by the score on the Hospital Anxiety and Depression Scale, a brief, well-validated, patient-administered questionnaire (Table 17–4), but should always be confirmed by *Diagnostic and Statistical Manual,* 4th ed. *(DSM-IV)* criteria. Depression is found in approximately one-third of patients with chest pain of undetermined etiology; it may antedate or coexist with panic disorder. Chest pain occurs primarily in women in the fifth or

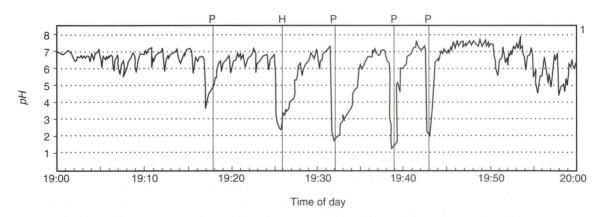

Figure 17–4. Ambulatory pH study in a patient with chest pain of undetermined etiology (time of day on horizontal axis; pH on vertical axis). One hour of the 24-hour record is displayed. The pH probe is placed in the distal esophagus, 5 cm above the lower esophageal sphincter. The normal esophageal pH fluctuates between 5 and 8. A fall in pH below 4 indicates an acid reflux event. In this recording, the chest pain (P) and heartburn (H) occurred during a documented acid reflux episode; this is evidence of reflux-induced chest pain.

Table 17–4. *DSM-IV* critieria for panic attack.[1]

A discrete period of intense fear or discomfort, in which four (or more) of the following symptoms developed abruptly and reached a peak within 10 minutes:

1. Palpitations, pounding heart, or accelerated heart rate
2. Sweating
3. Trembling or shaking
4. Sensations of shortness of breath or smothering
5. Feeling of choking
6. Chest pain or discomfort
7. Nausea or abdominal distress
8. Feeling dizzy, unsteady, light-headed, or faint
9. Derealization (feeling of unreality) or depersonalization (being detached from oneself)
10. Fear of losing control or going crazy
11. Fear of dying
12. Paresthesias (numbness or tingling sensations)
13. Chills or hot flushes

[1]Reproduced, with permission, from American Psychiatric Association: *Diagnostic and Statistical Manual of Mental Disorders,* 4th ed. text revision Washington, DC. American Psychiatric Press, 2000. Copyright 2000 American Psychiatric Assoc.

sixth decade of life, and a history of panic attacks can often be obtained.

Chest pain may also result from myocardial ischemia, even when coronary arteries are found to be anatomically normal (**microvascular angina or syndrome X**). This diagnosis should be considered in patients with typical anginal symptoms and normal coronary arteries, especially when abnormalities are present on noninvasive tests of cardiac function such as exercise radionuclide angiography or exercise thallium scintigraphy. Although mitral valve prolapse is frequently present in patients with chest pain of undetermined etiology, most investigators agree that it does not cause chest pain or panic disorder.

An array of musculoskeletal disorders may also cause chest pain, including "chest wall" (localized myofascial) pain, ankylosing spondylitis, fibromyalgia, Tietze's syndrome, rheumatoid arthritis, thoracic outlet syndrome, and "slipping rib" syndrome (via impingement of an intercostal nerve).

With the exception of achalasia, there is little evidence implicating esophageal motility disorders as a cause of chest pain for the following reasons:

1. Studies claiming a causal association are not well designed.
2. There is no "dose–response" between the severity of chest pain and the severity of the motility disorder.

3. There is poor temporal correlation between esophageal motility disorders (EMDs) found on **manometric** studies with episodes of chest pain.
4. Treatment of the EMD does not reliably relieve chest pain.

Clinical Findings

A. SYMPTOMS AND SIGNS

The history and physical examination should focus on the patient's description of the chest pain, any associated esophageal symptoms or behavioral disorders, and reproduction of the pain with chest wall palpation.

1. Gastroesophageal reflux—Most patients with gastroesophageal reflux and chest pain complain of typical reflux symptoms (eg, heartburn, regurgitation, water brash, or dysphagia). The chest pain may worsen after meals or when the patient is supine, and may improve with use of antacids. The absence of typical reflux symptoms, however, does not rule out gastroesophageal reflux, because 10–20% of patients who reflux will have chest pain alone.

2. Panic disorder—The diagnosis of panic disorder can be made in patients who have recurrent unexpected panic attacks (see Table 17–4) that have been followed by at least 1 month of (1) persistent concern about having further attacks, (2) worry about the implications of the attacks, or (3) change in behavior as a result of the attacks. The panic attacks must not be a result of drugs, other medical conditions, or other psychiatric diagnoses.

3. Musculoskeletal disorders—The diagnosis of a musculoskeletal cause of chest pain rests on the history and physical examination. Patients with thoracic outlet syndrome may complain of chest pain and arm paresthesias due to compression of the brachial plexus and subclavian vessels. The diagnosis of fibromyalgia is based on at least a 3-month history of widespread pain, with more than 10 of 18 sites of tenderness on digital palpation.

B. DIAGNOSTIC STUDIES

1. Ambulatory pH monitoring—The diagnosis of gastroesophageal reflux should be objectively confirmed in patients who do not respond to empiric treatment, are candidates for long-term treatment, or who lack typical reflux symptoms. The "gold standard" for diagnosis is ambulatory pH monitoring, which allows detection of increased esophageal acid contact as well as temporal correlation of chest pain episodes with reflux events. The ratio of chest pain episodes during reflux to total chest pain episodes is referred to as the symptom index. Although gastroesophageal reflux can be diagnosed with barium esophagography or endoscopy, the sensitivity of these tests is much lower than that of ambulatory pH monitoring.

2. Manometry—The diagnosis of an EMD in patients with central chest pain can be considered in those with complaints of dysphagia to solids and liquids. However, EMDs are found in a minority of patients with undetermined chest pain (UCP). Therefore, manometry should not be the initial test in the evaluation of UCP.

3. Provocative testing—The diagnosis of heightened visceral nociception is suggested by the reproduction of chest pain with any positive provocative test. Provocative tests include the acid perfusion test ("Bernstein" test), in which 0.1% hydrochloric acid is perfused by catheter into the distal esophagus, intraesophageal balloon inflation, and intravenous edrophonium administration ("Tensilon" test). Both the Bernstein and Tensilon tests have low sensitivities (20–35%) for diagnosing an esophageal cause of UCP. Additionally, although provocative testing may identify the esophagus as the source of symptoms, studies have not shown that results of testing can be used to direct subsequent therapy. Their use in clinical practice is, therefore, controversial and perhaps should be considered only in refractory cases with suboptimal response to therapy.

4. Noninvasive cardiac testing—The diagnosis of microvascular angina may be confirmed in clinical practice by observing (1) a functional abnormality during noninvasive cardiac testing in patients with normal coronary angiography, (2) a fall in the left ventricular ejection fraction or the development of a regional wall motion abnormality with exercise during radionuclide ventriculography, and (3) abnormal uptake or clearance of thallium on exercise scintigraphy. Sophisticated measurement of microvascular coronary resistance during provocative maneuvers, such as rapid atrial pacing and ergonovine infusion, is the province of specialized cardiac catheterization laboratories.

Differential Diagnosis

It is essential to exclude life-threatening conditions, usually significant coronary artery disease, in any patient who presents with chest pain. This should be accomplished using testing appropriate to the individual patient's probability of significant coronary artery disease. Once this has been done, the differential diagnosis can be expanded to include disorders of the esophagus and upper gastrointestinal tract, psychiatric disorders, cardiovascular disorders other than coronary artery disease, and musculoskeletal disorders. Clinicians should look for symptoms of achalasia, gastroesophageal reflux, peptic ulcer, biliary colic, anxiety, or depression. Pa-

tients with dysphagia should undergo endoscopy, barium esophagram, or manometry when appropriate (see the preceding section, "Clinical Findings"). A diagnosis of gastroesophageal reflux can be made in those patients with typical reflux symptoms who respond to empiric therapy for gastroesophageal reflux. In fact, recent studies have shown that the empiric use of potent antisecretory agents is more cost effective than using diagnostic tests in the initial evaluation of UCP. Patients with affective symptoms should be treated or referred to a psychiatrist or psychologist.

Complications

There are no complications of chest pain of undetermined etiology in the traditional sense. What may be viewed as complications, however, are the poor quality of life and overutilization of health care resources that may result when patients do not receive effective therapy.

Treatment

A. CHEST PAIN INDUCED BY GASTROESOPHAGEAL REFLUX

Patients with gastroesophageal reflux should be treated in a typical stepwise fashion. This begins with life-style modifications (eg, elevate the head of the bed, avoid fatty foods) and use of an H_2-receptor antagonist (eg, ranitidine, 150 mg twice daily, or famotidine, 20 mg twice daily). Patients with refractory chest pain and a confirmed diagnosis of gastroesophageal reflux may be treated with a proton-pump inhibitor (to be given 15–20 minutes before meals); if there is no response, the dose may be increased. An attempt to discontinue treatment should be made after 8 weeks, although many patients with moderate to severe GERD require life-long antisecretory therapy. Antireflux surgery may be considered for patients with severe chest pain and documented gastroesophageal reflux in whom a proton pump inhibitor has clearly improved chest pain.

B. ESOPHAGEAL MOTILITY DISORDERS

Patients with chest pain of undetermined etiology and EMDs often have an additional, more treatable condition, such as gastroesophageal reflux or panic disorder. These two disorders should be excluded before treatment directed specifically at the motility disorder is begun. In most cases, the EMD is a manometric epiphenomenon rather than a cause per se of the chest pain. Although it seems logical to presume that drugs relaxing smooth muscle might improve chest pain, only two of five randomized controlled trials concluded that calcium channel blockers were effective. Despite these results, it may be reasonable to try nifedipine,

10–20 mg orally four times daily (30 minutes before meals and at bedtime), in patients in whom an EMD is felt to play a predominant role in causing chest pain. Patients who respond can be switched to long-acting preparations. The antidepressant trazodone (100–150 mg/d), which has no direct effect on esophageal motility, has been effective in decreasing the distress of esophageal symptoms in patients with EMDs. This once again suggests that underlying psychiatric problems may play a significant role in patients with esophageal motility abnormalities. Use of trazodone in men is limited by the side effect of priapism. Surgical myotomy has no role in the management of patients with chest pain and EMDs other than achalasia.

C. Panic Disorder

The first step in the treatment of panic disorder is patient education. Patients should understand that they suffer from a common disorder that affects approximately 5% of the U.S. population. Although the cause of panic disorder is unknown, effective treatment exists in the form of antidepressants, anxiolytics, or behavioral cognitive therapy. Antidepressants are the treatment of choice for panic disorder without severe anxiety. Imipramine should be started at a low dose (eg, 10 mg before bedtime) to minimize troubling side effects. The dose should be increased slowly by 10 mg every 2–4 days until the dose is 50 mg. Thereafter, the dose may be increased by 25 mg every 2–4 days to a target dose of 150–200 mg before bedtime (2.5 mg/kg/d). Between 6 and 24 weeks of therapy may be needed for a response, and treatment should be continued for at least 6 months or as long as there is continued improvement. Unfortunately, up to 25% of patients discontinue therapy because of side effects. The dosage of imipramine should be gradually tapered by 25 mg every 3 days. Despite gradual tapering of the drug, 15–30% of patients will relapse within 2 years.

Patients with a severe anxiety component may benefit from the more rapid effects of an anxiolytic. Alprazolam, begun at 0.25–0.5 mg four times a day, will bring relief of anxiety within 1–2 weeks. The major drawback of the benzodiazepines is the risk for abuse of, or dependence on, the drugs and unpleasant withdrawal symptoms when they are discontinued. Patients with a personal or family history of drug or alcohol abuse should not be given benzodiazepines.

Preliminary reports regarding use of serotonin reuptake inhibitors in panic disorder have been promising. β-Blockers are useful for controlling associated autonomic symptoms. Lastly, behavioral therapy geared toward control of stress and improvement of coping skills brings about a level of improvement comparable to pharmacotherapy. The treatment of depression and somatoform disorder is beyond the scope of this chapter.

D. Heightened Visceral Nociception

A study by Cannon and colleagues suggests that imipramine is effective in patients with chest pain of undetermined etiology, regardless of the underlying diagnosis. Sixty consecutive patients who were referred to the National Institutes of Health for evaluation of chest pain were studied. The following disorders were diagnosed: esophageal motility disorders (41%), panic disorder (43%), and microvascular angina (22%). Eighty-seven percent of patients developed characteristic chest pain during catheterization with right ventricular stimulation or intracoronary adenosine infusion (markers of heightened visceral nociception). Patients were initially treated with a placebo for 5 weeks and then randomly given imipramine, 50 mg at bedtime; clonidine, 0.1 mg twice daily; or a placebo. Patients treated with imipramine had a 52% reduction in chest pain ($P = .03$) regardless of the underlying diagnosis; this suggests that imipramine was acting as a visceral analgesic. There are currently no studies comparing empiric therapy for GERD versus empiric therapy for visceral hyperalgesia in UCP. The search continues for other medications, such as the serotonin antagonists, which may act as visceral analgesics.

E. Microvascular Angina

Patients with microvascular angina may respond to treatment with a calcium channel blocker (eg, verapamil, 80 mg four times daily, or nifedipine, 10 mg four times daily).

F. Musculoskeletal Disorders

Patients with musculoskeletal chest pain should be treated with reassurance, local heat application, nonsteroidal antiinflammatory drugs (NSAIDs), and corticosteroid-lidocaine injection when appropriate. Patients with fibromyalgia may benefit from cyclobenzaprine, 2.5–10 mg four times daily, or amitriptyline, 10–50 mg at bedtime. Exercise is beneficial.

Prognosis

Although patients with chest pain of undetermined etiology have an excellent survival rate (cardiac survival exceeds 98% at 10 years), the quality of life and functional status are markedly impaired. Most patients continue to experience chest pain, and up to one-half cannot perform strenuous activities. One retrospective study has suggested that the diagnosis of an esophageal motility disorder may alleviate patient anxiety, leading to improvement in the functional status of patients with chest pain of undetermined etiology. Contradictory results were obtained from a more recent prospective study, in which chest pain improved only in patients *without* an esophageal motility disorder or positive provocative test.

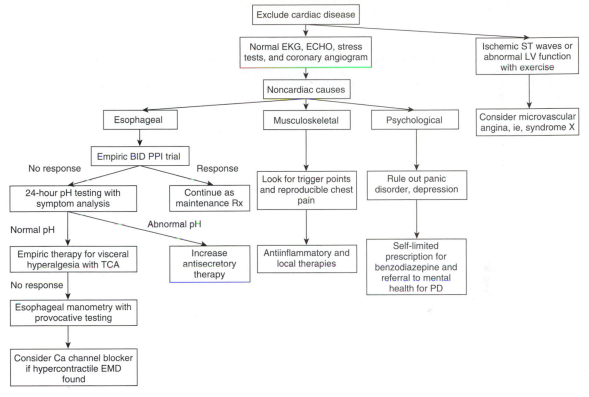

Figure 17–5. Algorithm for the approach to unexplained chest pain. EKG, electrocardiogram; LV, left ventricle; ECHO, echocardiogram; EMD, esophageal motility disorder; TCA, tricyclic antidepressant; BID PPI, proton-pump inhibitor twice a day; PD, panic disorder. (Reproduced, with permission, from Fang J, Bjorkman D: A critical approach to noncardiac chest pain: pathophysiology, diagnosis, and treatment. Am J Gastroenterol 2001;96:958.)

The outlook for patients with chest pain of undetermined etiology may be improved by (1) identification of subsets of patients with treatable causes of chest pain (eg, gastroesophageal reflux, panic disorder, or achalasia), and (2) treatment of the remaining patients with "visceral analgesics" such as imipramine.

An approach based on this strategy is shown in Figure 17–5.

REFERENCES

Barkin JS et al: Forceful balloon dilatation; an outpatient procedure for achalasia. Gastrointest Endosc 1990;36:123.

Cannon RO III: Imipramine in patients with chest pain despite normal coronary angiograms. N Engl J Med 1994;330:1411.

Clouse R et al: Low dose trazadone for symptomatic patients with esophageal contraction abnormalities: a double-blind, placebo-controlled trial. Gastroenterology 1987;92:1027.

Csendes A et al: Late results of a prospective randomized study comparing forceful dilatation and oesophagomyotomy in patients with achalasia. Gut 1989;30:299.

De Caestecker JA, Pryde A, Heading R: Comparison of intravenous edrophonium and esophageal acid perfusion during esophageal manometry in patients with noncardiac chest pain. Gut 1988;29:1029.

Fang J, Bjorkman D: A critical approach to noncardiac chest pain: pathophysiology, diagnosis, and treatment. Am J Gastroenterol 2001;96:958.

Fass R et al: The clinical and economic value of a short course of omeprazole in patients with non-cardiac chest pain. Gastroenterology 1998;115:42.

Goyal R, Sivaro DV: Functional anatomy and physiology of swallowing and esophageal motility. In: *The Esophagus,* 3rd ed. Castell DO, Richter JE (editors). Lippincott, Williams & Wilkins, 1999.

Hewson E, Dalton C, Richter J: Comparison of esophageal manometry, provocative testing, and ambulatory monitoring in patients with unexplained chest pain. Dig Dis Sci 1990; 35:302.

Hewson E et al: 24-hour esophageal pH monitoring: the most useful test for evaluating noncardiac chest pain. Am J Med 1991; 90:576.

Hunter J et al: Laparoscopic Heller myotomy and funduplication for achalasia. Ann Surg 1997;225:655.

Johnson D: Alterations in visceral perception represent primary pathophysiology in chest pain of unexplained etiology. Pract Gastroenterol 1999;Sept:70.

Kahrilas PJ: American Gastroenterological Association technical review on the clinical use of esophageal manometry. Gastroenterology 1994;107:1865.

Kahrilas PJ, Quigley EMM: Clinical esophageal pH recording: a technical review for practice guideline development. Gastroenterology 1996;110:1982.

Leite LP et al: Ineffective esophageal motility. Dig Dis Sci 1997; 42:1859.

Pasricha PJ et al: Botulinum toxin for achalasia: long-term outcome and predictors of success. Gastroenterology 1996;110:1410.

Prakash C, Clouse RE: Long-term outcome from tricyclic antidepressant treatment of functional chest pain. Dig Dis Sci 1999;44:2373.

Rao S et al: Unexplained chest pain: the hypersensitive, hyperreactive, and poorly compliant esophagus. Ann Intern Med 1996; 124:950.

Richter J, Bradley L, Castell D: Esophageal chest pain: current controversies in pathogenesis, diagnosis and therapy. Ann Intern Med 1989;110:66.

Tack J, Janssens J: The esophagus and noncardiac chest pain. In: *The Esophagus,* 3rd ed. Castell DO, Richter JE (editors). Lippincott Williams & Wilkins, 1999.

Vaezi M et al: Botulinim toxin versus pneumatic dilatation in the treatment of achalasia: a randomized trial. Gut 1999;44:231.

Van Peski-Oosterbaan A et al: Cognitive-behavioral therapy for noncardiac chest pain: a randomized trial. Am J Med 1999; 106:424.

Esophageal Tumors

18

James C. Chou, MD & Frank G. Gress, MD

ESOPHAGEAL CANCER

Demographics & Epidemiology

Esophageal cancer is a gastrointestinal malignancy with an insidious onset and a poor prognosis. The disease predominantly affects older age groups with a peak incidence between 60 and 70 years of age; it is rarely seen in children or young adults. There is also a predilection toward men with a ratio of at least 4:1. By far, the most common esophageal cancer worldwide is squamous cell carcinoma. Adenocarcinoma accounts for less then 15% of all esophageal cancers. Other malignant tumors of the esophagus, such as sarcomas, lymphoma, primary malignant melanoma, and small cell carcinoma, are very rare (Table 18–1). Although considered relatively uncommon, esophageal cancer is the seventh most common cause of cancer-related deaths in men in the United States and has ranked among the top 10 causes of cancer-related deaths worldwide.

The incidence of esophageal cancer also differs significantly by geographic region and race. The rates can vary between regions in a given country, demonstrating an important role for environmental and possibly dietary/nutritional factors. Worldwide, the highest incidence of esophageal cancer is observed in Linxian, China, with an annual rate of more than 130 per 100,000 population. Other regions with high incidences of esophageal cancer include areas of Iran, Russia, Colombia, and South Africa. In the Western Hemisphere, the incidence is approximately 5–10 per 100,000 population. In the United States, the estimated number of new cases of esophageal cancer for the year 2000 was 12,300, with estimated deaths of 12,100.

Over the past two decades, the patterns of esophageal cancer have changed dramatically in the United States. Parallel changes are also seen in other Western countries. The incidence of adenocarcinoma of the esophagus has risen sharply, especially among white males, whereas the rates of squamous cell carcinoma have remained essentially unchanged or have declined slowly. By the early 1990s, adenocarcinoma surpassed squamous cell carcinoma to become the most common type of esophageal cancer among white males, accounting for nearly 60% of all esophageal cancers, although squamous cell carcinoma remains the predominant cell type among African Americans. This change in the epidemiology of esophageal cancer is most likely multifactorial, involving a combination of factors and is not simply explained by the reclassification of gastric cardia carcinoma as esophageal adenocarcinoma or accounted for by the rising rate of Barrett's esophagus.

Etiology

Numerous studies have demonstrated that in developed countries cigarette smoking and alcohol consumption are the most important predisposing factors for esophageal cancer (Table 18–2). The carcinogenic effects of alcohol and tobacco are far more pronounced for squamous cell carcinoma than for adenocarcinoma of the esophagus. Although the mechanisms remain unclear, it is postulated that alcohol may act at several steps in the multiphase process of carcinogenesis, whereas the many tobacco-derived chemicals, such as nitrosamines, may affect the initiation of esophageal carcinoma or act as promotional agents.

It was previously thought that the total lifetime consumption of alcohol and amount smoked correlated with the risk of esophageal cancer. However, recent studies have shown the contrary; alcohol consumption and tobacco use do not affect the risk of esophageal cancer in the same way. For alcohol consumption, it is the mean intake (>200 g/week) rather than the duration, and for tobacco smoking, it is the duration (>15 years) rather than the mean intake that is more closely associated with the risk of esophageal cancer. In other words, a high intake of alcohol during a short period of time carries a higher risk than a moderate intake for a long time; a moderate consumption of tobacco for a long period carries a higher risk than a high intake for a short period. The risk of esophageal squamous cell carcinoma can be significantly reduced once patients achieve long-term smoking cessation (>10 years); however, the risk of esophageal adenocarcinoma may remain elevated for up to 30 years from the time of smoking cessation

Whereas alcohol consumption and tobacco use are the most significant risk factors for esophageal squamous cell carcinoma, Barrett's esophagus is the most important risk factor for esophageal adenocarcinoma. Barrett's esophagus, a known premalignant

299

Table 18–1. Malignant tumors of the esophagus.

Squamous cell cancer
Adenocarcinoma
Sarcoma
   Epidermoid carcinoma (carcinosarcoma and pseudo-
      sarcoma)
   Leiomyosarcoma
   Fibrosarcoma
   Rhabdomyosarcoma
   Kaposi's sarcoma
Mucoepidermoid carcinoma
Adenoid cystic carcinoma
Endocrine cell tumor (small cell carcinoma)
Lymphoma
Adenosquamous carcinoma
Primary malignant melanoma
Primary esophageal carcinoid tumor

lesion, is a consequence of chronic gastroesophageal reflux disease (GERD) in which the squamous epithelium of the distal esophagus is replaced by intestinal-type columnar epithelium. Patients with GERD who develop Barrett's esophagus may have a certain degree of esophageal dysmotility. This usually results in a hypotensive or inappropriately relaxed lower esophageal

Table 18–2. Risk factors for esophageal cancer.

Squamous cell carcinoma
   Chronic tobacco use
   Heavy alcohol consumption
   History of head and neck malignancy
   History of radiation therapy
   Chronic esophagitis (most common in Asia and Africa)
   Chronic stricture (lye ingestion and radiation)
   Tylosis (palmar and plantar hyperkeratosis)
   Plummer-Vinson syndrome
   Achalasia
   Dietary/nutritional
      Deficiency in carotene, vitamins C and E, riboflavin,
         selenium, and zinc
   Low intake of fruits and vegetables
   High intake of red meat and nitrate-containing foods
   Consumption of scalding hot beverages
Adenocarcinoma
   Barrett's esophagus and GERD
   Obesity
   Cigarette smoking
   Alcohol consumption
   Scleroderma
   History of colon cancer
   Medications: theophylline and β-agonists (long-term use
     >5 years)

sphincter (LES) allowing reflux of gastric contents into the esophagus and ineffective peristalsis prolonging contact of refluxate with esophageal mucosa, thus causing esophageal epithelial damage. It is postulated that esophageal cancer evolves through a similar temporal sequence of alterations seen in the dysplasia-to-carcinoma sequence in colonic neoplasm: metaplasia to low-grade dysplasia to high-grade dysplasia to adenocarcinoma. Barrett's esophagus is found in 10–15% of patients who undergo endoscopic evaluation for GERD. It is believed that this number probably underestimates the disease prevalence as many patients with Barrett's esophagus remain asymptomatic. The lifetime risk of esophageal adenocarcinoma in Barrett's esophagus is estimated to be 5%. In addition to its role in the pathogenesis of Barrett's esophagus, GERD is an independent risk factor for esophageal adenocarcinoma.

Recent epidemiologic studies have found that obesity (measured as body mass index) is another strong risk factor for esophageal adenocarcinoma. The elevated risk is mainly associated with excessive weight per se and is not related to weight changes over time. Although the mechanism by which obesity contributes to the increased risk of esophageal adenocarcinoma is unclear, it has been speculated that obesity promotes gastroesophageal reflux disease by increasing intraabdominal pressure, which in turn predisposes to developing a chronic GERD state and Barrett's esophagus. Other factors that may affect the cancer risk associated with obesity include body fat distribution, dietary practices, medications, and other conditions that may affect the severity of GERD.

Several esophageal motility disorders have been implicated in the development of esophageal cancer. Long-standing achalasia has been associated with increased risk of esophageal squamous cell carcinoma. On the other hand, scleroderma (systemic sclerosis) increases the risk of esophageal adenocarcinoma, perhaps through the development of Barrett's esophagus as the collagen deposits in the distal esophagus cause LES dysfunction. Other abnormalities or inflammatory lesions of the esophagus known to contribute to the development of esophageal squamous cell carcinoma include chronic esophagitis and strictures, tylosis, Plummer-Vinson syndrome, and lye ingestion.

In certain regions of the world, exceedingly high rates of esophageal cancer have been attributed to other environmental and dietary/nutritional factors. These include ingestion of hot foods and beverages, nitrate-containing preserved food, deficiencies in essential nutrients (carotene, riboflavin, vitamins C and E) and minerals (zinc and selenium), as well as infrequent consumption of fruits and vegetables. Human papillomavirus has also been implicated as a potential cause of esophageal squamous cell carcinoma.

Interestingly, colon cancer and breast cancer are found to be associated with an increased risk of esophageal cancer. More specifically, colon cancer is associated with adenocarcinoma, whereas breast cancer is associated with both adenocarcinoma and squamous cell carcinoma of the esophagus. The increased risk of esophageal squamous cell carcinoma in breast cancer is greater in those who have received radiation therapy as part of their treatment. Radiation may damage the genetic repair mechanisms or cause chronic esophagitis and strictures, both of which predispose to the development of squamous cell carcinoma.

Natural History

A. CLINICAL PRESENTATION

Approximately 15% of esophageal cancers arise in the upper one-third of the esophagus, 50% in the middle third, and 35% in the lower third and at the gastroesophageal junction. The presenting symptoms tend to correlate with the location of the tumor. Unfortunately, many of the symptoms experienced by patients with esophageal cancer occur late in the course of the disease, at which time the disease is already at an advanced stage, resulting in a very poor prognosis.

The most common presentation of esophageal cancer leading to its diagnosis is progressive dysphagia (Table 18–3). The esophagus is capable of accommodating to the partial obstruction initially because it lacks a serosal layer so that the smooth muscle can stretch. As a result, a patient may not manifest dysphagia until the lumen is more than 50–60% obstructed by the tumor mass. The narrowed esophageal lumen leads to solid food dysphagia first and later to liquid dysphagia with further disease progression and obstruction. Regurgitation may also occur as the enlarging tumor narrows the esophageal lumen.

Odynophagia is the second most common presenting symptom of esophageal cancer. It may be due to an ulcerated area in the tumor or involvement of mediastinal structures, although mediastinal invasion would more typically present as constant pain in the midback or midchest. Anorexia and weight loss often ensue with decreased nutritional intake. Hoarseness or voice change appears when the tumor invades the recurrent laryngeal nerve, causing vocal cord paralysis. Severe cough and aspiration are usually the result of tumor invasion into the airway or development of a fistula between the esophagus and the tracheobronchial tree.

Overt gastrointestinal bleeding as manifested by hematemesis or melena is rarely encountered. However, anemia is relatively common at presentation. Chronic subclinical bleeding is a major contributing factor for anemia. Massive hemorrhage can rarely occur and may require emergent surgical treatment if endoscopic therapy fails.

B. COMPLICATIONS

Esophageal cancer readily extends through the thin esophageal wall due to the absence of a serosa to invade adjacent structures. The vital mediastinal structures adjacent to the esophagus include the trachea, the right and left bronchi, the aortic arch and descending aorta, the pericardium, the pleura, and the spine. Tumor infiltration into these structures accounts for the most serious and, sometimes, life-threatening complications of esophageal cancer.

Most complications due to esophageal cancer are attributed to luminal obstruction and local tumor invasion. Patients often subconsciously adjust their diets to soft or liquid foods to avoid solid food dysphagia. The progressive inability to swallow solids leads to weight loss and nutritional deficiencies. Solid food impaction can result when there is severe stenosis, requiring endoscopic intervention for disimpaction. Regurgitation of food or oral secretions may also occur in the setting of significant luminal obstruction. Halitosis may be present due to food stasis and regurgitation.

Pulmonary complications from aspiration include pneumonia and pulmonary abscess. The tumor mass may cause compression and obstruction of the tracheobronchial tree, leading to dyspnea, chronic cough, and at times postobstructive pneumonia. Esophagoairway fistula may develop with tumor invasion of the trachea or bronchus. Airway fistulas are severely debilitating and are associated with significant mortality owing to the high risk of pulmonary complications such as pneumonia and abscess.

Although the aortic arch and descending aorta lie adjacent to the esophagus, extension into these structures is less frequent than airway invasion. Erosion through the aortic wall can result in severe hemorrhage and is often fatal. Tumor ingrowth of the pericardium has been reported as an infrequent cause of arrhythmias and conduction abnormalities. Pleural effusions are

Table 18–3. Signs and symptoms of esophageal cancer.

Dysphagia (most common)—solids then liquid
Odynophagia/retrosternal discomfort
Back pain/chest pain
Anorexia
Weight loss
Regurgitation
Hoarseness/voice change
Aspiration/cough/recurrent pneumonia
Hematemesis

usually small, but may signify pleural invasion when large effusions are present.

C. PROGNOSTIC FACTORS

1. Radiographic and endoscopic—Radiographic tests have been utilized to delineate the location and extent of esophageal involvement, as well as to stage the depth of tumor invasion, the presence of nodal involvement, and the presence of distant metastases. The length of esophageal involvement can be readily seen on barium esophagram and has been found to be a useful predictor of extraesophageal extension. Tumors measuring <5 cm are often confined to the esophageal wall whereas only 10% of those measuring >5 cm are localized. Computed tomography (CT) scan or magnetic resonance imaging (MRI) of the chest and abdomen are particularly useful in identifying distant metastases (most commonly to the liver and lung). The presence of metastases is a poor prognostic sign and is a contraindication to surgery.

For better evaluation of locoregional lymph node involvement and definition of depth of tumor penetration, endoscopic ultrasound (EUS) has emerged as the tool with the greatest accuracy (>80–90%). The primary advantage of EUS is as a staging modality. EUS is useful for identifying locally advanced disease after CT has ruled out metastatic disease. The presence of transmural invasion into adjacent organs such as the pericardium or trachea is associated with a poor prognosis. Evidence of lymph node involvement is also associated with a poor overall 5-year survival (<20%).

2. Pathologic—Typically, the clinical prognosis of any malignant neoplasm depends on the histologic type and grade and the clinical stage. Esophageal cancer is no exception. The vast majority of esophageal tumors are either squamous cell carcinomas or adenocarcinomas. The former usually arise in the middle and the lower third of the esophagus whereas the latter are typically seen in the lower third. When compared stage to stage, there seems to be very little difference in the prognosis between the two. Rare esophageal malignancies associated with a poorer prognosis are small cell carcinoma and primary malignant melanoma. The overall prognosis of a poorly differentiated tumor is worse than that of a well-differentiated tumor.

3. Clinical stage—The revised tumor, nodes, metastasis (TNM) classification of 1997 is currently recommended for staging of esophageal cancer. The older classification system in which tumors were staged based on size, circumferential involvement, and extent of obstruction was abandoned. The new system recognizes five major prognostic stages (stage 0 to IV) of tumor extent and clearly defines the cancer stage based on local invasion of the tumor, nodal involvement, and presence of metastases (Table 18–4). According to the current classification, a T1 tumor is limited to the mucosa or submucosa. In stage T2, tumor invasion extends into but not through the muscularis propria. In stage T3, adventitia invasion is present. In stage T4, there is evidence of tumor invasion into adjacent structures such as the trachea, pericardium, or aorta. The 5-year survival rates associated with the depth of tumor invasion (T1 to T4) are approximately 80%, 45%, 25%, and <20%, respectively.

In the present TNM system, all local lymph node involvement is classified as N1, whereas nodal metastases outside the regional nodes (eg, cervical or celiac) and distant organ metastases are classified as M1. Distant nodal involvement is less serious than the blood-borne metastases to distant organs such as liver or lung, although the higher the number of nodes involved the worse the prognosis.

The disadvantage of the current TNM system is the lack of reference to the presence of lymphatic or blood vessel invasion adjacent to the tumor mass. These are important independent adverse prognostic factors in esophageal squamous cell carcinoma. Blood vessel and lymphatic invasion should correlate with an advanced stage and presence of distant metastases.

Diagnosis

The initial diagnostic imaging test for most patients with dysphagia should be a barium esophagram (Figure 18–1). The study readily demonstrates narrowing of the esophageal lumen at the tumor site and dilatation proximally. Typical features of malignant obstruction on the barium esophagram include irregular mass lesions, irregular mucosal relief, and abrupt angulation of the esophageal contour (so-called **tumor shelf**). Benign lesions of the esophagus are typically associated with a smooth outline of the mucosa and symmetric narrowing without angulation or extrinsic compression.

All patients with abnormal barium esophagrams should undergo upper gastrointestinal endoscopy with biopsy to provide a definitive histologic diagnosis, assess the patency of the esophageal lumen, and confirm the endoscopic extent of the tumor. Endoscopy also offers important information regarding the feasibility of subsequent endoscopic therapeutic interventions such as dilation of a stenotic lumen, placement of prostheses (ie, stents), or ablation of an intraluminal tumor.

Routine chest x-ray may reveal an esophageal air–fluid level above the site of obstruction or a pulmonary infiltrate from aspiration. A pleural effusion or mediastinal mass may suggest mediastinal tumor extension. Electrocardiogram changes are unusual except in cases of advanced pericardial invasion in which the normal conduction pathways may be impaired.

Table 18–4. TNM staging system for esophageal cancers.[1]

Primary tumor infiltration (T)

TX	Primary tumor cannot be assessed
T0	No evidence of primary tumor
Tis	Carcinoma *in situ*
T1	Tumor limited to mucosa/submucosa
T2	Tumor involving muscularis propria
T3	Involvement of adventitia, no extraesophageal structures
T4	Extension into extraesophageal structures

Regional lymph nodes (N)

NX	Regional lymph nodes cannot be assessed
N0	No nodal involvement
N1	Regional nodes involved

Distant metastasis (M)

MX	Distant metastases cannot be assessed
M0	No distant metastases
M1	Distant metastases for tumors of the lower thoracic esophagus:
M1a	Metastases in celiac nodes
M1b	Other distant metastases for tumors of the cervical thoracic esophagus:
M1a	Metastases in cervical lymph nodes
M1b	Other distant metastases for tumors in the middle thoracic esophagus:
M1a	Not applicable
M1b	Nonregional lymph nodes or other distant metastases

Stage grouping

Stage 0	Tis	N0	M0
Stage I	T1	N0	M0
Stage IIA	T2–3	N0	M0
Stage IIB	T1–2	N1	M0
Stage III	T3	N1	M0
	T4	Any N	M0
Stage IV	Any T	Any N	M1
Stage IV A	Any T	Any N	M1a
Stage IV B	Any T	Any N	M1b

[1]1997 revision.

Staging Techniques

Once the diagnosis is made, defining the stage of the esophageal cancer is the next essential step for further patient management. Previously, a significant number of patients with esophageal cancer went for exploratory surgery to attempt curative resection and/or for final staging. Unfortunately, this approach was disappointing as the majority of these patients were found to be inoperable due to extensive tumor invasion. At present, with advances in imaging techniques, the task of tumor staging is best accomplished by a combination of multiple imaging modalities, including EUS and CT or MRI. The current TNM classification for esophageal cancer was revised to reflect the improved preoperative staging available through these imaging studies.

Additional imaging for staging is necessary as contrast x-ray studies and endoscopy alone are often inaccurate for staging esophageal cancer because the extent of local invasion and presence of regional nodal and distant metastases cannot be determined. CT imaging has provided a nonoperative way to stage esophageal cancer. The standard CT imaging protocol for esophageal cancer involves the use of oral and intravenous contrast with examination from the upper chest to the upper abdomen, including the entire liver. The overall accuracy of CT for staging esophageal cancer is excellent for advanced disease. Liver metastases and findings consistent with adjacent organ invasion can be reliably noted on CT scan as well as by MRI. The sensitivity and specificity for detecting bronchotracheal and pericardial invasion exceed

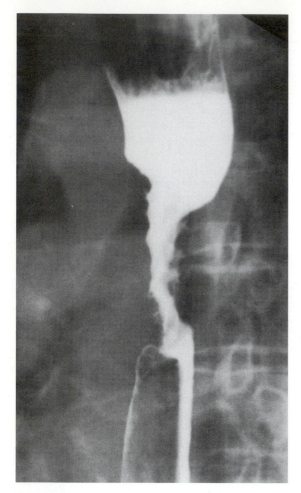

Figure 18–1. Barium esophagram showing mid-esophageal stricture. The abrupt change in caliber, irregular mucosa, and near circumferential narrowing are highly suggestive of an esophageal cancer.

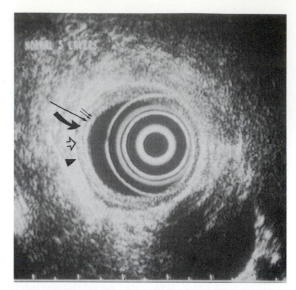

Figure 18–2. Endoscopic ultrasound image of the normal five-layered esophagus. ***Two small arrows:*** The inner-most layer corresponds to an interface echo and the mucosa. ***Single long arrow:*** The second layer corresponds to the mucosa (including the muscularis mucosa). ***Curved solid arrow:*** The third layer corresponds to the submucosa. ***Open arrow:*** The fourth layer corresponds to the muscularis propria. ***Solid arrowhead:*** The fifth outer-most layer corresponds to an interface echo and the adventitia (serosa equivalent). The five-layered appearance is essentially the same throughout the gastrointestinal tract. Because the esophagus lacks a serosa, the fifth echogenic layer in the esophagus represents the interface echo with the adventitia.

90–95% in most series. However, CT imaging does not reliably detect local and regional lymph node metastases and "early" (T1–T2) tumors.

The advent of EUS offers the most significant advance in the preoperative staging of esophageal cancer. EUS is performed using a modified upper endoscope with an ultrasound transducer housed within the tip. At frequencies ranging from 7.5 to 12 MHz, EUS depicts five layers of the esophageal wall corresponding to its distinct histologic layers (Figure 18–2). Malignant tumors are identified as hypoechoic masses with irregular margins that disrupt the normal esophageal architecture. The depth of tumor invasion is defined by the outermost margin of the hypoechoic mass (Figure 18–3). Suspi-

cious appearing lymph nodes are identified as hypoechoic rounded structures within the mediastinum and near the esophagus (Figure 18–4). Fine needle aspiration (FNA) biopsies of lymph nodes can be obtained through some EUS scopes for definitive diagnosis of malignant involvement (Figure 18–5). EUS can accurately diagnose early cancers, that is, those classified as T1–T2 (Figures 18–6 and 18–7). The overall accuracy of EUS for predicting the extent of esophageal cancers approaches 80–90% for T and 70–80% for N classification.

There are several limitations of EUS for staging esophageal cancer that need to be recognized. Overstaging of a T2 lesion can sometimes happen when there is significant peritumoral inflammation, whereas understaging sometimes occurs largely due to microscopic invasion beyond the muscularis propria. EUS is also very reliable in diagnosing adjacent organ invasion (ie, invasion to pleura or aorta) (Figures 18–8 and 18–9); how-

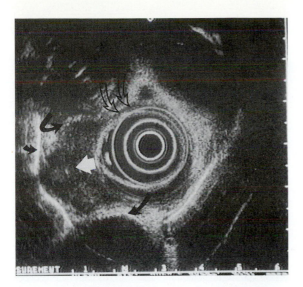

Figure 18–3. EUS image of an esophageal cancer in close proximity to mediastinal structures. ***Curved open black arrow:*** Muscularis propria, fourth hypoechoic layer. ***Solid white arrow:*** The tumor extending from the mucosa through the muscularis propria (T3). ***Angled arrow:*** Distinct fat plane between the tumor and right bronchus, indicating absence of bronchial invasion. ***Short curved arrow:*** Hyperechoic (bright white) plane between the tumor and right pleura. The tumor mass extends to the pleura but does not definitively invade. ***Curved arrow (bottom of image):*** Intact fat plane between the tumor and thoracic aorta.

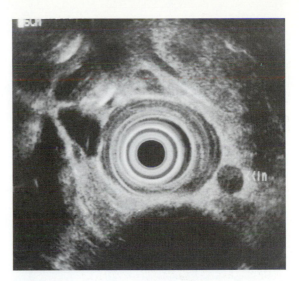

Figure 18–4. Suspicious appearing lymph nodes are identified as hypoechoic rounded structures within the mediastinum.

CT scan is still the better imaging study to detect distant organ metastases. Nonetheless, CT scan should be considered as complementary to EUS and should be combined with EUS to determine the extent of extra-esophageal invasion into the mediastinum and distant metastases. The ideal algorithm for managing these patients should include a CT scan of chest and abdomen, and, if negative for metastasis, an EUS should be done to rule out locally advanced disease.

ever, limited depth of penetration of EUS results in incomplete assessment for distant metastases. In addition, about 30% of esophageal cancers produce severe esophageal obstruction and cannot be traversed with the regular ultrasound endoscope at the time of presentation. Generally, these tumors can be accurately staged with EUS after dilation of the stricture; and when this occurs, they are almost always advanced tumors, that is, T3 or greater (Figure 18–10). Recently, the development of through-the-scope miniprobes and wire-guided small-diameter blind ultrasound probes has overcome the problems with tumor strictures in most cases. In addition, as these small caliber ultrasound probes utilize higher scanning frequencies (12–20 MHz), the detection and accuracy of staging for T2 tumors has improved significantly.

A large number of studies have looked into the staging accuracy of EUS and CT scan. It has been demonstrated that EUS is more accurate than CT scan for locoregional staging (both T and N classification). EUS appears to be superior in defining abdominal lymph node metastases (especially celiac axis nodes), although

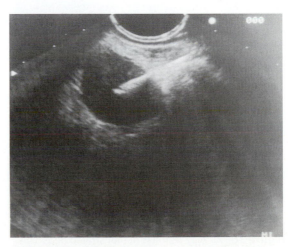

Figure 18–5. EUS-guided fine-needle aspiration biopsy of suspicious lymphadenopathy can be obtained during the staging process for definitive staging.

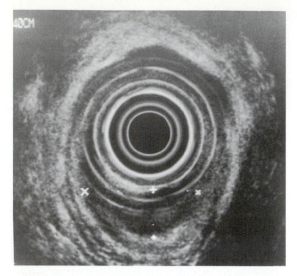

Figure 18–6. A T1 lesion is depicted. Note the hypo-echoic focal mass that involves the mucosal and sub-mucosal layers only.

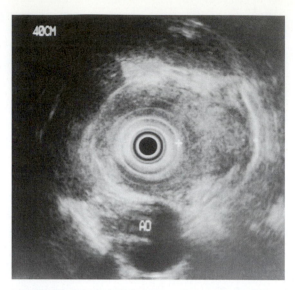

Figure 18–8. This EUS image demonstrates a large esophageal tumor invading the left pleura. AO, aorta.

A few other diagnostic tools have also been employed to assist in the staging of esophageal cancer. Bronchoscopy is widely used for assessment of bronchial invasion, primarily in mid-esophageal tumors. Although bronchial invasion is common, invasion into the bronchial lumen is rare. Therefore, bronchoscopy generally provides only indirect evidence of bronchial invasion, such as luminal indentation or narrowing. Diagnostic laparoscopy has been utilized in the assessment of peritoneal metastases. It offers the advantage of tissue biopsy under direct vision and an access for laparoscopic ultrasound. Thoracoscopy has also been used to better assess mediastinal and pulmonary metastases.

Differential Diagnosis

The differential diagnosis of patients with dysphagia or odynophagia includes esophageal mucosal diseases, motility disorders, and benign and malignant obstructing lesions. The insidious onset of progressive dysphagia to solids and then to liquids with associated weight loss in patients over 40–50 years of age almost invariably points to esophageal cancer. Patients with benign obstructing lesions of the esophagus, such as benign peptic strictures, webs and rings, and achalasia, may present with features resembling esophageal cancer. Barium esophagram offers indirect evidence for benign versus malignant processes; however, endoscopy with biopsies should still be employed to distinguish benign from malignant disease.

Achalasia is a motility disorder with impaired relaxation of the lower esophageal sphincter and aperistalsis of the esophageal body. The classic radiographic appearance on the barium esophagram is a smooth, tapered distal esophagus referred to as a "bird's beak" appearance. Tumors at the gastroesophageal junction may at times mimic the signs, symptoms, and manometric findings of achalasia. Hence, endoscopy is required in all patients

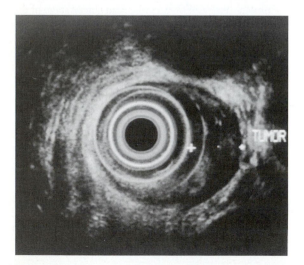

Figure 18–7. A T2 lesion is demonstrated here. This lesion is characterized by involvement of the mucosa and submucosa with invasion into the muscularis propria but not beyond the muscle layer.

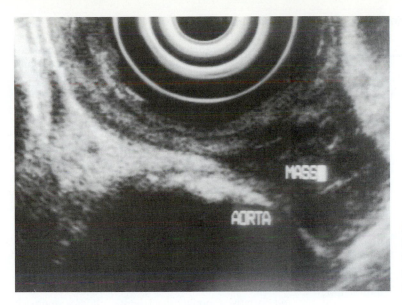

Figure 18–9. This EUS image demonstrates a large esophageal tumor that closely borders the aorta with focal involvement of the aortic wall.

with suspected achalasia to exclude undiagnosed malignancy ("pseudoachalasia").

Malignant tumors of the esophagus other than squamous cell carcinoma and adenocarcinoma are exceedingly rare. These tumors usually cannot be distinguished based on clinical grounds and require histologic confirmation. Mucoepidermoid carcinoma and cystic adenoid carcinoma of the esophagus are rare yet extremely aggressive and can be missed on endoscopic biopsy due to their primarily submucosal growth pattern.

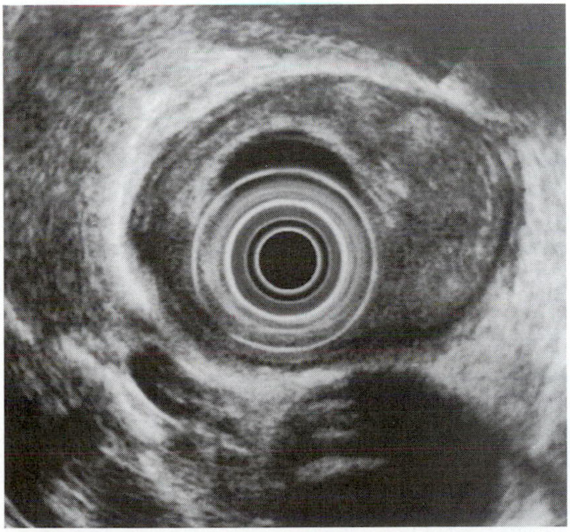

Treatment

The next step following the diagnosis of esophageal cancer is to determine whether the patient is a candidate for major curative surgery. Unfortunately, over 60% of patients with esophageal cancer are not candidates for surgery at the time of presentation due to the advanced stage of disease or significant comorbidity that would result in high perioperative mortality. The combination of a thin wall, absence of a serosa, and an extensive lymphatic drainage system facilitates early regional and distant metastases in esophageal cancer. Extensive medical problems, most commonly severe cardiopulmonary disease, are contraindications to surgery. These factors demand that treatment of esophageal cancer be based on a systematic evaluation (Table 18–5). Cancer staging is generally not required for patients who are not candidates for surgery.

Surgery

A. General Considerations

Surgical therapy has long been the preferred approach for both cure and palliation of patients with resectable tumors. Patients in the subgroup with limited local spread (T1–T2) and no regional nodal involvement are potentially curable by surgery. Patients who are deemed surgical candidates based on their good medical condition should undergo thorough staging to determine if they have cur-

Figure 18–10. A T3 tumor is depicted here. These lesions typically are large and invade into and through the muscularis propria without invasion into adjacent structures.

Table 18–5. Therapeutic interventions for palliation or cure of esophageal cancer.

Surgery
  Transhiatal
  Thoracoabdominal: right (Ivor Lewis) or left *en bloc*
Radiation
Combined modality chemoradiation
Dilation
Ablation
  Chemical sclerosant injection
  Electrocautery: monopolar or bipolar
  Argon plasma coagulation
  Nd:YAG laser
Photodynamic therapy
Endoscopic mucosal resection
Protheses/stents

able disease, incurable but resectable disease, or unresectable disease. Resectable tumors are characterized by the absence of extension into mediastinal structures and the absence of nodal or organ metastases. Direct invasion of the aorta, bronchi, pleura, or laryngeal nerve or distant organ metastases are evidence of nonresectable disease. Preoperative radiation with or without chemotherapy may sometimes downstage the cancer to a resectable or potentially curable stage.

Prior to surgery, it is important to confirm that the patient has sufficient cardiopulmonary reserve. Respiratory function is best assessed by the forced expiratory volume (FEV_1), which, ideally, should be 2 L or more. Any patient with an FEV_1 of less than 1.25 L is a poor surgical candidate due to the high risk of respiratory insufficiency postoperatively. Cardiac reserve should be assessed and a resting ejection fraction of less than 40% is an ominous finding.

Perioperatively, nutritional support should be provided to improve postoperative complications and recovery. A poor nutritional status affects the host resistance to infections and impairs anastomotic and wound healing. As oral intake is usually inadequate in patients with advanced disease, a feeding jejunostomy tube is the most reliable and safest method for nutritional support in those with a functional small bowel. A gastrostomy is inadvisable for these patients because it may interfere with the use of the stomach for reconstruction. The jejunostomy also minimizes the danger of regurgitation into the pharynx and possible aspiration. Total parenteral nutrition may also be indicated for some patients.

B. SURGICAL APPROACH

The surgical options available for esophageal tumor resection include (1) transhiatal, (2) combined right thoracic and abdominal (Ivor Lewis), (3) left thoracoabdominal, and (4) en bloc, either two field or three field. In a simple esophagectomy, whether by the transhiatal or the transthoracic route, there is no specific attempt to remove lymph node tissues in the mediastinum or upper abdomen. Cure is thus uncommon and occurs only by chance. En bloc resection involves a radical esophagectomy to include mediastinal, upper abdominal (two field), and/or cervical (three field) lymphadenectomy.

Transhiatal esophagectomy is currently the preferred surgical approach for palliation of esophageal cancer independent of its location. In patients with distal esophageal cancer, transhiatal esophagectomy may be curative when adequate inspection of the paraesophageal cancer tissue is provided by the abdominal incision. The operation consists of abdominal and cervical incisions and a cervical gastroesophageal anastomosis. This procedure does not allow visual inspection of the mediastinal bed, which theoretically is necessary to ensure removal of the locally invasive tumor, although it offers a slightly better 3-year survival and operative mortality than the transthoracic approach (25% versus 20% and 5% versus 10%, respectively).

En bloc resection remains the definitive surgical cure for esophageal cancer. The operation consists of removal of a tissue block completely surrounded by normal tissue. Two or three fields of lymphatic resection are included depending upon the tumor location: upper abdominal celiac and splenic nodes (field one), infracarinal posterior mediastinal nodes (field two), and upper mediastinal and cervical (field three). Recent studies encouraged inclusion of the surrounding mediastinal pleura, the azygos vein, the thoracic duct, and possibly the pericardium at the time of surgery to improve the overall survival. The overall 5-year survival of en bloc resection approaches 40% although the operative mortality still ranges from 5 to 10%.

Locally advanced tumors (T1N1, T2N1, T3N0, and T3N1) are resectable but incurable. These tumors are associated with a high recurrence rate following surgery. The optimal intervention in these patients remains controversial, and practices vary widely depending on the local surgical expertise and the assessment of the patient's preexisting medical condition.

Palliation Therapy

As the majority of patients present with incurable disease, pallative therapy remains the mainstay of treatment options for esophageal cancer. The options currently available include radiation therapy, chemotherapy, endoscopic dilation and ablation (chemical injection, electrocautery, argon plasma coagulation, and laser), photodynamic therapy, and esophageal prostheses/stents. They are all palliative procedures employed as adjuvant therapy to surgery or for patients who are not considered surgical candidates.

The treatment again varies according to availability and local expertise, patient preference, and cost.

A. RADIATION THERAPY

External beam radiation therapy alone provides reasonable palliation for esophageal cancer, especially for those who are medically unable to undergo surgery or chemotherapy. At the end of treatment, radiotherapy achieves palliation of dysphagia in 70–90% of patients. The 5-year survival curves are similar to those for surgery for patients with a comparable cancer stage (5–10%). It is recommended that for patients treated with curative intent, radiation therapy should be limited to tumors <10 cm with no evidence of distant metastasis. Contraindications to radiotherapy include tracheal or bronchial involvement, cervical esophagus location of the tumor, or stenosis that cannot be bypassed. The major complications of radiation therapy in esophageal cancer are airway fistulas (10–15%) and esophageal strictures (20–40%).

In an attempt to improve its effectiveness, radiotherapy has been given in a hyperfractionated manner. Several recent studies employing continuous hyperfractionated accelerated radiotherapy demonstrate a slightly improved median survival and prolonged relief of dysphagia, although there is no significant improvement in the 5-year survival rates. In addition, many studies have looked into the role of radiation therapy as an adjuvant to surgery to improve local tumor control and survival. Several randomized control studies comparing the benefit of preoperative and/or postoperative radiation in addition to surgery demonstrated disappointing results. There is no additional survival benefit, and there seems to be a higher rate of operative complications following radiation.

By combining external beam radiation with intraluminal irradiation using cobalt-60, cesium-137, or iridium-192, it is possible to increase the dose of radiation to the tumor without significantly increasing the dose of radiation to normal tissue. A major limitation of intraluminal irradiation is the effective treatment distance. Initial studies have demonstrated promising results with improved median survival and 5-year survival, and more clinical trials are underway.

B. CHEMOTHERAPY

1. Single agent—Despite the increasing choice of agents, chemotherapy alone has been of little benefit to patients with esophageal cancer. The most commonly employed classes of agents for treating esophageal cancer include (1) antibiotics—bleomycin and mitomycin C, (2) antimetabolites—5-fluorouracil (5-FU) and methotrexate, (3) alkaloids—vindesine and vinorelbine, (4) platinum analogs—cisplatin, carboplatin, and oxaliplatin, (5) taxanes—paclitaxel and docetaxel, and (6) topoisomerase inhibitors—etoposide and irinotecan. The clinical response rates for most single agents are very poor (5–15%), although cisplatin and the taxanes are exceptions and have been the focus of most combination chemotherapy. The response durations are also very brief, ranging from 2 to 4 months.

2. Combination chemotherapy—Combination chemotherapy has typically demonstrated better clinical response rates than single agent chemotherapy. Most trials of combination chemotherapy are based on cisplatin, as it alone has a response rate of 20–25%. In general, the cisplatin-based combination chemotherapy has yielded a response rate of 25–35%. The results are even more impressive in locoregional disease, yielding 45–75%. Unfortunately, the higher response rates do not translate into improved response duration or improved survival. In addition, the higher response rate of combination chemotherapy needs to be balanced against a higher systemic toxicity. To date, there is no role for chemotherapy, single agent or combination, as an adjuvant to surgery.

3. Combined-modality therapy—As primary management, combined-modality therapy of chemoradiation has achieved better median survival and 5-year survival when compared with radiation alone. In addition, there is much current interest in the role of chemoradiation as induction therapy prior to surgery. Theoretically, induction chemoradiation therapy has several advantages over primary surgery alone or postoperative chemoradiation. As the local blood circulation is not yet disrupted by surgical dissection, preoperative chemotherapy should result in better drug delivery to the tumor. Preoperative treatment also allows for identification of patients who may in turn benefit from further postoperative therapy if needed. In addition, concurrent chemoradiation can take advantage of the radiation-sensitizing properties of many chemotherapeutic agents (eg, paclitaxel, 5-FU, and cisplatin), resulting in a synergistic antitumor effect. Distant control should be enhanced as remote micrometastases are treated early in the course instead of having to wait for postsurgical recovery. Preliminary results from recent studies are encouraging, and many trials are currently underway to define the role of chemoradiation further.

C. ENDOSCOPIC THERAPY

Whereas endoscopy has mainly been used to diagnose cancers, new technologies such as photodynamic therapy and endoscopic mucosal resection have provided endoscopic treatments with the potential of curing early stage tumors of the esophagus.

1. Dilation—Esophageal dilation is most commonly performed with either expandable through-the-scope balloons or wire-guided polyvinyl bougies under fluoroscopy. A small percentage of patients can be successfully dilated to allow for soft diet consumption. However, the benefit from dilation is usually of short duration, and other methods are usually required for more prolonged symptom relief. One of the major complications of esophageal dilation is perforation.

2. Ablation—Tumor ablation treatments available for palliation include photodynamic therapy, chemical sclerosant injection, monopolar and bipolar electrocautery, argon plasma coagulation (APC), and neodymium:yttrium–aluminum–garnet (Nd:YAG) laser. The simplest and least expensive intervention for esophageal cancer ablation is the injection of a chemical sclerosant during endoscopy. Absolute alcohol is the most widely employed chemical agent. The method has been shown to be capable of results similar to laser therapy. The major problem with chemical injection relates to a lack of control as the sclerosant tracks along the tissue planes, causing damage to normal tissue and, sometimes, perforations. Patients may experience temporary worsening of symptoms until adequate tumor necrosis occurs.

Monopolar and bipolar electrocautery are falling out of favor and are rarely used as it is difficult to control the depth of treatment. A newer method, argon plasma coagulation, uses ionized argon gas to convey electrical energy to achieve thermal desiccation of tumor tissue. Unfortunately, the effect is generally superficial, and it is less efficient in relieving dysphagia in advanced esophageal cancer than the tissue ablation achieved using lasers.

High-power Nd:YAG laser can provide palliation of dysphagia by coagulating and vaporizing malignant tissue under endoscopic control. Tumors amenable to laser therapy are exophytic or polypoid, preferably located in a straight segment of the esophagus such as in the midesophagus or lower esophagus, and shorter than 5 cm. Multiple endoscopic laser treatment sessions may be required to reduce the size of the intraluminal tumor to improve swallowing. Periodic follow-up is performed to reduce any recurrent intraluminal tumor growth. Although more expensive, laser treatment is more widely available.

3. Photodynamic therapy (PDT)—PDT has emerged as an attractive palliative treatment for esophageal cancer and its complications. PDT has been successful in reducing tumor bulk and in opening the esophageal lumen in patients with complete obstruction, a situation in which Nd:YAG therapy was considered too risky. PDT has also been utilized as a salvage therapy in patients whose stents have failed because of tumor ingrowth/overgrowth.

The treatment begins with an intravenous injection of a photosensitive chemical, porfimer sodium (Photofrin). It is administered at a dose of 2 mg/kg of body weight and preferentially concentrates in the tumor tissue. After 40–50 hours following the injection, the area of the esophageal cancer is exposed to a red light at a wavelength of 630 nm, delivered from a continuous-wave dye laser via an optical fiber diffuser for a total cumulative light dose of 300 J/cm. The red light has been chosen for greatest depth of penetration (5 mm). The process initiates a photochemical reaction and the effect takes place over the ensuing hours to days, ultimately resulting in necrosis of the tumor. Improvement in the dysphagia is usually noted within 5–7 days, although some patients may experience worsening of dysphagia initially due to local tissue inflammation and edema. The major issue with PDT is retention of the photosensitive dye in the skin (up to 6 weeks), which requires patients to avoid direct sun exposure or risk severe sunburn. Other complications following PDT include fever, leukocytosis, nausea, and pleural effusion. Severe complications, which fortunately are uncommon, include atrial arrhythmias, stricture formation, hemorrhage, and perforation. The advantage of PDT in early esophageal cancer (T1 or T2 disease) is the overall greater than 80% cure rate.

4. Endoscopic mucosal resection (EMR)—The development of EMR, or mucosectomy, was sparked by the need to treat superficial flat and polypoid neoplasms of the mucosa of the gastrointestinal (GI) tract with minimally invasive procedures. Long-term studies have demonstrated that EMR outcomes are similar to those of surgery, which has led to acceptance of EMR as a standard treatment, especially in early stage GI cancers. The availability of endoscopic ultrasound to determine the depth of tumor invasion and lymph node metastases as well as chromoendoscopic techniques to reveal tumor borders otherwise not visible without staining further facilitate the ease and use of EMR.

Numerous EMR techniques have been described, such as injection and snare cautery, injection with precut, EMR with cap, or EMR with band ligation. Nevertheless, the general principles are the same. EMR involves expansion of the submucosal layer and lifting of the mucosa to allow for a safe longitudinal resection. Injection of an expansion solution (typically normal saline) into the submucosa creates a bleb and increases the distance between the mucosa and muscularis propia. This lifting of the mucosa is essential to prevent transmural burning or perforation. A snare is placed over the base of the "neopolyp" and the mucosa is resected with electrocautery. The cancerous lesion is removed en bloc and allows for a complete detailed histopathologic analysis.

In esophageal cancers, EMR has been applied mainly for squamous cell carcinoma and much less for Barrett's esophagus-related adenocarcinoma. EMR is indicated when the lesion is superficial and without evidence of lymph node metastasis. Although conventional EUS is accurate in determining tumor depth and lymph node metastasis of large or bulky lesions, it is less precise for small, flat, or depressed tumors. Therefore, in these instances, high-frequency ultrasound probes have been recommended. The application of Lugol's solution further assists in visual distinction between a cancerous lesion and normal mucosa (squamous cell carcinoma or dysplasia does not stain). Once the lesion is identified and staged, approximately 20 mL of saline is injected into the submucosa, causing more than half-circumferential mucosal lifting. EMR can then be safely performed. EMR should be avoided if the lesion cannot be lifted by submucosal saline injection (nonlifting sign), which does occur when a tumor has indeed invaded the muscularis propia or when there has been fibrosis due to prior polypectomy. There is no consensus on the maximal lesion size suitable for EMR in esophageal cancer. However, it is recommended that the lesion should be less than 3 cm in height and should not exceed one-third of the esophageal circumference in width to avoid the late complication of stenosis. For larger lesions, other alternatives, such as photodynamic therapy, should be considered.

The major complications of esophageal EMR are bleeding, perforation, and stenosis. Bleeding during EMR is almost always controllable by injection of a low-concentration epinephrine-saline solution, thermal coagulation, or endoscopic clipping. Large perforations invariably require immediate surgery, although small perforations may be manageable with more conservative measures. Stenosis can occur when circumferential resection has been attempted.

5. Esophageal prostheses—Placement of esophageal prostheses ("stents") is another appealing method for the palliation of malignant strictures and provides effective relief of dysphagia in most cases. The prostheses are usually inserted surgically or endoscopically with fluoroscopic guidance. A wide variety of stents have been developed and modified over the years that provide good mechanical support for maintaining esophageal lumen patency and reduce complications such as stent migration and tumor ingrowth. At present, the expandable metal stents are the most widely applied form of prostheses. The principal merits of such stents are the ease of insertion and the remarkably low risk of esophageal perforation. Covering the stent with a polymer sheet effectively reduces tumor ingrowth and provides for treatment of tracheoesophageal fistulas, while the outer flange diameters have been increased, thereby making a funnel-shaped stent that adheres to the esophageal wall to significantly lower the rate of migration. Early complications of expandable metal stents have included incomplete expansion, perforation, bleeding, and pain. Late complications include tumor overgrowth/ingrowth, ulceration, food impaction, and stent migration. Patients who have received prior radiation and chemotherapy are more prone to develop complications. Stents that cross into the gastric cardia may cause significant gastroesophageal reflux that can usually be controlled with proton-pump inhibitors; however, a new stent has been developed that prevents reflux via a valve mechanism. In cases in which patients developed an airway fistula, such as bronchoesophageal or tracheoesophageal fistula, stent placement is the optimum therapy. Furthermore, a second stent may be placed in the airway if there is significant stenosis causing dyspnea.

Prognosis

Despite the widespread use of endoscopy, significant advances in surgical techniques and neoadjuvant chemoradiation therapy, and improvements in postoperative care, the prognosis for patients with esophageal cancer remains poor. The reported overall 5-year survival rates are at best 10–15%. Delayed clinical manifestations and rapid intramural invasion and distant metastases account for the poor prognosis of this GI malignancy. Patients with an early stage of disease carry a better prognosis. For patients with T1 or T2 disease and no nodal involvement, the 5-year survival rate is greater than 40%. On the other hand, patients with T3 or T4 lesions have a 5-year survival of less than 25%.

Stage 0, I, and II tumors are considered resectable for cure. The 5-year survival for such patients who are sufficiently fit to undergo surgery ranges from greater than 85% for stage 0, to 50% for stage I, to 40% for stage II. On the other hand, stage III tumors are rarely resectable for cure, and stage IV cancers are considered incurable and nonresectable by most clinicians. The presence or absence of nodal involvement also has a significant prognostic impact. The 5-year survival for N0 disease is over 70%, whereas N1 disease is associated with a survival near 40%, independent of the T classification.

BENIGN ESOPHAGEAL TUMORS

General Considerations

A variety of benign mass lesions can arise from different wall layers in the esophagus (Table 18–6). These tumors are usually asymptomatic and slow growing, noted only as incidental findings during routine radiography or endoscopy. Occasionally, they may be discovered during the evaluation of dysphagia or vague chest discomfort. The most common benign esophageal tumor is the leiomyoma. Because the tumor arises from the muscularis propria, it is covered by an intact submucosa and mucosa, making it difficult to biopsy endoscopically.

Inflammatory polyps and granulomas can arise in the setting of esophagitis and may be confused with

Table 18–6. Benign esophageal tumors.

Leiomyoma
Hemangioma
Granular cell tumor
Congenital esophageal cyst
Fibrovascular polyp
Bronchogenic cyst
Inflammatory fibroid polyp (eosinophilic granuloma)
Lymphangioma
Squamous cell papilloma
Lipoma
Neurofibroma

---

malignant lesions from time to time. Endoscopic removal is possible, although usually not indicated. Endoscopic biopsy and regression with therapy for esophagitis clearly distinguish the clinical course of inflammatory polyps and granulomas from cancers.

Clinical Findings

A. SYMPTOMS AND SIGNS

Although the vast majority of benign esophageal tumors are clinically silent and go undetected, large or strategically located tumors may become symptomatic. Similar to their malignant counterparts, dysphagia is the most common presentation for patients with benign esophageal tumors. Less common presenting symptoms include odynophagia, retrosternal pain or thoracic pressure, food regurgitation, anorexia, and weight loss. Respiratory complaints such as cough, dyspnea, or sore throat may also contribute to the presentation. Occasionally, leiomyomas can outgrow their own blood supply, leading to necrosis and ulceration of the overlying mucosa and resulting in overt GI hemorrhage such as hematemesis or melena.

B. IMAGING

Endoscopic appearance and biopsy can identify some benign esophageal tumors. However, EUS provides high-resolution images that define the individual esophageal wall layers and can readily identify lesions in the deeper layers (ie, submucosa and muscularis propria) that elude endoscopic biopsy diagnosis. If necessary, EUS-guided FNA can be performed for diagnostic purposes. Leiomyomas are generally noted as hypoechoic mass lesions within the muscularis propria. Occasionally, the echopattern is more heterogeneous, which may indicate hemorrhage into the tumor. Cystic lesions may appear as anechoic structures within the mucosa and submucosa, whereas inflammatory growths are always superficial and localized to the mucosa.

Treatment

Small, mucosal-based and submucosal esophageal tumors can be removed endoscopically using EMR techniques or possibly obliterated by endoscopic injection of sclerosants or by APC. Larger mass lesions, especially leiomyomas, are generally removed surgically if they are associated with severe symptoms or other complications, eg, bleeding. In many instances, the resection can now be accomplished by minimally invasive techniques.

REFERENCES

Bancewicz J: Palliation in esophageal neoplasia. Ann R College Surgeons Engl 1999;81:382.

Blot W, McLaughlin J: The changing epidemiology of esophageal cancer. Sem Oncol 1999;26(5, Suppl 15):2.

Bollschweiler E et al: Preoperative risk analysis in patients with adenocarcinoma or squamous cell carcinoma of the esophagus. Br J Surg 2000;87:1106.

Brierley J, Oza A: Radiation and chemotherapy in the management of malignant esophageal strictures. Gastrointest Endosc Clin North Am 1998;8(2):451.

Bytzer P et al: Adenocarcinoma of the esophagus and Barrett's esophagus: a population-based study. Am J Gastroenterol 1999;94(1):86.

Chalasani N, Wo J, Waring J: Racial differences in the histology, location, and risk factors of esophageal cancer. J Clin Gastroenterol 1998;26(1):11.

Chow W et al: Body mass index and risk of adenocarcinoma of the esophagus and gastric cardia. J Natl Cancer Inst 1998;90(2):150.

Choy H: Taxanes in combined-modality therapy for solid tumors. Oncology 1999;13(10, Suppl 5):23.

DeCamp M, Swanson S, Jaklitsch M: Esophagectomy after induction chemoradiation. Chest 1999;116(6, Suppl):466S.

Devesa S, Blot W, Fraumeni J: Changing patterns in the incidence of esophageal and gastric carcinoma in the United States. Cancer 1998;83(10):2049.

Dolan K et al: New classification of esophageal and gastric carcinomas derived from changing patterns in epidemiology. Br J Cancer 1999;80(5/6):834.

Ell C et al: Endoscopic mucosal resection of early cancer and high-grade dysplasia in Barrett's esophagus. Gastroenterology 2000;118:670.

El-Serag H, Sonnenberg A: Ethnic variations in the occurrence of gastroesophageal cancers. J Clin Gastroenterol 1999;28(2):135.

Enzinger P, Ilson D, Kelsen D: Chemotherapy in esophageal cancer. Sem Oncol 1999;26(5, Suppl 15):12.

Greenlee RT et al: Cancer statistics, 2000. CA: Cancer J Clinicians 2000;50:7.

Hansen S et al: Esophageal and gastric carcinoma in Norway 1958–1992: incidence time trend variability according to morphological subtypes and organ subsites. Int J Cancer 1997;71:340.

Heath E et al: Adenocarcinoma of the esophagus: risk factors and prevention. Oncology 2000;14(4):507.

Kubba A, Poole N, Watson A: Role of *p53* assessment in management of Barrett's esophagus. Dig Dis Sci 1999;44(4):659.

Launoy G et al: Alcohol, tobacco and esophageal cancer: effects of the duration of consumption, mean intake and current and former consumption. Br J Cancer 1997;75(9):1389.

Lerut T et al: Treatment of esophageal carcinoma. Chest 1999;116 (6, Suppl):463S.

Lightdale C: Role of photodynamic therapy in the management of advanced esophageal cancer. Gastrointest Endosc Clin North Am 2000;10(3):397.

Mayoral W, Fleischer D: The esophacoil stent for malignant esophageal obstruction. Gastrointest Endosc Clin North Am 1999;9(3):423.

Meyenberger C, Fantin AC: Esophageal carcinoma: current staging strategies. Recent Results Cancer Res 2000;155:63.

Minsky B: Carcinoma of the esophagus. Part 1: Primary therapy. Oncology 1999;13(9):1225, 1235.

Minsky B: Carcinoma of the esophagus. Part 2: Adjuvant therapy. Oncology 1999;13(10):1415.

Noguchi H et al: Evaluation of endoscopic mucosal resection for superficial esophageal carcinoma. Surg Laparosc Endosc Percutan Tech 2000;10(6):343.

Patti M, Owen D: Prognostic factors in esophageal cancer. Surg Oncol Clin North Am 1997;6(3):515.

Ponchon T: Endoscopic mucosal resection. J Clin Gastroenterol 2001;32(1):6.

Pompili M, Mark J: The history of surgery for carcinoma of the esophagus. Chest Surg Clin North Am 2000;10(1):145.

Radu A et al: Photodynamic therapy of early squamous cell cancer of the esophagus. Gastrointest Endosc Clin North Am 2000; 10(3):439.

Rösch T: The new TNM classification in gastroenterology (1997). Endoscopy 1998;30(7):643.

Rudolph R et al: Effect of segment length on risk for neoplastic progression in patients with Barrett's esophagus. Ann Intern Med 2000;132(8):612.

Sharma V et al: Changing trends in esophageal cancer: a 15 year experience in a single center. Am J Gastroenterol 1998;93:702.

Soetikno R, Inoue H, Chang K: Endoscopic mucosal resection—current concepts. Gastrointest Endosc Clin North Am 2000; 10(4):595.

Streitz J et al: Endoscopic surveillance of Barrett's esophagus: a cost-effectiveness comparison with mammographic surveillance for breast cancer. Am J Gastroenterol 1998;93(6):911.

Miscellaneous Disorders of the Esophagus

19

Richard S. Bloomfeld, MD & Wallace C. Wu, MBBS

ESOPHAGEAL RINGS & WEBS

Lower esophageal ring (**Schatzki's ring**) is the most common cause of intermittent solid food dysphagia. Esophageal webs are uncommon. Both rings and webs are thin diaphragm-like structures that partially interrupt the lumen of the esophagus. Rings occur at the gastroesophageal junction and are covered by squamous epithelium proximally and columnar epithelium distally. A web refers to any ring-like structure along the entire length of the esophagus and is covered entirely by squamous epithelium.

1. Cervical Esophageal Web

Cervical esophageal webs are thin diaphragm-like structures usually located anteriorly in the immediate postcricoid area and covered with normal esophageal epithelium. They are more commonly found in females and are often associated with iron deficiency anemia (**Paterson-Kelly syndrome; Plummer-Vinson syndrome**). The pathogenesis is unknown, but it has been associated with thyroid diseases, Zenker's diverticulum, esophageal intramural diverticulosis, and ectopic gastric mucosa in the cervical esophagus. Cervical webs may be part of the syndrome of multiple esophageal webs, which may be idiopathic, associated with bone marrow transplantation, one component of a dermatologic disorder such as epidermolysis bullosa or benign mucous membrane pemphigoid, or may be an atypical manifestation of gastroesophageal reflux disease.

Clinical Findings

A cervical esophageal web may be an incidental finding in an asymptomatic patient. Most symptomatic patients are female and complain of intermittent solid food dysphagia. Signs and symptoms of pulmonary aspiration and iron deficiency anemia may be present.

Endoscopy may miss or disrupt webs in the cervical esophagus, and it is therefore less useful in the initial diagnosis than radiographic studies. Endoscopy may be warranted to distinguish cervical webs from other causes of cervical stenosis. Cine-esophagography is the study of choice in the diagnosis of this condition. A web is seen as a thin projection anteriorly in the postcricoid esophagus. The differential diagnosis includes extrinsic postcricoid impression, inflammatory stenosis, strictures from various causes, and carcinoma.

Treatment

A cervical web is frequently ruptured during diagnostic endoscopy, so that this procedure may in itself be curative. Esophageal bougienage may be necessary in some patients. Surgery may be indicated if a Zenker's diverticulum is present.

2. Lower Esophageal Ring

Lower esophageal ring (ie, lower esophageal mucosal ring; Schatzki's ring) is seen in 6–14% of routine upper gastrointestinal barium studies. It is usually asymptomatic but nevertheless is one of the most common causes of intermittent solid food dysphagia. It is located at the gastroesophageal junction. The pathogenesis of lower esophageal ring is unknown; it is speculated that it may be congenital or developmental in origin. Chronic gastroesophageal reflux may be an important contributing factor, however, particularly in symptomatic patients.

Clinical Findings

Intermittent solid food dysphagia with no dysphagia for liquids is the characteristic history in patients with symptomatic lower esophageal rings. The dysphagia tends to occur particularly when the patient is eating quickly. Inadequate mastication may be an important factor in precipitating symptoms. Daily symptoms are rare, and their presence should raise suspicion for other diagnostic possibilities. Symptoms of gastroesophageal reflux disease may also be present and should raise the possibility of a peptic stricture.

The caliber of the ring is clearly the most important factor in determining whether the patient is symptomatic. Rings with a diameter of 13 mm or less, as measured on radiologic studies, are always symptomatic, whereas rings greater than 20 mm rarely, if ever, produce symptoms. It is speculated that the dysphagia arises from a combination of inadequate ring caliber, a large bolus, inadequate mastication, and ineffective peristalsis.

A properly performed barium esophagogram is the most useful diagnostic tool. The lower esophagus must be fully distended before the ring can be visualized (Figure 19–1). Use of a marshmallow or a barium tablet is helpful in this regard. Barium esophagography is also useful in excluding other diagnostic possibilities such as esophageal motility disorders, peptic strictures, and other esophageal diseases. A small-caliber endoscope can miss a symptomatic ring. For the ring to be seen, the lower esophagus must be well distended with air.

Treatment

Esophageal dilation with a single large rigid dilator or balloom dilator (ie, 17 mm or more) is effective in providing initial symptomatic relief. The patient should also be reassured as to the benign nature of this problem and advised to chew properly. Unfortunately, only 35% of patients are free of dysphagia 2 years after the initial dilation. Most of these patients will require repeated dilation. Gastroesophageal reflux, if present, should be treated aggressively; this may decrease the likelihood of recurrence.

3. Midesophageal Web

All other ring-like structures in the esophagus are classified as midesophageal webs. These lesions are uncommon and may be multiple. Diseases that cause desquamation of the esophagus are associated with multiple esophageal webs, including some dermatologic disorders such as epidermolysis bullosa, mucous membrane pemphigoid, psoriasis, and Stevens-Johnson syndrome. Multiple webs may also form after bone marrow transplantation. Recent data suggest that multiple esophageal webs may be an atypical manifestation of gastroesophageal reflux disease.

Esophageal bougienage is effective in the treatment of these patients. Dilation should be done with extreme caution in patients with esophageal webs associated with bone marrow transplantation, as there appears to be a higher incidence of perforation in this group.

PILL-INDUCED ESOPHAGEAL INJURY

Pill-induced esophageal injury was first described in 1970. Since then, it has become common and may occur with a variety of medications. The prevalence is unknown, as most cases are not seen by a physician. The most common medications causing esophageal injury are alendronate, tetracycline, and doxycycline preparations, potassium chloride, quinidine, and nonsteroidal antiinflammatory drugs (NSAIDs). Sustained-release formulations may be more likely to cause injury.

Damage is caused by prolonged contact of the medication with the esophageal mucosa. Pill-induced injury is most common in patients who ingest medications in bed or just prior to reclining, without drinking adequate fluids. Some degree of partial esophageal obstruction such as left atrial enlargement or peptic stricture may also be present, retarding the passage of the pill. The most common area of injury occurs in the midesophagus, although both the proximal and distal esophagus may be affected. Stricture formation may occur as a complication of pill-induced esophageal injury.

Clinical Findings

The diagnosis can be made on the basis of the history alone. In an immunocompetent subject, the sudden onset of severe odynophagia with or without dysphagia after ingestion of medication is suggestive of pill-induced esophagitis. Many patients may be unable to provide a clear history. In patients with a suggestive history, further diagnostic studies may be necessary. In rare cases, pill-induced ulcers may cause hemorrhage or perforation.

The diagnosis may be confirmed by upper endoscopic studies, although radiologic studies may also be helpful (Figure 19–2). Endoscopic studies show an area of injury clearly surrounded by normal mucosa. Endoscopic biopsies can exclude infection or neoplasia. The

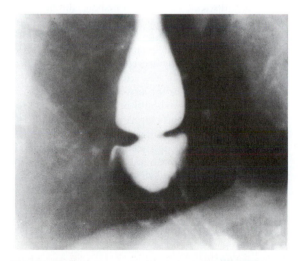

Figure 19–1. Lower esophageal mucosal ring or Schatzki's ring.

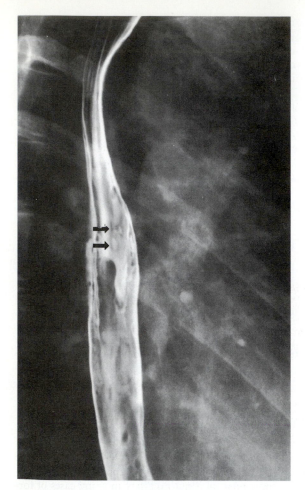

Figure 19–2. Focal erosions *(arrows)* in the mid-esophagus in a young woman with odynophagia being treated with tetracycline.

presence of a midesophageal stricture should always raise the possibility of pill-induced injury.

Treatment

The offending medication should be withdrawn; if this is not possible, liquid formulations should be given. If a liquid preparation is not available, the patient should be instructed to ingest the medication in an upright position, drink plenty of liquids, and remain upright for at least 10 minutes before lying down. Medications known to cause esophageal injury should be avoided in bedridden patients or those with esophageal compression or stricture. Most patients will recover uneventfully after several days or weeks without any specific

treatment. Complications such as hemorrhage, perforation, and stricture may require specific therapy.

CAUSTIC ESOPHAGEAL INJURY

In the United States, caustic injury to the esophagus is usually caused by ingestion of alkali (sodium or potassium hydroxide) contained in drain openers and cleaning preparations. Acids may also be ingested, including hydrochloric, sulfuric, and phosphoric acids, which are marketed in toilet bowl cleaners, battery fluids, and swimming pool cleaners. Of note, sodium hypochlorite (bleach) rarely causes severe esophageal injury. Ingestion is usually accidental in children but intentional in adults. Ingestion of alkali acutely results in a penetrating liquefaction necrosis of the epithelium. This is followed by sloughing of the mucosa, with subsequent fibrosis and reepithelialization. Acids typically produce a more superficial coagulation necrosis. In the acute phase, esophageal perforation and upper airway obstruction are the main causes of complications and death. Esophageal stricture is the most important chronic sequela of caustic ingestion.

Clinical Findings

Clinical features vary widely, and symptoms may not correlate with the extent of esophageal injury. Patients may complain of local pain, dysphagia, odynophagia, chest and abdominal pain, hoarseness, and respiratory difficulties. After the nature of the ingested material has been verified, it is important to assess the extent of injury. Patients with significant lip, mouth, and tongue injury should be monitored closely for the rapid development of airway obstruction. Stridor or other signs of respiratory distress warrant immediate attention to maintenance of airway patency. An initial ear, nose, and throat examination should be performed to exclude significant injury to the pharynx and larynx. If the epiglottis or vocal cords are edematous, endotracheal intubation is contraindicated and cricothyroidotomy is the procedure of choice for airway control. Upper gastrointestinal endoscopy should be done to evaluate the extent of damage to the esophagus and stomach. The presence or absence of oropharyngeal burns is not a reliable indicator of the presence of esophageal burns. If the esophagus and stomach are found to be normal or minimally involved, hospitalization is unnecessary, but the presence of second- or third-degree burns warrants close observation in a hospital setting, preferably in the intensive care unit. Chest and abdominal x-rays may be needed to rule out a perforated viscus.

Treatment

Immediate therapy is mainly supportive. Emetics should not be used, as their use may increase the extent of damage. Burns of the lips, mouth, and tongue can be cleaned with water and all visible granules removed carefully. Neutralization of ingested substances should not be attempted, because damage by the agent is almost instantaneous. Furthermore, neutralization results in exothermic release of heat, which may compound mucosal injury. Patients should be assessed for signs of shock or perforated viscus. When these are present, fluid resuscitation should be initiated and an immediate surgical consultation obtained.

When significant esophageal injury is evident at endoscopy, a controlled trial has demonstrated no benefit of steroid therapy on the development of stricture formation. Therefore, steroids are not recommended and may increase the risk of infectious complications. Antibiotics are not indicated in the absence of proven infection. Chronic strictures are usually treated by esophageal bougienage, but dilation may be extremely difficult, and surgery may be necessary. Barium swallows obtained in the third and fourth weeks following ingestion may detect strictures at a presymptomatic stage that may benefit from repeated dilation.

ESOPHAGEAL FOREIGN BODY

Ingestion of foreign bodies and large food boluses is extremely common, particularly in children. Most ingested foreign bodies pass readily through the gastrointestinal tract, but, occasionally, one will become impacted at an area of physiologic or pathologic narrowing. The esophagus has three areas of physiologic narrowing: (1) the upper esophageal sphincter, (2) the midesophagus at the points where the aortic arch and the left main bronchus cross the esophagus, and (3) the diaphragmatic hiatus. Esophageal strictures secondary to gastroesophageal reflux disease and lower esophageal rings are common pathologic factors that may cause foreign body or food impaction. Achalasia may rarely present with food impaction. Children and mentally impaired adults are more likely to have problems with a foreign body in the esophagus.

Clinical Findings

Whereas adults and older children may provide a clear history, younger children and mentally impaired patients may not be able to provide a history of foreign body ingestion. Patients usually complain of difficulties in swallowing, inability to handle oral secretions, and regurgitation. Respiratory symptoms are common in young children because the trachea is easily compressed by an esophageal foreign body. The inability to handle oral secretions is indicative of complete esophageal obstruction and warrants immediate endoscopic intervention to remove the impacted foreign body. Swelling or crepitation in the neck indicates a cervical esophageal perforation. A plain film of the neck, chest, and abdomen should be obtained to rule out complications such as perforation. In addition, the film may better define the location of radiopaque foreign bodies such as bones and coins. A negative radiograph does not rule out the presence of a radiolucent foreign body. Asymptomatic patients with negative plain radiographs need no further treatment. If the patient is symptomatic, upper endoscopy should be performed. Of note, a barium esophagogram should not be done, as this will interfere with visualization during endoscopy.

Treatment

Treatment is dependent on the type of foreign body and its location upon presentation. Meat impaction at the upper esophageal sphincter may compress the airway and can be dislodged in an emergency by the Heimlich maneuver. In managing foreign bodies at the level of the cricopharyngeus, the airway must be maintained at all times, preferably by endotracheal intubation. The foreign body may then be safely extracted by a rigid laryngoscope or flexible endoscope. Patients with a meat impaction in the esophageal body who appear uncomfortable and can manage their oral secretions may be given a trial of intravenous glucagon to promote relaxation of the esophagus. Intravenous glucagon is of questionable value but is usually safe. If the bolus does not pass or sialorrhea is evident, endoscopy should be performed to remove the bolus and to determine the cause of obstruction. Most other foreign bodies that remain in the esophagus should be removed by upper endoscopy. Endoscopic removal is not necessary in many cases of foreign bodies in the stomach, as most will pass uneventfully through the gastrointestinal tract. Objects that are more than 5 cm in length; sharp, pointed objects; and razor blades usually should be removed. Disk batteries usually pass readily through the gastrointestinal tract. If they lodge in the esophagus, they should be removed immediately. If they remain in the stomach for more than 48 hours, they may cause perforation and should be removed by endoscopy as well.

Instruments that may be useful during the endoscopic removal of a foreign body include forceps, snares, and baskets. An overtube should be used during the removal of a sharp or pointy object. Nonendoscopic methods such as blind passage of an esophageal bougie or Foley catheter extraction are not recommended.

ESOPHAGEAL PERFORATION

Esophageal perforation can occur spontaneously (**Boerhaave's syndrome**), from external trauma, or as a result of iatrogenic instrumentation. Spontaneous rupture arises from a combination of elevated intraesophageal pressure and negative intrathoracic pressure associated with vomiting and retching (Figure 19–3). A large meal and alcohol intake are contributory factors. Most cases occur at the distal esophagus within a few centimeters of the diaphragm.

Instrumentation of the esophagus is the most common cause of perforation. The risk of perforation with diagnostic endoscopy is extremely low. Perforations typically occur either in the cervical esophagus (at the cricopharyngeus) or at the site of a benign or malignant stricture. Perforations most commonly occur during therapeutic procedures such as esophageal dilation, sclerotherapy and banding for esophageal varices, palliation of esophageal carcinoma, and foreign body removal (Figure 19–4). Trauma is a rare cause of esophageal rupture.

Clinical Findings

The clinical presentation is dependent on the cause and location of involvement. Most cases of spontaneous perforation are characterized by severe retching and vomiting, followed by the onset of severe chest and ab-

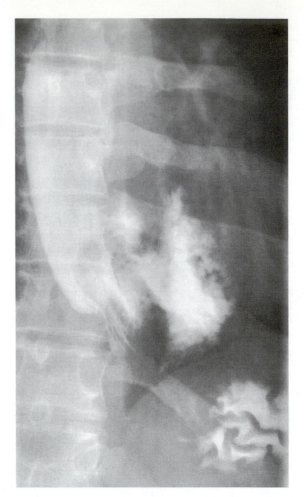

Figure 19–4. Rupture at the lower end of the esophagus following pneumatic dilation for achalasia.

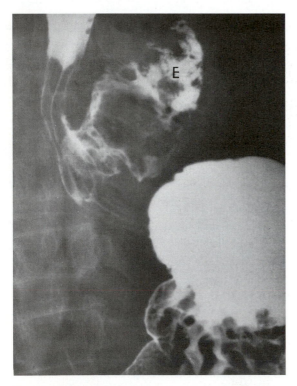

Figure 19–3. Extravasation (E) of contrast material from the lower esophagus from a patient with Boerhaave syndrome.

dominal pain. This may then be followed by the rapid development of fever, tachypnea, and shock. Subcutaneous emphysema is often present but may be absent in the initial 24 hours. With perforation of the thoracic esophagus, chest radiographs are abnormal, revealing pleural effusions, pneumomediastinum, pneumothorax, or subcutaneous emphysema in most cases. The location of the spontaneous laceration is most commonly on the left side of the distal esophagus.

The signs and symptoms of instrumental perforation of the esophagus vary with the site of injury. A contained cervical perforation may result in localized pain, dysphagia, and subcutaneous emphysema (with crepitus in the neck), without signs of significant infection. In contrast, free cervical or thoracic perforations result in clinical signs and symptoms similar to those of spontaneous rupture.

The diagnosis of esophageal perforation should be confirmed by a meglumine diatrizoate water-soluble contrast esophagogram. This will reveal the site and extent of perforation and will be of assistance in designing a therapeutic approach for the patient. If the meglumine diatrizoate study is negative, a barium study should be employed. Computed tomography (CT) scanning may be helpful in those patients with a negative esophagram in the setting of a high clinical suspicion, as this can detect extraluminal air.

Treatment

Esophageal perforation is traditionally treated within 24 hours by surgery, with primary closure and external drainage. In selected patients, conservative medical therapy may suffice. Medical therapy consists of parenteral feeding and intravenous antibiotics, nothing by mouth, and nasogastric suction. Conservative therapy may be indicated in the patient with an iatrogenic perforation who is clinically stable, as evidenced by minimal pain, the absence of shock or clinical sepsis, and only mild to moderate fever or leukocytosis. The perforation must be detected before major mediastinitis occurs and must be well contained within the mediastinum or cervical region with ready drainage into the esophagus on meglumine diatrizoate study.

ESOPHAGEAL DIVERTICULA

An esophageal diverticulum is an outpouching of the esophagus. Most lack a muscular wall and are usually caused by pulsion forces secondary to esophageal motility disorders. Diverticula are classified according to their anatomic location: hypopharyngeal or pharyngoesophageal (Zenker's) diverticula, midesophageal diverticula, epiphrenic diverticula, and intramural pseudodiverticulosis.

1. Zenker's Diverticulum

Zenker's (hypopharyngeal or pharyngoesophageal) diverticulum is a protrusion of the mucosa between the oblique fibers of the inferior pharyngeal constrictor and the transverse fibers of the cricopharyngeus muscles. It is the most common form of esophageal diverticulum. Its pathogenesis is uncertain, but speculations center on various forms of oropharyngeal discoordination and dysfunction of the upper esophageal sphincter. The sphincter may be in spasm, fail to relax, have early closure, or have a delay in relaxation. These conditions may result in increased pharyngeal pressure, with herniation of the mucosa in an area where the esophageal wall is the weakest.

Clinical Findings

Many Zenker's diverticula are asymptomatic and are found incidentally on an upper gastrointestinal series (Figure 19–5). Dysphagia and regurgitation are the most common presenting symptoms. Spontaneous regurgitation of food ingested up to several hours previously is characteristic in a patient with a large Zenker's diverticulum. Other symptoms include discomfort in the throat, a palpable mass in the neck area, recurrent pulmonary aspiration, and bad breath.

Barium esophagography is the optimal method for diagnosing Zenker's diverticulum. Endoscopy is not necessary; furthermore, it is relatively contraindicated due to the risk of inadvertent perforation of the diverticulum. If endoscopy is necessary, the instrument must be passed under direct vision through the cricopharyngeus.

Treatment

Surgery is often useful in the treatment of patients with a symptomatic Zenker's diverticulum. The operation usually consists of diverticulectomy with or without cricopharyngeal myotomy. Currently, endoscopic sta-

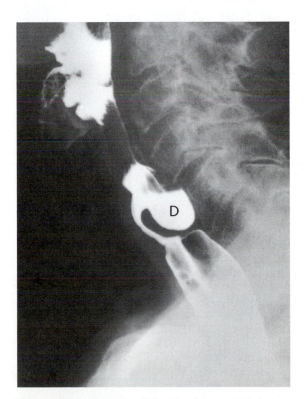

Figure 19–5. Lateral radiograph of the neck showing a Zenker's diverticulum (D).

pling and endoscopic division of the common wall between the cervical esophagus and the diverticulum are being evaluated.

2. Midesophageal & Epiphrenic Diverticula

Midesophageal diverticula are outpouchings of the middle third of the esophagus, and epiphrenic diverticula are outpouchings of the distal third (Figures 19–6 and 19–7). Esophageal motility disorders of all types, such as diffuse esophageal spasm, achalasia, and nonspecific esophageal motor disorders, occur in a high percentage of patients with both types of diverticula. It is speculated that abnormal motor activity in the body of the esophagus together with abnormal lower esophageal sphincter function contributes to their formation. "Traction" di-

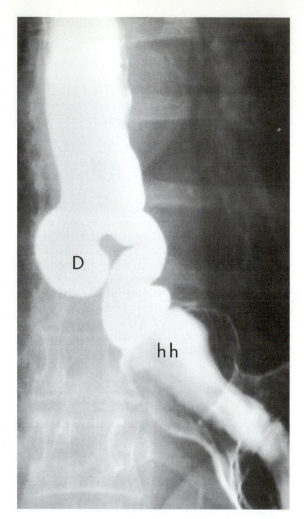

Figure 19–7. Epiphrenic diverticulum (D) of the lower esophagus associated with a hiatal hernia (hh).

verticula may occur in the midesophagus secondary to pathologic changes in the mediastinum.

Clinical Findings

Midesophageal diverticula are usually small and rarely cause symptoms, whereas epiphrenic diverticula are larger and may be symptomatic. Patients may complain of dysphagia and regurgitation, which may also be caused by the associated esophageal motility disorder.

Diagnosis of diverticula and the associated motor disorder is by barium esophagogram. Endoscopy is useful not only in confirming the diagnosis but also in

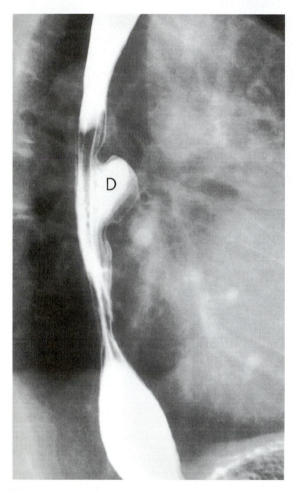

Figure 19–6. Midesophageal diverticulum (D).

excluding other structural abnormalities. Esophageal manometry is mandatory in defining the underlying esophageal motility disorder.

Treatment

Almost all patients with midesophageal diverticula and most patients with epiphrenic diverticula are asymptomatic and hence do not require any treatment. Symptomatic epiphrenic diverticula may be treated surgically by diverticulectomy and longitudinal myotomy for the underlying motor disorder.

RADIATION ESOPHAGITIS

Radiation damage to the esophagus is often seen in patients receiving radiation therapy to the mediastinum for bronchogenic carcinoma, metastatic breast carcinoma, lymphoma, testicular carcinoma, or esophageal carcinoma. Pathologic changes such as inhibition of mitosis, basal cell degeneration, and vascular damage occur early in the course of irradiation. Acutely, sloughing of the mucosa occurs, resulting in erosions and ulcerations. Regeneration of the epithelium occurs after cessation of radiation therapy, with submucosal fibrosis that may result in stricture formation.

Acute radiation esophagitis occurs during or shortly after radiation therapy. Patients usually complain of dysphagia, odynophagia, retrosternal burning, or chest pain. Contrast studies or endoscopy may show esophageal ulceration. Treatment consists of switching the patient temporarily to a liquid diet. If possible, the radiation treatment should be interrupted or modified until symptoms improve.

Chronic radiation esophagitis may occur from 3 months to years after radiation treatment. Patients report progressive dysphagia to both solids and liquids. Chronic radiation changes may result in fibrosis and stricture formation and may also impair esophageal peristalsis. Evaluation with barium esophagography reveals altered esophageal motility, with or without the presence of a fibrotic stricture. Treatment consists of dietary modification and esophageal bougienage, if a stricture is present.

SYSTEMIC DISEASES AFFECTING THE ESOPHAGUS

Many systemic diseases impair esophageal peristalsis. In most cases, the involvement is subclinical and asymptomatic (eg, in diabetes mellitus and hypothyroidism). In other diseases such as progressive systemic sclerosis (scleroderma), esophageal symptoms may be the predominant presentation.

1. Progressive Systemic Sclerosis (Scleroderma)

Progressive systemic sclerosis can affect the smooth muscle portion of the esophagus. Up to 75% of patients have esophageal involvement consisting of esophageal smooth muscle atrophy and collagen deposition. Patients with concurrent Raynaud's phenomenon are more likely to have esophageal involvement. Esophageal manometry may show low to absent lower esophageal sphincter pressure, with weak or absent peristaltic contractions in the distal esophagus. The upper esophagus is functionally normal. Due to the lack of a functional lower esophageal sphincter barrier and impaired esophageal clearance, patients with scleroderma commonly have severe gastroesophageal reflux disease.

Clinical Findings

Patients with progressive systemic sclerosis tend to have sclerodactyly, digital scars, and pulmonary fibrosis. About 75% have esophageal manometric abnormalities, and two-thirds have esophageal symptoms of gastroesophageal reflux disease (ie, heartburn and regurgitation). Patients may also have dysphagia, which may be due to abnormal esophageal peristalsis, severe esophagitis, or a benign reflux-induced peptic stricture.

An esophagogram may show absent or diminished peristalsis in the distal esophagus and erosive esophagitis with or without the presence of a stricture. Esophageal manometry will reveal low or absent lower esophageal sphincter pressure and weak to absent distal peristalsis. Endoscopy is most useful for the therapy of strictures.

Treatment

In patients with progressive systemic sclerosis with esophageal symptoms, standard antireflux measures such as elevation of the head of the bed and dietary measures should be instituted. Drug therapy with a proton-pump inhibitor usually is needed. Patients with severe erosive esophagitis should be treated aggressively with proton-pump inhibitors to prevent the onset of an esophageal stricture. Most strictures can be endoscopically dilated. Since the advent of proton-pump inhibitors, surgery has seldom been necessary.

2. Other Connective Tissue Diseases

Mixed connective diseases commonly have esophageal involvement, but most of these patients are asymptomatic. The manometric abnormalities are similar to those of progressive systemic sclerosis, but the upper esophageal sphincter may also be abnormal. Patients usually present with symptoms of gastroesophageal reflux. As in progressive systemic sclerosis, these symptoms should be treated aggressively to prevent stricture formation.

Esophageal involvement occurs with much less frequency in other types of connective tissue diseases. In rheumatoid arthritis, some patients have diminished peristalsis with decreased lower esophageal sphincter pressure, but most are asymptomatic. Similar changes may be seen in systemic lupus erythematosus. Patients with Sjögren's syndrome may have dysphagia and erosive esophagitis due to diminished esophageal motor function and decreased salivary secretion. In Behçet's syndrome, the characteristic aphthous ulcerations may occur in the esophagus.

Patients with polymyositis and dermatomyositis may have involvement of the skeletal muscle portion of the esophagus, with symptoms of oropharyngeal dysphagia, such as difficulty in initiating a swallow, aspiration, cough, and nasal regurgitation. Involvement of the smooth muscle portion of the esophagus can also occur, with decreased peristalsis and a hypotensive lower esophageal sphincter. Treatment of the underlying disorder results in improvement of esophageal function and symptoms.

3. Endocrine Diseases

Diabetic patients with evidence of autonomic dysfunction commonly have abnormalities on esophageal motility studies (usually motor abnormalities of the esophageal body and hypotensive lower esophageal sphincter pressure). Most patients are asymptomatic. Diabetic patients are also believed to be prone to esophageal candidiasis, although objective proof of this phenomenon is lacking.

Hypothyroidism may rarely affect the esophagus. Reduction of peristaltic pressure and low esophageal sphincter pressure may be observed.

4. Dermatologic Diseases

The autosomal recessive form of epidermolysis bullosa dystrophica is characterized by the formation of blebs, bullae, vesicles, and ulcers of the skin, mucous membrane, and any organ lined with squamous epithelium. Both the mouth and the esophagus may be involved, resulting in severe dysphagia. The lesions in the esophagus may result in scarring and stricture formation. Treatment is symptomatic, and esophageal bougienage should be avoided if possible, as trauma may result in more bulla formation. Esophagectomy and colonic interposition may be necessary in severe cases.

Other dermatologic diseases that may affect the esophagus include pemphigus vulgaris, bullous pemphigoid, and benign mucous membrane pemphigoid. These are diseases of varying cause in which bullae form in the squamous epithelium, and these may progress to esophageal lesions. Treatment of the underlying disorder is usually adequate.

5. Chronic Idiopathic Intestinal Pseudoobstruction

Intestinal pseudoobstruction is a syndrome in which patients present with recurrent episodes of nausea, vomiting, and intestinal distention without evidence of mechanical obstruction of the small or large intestine. It may be caused by connective tissue disease, endocrine disease, or neuromuscular disease, but in many instances, the cause is unknown. When there is no identifiable cause, the disease is known as chronic idiopathic intestinal pseudoobstruction. Esophageal motility is usually abnormal, with absent peristalsis and abnormal lower esophageal sphincter function that may be manometrically indistinguishable from achalasia. Most patients do not have symptoms of esophageal diseases and do not require therapy.

6. Infectious Esophagitis

Infectious esophagitis may occur with such pathogens as *Candida,* herpes simplex virus, or cytomegalovirus, usually in an immunocompromised host (see Chapter 2). These infections, particularly candidiasis, may occur occasionally in an immunocompetent host. Disorders that may be associated with these infections are diabetes mellitus, malnutrition, systemic lupus erythematosus, multiple myeloma, hypoparathyroidism, and esophageal obstructions such as achalasia.

REFERENCES

Anderson KD, Rouse TM, Randolph JG: A controlled trial of corticosteroids in children with corrosive injury of the esophagus. N Engl J Med 1990;323:637.

Chowhan NM: Injurious effects of radiation on the esophagus. Am J Gastroenterol 1990;85:115.

DeVault KR: Lower esophageal (Schatzki's) ring: pathogenesis, diagnosis, and therapy. Dig Dis 1996;14:323.

Eckardt VF, Kangler G, Williams D: Single dilation of symptomatic Schatzki rings: a prospective evaluation of its effectiveness. Dig Dis Sci 1992;37:577.

Kikendall JW: Pill esophagitis. J Clin Gastroenterol 1999;28:298.

Shaffer HA, Valenzuela G, Mittal RK: Esophageal perforation: a reassessment of the criteria for choosing medical or surgical therapy. Arch Intern Med 1992;152:757.

Walton S, Bennett JR: Skin and gullet. Gut 1991;32:694.

Webb WA: Management of foreign bodies of the upper gastrointestinal tract: update. Gastrointest Endosc 1995;41:39.

Younes Y, Johnson DA: The spectrum of spontaneous and iatrogenic esophageal injury: perforations, Mallory-Weiss tears, and hematomas. J Clin Gastroenterol 1999;29:306.

Peptic Ulcer Disease

20

William D. Chey, MD & James M. Scheiman, MD

From a histologic perspective, an **ulcer** is a loss of the surface epithelium that extends deeply enough to reach or penetrate the muscularis mucosae. From a clinical perspective, an ulcer is a loss of the mucosal surface, visible by endoscopy or radiography, which, in addition to having depth, is greater than 5 mm in diameter (Figure 20–1). Ulcers are distinguished from **erosions,** which are small (<5 mm) superficial mucosal lesions. Because the superficial mucosa contains only capillaries, erosions usually result in clinically mild bleeding (oozing) and are unlikely to give rise to clinically significant bleeding, scarring, or perforation. In contrast, ulcers may give rise to all of these complications.

Peptic ulcer disease (PUD) refers to the underlying tendency to develop mucosal ulcers at sites that are exposed to peptic juice (acid and pepsin). Most commonly, ulcers occur in the duodenum and stomach, but they may also occur in the esophagus, in the small intestine, at gastroenteric anastomoses, and, rarely, in areas of ectopic gastric mucosa, for example, in Meckel's diverticula.

PATHOPHYSIOLOGY

Etiology

In the past, peptic ulcer disease was thought to be of multifactorial etiology. Ulcers were believed to arise when one or more of a variety of biological influences noxious to the mucosa overwhelmed its capacity to resist, contain, and heal injury. Until recently, PUD was regarded as a life-long condition. This concept has been revised due to the recognition that two environmental factors appear to be of overwhelming importance in most persons with ulcer disease: *Helicobacter pylori* infection and the use of aspirin (acetylsalicylic acid, ASA) or nonsteroidal antiinflammatory drugs (NSAIDs). Much of the familial aggregation of ulcer disease that has been observed may reflect intrafamilial infection with *H pylori* rather than genetic susceptibility, although both factors likely play a role.

Other recognized risk factors, such as cigarette smoking, may interact with both *H pylori* infection and NSAID injury to increase the risk of PUD. In a minority of peptic ulcer patients, other factors—such as hypersecretory states (eg, Zollinger-Ellison syndrome), mucosal infection with viruses such as herpes simplex, cytomegalovirus, the use of cocaine or "crack," and emotional or psychiatric stress—may play a primary or supplementary etiologic role. Nevertheless, in most cases the prevention or "cure" of ulcer disease will result from eradication of *H pylori* [and the associated chronic active (type B) gastritis] or from the avoidance of ASA or NSAIDs.

Original reports suggested that over 90% of all duodenal and gastric ulcers in subjects not using ASA or NSAIDs occur in those with concurrent chronic active gastritis due to *H pylori* infection. Although *H pylori* infection can be identified in the majority of patients with PUD, more recent data suggest that the prevalence of *H pylori* in patients with PUD may be lower than originally reported. It is becoming clear that the prevalence of non-*H pylori,* non-NSAID ulcers varies geographically and may be as high as 48% in some parts of the United States. These ulcers presumably are due to the surreptitious use of ASA or NSAIDs, or some other agent of injury. Gastric stasis, duodenal reflux, and ischemia may all have some role in gastric ulcer pathogenesis.

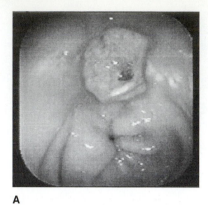 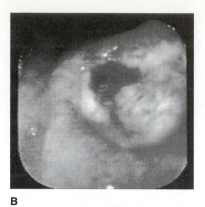

A   B

Figure 20–1. Endoscopic views of peptic ulcer disease. **A:** A large ulcer in the gastric antrum. The protuberant lesion in the center of the ulcer is a visible vessel that confers a high risk of ulcer bleeding. **B:** A large ulcer in the duodenal bulb that was actively bleeding at the time of endoscopy.

Great strides in the understanding of ulcer formation due to *H pylori* infection or ASA/NSAID ingestion has occurred in recent years. Although these appear to be independent risk factors, in some situations they may also be synergistic in causing ulcers and, especially, in the development of ulcer complications. Given the high prevalence of asymptomatic peptic ulcers in the general population, patients with occult ulcers may develop clinically relevant lesions when given ASA or NSAIDs, due to the adverse effects on hemostasis, as well as ulcer repair and healing.

The risk of complications may also be accentuated by the analgesic effects of NSAIDs, which may mask early symptoms of ulcers. These analgesic effects may account for the low prevalence of symptoms among NSAID users with clinically significant or complicated ulcers.

Pathogenesis

Despite the fact that *H pylori* and NSAIDs initiate damage by distinct mechanisms, the clinical consequences are closely correlated with the amount of acid (pH) and degree of activation of pepsinogen (peptic activity) within the gastric lumen. Suppression of acid secretion with pharmacologic agents results in an increase in the intragastric pH and inactivation of pepsinogen, which facilitate mucosal healing, a reduction in bleeding, and a reduction in other ulcer complications. Until recently, acid-suppressing drugs were the mainstay of antiulcer therapy, with antacids, mucosal-protective drugs, and surgery also playing minor roles. That ulcer healing occurred after reducing acidity essentially validated Schwartz's dictum—"No acid-peptic activity, no ulcer." However, there is no evidence that hypersecre-

tion of acid or pepsin is the principal factor in the pathogenesis of most ulcers.

Recent studies in *H pylori*-infected patients have shown that antibiotic therapy alone is as effective as treatment that combines an antibiotic with acid-suppressive therapy, both in promoting ulcer healing and in relieving ulcer symptoms. Thus, most ulcers are a manifestation of an infectious disease, *H pylori* gastritis, rather than acid per se. However, exactly how this chronic infection causes peptic ulcers—especially duodenal ulcers—remains unclear.

Effects of ASA & NSAIDs

ASA in particular and most other NSAIDs contribute to the manifestations of peptic ulcer disease in a number of ways. First, small doses of these drugs (eg, 30–80 mg/d of ASA) cause platelet dysfunction that may increase the risk of bleeding from any lesion within the gut, including peptic ulcers. Slightly higher doses may cause acute, usually superficial gastric erosions that result in gastric bleeding, which is generally occult or clinically minor except in patients with disorders of coagulation. Higher doses (eg, 14–21 tablets of ASA/week) taken long term (weeks) may lead to chronic ulcers.

About two of every three patients on long-term NSAIDs have some endoscopically visible gastroduodenal mucosal lesions, most of which are superficial (erosions, hemorrhages, etc). In prevalence studies, about one in four chronic ASA/NSAID users has an ulcer (gastric ulcers = 15%, duodenal ulcers = 10%). Based on information from several sources, however, it seems that only 1–2% of long-term NSAID users are hospitalized for an ulcer complication (such as hemorrhage, perforation, or obstruction).

The damaging effects of NSAIDs occur principally because of inhibition of prostaglandin synthesis. Prostaglandins are important mediators of defensive mechanisms that protect the gastroduodenal mucosa from acid and other potentially damaging luminal agents. Prostaglandins stimulate the secretion of mucus and bicarbonate and enhance surface hydrophobicity making the mucosa resistant to acid penetration. Prostaglandins and other cyclooxygenase products also increase mucosal blood flow and play an important part in healing, for example, the promotion of angiogenesis. The recognition of two isoforms of cyclooxygenase has resulted in the development of new antiinflammatory drugs, the *cox-2* specific inhibitors, which appear to cause significantly less damage to the upper gastrointestinal (GI) tract. These agents do not significantly affect upper GI prostaglandin levels, which derive mainly from the *cox-1* isoform. The *cox-2* selective inhibitors (eg, rofecoxib, celecoxib, meloxicam) are effective in relieving pain and inflammation (mediated by prostaglandins produced by *cox-2*), but cause little damage to the upper GI tract because mucosal prostaglandin production, mediated by *cox-1,* is spared.

Several factors increase the risk of ulcer complications in patients taking NSAIDs (Table 20–1): age, past history of ulcer disease, NSAID dose, use of anticoagulants,

Table 20–1. Relative risks and confidence intervals for ASA/NSAID gastrointestinal outcomes (case–control studies).[1]

Outcome	Relative Risk	Confidence Interval
Gastric ulcer (ASA)	4.67	3.06–7.14
Gastric ulcer (NSAIDs)	4.03	2.80–5.78
Gastrointestinal bleeding (ASA)	3.30	2.39–4.54
Gastrointestinal bleeding (NSAIDs)	3.09	2.26–4.40
Ulcer perforation (NSAIDs)	5.93	4.0–8.81
Ulcer perforation (ASA)	Similar	Not well studied
Duodenal ulcer (ASA)	1.71	0.69–1.98 (NS)
Duodenal ulcer (NSAIDs)	3.16	1.78–5.61
Death (ASA)[2]	Uncommon	Not well studied
Death (NSAIDs)[2]	7.62	6.17–9.41

[1]Reprinted from Nonsteroidal anti-inflammatory drugs—the clinical dilemmas. by McCarthy DM from Scand J Gastroenterol, www.tandf.no/gastro, 1992; 27(Suppl92):9, by permission of Taylor & Francis AS. Data from Hawkey CJ: Non steroidal anti-inflammatory drugs and peptic ulcers. Br Med J 1990;300: 278.
[2]Although the association of drug use and death is clear, given the fact that most deaths occur in very old people with multiple diseases, the percentages of deaths truly attributable to NSAID use, to chronic peptic ulcer disease, or to comorbidities remains unclear.

and use of corticosteroids. Several questions regarding the pathogenesis of NSAID damage remain unanswered: (1) Why do so few mucosal lesions become symptomatic ulcers? (2) What proportion of ulcers in ASA/NSAID users is actually caused by these drugs versus other factors (eg, *H pylori*)? (3) What percentage of ulcer complications arises from prior peptic ulcer disease that is exacerbated by ASA/NSAIDs and what percentage arises from ASA/NSAID-induced ulcers?

GENERAL CONSIDERATIONS

Peptic ulcer disease is a common disease, and both the direct costs of diagnosis and treatment and the indirect costs attributable to loss of work and impaired quality of life are significant. From the turn of the century until 1955, the incidence and prevalence of PUD in the United States increased. Since then, it has fallen steadily, however this decline cannot be attributed definitively to any medical intervention, such as antiulcer drugs or surgery. Factors that may be linked to the decline in ulcer disease are the pervasive use of antibiotics and better sanitation and water supplies, which are correlated with a decline in the prevalence of *H pylori* infection in the general population.

Despite the decline in incidence and prevalence of *H pylori* infection, PUD remains a major problem, resulting in direct costs approaching four billion dollars per year in the United States. About 200,000 hospitalizations and over three million outpatient visits for PUD are estimated to occur annually. Historical data suggest that the lifetime population prevalence of symptomatic ulcers is 10%. However, based on prospective endoscopic studies that indicate that more than one-half of patients with peptic ulcers are asymptomatic, the true prevalence of ulcers could be as high as one in five. Duodenal ulcers are now much more common than gastric ulcers (whereas the opposite was previously true). The ratio of males to females with ulcers has fallen from a high of 10:1 and is now nearly equal.

Despite the falling incidence and prevalence, the overall mortality rate from ulcer disease has changed little since 1930, but the disease-associated deaths now occur 20–30 years later in life, that is, in older patients. PUD now exerts its greatest impact on the elderly, being associated with 16% of hospitalizations and deaths in persons over age 65. Visits to physicians for ulcer disease increase with age.

The explanation for the rising incidence of complicated ulcer disease in the elderly remains unclear. Some of the trend may be due to increased longevity in the population, decreased death from other causes, and increased usage of ASA and NSAIDs in elderly persons. Over age 65, death from ulcer complications, surgery, and postoperative sequelae are greatly increased by the impact of comorbid conditions.

Only recently has medical therapy for ulcer disease been developed that is potentially curative, at least in those patients with *H pylori* infection. Whether this will alter morbidity and mortality of ulcer disease in those using ASA or other NSAIDs has not been determined. The recent developments of several types of newer NSAIDs that are less injurious to the gastrointestinal mucosa may in time lead to reductions in ulcer disease and associated morbidity and mortality in the population. However, the ubiquitous use of low-dose aspirin for its cardiovascular benefits may offset some of the safety of these new agents, as even low doses of aspirin (80–325 mg/d) are associated with a 2- to 4-fold increased risk of ulcer bleeding. Given the expected growth of the elderly population with their attendant comorbidities, there will be a significant rise in the population at greatest risk for ASA-associated gastrointestinal complications. As such, it is possible that rates of complicated ulcer disease may remain relatively stable.

CLINICAL FINDINGS
Symptoms & Signs
A. Typical Presentation

The cardinal symptom of peptic ulcer is epigastric pain or dyspepsia, which is often described as "gnawing," "aching," or "like a hunger pain." Classically, the pain of duodenal ulcer is rhythmic, that is, it is regularly relieved by food, milk, or antacids but returns 1.5–4 hours after eating. It may awaken the patient from sleep between 1:00 and 3:00 AM, especially if a snack at bedtime was taken. The pain may radiate into the right hypochondrium, or posteriorly into the back. This latter development, if it becomes persistent, may herald penetration of the ulcer through the posterior wall.

The other major characteristic of ulcer pain is periodicity. That is, ulcer symptoms tend to recur at intervals of weeks or months. During periods of exacerbation, the pain occurs daily for a period of weeks and then remits until the next recurrence. The classic pain of gastric ulcer is also periodic and rhythmic, but the pain pattern is different in its rhythmicity. Usually, the pain is least or absent during fasting, but occurs shortly after eating (5–15 minutes) and remains until the stomach empties, either naturally or by vomiting. For this reason, most gastric ulcer patients avoid food, reduce their dietary intake, and lose weight. Gastric ulcer pain may also occur at night, but this is less common than in duodenal ulcer patients. The pain may radiate posteriorly and sometimes to the left upper quadrant.

With duodenal ulcer or gastric ulcer, a marked increase in the pain or spread to the entire abdomen may indicate that the ulcer has perforated. This is usually followed rapidly by cessation of bowel sounds and the development of diffuse rebound tenderness. Similarly, a change from normal rhythmicity to constant pain may herald the development of penetration.

On physical examination, tenderness is classically said to occur at or to the left of the midline with gastric ulcer, and 1 inch or more to the right of the midline with duodenal ulcer.

Chronic peptic ulcers in either the stomach or duodenum may cause scarring and impair gastric emptying—a condition known as **gastric outlet obstruction.** This may cause nausea or vomiting, the latter bringing transient relief of pain or discomfort. The vomiting of gastric outlet obstruction may occur shortly after meals or up to several hours later. Otherwise, nausea and vomiting are very rare in uncomplicated duodenal ulcers and uncommon in gastric ulcers, although some gastric ulcer patients induce vomiting in an effort to relieve their pain. The stool may contain occult blood, and a minority of patients present with anemia because of acute or chronic gastrointestinal blood loss.

Symptoms of acid gastroesophageal reflux, such as heartburn or regurgitation, are not uncommon in ulcer patients, especially in those with some impairment of gastric emptying. However, it is the presence of gastroesophageal reflux and not the presence of peptic ulcer that causes the heartburn.

B. Atypical Presentation

Atypical presentations of ulcer disease are common. In fact, "classic presentations" are the exception rather than the rule. Thus, the history and physical examination alone cannot reliably lead either to the diagnosis of peptic ulcer or to a clear distinction between duodenal and gastric ulcers. In many cases, pain is absent or ill defined. Patients may be totally asymptomatic or complain only of "indigestion" or other vague dyspeptic symptoms. These symptoms are very nonspecific and in most cases are not due to ulcers.

Fewer than 1% of duodenal bulb ulcers and a higher percentage of postbulbar or jejunal ulcers are associated with the presence of an underlying hypersecretory disorder, such as Zollinger-Ellison syndrome, systemic mastocytosis, granulocytic leukemia, or hyperparathyroidism, or occur after small bowel resection. The clinical clues to the existence of such an underlying disorder are the presence of diarrhea, weight loss, and a gastric pH value consistently close to 1.0. In the documented presence of such hyperacidity or in those with refractory PUD despite adequate medical therapy, fasting serum gastrin and calcium concentrations should be measured. These are seldom indicated in clinical practice and are uninterpretable in patients taking a proton-pump inhibitor or in the absence of careful studies of gastric acid secretion. Complications of ulcer disease including hemorrhage, perforation, penetration, and obstruction are discussed later in this chapter.

Laboratory Findings

Laboratory findings have little or no role in the diagnosis and routine management of peptic ulcer disease, but may be involved in defining an underlying disorder or a complication. In uncomplicated disease, laboratory tests are typically normal.

Investigations

A. Empiric Treatment versus the Test-and-Treat Strategy for *H pylori*

Epigastric discomfort or dyspepsia is a common problem in general medical practice. Without diagnostic testing, it is virtually impossible for the clinician to distinguish between patients with PUD and the much larger group of dyspeptic patients suffering from nonulcer conditions such as nonulcer or functional dyspepsia, gastroesophageal reflux disease, and/or biliary tract disease. When confronted with a patient with a suspected ulcer, the clinician has a number of management options. Dyspeptic patients under the age of 45–50 years with classic symptoms of uncomplicated peptic ulcer disease may be treated empirically with H_2-receptor antagonists (H_2RAs) or proton-pump inhibitors and if they respond within 2–4 weeks, no further investigation is necessary. However, if symptoms persist or recur, some investigation is warranted. Recommendations as to the nature of these investigations are rapidly changing and controversial.

Another widely advocated approach in young dyspeptic patients with no warning signs is the "test-and-treat" strategy for *H pylori.* In this strategy, patients with suspected ulcer undergo a noninvasive test for *H pylori* (antibody test, urea breath test, fecal antigen test). Those patients with a positive test are treated for possible ulcer disease with triple- or quadruple-drug therapy designed to eradicate *H pylori.* In European trials, the test-and-treat strategy has been shown to reduce the utilization of expensive endoscopy without adversely affecting clinical outcomes. Further investigation with endoscopy is recommended in *H pylori*-positive patients with persistent symptoms despite a course of antibiotic therapy and in *H pylori*-negative patients who fail to respond to reassurance and empiric symptomatic treatment.

All patients with suspected ulcer who have warning symptoms (evidence of bleeding, weight loss, vomiting, severe or progressive symptoms) should be evaluated early with endoscopy. Patients with gastric ulcers should undergo biopsy to exclude a malignancy and

may require a subsequent endoscopy to document complete ulcer healing. The role of endoscopy is discussed in a subsequent section.

B. Radiologic Studies

Plain films of the abdomen are of little value in the diagnosis of peptic ulcer disease unless perforation is suspected. In this situation, upright or lateral decubitus x-rays may show the presence of free air. General physicians suspecting the presence of an ulcer may consider obtaining a barium upper gastrointestinal (UGI) examination, employing either single-contrast or preferably double-contrast ("air-contrast") techniques. These tests are widely available, safer and cheaper than endoscopy, well tolerated by patients, and provide a permanent record of the findings. Compared to endoscopy, however, the UGI series suffers from limited accuracy (20–30% error rate), the inability to obtain tissue for histologic examination, the lack of therapeutic potential in bleeding patients, and an inability to identify most superficial mucosal lesions. Further, despite its lower acquisition cost, UGI is less cost effective than the *H pylori* test-and-treat strategy for patients with suspected ulcer disease. Given its widespread availability and decreasing cost, endoscopy should be the preferred approach in patients with suspected ulcer who fail *H pylori* eradication therapy or a trial with empiric antisecretory therapy.

If a duodenal ulcer or a scarred duodenal bulb is identified on x-ray, endoscopy is unnecessary before treatment in most cases. This is also true for most radiographically diagnosed gastric ulcers in patients under the age of 40 years. However, if the radiologist is initially uncertain as to the nature of the ulcer or suspects that it may be malignant, endoscopy should not be delayed.

Repeat x-ray or endoscopy to confirm healing is unnecessary in duodenal ulcer if symptoms resolve and remain absent. In patients with gastric ulcer, endoscopy should be performed after 3 months of therapy to confirm healing, with biopsy of any residual ulcer to rule out malignancy. Among ulcers initially called "benign" on a barium study, about 2–6% eventually prove malignant. Patients with chronic symptoms in whom x-rays are reported as normal should also be referred for endoscopy: the false negative rate for gastric ulcer has been as high as 40% in some series.

C. Endoscopy

Upper gastrointestinal endoscopy has come to be the "gold standard" in diagnosing peptic ulcers, although it is less than perfect. In most series, more than of 90% of lesions present are diagnosed at endoscopy. Gastric ulcers or craters may be missed when gastric folds are very prominent, when secretions are copious, when there is food, blood, or clot in the stomach, when ulcers are high in the stomach or in a fundic pouch or hiatal hernia sac, when peristalsis or patient movement is excessive, or when the operator is inexperienced. Duodenal ulcers may be missed when the bulb is badly scarred, when ulcers are located in the lateral fornices of the cap, when the ulcer is bleeding, or when peristalsis is active.

Practitioners must realize that endoscopy is not infallible, and in critical cases, x-ray and endoscopy may be complementary. Duodenal ulcers are almost always benign and do not require biopsy, except in the setting of Crohn's disease, which rarely may affect the duodenum and mimic peptic ulcer. Duodenal ulcer patients undergoing endoscopy should have gastric biopsies to detect *H pylori* infection. Similar biopsies should be obtained in gastric ulcer patients, regardless of whether they are using ASA/NSAIDs. Findings of chemical or type C gastritis in this latter group occasionally lead to identification of unsuspected use of ASA/NSAIDs. However, these histologic appearances are by no means specific.

In gastric ulcer patients over 40 years old, whether or not they are using ASA/NSAIDs, the most important issue is to exclude the possibility of gastric cancer, whose presentation may be similar to that of ulcer. At least six biopsies of the ulcer and surrounding folds should be obtained, supplemented by brushings or irrigation cytology when adequate biopsies are not feasible. Endoscopies without such biopsies do not meet the standard of care. The endoscopic interpretation of benign versus malignant gastric ulcers based solely on visual inspection is subject to considerable error.

In patients with gastric ulcers diagnosed by upper gastrointestinal series in whom the suspicion of a gastric malignancy is deemed low (due to the patient's age or appearance of the ulcer) endoscopy and biopsy can be deferred for 12 weeks to verify complete ulcer healing. On the other hand, when clinical suspicion is high—even when initial endoscopic biopsies are negative or equivocal—endoscopy and biopsy should be repeated sooner. Patients with gastric ulcers first encountered in

the setting of active hemorrhage may not undergo ulcer biopsy while bleeding, especially if they are taking ASA/NSAIDs, heparin, anticoagulants, or other antiplatelet drugs. The risk of complications in this setting is unclear but most prudent endoscopists defer biopsy acutely. Ulcer biopsy in the setting of portal hypertensive gastropathy also is controversial.

D. IDENTIFICATION OF *H PYLORI* INFECTION

Because eradication of *H pylori* in infected subjects allows ulcers to heal and greatly reduces the chance of recurrence, identification of infection is of utmost importance in planning ulcer therapy. No single test can stand alone as a "gold standard" as none is 100% accurate. It is convenient to divide the diagnostic tests into those that do and those that do not require endoscopy. Nonendoscopic tests can be subdivided into those that identify the presence of an antibody response to *H pylori* infection (antibody testing) and those that identify active infection, either on the basis of the urease activity of *H pylori*'s or through the detection of fecal antigen. The endoscopic tests, including the rapid urease test, histology, and culture, identify only patients with active *H pylori* infection.

1. Nonendoscopic tests

a. Serology—There are quantitative and qualitative antibody tests. Quantitative tests or the enzyme linked immunosorbent assays (ELISAs) allow the determination of antibody titer. Qualitative tests utilize serum or whole blood obtained by a fingerstick to identify the presence or absence of immunoglobulin G (IgG) antibody to *H pylori* infection. Antibody tests are attractive because of their relatively low cost and widespread availability. Overall, quantitative tests have a sensitivity of 85% and specificity of 79%. Unfortunately, the currently available qualitative tests are probably less accurate than their quantitative counterparts. In addition, the pretest probability of *H pylori* infection has important effects on the positive predictive value of the anti-

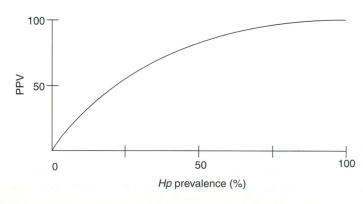

Figure 20–2. Effect of *H pylori* prevalence on the positive predictive value (PPV) of serology tests (assumes a sensitivity of 85% and specifity of 79%). (Reproduced, with permission, from Loy CT et al: Am J Gastroenterol 1996;91:380.)

body tests (Figure 20–2). For example, the antibody tests are less useful in situations in which the pretest probability of infection is low as is the case in patients with unevaluated dyspepsia. Conversely, antibody tests are more useful in situations in which the pretest probability of infection is high as would be expected in a patient with known PUD. It is important to realize that after successful cure of *H pylori* infection, antibody titers for *H pylori* gradually decline over months to years but do not always become negative. Therefore, a positive serologic test does not necessarily establish the presence of active infection.

b. Nonendoscopic urease tests (NUTs)—The urea breath or blood tests are noninvasive and unlike antibody tests, identify only patients with active *H pylori* infection. Furthermore, NUTs avoid the sampling error caused by patchy gastritis that may occur with endoscopic biopsies. The NUTs depend on the production by *H pylori* of large amounts of bacterial urease (a nonmammalian enzyme). When the patient is administered oral radioactive [^{14}C]- or nonradioactive [^{13}C]urea, urease from *H pylori* in the stomach metabolizes urea as follows:

$$NH_2 \, {}^*CO \, NH_2 + 3H_2O \rightarrow 2NH_4OH + {}^*CO_2$$

The CO_2 is rapidly absorbed across the gastric epithelium into the bloodstream and eventually excreted in exhaled breath. An increase in labeled bicarbonate in venous blood or labeled carbon dioxide in the breath identifies the presence of active *H pylori* infection. These tests have consistently been found to have a sensitivity and specificity exceeding 90%. The NUTs are also accurate as a means of establishing cure after treatment of *H pylori* infection. Versions of the [^{14}C]urea breath test and [^{13}C]urea breath or blood tests are commercially available in the United States. The NUTs can be performed in most clinical facilities and breath or blood samples mailed to a central laboratory for ${}^*CO_2$ measurement. The result is available to the doctor within a few days. More practical point of service NUTs have recently become available. NUTs may be falsely negative in patients in whom *H pylori* infection has been suppressed by the recent use of antibiotics or bismuth or treatment with proton-pump inhibitors (PPIs). For this reason, antibiotics and bismuth-containing compounds should be withheld for 4 weeks and PPIs for 1–2 weeks prior to the NUTs. Issues of availability, cost, and reimbursement have slowed the widespread use of these tests.

c. Fecal antigen test—The fecal antigen test (FAT) utilizes polyclonal anti-*H pylori* capture antibody adsorbed to microwells. In infected patients, enzyme–substrate binding leads to a color change that can be detected visually or spectrophotometrically. After collection, stool samples can be stored at 2–8°C for 3 days and at −20°C indefinitely.

Studies have reported sensitivity and specificity for the FAT of >90% in patients not previously treated for *H pylori* infection. Like the NUTs, the FAT identifies patients with active *H pylori* infection. Preliminary studies suggest that the FAT may be useful as a means of establishing cure after antimicrobial therapy. The sensitivity of the FAT is decreased by recent use of antibiotics, bismuth, or PPIs, although to a lesser degree than the NUTs. Issues that have slowed the widespread use of this test include the inherent unpleasantness associated with the handling and storing of stool, limited availability, and highly variable state-to-state reimbursement.

2. Endoscopic tests—In patients with a peptic ulcer diagnosed by endoscopy, biopsies can be performed to look for evidence of *H pylori*. Even in patients in whom another cause of peptic ulcer is apparent, such as ASA/NSAID use, *H pylori* status should be established at the time of endoscopy using a biopsy-based method or later, using a nonendoscopic test. The main methods by which *H pylori* can be diagnosed at the time of endoscopy include rapid urease testing, histology, and culture.

a. Rapid urease testing—As mentioned earlier, *H pylori* produces large amounts of the enzyme urease, which cleaves urea to ammonia and bicarbonate leading to a pH change in the microenvironment of the organism. The rapid urease tests (RUTs) utilize a gel matrix or reaction strip embedded with urea and a pH-sensitive indicator. Mucosal biopsies obtained at the time of endoscopy are placed into the gel or on the reaction strip. If *H pylori* is present, urease causes an increase in environmental pH and a consequent color change in the test medium.

The RUTs commercially available are equally sensitive (>89%) and specific (>90%) in the pretreatment setting. There are differences between the available tests in terms of time to yield a positive result (1–24 hours). This can be influenced by the amount of urease inoculated into the test medium. For this reason, it is recommended that two mucosal biopsies (one from the body and one from the antrum of the stomach) be obtained for rapid urease testing. The sensitivity of these tests can be influenced by the recent use of antibiotics, bismuth compounds, and PPIs. The RUTs are relatively inexpensive (~$5–10) and, therefore, the most cost-effective means of establishing the presence of *H pylori* infection at the time of endoscopy. However, the overall cost of this form of testing remains substantial because of the need for endoscopy. It should be noted that the RUTs render information only regarding the presence or absence of *H pylori* and do not allow the identification of concurrent histologic abnormalities such as gastric malignancy.

b. Histology—Routine hematoxylin and eosin staining typically allows recognition of the organism by an experienced pathologist. The finding of polymorphonuclear leukocytes (PMNs) in inflamed gastric tissue is highly suggestive of gastritis due to *H pylori*. Although other causes of gastric injury may be identified in the patient's history, such as the use of ASA or NSAIDs, none of these leads to significant PMN infiltration. Once PMNs are visualized, the experienced pathologist will search widely for *H pylori* organisms that may be harder to find. Modified Giemsa ("Diff-quick"), Warthin-Starry, Genta, and other stains can be used in situations in which *H pylori* is suspected (because of gastritis) but not readily identified. These stains also can help the less experienced pathologist to see the organisms. If all available diagnostic methods fail to reveal *H pylori* organisms but gastritis with PMNs is identified on histology, and the patient is not taking ASA or NSAIDs, a course of therapy aimed at *H pylori* eradication should be considered provided that the patient has an ulcer.

c. Culture—Although *H pylori* can be cultured from gastric biopsies, the process is slow, complicated by the need for special culture media, and expensive. In addition, culture is not as sensitive as many of the other diagnostic methods. For these reasons, culture is rarely used in routine clinical care in the United States. The main advantage that culture offers is the ability to determine the sensitivity of *H pylori* isolates to commonly used antibiotics such as metronidazole and clarithromycin. As the rate of antibiotic-resistant *H pylori* strains rises, it is conceivable that culture and antibiotic sensitivity testing could take on a more important role.

3. Testing to prove *H pylori* cure after treatment— It was previously recommended that testing to prove cure of *H pylori* infection was necessary in only selected clinical situations including recalcitrant or complicated (significant bleeding, perforation, penetration, obstruction) ulcers. However, the recommendations for testing following therapy for *H pylori* are broadening. Given the possibility of future ulcer-related morbidity and mortality in those with persistent infection, most clinicians would agree that all patients with *H pylori*-related PUD should undergo follow-up testing to establish cure. Another consideration is that many patients will want to know that *H pylori* infection has been eliminated. A recent study found that >70% of PUD patients would be willing to pay more than $50 to obtain the peace of mind provided by a test to prove cure of the infection.

DIFFERENTIAL DIAGNOSIS

Other conditions that may give rise to similar upper abdominal pain syndromes include gallstone disease and its complications, gastroesophageal reflux disease, chronic pancreatitis, cancers of the stomach and pancreas, postgastrectomy gastritis, and rarely, diseases of the transverse colon. In most cases, other features of these diseases will draw attention to their presence. However, when all such conditions have been excluded, >50% of all patients with recurrent upper abdominal discomfort or dyspepsia remain, whose symptoms cannot be explained by endoscopic or radiographic tests. These patients are often grouped under the diagnostic heading of "nonulcer or functional dyspepsia" (see Chapter 21).

Severe ulcer pain, although uncommon, also can mimic the pain of myocardial infarction, aortic dissection, biliary or ureteral/colic, acute pancreatitis, cholecystitis or diverticulitis, or mesenteric infarction. The physical findings, including the location of abdominal tenderness, may aid considerably in narrowing the differential diagnosis.

COMPLICATIONS

The complications of ulcer disease are principally hemorrhage, perforation, penetration, and obstruction, in that order, with hemorrhage being the most common and perforation the most lethal. Today, these constitute the main indications for ulcer surgery and account for most deaths from ulcer disease. When emergency surgery is needed, attention is focused on rapid correction of the immediate complication. Until recently, surgery for ulcer complications often included aggressive antiulcer operations (vagotomy with partial gastric resection or drainage procedures) that markedly altered normal gastric physiology. The modern trend is toward joint medical and surgical management of the patient, with early performance of the minimum surgical procedure needed for the patient to survive the complication. Specific therapy of the underlying ulcer diathesis can be rendered postoperatively in most patients with anti-*H pylori* eradication therapy, elimination of ASA/NSAID use, or long-term antisecretory therapy if required.

Hemorrhage

Classically, hematemesis is more common in gastric ulcers and melena in duodenal ulcers, although the combination of hematemesis and melena can occur with either ulcer when bleeding is brisk. In the patient with hematochezia, the absence of blood in gastric aspirates is good evidence against a gastric ulcer. In contrast, a negative gastric aspirate does not reduce the likelihood of bleeding from a duodenal ulcer (which may not reflux through the pylorus) unless it contains bile. Bleeding complications of peptic ulcers often are catastrophic in the elderly and may prove fatal, either in the home or while the patient is being transported to the hospital.

Ulcer hemorrhage may be recognized clinically in five patterns of increasing severity and clinical importance:

1. Occult blood in the stool with or without anemia.
2. Coffee grounds emesis.
3. Hematemesis.
4. Melena.
5. Sudden collapse and shock or focal dysfunction in a vital organ (eg, cerebrovascular accident, coronary ischemia), with or without obvious hemorrhage.

In ulcer patients who are not using ASA/NSAIDs, pain is the most common indication for endoscopy. In contrast, among those with NSAID-induced ulcers, the most common indication for endoscopy is acute blood loss or anemia.

Approximately 90% of clinically significant ulcer bleeds (3, 4, and 5 in the numbered list above) stop spontaneously, although blood transfusion may be required. The overall mortality is about 10%, but mortality is much higher in the elderly and in those with serious comorbid conditions. Bleeding ulcers account for about one-half of all upper gastrointestinal hemorrhages. Bleeding may be the first sign of an ulcer in 10–15% of clinically recognized cases.

Ulcer bleeding and rebleeding rates are greatly reduced in patients taking any kind of maintenance antiulcer therapy. Hence, maintenance antiulcer therapy (see the following discussion) traditionally has been given to almost all patients with a history of a bleeding ulcer. *H pylori* eradication also appears to decrease the risk of ulcer rebleeding dramatically. Because of the high risk of rebleeding in patients who have had one ulcer-related bleed, if *H pylori* cannot be eradicated, maintenance therapy (discussed below) should continue indefinitely.

Every effort should be made to avoid or minimize surgery in patients who have had a bleeding ulcer that is attributable to ASA/NSAIDs, as the course of their gastric disease may be exacerbated following surgery if drug use is resumed. Long-term prophylaxis with antiulcer drugs may be indicated in such patients. For additional information on the investigation and management of ulcer bleeding, see Chapter 3.

Perforation

Perforation is no longer common in peptic ulcer disease. In most contemporary series, admissions for hemorrhage are between four and six times more common than those for perforation. Perforation of an ulcer is usually a dramatic event, the onset of which may be accompanied by severe generalized abdominal pain, loss of bowel sounds, and board-like rigidity of the abdominal wall. The patient experiences a great reluctance to move and a feeling of impending doom. The development of perforation may be the first sign of the presence of an ulcer, particularly in those using ASA or NSAIDs or suffering from Zollinger-Ellison syndrome. The clinical picture may vary greatly. Elderly patients and those using ASA/NSAIDs or steroids may manifest minimal signs until late in the course of their illness, when peritonitis, bacteremia, and shock develop. In others, pain and tenderness may be localized because the perforation has occurred into the lesser sac, leaked contents have tracked into the subhepatic or subphrenic areas, or leaked contents have been limited by the omentum. Other intraabdominal catastrophic events, eg, dissection or rupture of an aortic aneurysm or mesenteric infarction, may cause similarly severe sudden pain but, unlike perforation, these events are usually accompanied by shock from the outset. Acute pancreatitis may closely mimic perforation and may even accompany perforation. However, its onset is not as explosive and it is usually accompanied by a high serum lipase concentration. Aortic and mesenteric vascular injuries, despite severe pain, usually present with a paucity of abdominal findings and rapidly progressing acidosis.

Laboratory tests usually reveal polymorphonuclear leukocytosis. Other findings are unpredictable. A mild rise in serum amylase may be caused by peritoneal absorption of pancreatic enzymes from leaked duodenal secretions. Plain x-ray of the abdomen, in most cases, shows free intraperitoneal air on upright or decubitus views. When x-rays are negative and perforation is suspected, administration of oral soluble radiographic contrast may demonstrate a leak. Barium studies should be avoided when perforation is suspected. Endoscopy should not be performed. In rare cases, urgent laparotomy is required to make the diagnosis.

All patients with suspected perforation should have a nasogastric tube placed in order to evacuate the stomach and minimize further peritoneal soilage. Fluid resuscitation should be aggressively pursued and broad-spectrum antibiotics should be administered. In most circumstances in which perforation is identified early, laparoscopy or laparotomy with closure of the perforation by an omental patch is sufficient, and more definitive antiulcer surgery is not required. Mortality is at least 5% but may be as high as 30–50% in elderly patients with bleeding or other comorbid conditions, particularly when the diagnosis is delayed. For this reason, an initial trial of conservative nonoperative management may be recommended in the frail patient with serious comorbid illness, especially if no leakage of water-soluble contrast can be demonstrated on an upper gastrointestinal series. Such patients may be followed closely over 12–24 hours for signs of regression of peritonitis, provided that the possibility of other surgical catastrophes can be excluded.

Penetration

Unlike perforation, ulcer penetration into an adjacent viscus, such as the liver, pancreas, or biliary system, is rarely dramatic. Rather, it presents with gradual exacerbation of pain, loss of rhythmicity, increase in local tenderness, increasing requirement for medication, or the development of features of an additional disease process, such as pancreatitis or cholangitis. Its most common manifestation is pancreatitis. The association of pancreatitis and duodenal ulcer is more common than can be accounted for by the presence of penetration. The complication of penetration is rarely catastrophic and responds, in most cases, to intensive medical therapy. Only a minority of cases require surgery.

Obstruction

The frequency with which contemporary patients develop gastric outlet obstruction is unknown, but in older studies 1–3% developed permanent narrowing over 10–20 years of follow-up. Patients may present with gastric outlet obstruction of two types. The first is due to edema and inflammation surrounding an acute ulcer, especially in the antrum or pyloric channel. The second is due to chronic, permanent scarring with fibrosis and outlet narrowing. Although intensive medical therapy may reverse the first type, it cannot resolve the second.

Gastric outlet obstruction is the least common complication of peptic (pyloric channel or duodenal) ulcer disease. Other causes aside from PUD include carcinomas of the stomach, pancreas, liver, and bile ducts as well as other extrinsic intraabdominal masses that may compress the stomach or duodenum.

Gastric outlet obstruction must be distinguished from gastroparesis, in which the stomach fails to empty despite the absence of mechanical obstruction. Patients with gastric outlet obstruction usually complain of postprandial epigastric fullness, early satiety, and vomiting of materials ingested hours to days previously. Vomiting may be worse toward the end of the day. The relationship of vomiting to the ulcer pain is variable. If gastric outlet obstruction is chronic, patients may develop hypochloremic alkalosis, tetany, weight loss, and, rarely, aspiration pneumonia.

With chronic obstruction, the stomach may become grossly dilated and contain 200–2000 mL of foul-smelling contents. A succussion splash may be audible on physical examination. The diagnosis may be confirmed using radiographic (barium), endoscopic, or scintigraphic (gastric-emptying) studies. The "saline-load test" is rarely employed, except as a means of following a patient's progress during conservative therapy. In this study, 700 mL of saline is instilled into a nasogastric tube that has been confirmed by radiography to be within the gastric body. After the patient has been kept for 30 minutes in the left lateral decubitus position, the remaining gastric fluid is aspirated, with care taken to roll the patient in several positions to verify complete aspiration. A residual volume of greater than 400 mL is indicative of significant gastric retention.

Most patients with gastric outlet obstruction require suction with a large orogastric tube to fully evacuate the stomach. Thereafter, nasogastric suction with a smaller tube (18 F) should be maintained for 4–7 days to allow pyloric edema and spasm to subside and gastric motility to return. Intravenous replacement of fluid and electrolytes is imperative. Intensive antisecretory therapy with intravenous H$_2$RAs or proton-pump inhibitors should be given to reduce nasogastric fluid losses and to promote ulcer healing. Patients with chronic obstruction and signs of malnutrition should be given parenteral nutrition. A saline load test or upper GI study using water-soluble contrast should be performed after 72 hours of gastric decompression. If this demonstrates significant improvement, a liquid diet may be tried. About one-half to two-thirds of patients fail to improve after 5–7 days of gastric aspiration. Up to 90% of cases of gastric outlet obstruction will come to either surgical or endoscopic dilatation within 1 year.

Where possible, short strictures (<5 mm long) that are wide enough to allow passage of a pediatric endoscope should be treated with endoscopic balloon dilatation sometimes over three or four sessions, combined with intensive acid-suppressive therapy. This drug therapy should be continued indefinitely after symptoms have resolved, especially in high-risk patients. Balloon dilatation therapy has been reported to provide short- and long-term relief of obstructive symptoms in over three quarters of suitable patients without the need for surgery. In patients in whom balloon dilatation therapy is not possible or is unsuccessful, surgical therapy is generally required. Surgical treatment is usually necessary when there is extensive scarring, a long stricture, a large ulcer, or a badly deformed bulb. Morbidity following surgery (dumping, diarrhea, stasis, etc) approaches 10–15%.

TREATMENT

In the age of *H pylori* infection, treatment has transitioned from control of PUD with long-term antisecretory therapy to cure of PUD by eradication of the offending organism. In the past, therapy consisted of acid-neutralizing or acid–secretory-inhibiting drugs that were useful in the control of symptoms but usually led only to transient healing of the ulcer crater. Although the traditional therapies of "acid-peptic" disease remain useful, they are now more relevant to the treatment of gastroesophageal reflux disease than to PUD. For PUD, these agents now play a secondary role, as supplemental therapy when measures addressing the primary cause of the ulcer are unsuccessful.

The two major underlying causes of peptic ulcers are chronic active gastritis due to *H pylori* infection and mucosal damage due to NSAIDs, or ASA. To what extent these independent etiologic factors are also interactive remains unclear. In particular, the issue of whether NSAIDs adversely affect the course of conventional peptic ulcer disease due to *H pylori* is unresolved. Eradication of *H pylori* is desirable in all *H pylori*-positive cases of ulcer disease, including patients in whom organisms cannot be identified on mucosal biopsy but who have prominent PMNs (highly suggestive of *H pylori*-associated gastritis). Eradication therapy should also be prescribed in *H pylori*-positive patients with NSAID-associated ulcers. Where possible, ASA or NSAID use should be discontinued in all ulcer patients. Nevertheless, there remain numerous patients who need to continue ASA/NSAID therapy.

Treatment of peptic ulcer will be discussed under three major headings: (1) treatment in *H pylori*-positive patients, (2) treatment in *H pylori*-negative, ASA/NSAID users, and (3) treatment in *H pylori*-negative patients who are not using ASA/NSAIDs.

Treatment of *H pylori*-Infected PUD

At the present time, *H pylori*-positive patients who have an active ulcer are treated simultaneously with antibacterial therapy to eradicate the *H pylori* and with traditional antiulcer drugs, such as antacids, H₂RAs, proton-pump inhibitors, or sucralfate to promote active ulcer healing. Although antimicrobial therapies against *H pylori* may be adequate to induce ulcer healing as well as to eradicate *H pylori,* there is a lack of sufficient studies involving adequate numbers of patients who have been treated solely with antimicrobial drugs. A few such studies suggest that antibiotics alone are as effective as combinations of these with antiulcer drugs, both in relieving symptoms and in healing ulcers. Pending further studies, most physicians continue to employ combination therapy with both classes of agents.

A. ANTIBACTERIAL THERAPY

Although numerous antibiotics have activity against *H pylori in vitro,* therapy with a single antibiotic is generally ineffective. This is likely related to factors including

the acid environment of the stomach, which can decrease the effectiveness of certain antibiotics, and the protection afforded by the gastric mucous gel in which *H pylori* resides. Successful therapies for *H pylori* consist of three to four drugs given for 7–14 days. To be considered useful, a therapeutic regimen should have an efficacy of >80% in clinical trials.

The original therapy used to cure *H pylori* infection consisted of tetracycline, bismuth, and metronidazole for a period of 14 days. In U.S. trials, so-called **bismuth triple therapy** has been found to have an eradication rate of 77–82% (Table 20–2). A 7-day course of traditional bismuth triple therapy may also be effective but has not been adequately validated in large U.S. trials. Adding a PPI appears to enhance the efficacy of bismuth triple therapy (known as *quadruple therapy*). Using amoxicillin in place of tetracycline results in lower rates of *H pylori* eradication. Side effects occur in 30–50% of patients, although fewer than 5% have to discontinue therapy.

The first regimens to achieve widespread use in the United States consisted of two drugs. At first glance, **dual therapy** appears an attractive option because of its simplicity and potential for improved medical compliance. The combination of clarithromycin and either a PPI or ranitidine bismuth citrate (RBC) has yielded eradication rates in the range of 64–84%. Unfortunately, RBC is no longer available in the United States. In general, dual therapy is better tolerated than bismuth triple therapy. Side effects are most often associated with clarithromycin and include altered taste, nausea, diarrhea, and headache. Despite being simple and well tolerated, the current dual regimens can no longer be recommended given their marginal efficacy.

PPI or RBC-based triple therapies (see Table 20–2) are effective in eradicating *H pylori* infection and reasonably well tolerated by patients. These regimens consist of a PPI or RBC in combination with two antibiotics (amoxicillin, clarithromycin, or metronidazole). Medications are given twice daily for periods of 7–14 days. Particularly notable are the combinations of a PPI or RBC, clarithromycin, and either amoxicillin or metronidazole, which have consistently achieved eradication rates of >80%. In the United States, regimens containing lansoprazole or omeprazole with clarithromycin and amoxicillin taken twice daily for 10–14 days have achieved FDA approval.

B. FACTORS INFLUENCING THE EFFECTIVENESS OF THERAPY

Perhaps the single most important factor influencing the success of therapy is compliance with the medical regimen. The secret of success with these regimens lies in having a physician who is knowledgeable about the effects of the drugs spend sufficient time with patients in advance of

Table 20–2. FDA-approved treatment regimens for *H pylori*.

Regimen	Dosage	Number of Pills/d	Eradication Rate (United States Studies) (%)
Bismuth triple therapy	Bismuth (525 mg four times daily for 14 days), tetracycline (500 mg four times daily for 14 days), metronidazole (250 mg four times daily for 14 days) *plus* H$_2$ blocker at approved dose (eg, Zantac, 150 mg twice daily for 28 days	18	77–82
RBC[1]	400 mg twice daily for 28 days		
Clarithromycin	400 mg three times daily for 14 days	5	73–84
Omeprazole	40 mg once a day for 14 days *plus* 20 mg once a day for 14 days		
Clarithromycin	500 mg three times daily for 14 days	4	64–74
Lansoprazole	30 mg three times daily for 14 days		
Amoxicillin	1 g three times daily for 14 days	9	61–77
Omeprazole	20 mg twice daily for 10 days *plus* 20 mg once a day for 18 days	8	69–90
or			
Lansoprazole	30 mg twice daily for 10 days	8	81–84
Clarithromycin	500 mg twice daily for 10 days		
Amoxicillin	1 g twice daily for 10 days		
Lansoprazole	30 mg twice daily for 14 days		
Clarithromycin	500 mg twice daily for 14 days		
Amoxicillin	1 g twice daily for 14 days	8	83–92

[1]RBC, ranitidine bismuth citrate.

therapy. The physician needs to educate the patient about possible side effects, advise the patient when to continue and when to terminate therapy, and be alert to the need to switch to an alternative regimen, if necessary.

Another important determinant of *H pylori* treatment success is the presence of preexisting or primary antibiotic resistance. The prevalence of *H pylori* strains resistant to antibiotics such as clarithromycin and metronidazole varies geographically. In the United States, 6–12% of *H pylori* isolates are resistant to clarithromycin and 13–50% are resistant to metronidazole. Resistance to amoxicillin or bismuth is currently quite rare.

Duration of therapy and antibiotic dosing also appear to influence the effectiveness of therapy. In Europe, the accepted duration of therapy for *H pylori* infection is 7 days based upon large trials reporting eradication rates of >85%. Unfortunately, currently available U.S. studies have not reproduced these results. As such, it is recommended that treatment be given for 10–14 days in the United States.

C. Considerations in Patients Who Remain Infected after Therapy

There are currently few data addressing the management of patients who fail an initial attempt at eradicating *H pylori* infection. As such, much of what is presented in this section is based upon common sense and the author's anecdotal experience. Dual therapy should not be used in the setting of treatment failure. In addition, a second course of therapy should be given for no less than 10–14 days.

When a regimen containing metronidazole and/or clarithromycin is used to treat *H pylori,* the development of resistance is likely in cases of treatment failure. If metronidazole or clarithromycin was used in the initial regimen, a second course of therapy should avoid these antibiotics. If clarithromycin was not used initially and there is no history of penicillin allergy, the combination of a PPI with clarithromycin and amoxicillin twice daily for 14 days can be quite useful.

If the initial therapy contained clarithromycin but not metronidazole, quadruple therapy (PPI, tetracycline, bismuth, and metronidazole) could be considered for 14 days. If both metronidazole and clarithromycin were included in the initial therapy, consider treating with a PPI, tetracycline, bismuth, and the synthetic nitrofuran antibiotic, furazolidone (100 mg four times daily) for 14 days. Furazolidone has been used instead of metronidazole in treatment regimens for *H pylori* and appears to be effective even for many *H pylori* strains resistant to metronidazole. When furazolidone is used, patients should be warned against using alcohol or monamine oxidase inhibitors.

D. TRADITIONAL ANTIULCER THERAPIES

Because of their excellent efficacy, safety, and relatively low cost, H_2RAs remain popular choices for healing peptic ulcers. There are four H_2RAs clinically available: cimetidine, ranitidine, famotidine, and nizatidine. All inhibit the secretory agonist effect of histamine on the parietal cell, but are less effective in inhibiting cholinergic or gastrin-mediated postprandial secretion. These four drugs are comparable in efficacy and safety.

For the treatment of duodenal ulcers, all are highly efficacious when administered as once-daily nocturnal doses. These agents can also be given twice daily (all agents) or even four times daily (cimetidine). For the treatment of uncomplicated duodenal ulcers, once-daily nocturnal dosing regimens appear equivalent in efficacy to the more frequent dosing regimens and are, therefore, recommended. For the treatment of gastric ulcers, once-daily regimens are also efficacious but the more frequent dosing regimens may afford better symptom relief.

Effective daily oral doses are cimetidine 800 mg at bedtime, 400 mg twice daily, or 300 mg four times daily; ranitidine or nizatidine 300 mg at bedtime or 150 mg twice daily; and famotidine 40 mg at bedtime or 20 mg twice daily. All of the drugs are safe; clinically significant side effects occur in fewer than 3% of patients. Serious side effects are very rare, except at higher doses and with intravenous administration. Duodenal ulcers should be treated for 8 weeks, and gastric ulcers for 12 weeks, unless healing is verified endoscopically or radiographically at an earlier time. At standard doses, ulcer healing rates of greater than 90% can be expected after 8–12 weeks of therapy.

Similar ulcer healing rates may be achieved with sucralfate 4.0 g/d (2 g twice daily or 1 g four times a day), a nonabsorbed, surface-active disaccharide bound to aluminum sulfate whose precise mode of action is unknown. Other "mucosal protective agents," such as bismuth salts, various prostaglandin analogs, carbenoxalone, and numerous other compounds, have not been proven to be as safe or effective in the United States and are not approved therapy.

Antacids have enjoyed widespread use for over 100 years in the treatment of peptic ulcers, with efficacy that is similar to other antiulcer agents. In the original U.S. trials, the very high doses of antacids that were employed (seven doses or 1008 mEq of neutralizing capacity per day) were associated with unacceptably high rates of diarrhea. However, in many other countries, studies of low doses of antacids of only 120–240 mEq/d have proven to be as effective as H_2RAs, with minimal side effects at a fraction of the cost.

The H^+/K^+-ATPase or "proton-pump" inhibitors are the most effective medical therapy for PUD. These drugs are concentrated in the acidified tubulovesicular membranes of parietal cells where they bind covalently to the enzyme H^+/K^+-ATPase, the final common pathway of acid secretion. Restoration of normal acid secretion is dependent on synthesis of new proton pumps, which have a half-life of approximately 18 hours.

Regardless of the agonist or stimulus, these agents induce profound long-lasting, dose-dependent inhibition of acid secretion. Because of the loss of normal acid feedback inhibition of antral gastrin release, fasting and postprandial serum gastrin rise in almost everyone who takes a proton-pump inhibitor. In up to 10% of people, the rise in serum gastrin may be dramatic (>500 pg/mL). To date, this drug-induced hypergastrinemia has not had serious adverse consequences in humans.

There are currently five PPIs (omeprazole, lansoprazole, rabeprazole, pantoprazole, and esomeprazole) that have been approved for the treatment of PUD in the United States. A single oral dose of omeprazole 20 mg daily achieves greater than 90% ulcer healing within 4 weeks in the case of duodenal ulcers and within 8 weeks in the case of gastric ulcers. Higher doses of omeprazole do not accelerate restoration of the deeper mucosal glandular architecture or benefit the patient clinically. PPIs are bactericidal to *H pylori in vitro. In vivo,* they reduce intragastric acidity so much that the organism cannot find enough acid to survive its own endogenous production of NH_4OH from urea.

Side effects of PPIs are clinically negligible. PPIs appear safe even for long-term use. In patients who cannot take a capsule or pill, these drugs can be given as a suspension or solution without adverse effects on their potent acid inhibitory effects. Only pantoprazole is currently available for parenteral administration. Recent studies suggest that early treatment with an intravenous PPI can reduce recurrent bleeding in patients with a duodenal ulcer.

For the past 15 years, the standard practice after an active ulcer has healed has been to continue the patient on a half dose of the antiulcer drug indefinitely to reduce the likelihood of ulcer recurrence. This "maintenance therapy" to prevent endoscopic or symptomatic ulcer recurrence has become largely obsolete, because most of the population that benefited from it can now be cured of their disease by eradication of *H pylori*. However, it is important to realize that eradication of *H pylori* significantly reduces but does not eliminate the risk of ulcer recurrence. A careful review of large ulcer healing trials from the United States reveals that eradication of *H pylori* reduces ulcer recurrence from 60–70% to ~20% at 1 year. As such, patients with recurrent symptoms despite successful eradication of *H pylori* need investigation and if found to have a recurrent ulcer, require maintenance therapy with acid suppression. In addition, there are insufficient data on the outcome of *H pylori* eradication in high-risk elderly persons, ie, those patients with a previous ulcer hemorrhage or perforation that was not attributable to ASA/NSAIDs—to warrant abandoning maintenance therapy in this group. Therefore, maintenance therapy is still recommended in high-risk patients with a prior ulcer complication, even if *H pylori* has been successfully treated. H_2RAs have been demonstrated to reduce the incidence of recurrent ulcer hemorrhage from almost 40% to less than 10%. The efficacy of half-dose therapy has not been validated in such high-risk cases, and full doses should be given indefinitely. In NSAID users with ulcer disease who must continue to use these ulcerogenic drugs, it also has not been shown that half-dose therapy is of any value in the prevention of recurrent NSAID-associated ulcers. There is some evidence that PPIs or higher doses of H_2RAs (eg, famotidine 40 mg twice daily) are needed for ulcer healing and for maintenance therapy of the NSAID ulcer in the healed state. Thus, classical maintenance (half-dose) therapy is now rarely used.

Treatment of *H pylori*-Negative ASA/NSAIDs-Associated PUD

A. INITIAL TREATMENT OF UNCOMPLICATED NSAID-ASSOCIATED ULCERS

The approach to treating *H pylori*-negative ulcers in NSAID users depends on the setting in which the ulcer is encountered. If diagnosed in an elective (nonemergency) setting, treatment is traditional antiulcer therapy, except that no eradication therapy is needed. Healing of the ulcer may be achieved with standard doses of a PPI, H_2RA, or sucralfate if the NSAID can be stopped entirely. Due to their effectiveness as once a day therapy and rapid healing rates, PPIs are usually the drug of choice. Numerous studies have shown that most people using NSAIDs need analgesic rather than antiinflammatory drugs. Therefore, the NSAID should be stopped whenever possible and replaced with adequate doses of a non-NSAID compound, such as acetaminophen at doses up to 1000 mg every 6 hours. Doses of 325–650 mg tablets

of acetaminophen are usually inadequate in chronic pain syndromes, such as osteoarthritis. The opiates or Tramadol, a nonaddictive, orally active, nonnarcotic agent, may also be needed for effective pain control.

For patients with uncomplicated NSAID-associated ulcers in whom it is deemed medically necessary to continue NSAID therapy, dosage should be reduced to the minimal dose necessary to achieve adequate antiinflammatory effects. Trials have shown that ulcer *healing* is more rapid when NSAID therapy is stopped than when continued. However, when NSAIDs are continued, ulcer healing eventually occurs in most cases treated with antacids, H_2RAs, sucralfate, misoprostol, or PPIs. With antacids, H_2RAs, and misoprostol in ordinary dosages, ulcer *healing* is delayed in those patients who continue using NSAIDs compared with those who stop using these drugs. However, clinical studies demonstrate that treatment with proton pump-inhibitors results in effective healing of >80% of duodenal ulcers and gastric ulcers despite continued NSAID therapy—and are superior to either H_2-antagonists or misoprostol. At present, it would appear prudent to use PPI therapy in patients with active NSAID ulcers who must remain on their NSAID during ulcer therapy.

B. INITIAL TREATMENT OF NSAID-ASSOCIATED PEPTIC ULCERS WITH ACUTE COMPLICATIONS

In patients presenting with complications of NSAID-associated ulcers such as hemorrhage or perforaction, it is advisable to stop ASA/NSAIDS for both medical and medical-legal reasons. Those who absolutely need antiinflammatory therapy should be treated initially with analgesics and low-to-moderate doses of either corticosteroids or second-line antiarthritic drugs whenever possible until the ulcer is fully healed. In those taking ASA for prophylaxis against cardiovascular or cerebrovascular thrombosis, the dosage should be reduced. It is likely that doses of 30–80 mg daily are sufficient to inhibit platelets. Use of enteric-coated ASA reduces superficial gastric erosive injury, but still results in systemic and mucosal prostaglandin inhibition with increased risk of peptic ulcers.

Use of *cox-2* selective NSAIDs (rofecoxib, celecoxib, meloxicam) can also be recommended for managing inflammation. A theoretical concern with these selective agents or "coxibs" is that they may interfere with ulcer healing (partly mediated by *cox-2*); however, this effect is likely ameliorated in the presence of potent acid suppression.

Patients with a history of NSAID-associated ulcer complications are at significantly increased risk of sustaining another NSAID-induced complication. Therefore, once ulcers have healed completely, if continued NSAID use is medically necessary, long-term antiulcer prophylactic therapy must be administered. The optimal ulcer prevention regimen in this high-risk setting is unclear although recent data with PPIs are encouraging. Trials of the prostaglandin E_1 (PGE_1) analog, misoprostol, have systematically excluded all such high-risk ulcer patients from study. Most prospective studies with H_2RAs are also flawed.

C. PREVENTION OF NSAID-INDUCED ULCERS AND COMPLICATIONS

There has been much interest in developing prophylactic therapy to prevent adverse outcomes in NSAID users. Cotherapy with a variety of antiulcer drugs has been evaluated in clinical trials, including sucralfate, H_2RAs, PPIs, and prostaglandin analogues. The optimal approach to the prevention of NSAID-induced ulcers or ulcer recurrences remains highly controversial.

In randomized controlled trials assessing the efficacy of prophylactic therapies to prevent NSAID-associated ulcers, patients placed on NSAIDs were given cotherapy with placebo or an active antiulcer agent (H_2RA, PPI, sucralfate, or misoprostol) and were followed for several weeks to determine the development of endoscopic or symptomatic ulcers. Importantly, most of these trials excluded patients with significant comorbid conditions, the elderly, and patients with a history of ulcers or ulcer complications, ie, the patients who are at greatest risk from NSAID complications and most likely to benefit from prophylactic therapy. Therefore, it is difficult to extrapolate from the results of these trials to patients at high risk of NSAID-induced complications. Furthermore, the end point of these studies was the development of endoscopically visible "ulcers," defined as mucosal lesions of at least 3–5 mm in diameter, rather than the development of symptomatic ulcers or ulcer complications. However, the development of these mucuosal lesions, most of which are small and not associated with symptoms, has not been shown to be clinically relevant or to predict serious adverse outcomes.

These shortcomings notwithstanding, the following may be concluded. Sucralfate is not an effective agent in preventing NSAID-related ulcers and should not be used for this indication. Misoprostol 100–200 μg four times daily significantly reduces the incidence of NSAID-induced, endoscopically visible duodenal and gastric lesions over a 3-month period but does not reduce the development of dyspeptic symptoms. H_2RA in conventional doses (eg, ranitidine 150 mg twice daily) are comparable in efficacy to misoprostol in the prevention of duodenal ulcers but inferior in the prevention of gastric ulcers. One study reported that high-dose famotidine (40 mg twice daily) was equally effective in reducing the development of NSAID-induced gastric ulcers. PPIs (eg, omeprazole 20 mg/d; lansoprazole 30 mg/d; pantoprazole 40 mg/d) are superior to standard dose H_2RAs (ranitidine 150 mg twice daily) and misoprostol (200 μg twice daily) in the prevention of NSAID-induced ulcers.

For the prevention of serious NSAID-induced gastrointestinal complications (eg, bleeding, perforation, obstruction), clinical trials have been performed only with misoprostol. The MUCOSA trial identified a 40% relative risk reduction in serious complications in NSAID users given cotherapy with misoprostol compared with placebo. Thus, although misoprostol has been shown in short-term endoscopic studies to reduce the incidence of endoscopic ulcers by >80–90% in patients taking NSAIDs for 2–3 months, the reduction in long-term significant gastrointestinal complications was far lower. Moreover, it is estimated that 264 chronic NSAID-using patients would need to be treated with misoprostol for 6 months to prevent a single upper gastrointestinal complication. Therefore, analyses indicate that misoprostol cotherapy is cost effective only if given to those patients at high risk of developing NSAID-associated ulcers (see below). Major drawbacks of misoprostol cotherapy are its failure to reduce NSAID-associated dyspepsia and a 10–20% incidence of diarrhea. For these reasons, cotherapy with misoprostol is used less frequently than cotherapy with PPIs or H_2RAs.

Despite a lack of long-term prospective outcome trials, PPIs enjoy widespread acceptance among clinicians as the preferred agent for the prophylaxis of NSAID-induced ulcers and complications. Compared with misoprostol, PPIs have demonstrated superiority and H_2RAs comparable efficacy in the incidence of NSAID-induced ulcers detected by endoscopy after 2–3 months. Furthermore, PPIs and H_2RAs both reduce dyspeptic symptoms in chronic NSAID users. Finally, from a clinical perspective, it would appear reasonable to assume that because PPIs are capable of healing active ulcers even in the face of continued NSAID therapy, they should be capable of maintaining remission and preventing NSAID-induced ulcer recurrence.

Recent prospective placebo controlled trials in arthritis patients demonstrate that compared with conventional NSAIDS, cox-2 specific inhibitors (celecoxib, rofecoxib) "coxibs" have a lower incidence of endoscopic ulcer as well as a reduction in clinically significant ulcers, ie, symptomatic and complicated ulcers. Therefore, NSAID treatment with coxibs alone may be a better alternative in high-risk patients than administration of a standard, nonselective NSAID plus cotherapy with misoprostol or a PPI. Treatment with coxibs alone may be justified in high-risk patients on both clinical and economic grounds, given the higher cost of cotherapy compared with coxib therapy and the lack of long-term outcome data with acid-suppressive medications.

Two patient subgroups merit further discussion. Among patients taking coxibs and low-dose aspirin (which inhibit cox-1), it appears the safety of coxibs is significantly reduced, suggesting the need for cotherapy.

Furthermore, because the long-term coxib outcome studies did not include significant numbers of patients with prior ulcer complications, it is unknown whether coxibs alone are safe in this high-risk subgroup. In patients with prior catastrophic NSAID-induced ulcer complications, it therefore may be prudent to prescribe a coxib and cotherapy with a PPI or misoprostol.

The following recommendations are provided. In patients without risk factors for the development of NSAID-associated complications, the risk of complications with standard, nonselective NSAIDs is approximately 1% per year. For this low-risk group, prophylactic cotherapy with a PPI or misoprostol is not indicated. Coxibs appear to reduce further the incidence of symptomatic ulcers and complications, but are significantly more expensive than nonselective NSAIDs. Patients at increased risk of NSAID-induced complications should be treated either with a coxib or with a nonselective NSAID plus cotherapy with a PPI or misoprostol. These high-risk patients include the elderly, patients with severe comorbid medical conditions, patients with prior NSAID-induced ulcers, patients taking corticosteroids, and patients taking anticoagulants. Patients with a prior history of NSAID-induced complications (bleeding, perforation) have a dramatically increased risk of recurrent NSAID-induced complications. Wherever possible, NSAIDS should be avoided in this subgroup. If ASA and/or NSAIDS must be administered, the optimal, cost-effective prophylactic strategy is unknown. Cotherapy with a coxib and either a PPI or misoprostol is recommended.

Treatment of PUD Not Associated with *H pylori* or ASA/NSAIDs

It has been suggested that only a small number (<5–10%) of patients with ulcers do not have infection with *H pylori* or a history of NSAID use. However, as the prevalence of *H pylori* infection falls in the United States and Europe, the proportion of *H pylori*-negative, NSAID-negative ulcers is likely to rise. Several recent studies have reported an *H pylori*-negative, NSAID-negative ulcer rate as high as 48% in some parts of the United States. However, many patients prove on further investigation to have been surreptitiously or unintentionaly taking ASA/NSAIDs. Plasma salicylate or thromboxane B_2 concentrations, platelet function abnormalities, abnormal bleeding time, or gastric biopsies showing marked foveolar hyperplasia in the absence of inflammatory change may alert the clinician to the possibility of covert or unintentional NSAID use. Asking the patient or a family member to bring in all the medications in the home may also prove revealing.

A minority of ulcer patients, particularly those with complicated duodenal, postbulbar, or jejunal ulcers,

truly have an underlying ulcer diathesis that is not attributable to *H pylori* or ASA/NSAIDs. Causes of ulcers in such patients may include sporadic Zollinger-Ellison syndrome, multiple endocrine neoplasia type I, primary or secondary hyperparathyroidism, uremia, primary polycythemia, systemic mastocytosis, hyperhistaminemia due to foregut carcinoid syndrome or granulocytic leukemia, hypersecretion following small intestinal resection, or idiopathic gastric hypersecretion. The role of *H pylori* infection has not been examined in most of these conditions, as descriptions of their associations with ulcer disease antedated appreciation of this pathogen's great importance.

A detailed discussion of the diagnosis and management of ulcers in all of these conditions is beyond the scope of this chapter. Zollinger-Ellison syndrome is addressed in the next section. Briefly, the presence of diarrhea, marked weight loss, poor response to healing, rapid or frequent recurrence, multiple or ectopic ulcers, or the presence of systemic symptoms are all atypical in conventional peptic ulcer disease and should prompt additional investigation. Where available, acid secretory studies should be obtained to demonstrate acid hyersecretion. If hypersecretion is present, fasting serum gastrin, calcium, and blood urea nitrogen (BUN) measurements are indicated, together with a complete blood count. The patient should be referred to a subspecialist who is an expert in ulcer disease. Special investigations, such as secretin stimulation testing, CT, angiography, magnetic resonance imaging (MRI), and endoscopic ultrasound, should be undertaken only in centers with expertise in the interpretation and implementation of related complex management strategies.

Pending this type of comprehensive investigation, the clinical symptoms of ulcer disease may be treated effectively with standard or increased doses of a PPI to control pain and diarrhea.

PROGNOSIS

In uncomplicated peptic ulcer disease associated solely with *H pylori* gastritis, the prognosis is excellent if the organism is eradicated. Reinfection is uncommon in the United States (<1% per year), except in conditions of low socioeconomic status, poor sanitation, or overcrowding. Therefore, once eradication is achieved, recurrent ulceration due to reinfection is relatively uncommon. Treatment of *H pylori*-positive household contacts who do not have symptomatic ulcers is not currently recommended.

Similarly, in patients with NSAID-associated ulcers, the prognosis is excellent if ASA or NSAIDs can be stopped. The development of the coxibs represents a major advance in providing effective antiinflammatory therapy with deceased ulcer risk and has the potential to reduce the need for cotherapy to prevent ulcers. On the whole, the prognosis is excellent in uncomplicated cases of ulcer disease but is often poor in those with complicated disease, because of advanced age, poor compliance, polypharmacy, and the presence of serious comorbid conditions. The statistical association of a poor ulcer outcome with death does not establish that the death was truly or solely attributable either to the ulcer or to its underlying cause. Prognosis in ulcer patients with some other underlying condition no longer depends on the ulcer disease, which can be controlled medically in nearly all cases given adequate doses of antisecretory drugs. With overall mortality rates relatively stable over the past 60 years, the prevention of ulcer complications in high-risk elderly patients remains a major challenge. Every effort should be made to avoid "ulcer surgery" in complicated peptic ulcer cases, other than oversewing perforations or bleeding vessels. Operations such as vagotomy, pyloroplasty, and gastroenterostomy should be avoided in all but the most difficult of ulcer cases.

ZOLLINGER-ELLISON SYNDROME (GASTRINOMA)

 ESSENTIALS OF DIAGNOSIS

- *Peptic ulcer disease; may be severe or atypical.*
- *Gastric acid hypersecretion.*
- *Diarrhea common, relieved by nasogastric suction.*
- *Most cases are sporadic; 25% with multiple endocrine neoplasia (MEN) 1.*

Zollinger-Ellison syndrome is caused by gastrin-secreting gut neuroendocrine tumors (gastrinomas), which result in hypergastrinemia and acid hypersecretion. Less than 1% of peptic ulcer disease is caused by gastrinomas. Primary gastrinomas may arise in the pancreas (25%), duodenal wall (45%), or lymph nodes (5–15%), and in other locations or of unknown origin in 20%. Approximately 80% arise within the "gastrinoma triangle," bounded by the porta hepatis, neck of the pancreas, and third portion of the duodenum. Most gastrinomas are solitary or multifocal nodules that are potentially resectable. Over two-thirds are malignant, and one-third have already metastasized to the liver at initial presentation. Approximately 25% of patients have small multicentric gastrinomas associated with MEN 1 that are more difficult to treat.

Clinical Findings

A. SYMPTOMS AND SIGNS

Over 90% of patients with Zollinger-Ellison syndrome (ZES) develop peptic ulcers. In most cases, the symptoms are indistinguishable from other causes of peptic ulcer disease and therefore may go undetected for years. Ulcers usually are solitary and located in the duodenal bulb, but they may be multiple or occur more distally in the duodenum. Isolated gastric ulcers are unusual. Diarrhea occurs in one-third of patients, in some cases in the absence of peptic symptoms. Gastric acid hypersecretion can cause direct intestinal mucosal injury and pancreatic enzyme inactivation, resulting in diarrhea, steatorrhea, and weight loss; nasogastric aspiration stops the diarrhea. Screening for ZES with fasting gastrin levels should be obtained in patients with ulcers that are refractory to standard therapies, giant ulcers (>2 cm), ulcers located distal to the duodenal bulb, multiple duodenal ulcers, frequent ulcer recurrences, ulcers associated with diarrhea, ulcers occurring after ulcer surgery, and patients with ulcer complications. Ulcer patients with hypercalcemia or a family history of ulcers (suggesting MEN 1) should also be screened. Finally, patients with peptic ulcers who are not taking NSAIDs and who are *H pylori* negative should be screened.

B. LABORATORY FINDINGS

The most sensitive and specific method for identifying ZES is demonstration of an increased fasting serum gastrin concentration (>150 pg/mL). Levels should be obtained with patients not taking H_2RA for 24 hours and PPI for 6 days. The median gastrin level in ZES is 500–700 pg/mL, and 60% have levels less than 1000 pg/mL. Hypochlorhydria with increased gastric pH is a much more common cause of hypergastrinemia than is gastrinoma. Therefore, measurement of gastric pH (and, where available, gastric secretory studies) is performed in patients with hypergastrinemia. Most patients have a basal acid output of over 15 mEq/h. A gastric pH of >3.0 implies hypochlorhydria and excludes gastrinoma. In a patient with a serum gastrin >1000 pg/mL and acid hypersecretion, the diagnosis of ZES is established. With lower gastrin levels (100–1000 pg/mL) and acid hypersecretion, a secretin stimulation test is performed to distinguish ZES from other causes of hypergastrinemia.

Intravenous secretin (2 U/kg) produces a rise in serum gastrin of over 200 pg/mL within 2–30 minutes in 85% of patients with gastrinoma. An elevated serum calcium suggests hyperparathyroidism and MEN 1 syndrome. In all patients with ZES, a serum parathyroid hormone (PTH), prolactin lutenizing hormone and follicle stimulating hormone (LH-FSH), and growth hormone (GH) level should be obtained to exclude MEN 1.

C. IMAGING

The approach to therapy is determined in large part by whether there is metastatic disease, and, if not, to identify the site of the primary tumor. Although conventional radiologic studies such as CT, MRI, and transabdominal ultrasonography are commonly obtained, their sensitivity is less than 50–70% for hepatic metastasis and 35% for primary tumors. These studies are being supplanted by somatostatin receptor scintigraphy (SRS) and endoscopic ultrasonography (EUS). The former should be the first study obtained because of its high sensitivity (>90%) for detecting hepatic metastases, although its sensitivity for detecting primary gastrinoma is much lower, particularly for tumors in the pancreas. If SRS is positive for tumor localization, further imaging studies are not necessary. In patients with negative SRS, EUS is indicated to localize the primary tumor. This study has a sensitivity of >90% for tumors of the pancreatic head and can visualize half the tumors in the duodenal wall or adjacent lymph nodes. With a combination of SRS and EUS, more than 90% of primary gastrinomas can now be localized preoperatively.

Differential Diagnosis

Gastrinomas are one of several gut neuroendocrine tumors that have similar histopathologic features and arise either from the gut or pancreas. These include carcinoid, VIPoma, insulinoma, glucagonoma, and somatostatinoma. These tumors are differentiated by the gut peptides they secrete; however, poorly differentiated neuroendocrine tumors may not secrete any hormones. Gut neuroendocrine tumors may present in a number of ways. Functional symptoms arise from the effects of the secreted hormones (eg, ZES, carcinoid syndrome). In other cases, patients may present with symptoms caused by tumor metastases (jaundice, hepatomegaly) rather than functional symptoms. Once a diagnosis of a neuroendocrine tumor is established from the liver biopsy, the specific type of tumor can subsequently be determined. Finally, both carcinoids and gastrinomas can be detected incidentally during endoscopy after biopsy of a submucosal nodule and must be distinguished by subsequent studies.

Hypergastrinemia due to gastrinoma must be distinguished from other causes of hypergastrinemia. Atrophic gastritis with decreased acid secretion is detected by gastric secretory analysis. Other conditions associated with hypergastrinemia (eg, gastric outlet obstruction, vagotomy, chronic renal failure) are associated with a negative secretin stimulation test.

Treatment

A. METASTATIC DISEASE

The most important predictor of survival is the presence of hepatic metastasies. In patients with multiple hepatic metastases, initial therapy should be directed at controlling hypersecretion. Proton-pump inhibitors are given at doses of 40–120 mg/d, titrated to achieve a basal acid output of <10 mEq/h. At this level, there is complete symptom relief and ulcer healing. In patients with isolated hepatic metastases, surgical resection may decrease the need for antisecretory medication and may prolong survival. Because of the slow growth of these tumors, 30% of patients with hepatic metastases survive 10 years.

B. LOCALIZED DISEASE

Cure is achievable only if the gastrinoma can be resected before hepatic metastatic spread has occurred. Lymph node metastases do not adversely affect prognosis. Laparatomy should be considered in all patients in whom preoperative studies fail to demonstrate hepatic or distant metastases. A combination of preoperative studies and intraoperative palpation and sonography allows successful localization and resection in the majority of cases. The 15-year survival of patients who do not have liver metastases at initial presentation is over 80%.

REFERENCES

Aalykke C et al: *Helicobactor pylori* and risk of ulcer bleeding among users of nonsteroidal anti-inflammatory drugs: a case-control study. Gastroenterology 1999;l116:1305.

Bombardier C et al: Comparison of upper gastrointestinal toxicity of rofecoxib and naproxen in patients with rheumatoid arthritis. N Engl J Med 2000;343:1520.

Chan FKL et al: Preventing recurrent upper gastrointestinal bleeding in patients with *Helicobacter pylori* infection who are taking low-dose aspirin or naproxen. N Engl J Med 2001;34: 967.

Chey WD: Diagnosis of *Helicobacter pylori.* Pract Gastroenterol 2001;25:28.

Cohen H: Peptic ulcer and *Helicobacter pylori.* Gastroenterol Clin North Am 2000;29:775.

Delvalle J, Scheiman J, Chey WD: Acid-peptic disorders. In: *Textbook of Gastroenterology,* 4th ed. Yamada T (editor). JB Lippincott Co., in press.

Jyotheeswaran S et al: Prevalence of *Helicobacter pylori* in peptic ulcer patients in greater Rochester, NY: is empirical triple therapy justified? Am J Gastroenterol 1998;93:574.

Kearney DJ: Retreatment of *Helicobacter pylori* infection after initial treatment failure. Am J Gastroenterol 2001;96:1335.

Laine L, Hopkins RJ, Giradi LS: Has the impact of *Helicobacter pylori* therapy on ulcer recurrence in the United States been overstated? A meta-analysis of rigorously designed trials. Am J Gastroenterol 1998;93:1409.

Megraud F, Marshall BJ: How to treat *Helicobacter pylori:* first-line, second-line, and future therapies. Gastroenterol Clin North Am 2000;29:759.

Norton J et al: Surgery to cure Zollinger-Ellison syndrome. N Engl J Med 1999;341:635.

Proye C et al: Noninvasive imaging of insulinomas and gastrinomas with endoscopic ultrasonography and somatostatin receptor scintigraphy. Surgery 1998;124:1143.

Rich M, Scheiman J: Nonsteroidal anti-inflammatory drug gastropathy at the new millennium: mechanisms and prevention. Sem Arthritis Rheum 2000;30:167.

Rostom A et al: Prevention of NSAID-induced gastroduodenal ulcers. Cochrane Database Syst Rev 2000;4:CD002296.

Silverstein FE et al: Gastrointestinal toxicity with celecoxib vs nonsteroidal anti-inflammatory drugs for osteoarthritis and rheumatoid arthritis. The CLASS study: a randomized controlled trial. JAMA 2000;284:1247.

Wolfe MM, Lichtenstein DR, Singh G: Gastrointestinal toxicity of nonsteroidal antiinflammatory drugs. N Engl J Med 1999; 340: 1888.

Dyspepsia & Nonulcer Dyspepsia

Kenneth R. McQuaid, MD

DYSPEPSIA

ESSENTIALS OF DIAGNOSIS

- *Pain or discomfort centered in the upper abdomen.*
- *Commonly associated with upper abdominal fullness, early satiety, bloating, nausea, vomiting, or heartburn.*
- *Clinical history of limited value in distinguishing possible causes.*
- *Signs or symptoms of organic disease ("alarm symptoms") warrant diagnostic investigation.*
- *Endoscopy is study of first choice.*

General Considerations

The word dyspepsia is a medical term that refers to a vague constellation of upper abdominal symptoms. Thus, dyspepsia is a symptom—not a disease. Patients often refer to these symptoms as indigestion, which is used synonymously.

Dyspepsia is prevalent in more than one-fourth of the general adult population and is a frequent cause for medical consultation. Based on population surveys, each year approximately 25% (8–54%) of adults have dyspepsia lasting several days. It accounts for up to 7% of office visits and over half of gastrointestinal complaints in general medical practice. The majority of patients have recurrent or intermittent life-long symptoms. It has a significant impact upon patient quality of life and results in enormous direct and indirect societal costs. The annual attributable medical costs per year to an HMO for a patient with dyspepsia is more than $400. The indirect costs due to decreased productivity and time lost from work are believed to be significant.

The lack of a uniform definition of dyspepsia has hampered efforts of clinical investigators to study patients and compare therapeutic efficacy. A consensus conference (known as "Rome II") has formally defined dyspepsia as *pain or discomfort in the upper abdomen.* Dyspepsia may be characterized by or associated with upper abdominal fullness, early satiety, bloating, nausea, or heartburn. The consensus group has attempted to distinguish patients with probable gastroesophageal reflux disease from other patients with dyspepsia. Patients with dyspepsia may have heartburn (ie, retrosternal burning) as part of their symptom constellation. However, when heartburn is the dominant symptom, it is highly predictive for gastroesophageal reflux and should not be labeled dyspepsia, even when other dyspeptic symptoms are present.

Less than half of patients with dyspepsia ever seek medical attention. The factors that influence patient self-referral are not always clear. The severity or frequency of symptoms, fear of underlying disease (especially cancer), response to over-the-counter medications, illness in a friend or family member, anxiety or psychological stress, and lack of adequate psychosocial support may all be important factors. The physician should attempt to determine the reason for seeking medical care at a given time in order to address the patient's concerns fully.

In evaluating patients with dyspepsia, the practitioner must distinguish between a wide spectrum of "organic" causes, such as peptic ulcer disease or cancer, and nonulcer (also known as "functional") dyspepsia. In making this distinction, the clinician is confronted with a number of potential diagnostic tests and empiric treatment strategies. Upper endoscopy is the "gold standard" test for the diagnostic evaluation of the upper gastrointestinal tract in patients with dyspepsia. However, in many cases an initial empiric treatment strategy may be preferred.

Pathophysiology

Dyspepsia may be caused by a host of foods, medications, diseases of the luminal gastrointestinal (GI) tract, and systemic disorders (Table 21–1). An organic cause is found however in only 40% of patients, most commonly peptic ulcer disease, gastroesophageal reflux disease, and gastric cancer. In over half of patients, no obvious cause of symptoms is found and the dyspepsia is labeled idiopathic or "functional."

A. FOOD INTOLERANCE

A number of foods are reported by patients to provoke dyspepsia, including tomatoes, spicy foods, excessive alcohol, fatty foods, and coffee. The mechanisms by

Table 21–1. Causes of dyspepsia and upper abdominal pain.

Luminal GI tract	Pancreatic disease
Peptic ulcer disease	Chronic pancreatitis
Gastroesophageal reflux	Pancreatic neoplasm
Gastric neoplasms	Systemic conditions
Gastroparesis	Diabetes mellitus
Gastric infiltrative	Thyroid disease
disorders (amyloidosis,	Hyperparathyroidism
Ménétrier's)	Chronic renal insufficiency
Malabsorption syndromes	Pregnancy
Lactose intolerance	Collagen vascular
Parasites (Giardia lamblia)	disorders
AIDS	Ischemic heart disease
Chronic intestinal	Intraabdominal
ischemia	malignancy
Functional gastrointestinal	Miscellaneous causes of
disorders	intermittent abdominal
Nonulcer dyspepsia	pain
Aerophagia	Acute intermittent
Irritable bowel	porphyria
syndrome	Familial Mediterranean
Medications	fever
Nonsteroidal anti-	C_1-esterase deficiency
inflammatory drugs	Diabetic radiculopathy
(NSAIDs)	Nerve entrapment
Theophylline	syndromes
Digitalis	Vertebral nerve
Potassium	compression
Iron	Intussusception or internal
Niacin	hernia
Quinidine	Intermittent small bowel
Antibiotics	obstruction
Alcohol	
Biliary tract disease	
Choleithiasis with biliary	
colic	
Acute cholecystitis	
Choledocholithiasis	
Sphincter of Oddi	
dysfunction	
Hepatobiliary neoplasms	

which food may cause dyspepsia include overeating, delayed gastric emptying (cholecystokinin induced), direct mucosal irritation, or provocation of gastroesophageal reflux. Patients who are lactose intolerant may experience abdominal pain with modest lactose intake, followed by flatulence or diarrhea with larger intake. True food allergies are believed rare in adults.

B. MEDICATIONS

A number of medications can cause severe gastrointestinal irritation and should not be overlooked. Common culprits include nonsteroidal antiinflammatory drugs (NSAIDs), aspirin, potassium supplement, iron, antibiotics, digitalis, corticosteroids, narcotics, colchicine, niacin, quinidine, estrogens, theophylline, ACE inhibitors, loop diuretics, nitrates, and levodopa. Symptom improvement when a patient is taken off a potential offending medication may obviate the need for expensive evaluation.

C. LUMINAL GASTROINTESTINAL TRACT DYSFUNCTION

A number of organic disorders of the upper gastrointestinal tract may cause dyspepsia.

1. Peptic ulcer disease—Approximately 15% of patients referred to primary practitioners with dyspepsia have peptic (gastric or duodenal) ulcers. That is, the majority of patients do *not* have ulcer disease, yet it is the first disease considered by most practitioners. Almost all peptic ulcers occur in patients who are taking NSAIDs and/or who are infected with *Helicobacter pylori*.

2. Gastric neoplasm—Gastric cancer is present in <2% of patients with dyspepsia, but is rare in patients under age 50. More than 98% of gastric cancers occur in patients 50 years of age or older. The risk of gastric cancer is increased in patients with *H pylori* infection, a prior history of gastric surgery, a family history of gastric cancer and immigrants from areas endemic for gastric malignancy. Most gastric cancers presenting with dyspepsia are advanced, with a 5-year survival of 10%. Less than 1:10,000 patients with dyspepsia have a potentially curable gastric malignancy. Over 40% of patients with dyspepsia who present for medical attention report concern about underlying malignancy.

3. Gastroesophageal reflux disease—There is a large overlap between dyspepsia and gastroesophageal reflux disease (GERD). Many patients with dyspepsia also report some heartburn, and up to half of patients with proven GERD experience both dyspepsia and heartburn; a small number may have dyspepsia alone. Overall, among patients presenting with upper GI symptoms (dyspepsia and heartburn), the clinical diagnosis of GERD is only 80% sensitive and 60% specific. However, when symptoms of heartburn and regurgitation dominate the clinical picture, GERD is the likely diagnosis. Given the limited accuracy of clinical diagnosis, a diagnosis of GERD should be considered in all patients with dyspepsia who also have symptoms of heartburn or regurgitation.

4. Other intestinal disorders—Uncommon causes of dyspepsia include malabsorption disorders, infiltrative disorders, and motility disorders of the stomach or small intestine (see Chapters 22 and 23). Chronic mesenteric ischemia may be characterized by postprandial discomfort, sitophobia, and weight loss. Recurrent gastric volvulus may cause dyspepsia and bloating, belching, retching, or vomiting.

D. Pancreaticobiliary Disorders

Chronic pancreatic diseases (chronic pancreatitis or pancreatic cancer) may cause epigastric or periumbilical pain that may be confused with other causes of dyspepsia. Biliary colic due to symptomatic cholelithiasis is usually distinguishable from dyspepsia. There is no evidence that cholelithiasis causes dyspeptic symptoms.

E. Systemic Conditions

Dyspepsia may be present in a number of conditions, including diabetes mellitus, thyroid disease, ischemic heart disease, adrenal insufficiency, and collagen vascular disorders.

F. Nonulcer Dyspepsia

Over half of patients have no apparent organic or biochemical cause of dyspepsia. In these patients, dyspepsia is a manifestation of a chronic functional gastrointestinal disorder and is labeled functional or nonulcer dyspepsia. Dyspepsia commonly is seen in association with other functional gastrointestinal disorders, such as irritable bowel disorder (see Chapter 6).

Clinical Findings

The clinical history is of limited utility in distinguishing among organic disorders, or in distinguishing organic from functional dyspepsia. In evaluating patients with dyspepsia who have not previously undergone diagnostic investigation ("uninvestigated dyspepsia"), the provider must decide whether immediate diagnostic studies (especially endoscopy) are warranted to diagnose organic disorders or whether a course of empiric treatment should first be pursued. The goal of the clinician is to distinguish those patients who have a high likelihood of having a serious organic disorder and therefore require definitive diagnosis from the majority of patients who may be treated initially with empiric antisecretory therapy and/or *H pylori* eradication therapy.

As will be discussed, there is ongoing controversy regarding the relative economic and medical costs of performing early (initial) endoscopy versus empiric medical management for patients with uninvestigated dyspepsia. The optimal strategy is not clear. Recent prospective outcome studies have failed to demonstrate convincingly a benefit of one strategy over another in reduction of overall health care costs, physician visits, and medication use, or in improvement of patient satisfaction. Simply put, there are no compelling data that early endoscopy leads to improved outcomes or that empiric treatment strategies are cost effective. Appropriate guidelines may vary depending upon the costs of

endoscopy, the costs of medical therapy, the prevalence of *H pylori* and peptic ulcer disease, and the prevalence of gastric cancer. The most appropriate strategy is the approach with which both the patient and physician are most comfortable. A suggested algorithm is presented in Figure 22–1.

A. Symptoms and Signs

A careful history and physical examination are mandatory in all patients presenting with dyspepsia that has not previously been investigated. The primary usefulness of the history and physical examination is in identifying patients at high risk for having serious organic disease. These include patients with dyspepsia who have "alarm symptoms": (1) dysphagia, (2) weight loss, (3) evidence of gastrointestinal bleeding (hematemesis, melena, hematochezia, iron deficiency anemia, or fecal occult blood), or (4) signs of upper gastrointestinal obstruction (marked early satiety, vomiting). Patients with "alarm symptoms" require urgent endoscopy to exclude complicated peptic ulcer disease, GERD, or malignancy.

It was previously believed that certain historic features of dyspepsia helped to distinguish gastric ulcer, duodenal ulcer, nonulcer dyspepsia, and other causes of dyspepsia. Clinicians were taught to ask about the location of abdominal pain, the site of pain radiation, and the pain's rhythmicity and periodicity. The classic symptoms of peptic ulcer disease (especially duodenal ulcers) are epigastric pain that is not severe, fluctuates in intensity throughout the day and night, is relieved by food or antacids, and may awaken the patient from sleep. Nonulcer dyspepsia patients are more likely to report exacerbation of symptoms after meals and seldom have nocturnal pain. With the advent of upper endoscopy, it has become apparent that these features have limited diagnostic value. Even seasoned clinicians are correct only half the time in distinguishing peptic ulcer disease from functional dyspepsia based on history alone (Table 21–2).

Some groups have tried to classify symptoms of dyspepsia into the subgroups *ulcer-like dyspepsia* and *dysmotility-like dyspepsia* in hopes that these would improve diagnostic accuracy, predict underlying pathophysiology, and guide empiric treatment. For example, ulcer-like dyspepsia (well-localized pain occurring at night or between meals and relieved by food) might predict a higher likelihood of peptic ulcer disease, whereas dysmotility-like dyspepsia (poorly localized symptoms aggravated by meals and accompanied by postprandial fullness, nausea, bloating, or vomiting) might predict underlying gastroparesis. Unfortunately, the subgroupings have proven to be of no clinical utility. They do not reliably predict findings on upper endoscopy or distinguish functional from organic dyspep-

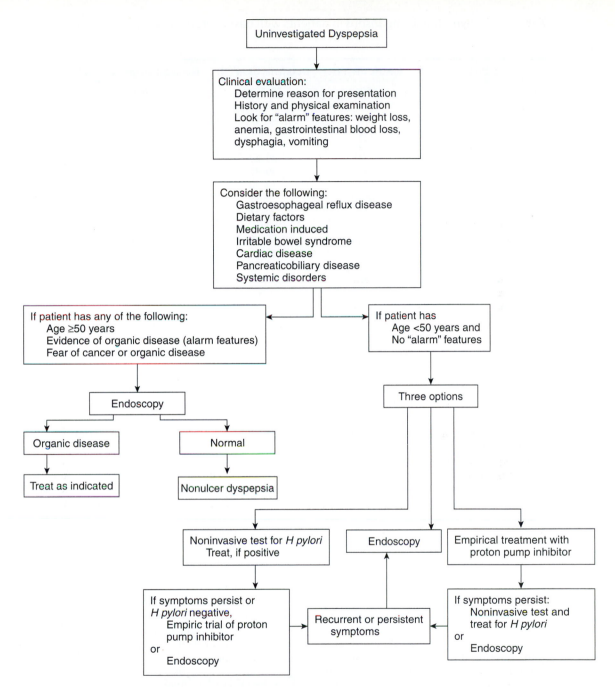

Figure 21–1. Suggested approach to the evaluation of dyspepsia.

Table 21–2. Symptom comparisons in patients with gastric ulcer, duodenal ulcer, and nonulcer dyspepsia.

Symptom	Gastric Ulcer (%)	Duodenal Ulcer (%)	Nonulcer Dyspepsia (%)
Age	>50 yr	30–60 yr	>20 yr
Features of pain			
Epigastric	67	61–86	52–73
Frequently severe	68	53	37
Within 30 minutes of food	20	5	32
Relieved by food	2–48	20–63	4–32
Relieved by antacids	36–87	39–86	26–75
Increased by food	24	10–40	45
Occurs at night	32–43	50–88	24–32
Radiation to back	34	20–31	24–28
Clusters (episodic)	16	56	35
Anorexia	46–57	25–36	26–36
Weight loss	24–61	19–45	18–32
Vomiting	38–73	25–57	26–34
Bloating	55	49	52
Belching	48	59	60
Heartburn	19	27–59	28

Modified, with permission, from Soll AH: Duodenal ulcers and drug therapy. In: *Gastrointestinal Diseases.* Sleisenger M, Fordtran J (editors). WB Saunders Co, 1989, p. 814.

sia. In contrast, approximately two-thirds of patients who have *heartburn* or *regurgitation* either as dominant symptoms or in concert with other dyspeptic symptoms ("reflux-like dyspepsia") should be given a presumptive diagnosis of gastroesophageal reflux, as half to two-thirds will respond to antisecretory therapies.

Certain historic features are important in distinguishing dyspepsia from other causes of upper abdominal pain. Severe pain or pain that radiates to the back suggests complicated ulcer disease (perforation or penetration), biliary tract disease, pancreatitis, or an abdominal aortic aneurysm. Pain in the right upper quadrant is unusual for ulcer disease or nonulcer dyspepsia and suggests biliary tract disease. Biliary colic begins abruptly, is steady, lasts for up to several hours, and subsides gradually. The pain of acute pancreatitis is epigastric or periumbilical, severe, and unrelenting, and radiates to the back. In contrast, the pain of chronic pancreatitis is less severe, waxes and wanes for days to weeks at a time, and may be misinterpreted as dyspepsia. Mild weight loss may occur in patients with gastric ulcer but is uncommon in duodenal ulcer or nonulcer dyspepsia. Significant weight loss is worrisome for complicated peptic ulcer disease with gastric outlet obstruction, gastric or pancreatic malignancy, or chronic pancreatitis with malabsorption. Occasional vomiting may occur with peptic ulcer disease or nonulcer dyspepsia, but severe vomiting of undigested food suggests gastric retention due to gastric outlet obstruction or impaired gastric motility (gastroparesis). Patients younger than 45 years of age with uncomplicated dyspepsia who also have lower abdominal pain or discomfort with altered bowel habits likely have irritable bowel syndrome.

B. PHYSICAL EXAMINATION

The physical examination should be normal in patients with uncomplicated dyspepsia, but it is mandatory to look for signs of serious organic disease. Furthermore, the "laying on of hands" may be reassuring to patients with functional dyspepsia, demonstrating to them that their symptoms are being taken seriously. Symptoms and signs of systemic disorders that may cause dyspepsia, such as cardiac disease, diabetes, and thyroid disease, should be considered. Mild, localized epigastric tenderness is found commonly in patients with peptic ulcers and nonulcer dyspepsia. Signs of serious organic disease, such as weight loss, organomegaly, abdominal mass, jaundice, or fecal occult blood, warrant immediate investigation.

C. LABORATORY FINDINGS

1. Routine laboratory tests—In patients over age 45–50 years, a complete blood count, routine electrolyte measurement, calcium, liver chemistries, and thyroid function studies should be considered. In younger patients with uncomplicated dyspepsia, these studies generally are unnecessary. Other studies such as amylase, stool for ova and parasites, and pregnancy tests are ordered as needed. Anemia may occur from acute or chronic upper gastrointestinal blood loss and requires prompt endoscopic evaluation. Elevated liver chemistries suggest hepatitis or biliary tract disease. Elevated amylase may suggest acute or chronic pancreatitis, penetrating ulcer, or choledocholithiasis.

2. Noninvasive "test and treat" for *H pylori* infection—Chronic infection with *H pylori* is associated with over 80% of peptic ulcers and 50% of gastric ulcers. Almost all other peptic ulcers are caused by NSAIDs or aspirin. The prevalence of *H pylori* infection in industrialized countries in patients with dyspepsia is 30–50%, but this is declining. Of patients with dyspepsia who are infected with *H pylori,* less than one-half have a peptic ulcer; most others have functional dyspepsia.

In patients younger than 45–50 years of age with uncomplicated dyspepsia (ie, those who have no "alarm features"), it has been the consensus opinion of a number of expert panels that noninvasive testing for *H pylori* infection should be performed using serologic tests, urease breath test, or fecal antigen testing (see Chapter 20). Patients testing positive for *H pylori* should be treated with an empiric course of antibiotics. Empiric *H pylori* eradication therapy of patients with dyspepsia and positive noninvasive tests for *H pylori* resolves dyspepsia in the majority of patients who have undiagnosed peptic ulcer disease, but does not have a significant impact upon symptoms in infected patients who have nonulcer dyspepsia. At least two-thirds of patients will not have evidence of *H pylori* infection and are unlikely to have peptic ulcer disease. Decision analytic models have suggested that this "test-and-treat" strategy is more cost effective than early endoscopy in young patients with uncomplicated dyspepsia. However, recent prospective randomized trials comparing empiric "test-and-treat" therapy with early endoscopy in primary care settings suggest that there may be no long-term differences between these strategies in overall costs, quality of life, or visits to physicians.

D. ENDOSCOPY

Upper endoscopy is the "gold standard" for evaluating the upper gastrointestinal tract in patients with dyspepsia because of its diagnostic accuracy and the ability to perform biopsies, as needed. It allows accurate diagnosis (or exclusion) of peptic ulcer disease, erosive esophagitis and Barrett's esophagus, and malignancy. For these reasons, it should be performed in all patients with dyspepsia who have "alarm features" (as defined above). Endoscopy also should be performed in patients with new-onset dyspepsia who are 50 years of age or older (due to increased risk of gastric malignancy) and immigrants from regions in which gastric cancer is endemic (eg, Japan, China, Chile). Endoscopy also should be employed to allay excessive patient anxiety about serious disease or "cancer phobia."

There is ongoing controversy pertaining to the role of endoscopy in patients with uncomplicated dyspepsia who are younger than 50 years of age. Specifically, there is debate as to whether patients first should undergo empiric "test and treat" for *H pylori* and/or a course of empiric antisecretory therapy. As discussed above, many expert panels have endorsed empiric strategies rather than endoscopy for the initial approach to such patients. However, prospective studies comparing empiric treatment strategies to early endoscopy in patients with uncomplicated dyspepsia have suggested that neither strategy is superior or more cost effective than the other. Thus, the decision to pursue empiric treatment or endoscopy should be determined jointly by the patient and physician. If an empiric treatment strategy is pursued, diagnostic endoscopy should be performed if symptoms persist or recur after treatment is discontinued. In patients with dyspepsia whose endoscopy is normal, endoscopists are discouraged from taking gastric biopsies to look for chronic *H pylori* infection. Such patients are presumed to have nonulcer dyspepsia, and there is no evidence that treatment of *H pylori* leads to symptomatic improvement in such patients (see section, "Nonulcer Dyspepsia").

E. OTHER IMAGING STUDIES

With the advent of upper endoscopy, the upper gastrointestinal series no longer plays a significant role in the evaluation of dyspepsia. Its use should be restricted to health care settings in which endoscopy is unavailable or in patients in whom endoscopy cannot be safely performed. An upper GI series is less sensitive and specific than endoscopy, and does not allow tissue biopsy. It has limited accuracy in distinguishing benign from gastric ulcers. Therefore, all patients with gastric ulcers identified on upper gastrointestinal (UGI) series should be fully evaluated by endoscopy after 8–12 weeks of therapy.

Abdominal ultrasonography and/or computed tomographic imaging are not indicated in patients with uncomplicated dyspepsia. They may be obtained in patients with suspected biliary tract disease, chronic pancreatitis, or intraabdominal malignancy.

Differential Diagnosis

The differential diagnosis of dyspepsia is discussed in the previous sections. Other causes of severe epigastric or periumbilical pain (which should not be confused with typical dyspepsia) include complicated peptic ulcer disease (penetration or perforation), acute pancreatitis, acute cholecystitis, chronic intestinal ischemia, gastric volvulus, intermittent small bowel obstruction, aortic dissection, ruptured aortic aneurysm, incarcerated hernia, ureteral colic, and myocardial infarction. Other causes of chronic abdominal pain (not to be confused with dyspepsia) include acute intermittent porphyria, lead poisoning, familial Mediterranean fever, C_1-esterase deficiency, diabetic radiculopathy, and vertebral nerve root compression.

Treatment

The treatment of dyspepsia is directed at the specific underlying cause, most commonly identified by endoscopy. However, in many cases, the physician or the patient may decide that initial diagnostic evaluation is not warranted and that a course of empiric management is warranted. Many patients present with mild symptoms of short duration that resolve spontaneously. Others may have symptoms that are mild and long-standing, for which an initial trial of dietary and lifestyle modifications may be reasonable. Careful history may reveal a correlation between initiation of a medication and symptom development, for which a trial off medications (especially aspirin and NSAIDs) may be warranted. The reasons for medical consultation at this time should be elicited so that specific fears and concerns can be addressed. Careful inquiry into the patient's social or family history may uncover stresses that are contributing to symptomatic worsening or current concern about chronic symptoms.

A. ANTACIDS OR BISMUTH SUBSALICYLATE

Both antacids and bismuth compounds are used widely as over-the-counter preparations for treatment of acute dyspepsia, although almost no studies have been performed that support their efficacy. Antacids (aluminum/magnesium hydroxide preparations; calcium carbonate) may be used in patients with infrequent dyspepsia, especially when attributable to dietary overindulgence or indiscretion. They are not suitable for chronic therapy. Bismuth subsalicylate (Pepto Bismol) may also be used on an infrequent basis for intermittent dyspepsia. Because small amounts of bismuth and salicylate are absorbed, chronic use is not recommended.

B. ANTISECRETORY AGENTS

Empiric therapy for 4–8 weeks with acid antisecretory agents (H_2-receptor antagonists or proton-pump inhibitors) may be expected to provide symptom improvement or relief to the subset of patients with dyspepsia caused by GERD or peptic ulcer disease. Antisecretory agents have little or no efficacy in the treatment of nonulcer dyspepsia (see section, "Nonulcer Dyspepsia"). For the empiric treatment of uncomplicated dyspepsia, antisecretory therapy may be given to all dys-

peptics, to those without evidence of *H pylori* infection on noninvasive testing, or to those with *H pylori* infection whose symptoms persist or relapse after antibiotic therapy.

H_2-receptor antagonists are available as over-the-counter formulations (ranitidine or nizatidine 75 mg; famotidine 10 mg; cimetidine 200 mg). Generic preparations of ranitidine and cimetidine are available by prescription, which in most situations are less expensive than proprietary agents or over-the-counter preparations. Patients may take H_2-antgonists on as an "as needed" basis, however onset of action may take 30–60 minutes. When used chronically, they are best administered in twice daily regimens: ranitidine or nizatidine 75–150 mg twice a day, famotidine 10–20 mg twice a day, or cimetidine 200–800 mg twice a day.

The proton-pump inhibitors afford potent (>95–99%) inhibition of gastric acid secretion. Five agents are available: omeprazole and rabeprazole 20 mg, lansoprazole 30 mg, and esomeprazole and pantoprazole 40 mg, all given on a once daily basis. In most health care settings, these agents are significantly more expensive than H_2-antagonists. Nonetheless, a 4-week course of a proton-pump inhibitor may be the preferred empiric therapeutic approach due to the potent acid inhibition afforded by these agents. Failure of symptoms to improve with acid inhibition is strong evidence that the patient does not have GERD or peptic ulcer disease—and most likely has functional dyspepsia.

C. *H PYLORI* ERADICATION THERAPY

In patients found to have *H pylori* infection on noninvasive testing, empiric eradication treatment is recommended. Suitable antibiotic regimens are discussed in Chapter 20. The most widely employed treatment consists of three agents: proton-pump inhibitor (lansoprazole 30 mg or omeprazole 20 mg), clarithromycin 500 mg, and either amoxicillin 1 g or metronidazole 500 mg. Each of these drugs is given twice daily for 10 days.

Prognosis

The prognosis for patients with dyspepsia is determined by the underlying cause. Patients with gastroesophageal reflux may be expected to experience excellent relief of symptoms with lifestyle changes and antisecretory medications. However, >80% will experience a symptomatic relapse within 1 year after discontinuation of therapy. Intermittent or continuous treatment usually is required. More than 80% of patients with peptic ulcer disease caused by *H pylori* are cured of their ulcers (and dyspepsia) after one course of appropriate antibiotic therapy. Symptom relapse may be attributable to recurrent ulcer caused by persistent *H pylori* infection or NSAIDs, or to gastroesophageal reflux or nonulcer dyspepsia. Upper endoscopy is required to distinguish among these possibilities. Recurrent ulcers may be treated with an additional course of eradication therapy or with a chronic proton-pump inhibitor. Approximately 1% of patients with dyspepsia ultimately are proven to have gastric malignancy, which generally is advanced. There is no evidence that empiric management for 2–3 months prior to definitive endoscopic diagnosis compromises patient outcome.

NONULCER DYSPEPSIA

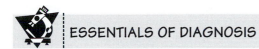

ESSENTIALS OF DIAGNOSIS

- *Dyspepsia of at least several weeks duration for which no obvious organic cause can be found.*
- *No abnormalities on physical examination or laboratory profile that explain symptoms.*
- *No focal or structural abnormalities at upper endoscopy.*

General Considerations

Half to two-thirds of patients with chronic dyspepsia do not have significant focal or structural lesions identified at upper endoscopy. These patients are labeled as having nonulcer or functional dyspepsia. A variety of other terms have been used more or less synonymously by clinicians, including nonorganic dyspepsia, essential dyspepsia, and dyspepsia of unknown origin. Even if further diagnostic studies are pursued in these patients to exclude mild (nonerosive) gastroesophageal reflux, irritable bowel syndrome, and pancreaticobiliary disorders, up to one-half of cases of chronic dyspepsia remain unexplained.

The costs of evaluating and treating nonulcer dyspepsia are enormous. It is estimated that the direct medical costs are $2 billion per year in the United States. The indirect costs due to time lost from work and decreased productivity may be even greater. Limited studies suggest that chronic dyspepsia impacts upon quality of life, interfering with daily activities, sleep, work, socializing, eating, and drinking, and contributes to emotional stress. Symptoms remain chronic in the majority, although symptom improvement or resolution may occur in up to half of patients over time.

Pathophysiology

The causes of nonulcer dyspepsia are poorly understood but appear to be heterogeneous. This disorder is part of a continuum of functional GI disorders that involves the entire gut, including functional heartburn, irritable bowel syndrome, noncardiac chest pain, and pelvic floor disorders. Patients with functional gut disorders often manifest a variety of GI symptoms as well as extragut symptoms, such as migraine headaches, fibromyalgia, and urinary or gynecologic complaints.

Patients with functional GI disorders may be best understood in the context of the biopsychosocial model of illness in which symptoms are postulated to arise out of a complex interaction between abnormal gastrointestinal physiology and psychosocial factors that affect how the individual perceives, interprets, and responds to the abnormal GI physiology. Higher neural centers may modulate GI sensation, motility, and secretion. Individuals with altered physiology who have a stable psychosocial profile either may not seek medical care or may respond to reassurance and lifestyle changes. Other patients with similar abnormalities in GI physiology who have psychological problems, increased life stress, or poor social support may be more likely to seek medical attention. Furthermore, the psychosocial stressors may exacerbate GI pathophysiology.

In evaluating the patient with functional dyspepsia, both the physiologic and psychosocial factors that have given rise to the symptoms must be considered. Pathophysiologic mechanisms may be identified in the majority of patients, however successful therapy is dependent upon an understanding of the patient's psychosocial variables.

A number of physiologic and psychological factors have been identified, but their relative importance is disputed. These factors are not mutually exclusive, and in many patients a number may be operative.

A. DIETARY AND ENVIRONMENTAL FACTORS

Patients with nonulcer dyspepsia often cite a number of dietary triggers. Many report that coffee, alcohol, tomatoes, citrus, fruits, spicy foods, and rich or fatty foods can exacerbate symptoms, however double-blind challenges dispute the importance of these claims.

B. ABNORMALITIES IN GASTRIC MOTILITY

Abnormalities in gastric motor function can be demonstrated in up to 60% of patients. Using a variety of tests, abnormalities can be demonstrated in gastric emptying, accommodation, and myoelectrical activity. However, the importance of these abnormalities in causing symptoms is debated.

A delay in gastric emptying of meals can be demonstrated in 40% of patients using scintigraphic studies or ultrasonography. Therapeutic trials, however, have shown poor correlation between symptom improvement and improvement in the rate of gastric emptying.

Ultrasonography and barostats have shown that up to half of patients have poor accommodation of the proximal stomach after a meal. After a meal, the fundus relaxes (accommodates) to decrease intragastric pressures, followed by a gradual redistribution of food to the antrum for mixing and emptying. Impaired accommodation of the proximal stomach leads to early antral filling with symptoms of early satiety and pain. Accommodation is controlled by vagal pathways mediated through release of nitric oxide and serotonin $5-HT_1$. Vagal autonomic dysfunction is demonstrated in some patients with impaired accommodation.

Gastroduodenal manometry is used to measure gastric contractile activity in the fasting and postprandial state. Electrogastrography can measure fasting and postprandial electrical activity. Gastric dysrhythmias can be demonstrated in 40% of patients with functional dyspepsia, but also in 20% of normal subjects. They do not appear to be associated with a specific symptom profile or to have a relation to abnormalities in gastric emptying.

C. Visceral Hypersensitivity

The majority of symptoms arising from the gastrointestinal tract are not consciously perceived. A lowering of the perception threshold for gastric distention can be demonstrated in over 50% of patients with functional dyspepsia. The cause of this visceral hypersensitivity is unknown, but may be due to sensitization of peripheral gastric mechanoreceptors (due to inflammation, injury, or inherited defect), dysfunction of descending spinal inhibitory pathways that normally modulate visceral sensation, or altered central nervous system (CNS) processing of afferent sensation resulting in increased patient vigilance for or amplification of visceral stimuli. Hypersensitivity is not related to abnormalities in gastric acid secretion, fundic accommodation, or gastric emptying. However, it is hypothesized that patients with visceral hypersensitivity are more likely to experience discomfort or pain when pathophysiologic abnormalities are present. Hypersensitivity is demonstrated in patients with functional dyspepsia as well as people with functional dyspepsia who have never consulted a physician. It does not appear to be related to the presence of psychological abnormalities.

D. Helicobacter pylori

Acute infection with *H pylori* causes transient symptoms of dyspepsia and vomiting. However, the overwhelming preponderance of data demonstrate that *H pylori* does not play a major role in causing chronic dyspepsia. A meta-analysis of 30 observational studies involving almost 4000 patients with functional dyspepsia concluded that there was no significant association between chronic *H pylori* infection and functional dys-

pepsia. Furthermore, studies have not found a relationship between *H pylori* infection and pathophysiologic abnormalities associated with functional dyspepsia. Specifically, infection has not been shown to affect gastric emptying, accommodation, or visceral sensation. The strongest evidence against the role of *H pylori* as a causative factor in functional dyspepsia comes from controlled therapeutic trials of *H pylori* eradication, which demonstrate no long-term improvement in symptoms. Three randomized, prospective, double-blind, placebo-controlled trials involving almost 900 infected patients with functional dyspepsia failed to demonstrate improvement of symptoms 1 year after successful *H pylori* eradication. A meta-analysis of 7 prospective therapeutic trials reported a nonsignificant odds ratio for symptom improvement of 1.29 (95% CI 0.89–1.89) with *H pylori* therapy compared with placebo. In sum, there is little evidence supporting an important causal role for *H pylori* in functional dyspepsia. Although the therapeutic trials do not exclude the possibility that a small number of patients (up to 10%) with functional dyspepsia derive some benefit from *H pylori* eradication therapy, it is clear that in the vast majority the organism plays no pathogenetic role.

E. Gastroesophageal Reflux

Although the symptoms of heartburn and regurgitation are specific for GERD, many patients with GERD do not present with such obvious symptoms. Approximately one-third of patients report both heartburn and dyspepsia. Whether the dyspeptic symptoms are due to acid reflux or to concomitant functional dyspepsia is not clear. In some patients with GERD, dyspepsia may dominate the picture or even be the sole symptom. A normal endoscopy is found in half of patients with proven GERD and therefore does not exclude the presence of GERD in patients with dyspeptic symptoms.

F. Psychosocial Factors

The degree to which psychosocial stressors contribute to chronic dyspepsia should be assessed. These factors may be an important determinant of health care-seeking behavior. Among people in the community with dyspepsia who have never sought medical attention, there is no increase in psychological abnormalities. However, patients with functional dyspepsia seeking medical attention score higher on personality inventories in areas of anxiety and neuroticism and have a higher incidence of psychiatric disorders, including depression, panic disorders, generalized anxiety disorders, and somatoform disorders. Psychosocial factors correlate with the number of gastrointestinal symptoms as well as extraintestinal complaints (fatigue, headaches).

The role of acute and chronic life stresses in dyspepsia is uncertain. Stress could perhaps cause symptoms by altering motility, autonomic regulation, or visceral pain threshold. Although painful physical and cognitive stressors can be shown to affect these factors in a laboratory setting, the relevance of these studies to acute and chronic life stresses is unknown. Studies of patients with functional dyspepsia who seek medical attention indicate that most patients are experiencing at least one chronic stressor (eg, marital, employment, financial, illness). Some studies also suggest that patients have impaired coping styles and less social support. It is hypothesized that life stressors may trigger the onset of symptoms and the decision to seek medical attention, but psychological factors, social support, and coping strategies determine the severity and duration of symptomatology.

Clinical Findings

As previously discussed, nonulcer dyspepsia cannot be reliably distinguished by history and physical examination from organic causes of dyspepsia. This difficulty may be contrasted with irritable bowel syndrome, another functional syndrome that can be diagnosed with a high degree of reliability from the clinical findings alone.

The diagnosis of functional dyspepsia is a diagnosis of exclusion. Other structural and organic causes of dyspepsia must first be excluded by physical examination, laboratory studies, upper endoscopy, and, in some cases, abdominal imaging studies. A full discussion of the approach to dyspepsia is given in the previous section.

A. SYMPTOMS AND SIGNS

Patients complain of vague abdominal discomfort that is described as gnawing, burning, aching, or heavy. Many may complain of bloating, early satiety, nausea, occasional vomiting, belching, heartburn, or exacerbation by meals. Nocturnal symptoms are uncommon. Symptoms tend to wax and wane, with periods of minimal symptomatology alternating with symptomatic episodes lasting days to weeks.

Some clinical investigators have tried to classify patients with functional dyspepsia into symptom subgroups: reflux-like (dyspepsia with heartburn or regurgitation), ulcer-like, or dysmotility-like. With the exception of "reflux-like dyspepsia," these symptom subgroups are of little utility. They do not correlate with pathophysiologic disturbances or clinical response to therapies. For example, "dysmotility-like" symptoms do not have a higher prevalence of gastroparesis or impaired accommodation and do not necessarily have a better response to promotility agents. In contrast, patients with "reflux-like" dyspepsia have a higher prevalence of gastroesophageal reflux and a better response to antisecretory therapies.

The physical examination in functional dyspepsia should be normal. Signs of serious organic disease (severe pain, weight loss, palpable abdominal mass, or fecal occult blood) cannot be attributed to nonulcer dyspepsia and mandate further investigation.

B. LABORATORY STUDIES

Laboratory studies (see section, "Dyspepsia") should be normal.

C. ENDOSCOPY

The indications for endoscopy are discussed in the section on "Dyspepsia." All patients with chronic unexplained dyspepsia and/or dyspepsia that does not respond to empiric medical therapy warrant upper endoscopic examination. By definition, patients with nonulcer dyspepsia have normal or nonspecific endoscopic findings. Careful attention should be given to the gastroesophageal junction to look for evidence of GERD. It is controversial as to whether gastric biopsies should be obtained to look for evidence of H pylori infection. Because chronic H pylori infection has not been shown to be a cause of functional dyspepsia, there would appear to be no reason to perform a biopsy. However, some clinicians believe that diagnostic biopsy is justified in view of the strong relationship of H pylori to peptic ulcer disease and gastric cancer.

D. ABDOMINAL IMAGING

Abdominal ultrasonography or computerized tomography commonly is ordered in patients with chronic symptoms and normal endoscopy to screen for pancreatic and biliary disorders or intraabdominal malignancy. The yield of these studies in patients with normal physical examination and normal laboratory data is low. Although they should not be obtained routinely, in difficult patients they may provide reassurance to the patient as well as the physician that no serious pathology has been overlooked.

E. OTHER STUDIES

Nuclear gastric scintigraphic emptying studies and gastroduodenal manometry are not useful in most patients and should not be obtained routinely. Although abnormal in up to half of patients, they do not help establish the diagnosis or guide therapy.

As discussed, neither the clinical history nor endoscopy reliably excludes gastroesophageal reflux in patients with dyspepsia. Ambulatory esophageal pH testing is a valuable tool to diagnose GERD in patients with atypical symptoms. In most cases however, it is more practical to treat patients with an empiric trial of a proton-pump inhibitor. Failure of symptoms of dyspepsia and/or heartburn to improve after 4 weeks of a proton-pump inhibitor is strong evidence that symptoms are not caused by acid reflux.

Differential Diagnosis

The differential diagnosis of dyspepsia and upper abominal pain is discussed in the section, "Dyspepsia." Patients with chronic dyspepsia should be distinguished from those with irritable bowel syndrome and chronic intractable abdominal pain (CIAP). Approximately one-third of patients with irritable bowel syndrome also report dyspepsia (see Chapter 6). Patients with CIAP report a long history of abdominal pain that is diffuse and tends to be described in vague or bizarre terms that do not conform to normal physiology. They commonly report a number of extraintestinal somatic complaints. The majority of CIAP patients have severe psychological problems, including depression and somatoform disorders. These patients tend to have little insight into their psychological condition and can be extremely difficult to manage. Referral to a multidisciplinary pain clinic is appropriate.

Treatment

A. GENERAL MANAGEMENT

The approach to the patient with functional gastrointestinal disorders is discussed in Chapter 6. In general, the most important aspect of therapy is the development of a therapeutic relationship between the patient and physician. The physician should foster the trust of the patient by taking a complete history and performing a thorough physical examination. An attempt should be made to determine the reason that the patient with chronic symptoms has presented at this time. The patient's fears (eg, cancer phobia) should be addressed and allayed. Life stresses should be explored, particularly those related to the patient's family, workplace, personal relationships, or living situation, that may have caused decompensation in a person previously coping adequately with chronic symptoms. Recent changes in diet and medications should be reviewed. The physician should take note of the patient's psychological state, as gastrointestinal symptoms may be somatic manifestations of serious psychiatric disease, such as depression, anxiety, or even psychosis.

After the initial evaluation, the differential diagnosis should be discussed with the patient, including the possibility of functional dyspepsia. A reasonable, cost-effective work-up should be proposed that addresses the patient's concerns and the physician's needs. Although in most cases this will include endoscopy (if not previously performed), an empiric trial of therapy may be appropriate in younger patients. After the diagnosis is established, the patient should be told that the diagnosis is

functional dyspepsia and that this is a recognized clinical entity. The tendency to "overinvestigate" should be resisted. Emphasis should shift from finding a cause of the dyspepsia to helping the patient cope with chronic symptoms.

Reassurance and education are extremely important. The pathogenesis of symptoms in functional disorders should be explained. It should be emphasized that the vast majority of patients with nonulcer dyspepsia have physiologic abnormalities—lest the patient infer that the physician is implying he or she is "crazy" or that "it's all in my head." Fear that the symptoms will progress or degenerate into ulcer or cancer should be allayed.

It is important for the physician to set reasonable goals and expectations for the patient. Symptoms tend to be chronic. It will be necessary for the patient to learn to cope with symptoms through lifestyle and behavioral changes. The majority of patients will be reassured by the above approach and require little or no ongoing care. A subset will require ongoing attention either for chronically or for symptomatic exacerbations. The value of the ongoing relationship in modifying symptoms cannot be overemphasized. In multiple clinical trials, symptomatic improvement occurs in over half of patients treated with placebo. Although most clinicians are not psychotherapists, patients clearly derive benefit from a stable therapeutic relationship. Over the course of time, life events that trigger symptoms may become evident. Similarly, psychological abnormalities that were not initially apparent may manifest. In some cases, referral to a trained psychologist, family counselor, or social worker is indicated. If a trusting relationship has been established, most patients will acquiesce to such a referral.

B. LIFE-STYLE CHANGES

Although the role of foods in chronic dyspepsia is unclear, many patients report symptomatic improvement with dietary alterations. Excessive coffee and alcohol should be eliminated. Smaller portions reduce postprandial symptoms. In some cases, a food diary in which patients record foods ingested, level of symptoms, and daily activities may be helpful. These chronicles may suggest foods or life stresses that precipitate symptoms. Patients should be counseled on stress reduction measures, such as exercise and good eating and sleeping habits. Classes in stress reduction or meditation may be suitable for some people.

C. MEDICATIONS

Drug therapy should be reserved for patients who fail to improve after reassurance and life-style changes. Results of drug treatment trials for functional dyspepsia have been disappointing. Meta-analyses of these trials have concluded that there is no unequivocal evidence of efficacy of any agent in the treatment of functional dyspepsia, with the *possible* exception of proton-pump inhibitors.

1. Antisecretory agents—The use of H_2-receptor antagonists (H_2RAs) is of dubious value. Response rates in controlled clinical trials range from 35 to 80% compared with placebo response rates of 30–60%. Some meta-analyses of these trials suggest that H_2RAs reduce the relative risk of dyspepsia by 30%, but the quality of these studies is poor. Any benefit that is seen appears to be confined to the subset of patients with dyspepsia and heartburn, that is, patients who most likely have undiagnosed GERD.

More recently, several well-designed, randomized, multicenter, double-blind trials have been performed comparing the efficacy of proton-pump inhibitors to placebo or H_2RAs in patients with functional dyspepsia. In four multicenter trials, symptom relief was achieved in 34–44% of patients treated with proton-pump inhibitors (omeprazole 10–20 mg/d or lansoprazole 15–30 mg/d) for 4–8 weeks compared with 26–33% of those treated with placebo—but in two of these studies this small difference was significant. In another multicenter trial, symptoms resolved in 20% more patients treated with a proton-pump inhibitor than with placebo, but there was little therapeutic gain compared with use of H_2RAs, which demonstrated 8–12% improvement compared with placebo. Subset analyses suggest that patients most likely to respond to proton-pump inhibitors are those with reflux-like dyspepsia (ie, heartburn and dyspepsia) and those with predominant epigastric pain (rather than discomfort). Proton-pump inhibitors are 30% more effective than placebo in patients with reflux-like symptoms and 10% more effective in patients with predominant epigastric pain. Symptoms of abdominal discomfort, nausea, and bloating are unimproved with proton-pump inhibitors.

In summary, proton-pump inhibitors are useful in a subset of patients with functional dyspepsia—primarily those with heartburn or predominant epigastric pain. It is unlikely that they afford any benefit to other patients with chronic dyspepsia. In the subset who benefit, it is not established that proton-pump inhibitors are superior to less expensive H_2-receptor antagonists.

2. Promotility agents—Promotility agents decrease gastroesophageal reflux, improve gastric emptying, and facilitate accommodation and might thereby be predicted to benefit patients with functional dyspepsia. Meta-analyses of small trials of promotility agents suggested that cisapride and domperidone achieved an impressive therapeutic gain of up to 40% above placebo, however, methodologic flaws in most of these studies precludes any legitimate conclusions. Several large well-

designed trials have failed to confirm significant benefit of cisapride in functional dyspepsia. At the present time, the issue of whether promotility agents benefit patients has been rendered moot by the lack of safe, available agents. Metoclopramide is the only agent available in the United States, but has undergone only limited testing for dyspepsia. The high incidence of adverse CNS effects and extrapyramidal effects associated with this drug makes it unsuitable for long-term use. Cisapride has been voluntarily withdrawn by the manufacturer due to a low but significant risk of QT prolongation and cardiac arrhythmias. Although domperidone is available in many countries, application for approval in the United States is not being pursued by the manufacturer at this time.

3. Antidepressants—Antidepressants are commonly used in the treatment of functional GI disorders, including functional dyspepsia, despite a dearth of controlled clinical trials demonstrating benefit. Benefit of these agents appears to be independent of their psychiatric effects, improvement in sleep, or reduction in visceral sensitivity. A neuromodulatory effect at the spinal cord or CNS level is hypothesized. Based upon uncontrolled, anecdotal experience, use of low doses of tricyclic antidepressants is favored. Experts recommend use of nortriptyline or desipramine, beginning at 10–25 mg/d, increasing slowly to 50–75 mg/d. Side effects are common, and it may be necessary to try several agents. Serotonin reuptake inhibitors may cause dyspepsia and are less commonly used for treatment of nonulcer dyspepsia.

4. Anti-*H pylori* eradication treatment—As discussed previously, meta-analyses of controlled trials do not indicate that eradication of *H pylori* leads to significant improvement in symptoms in patients with functional dyspepsia. Therefore, routine screening and treatment for *H pylori* are not recommended in patients with functional dyspepsia. Many patients, however, are aware of the relationship between *H pylori*, ulcer disease, and cancer, and request or insist upon noninvasive testing. In the patient with functional dyspepsia and proven *H pylori* infection, treatment is advisable.

5. Miscellaneous agents—Herbal and other nonprescription preparations are available for the treatment of nonulcer dyspepsia but have undergone little controlled testing. A combination of peppermint and caraway oil demonstrated symptomatic benefit in one placebo-controlled trial.

6. Recommendations for drug therapy—Drug therapy should be reserved for patients whose symptoms fail to improve after reassurance and life-style changes. Either H_2-receptor antagonists (ranitidine or nizatidine 150 mg; cimetidine 400 mg; famotidine 20 mg) twice daily, or proton-pump inhibitors (omeprazole or rabe-prazole 20 mg; lansoprazole 30 mg; or pantoprazole or esomeprazole 40 mg) once daily may benefit patients with reflux-like symptoms or epigastric pain. Responders should be treated with intermittent, short, 2–4 week courses for symptomatic episodes. In patients with other dyspeptic symptoms, the therapeutic options are limited. Metoclopramide may be tried, but long-term side effects must be considered. Antisecretory agents may be tried, but any benefit is likely due to a placebo effect. A trial of low-dose antidepressants may be considered even in patients who do not have evidence of anxiety or depression.

REFERENCES

Blum A et al: Lack of effect of treating *Helicobacter pylori* infection in patients with nonulcer dyspepsia. N Engl J Med 1998;339:1875.

Camilleri M, Coulie B, Tack J: Visceral hypersensitivity: facts, speculations, and challenges. Gut 2001;48:125.

Danesh J et al: Systematic review of the epidemiological evidence on *Helicobacter pylori* infection and nonulcer or uninvestigated dyspepsia. Arch Intern Med 2000;160:1192.

Delaney B et al: Initial management strategies for dyspepsia. Cochrane Database Syst Rev 2000;CD001961.

Drossman D et al: Psychosocial aspects of functional gastrointestinal disorders. Gut 1999;45:II25.

Hamilton J et al: A randomized controlled trial of psychotherapy in patients with functional dyspepsia. Gastroenterology 2000; 119:661.

Heading R: Prevalence of upper gastrointestinal symptoms in the general population: a systematic review. Scand J Gastroenterol 1999;34:3.

Hession P, Malagelada J: The initial management of uninvestigated dyspepsia in younger patients—the value of symptom-guided strategies should be reconsidered. Aliment Pharmacol Ther 2000;14:379.

Jackson J et al: Treatment of functional gastrointestinal disorders with antidepressant medications: a meta-analysis. Am J Med 2000;108:65.

Koloski N, Talley N, Boyce P: The impact of functional gastrointestinal disorders on quality of life. Am J Gastroenterol 2000;95:67.

Laine L, Schoenfeld P, Fennerty B: Therapy for *Helicobacter pylori* in patients with nonulcer dyspepsia. A meta-analysis of randomized, controlled trials. Ann Intern Med 2001;134:361.

Lassen A et al: *Helicobacter pylori* test-and-eradicate versus prompt endoscopy for management of dyspeptic patients: a randomized trial. Lancet 2000;356:455.

May B, Kohler S, Schneider, B: Efficacy and tolerability of a fixed combination of peppermint oil and caraway oil in patients suffering from functional dyspepsia. Aliment Pharmacol Ther 2000;14:1671.

Moayyedi P et al: Effect of population screening and treatment for *Helicobacter pylori* on dyspepsia and quality of life in the community: a randomised controlled trial. Lancet 2000;355:1665.

Ofman J, Rabeneck L: The effectiveness of endoscopy in the management of dyspepsia: a qualitative systematic review. Am J Med 1999;106:335.

Soo S et al: Pharmacological interventions for non-ulcer dyspepsia. Cochrane Database Syst Rev 2000;CD001960.

Stanghellini V, Corinaldesi R, Tosetti C: Relevance of gastrointestinal motor disturbances in functional dyspepsia. Baillieres Clin Gastroenterol 1998;12:533.

Tack J et al: Role of impaired accommodation to a meal in functional dyspepsia. Gastroenterology 1998;115:1346.

Talley N: Therapeutic options in nonulcer dyspepsia. J Clin Gastroenterol 2001;32:286.

Talley N et al: Efficacy of omeprazole in functional dyspepsia: double-blind, randomized, placebo-controlled trials (the Bond and Opera studies). Aliment Pharmacol Ther 1998; 12:1055.

Talley N et al: AGA technical review: evaluation of dyspepsia. Gastroenterology 1998;114:582.

Talley N et al: Functional gastroduodenal disorders. Gut 1999; 45:II37.

Talley N et al: Absence of benefit of eradicating *Helicobacter pylori* in patients with nonulcer dyspepsia. N Engl J Med 1999; 341:1106.

Talley N et al: Eradication of *Helicobacter pylori* in functional dyspepsia: randomised double blind placebo controlled trial with 12 months' follow up. BMJ 1999;318:833.

Talley N et al: Functional gastroduodenal disorders. In: *The Functional Gastrointestinal Disorders.* Drossman D (editor). McClean, Degnon Associates, 2000, p. 300.

Veldhuyzen van Zanten S et al: An evidenced-based approach to the management of uninvestigated dyspepsia in the era of *Helicobacter pylori.* CMAJ 2000;162:S3.

Veldhuyzen van Zanten S et al: Efficacy of cisapride and domperidone in functional (nonulcer) dyspepsia: a meta-analysis. Am J Gastroenterol 2001;96:689.

Motility Disorders of the Stomach & Small Intestine

Heather J. Chial, MD & Michael Camilleri, MD

In this chapter, we will provide an overview of the various motility disorders that can affect the stomach and small intestine. These disorders result from impaired control of the gut by the nervous and/or muscular systems. Associated symptoms include recurrent or chronic nausea, vomiting, bloating, and abdominal discomfort, which occur in the absence of intestinal obstruction. In addition to affecting the stomach and small bowel, gastroparesis and intestinal pseudoobstruction are sometimes associated with generalized disease processes that affect other regions of the gastrointestinal tract and extraintestinal organs including the urinary bladder. Other structural and rapid motility disorders affecting the stomach and small intestine are characterized by signs and symptoms of accelerated transit.

CONTROL OF GASTROINTESTINAL MOTOR FUNCTION

Motor function of the gastrointestinal tract is dependent on the contraction of smooth muscle cells and their integration and modulation by enteric and extrinsic nerves. Contractions that occur throughout the gastrointestinal tract are controlled by myogenic, neural and chemical mechanisms (Figure 22–1). Derangement of these mechanisms that regulate gastrointestinal motor function may lead to altered gut motility.

Neurogenic modulators of gastrointestinal motility include the central nervous system (CNS), the autonomic nerves, and the enteric nervous system (ENS). The ENS is an independent branch of the peripheral nervous system consisting of approximately 100 million neurons organized into two ganglionated plexuses (Figure 22–2). The larger myenteric plexus, also known as Auerbach's plexus, is situated between the longitudinal and circular muscle layers of the muscularis externa; this plexus contains neurons responsible for gastrointestinal motility and regulation of enzymatic output from adjacent organs. The smaller submucosal plexus is referred to as Meissner's plexus. The ENS directly interfaces with intestinal smooth muscle cells; it also plays an important role in visceral afferent function.

Myogenic control mechanisms include factors involved in regulating the electrical activity generated by smooth muscle cells of the gastrointestinal tract. An essential component of the myogenic control system is the electrical pacemaker activity that originates in the interstitial cells of Cajal (ICC). The ICC form a nonneural pacemaker system located at the interface of the circular and longitudinal muscle layers of the small intestine. The omnipresent slow waves of the small intestine, commonly referred to as electrical control activity (ECA) and the pacesetter potential (PP), originate in the network of ICC associated with Auerbach's plexus. In addition to generating pacemaker activity, the ICC appear to function as intermediaries between the neurogenic (ENS) and myogenic control systems as they are extensively innervated and are in close proximity to the gastrointestinal smooth muscle cells.

Chemical control refers to the observation that contraction of gastrointestinal smooth muscle during periodic depolarizations of membrane potential occurs only if an excitatory neurotransmitter such as acetylcholine is present. The distance over which a contraction is propagated depends on the length of the segment exhibiting electrical control activity and the length of the contiguous segment that is neurochemically activated.

Extrinsic neural control of gastrointestinal motor function can be subdivided into the cranial and sacral parasympathetic outflow and the thoracolumbar sympathetic supply. The cranial outflow is predominantly through the vagus nerve, which innervates the gastrointestinal tract from the stomach to the right colon and is composed of preganglionic cholinergic fibers that synapse with the ENS. The supply of sympathetic fibers to the stomach and small bowel arises from levels T5 to T10 of the intermediolateral column of the spinal cord. The prevertebral celiac, superior mesenteric, and inferior mesenteric sympathetic ganglia play important roles in the integration of afferent impulses between the gut and the CNS.

GASTRIC & SMALL BOWEL MOTILITY

The motor functions of the stomach and small intestine are characterized by distinct manometric patterns of activity in the fasting and postprandial periods (Figure 22–3).

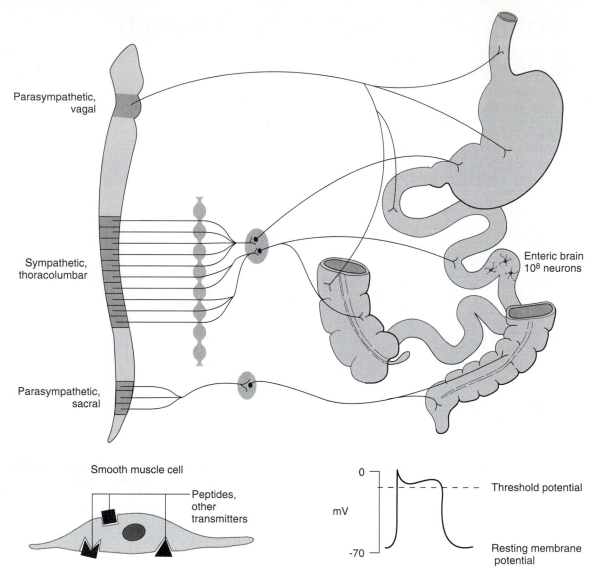

Figure 22–1. Control of gut motility. Interactions between extrinsic neural pathways and the intrinsic nervous system modulate contractions of gastrointestinal smooth muscle. Peptide–receptor interactions alter membrane potentials by stimulating bidirectional ion fluxes. In turn, membrane characteristics dictate whether muscle cell contracts.

The **fasting** or **interdigestive period** is characterized by a cyclic motor phenomenon, the interdigestive migrating motor complex (MMC). In healthy individuals, one cycle of this complex is completed every 60–90 minutes. The MMC has three phases: a period of quiescence (phase 1), a period of intermittent pressure activity (phase 2), and an activity front (phase 3) during which the stomach and small intestine contract at highest frequencies (3 per minute in the stomach and 11–12 per minute in the small intestine). The phase 3 interdigestive activity front migrates for a variable distance through the small intestine; the frequency of contractions ranges from 10–12 per minute in the duodenum to 5–8 per minute in the ileum. Another characteristic interdigestive motor pattern seen in the distal small intestine is the giant migrating complex

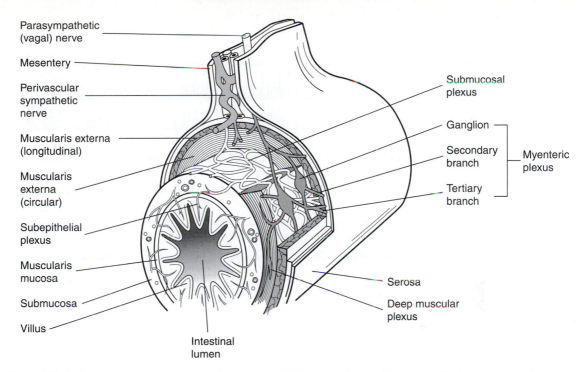

Figure 22–2. The enteric nervous system is composed of two ganglionated plexuses. The larger myenteric plexus is situated between the circular and longitudinal layers of the muscularis externa. The smaller submucosal plexus is located in the submucosa. (Reproduced, with permission, from Gershon MD: The enteric nervous system: a second brain. Hosp Pract 1999;34:37.)

(GMC) or power contraction; it serves to empty residue from the ileum into the colon in bolus transfers.

In the **postprandial period,** the interdigestive MMC is replaced by an irregular pressure response pattern of variable amplitude and frequency, which enables mixing and absorption. This pattern is observed in all stomach and small bowel regions in contact with food. The maximum frequency of contractions is lower than that noted during phase 3 of the interdigestive MMC. The duration of the postprandial motor activity is proportional to the number of calories consumed during the meal. Segments of the small intestine that are not in contact with food will continue to display interdigestive motor patterns.

Liquids empty from the stomach in an exponential manner. The half-emptying time for nonnutrient liquids in healthy individuals is usually less than 20 minutes. Solids are selectively retained in the stomach until particles have been triturated to a size of less than 2 mm in diameter; at this point, they are emptied in a linear fashion. Therefore, gastric emptying of solids is characterized by an initial lag period followed by a linear post-lag emptying phase. The small intestine transports solids and liquids at approximately the same rate. Due to the lag phase for the transport of solids from the stomach, liquids typically arrive in the colon prior to solids.

PATHOGENESIS

Although several factors may be involved in the development of gastric and/or small bowel motility disturbances, the underlying etiology can generally be characterized as neuropathic or myopathic (Figure 22–4). The exceptions include systemic sclerosis and amyloidosis, which can initially present with neuropathic patterns and later display myopathic characteristics with disease progression.

Neuropathic Processes

Processes involving the **extrinsic nervous system** include diabetic autonomic neuropathy, amyloidosis, paraneoplastic syndromes, and surgical vagotomy. Certain medications including α-adrenergic agonists, calcium channel blockers, anticholinergics, and opiate

A.

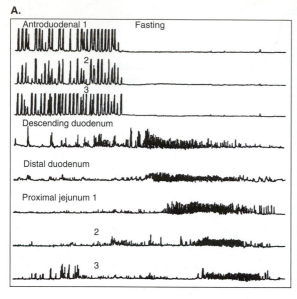
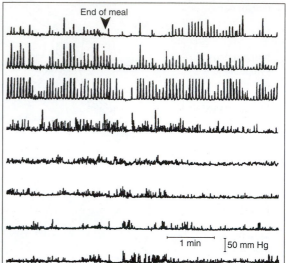

B.

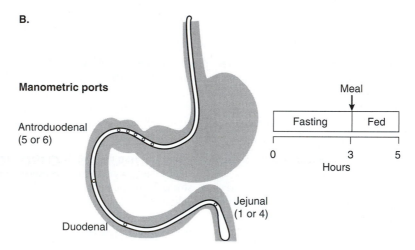

Figure 22–3. Experimental protocol for measuring upper gastrointestinal motility including a normal fasting and postprandial gastroduodenal manometric recording in a healthy volunteer. The patient has taken no medications for 48 hours and eats a 535-kcal meal during the study. Note the cyclic interdigestive migrating motor complex **(A)** and the sustained, high-amplitude but irregular pressure activity after meal **(B)**. *(A: Reproduced, with permission, from Malagelada J-R, Camilleri M, Stanghellini V: Manometric Diagnosis of Gastrointestinal Motility Disorders. Thieme, 1986. B: Reproduced by permission of Mayo Foundation for Medical Education and Research.)*

agents may cause motility abnormalities due to effects on extrinsic nerves.

Disorders of the **enteric nerves** or **ENS** are usually the result of degenerative, immunologic, or inflammatory processes. Although there are examples of gastroparesis and pseudoobstruction induced by Norwalk virus, cytomegalovirus, and Epstein–Barr virus, the un-

derlying etiology cannot be ascertained in the majority of cases. Studies using animal models of diabetic gastroparesis have shown structural abnormalities in ICC. Idiopathic gastroparesis and chronic intestinal pseudoobstruction are thought to occur in patients in whom there is no disturbance of extrinsic neural control and no underlying cause for the enteric neural abnormality.

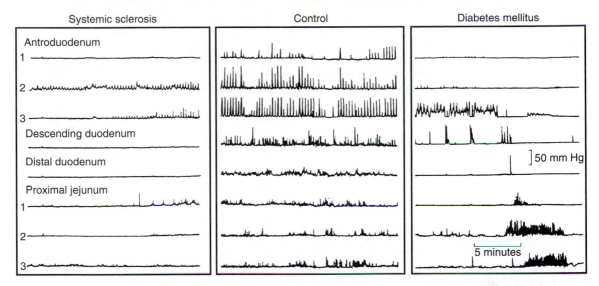

Figure 22–4. Postprandial manometric profiles in small bowel dysmotility secondary to myopathy (systemic sclerosis) and neuropathy (diabetes mellitus). Note the simultaneous, prolonged contractions of low amplitude during the fasting and postprandial periods in the setting of myopathy. Although the contraction amplitudes are normal in the setting of neuropathy, contractile activity is uncoordinated and contractile frequency is reduced. (Reproduced, with permission, from Camilleri M: Medical treatment of chronic intestinal pseudo-obstruction. Pract Gastroenterol 1995;15:10.)

Manometric characteristics of neuropathic processes include normal contraction amplitudes with uncoordinated contractile activity, a reduced frequency of contractions, abnormalities in propagation, and/or a lack of coordination between fasting and postprandial motor patterns. Full-thickness small bowel biopsy features of neuropathic disorders include degeneration in axons, dendrites, and/or neurons and may or may not include inflammatory changes; observation of these changes is enhanced with the use of silver-staining techniques.

Myopathic Processes

Diseases associated with myopathic processes, including progressive systemic sclerosis and amyloidosis, may result in significant gastric and small bowel dysmotility. Rarely, dermatomyositis, dystrophia myotonica, and metabolic muscle disorders such as mitochondrial myopathy may be causes. There may be a positive family history of these disorders. Rarely, myopathic disturbances may be the result of metabolic disorders such as hypothyroidism or hyperparathyroidism; these conditions tend to manifest as constipation.

Myopathic conditions are characterized by well-coordinated contractile activity with markedly reduced contraction amplitudes on manometric evaluation. Biopsy features of myopathic processes include fibrosis, muscle atrophy, and vacuolar degeneration of the muscularis propria.

GASTROPARESIS & CHRONIC INTESTINAL PSEUDOOBSTRUCTION

Clinical Findings

A. SYMPTOMS AND SIGNS

The clinical features of gastroparesis and chronic intestinal pseudoobstruction are similar and include nausea, vomiting, early satiety, abdominal discomfort and distention, bloating, and anorexia, which occur in the absence of intestinal obstruction. Weight loss and vitamin and mineral deficiencies may result when vomiting and stasis are significant. The severity of the motility problem may also be gauged by the degree of malnutrition and presence of electrolyte abnormalities. Prominent features of dysphagia, abdominal distention, diarrhea, and/or constipation may indicate that the motility disorder involves more than the stomach and/or small bowel.

Careful documentation of the patient's family history and medications may help to determine the underlying etiology. A thorough review of all organ systems will help to identify patients with underlying collagen vascular diseases including scleroderma and may identify patients with disturbances of extrinsic neural control. Important symptoms to screen for include orthostatic dizziness; difficulties with erection or ejaculation; recurrent urinary tract infections; dry mouth, eyes, or vagina; difficulties with visual accommodation in bright lights; or absence of sweating.

On physical examination, the presence of a succussion splash suggests there is a region of stasis within the gastrointestinal tract. The hands and mouth should be carefully examined for signs of Raynaud's phenomenon and features of systemic sclerosis. To assess for neurologic disturbance and oculogastrointestinal dystrophy, the following parameters should be evaluated: pupillary responses, extraocular movements, supine and standing blood pressures, and a complete neurologic examination including assessment for peripheral neuropathy.

B. DIAGNOSTIC STEPS

Four questions should be considered in the diagnosis of each patient:

1. Are the symptoms **acute or chronic**?
2. Is the disease due to a **neuropathy or a myopathy**?
3. What is the status of **hydration and nutrition**?
4. Which **regions** of the digestive tract are **affected**?

These questions can be answered by the thorough physiologic assessment described below (Figure 22–5).

1. Suspect and exclude mechanical obstruction— In patients with pseudoobstruction, plain radiographs of the abdomen taken at the time of symptoms typically show dilated loops of small bowel with associated air–fluid levels. Mechanical obstruction should be excluded by means of upper gastrointestinal endoscopy and barium studies including a small bowel follow-through. The presence of a motility disorder of the stomach or small bowel should be suspected whenever a large volume of material can be aspirated from the stomach, particularly after an overnight fast, for example, the presence of nondigested solid food or a large volume of liquid in the stomach during routine esophagogastroduodenoscopy. Barium studies may fortuitously suggest the presence of a motor disorder, particularly if there is gross dilatation, dilution of barium, or retained solid food within the stomach. However, these studies rarely identify the causative factor. The exception occurs in the setting of small bowel systemic sclerosis, which is characterized by megaduodenum and the presence of packed valvulae conniventes in the small intestine.

2. Assess gastric and small bowel motor activity— Once mechanical obstruction and alternative diagnoses such as Crohn's disease have been excluded, a transit profile of the stomach and/or small bowel should be performed. Efficiency in the emptying of solids is the most sensitive measurement of the upper gastrointestinal transit (Figure 22–6). Scans are typically performed

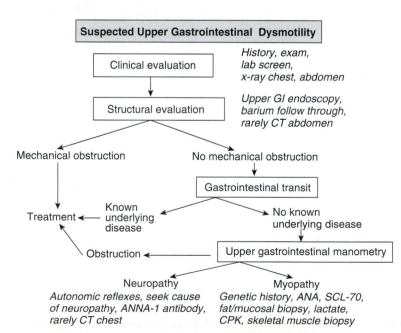

Figure 22–5. Flow diagram outlining steps involved in diagnosing gastroparesis and intestinal pseudoobstruction.

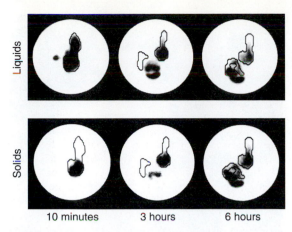

Figure 22–6. Transit of radiolabeled solids and liquids in a patient with chronic (neuropathic) intestinal pseudoobstruction. Note the prolonged retention of both phases of the meal in the stomach and small bowel. The upper outline depicts the stomach, and the lower outline depicts the right side of the colon on 3- and 6-hour scans. (Reproduced, with permission, from Camilleri M et al: Impaired transit of chyme in chronic intestinal pseudoobstruction: correction by cisapride. Gastroenterology 1986; 91:623.)

at 0, 1, 2, 3, 4, and 6 hours following ingestion of a radiolabeled meal. These tests can be easily performed at a fairly low cost.

If the cause of the motility disturbance is obvious, such as gastroparesis in a patient with long-standing diabetes mellitus, it is usually unnecessary to pursue further diagnostic testing. If the cause is unclear, **gastroduodenal manometry** using a multilumen tube with sensors in the distal stomach and proximal small intestine can differentiate between neuropathic and myopathic processes, as described previously. In general, manometric abnormalities associated with intestinal pseudoobstruction include (1) simultaneous wave forms or retrograde propagation of phase 3 activity, (2) bursts of high-amplitude and high-frequency pressure activity during the fasting and fed periods, (3) sustained pressure activity in an isolated segment of the small intestine, and/or (4) inability of a meal to initiate a fed pattern of activity.

Breath hydrogen testing is a noninvasive means of assessing gastric emptying and small bowel transit. The roles of other noninvasive tests such as electrogastrography, impedance tomography, and ultrasound are controversial, because it is still unclear whether they provide clinically useful information. Unlike gastroduodenal manometry, which enables assessment of both the stomach and small intestine, data from electrogastrography are limited to the stomach.

Gastric accommodation refers to the vagally mediated reduction in gastric tone that occurs in response to meal ingestion. Impaired gastric accommodation is a common phenomenon in diabetic vagal neuropathy as well as in a variety of other conditions including postvagotomy surgery, postfundoplication dyspepsia, and functional dyspepsia. Noninvasive means of assessing gastric accommodation using single-photon emission computed tomography (SPECT) have recently been developed (Figure 22–7). Such techniques may prove to be clinically useful in the assessment of symptoms associated with motility disorders of the upper gastrointestinal tract.

3. Identify the pathogenesis—Causes of gastroparesis and intestinal pseudoobstruction are outlined in Table 22–1. In the presence of a **neuropathic pattern** of motor activity in the small intestine, it is necessary to pursue further investigations including testing for autonomic dysfunction, type 1 antineuronal nuclear autoantibodies (ANNA-1) associated with paraneoplastic syndromes, and/or magnetic resonance imaging (MRI) of the brain. In certain cases, a laparoscopically obtained full-thickness biopsy of the small intestine may be required. Autonomic testing includes evaluation for orthostatic hypotension, assessment of supine and standing serum norepinephrine levels, measurement of the heart rate interval change during deep breathing, and plasma pancreatic polypeptide response to modified sham feeding. Such testing can identify sympathetic adrenergic and cholinergic neuropathies as well as vagal neuropathy.

The identification of a **myopathic disorder** on initial testing should lead to a search for amyloidosis (immunoglobulin electrophoresis, fat aspirate, or rectal biopsy), systemic sclerosis (SCL-70), and a family history of gastrointestinal motility disorders. Laboratory studies to consider include assessment of thyroid function, antinuclear antibody, creatine phosphokinase, aldolase, porphyrins, serologies for Chagas' disease, and an erythrocyte sedimentation rate. Special staining techniques of a full-thickness small bowel biopsy specimen may be needed to identify metabolic muscle disorders including mitochondrial myopathy. Genetic testing is now available to assess for certain mitochondrial myopathies.

4. Identify complications—It is important to look for complications of the motor disorder including nutritional deficiencies, inadequacies in essential elements and vitamins, and bacterial overgrowth in patients presenting with diarrhea. Due to the insufficient amplitude of contractions and an inability to clear residue from the small bowel, bacterial overgrowth is more common in myopathic than in neuropathic disorders.

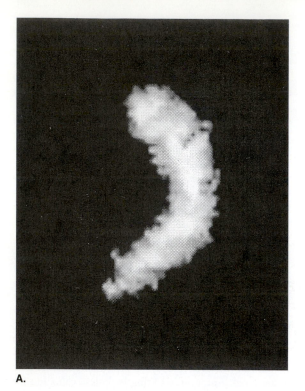

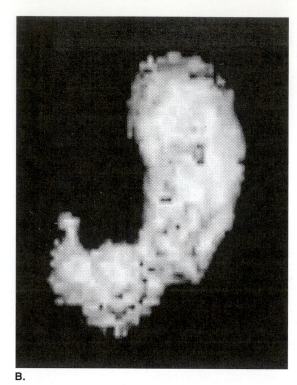

A.

B.

Figure 22–7. Gastric accomodation. SPECT images (based on transaxial views) outlining the stomach during fasting **(A)** and postprandial **(B)** periods in a healthy volunteer. Note the configuration of the stomach, which conforms to the appearance seen on barium radiography. The volume increase postprandially exceeds the fasting volume plus the meal volume indicating that reflex accommodation has occurred. (Reproduced, with permission, from Kuiken S et al: Development of a test to measure gastric accommodation in humans. Am J Physiol 1999; 277:G1217.)

Bacterial overgrowth may be difficult to detect using small bowel aspirates; on the other hand, breath H_2 after a glucose or lactose load is a nonspecific test that should be interpreted with caution and in conjunction with small bowel transit time. Often an empiric trial of antibiotics is used as a surrogate for formal testing.

Differential Diagnosis

The major conditions to be differentiated are mechanical obstruction, such as may occur because of peptic stricture or Crohn's disease in the small intestine, and eating disorders, particularly anorexia nervosa. There is impairment of gastric emptying in anorexia nervosa but to a minor degree compared with that of diabetic gastroparesis or postvagotomy gastric stasis.

Treatment

After completing the physiological assessment outlined in the preceding section, an individualized treatment

plan can be designed. The principal methods of management include (1) correction of hydration and nutritional deficiencies, (2) use of prokinetic and antiemetic medications, (3) suppression of bacterial overgrowth, (4) decompression, and (5) surgical treatment.

A. CORRECTION OF HYDRATION AND NUTRITIONAL DEFICIENCIES

Rehydration, electrolyte repletion, and nutritional supplementation are particularly important during acute exacerbations of gastroparesis and chronic intestinal pseudoobstruction. Restoration of nutrition can be achieved orally, enterally, or parenterally depending on the severity of the clinical syndrome. Initial nutritional measures include use of low-fiber supplements with the addition of iron, folate, calcium, and vitamins D, K, and B_{12}. In patients with more severe symptoms, enteral or parenteral supplementation of nutrition may be required. If enteral supplementation may be required for more than 3 months, it is usually best to provide

Table 22–1. Classification of gastroparesis and intestinal pseudoobstruction.

Type	Neuropathic	Myopathic
Infiltrative	Progressive systemic sclerosis	Progressive systemic sclerosis
	Amyloidosis	Amyloidosis
		Systemic lupus erythematosis
		Ehlers-Danlos syndrome
		Dermatomyositis
Familial	Familial visceral neuropathies	Familial visceral myopathies
		Metabolic myopathies
Idiopathic	Sporadic hollow visceral myopathy	Idiopathic intestinal pseudo-obstruction
Neurologic	Porphyria	Myotonia
	Heavy metal poisoning	Other dystrophies
	Brainstem tumor	
	Parkinson's disease	
	Multiple sclerosis	
	Spinal cord transection	
Infectious	Chagas' disease	
	Cytomegalovirus	
	Norwalk virus	
	Ebstein–Barr virus	
Drug-induced	Tricyclic antidepressants	
	Narcotic agents	
	Anticholinergic agents	
	Antihypertensives	
	Dopaminergic agents	
	Vincristine	
	Laxatives	
Paraneoplastic	Small cell lung cancer	
	Carcinoid syndrome	
Postsurgical	Postvagotomy with or without pyloroplasty/gastric resection	
Endocrine	Diabetes mellitus	
	Hypo/hyperthyroidism	
	Hypoparathyroidism	

feedings through a jejunostomy tube. Gastrotomy tubes should be avoided in the setting of gastroparesis. Many patients requiring long-term parenteral nutrition continue to tolerate some oral feedings.

B. PROKINETICS AND MEDICATIONS

Medications are being increasingly used for the treatment of neuromuscular motility disorders. Regrettably, there is little evidence that they are effective in myopathic disturbances except for the rare case of dystrophia myotonica affecting the stomach and for small bowel systemic sclerosis.

Erythromycin, a macrolide antibiotic that stimulates motilin receptors, results in the dumping of solids from the stomach. It has been shown to accelerate gastric emptying in gastroparesis; it also increases the amplitude of antral contractions and improves antral–duode-nal coordination. Erythromycin is most effective when it is used intravenously during acute exacerbations of gastroparesis or intestinal pseudoobstruction. The usual dose of intravenous erythromycin lactobionate is 3 mg/kg every 8 hours. The effect of oral erythromycin appears to be restricted by tolerance and gastrointestinal side effects, which often preclude its use for longer than 1 month. Use of the elixir formulation versus capsules may improve absorption in the setting of dysmotility. Although initial studies demonstrated effectiveness in patients with diabetic gastroparesis treated for 2 weeks, there is little evidence that continued therapy results in long-term improvement in gastric emptying or associated symptoms in these patients.

Metoclopramide is a dopamine antagonist with both prokinetic and antiemetic properties. Long-term use of metoclopramide is limited by the side effects of tremor and Parkinson-like symptoms, a consequence of anti-dopaminergic activity in the CNS. It is available in tablet or elixir form and is typically taken 30 minutes prior to meals and at bedtime. Usual doses range from 5 to 20 mg four times daily.

Serotonergic (5-HT) agents may prove to be beneficial in the treatment of gastroparesis and intestinal pseudoobstruction. The selective partial 5-HT$_4$ agonist tegaserod has been shown to promote peristaltic activity including orocecal transit and showed a tendency toward accelerated colonic transit. Tegaserod also improves abdominal pain and discomfort in females with constipation-predominant irritable bowel syndrome (IBS). Prucalopride, a full 5-HT$_4$ agonist, has been shown to accelerate small bowel and colonic transit in healthy volunteers and in patients with functional constipation. Clinical trials using tegaserod and prucalopride in patients with gastroparesis and pseudoobstruction are awaited.

Octreotide, a cyclized analog of somatostatin, has been shown to induce activity fronts in the small intestine that mimic phase 3 activity of the interdigestive MMC. Experience suggests that the small bowel motility is characterized by a simultaneous or very rapidly propagated activity front that is not well coordinated. The clinical effects of octreotide include an initial acceleration of gastric emptying, a decrease in postprandial gastric motility, and inhibition of small bowel transit. Therefore, the therapeutic efficacy of octreotide in patients with intestinal dysmotility associated with gastroparesis and pseudoobstruction requires further assessment in clinical trials. At this time, octreotide appears to be more useful in the treatment of dumping syndromes associated with accelerated transit. However, octreotide has been used at night to induce MMC activity and avoid bacterial overgrowth. If required during the day, octreotide is often combined with oral erythromycin to "normalize" the gastric emptying rate.

Antiemetics including diphenhydramine, trifluoperazine, and metoclopramide play an important role in the management of nausea and vomiting in patients with gastroparesis and intestinal pseudoobstruction. The more expensive serotonin 5-HT$_3$ antagonists (eg, ondansetron) have not proved to be of greater benefit than the less expensive alternatives.

Antibiotic therapy is indicated in patients with documented, symptomatic bacterial overgrowth. Although formal clinical trials have not been conducted, it is common practice to use different antibiotics for 7–10 days each month in an attempt to avoid development of resistance. Common antibiotics include doxycycline, 100 mg twice daily; metronidazole, 500 mg three times daily; ciprofloxacin, 500 mg twice daily; and double-strength trimethaprim-sulfamethoxazole, two tablets twice daily. Use of antibiotics in patients with diarrhea and fat malabsorption secondary to bacterial overgrowth results in significant symptomatic relief.

C. DECOMPRESSION

Decompression is rarely necessary in patients with chronic pseudoobstruction. However, venting enterostomy (jejunostomy) is effective in relieving abdominal distention and bloating. It has been shown to significantly reduce the frequency of nasogastric intubations and hospitalizations required for acute exacerbations of severe intestinal pseudoobstruction in patients requiring central parenteral nutrition. Access to the small intestine by enterostomy also provides a way to deliver nutrients enterally and should be considered in patients with intermittent symptoms. Currently available enteral tubes allow for aspiration and feeding by a single apparatus.

D. SURGICAL TREATMENT

Surgical approaches should be limited in patients with gastroparesis and intestinal pseudoobstruction. In patients who have had multiple abdominal operations, it becomes difficult to discern whether symptoms are associated with exacerbations of the underlying disease or are due to adhesions and mechanical obstruction. Surgical treatment should be considered whenever the motility disorder is localized to a resectable portion of the gut. Three instances that lend themselves to this approach include duodenojejunostomy or duodenoplasty for patients with megaduodenum or duodenal atresia in children; completion gastrectomy for patients with postgastric surgical stasis syndrome; and colectomy with ileoproctostomy for intractable constipation associated with chronic colonic pseudoobstruction.

E. NOVEL THERAPIES

Preliminary data suggest that gastric pacing may improve gastric emptying and symptoms in patients with severe gastroparesis. Gastric pacing is able to entrain gastric slow waves and normalize gastric dysrhythmias. However, data are inconclusive and further controlled clinical trials are needed to assess the long-term benefits, complications, and optimal treatment groups.

Small bowel transplantation is currently limited to patients with intestinal failure who have reversible total parenteral nutrition (TPN)-induced liver disease or life-threatening or recurrent catheter-related sepsis. Combined small bowel and liver transplantation is being performed in patients with irreversible TPN-induced liver disease. Complications following small bowel transplantation include infection, rejection, and lymphoproliferative disorders due to long-term immunosuppression. Studies have suggested that small bowel transplantation may improve quality of life and may be more cost effective than long-term TPN. In the future, improvements in immunosuppressive regimens, earlier detection of rejection, and treatment of cytomegalovirus based on polymerase chain reaction detection may enable small bowel transplantation to become the definitive treatment for short bowel syndrome or severe pseudoobstruction uncontrolled by TPN. In the meantime, parenteral nutrition will remain the treatment of choice for the majority of patients.

Prognosis

There has been no formal analysis of the natural history of gastroparesis and intestinal pseudoobstruction. Current impressions regarding prognosis are based upon case reports and data from clinical trials of medications studied in these disorders. In general, the long-term prognosis depends on the underlying disease process. Patients with suspected postviral gastroparesis appear to have an overall positive prognosis, with restoration of nutrition and reduction of symptoms occurring within 2 years. Patients with myopathic, dilated bowel tend to have persistent symptoms, are more prone to developing bacterial overgrowth, and usually require long-term parenteral nutrition. Between these two ends of the spectrum are patients with mild to moderately severe motility disorders. These patients can usually be managed as outpatients if dietary supplementation, medica-

tions, and decompression are instituted to provide symptomatic relief.

DUMPING SYNDROME & ACCELERATED GASTRIC EMPTYING

Dumping syndrome and accelerated gastric emptying typically follow truncal vagotomy and gastric drainage procedures. Now that highly selective vagotomy is being performed when surgical treatment of peptic ulcer disease is required, the prevalence of these problems is decreasing.

The pathophysiology of rapid gastric emptying is related to impaired gastric accommodation following ingestion of a meal. Intragastric pressure is relatively high and results in active propulsion of liquid foods from the stomach. A high caloric (usually carbohydrate) content of the liquid phase of the meal evokes a rapid insulin response with secondary hypoglycemia. These patients may also have impaired antral contractility and gastric stasis of solids, which may paradoxically result in a clinical picture of both gastroparesis (for solids) and dumping (for liquids). The most useful investigation is a dual-phase radioisotopic gastric emptying test (Figure 22–8).

The management of dumping syndrome includes patient education regarding dietary maneuvers (avoid-

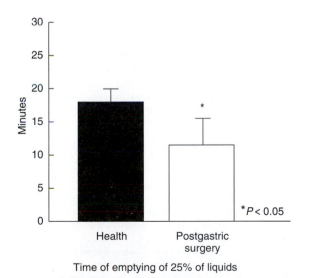
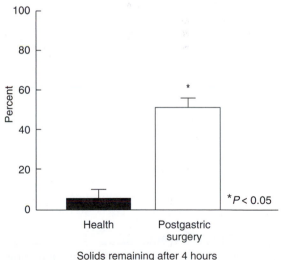

Figure 22–8. Gastric emptying of liquids and solids in healthy controls (***black bars;*** $n = 17$) and postgastric surgery patients (***white bars;*** $n = 16$). The time necessary for 25% of the liquids to empty is shorter in the postsurgical group; the proportion of solid radiolabeled material remaining in the stomach after 4 hours is larger in the postsurgical group. Data are means plus or minus standard error of the mean. (Modified, with permission, from Fich A et al: Stasis syndrome following gastric surgery: clinical and motility features of 60 symptomatic patients. J Clin Gastroenterol 1990;12:505.)

ance of high-nutrient liquid drinks and, possibly, addition of guar gum or pectin to retard emptying) and, rarely, pharmacologic treatment with a drug such as octreotide, 50–100 µg given subcutaneously before meals.

Accelerated gastric emptying of liquids can occur in patients with non-insulin-dependent diabetes mellitus without underlying autonomic dysfunction. This does not appear to be an important mechanism of postprandial hyperglycemia in these patients. The mechanism and clinical significance of accelerated liquid emptying are under investigation.

RAPID TRANSIT DYSMOTILITY OF THE SMALL BOWEL

Rapid transit of material through the small bowel may occur in the setting of postvagotomy diarrhea, short bowel syndrome, diabetic diarrhea, carcinoid diarrhea, and irritable bowel syndrome. With the exception of irritable bowel syndrome, these conditions may result in significant losses of fluid and electrolytes and may cause severe diarrhea. Idiopathic bile acid catharsis may represent an inability of the distal ileum to reabsorb bile acids because of rapid transit and reduced contact time with ileal mucosa; this condition may induce cholerrheic enteropathy with colonic secretion and secondary diarrhea.

Clinical Findings

These disturbances may be confirmed by scintigraphic studies or by the lactulose-hydrogen breath test. Manometric studies of the small bowel may reveal prolonged duration, high amplitude, and rapidly propagated contractions. Propagated spike bursts may be seen on intraluminal electromyographic studies in these patients. Similar myoelectric activity has been noted in a series of bacterial or toxic diarrheas induced in experimental animals.

Treatment

The objectives of treatment are restoration of hydration and nutrition and slowing of small bowel transit.

A. NUTRITIONAL THERAPY

Dietary interventions include the avoidance of hyperosmolar drinks and replacement with isoosmolar or hypoosmolar oral rehydration solutions. The fat content in the diet should be reduced to approximately 50 g to avoid delivery of unabsorbed fat to the colon. All nutritional deficiencies of calcium, magnesium, potassium, and water- and fat-soluble vitamins should be corrected.

In patients with less than 1 m of residual small bowel, it may be impossible to maintain fluid and electrolyte homeostasis without parenteral support. In patients with a longer residual segment, oral nutrition, pharmacotherapy, and supplements are almost always effective for this purpose.

B. DRUG THERAPY

The opioid agent loperamide (4 mg 30 minutes before meals and at bedtime) has been shown to suppress the gastrocolonic response and improve symptoms in these patients. Verapamil (40 mg twice daily) and/or clonidine (0.1 mg twice daily) may be used in addition to loperamide. Octreotide (50 µg three times daily) may be used in patients for whom these agents are ineffective or poorly tolerated. 5-HT$_3$ antagonists have demonstrated efficacy in the treatment of carcinoid diarrhea.

SUMMARY

Disorders of gastric and small bowel motility may result in either stasis or accelerated transit; understanding the mechanisms that control motility and pathophysiology in the individual patient is the key to optimal management. Simple, quantitative measures of transit and an algorithmic approach to identifying the underlying cause may lead to correction of abnormal function. Alternatively, correction of dehydration and nutritional abnormalities and providing symptomatic relief are important steps in the management of these patients. Patient education is essential to avoid aggravation of symptoms because of dietary indiscretions.

REFERENCES

Camilleri M: Appraisal of medium- and long-term treatment of gastroparesis and chronic intestinal dysmotility. Am J Gastroenterol 1994;89(10):1769.

Camilleri M et al: Towards a less costly but accurate test of gastric emptying and small bowel transit. Dig Dis Sci 1991;36(5):609.

Coulie B, Camilleri M: Intestinal pseudoobstruction. Annu Rev Med 1999;50:37.

DiBaise JK, Quigley EM: Tumor-related dysmotility: gastrointestinal dysmotility syndromes associated with tumors. Dig Dis Sci 1998;43(7):1369.

Di Lorenzo C: Pseudo-obstruction: current approaches. Gastroenterology 1999;116(4):980.

Farthing MJ: Octreotide in dumping and short bowel syndromes. Digestion 1993;54(Suppl 1):47.

Frank JW, Sarr MG, Camilleri M: Use of gastroduodenal manometry to differentiate mechanical and functional intestinal obstruction: an analysis of clinical outcome. Am J Gastroenterol 1994;89(3):339.

Hornbuckle K, Barnett JL: The diagnosis and work-up of the patient with gastroparesis. J Clin Gastroenterol 2000;30(2):117.

Richards RD, Davenport K, McCallum RW: The treatment of idiopathic and diabetic gastroparesis with acute intravenous and chronic oral erythromycin. Am J Gastroenterol 1993;88(2): 203.

Scolapio JS et al: Nutritional management of chronic intestinal pseudo-obstruction. J Clin Gastroenterol 1999;28(4):306.

Soudah HC, Hasler WL, Owyang C: Effect of octreotide on intestinal motility and bacterial overgrowth in scleroderma. N Engl J Med 1991;325(21):1461.

Sudan DL et al: Isolated intestinal transplantation for intestinal failure. Am J Gastroenterol 2000;95(6):1506.

Tougas G et al: Assessment of gastric emptying using a low fat meal: establishment of international control values. Am J Gastroenterol 2000;95(6):1456.

von der Ohe MR et al: Motor dysfunction of the small bowel and colon in patients with the carcinoid syndrome and diarrhea. N Engl J Med 1993;329(15):1073.

Wood JD, Alpers DH, Andrews PL: Fundamentals of neurogastroenterology. Gut 1999;45 Suppl 2:II6.

Malabsorption Disorders

Lawrence R. Schiller, MD

Each day, the average person consumes 2000–3000 kcal of food. Most of this caloric load is in the form of polymers or other complex compounds that must be broken down into smaller molecules, to be transported across the small intestinal mucosa. Thus, proteins are cleaved into dipeptides and amino acids, starches are split into monosaccharides, and fats are broken down into fatty acids and monoglycerides. The processes of digestion and absorption are complex and often go awry. Nearly 200 conditions are associated with defects in this process and can produce substantial disability.

General Considerations

Strictly speaking, **maldigestion** refers to impaired hydrolysis of luminal contents, and **malabsorption** refers to impaired transport across the mucosa. In clinical practice, malabsorption is used to describe the end result of either defect.

Malabsorption may involve a broad range of nutrients (**panmalabsorption**) or only an individual nutrient or class of nutrients (specific malabsorption). This distinction can be helpful in the differential diagnosis of malabsorption.

The many causes of malabsorption can be sorted pathophysiologically into conditions that are associated with (1) impaired luminal hydrolysis, (2) impaired mucosal function (mucosal hydrolysis, uptake, and packaging), and (3) impaired removal of nutrients from the mucosa (Table 23–1).

 ESSENTIALS OF DIAGNOSIS

- *Steatorrhea (foul-smelling, greasy stools with increased fat excretion) or chronic watery diarrhea.*
- *Increased flatus.*
- *Weight loss, signs of vitamin and mineral deficiencies (anemia, easy bruising, tetany, osteoporosis).*

Clinical Findings

A. SYMPTOMS AND SIGNS (TABLE 23–2)

Most patients with panmalabsorption have changes in their stools. Classically, steatorrhea (excess fat) is present. Typical characteristics of steatorrhea include a pale color, bulkiness, greasiness, and tendency to float (because of incorporated gas). Less commonly, patients with malabsorption present with watery stools resulting from the osmotic effects of unabsorbed carbohydrates and short-chain fatty acids.

Abdominal distention and gaseousness are common and most often a result of fermentation of unabsorbed carbohydrates by colonic bacteria. The presence of excess flatus may be the only finding in patients with some specific malabsorptive problems, such as lactase deficiency.

Weight loss is common in patients with severe panmalabsorption, but may not be seen in patients with more limited forms of malabsorption. It usually is substantial early in the course of the illness, but levels off with time as body weight and calorie absorption again come into balance. This is in contrast to the progressive weight loss seen with tuberculosis or cancer. If weight loss is progressive with malabsorption, conditions such as inflammatory bowel disease or lymphoma should be considered.

Vitamin and mineral deficiencies can lead to several problems. Anemia is common, but not universal. Iron deficiency anemia may be the only finding in some patients with celiac disease, for instance. More typically, anemia is part of a spectrum of findings. Microcytic anemia may also be seen in Whipple's disease (in which occult blood loss is frequent) and in lymphomas presenting with malabsorption. Macrocytic anemias complicate malabsorption when folate or B_{12} deficiency is present.

Deficiencies of the fat-soluble vitamins, D, K, and A, sometimes produce symptoms. Because substantial stores of these vitamins are maintained in the body, deficiency indicates longstanding malabsorption or inadequate intake. Vitamin D deficiency can produce osteomalacia, bone pain, cramps, and tetany resulting from hypocalcemia. Vitamin K deficiency can cause easy bruising and ecchymosis. Vitamin A deficiency sometimes produces night blindness.

Table 23–1. Causes of malabsorption or maldigestion.

Impaired luminal hydrolysis or solubilization
  Pancreatic exocrine insufficiency
  Bile acid deficiency
  Zollinger-Ellison syndrome
  Postgastrectomy malabsorption
  Rapid intestinal transit
  Small bowel bacterial overgrowth
  Autoimmune polyglandular failure
Impaired mucosal hydrolysis, uptake, or packaging
  Brush border or metabolic disorders
    Lactase deficiency
    Sucrase-isomaltase deficiency
    Glucose-galactose malabsorption
    Abetalipoproteinemia
  Mucosal diseases
    Celiac sprue
    Collagenous sprue
    Nongranulomatous ulcerative jejunoileitis
    Eosinophilic gastroenteritis
    Systemic mastocytosis
    Immunoproliferative small intestinal disease (IPSID)
    Lymphoma
    Crohn's disease
    Radiation enteritis
    Amyloidosis
  Infectious diseases
    Tropical sprue
    Whipple's disease
    Parasitic diseases
    Mycobacterium avium-intracellulare
    AIDS enteropathy
  After intestinal resection
Impaired removal of nutrients
  Lymphangiectasia
  Chronic mesenteric ischemia

Table 23–2. Symptoms and signs of malabsorption.

Changes in stools
  Pale, bulky, greasy stools
  Watery diarrhea
  Floating stools
Increased colonic gas production
  Abdominal distention
  Borborygmi
Weight loss, muscle wasting
Vitamin and mineral deficiencies
  Anemia
  Cheilosis
  Glossitis
  Dermatitis
  Neuropathy
  Night blindness
  Osteomalacia
  Paresthesia
  Tetany
  Ecchymosis
Fatigue, weakness
Edema

Deficiencies of water-soluble vitamins other than folate and B_{12} seldom produce identifiable clinical manifestations by the time patients seek medical attention. Glossitis and cheilosis are probably the most common manifestations; findings of overt beriberi, pellagra, scurvy, and other classic vitamin-deficiency syndromes are rarely seen unless a substantial period of malnutrition has been present.

Constitutional symptoms of chronic fatigue and weakness are often present. Appetite is typically well maintained until vitamin and other deficiencies develop. Edema is uncommon until late in the course, unless there is coexisting protein-losing enteropathy.

Abdominal pain is usually not present with malabsorption syndrome. Usually it involves only modest cramping associated with diarrhea. If pain is more severe, the physician should consider the possibilities of chronic pancreatitis, Zollinger-Ellison syndrome, lymphoma, Crohn's disease, or intestinal ischemia.

Signs and symptoms elsewhere in the body may also be related to malabsorption or to the disorder causing malabsorption. Aphthous ulcers in the mouth may be associated with celiac disease, Behçet's syndrome, or Crohn's disease. Iritis may be seen with Crohn's disease and conjunctivitis with Behçet's syndrome. Skin abnormalities may be seen in some conditions. Whipple's disease is associated with hyperpigmentation, and dermatitis herpetiformis (which produces a pruritic, blistering skin eruption) is associated with celiac disease. Tightening of the skin, digital ulceration, nail changes, and Raynaud's phenomenon suggest scleroderma. A history of chronic sinusitis, bronchitis, and pneumonia should raise the question of cystic fibrosis in a child or young adult.

Several systemic diseases can produce malabsorption (Table 23–3). Symptoms and signs suggesting these conditions may be present.

B. LABORATORY TESTS (TABLE 23–4)

1. Routine blood tests—Patients with established panmalabsorption typically have several laboratory abnormalities. Conversely, patients with isolated malabsorption may have no laboratory abnormalities.

The complete blood cell count may show a microcytic or macrocytic anemia depending on the specific

Table 23–3. Systemic diseases associated with malabsorption.

Endocrine diseases
    Diabetes mellitus
    Hyperthyroidism
    Hypothyroidism
    Addison's disease
    Hypoparathyroidism
Collagen-vascular diseases
    Scleroderma
    Vasculitis (systemic lupus erythematosus, polyarteritis
      nodosa)
Amyloidosis
AIDS

---

condition causing malabsorption. The white blood cell count and platelet counts are usually normal. Lymphopenia may be present in patients with acquired immunodeficiency syndrome (AIDS) or lymphangiectasia. High platelet counts can be seen with iron deficiency.

Biochemical screening tests often will show one or more abnormalities. Hypokalemia, chloride depletion, and acid–base abnormalities may be present, due to a combination of poor intake and excessive loss in stool. Renal function is well maintained in most conditions causing malabsorption; blood urea nitrogen may be low due to poor protein intake or absorption and serum creatinine concentration may be low due to reduction in muscle mass. Serum calcium concentration may be low as a result of malabsorption, vitamin D deficiency, or intraluminal complexing of calcium by fatty acids. In addition, concurrent hypomagnesemia may produce hypocalcemia that is resistent to intravenous repletion. Serum phosphorus, cholesterol, and triglyceride concentrations may be low because of poor intake or malabsorption. Liver tests [aspartate aminotransferase (AST), alanine aminotransferase (ALT), and bilirubin] remain normal in most individuals; refeeding (either enterally or parenterally) may be complicated by fatty infiltration and mild to moderate liver test abnormalities. Serum total protein and albumin levels are well maintained in most patients with malabsorption. Albumin levels may be depressed, if protein-losing enteropathy or a concurrent acute illness is present.

Prothrombin time and partial thromboplastin time are usually normal unless vitamin K malabsorption due to prolonged poor intake, chronic steatorrhea, antibiotic therapy, or colectomy has been present.

2. Blood levels of potentially malabsorbed substances—Additional circumstantial evidence of malabsorption can be obtained by measuring blood levels of several substances that may be reduced when malabsorption is present, including serum iron, vitamin B_{12}, folate, 25-hydroxyvitamin D, and carotene. The rationale is that generalized malabsorption will reduce serum concentrations of one or more of these substances. One problem with this concept, however, is that several of these substances have substantial body stores and thus depletion may take a long time. Another problem is that prolonged inadequate intake may also cause reduced serum levels. Thus, the sensitivity and specificity of low serum concentrations of these substances for malabsorption are poor. To make a firm diagnosis of malabsorption, more direct evidence of malabsorption should be obtained.

3. Tests of fat absorption—The simplest approach to detect the presence of fat malabsorption is a qualitative examination of stool. A spot specimen is smeared on a microscope slide and is gently heated with a drop of glacial acetic acid for a few seconds to allow fat droplets to form. A fat-soluble stain, such as Sudan III, is then applied and the slide is examined under the microscope. Stained fat droplets are sought and the number of droplets is assessed semiquantitatively.

This test is regularly positive (more than five droplets per high power field) when substantial steatorrhea is present, but may be equivocal if not done properly or with lesser degrees of steatorrhea. It has the additional advantage of being relatively simple and inexpensive. Light microscopy cannot be used to evaluate treatment (unless steatorrhea is completely eliminated) and is subject to false-positive results with some drugs and food additives (eg, mineral oil, orlistat, and olestra).

A more comprehensive evaluation of fat malabsorption can be obtained by chemical measurement of fat excretion. This test is best done as a 48-hour or 72-hour metabolic balance. Fat intake should be assessed by a dietician based on diet diaries to adjust for potentially large differences in fat intake. This works better than prescribing a 100 g fat diet or assuming that the patient is eating 100 g of fat each day. Stools need to be collected quantitatively; kits (consisting of a collection pan, preweighed containers, and coolant) can be made that simplify this task for outpatients. Once completed, the collected stools should be homogenized, weighed, and analyzed. Direct measurement of fat content by the VanderKamer (titrimetric) method or by gravimetric methods is preferable to indirect methods, such as near infrared spectroscopy. "False-positive" results can be due to ingestion of mineral oil, the lipase-inhibitor, orlistat, and the fat substitute, olestra.

Daily fecal fat output needs to be evaluated against stool weight. As stool weight increases, more fat is ex-

Table 23–4. Laboratory tests in malabsorption.

Routine blood tests	
Complete blood count	
Microcytic anemia	Blood loss, iron malabsorption
Macrocytic anemia	Vitamin B_{12} or folate deficiency
Lymphopenia	AIDS, lymphangiectasia
Thrombocytosis	Iron deficiency
Biochemical screening tests	
Hypokalemia	Poor potassium intake, excessive stool losses
Low blood urea nitrogen	Poor protein intake
Low serum creatinine	Muscle wasting
Low serum calcium	Calcium malabsorption, vitamin D deficiency, fat malabsorption, hypomagnesemia
Low serum albumin	Protein-losing enteropathy, concurrent acute disease
Prothrombin time	
Extended	Poor vitamin K intake, chronic steatorrhea, colectomy
Blood levels of potentially malabsorbed substances	
Serum iron, vitamin B_{12}, folate, 25-OH vitamin D, carotene	Reduced in malabsorption or prolonged inadequate intake
Tests of fat absorption	
Qualitative fecal fat	May be normal with mild or moderate steatorrhea
Quantitative fecal fat	Useful for follow-up, affected by stool weight
Tests of protein absorption	
Fecal nitrogen excretion	Adds little to assessment
α-antitrypsin clearance	Useful to identify protein-losing enteropathy
Tests of carbohydrate absorption	
Quantitative excretion (anthrone)	Does not account for colonic salvage
Stool pH <5.5	Characteristic for carbohydrate malabsorption
Osmotic gap in stool water	Not specific
Stool reducing substances	May be positive with reducing substances other than carbohydrates
D-Xylose absorption test	Measure urine and blood concentrations, low results suggest proximal intestinal dysfunction
Oral glucose, sucrose, lactose tolerance tests	May be misleading in patients with diabetes mellitus, bacterial overgrowth
Breath hydrogen tests	Simple and inexpensive test for malabsorption of a specific substrate
Schilling test with intrinsic factor	
Low urinary recovery	Suggests ileal dysfunction, may be abnormal with pancreatic exocrine insufficiency or bacterial overgrowth
Dual-labeled study	Corrects for pancreatic exocrine insufficiency
Tests of bile acid malabsorption	
Fecal bile acid excretion	"Gold standard," but difficult assay
Radiolabeled bile acid excretion	Correlates with fecal bile acid excretion
^{75}SeHCAT retention	Sensitive indicator of ileal bile acid malabsorption
[^{14}C] Glycocholic acid breath test	Abnormal with small bowel bacterial overgrowth or bile acid malabsorption
Tests for small bowel bacterial overgrowth	
[^{14}C] Glycocholic acid breath test	Sensitivity may be low
[^{14}C] Xylose breath test	Sensitivity may be low
Glucose breath hydrogen test	Inexpensive, some false negatives
Quantitative culture of jejunal aspirate (>10^5/mL)	"Gold standard" for this diagnosis
Tests for exocrine pancreatic insufficiency	
Stool chymotrypsin concentration	Low concentration in presence of steatorrhea highly suggestive of pancreatic insufficiency
Dual-labeled Schilling test	Complex test
Bentiromide test	May be abnormal if mucosal disease present
Secretin/CCK tests	Involve intubation, complex analysis

creted even without any mucosal pathology. Although normal fat excretion on an intake of 100 g/d is less than 7 g/d fat, outputs of up to 15 g/d may result solely from large stool weights. The stool fat concentration (grams of fat per 100 g stool) may also be helpful. Pancreatic exocrine insufficiency is associated with high stool fat concentrations (>10 g/100 g stool), since, unlike hydrolyzed fat, unhydrolyzed fat does not stimulate colonic water and electrolyte secretion that would dilute stool fat. Results can be affected by intake of mineral oil or other poorly absorbed lipids.

Measuring stool fat excretion is moderately difficult and somewhat expensive, but provides a reliable benchmark for the sequential assessment of therapy. It remains the gold standard for assessment of generalized malabsorption. Attempts to replace it with "cleaner" tests, such as the [^{14}C]triolein breath test, have not been successful.

4. Tests of protein absorption—Measuring fecal nitrogen excretion is not widely used to test for malabsorption. Although in theory the test can be conducted simultaneously with a quantitative stool fat collection, in practice it does not add much to the assessment of the patient.

When protein-losing enteropathy is suspected because of hypoalbuminemia, α_1-antitrypsin clearance can be measured. In this technique α_1-antitrypsin is used as a marker for serum protein loss into the intestine. It is about the same size as albumin, but is relatively resistant to hydrolysis by luminal enzymes. α_1-Antitrypsin is thought to leak into the intestine at the same rate as albumin, but passes into the stool with relatively little loss. By measuring α_1-antitrypsin concentration in serum and in a timed stool collection, clearance can be calculated by dividing stool output (concentration × volume) by serum concentration. This gives a result that can be interpreted as milliliters of serum leaked into the intestine each day. Values of more than 25 mL/d are associated with hypoalbuminemia.

5. Tests of carbohydrate absorption—Carbohydrate losses into the stool can be gauged by measuring total carbohydrate excretion in a quantitative stool collection by means of the anthrone method, but this does not measure small bowel malabsorption accurately because of fermentation of carbohydrate to short-chain fatty acids by colonic bacteria. The short-chain fatty acids can be absorbed by the colon, reducing the calorie loss and osmotic diarrhea that would otherwise occur with small intestinal carbohydrate malabsorption. This colonic salvage decreases the loss of carbohydrate calories, but the capacity for colonic short-chain fatty acid absorption is limited to about 80 g/d. Loss of unabsorbed short-chain fatty acids can be accounted for by

measuring their output in stool. This measurement can be converted back to carbohydrate fermented to short-chain fatty acids by applying an empiric fermentation formula. This calculated carbohydrate loss can be added to directly measured carbohydrate loss to give a better picture of overall carbohydrate malabsorption. Because of its complexity, such careful quantification is not often done for clinical purposes. Research studies on patients with chronic diarrhea have shown a wide range for carbohydrate malabsorption in various disorders.

More readily available, but indirect, tests for carbohydrate malabsorption are perfomed on routine stool chemical analysis. Because of carbohydrate fermentation in the colon, stool pH tends to be low when carbohydrate is malabsorbed. Stool pH less than 5.5 is characteristic, but may not always be present because other factors may alter stool pH. If a large amount of unfermented carbohydrate is present in stool water, an osmotic gap may be noted. The osmotic gap is an estimate of the amount of substances other than sodium, potassium, and their accompanying anions in stool water. The osmotic gap should be calculated by doubling the sum of the stool sodium and potassium concentrations (in mmol/L) and subtracting this from 290 mOsm, the osmolality of colonic contents within the body. Gaps greater than 50 mOsm suggest the presence of a substantial amount of some unmeasured solute, such as a simple sugar. Measured osmolalities in stool water should not be used for this calculation; they are often quite high due to fermentation of carbohydrate in the collection can in vitro. Another simple test on stool water is to measure reducing substances with a semiquantitative test, such as Glucotest tablets. If a substantial amount of unfermented reducing sugar is present, the test will be positive.

Another approach to evaluating carbohydrate malabsorption is an oral tolerance test in which a test sugar, such as glucose, sucrose, or lactose, is administered and blood glucose concentrations are measured over time. If no rise in blood sugar is seen, malabsorption is implied. A variant of this is the D-xylose test. In this test, D-xylose is given orally, usually in a dose of 25 g. Blood xylose concentration is measured after 1 and 3 hours and urinary excretion is measured for 5 hours after ingestion. Failure of blood xylose levels to rise above 20 mg/100 mL at 1 hour and above 22.5 mg/100 mL at 3 hours or failure of urinary output to exceed 5 g/5 h suggests malabsorption. For any of these oral tolerance tests a finding of malabsorption suggests mucosal dysfunction because none of these sugars depends on pancreatic enzymes or bile acids for absorption. These tests can be misleading if diabetes mellitus is present, if body fluid compartments are abnormal (ie, because of dehydration or ascites), or if renal function is impaired. They also can be abnormal in the presence of bacterial overgrowth in the upper intestine (or urinary tract infection for D-xylose) in which substrate may be destroyed.

Breath hydrogen tests are another approach to evaluating carbohydrate malabsorption. Substrates such as lactose or sucrose can be ingested orally. If these are not absorbed in the small intestine, they pass into the colon, where in most individuals the colonic bacteria can ferment the carbohydrate, producing hydrogen as a byproduct. This hydrogen is transported through the circulation to the lungs and exhaled, raising the hydrogen concentration in expired air. This can be measured with a simple gas chromatograph. Rises of more than 10–20 ppm after ingestion are consistent with malabsorption of the ingested substrate. This test is simple and inexpensive and is ideal for investigating patients in whom malabsorption of a specific carbohydrate is suspected (eg, due to disaccharidase deficiency). False-positive results can be due to small bowel bacterial overgrowth. (This produces an increase in breath hydrogen, but usually soon after ingestion.) False-negative results can be seen in individuals in whom the colonic flora does not produce hydrogen and in patients on antibiotic therapy.

6. Measurement of vitamin B_{12} absorption—In the context of evaluating malabsorption, vitamin B_{12} absorption is measured as an index of ileal function. Hence, part I of Schilling's test (measurement of B_{12} absorption in the absence of intrinsic factor) is not necessary, and part II (measurement of B_{12} absorption with intrinsic factor) can be done as the first step. In this test, radiolabeled B_{12} and exogenous intrinsic factor are given simultaneously by mouth, unlabeled B_{12} is given by injection to saturate internal B_{12} binding sites, and 24-hour urinary recovery of the radiolabel is measured. Recovery of less than 9% of the administered dose is abnormal and suggests ileal dysfunction. The test can be falsely positive for ileal dysfunction if pancreatic exocrine insufficiency is present (because endogenous R-protein may not be cleaved from R-protein–B_{12} complexes), if bacterial overgrowth is present, or if renal failure is present.

A dual-labeled Schilling test has been developed to investigate the possibility of exocrine pancreatic insufficiency as a cause for B_{12} malabsorption. In this study, two isotopes of cobalt are used to study the relative absorption of B_{12} coupled to R-protein and B_{12} coupled to intrinsic factor. Both complexes are labeled separately and given orally simultaneously. Urinary recovery of each isotope is measured. If pancreatic insufficiency is present, the B_{12} coupled with R-protein is malabsorbed and the ratio of isotopes in urine changes from the ratio that was administered. If bacterial overgrowth or ileal dysfunction is present, both B_{12} coupled to

R-protein and B_{12} coupled to intrinsic factor are malabsorbed equally and the ratio of the two isotopes is unchanged. Though not regularly performed because of its complexity, this test is becoming more available in large centers.

7. Evaluation of bile acid malabsorption—Selective malabsorption of bile acids by the ileum has been proposed as a common cause of chronic watery diarrhea and malabsorption of bile acid has been considered to be one factor contributing to chronic diarrhea in patients with ileal disease. Several tests have been developed to evaluate bile acid absorption.

The gold standard is to measure fecal bile acid concentration and output. This is difficult because of the complexity of the chemical analysis of bile acids, and therefore has been used mainly in research studies. Another test that has not been used widely is to feed radiolabeled bile and to measure recovery of the isotope in stool over several days. Results correlate with total fecal bile acid output, and the test is technically easier to perform.

More extensively used is the SeHCAT (selenium-75-labeled taurohomocholic acid) test. The radioactive taurocholic acid analog is administered orally and total body retention is measured over several days by repeated gamma scintigraphy. Retention of less than 50% after 3 days is abnormal and suggests bile acid malabsorption. Studies have suggested that this is a sensitive measure of bile acid malabsorption. Indeed, it may be too sensitive, producing a positive result when bile acid malabsorption may be too slight to produce diarrhea.

The [^{14}C]glycocholic acid breath test has also been used as a method of identifying bile acid malabsorption. This test was originally designed to evaluate small bowel bacterial overgrowth. ^{14}C is used to label the glycine residue of this conjugated bile acid and is liberated when the bile acid is deconjugated and glycine is metabolized by bacteria. Radioactive CO_2 is expired and measured. The test is positive when there is small bowel bacterial overgrowth or if glycocholic acid is malabsorbed by the ileum and enters the colon. The specificity and sensitivity of this test for ileal dysfunction have not been identified.

8. Tests for small bowel bacterial overgrowth—In addition to the [^{14}C]glycocholic acid breath test mentioned above, several other indirect tests have been developed. Each of these work on the principle that bacterial metabolism of a substrate will release some substance that is measurable in exhaled air. [^{14}C]Xylose is one of these substrates. In healthy individuals, xylose is absorbed from the small intestine and undergoes relatively slow metabolism in the body. If bacteria are present in the upper gastrointestinal tract or jejunum, xylose can be fermented and radioactive CO_2 will be exhaled in the breath. Recent studies indicate that the sensitivity of this test may be as low as 65%, making it of limited value.

A similar rationale is behind the glucose–breath hydrogen test. A bolus of glucose is ingested and breath hydrogen concentrations are measured sequentially. If no bacteria are present in the upper gastrointestinal tract or jejunum, the glucose is absorbed by the intestine and no hydrogen is generated since human metabolic pathways do not produce hydrogen gas as a byproduct. If bacteria are present, the glucose can be fermented before it can be absorbed and the hydrogen produced can be exhaled. This test also has sensitivity problems in some series, but is inexpensive and avoids exposure to radionuclides. Because of this, it is probably the indirect screening test of choice.

The gold standard for demonstrating bacterial overgrowth is quantitative culture of jejunal aspirate. A tube or long endoscope is inserted into the jejunum under radiographic or direct visual guidance and a sample of jejunal contents is aspirated and cultured quantitatively. Colony counts of more than 10^5/mL are abnormal. Care must be taken to avoid contamination of the specimen with oral flora or with antibacterials or bacteriostats that may have been used to clean the equipment.

9. Tests for exocrine pancreatic insufficiency— Whenever steatorrhea is present, exocrine pancreatic insufficiency needs to be considered. This insufficiency may result from pancreatic disease (eg, chronic pancreatitis) or lack of effective pancreatic stimulation (eg, because of mucosal atrophy in celiac disease, or as a sequela to gastric surgery that bypasses the duodenum). One of the simpler screening tests for exocrine pancreatic insufficiency is measurement of stool chymotrypsin concentration. In patients with steatorrhea, a low stool chymotrypsin concentration suggests the likelihood of exocrine pancreatic insufficiency, but does not prove it. Coupled with other information (eg, history of pancreatic disease, pancreatic calcification by x-ray), it may offer sufficient evidence to proceed with a therapeutic trial of high-dose pancreatic enzyme replacement. A low stool chymotrypsin concentration in the absence of steatorrhea does not have the same significance; most often this reflects dilution in a large stool volume.

Two other tubeless, indirect tests of pancreatic exocrine function are available. The dual-labeled Schilling test has already been discussed. The other test is the bentiromide test. In this technique, patients are fed an artificial substrate that can be hydrolyzed by chymotrypsin, N-benzoyl-L-tyrosyl-para-aminobenzoic acid (bentiromide). If adequate chymotrypsin activity is present, this substrate is hydrolyzed and the free para-aminobenzoic acid (PABA) is absorbed and excreted in the urine. Measurement of the amount of PABA recov-

ered provides an idea of the activity of chymotrypsin in the intestine. More than 50% reduction in enzymatic activity is necessary for PABA excretion to be reduced. The test can be "falsely" abnormal if mucosal disease, liver disease, or kidney disease alters the absorption, metabolism, distribution, or excretion of PABA. Attempts have been made to correct for some of this by simultaneously giving a tracer dose of [^{14}C]PABA or the closely related nonradioactive compound, para-aminosalicylate (PAS). Several drugs can interfere with analysis of PABA and these should be discontinued before the test.

The gold standard tests for exocrine pancreatic insufficiency involve duodenal intubation and stimulation of the pancreas with either secretin, secretin and cholecystokinin, or a test meal (Lundh meal). Duodenal contents are aspirated and volume, bicarbonate secretion, and enzyme secretion can be measured. Steatorrhea usually does not occur until less than 10–20% of pancreatic secretory capacity remains.

These tests are infrequently performed because of their complexity; therapeutic trials of exogenous enzyme therapy are used instead. If a therapeutic trial is undertaken, several precautions should be used to prevent misinterpretation: (1) give a large dose of an active enzyme preparation, (2) make sure that the patient knows exactly how to take the enzyme supplement, and (3) measure the response of stool fat to the trial. If these steps are not done, an equivocal trial may result.

C. IMAGING

Visualization of the absorptive surface of the small intestine by means of a small bowel follow-through study or by enteroclysis is an important step toward defining the cause of malabsorption. Table 23–5 details some of the many findings that have been associated with various conditions producing malabsorption. It is important to realize that differences in technique and contrast materials may accentuate or minimize some of these findings and therefore the reliability of some of the softer findings is questionable. It is also important to realize that severe malabsorption may be present despite no radiologic findings. Radiography cannot be used as a substitute for functional testing. Neither can the radiologist make a diagnosis of a malabsorptive disease with certainty. For example, the same findings could represent mucosal edema, lymphoma, or an acute viral syndrome. The radiologist can exclude some conditions and suggest others, but the definite diagnosis of these disorders depends on a clinical aggregation of history, laboratory findings, and pathology.

Use of computed tomography (CT) scans in patients with malabsorption disorders is frequently helpful. The CT scan allows visualization of the pancreas, lymph nodes, and mesentery in addition to the small

Table 23–5. Small bowel radiographic findings in malabsorption.

	Luminal Caliber	Luminal Fluid	Folds	Gut Wall	Extra-luminal Mass	Other
Celiac disease	Dilated	Increased	Thin, effaced ("moulage")	—	—	Segmentation of barium column, painless intussusceptions
Whipple's disease	Normal	—	Thick, wild pattern	—	—	Patchy micronodularity
Scleroderma	Dilated, especially the duodenum	—	—	—	—	Delayed peristalsis, hypomotility
Lymphoma	Variable	—	Coarse	Infiltrated, stiff	Often	—
Amyloidosis	Normal	—	Symmetric thickening, no edema	Stiff	—	Micronodularity
Lymphangiectasia	—	Increased	Thick, edematous	—	—	Micronodularity
Crohn's disease	Stenotic	—	Deformed	Rigidity, ulceration, thickening	Sometimes	—
Dysgamma globulinemia	—	—	Thick	—	—	Nodular lymphoid hyperplasia
Giardiasis	—	Increased	Thick in duodenum and jejunum	—	—	Spasm, rapid transit
Zollinger-Ellison syndrome	Dilated duodenum	Increased	Thick in duodenum	—	—	Peptic ulcers, reticulated small bowel pattern
Cystic fibrosis	Dilated duodenum	—	Thick in duodenum	—	—	Nodularity in duodenum
Abetalipoproteinemia	—	—	Thick	—	—	Fine mucosal graininess
Mastocytosis	—	—	—	Thick	—	Mucosal nodularity, "bull's eye" lesions

intestine. This often permits additional conditions to be considered or eliminated from consideration.

Some mucosal diseases produce gross changes that can be visualized by upper gastrointestinal endoscopy or enteroscopy. In general, it is not worthwhile doing endoscopic examination solely for the purpose of inspecting the intestine. However, endoscopy can be used to aspirate jejunal contents or to obtain mucosal biopsies.

D. PATHOLOGY

Most patients with panmalabsorption will require a small bowel biopsy to identify or exclude diffuse mucosal disease as a cause for their problem. Table 23–6 indicates conditions in which small bowel biopsy is use-

ful and offers diagnostic considerations for various findings.

For the pathologist to interpret the histology correctly, the gastroenterologist must provide enough tissue. In most cases, endoscopic biopsies from the distal duodenum can be interpreted, but it is important that multiple biopsies be obtained. Capsule biopsies provide larger samples of tissue and can be obtained more distally in the bowel, features that are important in some situations. When possible, biopsies should be oriented so that sections can be made perpendicular to the surface, since tangential sections are difficult to evaluate. When possible, the gastroenterologist should review the biopsy slides with the pathologist to ascertain both the

Table 23–6. Interpretatin of pathologic findings on small bowel biopsy in malabsorption.

Brush border abnormalities	
Sickle-shaped organisms	Giardiasis
Basophilic dots	*Cryptosporidium*
Inclusions	Microvillous inclusion disease
Abnormal enterocytes	
Intracytoplasmic organisms	Isosporiasis
Foamy vacuolation	Abetalipoproteinemia
Lack of enteroendocrine D cells	Autoimmune polyglandular syndrome
Abnormal basement membrane collagenous band	Collagenous sprue
Villous atrophy	
Total or partial	Celiac disease, tropical sprue, bacterial overgrowth, dysgamma-globulinemia, dermatitis herpetiformis, radiation enteritis, IPSID,[1] acute viral infection, ischemia, nongranulomatous ulcerative jejunoileitis, microsporidiosis
Lamina propria abnormalities	
Noncaseating granulomas	Crohn's disease
Infiltrating eosinophils	Eosinophilic gastroenteritis
Infiltrating malignant lymphocytes	Lymphoma, IPSID
Infiltrating mast cells	Mastocytosis
PAS-positive macrophages	Whipple's disease (bacilli on EM), *Mycobacterium avium-intracellulare* (acidfast bacilli)
Dilated lymphatics	Lymphanigiectasia

[1]IPSID, immunoproliferative small intestinal disease.

confidence of the pathologist in the diagnosis and the adequacy of the tissue provided.

Differential Diagnosis & Descriptions of Specific Entities

The differential diagnosis of malabsorption is quite broad (see Table 23–1). For clinical purposes, it is useful to divide these into five categories:

1. Mucosal disorders causing generalized malabsorption.

2. Infectious diseases causing generalized malabsorption.
3. Luminal problems causing malabsorption.
4. Postoperative malabsorption.
5. Disorders that cause malabsorption of specific nutrients.

A. MUCOSAL DISORDERS CAUSING GENERALIZED MALABSORPTION

1. Celiac sprue—Celiac disease is characterized by malabsorption usually of a variety of nutrients, villous atrophy of the small intestine, and clinical improvement following withdrawal of dietary gluten, a protein component of several grains.

The malabsorption is due to damage to the absorptive mucosa of the small intestine. Surface area is reduced substantially because of the villous atrophy, and the remaining absorptive cells are damaged, often lacking membrane-bound disaccharidases and peptidases, which are essential for mucosal hydrolysis. In contrast, the crypts undergo substantial hyperplasia and lengthen. The extent of malabsorption depends on the length of intestine affected. Patients with duodenal involvement only may have isolated iron deficiency, whereas those with more extensive involvement have panmalabsorption. Involvement is typically more severe proximally in the intestine and diminishes distally. In a few patients with celiac disease, the loss of the absorptive surface is so extensive that a secretory diarrhea is present even when the patient is fasting.

The current thinking about the cause of celiac disease is that it represents an abnormal immune response to gluten (specifically gliadin), a component of wheat, barley, rye, and some varieties of oats. Rice and corn do not contain gluten. The immune response is both humoral and cellular and can produce damage to the mucosa within hours of exposure to gluten. Genetic factors are important as in many immunologically mediated disorders. HLA-DQ2 or DQ8 is present in most European and North American patients with celiac disease. Environmental factors, such as prior exposure to type 12 adenovirus, the coat of which shares some homology to gluten, may also be important.

The clinical course of celiac disease is variable. Symptoms frequently develop in childhood and malabsorption may be severe enough to stunt growth. Children may be pale, thin, and spindly; often their symptoms subside in adolescence, only to reappear in middle age. Other patients first develop symptoms in adulthood.

The diagnosis of celiac sprue depends on the demonstration of malabsorption, typical histologic features on small intestinal biopsies, and response to a gluten-free diet. Serological tests such as antigliadin antibodies have not had sufficient specificity to preclude biopsy. Antiendomysial antibodies that are directed against tissue transglutaminase are highly specific and very sensitive. In cases with a classical presentation, a positive antitissue transglutaminase antibody may be sufficient for diagnosis.

Treatment of celiac disease consists of strict exclusion of gluten from the diet. This is more difficult than it seems, because gluten is present in a number of prepared foods that have no obvious connection to grains containing gluten. Initially, lactose intake should be restricted as well, because of the likelihood of secondary lactase deficiency. Patients need rigorous instruction by a dietician to ensure compliance with this diet. Symptoms should respond to gluten withdrawal within a few weeks. If they do not, adherence to the diet needs to be reevaluated. Failure to respond to a strict diet excludes celiac disease; other diagnoses then need to be considered.

Because adherence to the gluten-free diet is difficult and must be continued for a lifetime, objective evidence of improvement should be obtained. Ideally, the patient should undergo another small bowel biopsy to document a return to normal. If this is impossible, repeating the quantitative stool fat or some other test of absorption should be considered. In cases with equivocal biopsy results, a gluten challenge with repeat small bowel biopsy to document abnormality may be worthwhile.

The prognosis of patients with celiac disease is generally excellent with treatment. Absorptive defects resolve promptly and most deficiencies can be repaired with refeeding. Serious complications occur in a minority of patients. These include malignant neoplasms, progression to refractory sprue, and ulceration. Malignant disease may complicate the course of celiac sprue in up to one-eighth of patients. Most tumors are T cell lymphomas; there is also an excess incidence of small intestinal adenocarcinoma.

Refractory sprue is an unusual pattern of disease in which a patient responds to treatment, but then symptoms return despite continued adherence to a gluten-free diet. The cause for this is not clear. Some of these patients respond to corticosteroid therapy; others need to be maintained with parenteral nutrition. Ulceration occurs in very few patients and can be complicated by perforation or stricture formation.

2. Collagenous sprue—This rare condition of unknown cause presents with symptoms and signs of malabsorption, not unlike celiac sprue. Biopsy of the small intestine shows a flat mucosa with collagen deposition in the lamina propria and few crypts. It does not improve with a gluten-free diet and rarely with other therapy, such as corticosteroids or other immunomodulators. Without parenteral nutrition, it is invariably fatal.

3. Nongranulomatous ulcerative jejunoileitis—Patients with this disorder present with severe malabsorption and diarrhea related to extensive ulceration of the small intestine. The absorptive surface between ulcers is often abnormal with variable degrees of villous atrophy. The relationship to celiac disease is not clear, but some patients respond to gluten withdrawal or to corticosteroids. The disease is progressive and fatal. Enterectomy has been performed in a few patients with mixed results.

4. Eosinophilic gastroenteritis—Eosinophilic gastroenteritis is another rare condition that is associated with malabsorption. In this disorder, the wall of the intestine is infiltrated with eosinophils, which can disrupt absorptive function. It is most often a component of systemic eosinophilia, but 20% of cases may have no abnormality in the peripheral blood.

The cause of eosinophilic gastroenteritis is unknown. Food allergies have been implicated in one-half of cases and sensitivity to drugs or toxins in others. Eosinophils infiltrate the mucosa and submucosa and villous atrophy can be present. This is the form of the disease that is associated with malabsorption. Involvement of the muscular layers or serosa typically produces intestinal obstruction or ascites, respectively.

Laboratory tests may show peripheral blood eosinophilia (in 80% of patients), iron deficiency anemia (due to blood loss), and hypoalbuminemia (due to protein-losing enteropathy). In some patients, Charcot-Leyden crystals can be detected in stools, but the specificity of this for the diagnosis of eosinophilic gastroenteritis is unknown.

Intestinal biopsy is essential for diagnosis. The finding of increased eosinophils in the mucosa should prompt consideration of a diagnosis of eosinophilic gastroenteritis, but other conditions need to be considered as well. These include parasitic diseases, connective tissue diseases, vasculitis, systemic mastocytosis, inflammatory bowel disease, celiac disease, specific food allergies (eg, cow's milk, milk protein sensitivity), and hypereosinophilia syndrome. Local infiltration with eosinophils can be seen in some benign polyps (eosinophilic granuloma).

Treatment consists of an elimination diet (sequential elimination of individual sources of protein, such as milk, beef, or eggs) and corticosteroids. Experience with other immunosuppressive agents is quite limited. The prognosis for this disease is generally good with treatment.

5. Systemic mastocytosis—Some patients with mastocytosis have malabsorption in addition to other symptoms, such as nausea, vomiting, diarrhea, and flushing. In this disorder, mast cells infiltrate the intestinal wall and other organs and release mediators, such as histamine, eosinophil chemotactic factor, platelet-activating factor, and other cytokines. Release can be triggered by several different agents, such as exogenous and endogenous antigens.

Diagnosis of mastocytosis may be difficult because of the protean manifestations of this disease. If typical cutaneous involvement (urticaria pigmentosa), flushing, and gastrointestinal symptoms are present, only confirmatory tests may be necessary; measurement of plasma and urine histamine concentrations can provide indirect evidence for the presence of mastocytosis. Otherwise, intestinal biopsy can be useful. Mast cells are not well demonstrated by standard histochemical stains, such as hematoxylin and eosin, and impressive numbers may be overlooked with routine biopsy processing. Special stains, such as toluidine blue, may be necessary.

Treatment depends on the severity of the disease. For mild cases without much in the way of lymph node or splenic infiltration, therapy with oral sodium chromoglycate, H$_1$- and H$_2$-antagonists, and low-dose aspirin may be sufficient. For extensive disease, therapy with interferon may cause a marked reduction in mast cell burden. The outlook for patients with mastocytosis is generally good, if symptoms can be controlled and organ infiltration is not extensive.

6. Immunoproliferative small intestinal disease (IPSID)

—This disorder, once called alpha chain disease, is thought to be related to proliferation of the cells of the intestinal immune system in response to chronic antigenic stimulation, probably by bacteria. Signs include dense infiltration of the mucosa and submucosa of the entire small intestine with lymphocytes and plasma cells in association with flattening of the villi. The infiltrate may be benign appearing or have features consistent with a low-grade or intermediate-grade malignant lymphoma. Patients suffer from severe malabsorption and weight loss because of disruption of the absorptive surface of the small intestine.

The disease mainly affects adolescents and young adults in the Middle East, North Africa, and South Africa. Clinical manifestations include severe diarrhea, crampy abdominal pain, anorexia, and marked, progressive weight loss. Fever may be prominent in some patients. Organomegaly and abdominal mass are not seen early in the course, but may develop later.

Diagnosis depends on demonstration of diffuse intestinal involvement by radiography, the characteristic histologic findings by small bowel biopsy, and typical changes in serum proteins. Serum protein electrophoresis may show a broad band in the α_2 or β regions. This paraprotein is the Fc portion of immunoglobulin A (IgA). No light chains are present in the serum, and Bence Jones proteins are absent from the urine.

Treatment is empiric. For early stage disease, prolonged antibiotic therapy (tetracycline 250 mg four times a day or ampicillin plus metronidazole) may induce a remission within 6–12 months. Once malignant changes have occurred, combination cytotoxic chemotherapy can be tried; results have been variable. Surgery for cure is not feasible because of the extent of involvement.

7. Lymphoma

—Several types of lymphoma involve the small intestine. T cell lymphomas complicate the course of celiac disease. Tumors of the mucosa-associated lymphoid tissue (MALToma) affect the B lymphocytes associated with Peyer's patches. Multiple lymphoid polyposis is a multicentric polypoid mucosal tumor of B cells. The most common types are diffuse large cell lymphoma and small noncleaved lymphoma, in which involvement is initially segmental.

Malabsorption syndrome occurs with more extensive lymphomas, especially T cell lymphomas. Localized B cell lymphomas are more likely to produce pain, obstruction, and abdominal mass, unless bacterial overgrowth or terminal ileal involvement predisposes to malabsorption.

8. Lymphangiectasia

—Protein-losing enteropathy can complicate the course of several malabsorptive diseases, particularly when accompanied by mucosal ulceration or lymphatic obstruction (Table 23–7). It can also occur as an isolated phenomenon without generalized malabsorption. In such cases the only clinical finding may be hypoalbuminemia and lymphopenia.

Intestinal lymphangiectasia is a disease of children and young adults characterized by the formation of dilated lymphatic channels in the small bowel mucosa. These dilated channels are patchy and several biopsies may be necessary to make a diagnosis. The dilated lymphatics rupture easily and leak lymph containing a variety of plasma proteins, lymphocytes, and chylomicrons.

Table 23–7. Malabsorptive disorders associated with protein-losing enteropathy.

Mucosal diseases
  Celiac disease
  Tropical sprue
  Whipple's disease
  Eosinophilic gastroenteritis
  Small bowel bacterial overgrowth
  Ulcerative jejunoileitis
Lymphatic obstruction
  Congenital lymphangiectasia
  Lymphoma
  Crohn's disease
  Constrictive pericarditis

If the lesions are proximal, the processes of luminal digestion and mucosal absorption distally may remove most of the leaked protein and fat from the lumen so that measured stool protein or fat losses may be very low. When steatorrhea is present, it is typically mild (<10 g excretion per day). Diarrhea is usually not severe. Edema is the major sign at presentation.

Diagnosis depends on recognizing the possibility of protein-losing enteropathy and excluding other malabsorptive disorders associated with it (see Table 23–7). Measurement of α_1-antitrypsin clearance with a timed stool collection can confirm protein-losing enteropathy. Mucosal biopsy can show dilated lymphatic channels, but does not necessarily show the cause of the condition. Small bowel x-rays, abdominal CT scan, and cardiac catheterization may be needed to exclude primary causes.

Treatment of lymphangiectasia consists of dietary manipulation and supportive measures. Intestinal lymph flow varies with meal composition; a low-fat diet can reduce protein loss. Breakdown products of medium-chain triglycerides (MCT) are transported in portal blood and therefore do not increase lymph flow. MCT oil can be used to improve caloric intake without worsening enteric protein loss. Supportive measures include appropriate (limited) use of diuretics and elastic support hose to control edema. With these measures the prognosis for patients with intestinal lymphangiectasia is good.

9. Crohn's disease—Crohn's disease can produce malabsorption in four ways:

1. Extensive direct mucosal involvement.
2. Stricture formation and bacterial overgrowth.
3. Fistula formation leading to bacterial overgrowth.
4. Surgical resection of the small intestine.

Crohn's disease is discussed further in Chapter 7.

10. Radiation enteritis—Radiation therapy directed to the abdomen or pelvis routinely produces gastrointestinal dysfunction and often symptoms as well. These abnormalities can develop acutely or after many years. Whereas diarrhea may present acutely or chronically, and absorption tests may be abnormal acutely, clinically important malabsorption typically occurs only late after irradiation.

The pathogenesis of malabsorption involves several mechanisms. Acutely, subclinical malabsorption is due to mucosal damage, but this usually resolves as the mucosa regenerates. Chronic malabsorption can occur years after irradiation and may be due to (1) ileal dysfunction causing bile acid malabsorption and depletion, (2) bacterial overgrowth due to intestinal strictures, and (3) enteroenteral or enterocolic fistulas. Other contributing factors can be lymphatic obstruction, ischemia, and radiation-induced motility disorders.

Diagnosis depends on a careful history and typical radiographic findings. Because several mechanisms can contribute to diarrhea and malabsorption, it may be useful to define the mechanism of malabsorption so that the correct treatment can be selected. This may involve tests for bile acid malabsorption or bacterial overgrowth (see the section on "Tests for small bowel bacterial overgrowth").

Therapy is aimed at correcting malnutrition, maximizing absorption of nutrients, and correcting remediable processes, such as small bowel bacterial overgrowth. Parenteral nutrition and bowel rest may be needed to control symptoms and to allow time to institute other therapeutic measures. Maximizing absorption involves dietary manipulation (elemental diet if hydrolysis is impaired, medium-chain triglyceride if bile acid deficiency is present, frequent feedings to maximize exposure of the mucosa to nutrients), and antiperistaltic agents (opioids or anticholinergics) to slow transit and increase the contact time of luminal contents with the absorptive surface. Surgery should be limited to correction of obstruction or fistulous disease.

With adequate therapy the prognosis of malabsorption in radiation enteritis is good. Patients rarely need long-term parenteral nutrition.

11. Chronic mesenteric ischemia—Patients with chronic mesenteric ischemia often develop weight loss and evidence of malabsorption in addition to the cardinal feature of postprandial abdominal pain. Weight loss is frequently due to sitophobia, but many of these patients have mild to moderate steatorrhea, too.

This syndrome can occur when blood flow through two of the three mesenteric vessels is compromised. Audible bruits are heard in some of these patients, but diagnosis is prompted by history rather than physical or laboratory findings. Angiography shows vascular occlusion and collateral formation. In the presence of typical symptoms, such findings should prompt surgery. Revascularization can be accomplished by several methods and can produce a good long-term result with reversal of malabsorption and weight gain.

B. INFECTIOUS DISEASES CAUSING GENERALIZED MALABSORPTION

1. Small bowel bacterial overgrowth—The upper gastrointestinal tract ordinarily supports the growth of a very sparse bacterial flora ($<10^4$/mL). This is somewhat surprising in view of the large amount of nutrients and warm, dark environment that should be conducive to bacterial growth. This paradox is due to a series of defenses that limit bacterial proliferation, including gastric acidity, and immunologic, secretory, and motility mechanisms (migrating motor complex) that tend to clear the upper tract of luminal contents and prevent stasis.

When disease or therapy interferes with these protective mechanisms, bacteria can proliferate in the lumen and can produce malabsorption. Fat malabsorption results from bacterial deconjugation of bile acid. This allows the free bile acid to be reabsorbed, lowering luminal bile acid concentration and limiting micelle formation. In addition, patchy mucosal damage (villous blunting and increased lamina propria cellularity) due to bacterial toxins or the toxic effects of free bile acids may also contribute to fat malabsorption. Carbohydrate and protein malabsorption can also be related to mucosal damage or to intraluminal bacterial metabolism of these nutrients. To some extent bacteria can also compete for nutrients. For example, vitamin B_{12} is absorbed by gram-negative, anaerobic bacteria and is sequestered from ileal absorption sites. (Intrinsic factor protects vitamin B_{12} from uptake by aerobic bacteria.) In contrast, luminal bacteria release folate into the intestine, and deficiency of this vitamin is unlikely with bacterial overgrowth.

Conditions that predispose to bacterial overgrowth include achlorhydria or hypochlorhydria (due to atrophic gastritis or antisecretory drug therapy), motility disorders of the upper gut (diabetes mellitus, scleroderma, chronic intestinal pseudoobstruction), and anatomic problems, such as blind loops, diverticulosis, intestinal obstruction, afferent loop syndrome, and gastrocolic or enterocolic fistula. Although many of these predisposing conditions are "permanent," the severity of malabsorption and diarrhea may wax and wane as the bacterial population rises and falls.

The clinical features of bacterial overgrowth are those typical for malabsorption: steatorrhea or watery diarrhea, weight loss, and anemia. When present, anemia is macrocytic and is due to vitamin B_{12} malabsorption. Metabolic bone disease may complicate bacterial overgrowth in some patients.

Diagnosis is made by showing both evidence of malabsorption and direct or indirect evidence of bacterial overgrowth. A quantitative culture of luminal contents is the gold standard, but breath hydrogen testing and other indirect tests (see section, "Tests for small bowel bacterial overgrowth") may be sufficient if the clinical findings are very suggestive. Small bowel x-ray studies should be done in all of these patients to look for anatomic problems. Small bowel biopsies done in the course of evaluation of steatorrhea may show villous blunting and increased cellularity of the lamina propria, but these changes are not specific.

Treatment consists of antibiotic therapy, if no correctable anatomic problems are discovered. Tetracycline is no longer universally effective in these patients.

Amoxicillin with clavulinic acid, cephalosporins, chloramphenicol, ciprofloxacin, and metronidazole have been recommended in its place. Therapy should be given for 1–2 weeks and then discontinued. Patients should be retreated when symptoms recur. If symptoms recur quickly, intermittent expectant courses of antibiotic should be tried. Very few patients with this syndrome need to be on continuous antibiotic therapy. If anatomic problems are present, surgical correction should be considered. This may not be practical for some lesions (eg, duodenal diverticulum), but may be useful in others (eg, fistula).

2. Tropical sprue—Tropical sprue is a progressive, chronic malabsorptive disease occurring in people living in certain tropical countries. It is characterized by abnormalities in intestinal structure and function, symptoms related to malabsorption, and responsiveness to treatment with folic acid, tetracycline, or both. It must be differentiated from subclinical malabsorption, an endemic condition in tropical countries that may produce similar structural changes, but that does not produce symptoms. Subclinical malabsorption is quite common in indigenous populations in the Caribbean, Central America, northern South America, Equatorial and South Africa, the Indian subcontinent, and Southeast Asia. Tropical sprue occurs both in the indigenous population and in foreigners who reside in tropical places for extended periods.

It is unclear whether the incidence of tropical sprue is declining or not. Americans who fought in Vietnam and Peace Corps volunteers working in endemic areas did not have as much trouble with tropical sprue as expected. Whether improved nutrition, better sanitation, or prompt treatment of acute diarrhea with antibiotics is responsible for this is not known.

The leading hypothesis about the cause of tropical sprue is that it represents a form of small bowel bacterial overgrowth. Most individuals with tropical sprue have evidence of aerobic gram-negative bacterial overgrowth and at least some of these strains appear to secrete enterotoxins. What distinguishes individuals with tropical sprue from other patients with bacterial overgrowth (other than the obvious epidemiology) is not clear.

Tropical sprue typically begins as an acute diarrheal disorder that then develops into a chronic persistent diarrhea. Over the course of several months, evidence of more substantial malabsorption develops, associated with progressive weight loss. Megaloblastic anemia (due to folate or combined folate and B_{12} deficiency) then becomes prominent along with variable evidence of other deficiency states. Untreated tropical sprue can be fatal.

The basis for malabsorption is dysfunction of the mucosa. Histologically, the villi are shortened and thickened (partial villous atrophy); the flat mucosa of celiac sprue is not usually observed. The enterocytes themselves are abnormal with disruption of microvilli and reduced brush border enzyme levels. A chronic inflammatory infiltrate is present in the submucosa. Megaloblastic changes may be seen in the crypt epithelium.

Diagnosis of tropical sprue depends upon recognition of malabsorption in an individual complaining of diarrhea who was a resident of one of the endemic countries. The finding of B_{12} or folate deficiency and typical biopsy changes should suggest the diagnosis. It is important to exclude other infectious problems, such as giardiasis or cryptosporidiosis (see section, "Parasitic diseases"). Treatment of tropical sprue includes pharmacologic doses of folic acid (5 mg daily), injection of B_{12} (if deficient), and antibiotic therapy. Tetracycline (250 mg four times a day) or sulfonamide is the treatment of choice; newer antibiotics have not been extensively tested. Antibiotic therapy should be continued for 1–6 months. Optimal therapy includes both folate and an antibiotic; therapy with folic acid alone does not allow resolution of all of the structural changes in the intestine and therapy with antibiotic alone delays correction of the vitamin deficiencies until structural integrity is restored. Improvement should be seen with optimal therapy over the course of a few weeks.

The prognosis with treatment is excellent, but recurrences can occur, particularly in patients indigenous to endemic areas. There does not seem to be an excess risk for lymphoma or other cancers in patients with tropical sprue. Subclinical malabsorption may be associated with the development of low-grade lymphoma of the small intestine (MALToma) in some populations.

3. Whipple's disease—Whipple's disease is an uncommon chronic bacterial infection with multisystem involvement. The small bowel is usually involved and gastrointestinal symptoms are prominent. Typically, the intestinal mucosa is heavily infiltrated by foamy macrophages containing periodic acid–Schiff (PAS)-positive material, distorting the villi. Under electron microscopy or high-resolution light microscopy, bacteria can be visualized in the lamina propria. PAS-positive macrophages and bacteria have been demonstrated outside the intestine in lymph nodes, spleen, liver, central nervous system, heart, and synovium.

The bacterium responsible for Whipple's disease has been cultured with great difficulty. Genetic analysis shows that it is related to actinobacter and it has been named *Tropheryma whippleii*. It does not appear to be very contagious; no cases of direct person-to-person transmission have been published. Presumably, differences in host resistance or reaction to the organism allow proliferation without clearance of the bacteria.

Whipple's disease occurs mainly in older white men, but women and all races are susceptible. Most patients have diarrhea or other gastrointestinal symptoms of malabsorption, but some present with only joint or neurologic symptoms. Extraintestinal symptoms, including arthritis, fever, cough, dementia, headache, and muscle weakness, are common and can predate gastrointestinal symptoms. Unlike most other malabsorptive disorders, gastrointestinal bleeding, either gross or occult, can occur. Protein-losing enteropathy (and resultant hypoalbuminemia and edema) may occur due to blockage of lymphatic drainage by infiltrated lymph nodes.

When gastrointestinal symptoms predominate, diagnosis depends upon recognition of the clinical syndrome, proof of malabsorption, and small intestine biopsy. Diagnosis can be difficult if the patient presents with arthritis, fever, or neurologic symptoms and no intestinal symptoms.

Care must be taken to differentiate biopsies in Whipple's disease from those in infection with *Mycobacterium avium intracellulare* (MAI) in patients with AIDS. Both disorders have infiltration of the lamina propria with PAS-positive macrophages. MAI, however, is an acid-fast organism, whereas the Whipple's bacterium is not. Electron microscopy can also be used to differentiate the two conditions.

Antibiotic therapy produces an excellent response in most patients within days to weeks, but must be continued for months to years. Several different regimens have been recommended, including penicillin, erythromycin, ampicillin, tetracycline, chloramphenicol, or trimethoprim-sulfamethoxazole. Relapses are common with any of these regimens. If central nervous system involvement is present, chloramphenicol should be administered, and antibiotic therapy should be continued for a long time (if not permanently). The role of rebiopsy to confirm clearance of the organisms from the intestine is uncertain, but makes sense before discontinuing antibiotic therapy. PAS-positive macrophages may persist for years after bacteria disappear.

4. Parasitic diseases—Although many organisms parasitize humans on a regular basis, only a few produce malabsorption with any regularity (Table 23–8). Potential mechanisms producing malabsorption include competition for luminal nutrients, mechanical occlusion of the absorptive surface, and epithelial damage. It is also possible that immune responses to the organisms or their products alter intestinal motility or stimulate secretion.

Giardia lamblia is a cosmopolitan parasite that can be acquired from contaminated water in the United States. The organism can also be spread person to person by fecal–oral transmission, especially in daycare centers for

Table 23–8. Parasites associated with malabsorption.

Protozoa
  Giardia lamblia
  Coccidia
    Isospora belli
    Cryptosporidium
  Microsporidia (*Enterocytozoon bieneusi*)
Tapeworms
  Taenia saginata (beef tapeworm)
  Hymenolepis nana (dwarf tapeworm)
  Diphyllobothrium latum (fish tapeworm)

---

infants and in facilities for the mentally retarded. *Giardia* is found encysted and as trophozoites. The cysts are relatively resistent to environmental stresses, but can be killed by boiling or chemical disinfectants. Patients with dysgammaglobulinemia (decreased IgA and IgM levels) are particularly likely to be infected.

Patients with giardiasis complain of diarrhea, bloating, dyspepsia, fatigue, and weight loss. Symptoms can become chronic, but may be intermittent. Secondary disaccharidase deficiency can lead to flatulence and other symptoms of lactase deficiency.

Diagnosis depends on finding the *Giardia* organism or its antigens in stool, or by small bowel biopsy. Standard ova and parasite examination of stool is positive in only 50% of infected patients. Concentration and staining techniques can improve the yield somewhat, but the organism may never be seen in stool in up to 25% of patients. Immunologic studies [immunoelectrophoresis or enzyme-linked immunosorbent assay (ELISA)] for *Giardia* antigens in stool are better methods of detecting giardiasis and have a sensitivity of greater than 90%. Small bowel biopsy is another way to find the organism. Most patients with giardiasis have structurally normal small bowel mucosa and the organisms can be missed on casual inspection. Microscopic examination of duodenal contents or "touch preps" (in which a biopsy is pressed against a glass slide, leaving a layer of mucus that is then stained with Giemsa stain) may have a higher yield for the organisms than routine biopsies. Biopsies from patients with dysgammaglobulinemia may have changes resembling celiac disease and these patients may have more severe malabsorption.

Therapy consists of quinacrine 100 mg or metronidazole 250 mg three times a day for a week. Patients with immunodeficiency require longer courses of therapy (from 6 weeks to 6 months) to clear their infection. When clearance does not occur, combination therapy with quinacrine and high-dose metronidazole (750 mg three times a day) can be used. Furazolidone (100 mg four times a day) is an alternative.

Coccidia are protozoa that invade the epithelium, producing functional disruption. *Isospora belli* enters the enterocytes and reproduces within the cytoplasm. This can produce disruption of the cells, villous abnormalities, or even necrotizing enterocolitis. The onset is usually acute with diarrhea, weight loss, abdominal pain, and fever. Oocysts can be found on concentrated stool specimens and are pink with acid-fast stains. The parasites can also be seen on appropriately stained mucosal biopsies, but many sections may need to be examined. The disease is usually self-limited and runs its course over 1 week to 6 months. Treatment with trimethoprim-sulfamethoxazole or furazolidone may shorten the course.

Cryptosporidia are also classified as *Coccidia*. Unlike *Isospora*, *Cryptosporidia* do not enter cells, but instead attach to the brush border, destroying microvilli. This reduces absorptive capacity and produces a watery diarrhea associated with evidence of malabsorption of various nutrients. Acid-fast smears of stool or concentrated stool specimens can identify the organism. Mucosal biopsy with detection of basophilic bodies in the brush border is diagnostic. Normal subjects have a self-limited course lasting about 2 weeks. Patients with AIDS have a prolonged course that sometimes subsides with paromomycin 500 mg four times a day.

Microsporidia are intracellular protozoa that have been associated with diarrhea and malabsorption in patients with AIDS and other immunodeficiency diseases. They produce partial villous atrophy and may be difficult to see with light microscopy. Electron microscopy shows typical changes, however. Examination of stool with special trichrome stains has sometimes been helpful in finding the organism. No treatment has been shown to clear the organism reliably in AIDS patients. Metronidazole has been tried and may help some with symptoms.

Tapeworms compete with their hosts for nutrients in the lumen. In most cases substantial malabsorption does not occur. *Diphyllobothrium latum,* the fish tapeworm, can produce vitamin B_{12} deficiency. *Taenia solium,* the pork tapeworm, produces cysticercosis (from ingestion of eggs) more often than it produces tapeworms (from ingestion of larva in infected meat). *Taenia saginata* (beef tapeworm) is more commonly found in the United States and may produce weight loss. *Hymenolepis nana* (dwarf tapeworm) is the most common tapeworm in the United States. There is no intermediate host and infection results from ingestion of human feces containing embryonated eggs; autoinfection is possible. Diagnosis of any tapeworm infection depends on careful examination of stool for eggs and proglottids. Treatment of *Diphyllobothrium latum, Taenia solium,* or *Taenia saginata* is niclosamide 2 g in a single dose. Praziquantel 25 mg/kg or paromomycin

4 g can also be used. For the treatment of *Hymenolepis nana,* a single dose of praziquantel is preferred to niclosamide, which must be given for 7 days to prevent autoinfection. Paromomycin 45 mg/kg can also be given for 7 days.

5. Mycobacterium avium-intracellulare—Diarrhea and weight loss are common manifestations of AIDS. These symptoms may be due to any of a variety of infections, impaired oral intake, difficulty swallowing, or malabsorption. When malabsorption occurs in this setting, infection with *Mycobacterium avium-intracellulare* needs to be considered. Mucosal biopsy is diagnostic, but the changes can be confused with Whipple's disease (see previous discussion). Antibiotic therapy can reduce the intensity of infection in these patients, but rarely eradicates the organism.

C. LUMINAL PROBLEMS CAUSING MALABSORPTION

1. Pancreatic exocrine insufficiency—When pancreatic enzyme secretion is reduced by 90% or more, maldigestion and malabsorption will occur. There can be important clinical differences between the malabsorption of pancreatic exocrine insufficiency and that due to mucosal disease, like celiac sprue. When fat is not digested, it is transported through the gastrointestinal tract as triglyceride. When fat is digested, but not absorbed, it enters the colon as fatty acids and monoglyceride. This difference in chemical composition has several ramifications: (1) oil is seen in stool in pancreatic exocrine insufficiency, but not in celiac disease; (2) stool volumes are greater for equal fat outputs in celiac disease than in pancreatic exocrine insufficiency because of inhibition of colonic fluid absorption by fatty acids; (3) fecal fat concentration is accordingly higher with pancreatic exocrine insufficiency than with mucosal disease; and (4) hypocalcemia due to formation of complexes containing calcium and fatty acids (soap formation) is seen in celiac disease, but not pancreatic exocrine insufficiency. In addition, patients with pancreatic exocrine insufficiency tend to have fewer problems with vitamin deficiencies than those with celiac disease.

Carbohydrate malabsorption and protein malabsorption can be quite significant in pancreatic exocrine insufficiency. Symptoms related to carbohydrate malabsorption, such as bloating, flatulence, and watery diarrhea, may be prominent. Although protein malabsorption may be substantial, hypoproteinemia is usually not present until late in the course of the disease.

Tests to document pancreatic exocrine insufficiency have been discussed earlier in this chapter. The diagnosis and differential diagnosis of chronic pancreatitis are discussed in Chapter 31.

Treatment of pancreatic exocrine insufficiency involves replacing the missing enzymes with exogenous pancreatic enzymes. Adequate amounts of potent enzyme supplements (particularly enteric coated preparations that release the enzymes only when luminal pH is >5.5) are needed to reduce steatorrhea. Acid suppression with histamine-2 (H_2) receptor antagonists or with proton-pump inhibitors may improve the efficacy of orally administered enzyme preparations. The effectiveness of therapy should be judged by comparing fecal fat excretion before and after therapy.

2. Bile acid deficiency—Adequate concentrations of bile acids are necessary for micelle formation and fat digestion. If this critical concentration is not present, fat maldigestion ensues. Lack of micelle formation also impairs absorption of fat-soluble vitamins. Other nutrients continue to be absorbed normally.

Bile acid deficiency can develop in the course of chronic cholestatic liver disease, such as primary biliary cirrhosis, in patients with complete extrahepatic biliary obstruction or diversion, in patients after extensive terminal ileal resection, and in some patients with ileal dysfunction. As with pancreatic exocrine insufficiency, stools tend to have high fat concentration when bile acid deficiency is due to hepatic or biliary disease. With ileal resection or dysfunction, bile acid loss into the colon leads to a secretory diarrhea and dilution of fat by increased stool water.

Diagnosis of bile acid deficiency is made by measuring postprandial bile acid concentration in the duodenum. Feeding exogenous bile acid with meals can reduce fat malabsorption, but may worsen diarrhea if ileal bile acid malabsorption leads to sufficiently high colonic bile acid concentrations. This can be reduced to some extent by the concurrent use of opiate antidiarrheal drugs.

3. Zollinger-Ellison syndrome—The high rates of gastric acid secretion in Zollinger-Ellison syndrome produce malabsorption by several mechanisms. First, persistently low pH in the duodenum precipitates bile acid and can secondarily affect fat absorption. Second, low intraduodenal pH may inactivate pancreatic enzymes. Third, the excess acid and pepsin may damage the mucosal absorptive cells directly. Removal of acid by aspiration or by inhibitory drugs can promptly reduce the secretory diarrhea seen in some of these patients. Steatorrhea may take several days to weeks to respond to acid inhibition.

D. POSTOPERATIVE MALABSORPTION

1. After gastric surgery—Many patients operated upon for peptic ulcer disease lose weight after surgery. In most cases this results from reduced food intake due to early satiety and to the development of food-related symptoms (pain, nausea, vomiting, and diarrhea). In some patients malabsorption is responsible for weight loss.

Malabsorption after gastric surgery is multifactorial. Most operations for ulcer are designed to reduce gastric acidity. This also reduces pepsin secretion and may allow bacterial overgrowth in the stomach and small intestine. Truncal vagotomy or gastric resection impairs the grinding of solid food into small particles, reducing the surface area that can be attacked by digestive enzymes. Gastric emptying of liquid is somewhat more rapid after most traditional ulcer surgeries. This results in dilution of pancreatic enzymes and bile acid in the duodenum (when chyme has access to the duodenum) and mismatching of chyme delivery and absorptive capacity. Rapid transit through the intestine may reduce contact time with the absorptive surface, reducing absorptive capacity. In some patients gastrectomy brings out latent celiac sprue or lactase deficiency as independent causes of malabsorption. Malabsorption of specific nutrients, such as iron, calcium, or vitamin B_{12}, may also occur after gastric surgery.

Although there are many potential mechanisms of malabsorption after surgery, malabsorption is usually only mild to moderate unless complicating features such as small bowel bacterial overgrowth occur. Steatorrhea is typically less than 15–20 g daily.

Treatment depends on the specific findings of an evaluation for the mechanism of malabsorption. Bacterial overgrowth should be assessed, since it is readily treatable with antibiotics. Trials of antiperistaltic agents, such as anticholinergics or opiates, may reduce rapid gastric emptying and intestinal transit and redress some of the pathophysiology leading to malabsorption. In some patients exogenous pancreatic enzymes administered with food may improve intraluminal digestion and reduce steatorrhea. Reoperation is indicated in patients with anatomic problems causing malabsorption, such as blind loop syndrome, afferent loop obstruction, or gastrocolic fistula.

2. After intestinal resection—Short intestinal resections are usually well tolerated without symptoms. Extensive small bowel resections produce diarrhea and malabsorption of variable severity, commonly known as short bowel syndrome. The extent of resection necessary to produce malabsorption varies and depends upon the portion of the intestine removed, since functional capacity differs from segment to segment. Nutrient absorptive needs can generally be met if at least 100 cm of jejunum is preserved. However, fluid absorptive needs may not be met by this length of residual bowel. Moreover, the specific transport abilities of the ileum (eg, absorbing vitamin B_{12} or bile acid) will be lost if that segment of the intestine is removed. The issue of the extent of resection necessary to produce symptoms is further complicated by intestinal adaption. Absorptive capacity for some nutrients can increase with time;

thus, initially inadequate absorption may become adequate over weeks to months. The factors leading to hyperplasia and hypertrophy of the remaining intestine are not understood completely.

Malabsorption in short bowel syndrome is not due solely to loss of absorptive surface. Other factors contributing include (1) gastric acid hypersecretion, (2) bile acid deficiency, (3) loss of the "ileal brake," a neurohumoral mechanism slowing gastric emptying and intestinal transit when nutrients enter the ileum, and (4) bacterial overgrowth, particularly when the ileocecal valve has been compromised. It is claimed that small ileal resections (<100 cm) produce diarrhea due to bile acid malabsorption and that larger resections produce steatorrhea due to loss of absorptive surface.

Treatment of short bowel syndrome consists of maximizing absorptive capacity by slowing intestinal transit with antiperistaltic agents, ingestion of a diet designed to take advantage of remaining absorptive capacity, and correction of specific vitamin, mineral, and electrolyte abnormalities. Patients may need parenteral nutrition if they cannot be maintained with enteral intake (either orally or via continuous tube feeding). Attempts to improve nutrient absorption with octreotide or growth hormone treatment have not been consistently effective. Small bowel transplantation is a long-term solution for only some patients with short bowel syndrome.

Complications of short bowel syndrome include cholesterol gallstones, oxalate kidney stones, and lactic acidosis. Prognosis depends on the ability to maintain nutritional status, to prevent fluid and electrolyte depletion, and to avoid complications of therapy, such as sepsis or loss of venous access.

E. DISORDERS THAT CAUSE MALABSORPTION OF SPECIFIC NUTRIENTS

1. Disaccharidase (carbohydrase) deficiency—Ingested disaccharides, such as lactose or sucrose, and starch breakdown products, such as maltotriose and α-limit dextrins, are hydrolyzed by brush border enzymes into monosaccharides that can be transported across the apical membrane of the enterocyte. These enzymes include lactase, maltase, sucrase-isomaltase, and trehalase and are glycoproteins inserted into the brush border membrane of villous cells after intracellular processing. If these hydrolytic enzymes are not active because of defective synthesis or processing, or if the luminal surface of the villous cell is damaged, carbohydrate malabsorption results. Gaseousness occurs regularly and osmotic diarrhea can occur, if the load of carbohydrate entering the colon exceeds the capacity for colonic bacterial fermentation and short-chain fatty acid absorption.

Congenital deficiencies of these enzymes occur, but are rare diseases. For example, congenital lactase deficiency is an autosomal recessive trait (as are all of these genetic deficiencies) that has been described in fewer than 50 individuals. Symptoms begin as soon as milk is given to the newborn and disappear when milk is removed from the diet. Similar rare syndromes have been described for sucrase-isomaltase and trehalase, but symptoms do not begin until later in life when their substrates are introduced into the diet. (Trehalase, a disaccharide in mushrooms and insects, may never be consumed in large enough amounts to produce symptoms, even if trehalase activity is deficient.)

In contrast, secondary deficiency of lactase is quite common. In most human populations (as in most mammals) intestinal lactase activity declines to low levels after weaning. By early adulthood, most people have <10% of normal lactase activity and many develop symptoms with ingestion of milk or other lactose-containing foods. The one exception to this is the western European population, in which lactase activity is well maintained into adulthood. Thus, acquired lactase deficiency can be looked on as the rule and persistent lactase activity as the exception. Nevertheless, unrecognized hypolactasia may be the cause of symptoms when it develops in a person who previously could tolerate milk and must be considered when patients present with gaseousness or intermittent diarrhea. Secondary deficiencies of other disaccharidases also occur but are much less common unless there has been extensive compromise of the brush border membrane or ingestion of the α-glucosidase inhibitor, acarbose.

Symptoms of disaccharidase deficiency are diet dependent. They therefore vary widely from day to day, depending upon dietary intake of the malabsorbed substrate. Gaseousness, bloating, flatulence, and variable stool consistency are typical symptoms. Stools are usually acid and when diarrhea is profuse, an osmotic gap may be present in stool water. Diagnosis can be suggested by breath hydrogen testing after ingestion of the malabsorbed substrate and can be proven by assay for enzyme activity in mucosal biopsy specimens. Dietary management by elimination of substrate should be completely successful in abolishing symptoms, but dietary indiscretion is common, since many processed foods have fillers, such as nonfat dried milk, added to them. Pretreatment of food with exogenous lactase before ingestion may reduce symptoms, but is usually ineffective in completely relieving them.

2. Transport defects at the brush border—Glucose-galactose malabsorption is a rare congenital disease that presents like congenital lactase deficiency soon after birth. In this condition hydrolysis of lactose is intact, but the hexose transporter is defective, preventing entry of glucose and galactose into the cell. Transport of fructose is normal. Hexose transport in the renal tubule is

often abnormal also, producing glycosuria. Recognition of the disorder soon after birth is essential, since diarrhea is quite severe and dehydration occurs quickly. Feeding fructose and eliminating glucose and galactose from the diet prevent symptoms and allow normal development.

There are several other congenital transport defects producing malabsorption of specific nutrients, including Hartnup disease (neutral amino acid transport) and cystinuria. These do not produce prominent gastrointestinal symptoms.

3. Abetalipoproteinemia—This rare autosomal recessive disease is due to failure to produce apolipoprotein B and the lipoproteins containing apolipoprotein B (chylomicrons, very low-density lipoproteins, and low-density lipoproteins). Because long-chain triglyceride transport by enterocytes is linked to formation of chylomicrons, triglyceride "backs up" in the mucosal cells producing a foamy appearance under the microscope. Mild steatorrhea beginning in childhood, fat-soluble vitamin deficiencies, failure to gain weight, anemia with acanthocytosis, retinitis pigmentosa, and progressive peripheral neuropathy are the usual clinical manifestations. Several similar syndromes have been described, including normotriglyceridemic abetalipoproteinemia and chylomicron retention disease, which occur in patients with defects in apolipoprotein B-48 metabolism. A low-fat diet supplemented by medium-chain triglyceride (not requiring chylomicron formation for malabsorption) and fat-soluble vitamin replacement can reduce symptoms in all of these conditions.

Malabsorption in Specific Settings

A. MALABSORPTION IN CHILDHOOD

Malabsorption developing in infancy and childhood should bring to mind a distinct differential diagnosis (Table 23–9). For example, congenital enzyme deficiency states may become manifest as nutrients are added to the infant's diet. Other conditions may be more or less likely to occur in young individuals. Two conditions should be considered in particular, celiac disease and cystic fibrosis. Celiac disease can develop any time after wheat and other gluten-containing foods are added to the diet. Cystic fibrosis produces malabsorption when pancreatic insufficiency manifests itself. The diagnosis of cystic fibrosis should be considered when respiratory disease is accompanied by evidence of malabsorption.

The presentation of malabsorption may also be different than that in adults. Children may be less likely to complain of changes in stool consistency after toilet training is completed. Growth retardation may be more prominent than weight loss. Patients whose growth is

Table 23–9. Differential diagnosis of malabsorption in childhood.

Problem	Mechanism
Congenital	
Intestinal malrotation[1]	Blind loop syndrome
Intestinal duplication	Blind loop syndrome
Short small bowel[1]	Lack of absorptive surface
Lymphangiectasia	Lymphatic obstruction
Primary lactase deficiency[1]	Enzyme deficiency
Sucrase-isomaltase deficiency	Enzyme deficiency
Glucose-galactose malab- sorption	Transport protein dysfunction
Cystinuria	Transport protein dysfunction
Hartnup disease	Transport protein dysfunction
Abetalipoproteinemia	Metabolic disorder
Familial dysautonomia	Abnormal transit time
Cystic fibrosis[1]	Pancreatic exocrine insufficiency
Familial pancreatitis	Pancreatic exocrine insufficiency
Biliary atresia[1]	Bile acid deficiency
Immune deficiency syndromes	Small bowel bacterial overgrowth
Acquired	
Short bowel syndrome	Lack of absorptive surface
Giardiasis[1]	Parasitosis
Necrotizing enterocolitis[1]	Mucosal damage
Milk allergy[1]	Mucosal damage
Eosinphilic gastroenteritis	Mucosal damage
Celiac disease[1]	Mucosal damage
Tropical sprue	Mucosal damage
Dermatitis herpetiformis	Mucosal damage
Adrenal insufficiency[1]	Mucosal damage
Chronic pancreatitis	Pancreatic exocrine insufficiency
Neoplasm (ganglioneuroma, carci- noid, lymphoma)	Abnormal transit time, others
Crohn's disease[1]	Multiple

[1]More common diagnoses in North America.

slowed should be screened for malabsorption. Growth failure can be reversed if caught in time and adequate nutrition is provided.

B. Malabsorption in the Elderly

Almost any cause of malabsorption can present in old age. Several should be considered more prominently. These include small bowel bacterial overgrowth (due to hypochlorhydria, motility disorders, and jejunal diverticula), pancreatic exocrine insufficiency, and diabetes mellitus.

C. Systemic Diseases Causing Malabsorption

1. Diabetes mellitus and other endocrine disease— Gastrointestinal symptoms occur regularly in patients with diabetes mellitus and are usually attributed to the effects of autonomic neuropathy. These include nausea and vomiting, constipation, diarrhea, and fecal incontinence. In some diabetics, steatorrhea is prominent (usually with chronic diarrhea). The mechanism of diabetic steatorrhea is not always understood. Three conditions should be excluded: (1) small bowel bacterial overgrowth, (2) celiac disease, and (3) pancreatic exocrine insufficiency. These conditions occur with increased frequency in diabetics. Steatorrhea occurring in the absence of these conditions can sometimes be attributed to rapid intestinal transit. The mechanism of steatorrhea in diabetes is important to work out since it is likely to be a recurrent problem. Treatment depends on the cause of the malabsorption.

Both hyperthyroidism and hypothyroidism can be associated with malabsorption. In hyperthyroidism, rapid intestinal transit, hyperphagia, and altered intestinal secretion have all been implicated. Treatment of hyperthyroidism with drugs, radioiodine, or surgery corrects steatorrhea. In hypothyroidism, celiac disease or partial villous atrophy may occur. This seems to respond to gluten withdrawal.

Some patients with Addison's disease develop malabsorption that can be reversed by treatment with corticosteroids. Autoimmune adrenal insufficiency is associated with celiac disease; this responds to gluten withdrawal.

Hypoparathyroidism has been associated with malabsorption that may be due to villous atrophy, motility disorders, and lymphangiectasia.

2. Collagen-vascular diseases—Advanced scleroderma is often associated with small intestine problems. Replacement of the smooth muscle with fibrous tissue and the presence of small bowel diverticula predispose to bacterial overgrowth. This can produce steatorrhea of varying severity. Antibiotic therapy is quite helpful, but recurrence is the rule and episodic therapy may be necessary.

Vasculitis is sometimes associated with severe weight loss that has been attributed to small bowel ischemia.

3. Amyloidosis—Amyloidosis can produce malabsorption by several mechanisms. Infiltration of the mucosa can affect enterocyte function, but ischemia (from vascular compromise), pancreatic exocrine insufficiency, bacterial overgrowth, and dysmotility (from muscle infiltration) probably contribute as well. The diagnosis can be suggested by small bowel x-ray and confirmed by biopsy, but most experts advise avoiding intestinal biopsy, if possible, for fear of inducing bleeding. Biopsy of abdominal fat is easy, safe, and frequently positive.

4. AIDS—Chronic wasting is a common presentation of AIDS in Africa and is seen elsewhere as well. Diarrhea and malabsorption in AIDS are usually due to any of several opportunistic infections. Careful search for potential pathogens can result in improvement with therapy. The role of human immunodeficiency virus type 1 (HIV-1) in causing enterocyte dysfunction by itself is controversial. Pancreatic exocrine insufficiency can also occur in the course of this illness and may be readily treated. Lymphoma can produce malabsorption during the course of AIDS and is not amenable to treatment. *Mycobacterium avium-intracellulare* infection is frequent in patients with AIDS and probably accounts for many cases of malabsorption in this patient group (see section, *"Mycobacterium-avium intracellulare"*).

REFERENCES

Abdelshaheed NN, Goldberg DM: Biochemical tests in diseases of the intestinal tract: their contribution to diagnosis, management, and understanding the pathophysiology of specific disease states. Crit Rev Clin Lab Sci 1997;34:141.

Bai JC: Malabsorption syndrome. Digestion 1998;59:530.

Balasekaran R et al: Positive results on tests for steatorrhea in persons consuming olestra potato chips. Ann Intern Med 2000; 132:279.

Beebe DK, Walley E: Diabetic diarrhea. An underdiagnosed complication? Postgrad Med 1992;91:179.

Bonamico M et al: Radioimmunoassay to detect antitransglutaminase autoantibodies is the most sensitive and specific screening method for celiac disease. Am J Gastroenterol 2001;96: 1536.

Ciclitira PJ: AGA technical review on celiac sprue. Gastroenterology 2001;120:1526.

Craig RM, Ehrenpreis ED: D-xylose testing. J Clin Gastroenterol 1999;29:143.

DiMagno EP: Gastric acid suppression and treatment of severe exocrine pancreatic insufficiency. Baillieres Best Pract Res Clin Gastroenterol 2001;15:477.

Di Stefano M et al: Small intestine bacterial overgrowth and metabolic bone disease. Dig Dis Sci 2001;46:1077.

Dutly F, Altwegg M: Whipple's disease and *"Tropheryma whippelii."* Clin Microbiol Rev 2001;14:561.

Eckmann L, Gillin FD: Microbes and microbial toxins: paradigms for microbial–mucosal interactions. I. Pathophysiological aspects of enteric infections with the lumen-dwelling protozoan pathogen, Giardia lamblia. Am J Physiol Gastrointest Liver Physiol 2001;280:G1.

Eherer AJ, Fordtran JS: Fecal osmotic gap and pH in experimental diarrhea of various causes. Gastroenterology 1992;103:702.

Ehrenpreis ED et al: Histopathologic findings of duodenal biopsy specimens in HIV-infected patients with and without diarrhea and malabsorption. Am J Clin Pathol 1992;97:21.

Ehrenpreis ED, Salvino M, Craig RM: Improving the serum D-xylose test for the identification of patients with small intestinal malabsorption. J Clin Gastroenterol 2001;33:36.

Fernandez-Banares F et al: Sugar malabsorption in functional bowel disease: clinical implications. Am J Gastroenterol 1993;88:2044.

Fine KD, Fordtran JS: The effect of diarrhea on fecal fat excretion. Gastroenterology 1992;102:1936.

Fine KD, Schiller LR: AGA technical review on the evaluation and management of chronic diarrhea. Gastroenterology 1999; 116:1464.

Gruy-Kapral C et al: Conjugated bile acid replacement therapy for short-bowel syndrome. Gastroenterology 1999;116:15.

Gudmand-Hoyer E: The clinical significance of disaccharide maldigestion. Am J Clin Nutrit 1994;59(Suppl):735S.

Hammer HF et al: Carbohydrate malabsorption. Its measurement and its contribution to diarrhea. J Clin Invest 1990;86:1936.

Hofmann AF: The continuing importance of bile acid in liver and intestinal disease. Arch Intern Med 1999;159:2647.

Hogenauer C et al: Malabsorption due to cholecystokinin deficiency in a patient with autoimmune polyglandular syndrome type I. N Engl J Med 2001;344:270.

Holt PR: Diarrhea and malabsorption in the elderly. Gastroenterol Clin North Am 2001;30:427.

Layer P, Keller J, Lankisch AP: Pancreatic enzyme replacement therapy. Curr Gastroenterol Rep 2001;3:101.

Lee MF, Krasinski SD: Human adult-onset lactase decline: an update. Nutr Rev 1998;56:1.

Leus J et al: Detection and follow-up of exocrine pancreatic insufficiency in cystic fibrosis: a review. Eur J Pediatr 2000;159: 563.

Li-Ling, Irving M: The effectiveness of growth hormone, glutamine and a low-fat diet containing high-carbohydrate on the enhancement of the function of remnant intestine among patients with short bowel syndrome: a review of published trials. Clin Nutr 2001;20:199.

Lord LM et al: Management of the patient with short bowel syndrome. AACN Clin Issues 2000;11:604.

Lucas KH, Kaplan-Machlis B: Orlistat—a novel weight loss therapy. Ann Pharmacother 2001;35:314.

Naim HY: Molecular and cellular aspects and regulation of intestinal lactase-phlorizin hydrolase. Histol Histopathol 2001;16: 553.

Nehra V et al: An open trial of octreotide long-acting release in the management of short bowel syndrome. Am J Gastroenterol 2001;96:1494.

Poles MA et al: HIV-related diarrhea is multifactorial and fat malabsorption is commonly present, independent of HAART. Am J Gastroenterol 2001;96:1831.

Potter GD: Bile acid diarrhea. Dig Dis 1998;16:118.

Reyes J: Intestinal transplantation for children with short bowel syndrome. Semin Pediatr Surg 2001;10:99.

Riby JE, Fujisawa T, Kretchmer N: Fructose absorption. Am J Clin Nutrit 1993;58(Suppl):748S.

Rubesin SE, Rubin RA, Herlinger H: Small bowel malabsorption: clinical and radiologic perspectives. How we see it. Radiology 1992;184:297.

Rumessen JJ: Fructose and related food carbohydrates. Sources, intake, absorption, and clinical implications. Scand J Gastroenterol 1992;27:819.

Scheen AJ: Clinical efficacy of acarbose in diabetes mellitus: a critical review of controlled trials. Diabetes Metab 1998;24:311.

Schuppan D, Hahn EG: Celiac disease and its link to type I diabetes mellitus. J Pediatr Endocrinol Metab 2001;14(Suppl 1):597.

Strocchi A et al: Detection of malabsorption of low doses of carbohydrate: accuracy of various breath H_2 criteria. Gastroenterology 1993;105:1404.

Toskes PP: Bacterial overgrowth of the gastrointestinal tract. Adv Intern Med 1993;38:387.

Vanderhoof JA, Young RJ: Enteral nutrition in short bowel syndrome. Semin Pediatr Surg 2001;10:65.

Wahab PJ et al: Gluten challenge in borderline gluten-sensitive enteropathy. Am J Gastroenterol 2001;96:1464.

Tumors of the Stomach & Small Intestine

24

Samuel B. Ho, MD

 ESSENTIALS OF DIAGNOSIS

- *Common gastric and small intestinal malignancies include adenocarcinoma, lymphoma, metastatic carcinoma, gastrointestinal stromal tumors, and carcinoid. These must be differentiated from benign ulcerative lesions and polyps by endoscopic or surgical biopsy.*

- *Symptoms and signs include dyspepsia, weight loss, obstructive symptoms, and evidence of intestinal blood loss or iron deficiency anemia.*

- *Diagnosis of early stage gastric cancer requires a high index of suspicion for patients who are at increased risk, for example, new symptoms in patients aged over 40–45 years, history of prior gastric surgery, prior history of pernicious anemia, celiac sprue, immunodeficiency, or gastric polyps. Diagnosis requires referral for endoscopy and/or barium radiologic exams.*

- *Diagnosis of small bowel tumors often requires a barium enteroclysis examination performed by an experienced radiologist or endoscopy using small bowel enteroscopes.*

General Considerations

The stomach and less frequently the small intestine give rise to a variety of benign and malignant tumors (Table 24–1). In 5000 endoscopic examinations of the stomach conducted over a 7-year period at the University of Chicago, approximately 119 gastric malignancies (2.4%) and 125 benign gastric polyps (2.5%) were diagnosed. The most frequent gastric malignancy is adenocarcinoma, followed by primary gastric lymphoma, metastatic carcinoma, and less frequently leiomyosarcoma, carcinoid, and Kaposi's sarcoma. These present as ulcerated or polypoid lesions that must be differentiated from benign tumors by endoscopic or operative biopsies.

Gastric adenocarcinoma is the second most common malignancy worldwide. Gastric cancer is particularly common in Japan, China, Korea, Taiwan, Eastern Europe and countries of the former Soviet Union, Costa Rica, and South America. In Japan, the gastric cancer incidence is 100 per 100,000 persons and is the leading cause of cancer deaths. In the United States, the overall annual incidence of gastric cancer has declined from 33 cases per 100,000 population in 1935 to less than 6 cases per 100,000 in the 1990s. In the United States, it is estimated that 33,800 new cases of gastric cancer and 25,100 gastric cancer deaths occurred in the year 2000. Gastric cancer is currently the seventh leading cause of death due to malignancy among males and the eleventh among females in the United States. In contrast, the incidence of adenocarcinoma of the gastric cardia and gastroesophageal junction has been increasing in both the United States and Europe over the past 15 years.

Lymphoma is the second most common malignancy encountered in the stomach. Primary gastric lymphomas account for 3–5% of gastric neoplasms. The large majority of these lymphomas are B cell non-Hodgkin's lymphomas of the diffuse, large cell type. Gastric lymphoma is the most common extranodal lymphoma, accounting for 20–24% of primary extranodal lymphomas.

Less frequent primary gastric malignancies include carcinoid tumors and gastrointestinal stromal cell tumors (GISTs). The occurrence of carcinoids in the stomach is rare; approximately 95% of all carcinoid tumors occur in the rectum, appendix, and small intestine. GISTs represent the largest category of nonepithelial neoplasms of the gastrointestinal tract. They arise from the neoplastic degeneration of primitive mesenchymal cells and demonstrate considerable variability in their differentiation pathways. GISTs can be divided into several categories, including leiomyomas, schwannomas, and less differentiated tumors referred to as GIST. The GIST family may include most tumors labeled as leiomyomas, cellular leiomyoma, leiomyoblastomas, myofibroblastic tumors, and leiomyosarcomas. GISTs can occur in all segments of the intestine, with approximately 60% occuring in the stomach, 30% in

Table 24–1. Tumors of the stomach and small intestine.

Tumors	Percentage of Total	Benign Polyps	Percentage of Total
Gastric	**Endoscopic series**		**Endoscopic series**
Adenocarcinoma	86	Hyperplastic	71
Lymphoma	8	Adenomatous	11
Metastatic carcinoma	4	Leiomyoma	6
Leiomyosarcoma	<2	Pancreatic rest	<2
Carcinoid	<2	Myoepithelial hamartoma	<2
Kaposi's sarcoma		Peutz-Jeghers hamartoma, eosinophilic granuloma, no histologic diagnosis, neurogenic tumors, lipoma	5
Small intestine	**Surgical series**		**Surgical series**
Adenocarcinoma	29–40	Ademomas (polypoid, Brunner gland, islet cell)	25–38
Carcinoid	29–49	Leiomyoma	35
Leiomyosarcoma	15–22	Lipoma	4–20
Lymphoma	4–11	Hamartomas, fibromas, neurogenic	
Metastatic carcinoma		Angiomas, myxomas, other rare types	
Kaposi's sarcoma		Pseudotumors, lymphoid hyperplasia, hyperplastic inflammatory, pancreatic rests, Brunner gland hyperplasia, amyloidosis, endometrioma	

the small intestine, and 10% in the esophagus and colon. The clinical course of GISTs is heterogeneous and not easily predicted by standard clinicopathologic criteria. The most important prognostic features are size >5 cm, tumor necrosis, mitotic count >1 to 5 mitoses per 10 high power fields, and the presence of *c-kit* gene mutation.

Overall, tumors of the small intestine account for only 1–2% of all gastrointestinal malignancies. During a 20-year period at the Case Western Reserve University, 64 patients underwent surgical resection for primary small bowel tumors; of these 38 (59%) were malignant and 26 (41%) were benign. The relative frequencies of different histologic types of small bowel tumors are listed in Table 24–1. The majority of small bowel adenocarcinomas and leiomyosarcomas occur in the duodenum and jejunum. In contrast, the majority of small bowel carcinoids and lymphomas occur in the ileum.

Pathophysiology

Several case–control studies have suggested an association between *Helicobacter pylori* infection and gastric cancer, including gastric lymphomas and both intestinal and diffuse types of adenocarcinoma. A recent long-term, prospective study of 1246 patients with *H pylori* infection and 280 patients without *H pylori* infection in Japan was reported by Uemura et al. After a mean follow-up period of 7.8 years, gastric cancer was diagnosed in 2.9% of the infected patients and in none of the uninfected patients. Among the patients with *H pylori* infection, those with severe gastric atrophy, corpus-predominant gastritis, and intestinal metaplasia were at significantly higher risk for developing cancer.

The development of chronic atrophic gastritis in the corpus or gastric body and intestinal metaplasia leads to impaired gastric acid secretion, imbalanced cellular proliferation and apoptosis, and decreased gastric mucin synthesis. These histologic changes progress over long periods of time, and can eventually lead to the development of foci of dysplasia and cancer. Because only a small proportion of individuals infected with *H pylori* subsequently develop dysplasia or cancer, other carcinogenic factors are necessary. Numerous epidemiologic studies have identified other potential contributing factors for the development of gastric cancer. These include diets with low fat and protein intake, low vitamin

A and C intake, high intake of salted meat and fish, and high intake of nitrates. Low socioeconomic status is associated with increased cancer risk, which may be explained by poor food preparation, lack of refrigeration, and increased *H pylori* infection rates. Smoking increases the risk of gastric cancer, however alcohol intake does not. Investigators have speculated that the most important scenario leading to gastric cancer development is chronic gastritis in the corpus leading to impaired acid secretion in the stomach, which leads to bacterial overgrowth and increased bacterial production of carcinogenic nitrosamines from nitrates in the diet. The lack of ascorbic acid in the diet promotes the formation of *N*-nitroso mutagens in the gastric lumen.

Intestinal metaplasia is defined as the replacement of normal gastric epithelium with columnar epithelium similar to the small intestine or colon. Three types of intestinal metaplasia have been described based on morphologic criteria and mucin histochemistry. Type I intestinal metaplasia is characterized by straight crypts with well-developed goblet and absorptive cells. Goblet cells contain sialomucins and absorptive cells are nonsecretory. Type II intestinal metaplasia is characterized by less well differentiated small intestinal epithelium. Type III intestinal metaplasia is characterized by tortuous crypts with immature columnar cells and goblet cells containing sulfomucins. Several studies have shown that Type III intestinal metaplasia is most commonly associated with gastric cancer, usually of the intestinal type.

Other conditions associated with chronic gastritis have also been associated with increased risk for the development of gastrointestinal cancer. Chronic gastritis due to pernicious anemia is categorized as type A (autoimmune) and typically involves the body and fundus rather than the antrum. The increased risk attributable to pernicious anemia is considered to be small. In a recent large retrospective study of patients with pernicious anemia, the ratio of observed to expected gastric cancers was 3.2. Increased risk for gastrointestinal cancer is also found in patients with a previous partial gastrectomy with a Billroth II anastomosis and in patients who have had a Billroth I anastomosis or a vagotomy and pyloroplasty. The increased risk following gastric surgery occurs after a period of 10–15 years. In addition to atrophic gastritis, achlorhydria, a vagotomy, and duodenogastric reflux are factors contributing to the development of gastric cancer in this setting. Patients with congenital or acquired immunodeficiency states, including acquired immunodeficiency syndrome (AIDS), are at increased risk for the development of gastrointestinal lymphomas. Celiac sprue is a risk factor for intestinal lymphomas, which usually occur in the jejunum or may be multifocal. Inflammatory bowel disease is a risk factor for the development of adenocarcinoma and possibly lymphoma.

The increased risk for cancer in the patients described above is not considered to be high enough to warrant routine endoscopic screening.

Gastric cancer can be divided into two different histologic subtypes, with differing biologic characteristics that may reflect differing etiologic factors (Table 24–2). The first type is termed "intestinal" and is characterized by gland formation, and often appears similar to colon carcinoma. The second type is termed "diffuse" and is characterized by poorly differentiated cells that cluster in sheets or nodules and is devoid of gland-like structure. The intestinal type is the predominant form found in areas with epidemic gastric cancer and is associated with atrophic gastritis and intestinal metaplasia. This type is more common in males and the elderly. The diffuse type is more common in endemic areas and is not typically associated with precursor lesions in the stomach. This type is more common in women and in younger patients.

Aneuploidy is defined as an abnormal amount of DNA per cell and can be detected by flow cytometry in fresh or formalin-fixed specimens. A number of studies have determined that aneuploidy is present in 40–70% of gastric adenocarcinomas. The presence of aneuploidy correlates with increased pathologic stage and worse survival.

A number of specific genetic abnormalities have been described in gastric adenocarcinomas, which appear similar regardless of the country of origin. Chromosomal alterations include frequent deletions of portions of chromosomes 5q, 17p, and 18q, which are the sites of tumor suppressor genes APC and MCC, p53, and DCC, respectively. Abnormalitites of these tumor suppressor genes are found in 40–60% of gastric cancers. These sites are frequently altered in other cancers, such as adenocarcinoma of the colon. In general, more advanced cancers are associated with more numerous chromosomal abnormalities. The p53 gene product is a DNA binding phosphoprotein that plays a role in proliferation, apoptosis, and DNA repair, and is the most common genetic abnormality found in cancers. Altered p53 is found more frequently in advanced gastric cancers and is associated with a worse prognosis.

Several alterations of dominantly acting oncogenes have been described in gastric adenocarcinomas. Oncogenes related to fibroblast growth factor (*hst*-1/*int*-2) and fibroblast growth factor receptors (K-*sam*) are frequently amplified or overexpressed. Amplification or overexpression of *HER2/NEU* (*erb*B-2, a receptor related to the epidermal growth factor receptor) is associated with lymph node metastases and a worse prognosis, and is an independent predictor of survival in one multivariate analysis. In contrast to colon adenocarcinomas, mutations or overexpression of the *ras* family of oncogenes occur rarely in gastric adenocarcinomas. Precursor lesions such as su-

Table 24–2. Morphologic and histopathologic classification systems for gastric adenocarcinoma.

Classification	Characteristics	Associations	Prognosis (Compared with Average Survival)
Lauren			
Intestinal	Gland-like structures	Epidemic prevalence, associated with precursor lesions, men and older patients	Better
Diffuse	Poorly differentiated, unorganized sheets of cells	Endemic prevalence, younger patients and women	Worse
Broder's			
I	Well differentiated, tubular-like arrangement of cells		Better
II	Moderately differentiated, irregular tubules		
III	Poorly differentiated, irregular sheets of cells		
IV	Anaplastic		Worse
Ming			
Expansive	Discrete tumor nodules growing by expansion	Associated with intestinal metaplasia, M:F = 2:1, 6% under age 50	Better
Infiltrating	Tumor cells individually invade surrounding tissue	M:F = 1:1, 14% under age 50	Worse
Borrmann			
I	Polypoid or fungating		Better
II	Ulcerated with elevated borders		
III	Ulcerated and infiltrating gastric wall		
IV	Diffusely infiltrating		
V	Unclassifiable		Worse

perficial gastritis or gastric dysplasia may also demonstrate genetic alterations, such as altered expression of tyrosine kinase growth factor receptor *met, ras* oncogenes, and p53. However, the relationship of specific genetic abnormalities and progressive stages of gastric carcinogenesis has not been completely defined.

Prior *H pylori* infection has been associated with primary gastric lymphomas, but not with lymphomas of other sites. *H pylori*-induced gastritis is characterized by infiltration of the mucosa with lymphocytes. This is thought to give rise to the development of low-grade gastric lymphomas that resemble mucosa-associated lymphoid tissue (MALT) rather than lymphomas associated with lymph nodes. Low-grade MALT lymphomas and high-grade B cell lymphomas may be found together in patients with gastric lymphoma, and it is thought that low-grade MALT lymphomas may be a precursor to high-grade gastric lymphomas.

Chromosomal abnormalities play an important role in the pathogenesis of lymphocytic lymphomas of the gastrointestinal tract. More than 90% of lymphocytic lymphomas display cytogenetic abnormalities, and greater numbers of these abnormalities are associated

with higher grade tumors. Molecular genetics of lymphomas are characterized by translocation of DNA from one chromosome to another. Clinically important translocations appear to bring oncogene regions in proximity to immunoglobulin genes. The t(8;14) and t(8;22) translocations bring the *myc* oncogene on chromosome 8 close to immunoglobulin heavy chain or light chain loci, respectively. This results in upregulation of *myc* gene expression, which is a DNA-binding protein involved in control of proliferation. The t(14;18) trans-location juxtaposes the B cell leukemia lymphoma-2 gene (*BCL2*) and the immun-oglobulin heavy chain joining region on chromosome 14. These lead to increased *BCL2* protein expression, which is an inner mitochondrial membrane protein that contributes to tumor proliferation by blocking programmed cell death (apoptosis). Other genes that are implicated in translocations in lymphomas include *BCL1*, *PRAD1* (a cell-cycle regulatory protein or cyclin), and T cell receptor genes (*TCRα, TCRδ, TCRβ TCRγ*). Interestingly, low-grade MALT-type lymphomas of the stomach characteristically do not demonstrate rearrangement of the BCL2 gene. The differences in molecular alterations in gastrointestinal and nongastrointestinal lymphomas and the relationship of molecular changes in precursor and early stage lymphomas with late stage lymphomas have not been well characterized.

GISTs consistently express the *c-kit* gene, located on chromosome 4q11–21. The *c-kit* gene encodes a transmembrane receptor protein with an internal tyrosine kinase component. Gain-of-function mutations in exon 11 (and rarely exons 9 and 13) of the *c-kit* gene have been described in GISTs, which lead to ligand-independent tyrosine kinase activation. Studies have shown that 21–88% of predominantly malignant GISTs have *c-kit* mutations. The activated c-kit tyrosine kinase has recently been exploited as a target for chemotherapeutic inhibition, with good clinical response rates reported.

Clinical Findings

A. SYMPTOMS AND SIGNS

Symptoms associated with early gastrointestinal tumors are often minimal and/or nonspecific. The initial symptoms attributable to a tumor depend on the location of the tumor. Obstructing lesions of the lower esophagus and gastric cardia often cause dysphagia to solid foods. Because of this location, tumors of the lower esophagus and gastric cardia may be diagnosed at an earlier stage compared with tumors of the body or antrum. Early tumors in the body or antrum are asymptomatic or cause vague abdominal discomfort or "fullness," dyspepsia-like symptoms, nausea, or diminished appetite. Patients often will alter their diet in an attempt to ameliorate these symptoms. Symptoms of gastric outlet obstruction, early satiety, and weight loss are indicative of a large or advanced-stage tumor. Early satiety results from infiltration of the gastric wall and loss of distensibility. Gastric tumors may also cause occult gastrointestinal blood loss and the development of symptoms due to iron deficiency anemia.

Because the symptoms of early stage gastric tumors are minimal or mimic those of acid-peptic disease, the diagnosis is often delayed. Consequently, the proportion of patients diagnosed with advanced stage tumors is high. Diagnosis of operable gastric cancers requires a high index of suspicion and early referral for endoscopy or radiologic studies. If dyspeptic symptoms are accompanied by weight loss, vomiting, dysphagia, or evidence of gastrointestinal (GI) blood loss, endoscopy should be performed first before any therapeutic trials are initiated. Of particular concern are new "dyspeptic" symptoms that develop in patients over 40 years of age. Predisposing factors such as prior gastric resection, pernicious anemia, or prior gastric adenomas should also be taken into consideration and prompt early diagnostic studies.

The indications for endoscopy in patients presenting with dyspepsia and no other symptoms are evolving. Physicians may elect to treat simple dyspeptic symptoms with a course of H_2 blocker therapy and proceed to endoscopy only for persistent symptoms following a 1- to 2-month course of therapy. Many physicians will attempt to diagnose *H pylori* infection and associated ulcers prior to initiating treatment.

Tumors of the small intestine usually present with pain, obstructive symptoms, or bleeding. The pain is cramping and intermittent and results from partial lumenal obstruction. Other symptoms include nausea, vomiting, anorexia, altered bowel habits, and weight loss. Gastrointestinal bleeding is usually self-limited or occult. Patients presenting with melena or iron deficiency anemia should have a dedicated radiologic examination of the small intestine or enteroscopy if endoscopic studies of the gastroduodenum and colon do not reveal a cause. Similarly, occult fecal blood loss associated with anemia or symptoms should be evaluated in a similar fashion.

Less frequently, gastric and small intestinal tumors may present as a gastrointestinal emergency, such as massive hemorrhage, acute obstruction, intussusception, or perforation. Adenocarcinomas, lymphomas, and leiomyosarcomas may present with acute gastrointestinal hemorrhage and require management in intensive care units and blood transfusion. Diagnosis is initially attempted using endoscopic procedures. Injection or thermal endoscopic therapies that have been shown to be effective for bleeding peptic ulcers are often not successful if the bleeding is caused by a malignancy. Continued bleeding should be treated by urgent laparotomy or angiographic vessel occlusion. Leiomyosarcomas may present with acute bleeding into the peritoneal cavity with little intralumenal blood loss.

Patients with acute obstruction present with persistent nausea, vomiting, and abdominal pain. Flat and upright films of the abdomen may demonstrate dilated small intestine and air–fluid levels above the site of obstruction. Perforation should be considered if the pain is severe, constant, and associated with rebound tenderness, fever, and/or leukocytosis. The primary diagnostic and therapeutic procedure for patients presenting with acute obstruction or perforation is surgical; therefore early consultation with a surgeon is mandatory for patients presenting with these symptoms. Perforation is a sign of an advanced tumor and is associated with a worse prognosis.

Symptoms do not distinguish carcinoid from other tumors of the intestine unless the carcinoid is advanced and produces the carcinoid syndrome. The development of carcinoid syndrome depends on a large tumor mass with drainage into the caval circulation. This is found with hepatic metastases, with carcinoids developing in large teratomas of the ovaries or testes, or with large tumors that invade retroperitoneal vessels. Symptoms are thought to result from serotonin or other vasoactive substances synthesized by the tumor. The majority of patients complain of diarrhea and flushing episodes. Asthma and pellagra may occur in less than 10% of patients. Diagnosis of carcinoid syndrome is made by the demonstration of elevated urinary 5-hydroxyindoleacetic acid (5-HIAA) levels.

Physical examination often is not helpful in patients with early gastrointestinal tumors. Guaiac tests of stool obtained on rectal examination should be performed. Pallor and cachexia often indicate an advanced stage of gastric cancer. Palpation of the abdomen occassionally reveals an epigastric mass; however this is also evident only with advanced disease. Gastrointestinal lymphomas and leiomyomas may present with a palpable mass in 20–50% of cases. Advanced gastric adenocarcinomas may be associated with physical signs of distant metastases. These include hepatomegaly, ascites (due to peritoneal involvement or secondary to portal hypertension from extensive liver metastases), left supraclavicular lymphadenopathy (Virchow's node), left anterior axillary adenopathy (Irish's node), umbilical nodules (Sister Mary Joseph's node), a rigid rectal prominence above the prostate (Blumer's shelf), and ovarian metastases (Krukenberg tumor). Rare skin abnormalities associated with gastric cancer include acanthosis nigricans, dermatomyositis, metastatic nodules, or warty keratosis and pruritus (sign of Leser-Trelat).

B. LABORATORY FINDINGS

Evidence of iron deficiency anemia should always prompt an evaluation of the gastrointestinal tract, including upper and lower GI endoscopic procedures. If these procedures are negative a small bowel barium examination should be preformed. Abnormalities of liver function tests may suggest hepatic metastases. Asymptomatic patients without anemia who are found to have a positive stool guaiac on routine screening should have a colonoscopic or barium examination of their colon only, as the finding of gastric or small intestinal malignancies under these conditions (in North American patients) is exceedingly small.

C. ENDOSCOPY

Upper gastrointestinal endoscopy provides a sensitive and specific method for diagnosis of gastric tumors. The size and location of abnormalities should be carefully documented during endoscopy. All abnormal mucosal lesions such as ulcers, polyps, strictures, and thickened gastric folds should be biopsied. One study has shown that accurate histologic diagnosis of gastric adenocarcinoma is possible in 95% of cases when four biopsies are taken from a specific lesion. Diagnostic ac-

curacy increases to 98% when seven biopsies are taken, and if seven or eight biopsies and cytologic brushings or aspirates are taken diagnostic accuracy approaches 100%. Biopsies should be taken from both the margin and base of ulcer-like lesions. Because visual endoscopic assessment of malignancy is inaccurate, it is recommended that cytology and at least four to seven biopsies be obtained from all gastric mucosal lesions.

Several endoscopic features of gastric ulcers are more commonly associated with malignancies; however, differentiation of benign and malignant gastric ulcers by endoscopic appearance alone is not reliable. The size of an ulcer is an important risk factor for malignancy, as up to 20% of ulcers over 3 cm in diameter have been shown to be malignant. Other endoscopic features more frequently associated with malignancy include an irregular base, an irregular ulcer margin (which can be interrupted by tumor nodules), and disruption or abruptly cut-off folds adjacent to the ulcer. All gastric ulcers (with the possible exception of superficial ulceration associated with aspirin and nonsteroidal antiinflammatory drugs) should be followed with repeat endoscopy and biopsy until healed.

Gastric adenocarcinomas have been classified according to their gross appearance. The original classification system was proposed by Borrmann in 1926 and consisted of protruding and flat or depressed types of cancers, with the protruding type considered to have a better prognosis (see Table 24–2). This classification was modified by the Japanese Research Society for Gastric Cancer in 1981. The relationship of tumor contour and prognosis has not been consistent. The most common endoscopic appearance of gastric lymphoma is the presence of large folds in the body or antrum with diffuse ulceration. This is similar to the Bormann IV appearance of advanced gastric adenocarcinoma.

The majority of gastric polyps are benign, and again there are no reliable endoscopic features to differentiate benign from malignant. Polyp size >1 cm is a risk factor for the presence of neoplasia (adenoma) or malignancy (Figure 24–1). Biopsy of small polyps (<1 cm) is sufficient for diagnosis. Larger polyps should be biopsied to determine if neoplastic; however this may miss neoplastic foci within the polyp. Before removal of large polyps by endoscopic polypectomy or surgery, the physician must consider the histology obtained on biopsy, clinical symptoms attributable to the polyp, and the patient's age and medical status, in order to determine if polyp removal warrants the risk of the procedure. Endoscopic removal of large gastric polyps may be associated with a 4% risk of postpolypectomy bleeding, which may require surgery.

Submucosal polyps are less common than epithelial polyps (see Table 24–1). Because these lesions are submucosal, large forceps biopsies and double biopsies

Size (mm)	Lesion configuration I	II	III	IV	Total
≤ 4	○2	○8			10
5–9	○2	○13 ◐2	○24	○12	53
10–19	○7	◐2	○8 ◐4	○31	52
20–29	○1	○2	○1 ●1	○4 ◐2	11
≥ 30	○1	◐5 ●1	◐8 ●9	◐1 ●1	26
Total	13	33	55	51	152

○ Benign
◐ Early gastric cancer
● Advanced gastric cancer

Figure 24–1. The relationship of lesion size, shape, or configuration, and histology for 217 elevated lesions of the stomach diagnosed with double contrast radiography. Malignancy occurs more frequently in lesions over 1 cm in diameter. (Reproduced, with permission, from Yamada T, Ichikawa H: X-ray diagnosis of elevated lesions of the stomach. Radiology 1974;110:79.)

(biopsies within previous biopsy sites), especially in suspicious areas such as central ulcerations, should be performed. Infiltrating adenocarcinoma and lymphomas may also occur in the submucosa. Infiltrating adenocarcinoma (linitis plastica) may be difficult to recognize endoscopically. Subtle changes in gastric folds and areas with poor distensibility should be biopsied. Again, large biopsies and biopsies within biopsies may be required to make a diagnosis. If clinical and/or endoscopic findings suggest malignancy and biopsies and brushings are negative, large-particle snare biopsy or needle aspiration cytology during endoscopic ultrasound examination should be performed. Laparotomy may be required to obtain a histologic diagnosis.

Small bowel enteroscopes may be used to examine the small intestine, and have primarily been used in patients with gastrointestinal bleeding and no identifiable source on standard upper and lower GI endoscopies. "Push" enteroscopy entails the use of colonoscopes 135–160 cm in length or special 167-cm-long enteroscopes that are inserted through the mouth and into the proximal small intestine under direct visualization. Examination of 50–60 cm beyond the ligament of Treitz can be accomplished with this method. "Sonde-type" enteroscopes are more effective for examination of the distal small intestine. These contain a balloon at the tip that allows for peristalsis to propel the enteroscope into the ileum. Using "Sonde-type" enteroscopy, small intestinal lesions have been identified in one-quarter to one-third of patients examined for unexplained gastrointestinal blood loss. Small intestinal tumors have been found in 5% of patients examined by small bowel enteroscopy under these conditions. Diagnosis of small bowel tumors by small bowel enteroscopy has been reported in cases in which other imaging modalities, including enteroclysis and angiography, have been negative. The "Sonde" technique is limited by the length of time required for passage of the enteroscope (mean 4–8 hours) and lack of tip deflection and biopsy capabilities. Intraoperative endoscopy of the small bowel can also be performed. This involves passage of a colonoscope through the mouth or anus by the endoscopist. The surgeon then manually telescopes loops of bowel over the endoscope.

Routine surveillance endoscopy for gastric cancer is performed in Japan due to the high prevalence of cancer in that country. In the United States routine surveillance endoscopy for gastric cancer in asymptomatic patients with *H pylori* gastritis, pernicious anemia, or who have had a previous gastrectomy is generally not recommended.

D. IMAGING

Computed tomography (CT) scans of the chest and abdomen are the primary imaging modalities for preoperative staging of stomach and small intestine tumors. In stomachs that are well distended with contrast, wall thickness of >2 cm indicates transmural extension of the tumor (Figure 24–2). Evidence of direct invasion of perigastric fat, diaphragm, pancreas, transverse colon, and left lobe of the liver should be sought. Metastases to the liver, lung, and other organs can also be documented. For gastric adenocarcinoma overall accuracy of preoperative CT scans ranges from 61 to 72%. CT scans are particularly unreliable in assessing regional lymph nodes and invasion of adjacent organs, resulting

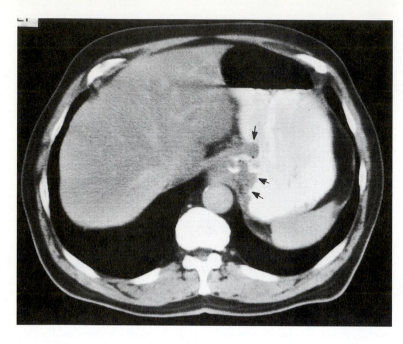

Figure 24–2. CT examination of the abdomen. Arrows denote tumor mass, a gastric adenocarcinoma of the cardia. (Courtesy of Dr. Howard Ansel.)

in understaging of the disease. CT scans may also overstage gastric adenocarcinoma, resulting in labeling the cancer as unresectable when in fact the tumor may be resectable. In one study comparing preoperative CT scanning with surgical staging it was found that 31% of patients were understaged and 16% were overstaged by CT. Careful review of preoperative CT scans by the gastroenterologist, surgeon, and radiologist is necessary before making a decision regarding resectability.

Endoscopic ultrasound is able to increase the accuracy of preoperative staging by determining the depth of invasion and possibly the involvement of regional lymph nodes. Several studies have compared endoscopic ultrasound, CT scans, and subsequent operative staging. Endoscopic ultrasound demonstrated 83–88% accuracy for determining depth of invasion compared with 35% accuracy for CT. For determining nodal involvement, endoscopic ultrasound is 66–72% accurate compared with 45% accuracy for CT.

Radiologic examination of the stomach can identify advanced gastric cancers; however it is less accurate than endoscopy for identification of early gastric cancer. All ulcers identified by x-ray examination should be referred for endoscopic biopsy. Radiologic criteria that suggest a benign ulcer include radiating folds and a normal-appearing mucosal surface around the crater. Linitus plastica is suggested by radiologic studies that demonstrate a nondistensible stomach.

Radiologic examination of the small bowel remains the most widely used method for diagnosis of small in-

testinal tumors (Figure 24–3). It is essential to communicate with the radiologist that a small bowel tumor is suspected, so that a dedicated small bowel examination can be performed. The "small bowel follow-though" that accompanies an upper GI x-ray is often inadequate for diagnosis of small bowel tumors. Enteroclysis, performed following placement of a nasoduodenal tube, is the most sensitive test for diagnosis of intestinal tumors, particularly if they occur in the jejunum. If an ileal lesion is suspected, a small bowel follow-through with air insufflated in the colon should be performed, which provides a clear air-contrast examination of the ileum. Patients actively bleeding from a suspected small bowel source should undergo a nuclear medicine tagged red blood cell (RBC) examination followed by angiography if the bleeding is continuous. Patients with gastrointestinal blood loss who are not actively bleeding and in whom a small bowel lesion is suspected should undergo a nuclear medicine Meckel's scan prior to barium studies. In addition to identification of Meckel's diverticula, this scan will occasionally identify leiomyomas or leiomyosarcomas, and can be followed by angiography or laparotomy to confirm the diagnosis.

A new and promising approach to imaging the small intestine to diagnose tumors and other sources of occult bleeding is a small capsule containing a light source and video chip camera, which can be swallowed. As the capsule passes through the small intestine, it transmits video images and information concerning its location to a recording device worn by the patient. These images

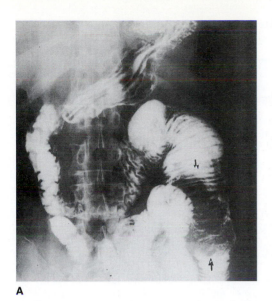
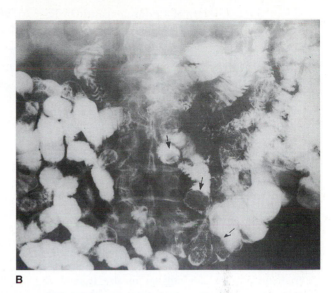

A

B

Figure 24–3. **A:** Primary jejunal adenocarcinoma *(arrows)* diagnosed with a small bowel follow-through barium examination. Bowel proximal to the tumor is dilated. **B:** Metastatic adenocarcinoma of the small bowel *(arrows)* diagnosed with a small bowel follow-through examination. (Courtesy of Dr. Howard Ansel.)

can then be reviewed, providing near-complete imaging of the small intestine.

Differential Diagnosis

Ulcerative and polypoid lesions of the stomach and intestine must be differentiated into benign and malignant. All ulcers found in the stomach require endoscopic biopsies and brushings at the time of initial diagnosis. A history of aspirin or nonsteroidal antiinflammatory drug use should be sought. Ulcers should also be followed with repeat endoscopy after a course of therapy in order to determine if they have healed, and repeat biopsies should be taken if nonhealing is demonstrated. Occasionally, malignant ulcers may appear to heal or partially heal following acid supression therapy and therefore repeated biopsies and brushings are important.

Most polyps found in the stomach represent hyperplastic polyps and usually occur in response to inflammation (see Table 24–1). Adenomatous polyps are the second most frequent type of gastric polyp and are considered precancerous. Adenomas should be removed by endoscopic polypectomy or surgical removal. The risk of malignancy increases in polypoid lesions greater than 1 cm in diameter, and surgical resection should be considered if a definitive diagnosis cannot be made by endoscopic biopsy. Less frequently, benign gastric polyps may represent carcinoid, leiomyoma, lipoma, and pan-

creatic rests. The latter represent ectopic pancreatic tissue, usually located in the submucosa of the antrum. Pancreatic rests may have a central umbilication or ulceration, and may present with bleeding, obstruction, or rarely clinical pancreatitis.

Gastric polyps frequently occur in patients with familial polyposis coli. Typically, hyperplastic polyps are found in the fundus and adenomatous polyps in the distal stomach and duodenum. Duodenal and periampullary adenocarcinoma can occur in 1 of 21 patients with familial polyposis coli over a lifetime. Screening endoscopy with careful attention to the duodenal ampulla and removal of all polyps has been recommended for these patients every 4 years. Peutz-Jeghers syndrome is an autosomal dominant condition characterized by intestinal polyps and pigmentation of the lips, buccal mucosa, hands, feet, or eyelids. Gastric hamartomas occur in 25% of patients with Peutz-Jeghers syndrome. Large folds (>1 cm in height) in the stomach that may resemble infiltrative malignancy may occur with hypertrophic gastritis and Menetrier's disease. The latter is a very rare condition characterized by mucosal hyperplasia and cystic dilation of gastric glands. Gastric folds in the fundus, body, and occasionally antrum appear enlarged, erythematous, and convoluted. Patients present with abdominal pain and hypoproteinemia.

Metastatic cancers may occur in the stomach and should be considered in any patient with gastrointestinal symptoms and history of a prior nongastric malignancy. The most common metastatic cancers to the stomach or small intestine include lung, breast, and melanoma (Figure 24–3B). These may appear as polypoid lesions with or without erosions or ulceration. Metastatic melanoma characteristically may appear as target or "bull's eye" lesions on a barium x-ray of the stomach, and at endoscopy often appear as small, discrete brown tumor nodules. Larger melanomas may appear as plaques with peripheral pigmentation, submucosal tumors with central ulceration, or large amelanotic masses. Metastatic breast carcinoma may present with a linitus plastica-type appearance. Other cancers that may metastasize to the stomach include cancer of the ovary, testes, liver, colon, and parotid gland.

Kaposi's sarcoma is a common tumor in patients with AIDS, and may be found in the gastrointestinal tract in up to 50% of patients with AIDS-related Kaposi's sarcoma. The endoscopic appearance may consist of erythematous nodules ranging in size from 1 to >5 mm, with or without central erosions. The appearance may also resemble gastric lymphoma with polypoid-type lesions.

Pseudotumors are lesions that simulate common tumors in the intestine. These include inflammatory pseudotumors or fibroid polyps (accumulation of fibroblasts), invasion of the gut wall by nematodes (helminthic pseudotumor), intestinal endometrioma, and amyloidosis.

Staging

A. GASTRIC ADENOCARCINOMA

Initial staging of gastric adenocarcinoma includes determination of operative resectibility. This requires a complete history and physical examination to evaluate for concomitant medical problems and ability to undergo abdominal surgery. Local staging of the actual tumor includes determination of the size and location of the tumor by endoscopy. Biopsies should be taken of apparently normal mucosa distal and proximal to the lesion to rule out infiltrative or submucosal spread. CT scans of the abdomen and chest are required to determine extent of disease into adjacent organs, possible lymph node involvement, and distant metastases. Careful questioning for new skeletal symptoms may direct x-ray or bone scan evaluations for osseous metastases. Patients with gastric tumors are generally considered operative candidates if they have no serious concurrent medical problems and when there is no evidence of distant metastases to liver, lung, or other organs.

The most commonly used staging system in the United States is the American Joint Committee on Cancer Staging System (Table 24–3). This system in-

Table 24–3. American Joint Committee on Cancer staging of gastric cancer.

Stage	Primary Tumor	Classification		5-Year Survival Rate
0	Tis	N0	M0	>90%
IA	T1	N0	M0	70–80%
IB	T1	N1	M0	55–70%
	T2	N0	M0	
II	T1	N2	M0	40–50%
	T2	N1	M0	
	T3	N0	M0	
IIIA	T2	N2	M0	10–20%
	T3	N1	M0	
	T4	N0	M0	
IIIB	T3	N2	M0	
	T4	N1	M0	
IV	T4	N2	M0	<1%
	Any T	Any N	M1	

Primary tumor (T)

TX	Primary tumor cannot be assessed
T0	No evidence of primary tumor
Tis	Carcinoma *in situ*
T1	Tumor invades lamina propria or submucosa
T2	Tumor invades muscularis propria
T3	Tumor invades adventitia
T4	Tumor invades adjacent structures

Regional lymph nodes (N)

NX	Regional nodes cannot be assessed
N0	No regional lymph node metastases
N1	Metastasis in perigastric lymph nodes within 3 cm of edge of primary tumor
N2	Metastasis in perigastric lymph nodes more than 3 cm from edge of primary tumor, or in lymph nodes along left gastric, common hepatic splenic or celiac arteries

Distant metastasis (M)

MX	Presence of distant metastasis cannot be assessed
M0	No distant metastasis
M1	Distant metastasis present

corporates depth of invasion (T), location of nodal metastases (N), and distant metastases (M). This staging system is similar to the Union Internationale Contre le Cancer (UICC) TNM system used in Europe. Japanese surgeons have developed a rigorous staging system that requires extensive nodal dissection at the time of surgery. This staging system also incorporates gross (Bormann's classification) and microscopic (Lauren's classification) pathologic characteristics of the cancers. As a consequence, comparison of cancers by stage from Japan and other countries is not often accurate.

"Early" gastric cancers are characterized by their location in the mucosa and submucosa (T1), and may or may not have nodal metastases. By definition, early gastric cancers include stage IA (T1N0), stage IB (T1N1), and stage II (T1N2) tumors. Not surprisingly, early gastric cancers are associated with excellent survival from surgical resection. Early gastric cancers account for only 15% of the cases in the United States. In contrast they comprise 40% or more of cancers reported in Japan, most likely due to extensive endoscopic surveillance programs. In Western countries 70–80% of resected gastric cancer specimens have advanced disease with metastases in the regional lymph nodes.

B. Lymphoma

Primary gastrointestinal lymphoma staging is adapted from the Ann Arbor staging system for lymphoma (Table 24–4). This staging system does not take into account several other criteria that have been shown to be associated with an adverse prognosis. These include size of tumor at presentation >7 cm, B-type symptoms (fever, sweats, weight loss), elevated serum lactate dehydrogenase and β_2-microglobulin, advanced depth of invasion and level of lymph node involvement, abdominal perforation, increased number of sites, nonresectability, advanced age, and the presence of comorbid disease. In addition to a physical examination, staging can be accomplished by intestinal barium studies, CT scans of the chest, abdomen, and pelvis, indirect laryngoscopy, and bilateral bone marrow biopsy and aspirates. Gallium scanning, bipedal lymphangiography, and a laparoscopic liver biopsy may also be used to complete the work-up. One-third of patients are diagnosed with stage IE lymphoma, one-third to one-half are diagnosed with stage IIE, and less than one-quarter are diagnosed with stage IV disease.

Treatment & Prognosis

The primary mode of treatment of most gastric and small intestinal tumors is surgical. Prognosis is directly related to the type and stage of the tumor and the completeness of the surgical resection.

A. Gastric Adenocarcinoma

The overall 5-year survival for gastric adenocarcinoma has changed little in the last several decades in the United States and currently remains at 10–15%. Early gastric cancer is curable with surgical resection, however this type comprises only 5–16% of patients undergoing resection for gastric cancer. In the United States, approximately 60% of patients with gastric cancer will have nonresectable disease at the time of diagnosis. Of the remaining 40% who have a "curative" resection (termed R0 resection), only 25–35% will survive 5 years (Figure 24–4).

Gastric adenocarcinomas are optimally resected using wide margins and with extensive lymph node dissections. Total gastrectomies are not routinely performed due to the increased morbidity associated with this procedure, but may be required if the tumor is extensive or multifocal. The Japanese Research Society for Gastric Cancer groups gastric lymph nodes (D1–D4) according to their proximity to the stomach. Curative resection requires resection of tumor-free lymph nodes in at least one group distant to involved lymph nodes and also often includes removal of the omentum and spleen. Extended or radical lymph node dissections have long been performed in Japan and may contribute to the extended survival found in Japanese patients with early stage cancer. The use of extended lymphadenectomies in Western countries is controversial, and several studies have not demonstrated a survival advantage with this procedure. Recent European studies have shown that extended D2 level lymph node resections result in higher morbidity and mortality than D1 level lymph node resections, with no survival advantage. Extended D2 level lymphadenectomies may benefit patients with serosal invasion or limited regional node disease; however, it most likely is not beneficial for patients with D3 node involvement, linitus plastica, and extensive invasion of adjacent organs.

Surgical resection should be considered even if CT scans suggest locally advanced disease. Occasionally a curative resection can be performed by en bloc resection of the tumor and adjacent involved organs. If the lesion is extensive and complete removal does not ap-

Table 24–4. Modified Ann Arbor staging system for primary gastrointestinal lymphoma.

Stage	Extent of Involvement
IE	Limited to one area of the GI tract with no other site
IIE	Localized involvement of an extranodal GI site and its lymph node chain
II$_1$E	Limited to the GI site and immediately draining lymph nodes
II$_2$E	A primary GI extranodal site and involvement of immediate and noncontinuous subdiaphragmatic lymph node groups
IIIE	Involvement of lymph nodes on both sides of the diaphragm and localized involvement of a dominant extranodal GI site
IV	Diffuse or disseminated involvement

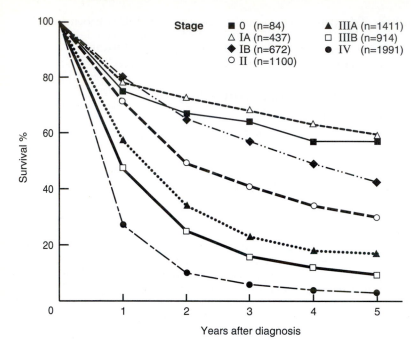

Figure 24–4. Survival by TNM classification and staging of 6609 patients with gastric adenocarcinoma. Stage IA versus IB, *P* < .01; stage II versus IB, IIIA, or IIIB, *P* < .01. (Reproduced, with permission, from Thompson GB, van Heerden JA, Sarr MG: Adenocarcinoma of the stomach: are we making progress? Lancet 1993;342:713. © by The Lancet Ltd., 1993.)

pear possible, a palliative resection can be planned. Survival and symptoms are improved if a palliative resection is performed instead of a simpler bypass procedure. Bypassing obstructing lesions with a gastrojejunal anastomosis may be the only surgical option for maintenance of fluid intake in some cases of advanced gastric cancer. Laparoscopic staging of patients with apparent locoregional carcinoma should also be considered.

Treatment guidelines for patients with gastric cancer have been published by the National Comprehensive Cancer Network (NCCN). Current recommendations indicate that patients with negative surgical resection margins and no evidence of metastases (R0 resection) be observed and receive no further therapy. Results of multicenter adjuvant therapy studies are pending for this type of patient. Patients with positive surgical resection margins (R1 resection) should be offered radiotherapy (45–50 Gy) with concurrent 5-fluorouracil (5-FU) chemotherapy. Patients with gross residual disease (R2 resection) and no metastases after surgery can be offered 5-FU chemotherapy with or without radiation therapy, cisplatin-based chemotherapy, or enrollment in a clinical trial. For inoperable patients with locoregional carcinoma, radiation therapy with concurrent 5-FU treatment, "salvage" chemotherapy with 5-FU or cisplatin-based therapy, or participation in a clinical trial can be recommended. Patients with a poor perfomance status (Karnofsky score ≤ 60 or ECOG score ≥ 2) should be offerred supportive care only. Following completion of chemotherapy the patients should be restaged, and if there is evidence of residual or metastatic disease then salvage therapy can be considered.

Chemotherapies in the adjuvant, primary treatment, or salvage setting are based on chemotherapeutic agents that have demonstrable activity in gastric carcinomas. A positive tumor response is defined as a 50% or greater reduction in the size of a measurable tumor. Single chemotherapeutic agents with response rates of 20–25% include 5-FU, mitomycin C, doxorubicin, nitrosoureas, and cisplatin. Combination chemotherapy with 5-FU, doxorubicin (Adriamycin), and mitomycin C (FAM) or etoposide, Adriamycin, and cisplatin (EAP) has a response rate of 22–50%. Several combinations have been described that demonstrate response rates of up to 50% in a limited number of trials. These include 5-FU, Adriamycin, and cisplatin (FAP); etoposide, leucovorin, and 5-FU (ELF); and 5-FU, Adriamycin, and methotrexate (FAMTx). Significant toxicities may occur with these regimes.

Palliation of obstructive or bleeding complications due to disseminated or recurrent gastric cancer represents a difficult management problem. For obstruction of the distal esophagus, endoscopic laser therapy or prosthetic wire mesh stents have been used successfully, or percutaneous endoscopic gastrostomy (PEG) tubes can be placed. For obstruction of the distal stomach a simple gastrojejunostomy or partial gastrectomy can be performed. Palliative resection may provide superior results compared with palliative bypass, however, at the expense of increased morbidity. Palliation of obstructing cancer at the gastric outlet may also be managed by wire mesh stents placed by endoscopy. Laser or thermal cautery therapy may be used for persistently bleeding lesions. Occasionally an obstructing tumor may respond to localized radiation therapy. However, the dose of radiation is often limited by the low tolerance of surrounding tissues.

B. Lymphoma

Definite data regarding the best treatment strategies for each stage of gastrointestinal lymphoma are lacking, and recommendations for therapy are made on the basis of the experience of a small, retrospective series of patients that used varying staging criteria. Patients with apparent stage IE or IIE disease should have surgical excision of the tumor and lymph nodes. Stage IE patients do well with surgical therapy alone, with long-term survival rates of 62–86%. The addition of adjuvant radiation therapy in this setting has not been shown to be beneficial; however most recommend postoperative radiation for extensive stage IE lesions. Patients with stage IIE lesions are often treated with adjuvant combination chemotherapy. For patients with significant residual disease after initial surgery, adjuvant radiation therapy is often used in addition to chemotherapy. Stage II_1E patients demonstrate survivals similar to stage IE, whereas stage II_2E patients usually develop progressive lymphoma within 3 years of diagnosis. Patients with stage III or IV disease should undergo radiation and/or combination chemotherapy as a primary treatment modality, with or without surgical debulking. Evidence exists to indicate that surgical debulking of stage III or stage IV disease may enhance survival and prevent the infrequent complications such as perforation or bleeding that may occur during chemotherapy. Very few 5-year survivals occur with stage III or IV disease.

C. Carcinoid

Carcinoid tumors are characterized by a slow rate of invasion and metastases. Carcinoid localized to the intestine will be cured by surgical resection in over 90% of patients. Patients with carcinoid tumors with nodal metastases at the time of surgery will have an 80% recurrence-free rate at 5 years; however after 25 years only 23% of patients will be recurrence free. Patients with unresectable abdominal tumors and patients with unresectable hepatic metastases will have a 50% and 30% survival rate at 5 years, respectively (Figure 24–5). Current therapies for treating hepatic metastases may extend these survivals and include a multispecialty approach using surgical debulking, cryoablation, hepatic artery embolization, octreotide, and possibly combina-

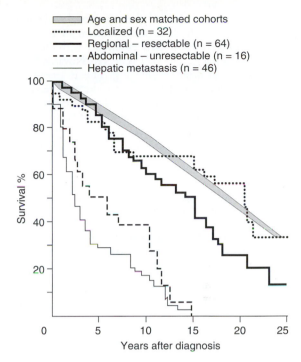

Figure 24–5. Carcinoid tumors of the small bowel. Survival is according to the stage at initial surgical diagnosis. (Reproduced, with permission, from Moertel CG: An odyssey in the land of small tumors. J Clin Oncol 1987;5:1503.)

tion chemotherapy. For example, promising results have been obtained by treatment of unresectable hepatic carcinoid by hepatic artery occlusion with or without adjuvant chemotherapy. Patients with advanced carcinoid and the carcinoid syndrome can be palliated by treatment with octreotide, a somatostatin analogue. Chemotherapy is generally ineffective and is often not recommended except on an experimental basis. Active agents include 5-FU, doxorubicin, dacarbazine, cyclophosphamide, or streptozotocin. The response rate to these drugs is poor (approximately 20%) and the median duration of tumor regression has been reported to be 4 months.

D. Gastrointestinal Stromal Tumors (Leiomyoma, Leiomyosarcoma)

Preoperative staging is necessary to identify disseminated disease. Approximately 67% of patients with leiomyosarcoma will have extragastric extension at laparotomy, and surgical resection with curative intent is successful in up to one-half of patients. Overall, the 5-year survival for leiomyosarcoma is 25–30%. Little efficacy has been reported for traditional radiation, chemotherapy, or both in the treatment of gastrointestinal stromal tumors. Early experience with the tyrosine kinase inhibitor, STI-571 (Gleevec, Novartis Pharmaceuticals) has been encouraging. This is a nontoxic chemotherapeutic agent that targets the *c-kit* receptor tyrosine kinase protein. This agent was recently approved by the FDA and is currently the treatment of choice for all patients with malignant GIST who have not had curative surgical therapy.

REFERENCES

Ajani JA et al: NCCN practice guidelines for upper gastrointestinal cancer. National Comprehensive Cancer Network. Oncology 1998;12:226.

Blackstone MO: *Endoscopic Interpretation. Normal and Pathologic Appearances of the Gastrointestinal Tract.* Raven Press, 1984.

Blanchard DK et al: Tumors of the small intestine. World J Surg 2000;24:421.

Bonenkamp JJ et al: Randomized comparison of mortality after D1 and D2 dissection for gastric cancer in 996 Dutch patients. Lancet 1995;345:745.

Correa P: Human gastric carcinogenesis: a multistep and multifactorial process. Cancer Res 1992;52:6735.

Correa P et al: Chemoprevention of gastric dysplasia: randomized trial of antioxidant supplements and anti-*Helicobacter pylori* therapy. J Natl Cancer Inst 2000;92:1881.

Cuschieri A et al: Patient survival after D1 and D2 resections for gastric cancer: long-term results of the MRC randomized surgical trial. Surgical Co-operative Group. Br J Cancer 1999; 79:1522.

Davis GR: Neoplasms of the stomach. In: *Gastrointestinal Disease. Pathophysiology, Diagnosis and Management,* 5th ed. Sleisenger MH, Fordtran JS (editors). W.B. Saunders Co., 1993.

Frazee RC, Roberts J: Gastric lymphoma treatment: medical versus surgical. Surg Clin North Am 1992;72:423.

Joensuu H et al: Effect of the tyrosine kinase inhibitor ST1571 in a patient with metastatic gastrointestinal stromal tumor. N Engl J Med 2001;344:1052.

Karpeh MS, Kelsen DP, Tepper JE: Cancer of the stomach. In: *Cancer: Principles and Practice of Oncology,* 6th ed. DeVita VT, Hellman S, Rosenberg SA (editors). Lippincott Williams & Wilkins, 2000.

Miettinen M, Sarlomo-Rikala M, Lasota J: Gastrointestinal stromal tumors: recent advances in understanding of their biology. Human Pathol 1999;30:1213.

Moertel CG: Gastrointestinal carcinoid tumors and the malignant carcinoid syndrome. In: *Gastrointestinal Disease. Pathophysiology, Diagnosis and Management,* 5th ed. Sleisenger MH, Fordtran JS (editors). W.B. Saunders Co., 1993.

Morris JC, Bruckner HW: Gastric cancer: molecular and cellular abnormalities. In: *Enclycopedia of Cancer.* Bertino JR (editor). Academic Press, 1997.

Thompson GB, van Heerden JA, Sarr MG: Adenocarcinoma of the stomach: are we making progress? Lancet 1993;342:713.

Uemura N et al: *Helicobacter pylori* infection and the development of gastric cancer. N Engl J Med 2001;345:784.

Zollinger RM, Sternfeld WC, Schreiber HS: Primary neoplasms of the small intestine. Am J Surg 1986;151:654.

Miscellaneous Disorders of the Stomach & Small Intestine

25

James H. Grendell, MD

A variety of "miscellaneous" disorders can involve the stomach and small intestine. Although these diseases are not as common as most of those described in other chapters, it is important that clinicians have some basic familiarity with their presentation.

STOMACH

Gastric Volvulus

Gastric volvulus is the twisting of the stomach. Most commonly, the stomach rotates on its longitudinal axis, a condition associated with paraesophageal hernia, although other patterns of rotation can occur.

Acute gastric volvulus presents with sudden, severe pain of the upper abdomen or chest, persistent retching producing only a little vomitus, epigastric distention, and the inability to pass a nasogastric tube. Upper gastrointestinal series demonstrates an abrupt obstruction at the site of the volvulus. Acute gastric volvulus requires emergency surgical evaluation because of the substantial risk of mortality related to gastric ischemia or perforation.

Chronic gastric volvulus may be asymptomatic or present with nonspecific symptoms of dyspepsia, heartburn, or postprandial bleeding. Diagnosis is made by performing an upper gastrointestinal series, and treatment consists of gastropexy and repair of any associated paraesophageal hernia.

Gastric Diverticula

Gastric diverticula are uncommon and typically asymptomatic, although the clinician may have difficulty in differentiating them from gastric ulcers on upper gastrointestinal series. Usually, no treatment is required, although diverticulectomy rarely may be necessitated owing to inflammation or hemorrhage.

Gastric Rupture

Gastric rupture may occur following blunt trauma, gastroscopy, vomiting, and overdistention of the stomach by massive overeating or ingestion of large doses of sodium bicarbonate. Patients usually present with abdominal pain and distention, and on examination usually have tympany and may have subcutaneous emphysema. Chest x-ray or upright or lateral abdominal x-rays typically demonstrate free intraperitoneal air. Emergency surgical repair is mandatory, and morbidity (eg, fistula, intraabdominal abscess) and mortality rates are high.

Bezoars

Bezoars are persisting accumulations of foreign material in the stomach. Although they can occur as a result of unusual eating habits (eg, trichobezoars from ingesting hair or persimmon bezoars), most bezoars in adults consist mainly of plant material in patients who have undergone surgery affecting gastric motor function (eg, vagotomy, particularly when associated with antrectomy or partial gastrectomy).

Patients typically present with abdominal pain, nausea, vomiting, and early satiety. Less commonly bezoars may result in mucosal ulceration, which may lead to acute or chronic gastrointestinal blood loss or perforation. The diagnosis may be made by upper gastrointestinal series or endoscopy.

Most gastric bezoars can be mechanically disrupted and can either be removed or will pass spontaneously from the stomach. This is accomplished using endoscopic tools or lavage either through the endoscope or through a large-bore gastric tube. Bezoars that cannot be removed in these ways or that result in serious complications may require surgery.

Following successful treatment of a bezoar, patients should be advised to avoid raw citrus fruits and persimmon. Prokinetic agents such as metoclopramide may also help prevent recurrence. Habitual ingestion of hair or other foreign indigestible material requires psychiatric evaluation and therapy.

Eosinophilic Gastroenteritis

This rare disease results from eosinophilic infiltration of the gut wall that can occur anywhere in the gastrointestinal tract, but it most commonly involves the stomach and small intestine. The cause of this disorder in most patients is unknown; however, allergies (eg, to foods) or drug or toxin exposures are thought to play a role in some cases.

There are three main patterns of involvement:

1. Mucosal and submucosal disease: These patients typically have cramping or colicky abdominal pain, nausea, vomiting, weight loss, and diarrhea.
2. Muscle layer disease: These patients have symptoms and signs of pyloric or intestinal obstruction.
3. Serosal layer disease: These patients usually present with eosinophilic ascites.

Peripheral blood eosinophilia is found in about 75–80% of patients and ranges from about 1000/µL in patients with muscle layer disease to 8000/µL in patients with serosal disease.

Upper gastrointestinal series or abdominal computed tomography may show thickened folds in the stomach or small intestine with or without nodules. These findings, however, are nonspecific. Endoscopy usually demonstrates prominent mucosal folds, nodularity, erythema, and, in some cases, ulcerations. However, endoscopic abnormalities may be subtle. Endoscopic biopsy of involved areas is the best way of making the diagnosis. In patients with disease that primarily involves the muscle layer or serosa, endoscopic biopsies may be negative, and the diagnosis is made on the basis of clinical, laboratory, and radiologic findings, or on full-thickness operative biopsy.

Patients with disease involving the mucosa may respond to dietary manipulation if they have a history suggestive of a specific food allergy or intolerance. Patients with mucosal disease failing to respond to elimination diets and those with muscle layer or serosal disease usually respond to treatment with corticosteroids. In some patients requiring high doses of steroids to keep them symptom free, azathioprine can be added in an attempt to reduce the maintenance corticosteroid dose. Because obstructive symptoms usually respond to medical therapy, surgery is generally not necessary and should be avoided unless it is required to confirm the diagnosis and exclude cancer.

SMALL INTESTINE

Small Bowel Obstruction

Mechanical obstruction of the small intestine is a common problem that usually is due to adhesions resulting from previous abdominal surgery. However, a variety of other causes can be found (Table 25–1).

The presentation depends on the level of the obstruction in the small intestine. High or proximal small bowel obstruction results in variable upper abdominal

Table 25–1. Causes of mechanical small bowel obstruction.

Postoperative adhesions
Congenital adhesive bands
External or internal hernias
Tumors
Strictures (eg, from Crohn's disease, ischemia, radiation injury)
Intussusception
Volvulus
Gallstones
Foreign bodies
Hematomas (eg, from trauma or spontaneously in patients on anticoagulants)

pain and profuse vomiting. Mid- or distal small bowel obstruction presents with cramping or colicky periumbilical or diffuse abdominal pain, abdominal distention, and episodic vomiting frequently associated with crescendos of pain. The more distal the obstruction, the greater the abdominal distention and the more feculent the vomitus or nasogastric drainage. When small bowel obstruction is complete, obstipation results.

Physical examination may demonstrate postural or resting changes in pulse and blood pressure owing to hypovolemia and dehydration. On abdominal examination, mild diffuse tenderness often is present and high-pitched "tinkling" bowel sounds and peristaltic "rushes" may be noted on auscultation of the abdomen. The patient should be evaluated carefully for incarcerated external hernias.

Depending on the duration of obstruction and degree of hypovolemia, patients may demonstrate leukocytosis, hemoconcentration, and varying degrees of electrolyte abnormalities. Supine and upright (or lateral) abdominal x-rays strongly suggest the diagnosis with a paucity of air in the colon and a ladderlike arrangement of small bowel loops with air–fluid levels (Figure 25–1). A radiologic examination of the small intestine with contrast or abdominal computed tomography may provide additional information concerning the level and cause of obstruction.

The differential diagnosis includes colonic obstruction, intestinal ileus, and intestinal pseudoobstruction. In colonic obstruction, abdominal x-rays demonstrate dilated colon proximal to the site of obstruction. Intestinal ileus may occur as a result of an intraabdominal inflammatory process (eg, acute pancreatitis, acute appendicitis), following abdominal surgery or as a multifactorial process in the hospitalized patient related to immobility, electrolyte abnormalities, and the administration of drugs (eg, narcotics and anticholinergics). Both symptoms and abdominal findings in intestinal

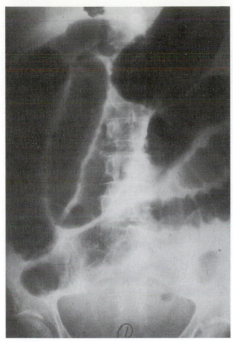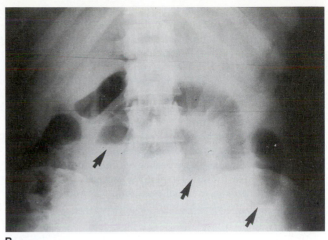

Figure 25–1. **A:** Dilated loops of intestine on a supine abdominal x-ray of a patient with small bowel obstruction. **B:** Air–fluid levels *(arrows)* on an upright abdominal x-ray of a patient with small bowel obstruction.

ileus tend to be milder than in small bowel obstruction, and abdominal x-rays typically show gas mainly in the colon without a pattern of numerous air–fluid levels. Patients with intestinal pseudoobstruction due to neuromuscular disease of the gastrointestinal tract have chronic or recurring symptoms that may involve one or more of the hollow digestive organs. In cases in which the differential diagnosis is in doubt, contrast radiographic studies of the small intestine, colon, or both need to be performed to determine if mechanical obstruction is present.

The initial treatment of small bowel obstruction is fluid and electrolyte resuscitation and nasogastric decompression. Partial small bowel obstruction will usually resolve spontaneously within a few days. Operative therapy is required for cases of partial obstruction that fail to resolve with expectant management and for most cases of complete obstruction.

Diverticular Disease of the Small Intestine

Diverticula may occur throughout the small intestine but are most commonly found in the duodenum or jejunum. In the duodenum about three-fourths of the diverticula are within 2 cm of the ampulla of Vater and

are termed **juxtapapillary.** These duodenal diverticula are usually asymptomatic and require no treatment, but can occasionally bleed or perforate. Furthermore, it has been suggested that juxtapapillary diverticula contribute to gallstone disease or acute pancreatitis in some patients.

Jejunal diverticula (other than Meckel's diverticulum) are acquired and are associated with disorders of impaired intestinal motility such as progressive systemic sclerosis and intestinal pseudoobstruction. Symptoms are usually related to the underlying motility disorder, although bacterial overgrowth leading to malabsorption, bleeding, and perforation has been reported.

Enteropathy from Radiation & from Nonsteroidal Antiinflammatory Drugs

Radiation therapy to the abdomen frequently produces acute intestinal mucosal injury characterized by self-limited abdominal pain, nausea, vomiting, and diarrhea (at times, bloody). In addition, radiation can injure blood vessels in the intestinal wall, causing a chronic fibroproliferative response leading to obliteration of the vessels and chronic intestinal ischemia. This process may result in symptomatic disease presenting anytime from several months to many years after completion of the course of radiation therapy with bleeding, stricture formation with obstruction, and, occasionally, perforation with abscess or fistula formation. Depending on the presentation and the patient's overall condition, the treatment is usually operative resection or bypass of the involved segment of intestine.

Long-standing use of nonsteroidal antiinflammatory drugs (NSAIDs) can produce mucosal injury to the small intestine leading to chronic gastrointestinal blood loss. In a small number of patients, overt intestinal ulcerations or transmural injury occurs and this can result in diaphragm-like intestinal strictures. Withdrawal of NSAIDs will result in eventual resolution of intestinal mucosal inflammation, although strictured areas may require resection.

Pneumatosis Cystoides Intestinalis

Pneumatosis cystoides intestinalis is an uncommon condition in which gas-filled cysts are found in the small intestine, colon, and occasionally in the stomach or mesentery. Cysts are subserosal and range from a few millimeters to several centimeters and can be single or in clusters. About 15% of cases are considered to be primary (idiopathic) and usually involve only the left colon. The remaining 85% of cases termed **secondary pneumatosis** are associated with a variety of gastrointestinal diseases, endoscopic and operative procedures, and pulmonary disease.

Patients with pneumatosis intestinalis are usually asymptomatic, with the diagnosis being an unexpected finding on a radiologic study. When present, symptoms are more likely related to the gastrointestinal process presumably producing the pneumatosis. Patients with gas in the bowel wall in other settings such as intestinal ischemia or a severe infectious process (eg, *Clostridium difficile* colitis) typically have obvious manifestations of sepsis.

Most patients with pneumatosis require treatment only of any associated disease process. Patients with symptomatic disease (usually colonic) can be treated with oxygen therapy by mask or in a hyperbaric chamber. Avoidance of nonabsorbable carbohydrates (eg, sorbitol, lactulose) and correction of any carbohydrate malabsorption (eg, lactase deficiency) may also be helpful.

REFERENCES

Bjarnason I et al: Side effects of nonsteroidal anti-inflammatory drugs on the small and large intestine in humans. Gastroenterology 1993;104:1832.

Chiu KW, Changchien CS, Chuah SK: Small-bowel diverticulum: is it a risk for small-bowel volvulus. J Clin Gastroenterol 1994;19:176.

Cho KC, Baker SR: Extraluminal air. Diagnosis and significance. Radiol Clin North Am 1994;32:829.

Galandiuk S, Fazio VW: Pneumatosis cystoides intestinalis: a review of the literature. Dis Colon Rectum 1986;29:358.

Hughes W, Pierce WS: Surgical implications of gastric diverticula. Surg Gynecol Obstet 1970;131:99.

Milne LW et al: Gastric volvulus: two cases and a review of the literature. J Emerg Med 1994;12:299.

Palder SB, Frey CB: Jejunal diverticulosis. Arch Surg 1988;123:889.

Psathakis D et al: Clinical significance of duodenal diverticula. J Am Coll Surg 1994;178:257.

Robles R et al: Gastrointestinal bezoars. Br J Surg 1994;81:1000.

Talley NJ et al: Eosinophilic gastroenteritis: a clinicopathological study of patients with disease of the mucosae, muscle layer, and subserosal tissue. Gut 1990;31:54.

Tsiotis GG, Farnell MB, Ilstrup DM: Nonmeckelian jejunal or ileal diverticulosis: an analysis of 112 cases. Surgery 1994;116:726.

Velanovich V: Gastric diverticulum: endoscopic and radiologic appearance. Surg Endosc 1994;8:1338.

Welch JP: *Bowel Obstruction. Differential Diagnosis and Clinical Management.* Saunders, 1990.

SECTION IV

Diseases of the Colon & Rectum

Malignant & Premalignant Lesions of the Colon

26

Robert S. Bresalier, MD

ESSENTIALS OF DIAGNOSIS

- *Ninety percent of colorectal cancers occur in patients over 50 years of age.*
- *Adenomas precede most carcinomas.*
- *Early cancers are asymptomatic.*
- *Screening tests can detect preneoplastic lesions and early cancers.*
- *Microcytic anemia in the elderly suggests the presence of colorectal cancer.*
- *Hematochezia may be a sign of colorectal cancer (especially of the distal colon and rectum).*
- *Weight loss and obstructive symptoms are late findings.*

GENERAL CONSIDERATIONS

Cancers of the colon and rectum (colorectal cancers) are a major cause of illness and death in patients living in the United States and other Western countries. There were an estimated 135,000 new cases of colorectal cancer in the United States in 2001, accounting for 57,000 cancer-related deaths (second only to lung cancer). Because these cancers arise over a long period of time as the result of interactions between genetic predisposition and environmental influences, it is possible to identify preneoplastic and early neoplastic lesions and improve survival rates. Rapidly evolving knowledge of the pathogenesis of colorectal cancer, especially in high-risk groups, is leading to the development of new tools for identifying people who will most benefit from cancer surveillance and adjuvant therapy following potentially curative surgery.

A rapid proliferation of knowledge about the molecular biologic characteristics of colorectal cancers and the molecular pathways involved in their evolution has provided useful insights into the pathogenesis of not only colonic neoplasia but of cancer in general. "Molecular diagnosis" of at-risk individuals is now clinically possible in families with familial adenomatous polyposis and for hereditary nonpolyposis colorectal cancer patients. A panel of molecular markers may in the future allow for identification of those in the general population at risk for sporadic cancer as well.

Screening for colorectal cancer has been advocated for some time because of the high prevalence of the disease in the United States and the potential for cure if preneoplastic or early neoplastic lesions are removed endoscopically or surgically. Although screening has been advocated by all major medical societies, compliance has been poor. Fecal occult blood testing (FOBT) is associated with false negative and false positive rates that have limited enthusiasm for its use. Recent prospective and case–control studies, however, clearly demonstrate improved survival rates in those screened with FOBT and sigmoidoscopy; these observations will no doubt increase the acceptance of screening of persons in the general population who are over 50 years of age, but more specific, cost-effective methods are clearly needed. Several recent studies confirm the high sensitivity of colonoscopy as a screening tool, and suggest its cost effectiveness. It is hoped that the growing menu of options for colorectal cancer screening, increased recognition of its effectiveness, and the willingness of Medicare and third-party insurers to pay for colorectal cancer screening will, further increase its use.

Removal of preneoplastic adenomatous polyps and early colorectal cancers improves survival rates. Hence, screening methods to date have focused on eliminating preexisting lesions. The ideal goal, however, would be to prevent the development of cancer in the general population (primary prevention). Ongoing clinical trials are concentrating on dietary manipulation (eg, decreased amount or altered composition of fat, increased fiber), use of antioxidants, dietary calcium supplementation, and use of aspirin and nonsteroidal antiinflammatory agents (NSAIDs), which affect prostaglandin synthesis (based on studies of familial adenomatous polyposis). At present, the efficacy of any such manipulation remains unproved, for prevention of cancer in the general population.

PATHOPHYSIOLOGY

Colorectal cancers arise through complex interactions between genetic and environmental influences. The relative contribution of each varies. Genetic factors predominate in defined hereditary syndromes such as familial adenomatous polyposis and hereditary nonpolyposis colorectal cancer. Sporadic colon cancers develop over longer periods of time as environmental influences produce genotoxic events eventually leading to cancer. In both types, tumors do not develop all at once but rather evolve from progressive identifiable changes in the colonic mucosa (eg, dysplasia, adenoma).

Environmental Influences

Several pieces of evidence suggest that the environment plays a role in the development of colorectal cancers. The frequency of colorectal cancer varies remarkably worldwide, with the highest rates in North America, Australia, and Europe, and much lower rates in regions of Asia, South America, and sub-Saharan Africa. The risk of cancer rises rapidly in populations migrating from low-risk to high-risk areas, again suggesting that environmental factors, especially dietary differences, are important in its development. Environmental influences that may potentially influence carcinogenesis in the colon are listed in Table 26–1.

Descriptive epidemiologic studies and studies of experimental carcinogenesis both suggest that diets containing high amounts of fat predispose to colorectal cancers, especially those arising in the descending and sigmoid colon. Total dietary fat accounts for 40–45% of

Table 26–1. Environmental factors that may influence colorectal carcinogenesis.[1]

Probably related
High dietary fat consumption[2]
Low dietary fiber consumption[2]
Possibly related
Environmental carcinogens and mutagens
Heterocyclic amines (from charbroiled or fried foods)
Products of bacterial metabolism
Beer and ale consumption (rectal cancer)
Low dietary selenium
Probably protective
Dietary fiber consumption (wheat bran, cellulose, lignin)
Dietary calcium
Aspirin and NSAIDs[3]
Physical activity/low body mass
Possibly protective[4]
Yellow-green cruciferous vegetables
Foods rich in carotene (vitamin A)
Vitamins C and E
Selenium
Folic acid
Cyclooxygenase-2 (COX-2) inhibitors
Hormone replacement therapy (estrogen)

[1]Based on epidemiologic observations.
[2]Dietary fats and fiber are heterogeneous in composition and which individual components are causative or protective remains to be determined.
[3]NSAIDs, nonsteroidal antiinflammatory drugs.
[4]Data are limited.

total caloric intake in countries with high incidence rates of colorectal cancer, whereas in low-risk populations, it accounts for only 10–15%. Several case–control and cohort studies also suggest a relationship between dietary fat intake and the incidence and mortality rates of colorectal cancer, but these are less convincing than data from descriptive epidemiologic studies. Experimental animals fed diets high in polyunsaturated and saturated fats develop greater numbers of carcinogen-induced colonic adenocarcinomas than those on low-fat diets. Dietary fat enhances cholesterol and bile acid synthesis by the liver. These substances are converted by colonic bacteria to secondary bile acids, cholesterol metabolites, and other potentially toxic compounds that may damage the colonic mucosa, leading to increased cellular proliferation (Figure 26–1). Actively proliferating cells are most susceptible to the effects of carcinogens and other genotoxic influences. Such carcinogens may result from the processing or cooking of foods or from the action of colonic bacteria on dietary components.

Whereas dietary fat may promote carcinogenesis in the colon, dietary fiber appears to have the opposite effect. Dietary fiber consists of plant material resistant to digestion, which includes a heterogeneous mix of carbohydrate and noncarbohydrate components. Cereals such as bran cereals may increase stool bulk, thereby diluting carcinogens and tumor promoters, decreasing their contact with the mucosa, and enhancing their elimination. Cellulose and hemicellulose decrease the level of bacterial enzymes, and may diminish the activation of carcinogens and cocarcinogens. The majority of both observational epidemiologic and case–control studies support the protective effect of fiber-rich diets. Recent randomized controlled trials have not, however, been able to confirm the ability of fiber supplementation to prevent recurrence of precancerous adenomas in the colon. This may be explained, in part, by the inability of existing data to define the relationships between fiber-rich foods, and the importance of nonfiber vegetable components, nutrients, and micronutrients in fruits and vegetables.

Dietary calcium may also have a protective role in preventing colonic carcinogenesis. Epidemiologic studies indicate that men who consume the least amount of calcium and vitamin D have twice the cancer risk of those who consume high amounts of these compounds. Calcium increases the fecal excretion of bile acids and decreases the ratio of dihydroxy to trihydroxy bile acids in duodenal bile. Supplemental calcium also decreases proliferation of the colonic mucosa, both in humans and experimental animals, by mechanisms that appear to be independent of its effects on bile acids. A recent prospective placebo-controlled trial demonstrated the ability of dietary calcium supplementation to reduce the incidence and number of recurrent adenomatous polyps in individuals chosen for a history of such lesions. Epidemiologic studies also suggest a lower incidence of colorectal cancer in those consuming diets high in folate or with folate supplementation. Folic acid and its metabolites play an important role in DNA synthesis and integrity and DNA methylation.

Although high dietary intake of yellow-green cruciferous vegetables, micronutrients such as selenium salts, and vitamins A, C, and E (antioxidants) has been linked to a reduction in colon cancer development, the influence of these foods in preventing colonic carcinogenesis remains controversial. Epidemiologic, case–control, and prospective cohort trials suggest a protective effect against development of colorectal cancer in women taking hormone (estrogen) replacement therapy. Increased physical activity and low body mass may also be protective.

The risk for development of both colonic adenomas and carcinomas may be substantially reduced (40–50%) among long-term users of aspirin and other NSAIDs as compared with controls. In familial adenomatous polyposis (FAP) where hundreds of adenomas occur in the colon and rectum, a significant decrease in the mean number and size of polyps has been demonstrated in those treated with NSAIDs compared with control patients in short-term trials. The mechanism for adenoma and cancer protection is unknown but may relate to altered synthesis of arachidonic acid metabolites (eicosanoids) that include prostaglandins, thromboxanes, leucotrienes, and hydroxyeicosatetraenoic acids. These compounds modulate a number of pathways involved in signaling between the cell surface and the nucleus that affect cellular adhesion, growth, differentiation, and programmed cell death (apoptosis). Cyclooxygenase is a key enzyme responsible for production of prostaglandins and other eicosanoids, and is inhibited by NSAIDs. One form of this enzyme, cyclooxygenase-2 (COX-2), is induced by cytokines, mitogens, and growth factors and is elevated in colorectal tumors (adenomas and carcinomas). COX-2 inhibition leads to prevention of colorectal cancer development in experimental models, and reduces polyp recurrence in patients with FAP. Trials are ongoing to determine the usefulness of NSAIDs and specific inhibitors of COX-2 in preventing adenoma recurrence in individuals with sporadic adenomas and carcinomas of the colon.

Genetic Influences

Although it is convenient to categorize colorectal cancers as hereditary (familial) and nonhereditary (sporadic), it is more appropriate to consider all colorectal cancers as having genetic components that are inherited or acquired to varying degrees. Individuals with familial adenomatous polyposis, hereditary nonpolyposis colorectal cancer, and other familial syndromes are born with genetic alterations that make them susceptible to the development of colonic neoplasia. Environmental factors then contribute additional "hits," leading to malignant transformation. In the case of "sporadic" cancers, multiple somatic mutations are contributed by the environment.

Genetic changes that may lead to the development of colorectal cancer can be organized into three major classes: alterations in protooncogenes, loss of tumor-suppressor gene activity, and abnormalities in genes involved in DNA repair. Although much of what is known about the molecular genetics of colorectal cancer has come from the study of familial syndromes, similar changes are associated with the development of sporadic cancers (Table 26–2).

Cellular protooncogenes are human genes containing a DNA sequence homologous to that of acute transforming retroviruses. Many of these genes play a role in the normal regulation of cell growth, and their altered expression contributes to abnormal proliferation

Risk factors: diets high in fats, cholesterol, and fried foods and foods low in fiber

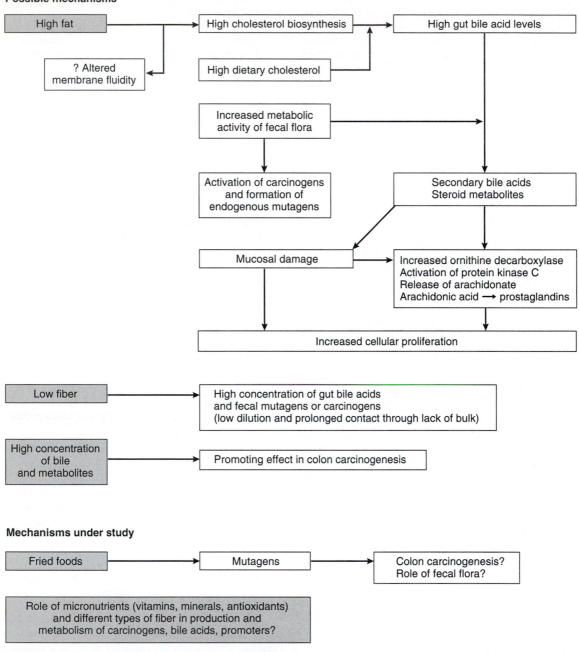

Table 26–2. Genes altered in sporadic colorectal cancer.

Gene	Chromosone	Tumors with Alterations (%)	Class	Function
K-*ras*	12	50	Protooncogene	Encodes guanine nucleotide-binding protein that regulates intracellular signaling
APC	5	70	Tumor suppressor	Regulation of β-catenin involved in activation of Wnt/TcF signaling (activates c-*myc*, cyclin D1)[1]; regulation of proliferation, apoptosis; interaction with E-cadherin (? cell adhesion)
DCC	18	70	? Tumor suppressor	Neutrin-1 receptor; caspase substrate in apoptosis; cell adhesion
SMAD4 (DPC4, MADH4)	18	?	Tumor suppressor	Nuclear transcription factor in TGF-β1 signaling; regulation of angiogenesis; regulator of WAF1 promoter; downstream mediator of SMAD2
p53	17	75	Tumor suppressor	Transcription factor; regulator of cell cycle progression after cellular stress, of apoptosis, of gene expression, and of DNA repair
hMSH2	2	—[2]	DNA mismatch repair	Maintains fidelity of DNA replication
hMLH1	3	—[2]	DNA mismatch repair	Maintains fidelity of DNA replication
hMSH6	2	—[2]	DNA mismatch repair	Maintains fidelity of DNA replication
TGF-β1 RII	3	—[3]	Tumor suppressor	Receptor for signaling in the TGF-β1 pathway; inhibitor of colonic epithelial proliferation, often mutated in tumors with MSI

[1]β-Catenin mutations (downstream of APC) are found in 16–25% of microsatellite instability (MSI) colon cancers, but not in microsatellite stable (MSS) cancers.
[2]Approximately 15% of sporadic colorectal cancers demonstrate microsatellite instability associated with alterations in mismatch repair genes (principally *hMSH2* and *hMLH1* but also *hMSH3, hMSH6, hPMS1,* and *hPMS2*).
[3]Mutated in 73–90% of MSI colon cancers. Up to 55% of MSS colon cancer cell lines may demonstrate a TGF-β signaling blockage distal to TGF-β1 RII.

and eventual carcinogenesis. Mutations of the K-*ras* gene, for example, can be found in approximately 50% of sporadic colon cancers.

Allelic losses in chromosomes 5q, 18q, and 17p are commonly found in colorectal cancers (Table 26–2). Originally described in association with familial adenomatous polyposis, alterations of the *APC* (adenomatous polyposis coli) gene on chromosome 5 can be found in at least 70% of sporadic adenomas, indicating that this is an early event in colonic carcinogenesis. APC is important in modulating extracellular signals that are transmitted to the nucleus through the cytoskeletal protein β-catenin. It is a tumor suppressor gene that binds to this protein and causes its degradation. Loss of APC, therefore, leads to

accumulation of β-catenin, which is translocated to the nucleus where it binds to transcription factors affecting cell cycling and growth. APC abnormalities may also lead to disruption of normal cell-to-cell adhesion through altered association with the cellular adhesion molecule E-cadherin. Other genetic changes occur later in the adenoma-to-carcinoma sequence. Tumor progression is associated in more than 75% of cases with loss of tumor suppressor activity located on chromosome 18q. The *DCC* (deleted in colon cancer) gene, found on chromosome 18q, was originally thought to be important because its loss from colon cancers is associated with a worse prognosis. Recent studies have questioned its role as an important tumor suppressor gene. *DPC4* (also known as

Figure 26–1. Scheme of current concepts of the environmental causation of colon cancer, based on epidemiologic considerations and experimental models of carcinogenesis. Many of the relationships depicted remain speculative. [Reproduced, with permission, from Bresalier RS, Kim YS: Malignant neoplasms of the large intestine. In: *Gastrointestinal Disease,* 5th ed. Sleisenger MH, Fordtran JS (editors). Saunders, 1993.]

SMAD4) is another candidate gene located on chromosome 18 whose inactivation may play a role in the development of colorectal cancer. This molecule is involved in cell signaling pathways activated through the transforming growth factor-β (TGF-β) family receptors. Mutations in *SMAD4* and a related gene *SMAD2* have been reported in some colorectal cancers. Deletions of chromosome 17p, present in approximately 75% of colorectal cancers, involve the *p53* gene, which normally prevents cells with damaged DNA from progressing beyond the G₁–S boundary in the cell cycle. This is a late, important event in colonic carcinogenesis.

Genes designated *hMSH2* and *hMLH1* play a role in repairing base pair mismatches occurring during DNA replication. Alterations in these genes (and in related genes, *hPMS1* and *hPMS2*, *hMSH3* and *hMSH6*) lead to DNA replication errors and increased mutation. Microsatellite instability (MSI) involves mutations or instability in short repeated DNA sequences. Affected DNA sequences are found in several key genes that are important in maintaining normal cellular function such as the receptor for transforming growth factor-b (TGF-bRII). The TGF-b pathway is an important tumor-suppressing pathway, and alterations in this pathway lead to tumor development. Alterations in mismatch repair genes play a major role in hereditary nonpolyposis colorectal cancers, but similar alterations may be found in approximately 15% of sporadic cancers.

Colorectal cancers thus arise as the result of complex interactions between hereditary and environmental factors. A proposed sequence of genetic events is outlined in Figure 26–2. Cancers develop from an accumulation of events in a multistep process.

Progression of Dysplasia to Carcinoma

Colorectal cancers do not arise *de novo*, rather the colonic mucosa progresses through a sequence of morphologic events that eventually culminates in invasive carcinoma. **Dysplasia** refers to abnormalities in crypt

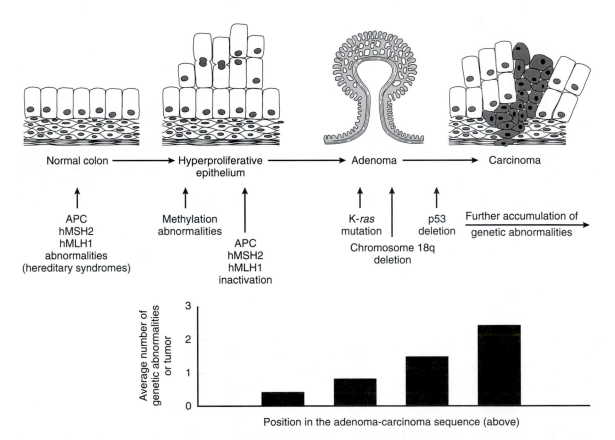

Figure 26–2. Proposed sequence of molecular genetic events occurring during the evolution of colorectal cancer. [Modified, with permission, from Bresalier RS, Toribara NW: Familial colon cancer. In: *Premalignant Conditions of the Gastrointestinal Tract.* Eastwood GL (editor). Elsevier, 1990.]

architecture (ie, reduced number, irregular branching, crowding resulting in a "back-to-back" appearance) and cytologic detail (ie, enlarged, hyperchromatic nuclei with multiple mitoses and pseudostratification) (Figure 26–3). In nearly all cases, dysplasia is manifested in macroscopic adenomatous polyps. Sometimes, as in ulcerative colitis, dysplasia may occur as a microscopic lesion in the mucosa (see the discussion following).

Risk Factors for Development of Colorectal Cancer

A. Age

Colorectal cancer is predominantly a disease of older age groups. Ninety percent of cancers occur in persons over 50 years of age, with the peak incidence in the seventh decade (Figure 26–4). A person who is 50 years of age has an approximately 5% chance of developing colorectal cancer by age 80 years, and a 2.5% risk of dying from the disease. Although the risk of developing colorectal cancer rises sharply after age 50 years in the general population, these cancers also occur in younger individuals, especially those with a family history of the disease (see the discussion following).

B. Adenomatous Polyps

The vast majority of colorectal cancers in the general population arise in adenomatous polyps. These are macroscopic lesions made up of dysplastic epithelium. They may be pedunculated, attached to the colonic wall through a fibrovascular stalk (Figure 26–5), or sessile with a broad base attachment. Tubular adenomas are characterized by a complex network of branching adenomatous glands (Figure 26–6A). Villous adenomas have glands extending straight down from the surface toward the base of the polyp (Figure 26–6B). Many polyps are tubulovillous adenomas, having characteristics of both types (Figure 26–6C). All adenomas by definition contain dysplastic epithelium. These are benign neoplasms that have the potential for malignant degeneration. The risk of evolution from adenoma to carcinoma is related to polyp size and histologic characteristics (Figure 26–7). Large polyps and those with a higher proportion of villous architecture are more likely to contain carcinoma. Likewise, polyps containing higher degrees of architectural distortion and cellular atypia (moderate to severe dysplasia) will more often contain coincident cancer. These features are interdependent. Large polyps often have higher degrees of villous architecture and dysplasia.

Adenomatous polyps are associated with abnormal cellular proliferation. In the normal colon, DNA synthesis and cellular proliferation occur only in the lower and middle regions of the crypt. Cells that have migrated to the upper crypt become terminally differentiated and can no longer divide. Disordered proliferative activity is characteristic of adenomas and a hallmark of neoplasia. Abnormal proliferation can be detected even in the normal-appearing mucosa of some individuals at especially high risk for cancer development (eg, members of kindreds with familial adenomatous polyposis, and nonpolyposis hereditary colorectal cancer). These abnormalities may be associated with alterations in biochemical markers of cellular proliferation such as ornithine decarboxylase and protein kinase C activity, and molecular markers such as *APC* gene inactivation and K-*ras* protooncogene mutations. Clinical studies suggest that the evolution of colon cancer may take as

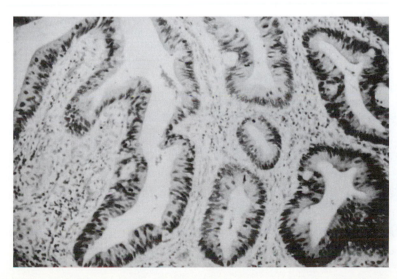

Figure 26–3. Dysplastic changes in the colonic mucosa are precursors to the development of invasive cancer. Glands are branched, irregular, and crowded together. Nuclei are hyperchromatic and do not line up on the basement membrane but are arranged in pseudopalisades (pseudostratification). Adenomatous polyps by definition contain dysplastic changes.

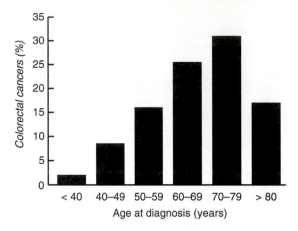

Figure 26–4. Colorectal cancer incidence by age at diagnosis, based on the United States population.

long as a decade, and as much as 5 years for progression from recognizable adenoma to invasive carcinoma. This has implications for screening, as will be discussed in later sections.

Several pieces of evidence support the view that colonic adenomas are the precursors to carcinoma. The epidemiologic description of colonic adenomas parallels that of carcinomas. Adenomatous polyps are rare in geographic regions with low colon cancer prevalence, and the distribution of adenomas in different segments of the colon mimics that of carcinomas. Adenomas often occur in anatomic proximity to colon cancers **(sentinel polyps),** and cancer risk is proportional to the number of adenomas present synchronously (at the same time)

or metachronously (at different times) in the colon. Cancer is often present in polyps removed endoscopically or surgically, and the risk of cancer is proportional to the degree of dysplasia in the polyp. Most importantly, several clinical studies now indicate that removal of adenomatous polyps in the context of surveillance sigmoidoscopy or colonoscopy decreases the risk of death from colon cancer.

C. FAMILY HISTORY

1. Sporadic cancer—It has become increasingly clear that there exists an inherited susceptibility to the development of colon cancer. This is true not only of well-defined hereditary syndromes such as familial adenomatous polyposis and hereditary nonpolyposis colorectal cancer, but also of so-called sporadic, or common, colorectal cancers. Cancer incidence and mortality studies suggest that the incidence of colon cancer in first-degree relatives of those with the disease is two to three times higher than that of the general population. This is echoed by more recent case-control and prospective family analyses, which demonstrated a risk 1.8 times higher for those with one affected relative, and 2.75–5.7 times higher for those with two affected relatives. The risk is greater if an affected relative has cancer diagnosed before age 45 years. Similar trends have been demonstrated for adenomatous polyps.

2. Familial adenomatous polyposis (FAP)—Familial adenomatous polyposis is inherited in an autosomal dominant fashion, with inactivation of the *APC* gene located on chromosome 5q. This syndrome have served as a model for the study of the sequence of events in which adenoma develops into carcinoma in the large bowel. Hundreds to thousands of adenomatous polyps

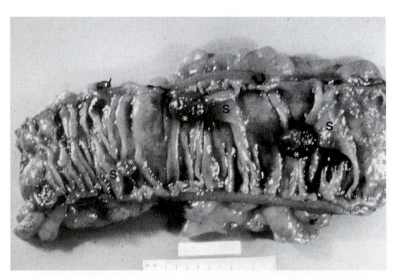

Figure 26–5. Colectomy specimen containing multiple pedunculated polyps *(asterisks).* S, polyp stalk.

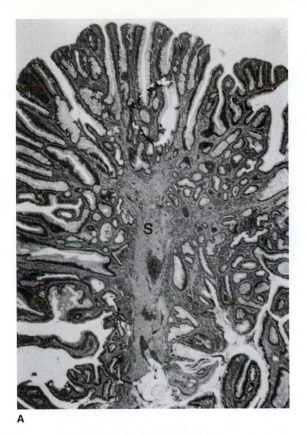

A

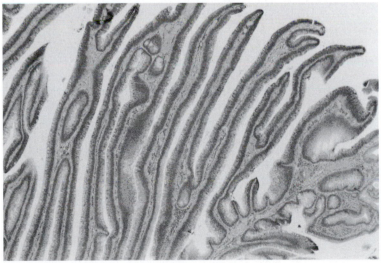

B

Figure 26–6. Adenomatous polyps contain various degrees of tubular and villous components. **A:** Tubular adenomas are characterized by a complex network of branching glands. S, stalk. **B:** Villous adenomas contain adenomatous glands that extend straight down from the surface to the center of the polyp.

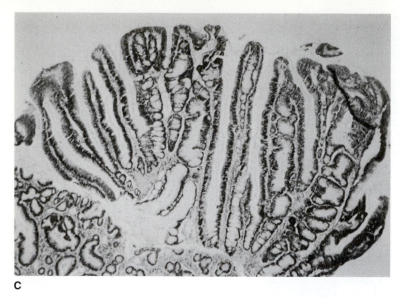

Figure 26–6. C: Many adenomas are mixed villotubular adenomas.

progressively develop in the colon and rectum of affected individuals (Figure 26–8). Polyps often begin to appear by 15–20 years of age. If the colon is not removed, cancer development is inevitable, usually within a decade of the appearance of adenomas. Histologic examination reveals numerous microadenomas, which may not yet be evident on gross examination. Hyperproliferation of the colonic mucosa can be detected by labeling with tritiated thymidine and as an increase in

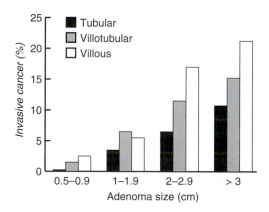

Figure 26–7. The risk that an adenoma will evolve into carcinoma is related to polyp size and histologic characteristics. Shown here is the percentage of adenomas containing invasive cancer by size and histologic findings, based on an analysis of 7000 endoscopically removed polyps.

the polyamine biosynthetic enzyme ornithine decarboxylase. Abnormalities can be detected on *in vitro* studies of skin fibroblasts, including abnormal responses to tumor promoters. Importantly, it is now possible to detect at-risk individuals in kindreds of familial adenomatous polyposis patients by means of practical, sensitive assays, which detect truncated *APC* gene products in patients who will manifest the disease (ie, molecular diagnosis). Once at-risk individuals develop adenomas, colectomy should be performed. Subtotal colectomy with ileorectal anastomosis, combined with frequent endoscopic surveillance plus medical management with NSAIDs, has been advocated by some, but the possibility of subsequent development of rectal cancer exists (see section on "Treatment").

Extracolonic manifestations occur in patients with FAP in conjunction with polyposis. Although the association of colonic polyposis with extracolonic manifestations was originally termed Gardner's syndrome, it is now recognized as a variant of FAP. The small intestine as well as the colon is at risk for neoplastic growth. Duodenal adenomas occur, and the periampullary region is especially susceptible to neoplastic degeneration. Extracolonic manifestations include osteomas of the mandible, skull, and long bones (Figure 26–9), epidermoid cysts, fibromas, lipomas, mesenteric fibromatosis, and desmoid tumors. Fundic gland hyperplasia of the stomach is common. Congenital hypertrophy of the retinal pigmented epithelium occurs in over 90% of patients with extracolonic manifestations of FAP.

3. Hereditary nonpolyposis colorectal cancer— Hereditary nonpolyposis colorectal cancer (**Lynch syn-**

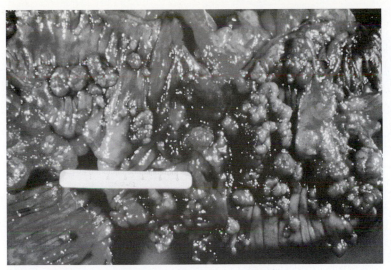

A

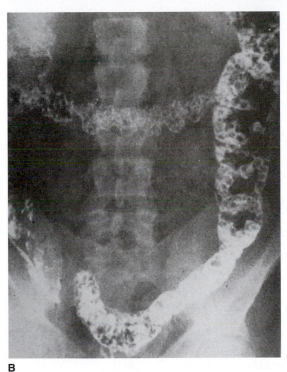

B

Figure 26–8. **A:** Colectomy specimen from a patient with familial adenomatous polyposis. Hundreds of polyps of varying size can be seen arising from the colonic mucosa. **B:** Barium enema study in a patient with familial adenomatous polyposis. Numerous filling defects represent polyps throughout the colon.

drome) is a disease of autosomal dominant inheritance in which colon cancers arise in discrete adenomas, but polyposis (ie, hundreds of polyps) does not occur. Table 26–3 lists the criteria for this disease, as defined by the International Collaborative Group on Hereditary Nonpolyposis Colorectal Cancer. Families must have at least three relatives with colorectal cancer, one

of whom is a first-degree relative of the other two (FAP excluded). Colorectal cancer must involve at least two generations, and at least one case must occur before age 50 years. Clinical features of cancers arising in hereditary nonpolyposis colorectal cancer are compared with those of sporadic cancer in Table 26–4. Cancers arising in hereditary nonpolyposis colorectal cancer occur at an

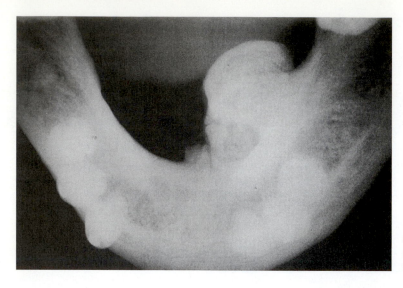

Figure 26–9. Radiograph demonstrating mandibular osteoma in a patient with Gardner's syndrome.

earlier age (age 40–50 years), are often proximal in location and multiple, and are more commonly mucinous or poorly differentiated. Patients with hereditary nonpolyposis colorectal cancer (HNPCC) are prone to develop cancers of the female genital tract (eg, ovary, endometrium) and other sites in addition to the colon. This has led to the development of broader clinical criteria for HNPCC. Colon cancers sometimes arise in flat, slightly raised lesions in the proximal colon, with foci of adenomatous change confined to the upper crypt ("flat" adenomas). People who develop colorectal cancer in the setting of HNPCC may have a better prognosis than individuals with sporadic colorectal cancers. Hereditary nonpolyposis colorectal cancer appears to account for at least 4–6% of colorectal cancers in the population. Genes that play a role in DNA repair are altered in this type of cancer. Loss of the *hMSH2* and *hMLH1* genes (additional genes, *hPMS1* and *hPMS2* and *hMSH6,* may also be involved) leads to increased susceptibility to mutation from failure to repair base pair mismatches. This is manifested in DNA replication errors (microsatellite instability), whose detection may eventually be important in clinical screening.

Table 26–3. Hereditary nonpolyposis colorectal cancer.

Three or more relatives with colorectal cancer (one must be a first-degree relative of the other two)
Colorectal cancer involving at least two generations
One or more colorectal cancer cases before age 50 years

4. Other hereditary syndromes

a. Peutz-Jeghers syndrome—Peutz-Jeghers syndrome (mucocutaneous pigmentation and hamartomas of the gastrointestinal tract) has been associated with an increased risk of large and small bowel cancer. Scattered adenomas may coexist with nonneoplastic hamartomas. Peutz-Jeghers syndrome is an autosomal dominant disease, which in most families has been mapped to chromosome 19 p13.3 and the *STK11* gene. Extracolonic cancers may occur in 15% of individuals with this syndrome.

Table 26–4. Clinical features of herediatary nonpolyposis colorectal cancer and sporadic colon cancer.

	Hereditary Nonpolyposis Colorectal Cancer	Sporadic Cancer
Mean age at diagnosis	44.6 years	67 years
Multiple colon cancers	34.5%	4–11%
Synchronous	18.1%	3–6%
Metachronous	24.3%	1–5%
Proximal location	72.3%	35%
Excess malignant tumors at other sites	Yes	No
Mucinous and poorly differentiated cancers	Common	Infrequent
Microsatellite instability	79%	17%
Prognosis	Favorable	Variable

b. Familial juvenile polyposis syndrome (JPS)— Familial juvenile polyposis is a rare autosomal dominant disease that may be associated with polyps limited to the colon, limited to the stomach, or throughout the gastrointestinal tract. Individuals with JPS develop juvenile hamartomatous polyps and gastrointestinal cancer, with a 15% incidence of colorectal cancer in young patients and a 68% incidence by age 60. Mixed juvenile and adenomatous polyps may occur. This syndrome has been associated with alterations in several different genes including *SMAD4* on chromosome 18 and *PTEN* on chromosome 10.

c. Torres's syndrome (Muir's syndrome)— Torres's syndrome is a variant of hereditary nonpolyposis colorectal cancer in which adenomas of the colon occur in conjunction with multiple skin lesions (eg, sebaceous adenomas and carcinomas, basal cell and squamous cell carcinomas, keratoacanthomas).

d. Turcot's syndrome— Turcot's syndrome is defined by a combination of inherited adenomatous polyposis and malignant brain tumors. Families have been described with germline mutations in the *APC* gene, or mutations in *hMLH1* and *hPMS2* characteristic of HNPCC. Inheritance is autosomal dominant.

D. INFLAMMATORY BOWEL DISEASE

1. Ulcerative colitis—Patients with inflammatory bowel disease are at increased risk for developing colorectal carcinoma; this is best documented in idiopathic ulcerative colitis. The risk of cancer correlates most closely with the duration of the colitis; the risk is lowest in patients who have had the disease for less than 7–10 years and rises 0.5–1% for each additional year of disease. Cancer risk is greatest in those who have pancolitis involving the entire bowel, but those with left-sided colitis (distal to the splenic flexure) are also at risk. Cancer develops in dysplastic epithelium. Unlike the general population, in which dysplasia occurs in adenomatous polyps, dysplasia associated with ulcerative colitis often occurs in flat mucosa. The risk of cancer is highest when dysplasia arises in visible plaques or masses (dysplasia-associated mass lesion). Dysplasia in ulcerative colitis is divided into low-grade and high-grade categories. The presence of high-grade dysplasia is associated with a significant risk of synchronous cancer or subsequent cancer development. Colonoscopic screening programs are therefore aimed at identifying dysplasia through multiple biopsies of the colonic mucosa. If high-grade dysplasia is detected or dysplasia occurs in a macroscopic lesion (ie, dysplasia-associated mass lesion), total colectomy is advised. Although the significance of low-grade dysplasia is less clear, its presence mandates frequent surveillance.

2. Crohn's disease—An increased risk for development of colorectal cancer has been reported in the setting of Crohn's disease. The exact risk of cancer in Crohn's disease patients remains unclear, but as in ulcerative colitis, dysplasia appears in diseased segments and its presence correlates with duration of disease.

Pathologic Findings

A. GROSS FEATURES

Colorectal cancers most often present as mass lesions. Carcinomas of the cecum and ascending colon are often polypoid and may become large and bulky prior to presentation because of the larger circumference of the right colon. Bulky mass lesions occur elsewhere in the colon as well. In the distal colon and rectum, where the bowel circumference is smaller, tumors may involve the entire circumference of the bowel to produce an annular constricting ("napkin ring") lesion, which may obstruct the lumen (Figure 26–10). Cancers occasionally have a flatter appearance, spreading intramurally. This feature is more common in the setting of inflammatory bowel disease. As tumors expand, they outgrow their blood supply, undergo necrosis, and ulcerate. This is a common feature of larger cancers.

B. MICROSCOPIC FEATURES

Carcinomas of the colon and rectum are adenocarcinomas that form glandular structures of varying degrees of differentiation. Most are moderately well to well differentiated in appearance (Figure 26–11) and secrete variable amounts of mucin. In poorly differentiated tumors, gland formation is less prominent or absent. Mucinous or colloid cancers contain scattered collections of tumor cells floating in "lakes" of mucin, whereas signet-ring cell carcinomas contain cells in which large vacuoles of mucin displace the nuclei. Poorly differentiated, colloid, and signet-ring cell carcinomas tend to have a poorer prognosis than well-differentiated cancers. Although it is convenient to categorize tumors in this fashion, most cancers are actually heterogeneous in their microscopic appearance, and may contain multiple populations of cells (Figure 26–12). Other pathologic features, such as venous, lymphatic, or neural invasion, may also affect the prognosis (see the discussion following). Tumors that are not adenocarcinomas represent less than 5% of malignant tumors in the large intestine. Primary lymphomas and carcinoid tumors together make up less than 0.1% of colorectal neoplasms. Other rare tumors include squamous cell, cloacogenic, and transitional cell carcinomas and melanocarcinomas at the anorectal junction.

Tumor Progression, Natural History, & Staging

Colorectal cancers evolve over long periods of time, beginning as intraepithelial lesions arising in dysplastic or

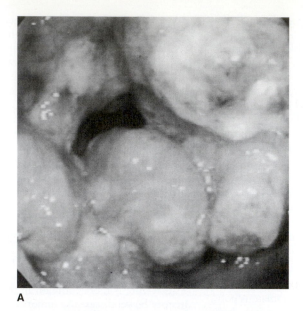

A

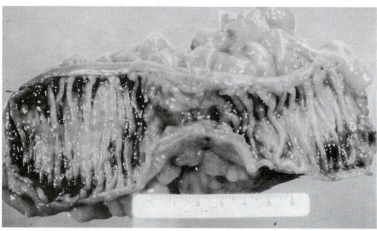

B

Figure 26–10. Obstructing carcinomas of the sigmoid colon. **A:** Endoscopic view showing bulky tumor mass nearly obstructing the lumen. **B:** Resected surgical specimen showing circumferential constricting lesion.

adenomatous tissue. Microscopic analyses of biopsy or surgical specimens have demonstrated adenomatous change in even single glands. In most cases, the growth of adenomatous epithelium gives rise to macroscopic polyps. Further evolution is associated with increasing degrees of cellular atypia and glandular disorganization, eventuating in intraepithelial carcinoma (carcinoma *in situ*). Further growth leads to invasion of the muscularis mucosa and eventual penetration of the bowel wall. Invasion of lymphatic and vascular structures gives rise to regional lymph node and distant metastases. This process occurs over a period of years. Approximations based on clinical observations indicate that it may take as long as a decade for the initial molecular changes to become inva-

sive carcinoma, and half that time for adenoma to become carcinoma. Patterns of spread of the tumor depend to some extent on its location. Rectal cancers tend to spread locally to involve lymph nodes and adjacent structures, whereas colon cancer spreads to regional lymph nodes and more distant sites (eg, liver, lung). Metastasis is a complex multistep process involving numerous biologic events (Figure 26–13). The long natural history of cancer evolution in the colon and rectum has significant implications for screening and diagnosis, and affects the ability to improve survival rates and achieve cure (see the discussion of diagnosis following).

Staging systems for colorectal cancer are based on the assumption that invasion and metastasis of colorec-

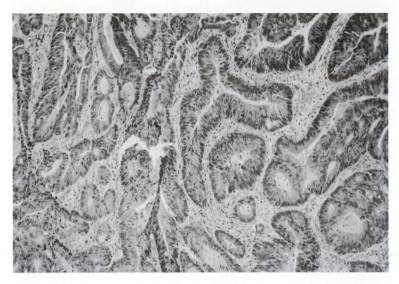

Figure 26–11. Photomicrograph of a well-differentiated adenocarcinoma of the colon.

tal neoplasms occur as an orderly progression. Clinical and pathologic correlations confirm that the prognosis depends on the depth of bowel wall invasion at the time of diagnosis. Lymph node involvement is associated with further decreased survival rates, whereas distant metastases are associated with the worst prognosis of all (see section on "Prognosis"). The two major staging systems used are modifications of the Dukes' classification (Table 26–5) and the TNM classification of the American Joint Committee on Cancer Staging for Colorectal Cancer (Table 26–6).

CLINICAL FINDINGS

Symptoms & Signs

Adenocarcinomas of the colon and rectum grow slowly and remain asymptomatic for long periods of time. When symptoms do occur, they depend to some degree on the location of the tumor in the large intestine. Cancers of the proximal colon and cecum usually attain a large size before becoming symptomatic because of the diameter of the bowel in this region. It is common for

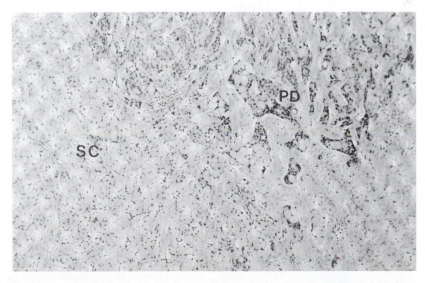

Figure 26–12. Photomicrograph of colonic carcinoma demonstrating heterogeneity in histologic morphologic study. This tumor contains areas of signet-ring cell (SC) as well as poorly differentiated (PD) carcinoma.

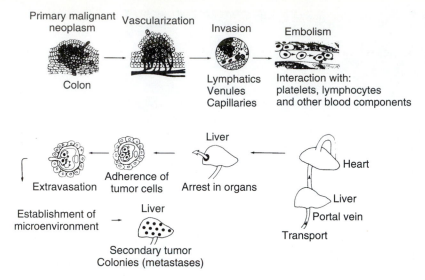

Figure 26–13. Metastasis is a multistep process involving numerous biologic events.

such right-sided cancers to present with microcytic anemia secondary to chronic blood loss.

Constitutional symptoms resulting from anemia may be the first indication of a problem when elderly patients present with fatigue, shortness of breath, or even angina. Occasionally, more acute bleeding results in the presentation of dark red blood admixed with stool. Vague abdominal discomfort or even a palpable mass may be late findings. Cancers of the descending and sigmoid colon often involve the bowel circumferentially. As they grow into the lumen, patients present with obstructive symptoms such as cramping, abdominal pain, or a change in bowel habits. Constipation may alternate with postobstructive diarrhea as stool moves beyond the obstructing lesion. Rectal cancers often present with hematochezia (red blood per rectum) or obstruction. These tumors may invade locally to involve surrounding structures such as the bladder or female genital tract. Pain due to involvement of the sacral plexus is a late occurrence.

Diagnostic Studies

A. DIAGNOSTIC PROCEDURE IN SYMPTOMATIC PATIENTS

When the presence of colorectal cancer is suggested by clinical signs and symptoms such as microcytic anemia, hematochezia, abdominal pain, weight loss, or change in bowel habits (see preceding section, "Symptoms & Signs"), prompt diagnostic evaluation should be undertaken endoscopically or radiographically (Figure

26–14). The finding of occult blood in the stool heightens the suspicion that neoplasia may be present, but its absence does not rule out a significant lesion and should not deter evaluation when cancer is suspected.

1. Colonoscopy—Colonoscopy is the most accurate means of evaluating the colonic mucosa, and allows biopsy of suspicious lesions. Colonoscopes have flexible shafts that accommodate the curves of the colon, high-resolution optics with magnification at close range, and instrument and suction channels that allow washing, mucosal biopsy, and electrocauterization. Video imaging and instant printing make a permanent record available. Complete examination of the colon to the cecum can be accomplished in over 95% of patients. The potential discomfort of the procedure is somewhat dependent on the operator, but in most cases the procedure can be comfortably performed with modest intravenous conscious sedation. Although the risk of colonic perforation or bleeding exists, complication rates for diagnostic procedures are less than 0.5%. The combined diagnostic accuracy is 90–95% for detecting polypoid lesions. Small polyps located behind folds, intramucosal lesions in the setting of ulcerative colitis, and abnormalities present in areas of extensive diverticulosis, stricture, or spasm account for missed lesions. Colonoscopy is approximately 12% more accurate than air contrast barium enema, especially in detecting small lesions such as adenomas (studies claim both lower and higher rates). The cost of the examination is an important issue, especially in reference to the value of screening examinations (see the discussion following). Colonoscopy is

Table 26–5. Dukes classification for carcinoma of the rectum and its modifications for colorectal carcinoma.

Stage	Dukes, 1932 (Rectum)	Gabriel, Dukes, Bussey, 1935 (Rectum)	Kirklin et al, 1949 (Rectum and Sigmoid)	Astler-Coller, 1954 (Rectum and Colon)	Turnbull et al, 1967 (Colon)	Modified Astler-Coller (Gunderson & Sosin, 1974) (Rectum and Colon)	GITSG, 1975 (Rectum and Colon)
A	Limited to bowel wall	Limited to bowel wall	Limited to mucosa	Limited to mucosa	Limited to mucosa	Limited to mucosa	Limited to mucosa
B	Through bowel wall	Through bowel wall	—	—	Tumor extension into pericolic fat	—	—
B1	—	—	Into muscularis propria	Into muscularis propria	—	Into muscularis propria	Into muscularis propria
B2	—	—	Through muscularis propria	Through muscularis propria (and serosa)	—	Through serosa (m = microscopic, m + g = gross)	Through serosa
B3	—	—	—	—	—	Adherent to or invading adjacent structures	—
C	Regional nodal metastases	—	Regional nodal metastases	—	Regional nodal metastases	—	—
C1	—	Regional nodal metastases near primary lesion	—	Same as B1 plus regional nodal metastases	—	Same as B1 plus regional nodal metastases	One to four regional nodes positive
C2	—	Proximal node involved at point of ligation	—	Same as B2 plus regional nodal metastases	—	Same as B2 plus regional nodal metastases	More than four regional nodes positive
C3	—	—	—	—	—	Same as B3 plus regional nodal metastases	—
D	—	—	—	—	Distant metastases (liver, lung, bone) or due to parietal or adjacent organ invasion	—	—

Reproduced, with permission, from Bresalier RS, Kim YS: Malignant neoplasms of the large intestine. In: *Gastrointestinal Disease*, 6th ed. Sleisenger MH, Fordtran JS (editors). Saunders, 2001.

Table 26–6. Staging of colorectal cancer by the American Joint Committee on Cancer (TNM classification).[1]

Stage 0	Carcinoma *in situ* Tis N0 M0
Stage I	Tumor invades submucosa T1 N0 M0
Stage II	Tumor invades through muscularis propria into subserosa, or into nonperitonealized pericolic or perirectal tissues T3 N0 M0
	Tumor perforates the visceral peritoneum or directly invades other organs or structures T4 N0 M0
Stage III	Any degree of bowel wall perforation with regional hymph node metastasis
	N1 1–3 pericolic or perirectal lymph nodes involved
	N2 4 or more pericolic or perirectal lymph nodes involved
	N3 Metastasis in any lymph node along a named vascular trunk
	Any T N1 M0
	Any T N2, N3 M0
Stage IV	Any invasion of bowel wall with or without lymph node metastasis, but with evidence of distant metastasis
	Any T Any N M1

[1]Based on American Joint Committee on Cancer Staging for Colorectal Cancer (5th ed). Lippincott, 1997. Dukes B (Corresponds to stage II) is a composite of better (T3, N0, M0) and worse (T4, N0, M0) prognostic groups, as is Dukes C (corresponds to stage III) (any T, N1, M0) and (any T, N2, N3, M0).

most accurate and highly cost effective in the evaluation of symptomatic patients, however.

2. Barium enema examination—Air contrast barium enema is an alternative to colonoscopy, but may miss small lesions. Nonetheless, if colonoscopy is unavailable, technically difficult, or refused by the patient, this examination is still highly accurate in detecting carcinomas and larger adenomas. Barium enema may also be effective in visualizing areas beyond strictures not accessible to the colonoscope. Full column barium enemas detect most large mass lesions, but are less accurate than air contrast examinations for detecting smaller lesions. Distal lesions, especially those in the rectum, are sometimes difficult to detect radiographically, and flexible fiberoptic sigmoidoscopy with retroflexion should complement the barium enema.

B. Screening Procedures in Asymptomatic Patients

Because colorectal cancer is curable if detected at an early stage, screening for preneoplastic adenomas and early cancers has received a great deal of attention. Screening pertains to detection in large asymptomatic populations. Screening in the general population has concentrated on fecal occult blood testing (FOBT) and sigmoidoscopy. For greater flexibility in achieving better compliance with screening, several major societies have recently offered a broader set of screening choices for different levels of colon cancer risk. Screening options for average-risk individuals include FOBT annually, flexible sigmoidoscopy every 5 years, annual FOBT plus flexible sigmoidoscopy every 5 years (preferred to either alone), double contrast barium enema every 5 years, or colonoscopy every 10 years (Table 26–7). It has been known for some time that colorectal cancer screening with these modalities can detect early cancers. Importantly, recent studies now confirm improved survival rates in patients in colorectal cancer screening programs.

1. Fecal occult blood testing—Annual fecal occult blood testing in persons over 50 years of age has been recommended for several years by numerous societies and organizations. Standardized slide tests, such as Hemocult II, employ guaiac-impregnated paper. In the presence of the pseudoperoxidase activity of hemoglobin (blood) and hydrogen peroxide (supplied in the developing solution), the colorless phenolic guaiac is converted to a blue-pigmented quinone that is visually apparent. Adequate performance of the examination (Table 26–8) requires that the patient avoid red meat and peroxidase-rich foods for 3 days before the test to prevent false-positive results, and that two samples from each of three consecutive stools be supplied. Slides should be developed within 4–6 days, since low levels of peroxidase activity may be degraded by fecal bacteria. Although adding a drop of water to the slide (rehydration) increases sensitivity and has been utilized in some screening trials, this is usually not recommended because of the excess cost of evaluating false-positive tests. Immunologic tests for fecal occult blood that are more specific for human hemoglobin have recently become available, and have demonstrated a high degree of sensitivity and specificity for detecting colonic lesions in preliminary trials.

Five major controlled trials have examined the potential benefit of fecal occult blood testing in screening asymptomatic individuals for colorectal neoplasms (Table 26–9). Compliance in these studies ranged from 50% in a clinical practice setting to 75% at a tertiary care center. Positive tests were obtained in approximately 2% of individuals. This was remarkably similar in all studies. The predictive value of a positive test (the proportion of positive results in persons who actually have the disease) for colonic neoplasms (adenomas plus carcinomas) ranged from 22 to 58%, whereas the predictive value for carcinomas was much lower, ranging from 5.6 to 18% for unrehydrated slides. In all five

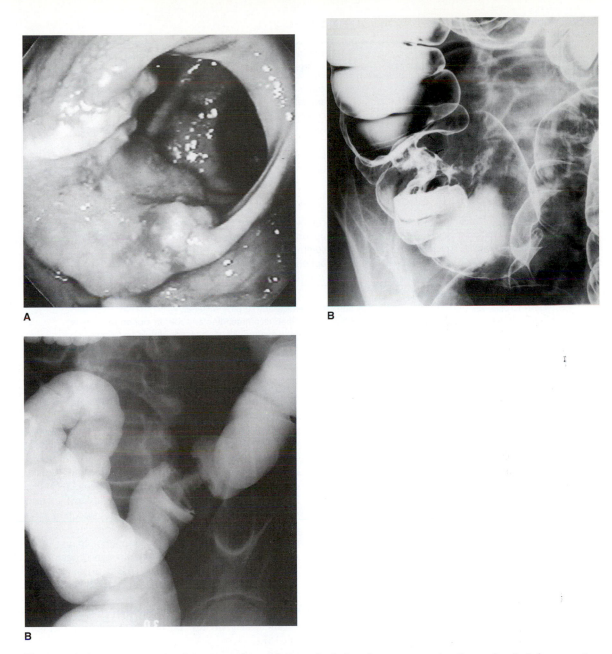

Figure 26–14. Modalities for detecting colorectal cancer include colonoscopy and radiography. **A:** Colonoscopic view of cancer of the ascending colon. Cancer is seen infiltrating a colonic fold and growing semicircumferentially and into the lumen. **B:** Air contrast barium enema demonstrating cancer similar to that seen in **A. C:** Constricting "apple core" lesion of the left colon seen on full column barium enema.

Table 26–7. Average-risk screening guidelines.

Screening Tool	USPSTF[1]	Multidisciplinary Expert Panel[2]	American Cancer Society[3]
FOBT[4]	Recommended annually	Recommended annually	Recommended annually as an option
Flexible sigmoidoscopy	Recommended "periodicity unspecified"	Recommended every 5 years	Recommended every 5 years as an option
FOBT + flexible sigmoidoscopy	Recommended as an option	Recommended as an option	Annual FOBT plus flexible sigmoido-scopy every 5 years recommended as an option
Colonoscopy	Insufficient evidence	Recommended as an option every 10 years	Recommended as an option every 10 years
Double-contrast barium enema	Insufficient evidence	Recommended as an option every 5–10 years	Recommended as an option every 5 years

[1]U.S. Preventative Services Task Force.
[2]Gastroenterology 1997;112:594. Endorsed by numerous medical and surgical societies.
[3]Updated guidelines 2001 provide menu of options rather than recommending any specific option to increase compliance with screening. FOBT should use take home sample method. All positive tests should be followed up with colonoscopy.
[4]FOBT, fecal occult blood testing.

trials, cancers at an earlier stage of development (Dukes' A and B cancers) were found in the screened group compared with those in the control group. Four of the trials have now demonstrated significant reductions in colorectal cancer-related mortality associated with FOBT. One study demonstrated that annual fecal occult blood testing decreased the 18-year cumulative mortality rate from colorectal cancer by 33%, with a 21% reduction for biennial testing.

Table 26–8. Performance of the slide guaiac test for fecal occult blood.

1. For 3 days prior to and during testing, patients should avoid
   a. Rare red meat
   b. Peroxidase-containing vegetables and fruits (eg, broccoli, turnips, cantaloupe, cauliflower, radishes)
   c. The following medications:
      Vitamin C (antioxidant)
      Aspirin
      NSAIDs
2. Two samples of each of three consecutive stools should be tested (it is proper to sample areas of obvious blood)
3. Slides should be developed within 4–6 days
4. Slides should not be rehydrated prior to developing (for average-risk screening)

2. Sigmoidoscopy—Routine proctosigmoidoscopy and removal of adenomatous polyps detected by this method can reduce the incidence and mortality rates due to colorectal cancers found within reach of the sigmoidoscope by as much as 70%. The 60-cm flexible sigmoidoscope has supplanted the rigid scope, because it causes less discomfort to the patient, visualizes at least 2.5 times more surface area, and detects two to three times more adenomas. Flexible sigmoidoscopy can be learned by paramedical personnel, and has been successfully used in screening programs employing nurse-practitioners. Current recommendations suggest that screening flexible sigmoidoscopy be performed every 5 years in asymptomatic individuals over 50 years of age. This should be combined with yearly fecal occult blood testing, since only half of carcinomas will be found within reach of the flexible sigmoidoscope (Figure 26–15).

3. Colonoscopy—Colonoscopy may be the most effective screening tool for detecting adenomatous polyps and colorectal cancers, but data from prospective randomized trials are lacking. Data from the National Polyp Study strongly suggest a reduction in colorectal cancer mortality as the result of removing adenomatous polyps found at colonoscopy. Recent trials suggest that sigmoidoscopy alone or sigmoidoscopy combined with FOBT may miss a large number of advanced proximal

Table 26–9. Controlled trials of fecal occult blood testing in screening asymptomatic persons for colorectal cancer.

Site	Cohort	Screening Interval	Rehydrated	Positive Predictive Value Cancer	Mortality Reduction
New York	22,000	—	No	10.7%	43%
Minnesota	46,000	1 and 2 years	Yes (most)	5.6% (unrehydrated) 2.2% (rehydrated)	Annual 33% Biennial 21%
England	152,850	2 years	No	First round 9.9% Second round 11.9%	15%
Sweden	28,000	14–22 months	Yes (most)	First round 5.0% (unrehydrated) Second round 4.2% (rehydrated)	No yet available
Denmark	61,933	2 years	No	First round 17.7% Second round 8.4%	18%

neoplasms (large adenoma, adenoma with villous features or dysplasia, cancer) in the proximal colon. Given the need for colonoscopic follow-up should FOBT or sigmoidoscopy be positive, colonoscopy may also be cost effective. The availability of adequate resources including funding and sufficient trained colonoscopists remains an issue with respect to routine use of colonoscopy for colon cancer screening.

4. Air contrast barium enema—Air contrast barium enema has been included as an option for colon cancer screening in a variety of guidelines. Several studies have indicated that the sensitivity of air contrast barium is less than that of colonoscopy, especially for detecting lesions less than 1 cm.

5. Other screening methods—"Virtual colonoscopy" involves the use of helical computed tomography (CT) to generate high-resolution, two-dimensional images of the abdomen and pelvis. Three-dimensional images are then reconstructed by computer. This method has the potential of being a rapid and safe method for evolution of the colon, but low sensitivity and specificity for polyps <1 cm in size and the need for special equipment currently limit its usefulness. Detection of shed cancer cells by cytometry, biochemical and immunologic detection of fecal cancer-associated antigens, and detection of mutated protooncogenes such as K-*ras* in stool may be possible, but the feasibility of such methods for screening programs remains unproved.

C. LABORATORY FINDINGS

Laboratory findings are most often absent until colorectal cancers are advanced. Microcytic anemia and iron deficiency with low transferring saturation results from chronic blood loss. Abnormalities in liver function tests are rare accompaniments to extensive metastatic disease. Elevated serum levels of tumor-associated glycoprotein antigens such as carcinoembryonic antigen also occur late in the course of disease and have negative prognostic implications. Because mutations in the *APC* gene are germline mutations in patients with familial adenomatous polyposis, these may be detected in at-risk individuals in kindreds through examination of peripheral blood leukocytes (see the discussion following). This is not possible, however, in sporadic colon cancer, where epithelial cell mutations are somatic (acquired). The expression of certain glycoprotein antigens in resected tumors or deletions in tumor suppressor genes such as *DCC* and *p53* have prognostic implications that will be further discussed (see section, "Prognosis").

D. DIAGNOSTIC AND IMAGING STUDIES

The general roles of colonoscopy, flexible sigmoidoscopy, and radiology in diagnosing colorectal cancer in symptomatic patients and in screening asymptomatic

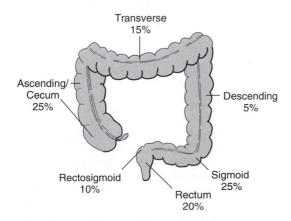

Figure 26–15. Distribution of colorectal cancers within the large intestine. Only half of the cancers are found within reach of the flexible sigmoidoscope.

individuals have been discussed earlier. The specific roles of these modalities in screening patients who are at average or high risk will now be discussed.

1. Individuals with average risk—Because colorectal cancer occurs in an older age group in the general population, individuals over age 50 years should be targeted for screening. This should at present include annual fecal occult blood testing and flexible sigmoidoscopy every 5 years after age 50 years (in keeping with the recommendations of the American Cancer Society and other groups), colonoscopy every 10 years, or air contrast barium enema every 5 years. Colonoscopy has the advantage of examining the entire colon and rectum, and providing the opportunity to biopsy or remove lesions should they be found. The presence of fecal occult blood dictates a diagnostic evaluation. Colonoscopy or air contrast barium enema combined with flexible sigmoidoscopy should be performed in those with positive fecal occult blood tests to rule out colonic lesions. Screening programs should include educational components to heighten the awareness of both patients and physicians as to the frequency and curability of colorectal cancer. Given the high cost of colorectal cancer screening in the general population and the long natural history of the disease, some have advocated the performance of a single barium enema or even colonoscopy at age 50 years, with no further evaluation in asymptomatic individuals with negative examinations. The appropriateness of such an approach has not, however, gained wide acceptance.

2. Patients with a family history of colorectal cancer—The familial pattern of colorectal cancer has already been discussed. Obtaining an accurate family history is an important component of evaluating patients at risk for this disease. Screening procedures are controversial for someone with only one first-degree relative who has had colon cancer. Some experts do not believe that the increased risk (two to three times that of the general population) warrants the added cost of screening modalities beyond those recommended for those with no family history. Others, however, feel that routine colonoscopy every 5–10 years beginning at age 40–45 years is indicated in this group, especially if the index case had colon cancer before age 60 years. When two first-degree relatives have had colon cancer, colonoscopic examination at periodic intervals (eg, every 5 years) is suggested (beginning at age 40 or 10 years younger than that of the youngest affected relative). The effectiveness of such a program remains to be determined. If three or more relatives have had colorectal cancer, a familial syndrome should be suspected.

a. Hereditary nonpolyposis colorectal cancer—Hereditary nonpolyposis colorectal cancer is defined by three relatives with colon cancer (one of whom is a first-degree relative of the other two), colorectal cancer involving at least two generations, and one case of cancer occurring before age 50 years. At present, members of such families should be screened by colonoscopy every 2 years, beginning at age 21 years (or at an age 10 years younger than the youngest case) until age 40, then annually. Counseling to consider genetic testing is recommended.

b. Familial adenomatous polyposis—Family members of kindreds with familial adenomatous polyposis should be screened for colonic polyposis by colonoscopy beginning at puberty. The recent availability of sensitive methods for detecting *APC* gene product abnormalities in at-risk individuals may supplant the need for routine colonoscopy in all family members in the future. Molecular diagnosis should be performed in all family members of kindreds to help determine who is at risk and facilitate genetic counseling.

3. Patients with a history of adenoma—The vast majority of colorectal cancers arise in adenomatous polyps. Substantial clinical evidence indicates that patients who have one adenoma are not only likely to have additional adenomas elsewhere in the colon, but to develop subsequent adenomas in the future (32% at 3 years after initial polypectomy in one study, and 42% in a second study). It is therefore suggested that patients with a history of adenomatous polyps undergo routine surveillance colonoscopy. It has become clear, however, that due to the slow growth of adenomas and their progression to carcinoma, repeat colonoscopy need not be performed at intervals less than every 3 years in patients whose index polyp demonstrates no evidence of high-grade dysplasia or carcinoma. After a normal examination, this interval may be extended to at least 5 years. Patients with multiple adenomas, large adenomas, and adenomas occurring before 60 years of age are more likely to develop recurrent adenomas. Multiplicity, however, seems to be the major risk factor for development of recurrent adenomas with advanced pathologic features (ie, large adenomas and those with high-grade dysplasia or invasive cancer). It should be borne in mind that although most cancers arise in adenomatous polyps, only a small percentage of adenomas will eventually demonstrate malignant degeneration. A case in point is "diminutive polyps" less than 5 mm in size. The chance of these polyps containing cancer and the long-term risk of development of cancer after excision of such polyps are low. Some have therefore advocated that persons whose index polyp is a single tubular adenoma under 1 cm in size with only mild to moderate dysplasia need not be routinely screened for polyp recurrence after a negative follow-up examination at 3 years.

4. Patients with a history of colorectal cancer—
Patients who have had resection of colon cancer for cure require surveillance for two reasons: to detect cancer recurrence and to screen for new metachronous cancers, which occur in 1–5% of patients. Such patients should have colonoscopy within 1 year after surgery and at 3 years to rule out local recurrence. Screening colonoscopy should then be performed every 5 years.

Elevated serum carcinoembryonic antigen levels may signal recurrence and should be measured at regular intervals following surgery. The ideal frequency of such testing is unclear, but one reasonable approach is 2-month intervals for 2 years and then 4-month intervals for an additional 3 years. If levels of carcinoembryonic antigen are elevated, "second-look" operations may improve survival rates in selected persons, and may help identify isolated hepatic metastases that are amenable to surgical resection.

The use of computed tomography (CT) scanning of the pelvis to detect local recurrence of rectal cancer and of the abdomen to detect distant liver metastasis has been suggested by some, but the cost effectiveness of such an approach compared with that of physical examination plus serial carcinoembryonic antigen determinations is unproved.

5. Patients with inflammatory bowel disease

a. Ulcerative colitis—Patients with long-standing ulcerative colitis (>7 years duration) should undergo routine surveillance colonoscopy with serial biopsies of the colonic mucosa, since dysplasia in this setting may occur in flat, normal-appearing mucosa. Biopsy specimens should be taken throughout the colon at 10-cm intervals. Any macroscopic lesion should be biopsied, since dysplasia occurring in polypoid masses or plaques suggests a high likelihood of coincident cancer. Common recommendations as to the interval between examinations vary from yearly to every 3 years. Given that the mucosa in ulcerative colitis must still undergo transition from dysplasia to carcinoma, colonoscopy every 2 years seems reasonable in such patients.

b. Crohn's disease—The need for routine surveillance in Crohn's disease is less clear. Patients undergoing colonoscopy for other reasons should of course have any suspicious lesions and all strictures biopsied. Some agencies recommend routine surveillance similar to that for ulcerative colitis.

DIFFERENTIAL DIAGNOSIS

Symptomatic patients with colorectal cancer are often initially misdiagnosed. Abdominal pain, bleeding, or a change in stool caliber may be wrongly diagnosed as diverticular disease, and rectal bleeding is often attributed to hemorrhoids. A high index of suspicion is necessary, especially in those over 50 years of age. Anyone in this age group presenting with microcytic anemia, hematochezia, or new onset of cramping abdominal pain should be properly evaluated for the presence of colorectal cancer. Table 26–10 lists some clinical situations that may be confused with colorectal cancer.

COMPLICATIONS

Complications of colon cancer include chronic and acute blood loss, bowel obstruction, bowel perforation, and the illness (ie, cachexia) and death associated with metastatic disease. Rectal cancers may invade locally to involve adjacent structures, creating rectovesical or rectovaginal fistula, ureteral obstruction, or neurologic symptoms referable to invasion at the sacral plexus.

Table 26–10. Differential diagnosis of colorectal cancer.[1]

Mass lesions
Benign tumors (mucosal and submucosal)
Diverticulosis
Inflammatory masses
Diverticulitis
Inflammatory bowel disease
Ischemia
Infections (tuberculosis, amebiasis, fungal infection)
Fatty infiltration of the ileocecal valve
Endometriosis
Strictures
Inflammatory bowel disease (Crohn's colitis)
Ischemia
Radiation (late sequelae)
Rectal bleeding
Diverticulosis
Ulcerative colitis
Infectious colitis
Ischemic colitis
Solitary rectal ulcer
Hemorrhoidal bleeding
Abdominal pain
Ischemia
Diverticulitis
Inflammatory bowel disease
Irritable bowel syndrome
Change in bowel habits
Inflammatory bowel disease
Infectious diarrhea
Medications (constipation or diarrhea)
Irritable bowel syndrome

[1]This list includes common clinical situations that may be initially confused with signs or symptoms of colorectal cancer, but it is not meant to be inclusive.

TREATMENT

Polypectomy

Endoscopic polypectomy (Figure 27–16) is adequate treatment for an adenomatous polyp that contains carcinoma if it can be demonstrated to be confined to the mucosa in the head of the polyp (carcinoma *in situ*; Figure 26–17). The adequacy of simple polypectomy remains controversial in cases in which malignant cells have invaded the polyp stalk, but most studies indicate that this is adequate treatment, provided that a margin of more than 2 mm is present, there is no vascular or lymphatic invasion, and the cancer is not poorly differentiated. These criteria are more difficult to assess in sessile than pedunculated polyps. If an adequate margin cannot be demonstrated or negative histologic indicators are present, surgery is recommended to rule out regional metastases.

Surgical Resection

A. PRIMARY TUMOR RESECTION

Surgical resection of primary colorectal cancer with curative intent is the treatment of choice in most patients.

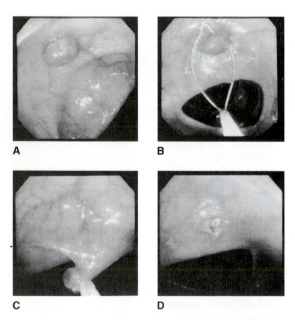

Figure 26–16. Endoscopic polypectomy prevents eventual malignant degeneration to carcinoma, and is adequate treatment when carcinoma is confined to the mucosa of the polyp (carcinoma *in situ*). **A:** Pedunculated polyp. **B:** The polypectomy snare is placed around the neck of the polyp. **C:** The polyp is brought into the lumen. **D:** The polypectomy site after removal of the polyp.

This involves wide resection of the involved bowel segment and removal of its lymphatic drainage (Figure 26–18). The extent of colonic resection is determined in part by the vascular supply of the large bowel and the distribution of regional lymph nodes. A minimum surgical margin of 5 cm on either side of the tumor is required, although segmental resection is not always possible, due to compromise of the vascular supply to portions of the colon. Rectosigmoid and many rectal lesions can be removed with a low anterior resection through an abdominal incision, combined with primary anastomosis of the remaining bowel. Primary anastomoses can now be performed even for low rectal lesions using end-to-end stapling devices and sphincter-saving operations. If an adequate uninvolved distal margin (usually at least 2 cm) cannot be obtained, the tumor is large and bulky, or the pelvis is involved by extensive local tumor spread, an abdominoperineal resection with ileostomy may be necessary for cancer of the distal rectum.

B. RESECTION OF LIVER METASTASES

Synchronous metastases to the liver are grossly evident at the time of initial surgery in 10–25% of patients with colorectal cancer. If adequate surgical margins have been obtained at resection of the primary tumor and there is no evidence of extrahepatic disease, resection of isolated hepatic lesions with curative intent is possible. Resection is usually confined to those with no more than four hepatic lesions, although even those with bilobar metastases may be resected for cure. Five-year survival rates exceed 25% in selected patients, with a low operative mortality rate of less than 2% in experienced hands. Seventy to eighty percent of hepatic metastases appear within 2 years following primary resection. Hepatic resection of isolated lesions subsequent to initial surgery follows the same principles as those for resection of synchronous lesions, and repeat hepatic resection can result in long-term survival times in selected individuals. Those with extrahepatic disease at presentation or bilobar metastases are at increased risk for recurrence after hepatic resection. Patients with underlying liver disease are poor candidates for hepatic resection because of limited functional hepatic reserve.

Adjuvant Chemotherapy

Chemotherapy of colon cancer can be divided into adjuvant chemotherapy and chemotherapy of advanced disease. Adjuvant therapy is aimed at eradicating microscopic metastases in patients who have undergone resection with curative intent but are at high risk for recurrence due to the presence of lymph node metastases or poor prognostic features. Adjuvant chemotherapy with 5-fluorouracil (5-FU, a fluoropyrimidine) plus lev-

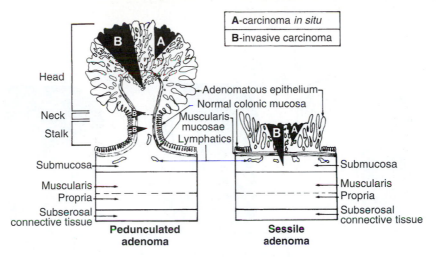

| **A**-carcinoma *in situ* |
| **B**-invasive carcinoma |

Figure 26–17. Diagrammatic representation of carcinoma within a polyp. Endoscopic polypectomy is adequate treatment for carcinoma *in situ* (**A**). If submucosal invasion occurs in a pedunculated polyp (**B**), polypectomy may be adequate if a sufficient margin (>2 mm) can be demonstrated and histologic features are favorable (see text). The depth of invasion in sessile polyps is often difficult to determine, and surgery may be required to rule out lymph node metastases. (Adapted, with permission, from Haggitt et al: Prognostic factors in colorectal carcinomas arising in adenomas: implications for lesions removed by endoscopic polypectomy. Gastroenterology 1985;89:328.)

amisole (an agent with possible immunomodulatory activity) decreases cancer recurrence by 40% and mortality rates by 33% after surgery in patients with Dukes C (stage III) tumors. Data for Dukes B2 (stage II) disease are equivocal, but if the primary tumors are poorly differentiated; demonstrate lymphatic, vascular, or perineural invasion; or demonstrate invasion into adjacent structures, patients should receive adjuvant therapy as well. Recent data suggest that the combination of 5-FU and leucovorin is superior with regard to convenience and efficacy compared with 5-FU plus levamisole. A great deal of ongoing research is aimed at defining prognostic variables that will help determine who will most benefit from adjuvant chemotherapy (see section, "Prognosis").

Although cancers of the colon tend to recur at distant sites, rectal cancers often recur both locally and distantly. Patients with rectal cancer who are treated with postoperative irradiation have a decreased incidence of local tumor recurrence, but die from metastatic disease. It has been demonstrated that combined adjuvant therapy with postoperative irradiation plus fluorouracil chemotherapy reduces cancer-related deaths in stage II and III rectal cancers (Dukes B2 and C disease) by 36% compared with tumors treated by surgery alone. The effect of combined treatment as postoperative adjuvant therapy in patients with high-risk rectal cancer is enhanced by administering fluorouracil as a protracted infusion during pelvic irradia-

tion rather than as an intermittent bolus. A variety of other regimens including 5-FU with leucovorin or levamisole are currently under investigation. Several trials are also underway to evaluate the efficacy of preoperative versus postoperative multimodality adjuvant therapy (radiation and chemotherapy) for rectal cancer.

Chemotherapy for Advanced Disease

Chemotherapy of advanced colorectal cancer is usually associated with short-lived responses and lack of improvement in survival rates. The fluoropyrimidines (fluorouracil and fluorodeoxyuridine) inhibit DNA synthesis by interacting with thymidylate synthase and inhibiting the methylation of deoxyuridylic to thymidylic acid. These agents may be administered by bolus or continuous intravenous infusion, with response rates as single agents of approximately 20%. Combinations of fluorouracil plus high-dosage intravenous leucovorin (tetrahydrofolate) are superior to fluorouracil alone, with response rates of up to 50%, but prolongation of survival rates has not been convincingly demonstrated. Addition of recombinant α_2-interferon increases response rates but not survival rates, and also increases toxicity. Irinotecan (CPT-11), an analogue of camptothecin, is a potent inhibitor of topoisomerase I, an enzyme involved in DNA replication. Treatment with irinotecan plus 5-FU and leucovorin may be superior to 5-FU plus leucovorin alone. Other drugs under

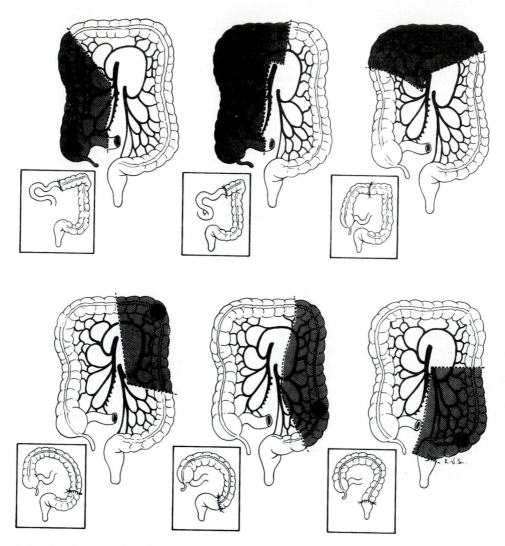

Figure 26–18. Surgical resection of colorectal cancer based on location of the primary tumor, blood supply, and lymphatic drainage. [Reproduced, with permission, from Schrock T: Large intestine. In: *Current Surgical Diagnosis and Treatment,* 10th ed. Way LW (editor). Lange, 1994.]

investigation include other anologues of camptothecin (topotecan and 9-aminocamptothecin), tomudex, a thymidylate synthase inhibitor, oxaliplatin, and UFT, an oral 5-FU prodrug. Selective infusion of chemotherapeutic agents such as fluorodeoxyuridine into the hepatic arterial system achieves objective response rates of

50–80% for liver metastases, but, again, the impact on survival rates is unclear. Selective infusion of fluoropyrimidines combined with hepatic arterial occlusion has also been advocated as treatment of hepatic metastases, with promising preliminary results. Others have attempted to deliver chemotherapeutic agents through liposomes linked to monoclonal antibodies that recognize tumor-associated antigens (immunotargeted therapy). Although conceptually appealing, this approach must be considered experimental.

Postoperative irradiation decreases local recurrence in patients with high-risk rectal cancers. The incidence of local recurrence in stage II or III disease is 40–50%, and these patients should receive postoperative irradiation. As previously noted, postoperative irradiation combined with chemotherapy improves survival rates when used in an adjuvant setting. Irradiation may also be used preoperatively in an attempt to convert large bulky tumors or those with fixation to pelvic organs to resectable lesions.

Endoscopic therapy using the neodymium:yttrium-aluminum-garnet (Nd:YAG) laser can be used for palliation of patients with obstructing rectal cancer or persistent bleeding who are poor surgical candidates. Photodynamic therapy, in which a hematoporphyrin derivative is used to sensitize tumor cells to phototherapy with a tunable dye laser, has also been used as experimental therapy in patients who are poor surgical risks.

PROGNOSIS

The prognosis of patients with colorectal cancer is most closely related to tumor stage at the time of diagnosis (see section, "Pathophysiology"). Tumor stage, in turn, is related to the degree of bowel wall penetration and presence or absence of involved lymph nodes or distant metastases. Thus, patients whose tumors are confined to the mucosa or submucosa (Dukes A, or T1 N0 M0, disease) or extend beyond the submucosa but are confined to the bowel wall (Dukes B1, or T2 N0 M0, disease) have excellent survival rates (Figure 26–19). Survival rates decrease with bowel wall penetration (Dukes B2, or stage II, disease) and lymph node involvement (Dukes C, or stage III, disease). The number of involved lymph nodes also has an impact on prognosis; patients having one to three involved nodes have better survival rates than those with four or more involved nodes. Distant metastatic disease (Dukes D, or stage IV, disease) is associated with a poor prognosis, with 5-year survival rates of only 5–10%.

Other histologic and clinical features may have an impact on the prognosis but are less important than the surgical and pathologic stage (Tables 26–11 and 26–12). Patients with poorly differentiated, colloid, or signet-ring cell cancers tend to have a poorer prognosis than those with moderately well or well-differentiated tumors. Tumor size (independent of penetration) seems to have less impact on prognosis. Venous, lymphatic, and perineural invasions indicate a diminished prognosis, whereas evidence of local inflammation and im-

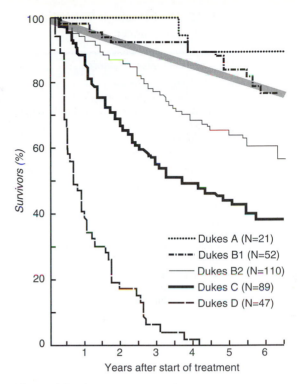

Figure 26–19. Survival rates after surgical resection, according to modified Dukes' staging system for colorectal cancer. Expected survival times of age- and gender-matched individuals in the general population are indicated by the shaded area. (Reproduced, with permission, from Moertel CG et al: The preoperative carcinoembryonic antigen test in the diagnosis, staging, and prognosis of colorectal cancer. Cancer 1986;58:603. Copyright © 1986 American Cancer Society. Reprinted by permission of Wiley-Liss, Inc., a subsidiary of John Wiley & Sons, Inc.)

munologic reaction (peritumoral lymphocytes) seems to indicate a better prognosis. Certain clinical features such as bowel obstruction or perforation, young age at diagnosis (in those without familial syndromes), and high preoperative serum carcinoembryonic antigen levels are associated with a poor prognosis.

In a search to better understand the natural history of tumor progression and identify patients who will most benefit from potentially toxic adjuvant therapies, molecular analysis of colorectal cancers has been recently employed. Patients whose tumors have abnormal chromosome numbers and, specifically, deletions of chromosomes 17p (*p53*), 18q (*DCC, DPC4*), and 8p have been demonstrated to have a worse prognosis than those whose tumors do not contain such allelic deletions. Patients with tumors demonstrating microsatel-

Table 26–11. Pathologic features that may affect prognosis in patients with colorectal cancer.

Pathologic Features	Effect on Prognosis
Surgical or pathologic stage	Increased penetration dimishes prognosis;
Depth of bowel wall penetration	1–4 nodes better than >4 nodes
Number of regional lymph nodes involved by tumor	
Histologic findings	
Degree of differentiation	Well-differentiated better than poorly differentiated
Mucinous (colloid or signet-ring cell histologic findings	Diminished prognosis
Scirrhous histologic findings	Diminished prognosis
Venous invasion	Diminished prognosis
Lymphatic invasion	Diminished prognosis
Perineural invasion	Diminished prognosis
Local inflammation and immunologic reaction	Improved prognosis
Tumor size	No effect in most studies
Tumor morphologic findings	Polypoid or exophytic better than ulcerating or infiltrating
Tumor DNA content	Increased DNA content (aneuploidy) diminishes prognosis
Molecular markers	
Deletinos in chromosome 18q (DCC, DPC4), 17p (*p53*), or 8p	Diminished prognosis
Mutation in *BAX* gene	Diminished prognosis
Microsatellite instability	Improved prognosis
Increased labeling index of p21[WAF/CIP1] protein	Improved prognosis

lite instability, on the other hand, may have an improved prognosis. Molecular changes can be detected clinically after microdissection of even formalin-fixed, paraffin-embedded tumors using the polymerase chain reaction to amplify polymorphic microsatellite markers. These assays can be readily adapted for clinical use and may be used in the future to help determine who should receive adjuvant therapy after surgical resection.

Table 26–12. Clinical features that may affect prognosis in patients with colorectal cancer.

Clinical Features	Effect on Prognosis
Diagnosis in asymptomatic patients	?Improved prognosis
Duration of symptoms	No demonstrated effect
Rectal bleeding as presenting symptom	Improved prognosis
Bowel obstruction	Diminished prognosis
Bowel perforation	Diminished prognosis
Tumor location	?Colon better than rectum
	?Left colon better than right colon
Age less than 30 years	Diminished prognosis
Preoperative serum carcinoembryonic antigen	Diminished prognosis with high level of carcinoembryonic antigen
Distant metastases	Markedly diminished prognosis

REFERENCES

Ahlquist DA et al: Colorectal cancer screening by detection of altered human DNA in stool: feasibility of a multitarget assay panel. Gastroenterology 2000;119:1219.

Baron JA et al: Calcium supplements for the prevention of colorectal adenomas. N Engl J Med 1999;340:101.

Burt RW: Colon cancer screening. Gastroenterology 2000;119: 837.

Fenlon HM et al: A comparison of virtual and conventional colonscopy for the detection of colorectal polyps. N Engl J Med 1999;341:1496.

Giardiello FM et al: The use and interpretation of commercial APC gene testing for familial adenomatous polyposis. N Engl J Med 1997;336:823.

Grady WM, Markowitz S: Genomic instability and colorectal cancer. Current Opin Gastroenterol 2000;16:62.

Grady WM et al: Mutational inactivation of transforming growth factor b receptor type II in microsatellite stable colon cancers. Cancer Res 1999;59:320.

Imperiale TF et al: Risk of advanced proximal neoplasms in asymptomatic adults according to the distal colorectal findings. N Engl J Med 2000;343:169.

Jarvinen HJ, Mecklin J-P, Sistonen P: Screening reduces colorectal cancer rate in families with hereditary nonpolyposis colorectal cancer. Gastroenterology 1995;108:1405.

Lieberman DA, Weiss DG: One time screening for colorectal cancer with combined fecal occult-blood testing and examination of the distal colon. N Engl J Med 2001;345:555.

Lippman SM, Lee JJ, Sabichi AL: Cancer chemoprevention: progress and promise. J Natl Cancer Inst 1998;90:1514.

Mandel JS et al: Reducing mortality from colorectal cancer by screening for fecal occult blood. N Engl J Med 1993;328: 1365.

Martinez-Lopez E et al: Allelic loss on chromosome 18q as a prognostic marker in stage II colorectal cancer. Gastroenterology 1998;114:1180.

Moertel CG et al: Fluorouracil plus levamisole as effective adjuvant therapy after resection of stage III colon carcinoma: a final report. Ann Intern Med 1995;122:321.

O'Connell MJ et al: Improving adjuvant therapy for rectal cancer by combining protracted-infusion fluorouracil with radiation therapy after curative surgery. N Engl J Med 1994;331:502.

Oshima M et al: Suppression of intestinal polyposis in APC^{D716} knockout mice by inhibition of cyclooxygenase 2 (COX-2). Cell 1996;87:803.

Potter JD: Colorectal cancer: molecules and populations. J Natl Cancer Inst 1999;91:916.

Rodriguiz-Bigas MD et al: A National Cancer Institute workshop on hereditary nonpolyposis colorectal cancer syndrome: meeting highlights and Bethesda guidelines. J Natl Cancer Inst 1997;89:1758.

Saltz LB et al: Ironotecan plus fluorouracil and leucovorin for metastatic colorectal cancer. N Engl J Med 2000;343:905.

Selby JV et al: A case-control study of screening sigmoidoscopy and mortality from colorectal cancer. N Engl J Med 1992;326: 653.

Smith RA et al: American Cancer Society Guidelines for early detection of cancer: update of early detection guidelines for prostate, colorectal and endometrial cancers. CA Cancer J Clin 2001;1:51.

Sonnenberg A, Delco F, Inadomi JM: Cost-effectiveness of colonoscopy in screening for colorectal cancer. Ann Intern Med 2000;133:573.

Steinbach G et al: The effect of celecoxib, a cyclooxygenase-2 inhibitor, in familial adenomatous polyposis. N Engl J Med 2000;342:1946.

Syngal S et al: Interpretation of genetic tests for hereditary nonpolyposis colorectal cancer. JAMA 1999;282:247.

Watanabe T et al: Molecular predictors of survival after adjuvent chemotherapy for colon cancer. N Engl J Med 2001;344: 1196.

Winawer SJ et al: Prevention of colorectal cancer: guidelines based on new data. Bull WHO 1995;73:7.

Winawer SJ et al: Risk of colorectal cancer in families of patients with adenomatous polyps. N Engl J Med 1996;334:82.

Winawer SJ et al: Colorectal cancer screening: clinical guidelines and rationale. Gastroenterology 1997;112:594.

Wolmark N et al: Clinical trial to assess the relative efficacy of fluorouracil, fluorouracil and leucovorin, fluorouracil and levamisole, and fluorouracil, leucovorin, and levamisole in Dukes' B and C carcinoma of the colon: results from the National Adjuvent Breast and Bowel Project C-04. J Clin Oncol 1999;17:3553.

Diverticular Disease of the Colon 27

Bruce E. Stabile, MD & Tracey D. Arnell, MD

Since Littre's initial description of saccular outpouchings of the colon in 1700, the incidence of diverticular disease, especially in Westernized areas, has steadily increased. It is among the most common diseases in the United States, affecting more than 30 million Americans annually. Nearly one-third of the population develops diverticulosis by age 50 years and two-thirds by age 80 years, with diverticular disease accounting for more than 130,000 hospital admissions per year in the United States. Only 10% of people under the age of 40 and less than 2% of people under the age of 30 are affected. There is no significant gender difference except in patients under the age of 40 years in whom there is a male preponderance.

The vast majority of cases do not involve true diverticula because the lesions do not contain all layers of the intestinal wall. They are false, or pseudodiverticula, and represent a herniation of the mucosa and submucosa through a defect in the muscular layer of the intestine being covered only by serosa. True diverticula are rare, probably congenital, occur almost exclusively in the cecum or ascending colon, are typically single, and may be quite large. The term **diverticulosis** usually refers to pseudodiverticula, which are common, acquired, occur largely in the sigmoid colon, are multiple, and are usually small.

The majority of people with diverticula of the colon remain asymptomatic. Symptoms attributable to diverticulosis develop in less than 30% of affected individuals. The broad spectrum of clinical presentations of colonic diverticula is termed **diverticular disease.** The range of symptoms includes localized abdominal pain and irregular bowel habits without evidence of inflammation, perforation with resultant infection and **diverticulitis,** and **diverticular hemorrhage.** The diagnosis and management of each clinical entity are quite different despite their shared origin.

Pathophysiology

Diverticula occur more commonly in the colon than in any other segment of the gastrointestinal tract. Additionally, among patients with diverticulosis in Western populations, 95% have involvement of the sigmoid colon. This is in contradistinction to Asian populations in which right-sided diverticula predominate. This suggests that something intrinsic to the sigmoid colon predisposes the mucosa and submucosa to herniation. Epidemiologic studies show evidence of an increasing incidence of diverticulosis with aging and the consumption of a highly refined, low fiber diet. Therefore, environmental factors contribute as well.

Diverticula occur where the vasa recta penetrate the circular muscle layer between the taenia coli (Figure 27–1). This explains the absence of diverticula in the rectum where the taenia coalesce to form the circumferential longitudinal muscle layer. Most colonic diverticula are presumed to be of the pulsion type resulting from segmentation. Segmentation refers to nonpropulsive muscular contractions that occur in a short segment of colon and likely function to increase water and electrolyte absorption (Figure 27–2). Proximal and distal simultaneous contractions occur producing a closed segment with increased intraluminal pressures. Ultimately, this may lead to herniation of the mucosa and submucosa. Manometric studies have confirmed that patients with diverticulosis have elevated colonic pressures that may be due to the more vigorous contractions needed to propel noncompressible fiber-deficient diets. Colonic work hypertrophy results in changes in the bowel wall that may be appreciated grossly as well as microscopically. Thickening of the bowel can be palpated. When viewed microscopically, the thickening is not due to fibrosis or hypertrophy of the muscle wall as might be expected. Instead, there is longitudinal foreshortening of the taenia coli with thickening of the circular muscle layer known as myochosis coli. Increases in type III collagen and deposition of elastin as seen with aging have also been observed. Recent studies suggest that the intrinsic innervation of the sigmoid colon in patients with diverticulosis may be different. Excitatory cholinergic nerves may be more prevalent, and the inhibition of nonadrenergic, noncholinergic nerves by nitric oxide may be relatively less. The colons of affected individuals demonstrate an exaggerated response to agents such as neostigmine and morphine. Based on the Law of Laplace, the resulting high pressures affect the sigmoid colon preferentially because of its smaller radius.

The pericolic fat of the mesocolon and the appendices epiploicae frequently obscures colonic diverticula. This explains the greater sensitivities of barium enema and colonoscopy in identifying diverticula compared

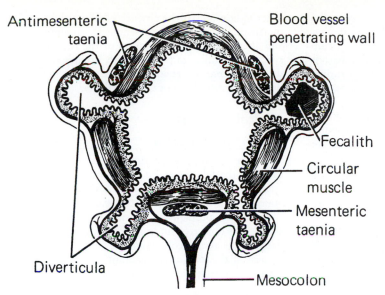

Antimesenteric taenia

Blood vessel penetrating wall

Fecalith

Circular muscle

Mesenteric taenia

Diverticula

Mesocolon

Figure 27–1. Cross section of the colon illustrating pseudodiverticula formation at sites of penetration of nutrient blood vessels through the circular muscle layer between the taenia coli. The presence of a fecalith within the lumen of a diverticulum may predispose to development of diverticulitis.

with direct visual inspection of the external surface of the bowel.

The derangements of colonic muscular anatomy and motility observed in diverticulosis result in symptoms in one-quarter of patients. Additionally, similar findings are present in patients with the irritable bowel syndrome. To a degree, some view the two conditions as different parts of a spectrum of colonic dysmotility; at one end are irregular muscular contractions causing severe pain; at the other end of the spectrum are intense muscular contractions and weakness of the bowel wall with mucosal and submucosal herniation. However, manometric studies have not confirmed segmentation and elevated luminal pressures in the irritable bowel syndrome.

Clinically, there is poor correlation between symptoms and location, size, or number of diverticula. The most common presentations of diverticular disease are diverticulitis and diverticular hemorrhage, which occur in 10–20% of patients. Diverticulosis may be the "hiatal hernia of the colon"; its presence does not necessarily equate with symptoms.

Diverticulitis describes the complication of perforation of a diverticulum resulting in acute infection. The pathogenesis of perforation may be twofold. A fecalith

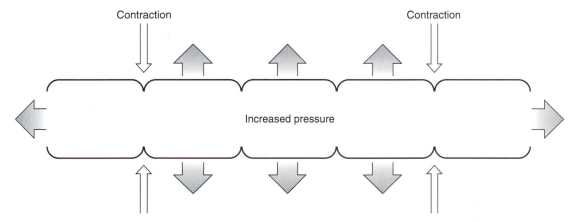

Contraction

Contraction

Increased pressure

Figure 27–2. Schematic diagram depicting segmentation resulting from nonpropulsive muscular contractions causing high intraluminal pressures that lead to pulsion-type pseudodiverticula.

within a diverticulum may erode the attenuated wall of the diverticulum, or high intraluminal pressure may cause rupture of the diverticulum. In either circumstance, an infectious process ensues that may be only pericolonic or may widely contaminate the peritoneal cavity. Thus, diverticulitis, by definition, is a perforation of one or more diverticula that manifests as localized peritonitis secondary to a pericolic phlegmon or abscess, or as generalized purulent or fecal peritonitis. Again, the sigmoid is the most commonly affected area of the colon. Infection of a solitary cecal diverticulum is an infrequent though well-recognized entity that is clinically indistinguishable from acute appendicitis.

Other sequelae of diverticulitis include fistula, acute obstruction, and chronic stricture. With infection and inflammation of the involved colon, fistulization to adjacent structures may occur. Fistulas have been described between the colon and nearly every intraabdominal structure but most commonly develop between the sigmoid colon and the bladder, the vagina in women who have had a hysterectomy, or occasionally the small intestine or skin. Coloenteric and colocutaneous fistulas more often occur after operative or radiologic interventions. Obstruction may be acute from edema, compression by an adjacent abscess, or chronic from repeated episodes leading to stricture.

Diverticular hemorrhage develops in approximately 5–10% of patients with colonic diverticulosis. The bleeding is thought to result from the close anatomic relationship between diverticula and the penetrating arterioles of the vasa recta. Although the exact mechanism precipitating hemorrhage is unknown, evidence suggests that a slow development of chemical or mechanical damage to the vessel wall results in rupture into the lumen of the colon. The bleeding is typically massive but self-limited. Chronic occult blood loss is atypical of diverticular bleeding.

DIVERTICULOSIS

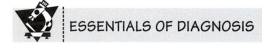

ESSENTIALS OF DIAGNOSIS

- *Characteristic radiologic or endoscopic signs.*
- *Absence of diverticulitis or bleeding.*
- *No fever or leukocytosis.*

General Considerations

Diverticulosis uncomplicated by perforation or bleeding is usually asymptomatic and diagnosed incidentally on barium enema or colonoscopy obtained for some other indication. In the absence of diverticulitis or hemorrhage, patients may present with abdominal pain and altered bowel habits typical of the irritable bowel syndrome. Similar to patients with irritable bowel syndrome, symptoms are likely related to the underlying dysmotility disorder, not the diverticula.

Clinical Findings

A. SYMPTOMS AND SIGNS

The pain of symptomatic diverticulosis is typically located in the left lower quadrant, is intermittent and cramping in nature, and may be associated with alterations in bowel movements. Muscular contractions of the colon are probably responsible for the pain, hence the lack of objective findings. Examination of the abdomen may reveal voluntary guarding with mild tenderness in the left lower quadrant. Alterations in vital signs such as tachycardia and fever are absent.

B. LABORATORY FINDINGS

Because of the absence of bleeding or infection, the hematocrit, hemoglobin, and white blood cell count are normal. The stool hemoccult blood test is negative.

C. IMAGING

Plain abdominal x-rays are unremarkable, without ileus or distention. A contrast enema reveals multiple diverticula, most commonly involving the sigmoid and descending colon (Figure 27–3). Segmental spasm with a sawtooth pattern may be present, but is not persistent. Evidence of contrast extravasation, fistula, stricture, or unremitting spasm indicates diverticulitis. Abdominal computed tomography (CT) in uncomplicated diverticulosis is normal without stricture or inflammatory changes. Luminal narrowing or stricture is evidence of diverticulitis, although the clinical episode may be remote.

D. ENDOSCOPY

Endoscopic evaluation is relatively contraindicated if there is any suspicion of diverticulitis. When performed, flexible sigmoidoscopy or colonoscopy may reveal diverticula, although mucosal folds may obscure them. Diverticula are not present in the rectum so rigid proctoscopy is less reliable because of the limited length (25 cm) of bowel examined. If spasm is present on endoscopic exam, it is not persistent.

Differential Diagnosis

Differentiation of symptomatic diverticulosis from mild diverticulitis may be quite difficult. The absence of fever, leukocytosis, and other systemic signs of infection does not exclude diverticulitis. If findings such as persistent colonic spasm on contrast enema or pericolic inflamma-

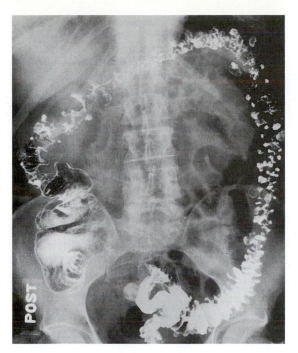

Figure 27–3. Barium enema demonstrating extensive diverticulosis of the left hemicolon. (Reproduced, with permission, from Stabile BE: Therapeutic options in acute diverticulitis. Comp Ther 1991;17:26.)

tion on CT are found, the diagnosis of diverticulitis should be made. In instances where symptomatic diverticulosis cannot be distinguished from mild diverticulitis, observation of the clinical course may be revealing.

Consideration of a number of conditions of the pelvis and lower abdomen should be given in patients presenting with symptoms of lower abdominal pain. These include appendicitis, colitis (infectious, inflammatory, ischemic), colorectal cancer, endometriosis, ovarian pathology, and pelvic inflammatory disease. A complete physical examination and appropriate ancillary studies should be performed in all patients.

The irritable bowel syndrome is particularly difficult to distinguish from symptomatic diverticulosis based on clinical presentation. In fact, the two may coexist in the same patient. As opposed to irritable bowel syndrome, which commonly causes diffuse abdominal pain, symptomatic diverticulosis is more likely when pain is limited to the left lower quadrant and associated with demonstrated diverticula.

Complications

Perforation of a diverticulum may lead to diverticulitis. Erosion of the penetrating nutrient arteriole associated

with a diverticulum results in colonic hemorrhage. Unlike simple diverticulosis, both of these complications are potentially life threatening.

Treatment

A. MEDICAL

Once diverticulosis is present, there is no medical therapy that causes regression. Medical therapy is aimed at decreasing pain and bowel irregularity, and preventing progression. Such therapy currently is based on increasing dietary fiber. The use of anticholinergics, motility-altering drugs, antispasmodics, narcotics, and sedatives is of no proven benefit and may be harmful. Unfortunately, although a diet low in fiber is thought to be a causative factor in diverticulosis, there is no convincing evidence that high fiber diets are effective in preventing symptoms, progression, or the development of complications. However, patients with pain and bowel dysfunction attributable to diverticulosis do appear to benefit from increased fiber intake. In animal models, progressive decreases in intracolonic pressures with increasing dietary fiber have been shown. Increasing stool bulk and water content has a salutary effect on the ease and regularity of bowel movements and ameliorates painful spasms. In general, the least expensive and most widely recommended dietary source of added vegetable fiber is unprocessed wheat bran. The relative effectiveness of various brans may be related to their particle size and hydrophilia. Increasing the bran content of the diet typically gives rise to abdominal distention and increased flatus. Therefore, it is recommended that the dosage be slowly increased over a period of 1–2 months to 10–25 g/d in divided portions with meals.

Avoiding seeds, nuts, and popcorn has never been shown to decrease the complications of diverticulosis. In fact, impaction of diverticula with fecaliths is commonly observed endoscopically and there are no reports of finding intraabdominal seeds in macroperforated diverticulitis.

B. SURGICAL

In general, surgical therapy is not indicated for uncomplicated diverticulosis. Most symptomatic patients will continue to have pain and alteration in bowel movements. Of historical interest are operations aimed at disrupting the longitudinal muscle of the colon to decrease painful spasms. The postoperative complication rates were unacceptably high and the beneficial results were minimal.

Prognosis

Despite its high prevalence, diverticulosis is most often unattended by complications. Nevertheless, an occasional patient with severe pain and colonic dysmotility may be disabled. Such symptoms, however, are not predictive of life-threatening complications. For the 10–20% of patients who develop diverticulitis or lower intestinal bleeding, the prognosis is more worrisome. Three-quarters of patients who develop complications do so in the absence of preceding symptoms. Diverticulitis or hemorrhage is often the initial manifestation of diverticular disease. Although most episodes of diverticulitis and hemorrhage are self-limited or can be managed medically, considerable morbidity and mortality may occur among the elderly and the immunocompromised.

ACUTE DIVERTICULITIS

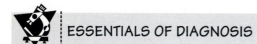 **ESSENTIALS OF DIAGNOSIS**

- *Acute abdominal pain.*
- *Abdominal tenderness.*
- *Fever and/or leukocytosis.*
- *Characteristic radiologic signs.*

General Considerations

Diverticulitis occurs in 15–20% of individuals with diverticulosis. It demonstrates a male preponderance in patients younger than 40 years of age, but no gender difference over the age of 60. As discussed earlier, high fat and low fiber intake likely predispose to diverticulitis. The intake of caffeine, alcohol, and tobacco does not appear to increase the risk of diverticulitis.

Diverticulitis is, by definition, a result of perforation of a diverticulum with subsequent infection and inflammation extending into the colon wall, epiploic appendages, mesentery, adjacent organs, or freely into the peritoneal cavity. As such, diverticulitis is more accurately termed peridiverticulitis, as the inflammatory response extends beyond the diverticulum itself. The Hinchey classification (Table 27–1) of diverticulitis is

frequently used to describe severity and can aid in decision making regarding surgical options. Briefly, the most common manifestation of diverticulitis is that of an indolent microperforation of a diverticulum by a contained fecalith. This typically results in phlegmonous swelling of the bowel wall with resulting microabscesses, sinus tracts, and intramural fistulas (Hinchey stage I). If the infectious process penetrates the bowel serosa but is confined locally, pericolic or pelvic macroabscesses occur (Hinchey stage II). If the infectious process is not contained, purulent peritonitis (Hinchey stage III) ensues. With free perforation, a severe diffuse feculent peritonitis (Hinchey stage IV) is encountered.

Other complications of diverticulitis include fistula formation and colonic obstruction. Fistulas occur by direct extension of peridiverticular abscesses that rupture into adjacent organs such as the bladder, vagina, or skin. Once fistulization has occurred, the acute sepsis usually subsides because it is alleviated by the decompression. Obstruction may occur acutely as a result of edema of the bowel wall during an episode of diverticulitis, or chronically if fibrosis develops due to repeated episodes. The chronic form often requires surgery for relief.

Clinical Findings

A. SYMPTOMS AND SIGNS

In concordance with the gradual development of the inflammatory process, patients with diverticulitis generally present with left lower quadrant abdominal pain of gradual onset. The pain is constant and unrelenting and may be accompanied by intermittent exacerbations associated with colonic spasms followed by loose bowel movements. In contrast to symptomatic diverticulosis, the pain of diverticulitis does not subside within minutes or hours, but persists if untreated.

Patients with stage I and II disease confined to the pericolonic tissues present with localized pain and tenderness, usually in the left lower quadrant, although they may extend to the mid or right abdomen if the sigmoid loop is large. With stage II disease, anorexia, nausea, and emesis may occur, particularly in patients with large abscesses or severe localized peritonitis. Nonspecific urinary symptoms such as urgency and frequency suggest proximity of the inflammatory process to the urinary bladder. Localized tenderness, swelling, and erythema of the abdominal wall suggest the presence of an underlying abscess with imminent colocutaneous fistulization.

In patients with diffuse peritonitis due to stage III and IV disease, the abdominal pain is severe and generalized, and may inhibit movement. There is usually as-

Table 27–1. Hinchey clinical stages of acute diverticulitis.

Stage	Description
I	Peridiverticular phlegmon with microabscesses
II	Pericolic or pelvic macroabscess
III	Generalized purulent peritonitis
IV	Generalized feculent peritonitis

sociated ileus, bloating, nausea, and emesis. Patients with stage IV disease may present with a precipitous illness characterized by the acute onset of severe abdominal pain consistent with a large, free perforation and fecal peritonitis. Physical examination may reveal high fever, hemodynamic compromise as a result of sepsis, and generalized abdominal rigidity. The presence of ileus is suggested by abdominal distention and hypoactive bowel sounds.

B. LABORATORY FINDINGS

The diagnosis of acute diverticulitis is largely a clinical exercise; laboratory investigations are not particularly useful in refining the diagnosis. Leukocytosis is commonly present although one-half of patients with mild diverticulitis have normal white blood cell counts. Marked leukocytosis is usually present only with abscess formation or peritonitis. If the urinary bladder is involved in the acute process, there may be red and/or white cells in the urine. In the case of a colovesical fistula, the urinalysis may be consistent with a polymicrobial infection. With severe episodes of diverticulitis, there may be hyponatremia, acidosis, and impaired renal function consistent with sepsis.

C. IMAGING

Three-quarters of patients with diverticulitis present with the classic findings of left lower quadrant pain and tenderness, fever, and leukocytosis. In these patients, further imaging may be unnecessary in the acute setting. In those patients undergoing imaging, the findings depend on the stage of the disease.

Plain abdominal radiographs are often normal in mild diverticulitis. In the presence of severe infection or significant obstruction, there may be an ileus pattern or bowel dilation proximal to the narrowing. An air–fluid level may be seen with a large abscess on an upright plain radiograph. Retroperitoneal air can diffuse along the psoas muscle and obliterate the psoas shadow. A significant amount of free air often accompanies feculent peritonitis.

Ultrasound, contrast enemas, and CT scans can confirm and better delineate the extent of acute diverticulitis. They are useful if the diagnosis is in doubt, in patients who fail to respond to medical therapy, and in the immunocompromised and elderly who often fail to manifest the usual signs and symptoms of inflammation and infection.

Traditionally, contrast enemas have been used to diagnose acute diverticulitis. The most common finding is that of persistent spasm and a sawtooth pattern of the involved segment. Additional possible radiologic findings are listed in Table 27–2. Included among these are the presence of an intramural fistula, sinus tract (Figure 27–4), and demonstration of an extraluminal collection

Table 27–2. Radiographic signs of diverticulitis seen on contrast enema.

Sinus tract
Fistula
Extravasation
Abscess
Deformed diverticulum
Stricture
Spasm
Obstruction
Extraluminal mass effect
Pneumoperitoneum

of contrast medium (Figure 27–5). Contrast enemas can also differentiate a cancer from diverticulitis. Acute diverticulitis is a relative contraindication to contrast enema because of the danger of precipitating or exacerbating bowel perforation. It should be reserved for those cases that are equivocal or until the acute episode has resolved. If performed acutely, water-soluble contrast should be used with minimization of the amount of contrast instilled and the pressure used.

CT scanning has largely replaced the contrast enema in the setting of acute diverticulitis. Rectal contrast is unnecessary, although oral contrast is very useful in separating bowel from intraabdominal fluid collections. It is superior to a contrast enema in evaluating the pericolonic tissues and structures frequently involved in the diverticulitis process. Findings on CT scan include inflammation of surrounding tissues including mesentery, retroperitoneum, and abdominal wall described as stranding, fatty infiltration, streaking, "dirty fat," or phlegmon. The bowel wall may be thickened and involvement of adjacent structures and abscesses may be visible. Identification of fluid collections or abscesses by CT is superior to that by contrast enemas, especially with the use of oral contrast (Figure 27–6). Inclusion of the rectum in the process generally excludes the diagnosis of diverticulitis.

Ultrasound can identify a large inflammatory process or phlegmon, abscesses, and bowel wall thickening. It is very operator dependent and is limited in the setting of an ileus because of gas distention of the bowel. It offers the advantages of being noninvasive and may be performed at the bedside. Its greatest utility may be in guided drainage of intraabdominal abscesses.

D. ENDOSCOPY

Endoscopic evaluation including rigid proctoscopy, flexible sigmoidoscopy, and colonoscopy are generally contraindicated in suspected acute diverticulitis. Insufflation of air is required and has the potential of wors-

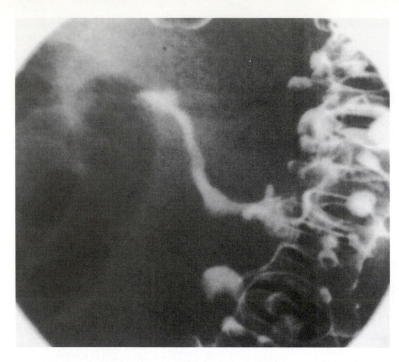

Figure 27–4. Barium enema illustrating extraluminal contrast in a sinus tract due to diverticular perforation into the sigmoid mesocolon. This radiographic sign is diagnostic of diverticulitis.

ening or unsealing a perforation. Usually a period of 6–8 weeks is allowed to pass after resolution of an acute attack before endoscopy is attempted. If emergent operation is necessary, endoscopy should be performed by an experienced endoscopist to differentiate diverticulitis from a mucosal process such as carcinoma or colitis. Findings include edema, erythema, stricture, and rarely, purulent discharge from a diverticulum. When performed after complete resolution of the episode, findings are frequently minimal. The primary purpose of delayed endoscopy is to exclude another diagnosis such as colitis or cancer.

Differential Diagnosis

The differential diagnosis of acute diverticulitis encompasses a wide range of inflammatory, mechanical, vascular, and neoplastic processes with the pertinent inclusions being dictated by the stage of acute diverticulitis under consideration. Thus, patents with very mild diverticulitis associated with only minimal abdominal findings and no radiographic abnormalities, fever, or leukocytosis, might be misinterpreted as having irritable bowel syndrome or uncomplicated symptomatic diverticulosis. In general, the duration of acute symptoms, the degree of abdominal tenderness, and the ultimate development of fever and leukocytosis make the diagnosis of diverticulitis apparent. In more severe cases of phlegmonous diverticulitis, the differential diagnosis includes appendicitis, in-

flammatory bowel disease, pelvic inflammatory disease, ischemic colitis, infectious colitis, and colorectal carcinoma. The differentiation of cecal diverticulitis from appendicitis is virtually impossible preoperatively. Similar confusion arises in instances of sigmoid diverticulitis when an elongated, inflamed sigmoid loop resides in the right lower quadrant of the abdomen.

In cases of diverticular pericolic or pelvic abscess, the differential diagnosis includes a variety of other causes of hollow viscus perforation such as appendicitis, tuboovarian and inflammatory bowel disease abscesses, colorectal and other intraabdominal cancers, foreign body and iatrogenic perforations, as well as perinephric and pancreatic abscesses. The symptoms and clinical course prior to appearance of the abscess, together with imaging studies and endoscopy, clarify its cause. Aspiration of the abscess with culture of the fluid may differentiate noncolonic causes from the other possibilities. In some cases, endoscopy or contrast enema examination is necessary to settle the issue of diverticulitis versus colonic Crohn's disease or carcinoma.

The differential diagnosis for patients presenting with peritonitis includes all variety of gastrointestinal perforations including peptic ulcer disease, Crohn's disease (although free perforation is unusual), appendicitis, and perforated intestinal malignancies. In addition, pelvic inflammatory disease, ischemic bowel, severe pancreatitis, and bacterial peritonitis in patients with ascites should be considered. If a significant pneumoperito-

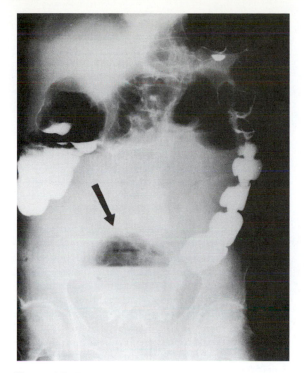

Figure 27–5. Barium enema demonstrating a large diverticular pelvic abscess **(arrow)** containing an air–fluid level. (Reproduced, with permission, from Stabile BE: Therapeutic options in acute diverticulitis. Comp Ther 1991;17:26.)

neum is evident, the source is almost invariably colonic or gastroduodenal. In patients with acquired immunodeficiency syndrome (AIDS), perforation of the small or large intestine as a result of cytomegalovirus infection or Kaposi's sarcoma warrants serious consideration.

Among patients with colovesical, colovaginal, coloenteric, or colocutaneous fistulas, the differential diagnosis includes Crohn's disease and malignancies. Endoscopy with biopsy of any mucosal abnormalities is necessary.

In cases of large bowel obstruction, the differential diagnosis includes all potentially obstructing lesions, but most prominently, colorectal carcinoma. Crohn's disease, ischemic strictures, endometriosis, colonic tuberculosis, and ameboma, as well as atypical presentation of sigmoid volvulus, are occasional causes. CT, endoscopy, and contrast enema generally clarify the issue.

Complications

The serious complications of acute diverticulitis include pericolic and pelvic macroabscesses, purulent or feculent peritonitis, fistulization to adjacent organs, and colonic obstruction. All of these complications represent a virulent extension of the disease beyond the colonic wall. Abscesses may rupture to cause purulent peritonitis, they may involve adjacent organs and lead to fistula formation, or they may slowly lead to systemic sepsis. Peritonitis almost inevitably progresses to septic shock and death if untreated. Among survivors, it is often the source of recurrent small bowel obstructions due to adhesions. Fistulas to the urinary bladder are frequently complicated by urosepsis, whereas those involving the small intestine can lead to bacterial overgrowth with associated malabsorp-

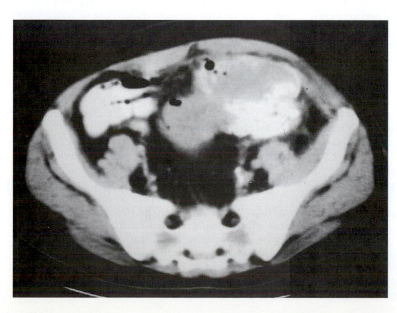

Figure 27–6. Abdominal CT scan demonstrating large pericolic diverticular abscess containing gas bubbles.

tion and diarrhea. Colovaginal and colocutaneous fistulas are less dangerous but may be responsible for fluid losses and significant local irritation of the perineum or abdominal wall skin. Colonic obstruction due to diverticular disease is typically partial but may precipitate acute colonic dilatation and perforation.

Treatment

A. MEDICAL THERAPY

Many patients with diverticulitis require hospitalization for intravenous antibiotics, rehydration, and pain control. If a significant component of paralytic ileus is present, nasogastric decompression should be instituted. Patients with mild pain, minimal evidence of systemic infection, lack of paralytic ileus, and good functional status may be treated as outpatients with clear liquid diet, oral antibiotics, and close follow-up. Patients who fail to improve after 48 hours should be admitted to the hospital. The choice of antibiotics must include anaerobic and aerobic coverage. Because diverticulitis is by definition infection extending beyond the colonic mucosa, nonabsorbable intraluminal antibiotics are ineffective. Anticholinergic agents, glucagon, and other smooth muscle relaxing agents have not been found to be beneficial in the acute setting.

In most cases, aggressive medical therapy results in rapid and dramatic clinical improvement with resolution of pain, tenderness, fever, and ileus within 48–72 hours. Broad spectrum antibiotics should be continued for 7–10 days. An oral antibiotic regimen may be begun when the patient shows signs of improvement, and there is resolution of the ileus. Oral intake is gradually reintroduced as tolerated. Upon discharge, the patient should begin a high fiber diet and psyllium supplementation. There is some evidence that this decreases the incidence of recurrence. If patients do not improve during the initial 48–72 hours, consideration should be given to broadening antibiotic coverage to include organisms such as *Enterococcus,* and abdominal imaging should be performed to evaluate for an abscess.

Longitudinal studies of patients following resolution of the initial attack of diverticulitis suggest that nearly two-thirds to three-fourths have no further problems. The incidence of recurrent attacks is approximately 2% per year. After two attacks of diverticulitis, it is reported that only 6% of patients will resolve with further medical management. About 10–20% of affected individuals experience repeated episodes and require surgical resection of the involved colon.

B. SURGICAL THERAPY

Operation for diverticulitis and its complications may be required as either an elective or emergency procedure (Table 27–3). Indications for elective operation include

Table 27–3. Indications for operation in diverticulitis.

Diffuse peritonitis
Unresolving obstruction
Fistula
Symptomatic stricture
Failure to improve or progression on medical therapy
Recurrent attacks
Younger than 40 years old
Inability to exclude carcinoma
Immunosuppressed patient

(1) two or more well-documented episodes of diverticulitis successfully treated medically; (2) one attack with evidence of macroperforation, colonic obstruction, or fistula formation; (3) one attack in a patient who is immunosuppressed; and (4) the inability to exclude carcinoma. Because a second episode of diverticulitis portends a clinical course of recurrences, often each more complicated than the last, elective operation is advised unless the patient's overall medical condition precludes safe elective operation. Several studies suggest that patients 50 years of age or younger present with more complicated disease, and require emergent surgery more frequently at their initial hospitalization. This has led to the recommendation that patients younger than 40 years of age undergo resection after a single episode. Subsequent studies have not found recurrent episodes to be more complicated or more frequent in these younger patients compared with the elderly, though. Therefore, the recommendation for resection in the young patient should not be considered absolute. Regardless of age, patients with an episode of complicated diverticulitis should undergo resection as they are prone to recurrences and further complications.

Because the overwhelming majority of patients with acute diverticulitis have sigmoid involvement, resections of other portions of the colon are infrequent. Patients deemed to be candidates for elective operation following successful medical treatment of an acute attack should be evaluated for surgery 6–8 weeks after the most recent episode. There are recent reports of resection for mild disease during the same hospitalization without increased morbidity, and this may be considered. Other than the standard preoperative work-up, full colonic evaluation either by colonoscopy or contrast enema should be performed. This is done to exclude other causes of inflammation (ie, cancer, Crohn's disease) and to assess for synchronous neoplastic lesions in the remainder of the colon.

Elective operation for diverticular disease is preceded by mechanical and oral nonabsorbable antibiotic bowel preparation followed by parenteral antibiotics immediately prior to incision. Generally, the patient is placed in the lithotomy position if a stapled anastomosis is planned. After initial exploration of the abdomen, the colon is examined. In sigmoid diverticular disease, the proximal extent of resection is to normal, soft, colon. Involved colon is usually thickened on palpation and there may be evidence of inflammation in the surrounding tissues. The distal resection margin is the upper rectum because anastomosis to the sigmoid is associated with a doubling of the recurrence rate of diverticulitis. The extent of resection of other parts of the colon for diverticulitis should also include all areas of abnormal, thickened colon. It is unnecessary to resect all diverticula, as recurrence proximal to the anastomosis is distinctly uncommon. Frequently, the colon is adherent to adjacent structures such as the small bowel, abdominal wall, bladder, or uterus. Gentle pinching of the colon and careful sharp dissection are usually successful in separating the tissues without injuring the adherent organs. Rarely is resection of these other structures necessary. A primary anastomosis is performed without diversion or stoma formation and is termed a single stage colectomy (Figure 27–7). If an unexpected abscess or severe active inflammation is encountered (Hinchey grade I or II), primary anastomosis is still feasible if the patient is otherwise healthy and well nourished.

For patients who fail to improve during their hospitalization after 48–72 hours, a CT scan of the abdomen should be performed to evaluate for an abscess. The presence of an abscess does not mandate drainage per se, as many will resolve spontaneously. Drainage is recom-

mended if the patient demonstrates clinical signs of continuing systemic infection, or failure to resolve an obstruction. Previously, the presence of a large abscess required surgical exploration and drainage. Presently, CT or ultrasound-guided percutaneous drainage is successful in 70–90% of cases and may convert a potential emergent operation to an elective one. Drainage is more likely to fail in patients with multiple abscesses or feculent drainage. The catheter is removed when the abscess is collapsed and drainage is minimal (Figure 27–8).

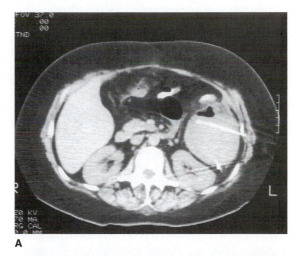

A

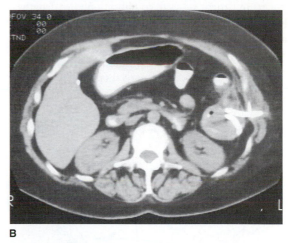

B

Figure 27–8. **A:** Abdominal CT scan showing aspirating needle in a large left pericolic diverticular abscess. **B:** Repeat CT scan showing coiled percutaneous drainage catheter in collapsed abscess cavity. (Reproduced, with permission, from Stabile BE et al: Preoperative percutaneous drainage of diverticular abscesses. Am J Surg 1990;159:99.)

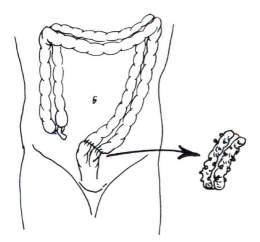

Figure 27–7. Single-stage sigmoid colectomy with primary anastomosis. (Reproduced, with permission, from Stabile BE: Therapeutic options in acute diverticulitis. Comp Ther 1991;17:26.)

Patients who present with peritonitis or fail to improve with medical management require emergent operation after fluid resuscitation and intravenous antibiotics. Prior to surgery, limited endoscopy by an experienced examiner is performed, often in the operating room. This is to exclude carcinoma as a cause of the inflammation. This should be done because the accuracy of distinguishing diverticulitis from cancer at the time of operative exploration and external examination of the bowel is only 50%. In cases of cancer, any adherent organs should be resected en bloc rather than separated as previously described.

If purulent or feculent peritonitis (Hinchey grade III or IV) is found, resection with end colostomy and Hartmann pouch should be performed in the case of sigmoid diverticulitis (Figure 27–9). Leaving the rectal stump long enough to create a mucous fistula precludes resection to the rectum and should be avoided if possible. In the unusual case of cecal or right-sided diverticulitis, a right colectomy is performed with an ileostomy and mucous fistula. Subsequently, the patient may have the colostomy taken down and an anastomosis performed resulting in a two-stage procedure. The three-stage procedure of proximal colostomy and drainage followed by resection and subsequent closure has lost favor because of the high morbidity and mortality associated with this approach (Figure 27–10). Leaving the septic focus in place appears to worsen the clinical course, and the necessity of two additional operations is generally unwarranted. Numerous studies have documented substantial improvements in patient survival, complication rates, lengths of hospitalization, and disability with the two-stage rather than three-stage procedure.

When medical management fails and urgent surgery is required, or an unexpected finding of active diverticulitis is found at operation, several options are available.

The previously described technique of resection with end colostomy and Hartmann closure of the rectum may be performed. This is time tested and carries a mortality of less than 5%.

With the recognition that the morbidity from the colostomy and subsequent colostomy closure is significant and that only two-thirds of patients undergo closure, alternatives to this approach have been tried. In the urgent setting when a bowel prep has not been performed, an on-table lavage may be utilized. The technique involves mobilizing the portion of colon to be resected, and splenic and hepatic flexures. The bowel is divided proximal to the specimen. Corrugated tubing is placed in this distal colon and secured with a dacron tape. The corrugated tubing is run from the table to a bucket off of the field. A large foley catheter is placed into the base of the appendix after appendectomy or into a cecostomy using a purse-string suture. Then 3–6 L of warm saline is run from the cecum to the distal bowel. Ten percent povidone-iodine is added to the last liter of irrigant. The tubing and foley are removed and the purse-string suture is tightened. The resection is completed and the anastomosis is performed in the standard manner. Using this technique, the wound infection rate has been demonstrated to be less than 20% and the anastomotic leakage rate less than 6%. Generally, it can safely be performed in patients with obstruction, Hinchey stages I and II, and otherwise healthy, hemodynamically stable patients with Hinchey stage III diverticulitis.

Diverticulitis complicated by a fistula rarely requires emergent operative intervention. Development of a fistula represents spontaneous decompression of an abscess and usually results in resolution of the inflammation. Patients with fistulas are best treated medically first, and subsequently by elective operation. Again, preopera-

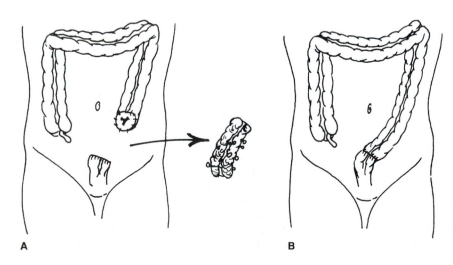

Figure 27–9. **A:** Sigmoid colectomy, descending end colostomy, and Hartmann closure of the rectal stump. **B:** Colostomy takedown and anastomosis as a second procedure. (Reproduced, with permission, from Stabile BE: Therapeutic options in acute diverticulitis. Comp Ther 1991;17:26.)

A

B

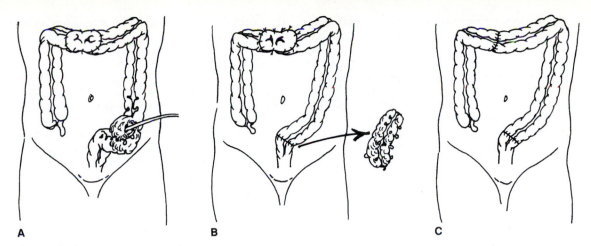

Figure 27–10. A: Transverse loop colostomy with catheter drainage. **B:** Sigmoid colectomy and anastomosis as a second procedure. **C:** Closure of transverse colostomy as a third procedure. (Reproduced, with permission, from Stabile BE: Therapeutic options in acute diverticulitis. Comp Ther 1991;17:26.)

tively, the colon should be evaluated to assess for the presence of a neoplasm. At surgery the colon can be separated from the adherent organs or abdominal wall without resecting the involved structures. When the bladder is involved and the defect is large, simple closure with catheter drainage for 7 days is all that is necessary.

The role of laparoscopic surgery for diverticular disease is expanding as experience is gained. Laparoscopic surgery has been used in elective resections, complicated diverticulitis including those with fistulas and abscesses, and colostomy reversal with excellent results. With the addition of hand-assisted techniques to mobilize fistulas and areas of inflammation not amenable to customary laparoscopic dissection, the role is broadening. Several studies have attempted to identify factors that may predict conversion from laparoscopic to open surgery. Patient obesity, surgeon inexperience, presence of fistulas, and severity of diverticulitis are the factors most often sited. With experience, operative time has decreased and outcomes have improved. Recent studies report conversion rates of less than 10%, complication rates less than 8%, and average hospital stay of 4 days. The greatest benefit of the laparoscopic over the open procedure appears to be in the time to return of regular activity and work. As long as the same principles of complete resection of thickened bowel and tension-free anastomosis are applied, the long-term outcomes will likely be the same for the two techniques.

Prognosis

Approximately 15–20% of patients presenting with an initial attack of diverticulitis require surgical interven-

tion because of peritonitis, obstruction, or failure of medical management. Among patients whose initial attack is successfully treated medically, 10–20% recur. The mortality rate for elective colon resection and primary anastomosis is approximately 1%, as compared with 30% if free perforation has occurred. Following resection, the recurrence rate is less than 5% if a complete resection of all thickened or inflamed colon has been accomplished.

DIVERTICULAR HEMORRHAGE

 ESSENTIALS OF DIAGNOSIS

- *Elderly patient.*
- *Hematochezia or melena.*
- *Gastric aspirate positive for bile and negative for blood.*
- *Transfusion often required.*

General Considerations

It is estimated that 5–15% of patients with known diverticulosis develop the complication of acute hemorrhage and 5% can be characterized as severe. Diverticular hemorrhage is likely responsible for approximately 50% of episodes of lower gastrointestinal bleeding. Progressive enlargement of a colonic diverticulum leads to stretching and splaying of the small associated arteriole over the dome of the lesion. Hemorrhage results from weakening and finally rupture of the vessel with decompression into the bowel lumen. Histopathologic observations have confirmed changes in the intima and media of the arteriole. Thus owing to its arterial nature, the hemorrhage associated with diverticulosis tends to be massive. Right-sided colonic diverticula, although much less common than left-sided colonic diverticula, are likely responsible for 60% of cases of diverticular bleeding. It is difficult to confirm this impression, though, because it is unusual to identify a bleeding diverticulum and the same patient population has a high prevalence of angiodysplastic lesions that also may bleed. In some instances diverticular hemorrhage is associated with the use of anticoagulants such as warfarin or aspirin.

Clinical Findings

A. SYMPTOMS AND SIGNS

The presentation of diverticular bleeding is dark to bright red blood per rectum in moderate to large amounts. The more distal the source in the colon, the more likely the hematochezia is to be bright red and contain clots. Occasionally, slow right colonic diverticular bleeding produces melena, thus mimicking an upper gastrointestinal bleeding source. Because of the cathartic effect of blood in the intestine, some abdominal cramping may be present, but otherwise, bleeding is painless. In approximately 80–90% of patients, the bleeding stops spontaneously, often by the time of patient presentation. In the remaining 10–20% of patients whose bleeding is massive and unrelenting, pallor, tachycardia, and orthostatic hypotension or shock may be present. Significant bleeding can occur in the absence of hemodynamic instability, though. In one reported series, 90% of patients with a positive arteriogram were normotensive and only 30% had tachycardia. The abdominal examination may reveal slight distention and active bowel sounds and a lack of tenderness or a mass. The rectal examination demonstrates gross blood ranging from bright red to melena. Passage of a nasogastric tube reveals no blood in the stomach aspirate with return of bile.

B. LABORATORY FINDINGS

It is important to note that a normal hematocrit or hemoglobin level does not negate the diagnosis of acute diverticular hemorrhage. Sufficient time must elapse with hemodilution and intravascular equilibration before there is laboratory evidence of bleeding. A low initial hematocrit or hemoglobin level suggests bleeding that has been ongoing for hours or days, or the presence of a chronic anemia. A hypochromic, microcytic anemia specifically suggests chronic blood loss. Abnormali-

ties of platelet count, coagulation parameters, or liver function tests suggest specific associated medical conditions or drug therapy that may contribute to the severity of bleeding.

C. IMAGING

Plain abdominal x-rays reveal no diagnostic clues. Nuclear scintigraphy bleeding scans incorporating technetium sulfur colloid or ^{99m}Tc-labeled red blood cells utilize external gamma counters to detect intraluminal extravasation of blood. The sulfur colloid scans can detect bleeding as slow as 0.1 mL/min and can be completed in less than 1 hour. The labeled red blood cell scans allow repeated scanning up to 36 hours and are able to detect intermittent bleeding. They also provide better bleeding site localization by demonstration of anatomic contours within the gastrointestinal tract. The specificity for identifying the location of the bleeding site is only 60–70%, making operation based on a positive bleeding scan alone somewhat unreliable.

Because of the intermittent nature of lower gastrointestinal bleeding, angiographic examination should be performed only on actively bleeding, hemodynamically stable patients. A bleeding rate of greater than 0.5 mL/min is necessary for a positive angiogram. Selective injection of the mesenteric vessels beginning with the superior mesenteric artery followed by the inferior mesenteric artery and then celiac artery is performed. The rate of identifying the bleeding site varies from 35 to 85% depending on when the angiogram is obtained. If the initial study is negative, an angiography catheter may be left in place for a short period to allow for repeating the study if bleeding recurs. A positive arteriogram demonstrates accumulation of contrast material at the sight of the bleeding diverticulum (Figure 27–11).

Traditionally, nuclear medicine scans have been used as a screening tool to identify those patients actively bleeding who will subsequently undergo angiography. Unfortunately, no study has demonstrated that bleeding scans reduce the number of negative angiograms. The roles of the angiography and the bleeding scans vary from hospital to hospital based on local availability and expertise.

Barium enema no longer plays a role in the evaluation of the acutely bleeding patient. Diagnostically, the detection of diverticula by contrast enema implies neither causality nor localization of the bleeding episode. Therapeutically, retention of barium within the bowel lumen may preclude angiography and colonoscopy, both of which are better for localization and treatment of the bleeding site. After resolution of the acute bleeding episode, contrast enema may have a role in diagnosis of neoplastic lesions and confirmation of the presence of diverticulosis.

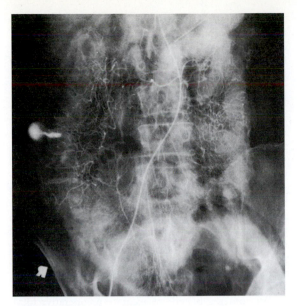

Figure 27–11. Superior mesenteric arteriogram demonstrating extravasated contrast material in a bleeding diverticulum of the ascending colon. This angiographic sign is diagnostic of diverticular hemorrhage.

D. ENDOSCOPY

Whenever the nasogastric aspirate is negative for blood and the clinical presentation suggests a lower gastrointestinal source, the first specific diagnostic maneuver should be rigid proctosigmoidoscopy. Although most lower gastrointestinal hemorrhages are found to be emanating from more than 25 cm above the anal verge, proctosigmoidoscopy allows accurate evaluation for the presence of bleeding internal hemorrhoids, rectal neoplasms, hemorrhagic mucosal disorders, and ulcerations. These sources must be ruled out prior to pursuit of more proximal intestinal bleeding with more invasive procedures.

The utility of colonoscopy in patients with lower gastrointestinal bleeding remains controversial. Direct visualization of actual bleeding is relatively uncommon and indirect indicators such as adherent clots and mucosal lesions must often be relied upon. Endoscopy in the acute setting can be extremely difficult because of the large amount of blood in the colon obscuring the lumen and mucosa. Additionally, the blood adversely affects the fiberoptics. The patient is often hemodynamically unstable and administration of sedatives is ill advised.

Colonoscopy in the acute setting—even in the setting of active bleeding—has its proponents. With the use of large volume (4–8 L of polyethylene glycol solution) lavage administered orally or by nasogastric tube the colonic lumen can be cleared adequately of blood in most patients and colonoscopy safely performed. A probable or definite bleeding site can be visualized in more than 75% of patients with lower gastrointestinal bleeding, of which approximately half of cases are attributed to diverticulosis. In the hands of dedicated and experienced endoscopists, findings or "stigmata" of a definite site of diverticular hemorrhage may be found in up to 40% of cases of presumed diverticular hemorrhage. These findings include visualization of a bleeding diverticulum, accumulation of fresh blood after clearing the colon, a visible vessel at the mouth of a diverticulum, and an adherent clot that persists despite vigorous irrigation of the mucosa. Injection or coagulation therapy (bipolar or heater probe) of the actively bleeding site or a nonbleeding visible site has been reported to arrest acute bleeding and reduce the recurrence of rebleeding. Tattooing of the bleeding with a pigmented dye can also be performed to assist with subsequent localization of the bleeding site at surgery, if needed. It must be emphasized that thus far this high efficacy of colonoscopic therapy for actively bleeding diverticular hemorrhage is reported only at certain institutions.

Differential Diagnosis

In the majority of cases massive lower gastrointestinal hemorrhage derives from one of two causes: colonic diverticula or arteriovenous malformations (angiodysplasia). It is debatable which of these lesions is more common, but both are prevalent in the aged population. As is the case with colonic diverticula, a disproportionate number of bleeding episodes attributable to angiodysplasia derive from the right colon. Also, like diverticula, the pattern of bleeding from angiodysplasia is typically one of recurrent episodes. The intermittent nature of the bleeding frequently foils attempts at definitive localization if they are not performed in a timely manner. Visceral angiographic criteria that identify bleeding angiodysplastic lesions include (1) early and prolonged filling of a draining vein, (2) tufts of small arteries, and (3) evidence of active extravasation into the lumen.

Inflammatory bowel disease and ischemic colitis occasionally present with massive lower intestinal bleeding. Although in ulcerative colitis there is a tendency to bleed more frequently, severe bleeding is more commonly a result of Crohn's disease. This is because ulcerative colitis is a mucosal disease, involving smaller blood vessels, and Crohn's may involve the larger submucosal vessels. Patients with colitis as a source of bleeding usually have significant abdominal pain and tenderness. Proctoscopic examination may be helpful in ulcerative colitis, and occasionally in Crohn's disease, in identifying the lesions. The rectum is usually spared in ischemic colitis because of its dual blood supply.

Colorectal neoplasms account for less than 10% of lower intestinal hemorrhage. The majority of symptomatic bleeds are due to malignant tumors rather than polyps, and are associated with slow, chronic blood loss. Rectal causes of severe bleeding include varices, radiation proctitis, and ulcers. An appropriate history and proctoscopy will identify these patients. Occasionally, a patient will present with a Meckel's diverticulum that contains gastric mucosa responsible for ulceration and bleeding. They are more common in younger patients and can be identified with a Meckel's technetium scan.

Complications

The complications associated with diverticular bleeding include all of those associated with acute massive blood loss. Myocardial ischemia, cerebral vascular accidents, and acute oliguric renal failure are the principal organ injuries that account for the major morbidity in the elderly population predisposed to diverticular hemorrhage.

Treatment

A. MEDICAL THERAPY

The medical therapy for diverticular hemorrhage initially is largely supportive and consists of intravenous fluid administration, correction of coagulopathies, and blood transfusion as necessary. Anticoagulants and antiplatelet agents are discontinued. Hemodynamically unstable patients and those with evidence of cardiac ischemia are resuscitated and monitored in an intensive care unit.

Options for medical treatment of identified diverticular bleeding include angiographic and endoscopic interventions. If the bleeding site is identified on angiography, superselective embolization may be performed. The patient must be closely followed, though, because ischemia with full thickness bowel necrosis may develop. More commonly, vasopressin infusion with a selective catheter can be carried out. The infusion is begun at 0.2 units/min and doubled to 0.4 units/min if needed. The catheter is left in place for 12 hours, after which the vasopressin is tapered. Approximately 50% of patients will rebleed and require surgical intervention. The temporary cessation of bleeding allows for resuscitation and conversion of an emergent operation to a more elective one. Potential complications of vasopressin include cardiac ischemia and fluid and electrolyte disturbances.

When visualized endoscopically, bicap electrocautery, heater probe coagulation, injection sclerotherapy, epinephrine injection, and laser photocoagulation may be performed. Coagulation carries a significant risk of perforation and patients must have close follow-up.

B. SURGICAL THERAPY

Despite optimal medical therapy a small subset of patients requires operative intervention. This includes patients who have unremitting bleeding and those presenting with recurrent episodes of bleeding. For all patients every attempt possible should be made to identify the location of the bleeding lesion preoperatively. If localization has been possible, a segmental colectomy is performed. A primary anastomosis can be performed in the majority of cases because of the cathartic effect of the blood. The same surgical options apply for emergent surgery in diverticular bleeding as for diverticulitis, including stoma creation and on-table lavage if necessary.

Without the benefit of accurate preoperative localization of the bleeding site, blind segmental colectomy has no place in the treatment of lower intestinal bleeding as it is associated with a 30% rebleeding rate. The patient should undergo operative exploration after a proctosigmoidoscopy has been performed to rule out a rectal source of bleeding. Upon exploration, the small bowel is examined for evidence of intraluminal blood. It is not uncommon for blood to backwash a short distance into the ileum from the ileocecal valve and this should not be misinterpreted as small bowel hemorrhage. If a significant portion of the small bowel is blood filled, on-table enteroscopy should be done. In the absence of an identified noncolonic source, an abdominal colectomy should be performed. A primary iliorectal anastomosis can be safely done in most cases. The procedure has an acceptable mortality rate of less than 10%, a rebleeding rate of less than 10%, and acceptable postoperative bowel function. The majority of patients will have two to four bowel movements per day and can be controlled with fiber and antimotility agents.

Prognosis

Approximately 80–90% of patients with acute diverticular bleeding will have spontaneous cessation of hemorrhage. The risk of rebleeding after the initial event is 25% and increases to 50% with a second episode. Among the minority of patients who require surgical intervention to control exsanguinating or persistent hemorrhage, the operative mortality rate is 5–10% and far less than those of other treatment modalities in this subset of patients.

REFERENCES

Ambrosetti P et al: Acute left colonic diverticulitis-compared performance of computed tomography and water-soluble contrast enema: prospective evaluation of 420 patients. Dis Col Rect 2000;43:1363.

Gordon PH: Diverticular disease of the colon. In: *Principles and Practice of Surgery for the Colon, Rectum and Anus,* 2nd ed. Gordon PH, Nivatvongs S (editors). Quality Medical Publishing Inc., 1999.

Gordon RL et al: Selective arterial embolization for the control of lower gastrointestinal hemorrhage. Am J Surg 1997;174:24.

Hinchey EF, Schaal PG, Richards GK: Treatment of perforated diverticular disease of the colon. Adv Surg 1978;12:85.

Jensen DM et al: Urgent colonosocopy for the diagnosis and treatment of severe diverticular hemorrhage. N Engl M Med 2000;342:78.

Schlachta CM et al: Determinants of outcomes in laparoscopic colorectal surgery: a multiple regression analysis of 416 resections. Surg Endosc 2000;14:258.

Schoetz DJ: Diverticular disease of the colon: a century-old problem. Dis Col Rect 1999;42:703.

Schoetz DJ et al: Controversies in diverticular disease. Sem Col Rect Surg 2000;11:196.

Schwesinger WH et al: Operative management of diverticular emergencies: strategies and outcomes. Arch Surg 2000;135:558.

Stabile BE: Preoperative percutaneous drainage of diverticular abscesses. Am J Surg 1990;159:99.

Wong DW et al: Practice parameters for the treatment of sigmoid diverticulitis—supporting documentation. Dis Col Rect 2000;43:290.

Young-Fadok TM et al: Colonic diverticular disease. Curr Probl Surg 2000;37:457.

Zuckerman GR, Prakash C: Acute lower intestinal bleeding. Part H: etiology, therapy and outcomes. Gastrointest Endosc 1999;49:228.

Anorectal Diseases[1]

Mark Lane Welton, MD

■ GENERAL ANATOMIC CONSIDERATIONS

Embryologic considerations are important when considering the epithelium, innervation, vascular supply, and venous and lymphatic drainage of the anorectum. The rectum, endodermal in origin, is derived from the dorsal component of the cloaca, which is partitioned by the anorectal septum. The anal canal arises from an invagination of ectodermal tissue. The anorectum develops in the 8-week embryo from the fusion of the rectum and the anal canal, which occurs when the anal membrane ruptures. The dentate line marks the point of fusion and the transition from endodermal to ectodermal tissue.

The rectum is approximately 12–15 cm long. It extends from the rectosigmoid junction, marked by the fusion of the tenia, to the anal canal, marked by the passage into the pelvic floor musculature (Figure 28–1). The rectum lies in the sacrum and has three distinct curves resulting in folds that are visible on endoscopy and known as the **valves of Houston.** The proximal and distal curves are convex to the left, and the middle curve is convex to the right. The middle curve roughly marks the anterior peritoneal reflection, which is generally 6–8 cm above the anus. Viewed from the abdomen, the rectum is seen to gradually transition from intraperitoneal to extraperitoneal beginning posteriorly at 12–15 cm from the anus. It becomes completely extraperitoneal at 6–8 cm from the anus. The rectum is "fixed" posteriorly, laterally, and anteriorly by the presacral or Waldeyer's fascia, the lateral ligaments, and Denonvilliers' fascia, respectively.

The anatomic anal canal starts at the **dentate line,** the junction of colorectal mucosa and anal mucosa, and ends at the **anal verge,** the junction of the anal mucosa with the perianal skin. However, the surgical anal canal is more clinically relevant. It extends from the muscular diaphragm of the pelvic floor to the anal verge. The **anal canal** is a 3- to 4-cm-long collapsed slit that tilts posteriorly from the anal verge. The anal canal is "supported" by the surrounding **anal sphincter mechanism,** composed of the internal and external sphincters. The **internal sphincter** is a specialized continuation of the circular muscle of the rectum. It is an involuntary muscle that is normally contracted at rest. The structure and function of the **external sphincter** are controversial; however current evidence suggests that the external sphincter is the spout on a muscular funnel of continuous circumferential functional muscle mass that includes the external sphincter caudally and extends cranially to the conical puborectalis and levator ani muscles. The external sphincter is composed of voluntary striated muscle. The conjoined longitudinal muscle separates the internal and external sphincter. It is created by the aggregation of fibers from the longitudinal muscle of the rectum, fibers from the levator ani, and fibers from the puborectalis. Some fibers from this muscle become the corrugator cutis ani and insert on the perianal skin creating rugal folds and a puckered appearance. Other fibers traverse the internal sphincter and support the internal hemorrhoids as the mucosal suspensory ligaments.

The histologies of the rectum and anus are distinct. The rectum is composed of an innermost layer of mucosa that overlies the submucosa, the circular and longitudinal muscles, and in the proximal rectum, serosa. The mucosa is subdivided into three layers: (1) epithelial cells, (2) lamina propria, and (3) muscularis mucosa. The **muscularis mucosa** is a fine sheet of muscle containing a network of lymphatics. Lymphatics are essentially absent above this level, making the muscularis mucosa critical in defining metastatic potential of malignancies.

As the rectum enters the narrow musculature of the pelvic floor and becomes the anal canal, the tissue is thrown into folds known as the **columns of Morgagni.** At the lower end of the columns lie small pockets called crypts, some of which communicate with anal glands lying in or near the intersphincteric plane. The epithelium of the anal canal is composed of three types: colorectal mucosa is present in the proximal 2–3 cm; tran-

[1]Portions of this chapter are reprinted from Way LW, Doherty GM (eds): *Current Surgical Diagnosis & Treatment,* 11th ed. New York: McGraw-Hill, 2003.

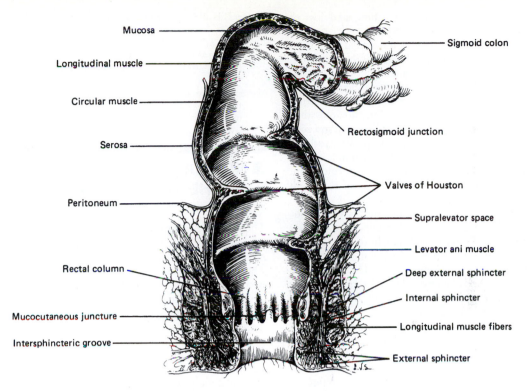

Figure 28–1. Anatomy of the anorectum. [Reproduced, with permission, from Welton ML: Anorectum. In: *Current Surgical Diagnosis & Treatment,* 11th ed. Way LW, Doherty GM (editors). McGraw-Hill, 2002.]

sitional epithelium is at and just above the dentate line; and anoderm, a squamous mucosa, is below the dentate line. The anoderm is a squamous mucosa rich in nerve fibers but lacking in secondary appendages (hair follicles, apocrine glands, and sweat glands). The anal verge marks the true mucocutaneous junction.

The pelvic floor is a consortium of funnel-shaped muscles that separates the pelvis and the perineum. It is composed of the levator ani and puborectalis muscles. The levator ani consists of two broad, thin, symmetric muscular sheets that originate around the pelvic sidewall and in the sacrospinous ligament that forms the principal support of the pelvic viscera. The puborectalis muscle originates on the posterior aspect of the pubis, forms a sling around the rectum, and returns to the posterior aspect of the pubis. The fibers of the puborectalis are situated immediately adjacent to and below the innermost component of the levator ani muscle, where they are intimately associated with the upper posterolateral fibers of the deep external anal sphincter. Thus, the puborectalis serves as a bridge between the broad sheet-like component of the funnel created by the leva-

tors and the narrow spout of the funnel created by the external anal sphincter. The puborectalis in the contracted state is responsible for the normal acute anorectal angle between the levators and the external sphincters. It is also responsible for the shelf that is normally palpable on digital examination as one passes from the distal narrow lumen of the "anus" to the more proximal capacious lumen of the "rectum."

The innervation of the rectum is via the sympathetic and parasympathetic nervous systems. The sympathetic nerves originate from the lumbar segments L1–3, form the inferior mesenteric plexus, travel through the superior hypogastric plexus, and descend as the hypogastric nerves to the pelvic plexus.

The parasympathetic nerves arise from the second, third, and fourth sacral roots and join the hypogastric nerves anterior and lateral to the rectum to form the pelvic plexus, from which fibers pass to form the periprostatic plexus. Sympathetic and parasympathetic fibers pass from the pelvic and periprostatic plexi to the rectum and internal anal sphincter as well as the prostate, bladder, and penis. Injury to these nerves or plexi can lead to impotence, bladder dysfunction, and loss of normal defecatory mechanisms.

The internal anal sphincter is innervated with sympathetic and parasympathetic fibers. Both are inhibitory and keep the sphincter in a constant state of contraction. The external sphincters are skeletal muscles innervated by the pudendal nerve with fibers that originate from S2–4. Above the dentate line, noxious stimuli are experienced as ill-defined dull sensations conducted through afferent fibers of the parasympathetic nerves. Below the dentate line, the epithelium is exquisitely sensitive. Cutaneous sensations of heat, cold, pain, and touch are conveyed through the inferior rectal and perineal branches of the pudendal nerve.

The arterial supply of the anorectum is via the superior, middle, and inferior rectal arteries. The superior rectal artery is the terminal branch of the inferior mesenteric artery and descends in the mesorectum. It supplies the upper and middle rectum. The middle rectal arteries arise from the internal iliac arteries and enter the rectum anterolaterally at the level of the pelvic floor musculature. They supply the lower two-thirds of the rectum. Collaterals exist between the middle and superior rectal arteries. The inferior rectal arteries, branches of the internal pudendal arteries, enter posterolaterally, do not anastomose with the blood supply to the middle rectum, and provide blood supply to the anal sphincters and epithelium.

The venous drainage of the anorectum is via the superior, middle, and inferior rectal veins draining into the portal and systemic systems. The superior rectal veins drain the upper and middle third of the rectum. They empty into the portal system via the inferior mesenteric vein. The middle rectal veins drain the lower rectum and upper anal canal into the systemic system via the internal iliac veins. The inferior rectal veins drain the lower anal canal, communicating with the pudendal veins and draining into the internal iliac veins. There is communication between the venous systems. This allows low rectal cancers to spread via the portal and systemic systems.

Lymphatic drainage of the upper and middle rectum is into the inferior mesenteric nodes. Lymph from the lower rectum may also drain into the inferior mesenteric system or into the systems along the middle and inferior rectal arteries, posteriorly along the middle sacral artery, and anteriorly through channels in the retrovesical or rectovaginal septum. These drain to the iliac nodes and ultimately to the periaortic nodes. Lymphatics from the anal canal above the dentate line drain via the superior rectal lymphatics to the inferior mesenteric lymph nodes and laterally to the internal iliac nodes. Below the dentate line, drainage occurs primarily to the inguinal nodes but can occur to the inferior or superior rectal lymph nodes.

Kodner IJ et al: Colon, rectum, and anus. In: *Principles of Surgery,* 7th ed. Schwartz SI (editor). McGraw-Hill, 1999.

Nivatvongs S, Gordon PH: Surgical anatomy. In: *Principles and Practice of Surgery for the Colon, Rectum, and Anus.* Gordon PH, Nivatvongs S (editors). Quality Medical Publishing, 1999.

Welton ML, Varma MG, Amerhauser A: Colon, rectum and anus. In: *Surgery. Basic Science and Clinical Evidence.* Norton et al (editors). Springer, 2000.

■ NORMAL FUNCTION OF THE ANORECTUM

The normal function of the anorectum is storage and appropriate release of intestinal waste products. The rectum functions mainly as a capacitance storage vessel. The normal rectum holds 650–1200 mL of waste. Resting rectal pressure is approximately 10 mm Hg. Changes in intrarectal pressure are primarily a reflection of intraabdominal pressure changes, as the rectum itself has little peristaltic function.

The function of the pelvic floor is complex and poorly understood. The levator ani create a broad muscular funnel suspending the rectum in a muscular sling that pulls the rectum forward at the anorectal junction creating an acute anorectal angle. The acuity of the angle created by the puborectalis is critical for maintaining continence. The puborectalis contracts (increasing the anorectal angle) during maneuvers that increase intraabdominal pressure (such as coughing, laughing), maintaining continence, but relaxes, opening the angle, when a Valsalva maneuver is performed as part of normal defecation. The levators also contain sensory fibers that detect pelvic fullness and therefore are believed to be important in the sensation of the urge to defecate.

The internal sphincter generates 85% of the resting anal sphincter tone. It is innervated with sympathetic and parasympathetic fibers that are both inhibitory and keep the sphincter in a constant state of contraction. The external sphincters are skeletal muscles innervated by the pudendal nerve with fibers that originate from S2–4. The external sphincter provides 15% of the resting anal sphincter tone and 100% of the voluntary squeeze pressures. Voluntary contraction of the external sphincter can double the resting anal sphincter pressure but voluntary contraction cannot be sustained for more than 3 minutes.

Hemorrhoids are important participants in maintaining continence and minimizing trauma during defecation. They function as protective pillows that engorge with blood during the act of defecation molding the stool and protecting the anoderm from direct trauma when stool passes. They also act as cushions that help seal the anal canal and prevent leakage of gas and stool. Hemorrhoidal tissues become engorged during defecation and lifting, and with other conditions that increase intraabdominal pressure such as obesity and pregnancy.

Defecation is a complex event involving multiple steps for successful evacuation. The anal sphincters function in concert with the levator ani, the puborectalis, and the rectum to promote defecation at socially acceptable times. Continence is maintained so long as intrarectal pressures are lower than internal and external sphincter pressures. In the resting state the rectum is not completely empty, however residual contents are not sensed. The rectum relaxes (accommodates) and sensory fibers in the levators adapt to the sense of pelvic fullness allowing these contents to remain. Periodically, the internal sphincter relaxes, allowing the rectal contents to drop down into the anal canal where they are sampled by the sensitive anoderm. After sampling, the external sphincter contracts and the contents are pushed back into the rectum. This "sampling reflex" or **rectoanal inhibitory reflex** also occurs up to seven times daily during periods of rectal distention. Progressive distention of the rectum eventually causes continuous inhibition of the internal sphincter and relaxation of the external sphincter causing an urge to defecate. If one wishes to evacuate, a sitting/squatting position is assumed (straightening the anorectal angle), intraabdominal pressure is increased by a Valsalva maneuver, the puborectalis relaxes (further shortening the anal canal and promoting formation of a muscular funnel), and reflex relaxation of the internal sphincter occurs as fecal contents enter the anal canal. The Valsalva maneuver primarily accomplishes evacuation.

Kodner IJ et al: Colon, rectum, and anus. In: *Principles of Surgery,* 7th ed. Schwartz SI (editor). McGraw-Hill, 1999.

Lestar B et al: The internal anal sphincter can not close the anal canal completely. Int J Colorectal Dis 1992;7(3):159.

Loder PB et al: Haemorrhoids: pathology, pathophysiology and aetiology. Br J Surg 1994;81(7):946.

Madoff RD et al: Fecal incontinence. N Engl J Med 1992;326(15):1002.

Schouten WR, Gordon PH: Physiology. In: *Principles and Practice of Surgery for the Colon, Rectum, and Anus.* Gordon PH, Nivatvongs S (editors). Quality Medical Publishing, 1999.

Sjodalil R, Ralibook O: Incontinence and normal sphincter function. In: *Colorectal Physiology: Fecal Incontinence.* Kuijpers HC (editor). CRC Press, 1994.

Welton ML, Varma MG, Amerhauser A: Colon, rectum and anus. In: *Surgery. Basic Science and Clinical Evidence.* Norton et al (editors). Springer, 2000.

■ DYSFUNCTION OF THE ANORECTUM

INCONTINENCE

 ESSENTIALS OF DIAGNOSIS

- *Inability to control elimination of rectal contents.*
- *Characterization of rectal contents that are uncontrolled.*
- *Characterization of timing of incontinence.*

General Considerations

Continence is dependent upon rectal compliance, anorectal sensation, anorectal reflexes, and anal sphincter function. The stool consistency (liquid versus solid) and quantity of stool also affect continence. The incidence of fecal incontinence is difficult to assess due to underreporting and lack of agreement as to what constitutes incontinence (eg, minor seepage versus complete incontinence). Although it is well accepted that incontinence is more commonly found in parous women, a high prevalence also occurs in men.

In women, the external sphincter is a thin band of muscle anteriorly, and thus especially susceptible to complete transection in this location resulting in incontinence. Obstetrical trauma during delivery may cause mechanical injury to the external sphincter. There is an increased incidence of incontinence after third-degree perineal tears, multiple vaginal deliveries, and infection of an episiotomy repair.

Neurogenic causes of incontinence include pudendal nerve stretch secondary to prolonged labor or to chronic straining during defecation. Vaginal deliveries are associated with reversible pudendal nerve injury in 80% of primagravida births. The injury may be unilateral or bilateral. If the nerve injury is permanent or is repeated multiple times, denervation and weakening of the external sphincter and pelvic floor result. The neuropathy and sphincter dysfunction progress because a weakened pelvic floor is unable to withstand increased intraabdominal pressure leading to further perineal descent and stretch injury. Similarly, descending perineum syndrome leads to cumulative stretch injury. Straining causes descent of the pelvic floor resulting in stretch of the pudendal nerve over the ischial spine.

Incontinence may also result from the treatment of perianal abscesses, fistula-in-ano, or perianal Crohn's disease due to disruption or division of the external sphincter.

Other causes of incontinence include systemic diseases affecting either the muscular or neurologic systems (eg, scleroderma, multiple sclerosis, dermatomyositis, and diabetes) or local anorectal problems (eg, radiation proctitis with fibrosis and decreased rectal compliance and tumors of the distal colon and rectum). Incontinence may also occur in people with normal anorectal neuromuscular function due to diarrhea or fecal impaction with overflow incontinence.

Clinical Findings

A. SYMPTOMS AND SIGNS

It is important to distinguish complete incontinence (which has major social consequences and virtually always denotes a significant neurologic or muscular disorder) from partial incontinence. **Complete incontinence** results in lack of control of gas, liquid, and solid stool. By contrast patients with **partial incontinence** have the ability to control solid stool but varying inability to control liquid stool and/or gas. Urgency, seepage, and soiling may occur regularly or intermittently, depending on the nature of the stool presenting to the rectum. Seepage of small amounts of fecal-stained mucus is extremely common with aging due to prolapsed hemorrhoidal tissue and inadequate dietary fiber. Soiling with urgency may be seen in patients with normal sphincteric function but a poorly distensible rectum due to proctitis or irritable bowel syndrome. However patients complaining of gross incontinence of solid fecal matter or an inability to sense stool until after incontinence has occurred often have a neurologic or muscular injury. Physical examination should include inspection and digital examination. On inspection, one should look for evidence of seepage or maceration of the perianal skin. The presence of external hemorrhoids or prolapsed internal hemorrhoids should be noted. Patients with gross incontinence may have a patulous anus. The anus should be inspected when the patient is instructed to squeeze: damage to the external sphincter may result in asymmetry or focal loss of corrugation of the anal verge. The patient should be instructed to perform a Valsalva to look for exaggerated descent of the perineum with straining or prolapse of hemorrhoidal tissue. Neurologic function is assessed grossly by looking for an anal wink and by testing for cutaneous pinprick sensation on both sides of the perianal gluteal region. Digital examination may detect a reduction in resting sphincter tone (primarily internal sphincter) or diminished voluntary squeeze pressures (primarily external sphincter).

B. LABORATORY AND IMAGING STUDIES

Patients with incontinence warrant anoscopy and proctoscopy to exclude fissures, fistula, hemorrhoidal disease, proctitis, and anorectal neoplasms. Further evaluation usually is not required in patients with minor seepage alone. Patients with complete or partial incontinence usually warrant further evaluation. Anorectal manometry, transrectal ultrasound, and pudendal nerve latency studies may all be part of the evaluation of the incontinent patient.

Anorectal manometry defines the presence of sphincteric injury by measuring the resting pressure, maximum squeeze pressure, sphincter length and symmetry, minimum sensory volume, presence or absence of the rectoanal inhibitory reflex, and ability to relax the puborectalis muscle. Normal resting pressures generally range from 40–80 mm Hg and maximal squeeze pressures range from 80–160 mm Hg. The minimum sensory volume is approximately 10 mL. The rectoanal inhibitory reflex is seen as a decrease in resting anal pressure when an air-filled balloon distends the rectum. The ability of the patient to relax the pelvic floor appropriately during defecation is assessed with the balloon expulsion test, which requires the patient to expel a fully inflated 60-mL latex balloon.

Transrectal ultrasound of the internal and external sphincters can provide imaging of anal sphincter defects. Transrectal ultrasound has largely replaced electromyography (EMG) for documentation of sphincter injury.

Pudendal nerve latency studies define the presence of neurologic injury in incontinent patients. If one or both nerves are injured success in surgical or nonsurgical treatment of incontinence may be diminished. The study is performed by placing a gloved finger with a stimulating electrode at the tip of the finger in the rectum and stimulating the pudendal nerve as it traverses the ischial spine. An electrode at the base of the examining finger records the delay between stimulation and contraction of the external sphincter. A normal "delay" is 2.0 ± 0.2 seconds. This may be prolonged with age, after childbirth, in individuals with a history of excessive straining to defecate and perineal descent, and in certain systemic disease states such as diabetes and multiple sclerosis.

Differential Diagnosis

The causes of incontinence are discussed above. In addition, incontinence may result from obstructed defecation secondary to tumor or intussusception. Rare patients with straining to defecate may develop intussusception, causing obstruction and apparent constipation. After straining is stopped, there is uncontrolled release of fluid. This may be detected by defecography.

Chronic straining at defecation stretches the pudendal nerve over the ischial spine, leading to "idiopathic fecal incontinence" in the elderly.

Treatment

Patients with seepage or minor incomplete incontinence may be treated with conservative measures. Patients should be given fiber supplements to reduce stool liquidity and mucus seepage after bowel movements. Symptomatic hemorrhoids should be treated. Patients should be instructed to cleanse the perinal area with Tucks™ or nonperfumed lanolin wipes but should avoid excessive cleansing with water or soaps, which may lead to irritation and dermatitis. Application of a cotton ball adjacent to the anus after bowel movements may absorb small amounts of seepage. Patients with urgency due to irritable bowel syndrome or proctitis may benefit from use of loperamide. Partial incontinence caused by weakness of the external sphincter or decreased rectal sensation secondary to incomplete neurologic injury or aging may respond to retraining with biofeedback and sphincteric muscle exercises.

The algorithm for the diagnosis and treatment of complete incontinence is summarized in Figure 28–2. If a sphincteric defect is limited and there is no neurologic injury, surgical correction with an overlapping sphincter reconstruction restores continence by reestablishing a complete ring of muscle. However, if there is extensive loss of sphincter muscle or severe neurologic injury, simple overlapping repair is not as successful, and consideration must be given either to colostomy or to muscle flap or encirclement procedures. The stimulated gracilis, gracilis, and gluteal muscle flap procedures have been reserved for those patients with complete neurologic injury or extensive muscle loss who wish to avoid a colostomy. Success with these muscle wrap procedures is limited. A new artificial sphincter is under trial and early reports are promising.

Anal encirclement procedures with foreign material have been reserved for the critically ill or patients with a short life expectancy. The anal canal is encircled with either a synthetic mesh or a silver wire. Patients are given daily enemas to evacuate the rectum providing a form of continence with artificial obstruction and stimulated evacuation. The foreign body is prone to infection and erosion into the rectum, which often necessitates removal.

Incontinence associated with rectal prolapse resolves after repair of the prolapse if there has not been significant nerve injury. Prior to repair, the prolapsing segment stimulates the rectoanal inhibitory reflex decreasing internal sphincter pressure, and impairing the external sphincter. The incontinence resolves with surgical repair in roughly 70% of patients.

Johanson JF, Lafferty J: Epidemiology of fecal incontinence: the silent affliction. Am J Gastroenterol 1996;91(1):33.

Ko CY et al: Biofeedback is effective therapy for fecal incontinence and constipation. Arch Surg 1997;132(8):829; discussion 833.

Lehur PA et al: Artificial anal sphincter: prospective clinical and manometric evaluation. Dis Colon Rectum 2000;43(8):1100.

Nelson R et al: Community-based prevalence of anal incontinence. JAMA 1995;274(7):559.

Nivatvongs S, Gordon PH: Surgical anatomy. In: *Principles and Practice of Surgery for the Colon, Rectum, and Anus.* Gordon PH, Nivatvongs S (editors). Quality Medical Publishing, 1999.

Osterberg A et al: Results of neurophysiologic evaluation in fecal incontinence. Dis Colon Rectum 2000;43(9):1256.

Ryhammer AM et al: Long-term effect of vaginal deliveries on anorectal function in normal perimenopausal women. Dis Colon Rectum 1996;39(8):852.

OBSTRUCTED DEFECATION

 ESSENTIALS OF DIAGNOSIS

- *Inability to voluntarily evacuate rectal contents.*
- *Normal colonic transit time.*

General Considerations

Obstructed defecation may result from anal stenosis, pelvic floor dysfunction, or abnormal rectal fixation. The most common cause of anal stenosis is scarring after anal surgery, in particular, inexpertly performed hemorrhoidectomies. Other causes include anal tumors, Crohn's disease, radiation injury, recurrent anal ulcers, infection, and trauma.

Pelvic floor dysfunction, alternatively referred to as nonrelaxing puborectalis syndrome, anismus, or paradoxical pelvic floor contraction, is a functional disorder in which the neuromuscular function of the pelvic floor and anus is normal but voluntary control is dysfunctional. In health, the puborectalis is contracted "at rest" maintaining the anorectal angle. During defecation, the muscle relaxes and evacuation occurs. In nonrelaxing puborectalis syndrome the patient does not relax the puborectalis and instead maintains or increases (paradoxical contraction) the anorectal angle. Thus, the patient performs a Valsalva maneuver against an obstructed outlet and elimination does not occur or is significantly diminished.

Patients who chronically strain at stool whether from chronic constipation or pelvic floor dysfunction may develop lengthening of the attachments of the rec-

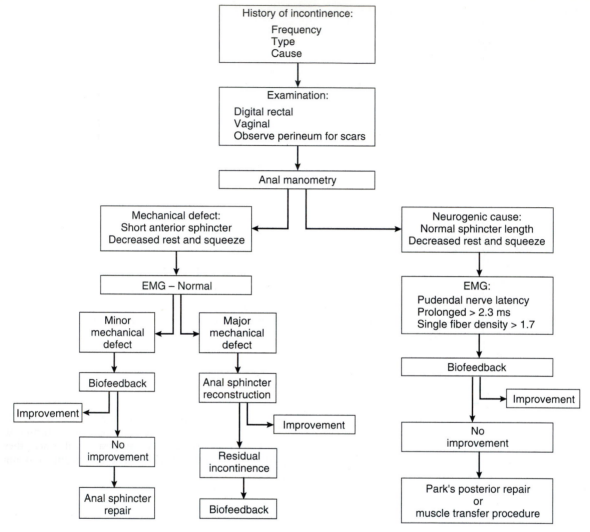

Figure 28–2. Algorithm for work-up and treatment of fecal incontinence.

tum to the sacrum leading to descending perineum syndrome. The increased mobility allows for internal rectal prolapse (intussusception) and in some cases formation of solitary rectal ulcer and rectal procidentia. Intussusception causes outlet obstruction because the upper rectum moves away from the sacrum and telescopes into the more distal rectum.

Clinical Findings

A. SYMPTOMS AND SIGNS

Anal stenosis presents with increasing difficulty with defecation, thin and sometimes painful bowel movements, and bloating. Patients with nonrelaxing pub-

orectalis syndrome similarly complain of straining and anal or pelvic pain, but also complain of constipation, incomplete evacuation, and a need to perform digital maneuvers to evacuate rectal contents. Patients with internal intussusception also complain of constipation, sensations of rectal fullness, or incomplete evacuation, but also note mucous discharge, rectal bleeding, and tenesmus.

Examination of the patient with anal stenosis may reveal postsurgical changes and a stenotic anal canal. Digital examination may be quite painful or impossible. Digital examination of the patient with nonrelaxing puborectalis syndrome may reveal a tender pelvic muscular diaphragm. During the digital examination if the patient is directed to squeeze to mimic holding in flatus, a paradoxical relaxation and Valsalva may occur. Similarly, if the patient is asked to "bear down" to simulate a bowel movement they may paradoxically contract the external sphincters and puborectalis muscles. Digital examination of the patient with internal intussusception may be much the same as that for nonrelaxing puborectalis but with the additional findings of a mass. The mass is the lead point of the intussusceptum. It may be anterior and ulcerated (solitary rectal ulcer) or circumferential. The ulcer is 4–12 cm from the anal verge and is the ischemic traumatized lead point of the internal intussusception. Sigmoidoscopy may reveal the circumferential intussusceptum or an ulcerated mass that appears malignant. Pathologic examination reveals diffuse submucosal cysts with a characteristic fibrosis pattern distinguishing it from colorectal malignancy.

B. LABORATORY AND IMAGING STUDIES

No additional studies of the patient with anal stenosis are required, but patients with nonrelaxing puborectalis syndrome and internal intussusception should have defecography, colonic transit studies, anorectal manometry with the balloon expulsion test, and barium enema or colonoscopy.

Patients with nonrelaxing puborectalis syndrome or internal intussusception will have a normal colon on barium enema or colonoscopy and normal colonic transit to the rectosigmoid. On balloon expulsion test, they will be unable to expel the balloon.

With nonrelaxing puborectal syndrome, cinedefecography will demonstrate persistent anterior displacement of the rectum on the lateral view and paradoxic contraction of the puborectalis with attempted defecation. In the patient with internal intussusception, defecography will document intussusception.

Differential Diagnosis

Causes of anal pain include a fissure, thrombosed external hemorrhoids, perirectal abscess, malignancy, foreign body, and proctalgia fugax. Proctalgia fugax (levator syndrome), a diagnosis of exclusion, is suggested when a patient complains of pain that awakens him or her from sleep. The pain is generally left-sided, short-lived, and relieved by heat, dilation, or muscle relaxants. The patient often has a history of migraines and may report the occurrence of pain in relation to stressful events.

Other causes of obstructed defecation include fecal impaction, rectal or anal cancer, descending perineum syndrome, and rectocoele. The work-up of these complex patients is diagrammed in Figure 28–3. Fecal impaction may occur as a result of nonrelaxing puborectalis syndrome, and therapy is therefore directed toward that disorder.

Treatment

A. MEDICAL

Mild anal stenosis may be treated successfully with gentle dilation and bulk agents. Nonrelaxing puborectalis syndrome is best treated with biofeedback. The puborectalis is retrained to relax during the act of defecation, which allows the act to proceed without obstruction. Mild to moderate intussusception is treated with bulk agents, modification of bowel habits, and reassurance. The patient is instructed to stimulate a bowel movement in the morning and avoid the urge to defecate the remainder of the day because the fullness they sense is the proximal rectum intussuscepting into the distal rectum. The urge to defecate resolves with time, as does the intussusception.

B. SURGICAL

Severe anal stenosis is treated surgically if there is no evidence of active disease (ie, Crohn's disease) and healthy tissue is available to perform the anoplasty. Both procedures involve incision of the stenotic anus, mobilization of the surrounding skin, and advancement of the healthy tissue into the closure relieving the stenosis.

Prognosis

The prognosis for anal stenosis is excellent if there is no evidence of active disease. Patients with nonrelaxing puborectalis have excellent results with biofeedback, but may require retraining. Most patients with mild to moderate intussusception do quite well once they are reassured that an abnormality exists and it is not malignant.

Glia A et al: Constipation assessed on the basis of colorectal physiology. Scand J Gastroenterol 1998;33(12):1273.

Mertz H et al: Symptoms and physiology in severe chronic constipation. Am J Gastroenterol 1999;94(1):131.

Nyam DC et al: Long-term results of surgery for chronic constipation [published erratum appears in Dis Colon Rectum 1997 May;40(5):529]. Dis Colon Rectum 1997;40(3):273.

ABNORMAL RECTAL FIXATION

 ESSENTIALS OF DIAGNOSIS

- *Increased mobility of the rectum.*
- *Altered defecation (constipation, incontinence, or both).*
- *Digital maneuvers to defecate.*

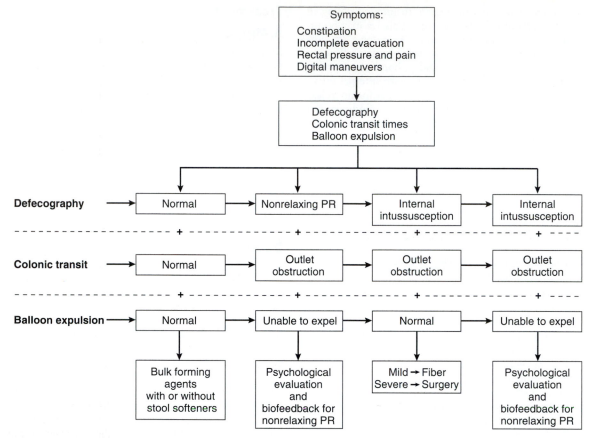

Figure 28–3. Algorithm for work-up and treatment of obstructed defecation. PR, puborectoris.

General Considerations

Abnormal rectal fixation is a group of diseases in which the attachment of the rectum to the sacrum has lengthened, allowing the rectum to block the act of defecation, to protrude into the vagina, or to prolapse through the anus. The reason for the increased mobility appears to be related to chronic straining. This may be secondary to colonic dysmotility or nonrelaxing puborectalis syndrome.

Clinical Findings

A. SYMPTOMS AND SIGNS

Internal intussusception leads to complaints of rectal fullness, urge to defecate, and if associated with solitary rectal ulcer syndrome, complaints of rectal bleeding, mucous discharge, or tenesmus. Patients with rectal prolapse complain of mucous discharge, progressive incontinence, pain, and bleeding, and upon direct questioning, report the rectum "falls out."

Digital examination of the patient with internal intussusception may reveal a mass. This is the lead point of the intussusceptum and may be mistaken for a malignancy. The mass may be anterior and ulcerated (solitary rectal ulcer) or circumferential. The ulcer is 4–12 cm from the anal verge and is the ischemic traumatized lead point of the internal intussusception. Sigmoidoscopy may reveal the circumferential intussusceptum or an ulcerated mass that appears malignant.

Physical examination of the patient who presents with an acute episode of rectal prolapse is not difficult. A large mass of prolapsed tissue with concentric mucosal rings will be apparent. However, the diagnosis in the patient with a history of prolapse but without active prolapse may be more difficult. It may be necessary to give the patient an enema and allow evacuation. This often induces prolapse and confirms the diagnosis. Prolapse may also be demonstrated on defecography. Digital examination may reveal decreased or absent sphincter tone.

B. LABORATORY AND IMAGING STUDIES

Patients with internal intussusception and rectal prolapse need anorectal manometry, pudendal nerve latency studies, defecography, and barium enema or colonoscopy. Defecography will document the intussusception or prolapse and may reveal the cause. Evaluation of the entire colon with either barium enema or colonoscopy is necessary to rule out a malignancy.

Differential Diagnosis

Internal intussusception must be differentiated from adenocarcinoma. The patient presentation, physical appearance, and histologic characteristics of the ulcer may be confused with malignancy. However, pathologic examination reveals diffuse submucosal cysts with a characteristic fibrosis pattern that distinguishes it from colorectal malignancy.

Rectal prolapse should be distinguished from hemorrhoidal disease. Rectal prolapse is seen as uninterrupted circumferential rings of mucosa, whereas hemorrhoidal prolapse will be seen as prolapsing tissue with deep grooves between areas of prolapsing edematous tissue.

Complications

The complications of intussusception and prolapse include progression of intussusception to prolapse, nerve injury from prolapse or chronic straining, descending perineum syndrome, bleeding, and incontinence. Severe cases of rectal prolapse may become too edematous to allow reduction and may progress to ischemia and gangrene.

Treatment

A. MEDICAL

Treatment of mild to moderate intussusception is discussed above.

B. SURGICAL

Severe intussusception or rectal prolapse is treated surgically. There are two general categories of operations for severe intussusception or rectal prolapse, abdominal or perineal. The abdominal procedures have a lower recurrence rate and preserve the reservoir capacity of the rectum but submit the patients to a higher risk intraabdominal procedure. The perineal procedures do not require an abdominal incision or an intraabdominal anastomosis but remove the rectum eliminating the rectal reservoir and have a higher recurrence rate. Thus, the abdominal procedures may be preferred over the perineal procedures in low-risk active patients less than 50 years of age and in those who are undergoing other abdominal procedures simultaneously.

The abdominal procedures for patients with severe intussusception or rectal prolapse with normal sphincter function are sigmoid resection with or without rectopexy and rectopexy alone. Both operations require complete mobilization of the entire rectum to the pelvic floor to avoid distal intussusception.

The rectopexy secures the rectum to the sacral hollow. The addition of a sigmoid resection at the time of rectopexy appears to lower the recurrence rate and the incidence of postoperative constipation and does not increase operative morbidity. Rectopexy corrects the mobility of the rectum but does not correct the underlying disorder in patients with pelvic floor dysfunction or chronic constipation. Sigmoid resection removes the site of intussusception and the mobile portion of colon. Thus, in the constipated patient or the patient with a redundant sigmoid colon, resection is preferable to fixation alone. Laparoscopic approaches for the repairs of rectal prolapse are directed at fixation and generally do not include resection. Therefore although no long-term follow-up data are available, one would suspect a higher recurrence rate might be seen.

The perineal approaches to rectal prolapse include anal encirclement and the transanal Delorme procedure and Altemeier procedure. In patients with prolapse with either prohibitively high operative risk or limited life expectancy, an anal encirclement procedure with synthetic mesh or silicone tubes may be performed. This procedure now is utilized less frequently.

The Delorme procedure is essentially a mucosal proctectomy with imbrication of the prolapsing rectal wall. The dissection is started 1–2 cm above the dentate line and is carried to the apex of the prolapsing segment where the mucosa is amputated. The muscle is reefed in with 4–8 heavy absorbable sutures and the mucosa is reapproximated with suture (running or interrupted) or a circular stapler.

The Altemeier procedure is a complete proctectomy and often partial sigmoidectomy. The apex of the prolapsing segment is delivered, placed on traction, and a full thickness incision is made approximately 1 cm above the dentate line. The rectum is everted. The dissection is carried into the deep cul-de-sac anteriorly. The dissection is carried up onto the midline mesorectum and sigmoid mesentery until the redundant segment of bowel has been mobilized. A levatoroplasty plicates the pelvic floor musculature and adds to improved continence by increasing the anorectal angle. The bowel is transected proximally encompassing the redundant bowel and a hand-sewn (heavy absorbable suture) or stapled anastomosis may be performed. The long-term follow-up of patients repaired by the perineal approach is not available, but this approach appears promising, especially in the high-risk patients in whom an abdominal operation is undesirable.

Prognosis

The prognosis for patients with mild to moderate intussusception who are treated with bulk agents is excellent. Those individuals with severe intussusception and those who have rectal prolapse without sphincter dysfunction should do well with either abdominal or perineal approaches. Those with sphincter dysfunction have a 60–70% chance of regaining function. Those who do not have return of sphincter function will not tolerate sigmoid resection. Therefore perineal proctectomy and posterior sphincter enhancement are recommended in these patients because the posterior reconstruction may alter the angle of the rectum or obstruct the outlet sufficiently to allow for continence.

Athanasiadis S et al: The risk of infection of three synthetic materials used in rectopexy with or without colonic resection for rectal prolapse. Int J Colorectal Dis 1996;11(1):42.

Graf W et al: Laparoscopic suture rectopexy. Dis Colon Rectum 1995;38(2):211.

Jacobs LK et al: The best operation for rectal prolapse. Surg Clin North Am 1997;77(1):49.

Mollen RM et al: Effects of rectal mobilization and lateral ligaments division on colonic and anorectal function. Dis Colon Rectum 2000;43(9):1283.

Wexner SD et al: Laparoscopic colorectal surgery: analysis of 140 cases. Surg Endosc 1996;10(2):133.

HEMORRHOIDS

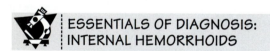

ESSENTIALS OF DIAGNOSIS: INTERNAL HEMORRHOIDS

- *Bright red blood per rectum.*
- *Mucous discharge.*
- *Rectal fullness or discomfort.*

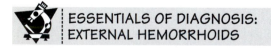

ESSENTIALS OF DIAGNOSIS: EXTERNAL HEMORRHOIDS

- *Sudden, severe perianal pain.*
- *Perianal mass.*

General Considerations

Hemorrhoidal tissues are part of the normal anatomy of the distal rectum and anal canal (see Figure 28–1). **Internal hemorrhoids** are vascular and connective tissue cushions that originate above the dentate line and are lined with rectal or transitional mucosa. **External hemorrhoids** are vascular complexes underlying the richly innervated anoderm.

The disease state of "hemorrhoids" may involve the internal complex, external complex, or both. Internal hemorrhoids become symptomatic when the internal complex becomes chronically engorged or the tissue prolapses into the anal canal due to laxity of the surrounding connective tissue and dilation of the veins. The external hemorrhoids become symptomatic with thrombosis, which leads to acute onset of severe perianal pain. When the thrombosis resolves, the overlying skin may remain enlarged, creating a skin tag.

Internal hemorrhoids may have two main pathophysiologic mechanisms seen most commonly in two distinct groups: older women and younger men. In older women the pathophysiologic mechanism may relate to chronic straining with vascular engorgement and dilatation. This results in disruption of the supporting connective tissue surrounding the vascular channels. The most common cause of prolonged straining is the act of defecation. The stool may be liquid or solid. There is no correlation between hemorrhoids and constipation (infrequent passage of stool), or hemorrhoids and portal hypertension. Hemorrhoids are not dilated vascular channels. Another mechanism, possibly more important in younger men, is that of increased resting pressures within the anal canal leading to decreased venous return, increased venous engorgement, and disruption of the supporting tissues. No precipitating causes have been identified for disease of the external hemorrhoids.

Internal hemorrhoids are traditionally classified by the following scheme: first-degree hemorrhoids—bleedng alone; second-degree hemorrhoids—bleeding and prolapse, but reduce spontaneously; third-degree hemorrhoids—bleeding and prolapse that requires manual reduction; fourth-degree hemorrhoids—bleeding with incarceration that cannot be reduced.

Clinical Findings

A. SYMPTOMS AND SIGNS

Internal hemorrhoids typically do *not* cause pain, but rather, bright red bleeding per rectum, mucous discharge, and a sense of rectal fullness or discomfort. Infrequently internal hemorrhoids will prolapse into the anal canal, incarcerate, thrombose, and necrose. In this instance, patients may complain of pain. Visual inspection of the perineum may reveal a normal-appearing perineum, edema near the involved hemorrhoid, a prolapsed hemorrhoid, or an edematous, gangrenous, incarcerated hemorrhoid. The perineum may be macerated from chronic mucous discharge, the resulting moisture, and local irritation. Anoscopy may reveal tissue with evidence of chronic vascular dilatation, friability, mobility, and squamous metaplasia.

External hemorrhoids may develop suddenly from acute intravascular thrombus. This is associated with acute onset of extreme perianal pain. The pain usually peaks within 48 hours. Repeated episodes of thrombosis may lead to enlargement of the overlying skin, which is seen as a skin tag on physical examination. The acutely thrombosed external hemorrhoid is seen as a purplish, edematous, tense subcutaneous perianal mass that is quite tender. The thrombus occasionally may cause ischemia and necrosis of the overlying skin resulting in bleeding.

B. Laboratory and Imaging Studies

Hemorrhoids are readily diagnosed with anoscopy. Chronic bleeding from internal hemorrhoids rarely results in anemia. Therefore, until all other sources of gastrointestinal blood loss have been ruled out by endoscopy and/or barium radiography, anemia must not be attributed to hemorrhoids, regardless of a patient's age. Defecography is helpful in evaluating patients when obstructed defecation or rectal prolapse is suspected.

Differential Diagnosis

Patients with perianal pathology often present, or are referred, with a chief complaint of "hemorrhoids." A thorough history frequently suggests the correct diagnosis. Painless bleeding due to hemorrhoids must be distinguished from rectal bleeding from colorectal malignancy, adenomatous polyps, inflammatory bowel disease, or diverticular disease. Painful bleeding associated with a bowel movement is more often due to an ulcer or fissure. Straining at stool may be attributed to hemorrhoids but is likely secondary to obstructed defecation. Similarly, rectal prolapse must be distinguished from hemorrhoids because it is safe to band a hemorrhoid but not a prolapsed rectum. Moisture or maceration may be secondary to hemorrhoids or condylomata acuminata.

Complications

The complications of internal or external hemorrhoids are the indications for medical or surgical intervention. They are bleeding, pain, necrosis, mucous discharge, moisture, and, rarely, perianal sepsis.

Treatment

A. Medical

Initial medical management for all but the most advanced cases is recommended. Dietary alterations, in-

cluding elimination of constipating foods (eg, cheeses), addition of bulking agents, stool softeners, and increased intake of liquids are advised. Changing daily routines by adding exercise and decreasing time spent on the commode is often beneficial.

B. Surgical

First- and second-degree hemorrhoids generally respond to medical management. Hemorrhoids that fail to respond to medical management may be treated with elastic band ligation, sclerosis, photocoagulation, cryosurgery, excisional hemorrhoidectomy, and many other local techniques that induce scarring and fixation of the hemorrhoids to the underlying tissues. The three most common techniques—elastic band ligation, sclerosis, and excisional hemorrhoidectomy—will be discussed.

Elastic band ligation is safe and effective in the treatment of first-, second-, third-, and selected fourth-degree hemorrhoids. Hemorrhoidal tissue 1–2 cm above the dentate line is pulled into the barrel of an elastic band applicator and two bands are placed at the base of the hemorrhoidal complex. After 7–10 days, the hemorrhoid itself sloughs removing a portion of the offending redundant tissues and leaving a scar that inhibits further prolapse and bleeding of the remaining tissue. If the band is placed in the transitional zone or below, patients may experience sudden severe pain as this mucosa and skin are highly innervated. The band should be immediately removed. Immune compromised patients or those with unrecognized rectal prolapse have developed severe sepsis after banding. Inordinate pain, fever, and urinary retention herald this complication. Treatment requires intravenous antibiotics, band removal, and debridement of necrotic tissue and observation. Patients are advised to avoid nonsteroidal antiinflammatory agents and aspirin for 10 days after ligation as significant bleeding may otherwise occur when the hemorrhoid sloughs.

Injection sclerotherapy is often tried for first-degree and second-degree hemorrhoids that continue to bleed despite medical measures. One to two milliliters of sclerosant is injected into the loose submucosal connective tissue above the hemorrhoidal complex causing inflammation and scarring. This inhibits prolapse and bleeding of the remaining hemorrhoidal tissue. The depth of injection is critical, as mucosal sloughing infection and full thickness injury have been reported.

Excisional hemorrhoidectomy is reserved for the larger third- and fourth-degree hemorrhoids, mixed internal and external hemorrhoids not amenable to banding of the internal component, and incarcerated internal hemorrhoids requiring urgent intervention. The base of the hemorrhoid is visualized with an anoscope. The vascular pedicle is suture ligated with an absorbable suture. The hemorrhoidal tissue is excised using the "knife" (scalpel, scissors, cautery, laser) preferred by the surgeon. Care must be taken to avoid the underlying internal sphincter while dissecting free the vascular cushion and overlying mucosa. The mucosal and skin defect may be left open, partially closed, or closed in a running fashion with the suture used for control of the vascular pedicle.

Severe pain, urinary retention, bleeding, and fecal impaction are the most common complications of excisional hemorrhoidectomy. The incidence of these complications can be minimized with improved postoperative pain control, limited intraoperative intravenous fluid administration, attention to surgical technique, and stool bulking agents and stool softeners. Anal stenosis is a long-term complication that may be avoided by leaving adequate anoderm between excised hemorrhoidal complexes.

The acutely thrombosed external hemorrhoid may be treated with excision of the hemorrhoid or clot evacuation if the patient presents less than 48 hours after onset of symptoms. Excision removes the clot and hemorrhoidal tissues, significantly decreasing the incidence of recurrence. However, many surgeons simply evacuate the thrombus, relieving the pressure and pain. If the patient presents over 48 hours after onset of symptoms, the thrombus has begun to organize and evacuation will not be successful. Conservative management with warm sitz baths, high-fiber diet, stool softeners, and reassurance is advised.

Prognosis

The prognosis for recurrence of hemorrhoidal disease is most related to success in changing the patient's bowel habits. Increasing dietary fiber, decreasing constipating foods, introducing exercise, and decreasing time spent on the toilet all decrease the amount of time spent straining in the squatting position. These behavioral modifications are the most important steps in preventing recurrence.

Arbman G, Krook H, Haapaniemi S: Closed vs. open hemorrhoidectomy—is there any difference? Dis Colon Rectum 2000;43(1):31.

Galizia G et al: Lateral internal sphincterotomy together with haemorrhoidectomy for treatment of haemorrhoids: a randomised prospective study. Eur J Surg 2000;166(3):223.

Hayssen TK et al: Limited hemorrhoidectomy: results and long-term follow-up. Dis Colon Rectum 1999;42(7):909; discussion 914.

Ho YH et al: Randomized controlled trial of open and closed haemorrhoidectomy [see comments]. Br J Surg 1997;84(12):1729.

Johanson JF: Association of hemorrhoidal disease with diarrheal disorders: potential pathogenic relationship? Dis Colon Rectum 1997;40(2):215; discussion 219.

Komborozos VA, Skrekas GJ, Pissiotis CA: Rubber band ligation of symptomatic internal hemorrhoids: results of 500 cases. Digest Surg 2000;17(1):71.

Konsten J, Baeten CG: Hemorrhoidectomy vs. Lord's method: 17-year follow-up of a prospective, randomized trial. Dis Colon Rectum, 2000;43(4):503.

MacRae HM, McLeod RS: Comparison of hemorrhoidal treatments: a meta-analysis. Can J Surg 1997;40(1):14.

Pescatori M: Urinary retention after anorectal operations [letter; comment]. Dis Colon Rectum 1999;42(7):964.

ANAL FISSURE & ULCER

 ESSENTIALS OF DIAGNOSIS

- *Tearing pain upon defecation.*
- *Blood on tissue or stool.*
- *Persistent perianal pain or spasm following defecation.*
- *Sphincter spasm.*
- *Disruption of anoderm.*

General Considerations

An anal fissure is a split in the anoderm. An ulcer is a chronic fissure. When mature, an ulcer is associated with a skin tag (**sentinel pile**), and a hypertrophied anal papilla (Figure 28–4). Fissures occur in the midline just distal to the dentate line. Goligher's rule is that 90% of fissures are posterior, 10% are anterior, and less than 1% occur simultaneously anteriorly and posteriorly. Recent studies suggest anterior fissures may be more common than predicted.

Fissures result from a vigorous stretching of the anal canal, most commonly caused during defecation by a large, firm bowel movement. However, fissures are less commonly caused by digital insertion, sexual trauma, or foreign body insertion. Factors that may predispose to fissure formation are previous anorectal surgery (hemorrhoidectomy, fistulotomy, condylomata ablation) resulting in scarring of the anoderm and loss of anoderm elasticity. Tearing of the anoderm exposes the underlying internal sphincter muscle causing muscular spasm. The internal sphincter may fail to relax with the bowel movement, leading to further tearing, deepening of the fissure, and further spasm. Persistent muscle spasm leads to relative ischemia of the overlying anoderm inhibiting healing.

Fissures are associated with severe anal pain, especially during bowel movements. As a result, patients may ignore the urge to defecate for fear of experiencing

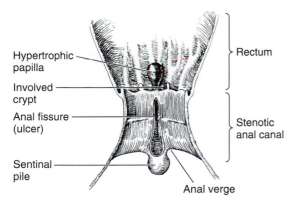

Hypertrophic papilla

Involved crypt

Anal fissure (ulcer)

Sentinal pile

Rectum

Stenotic anal canal

Anal verge

Figure 28–4. Diagram of the anorectum showing the fissure or ulcer triad. [Reproduced, with permission, from Welton ML: Anorectum. In: *Current Surgical Diagnosis & Treatment,* 11th ed. Way LW, Doherty GM (editors). McGraw-Hill, 2002.]

further pain. This ultimately results in passage of a large, hard stool that traumatizes the anoderm due to its size and the poor relaxation of the sphincter. A self-perpetuating cycle of pain, poor relaxation, and tissue reinjury results.

Clinical Findings

A. SYMPTOMS AND SIGNS

Fissures cause pain and bleeding with defecation. The pain is often tearing or burning, is most severe during defecation, and subsides over a few hours. Blood may be noted on the tissue, streaking the outer aspects of the stool, or dripping into the toilet water, but it is not mixed in the stool. Constipation may develop secondarily because of fear of recurrent pain. Less commonly, fissures may present as painless nonhealing wounds that bleed intermittently.

Physical examination with simple gentle traction on the buttocks will evert the anus sufficiently to reveal a linear tear of the anoderm in the midline at the mucocutaneous junction with a white ulcerated base. In patients with chronic fissure, an external hemorrhoid or "sentinel pile" may be visualized at the inferior margin of the fissure. Gentle, limited, digital examination confirms internal sphincter spasm. Anoscopy and sigmoidoscopy should be performed during a subsequent visit because the presence of associated anorectal malignancy or inflammatory bowel disease must be excluded. In the acute setting, anoscopy and proctosigmoidoscopy may be deferred until sufficient healing has occurred to allow comfortable examination or until these procedures can be performed under anesthesia. Anoscopy

may reveal a triad of a fissure with a hypertrophied anal papilla located above the fissure and a sentinel pile located at the anal verge. Biopsies of anal tissue are painful and not warranted for most patients with acute midline fissures. However, fissures that occur laterally and midline fissures that fail to heal should be biopsied to exclude Crohn's disease or malignancy.

B. LABORATORY AND IMAGING STUDIES

Anal manometry is unhelpful. Studies have shown increased pressures in patients with ulcers, but patients with high anal pressures have not been found to have an increased risk for developing anal fissure.

Differential Diagnosis

Most anal fissures/ulcers occur in the anterior or posterior midline and involve the mucosa immediately distal to the dentate line. Ulcers occurring off the midline, or away from the dentate line, are suspicious. Crohn's disease, anal tuberculosis (TB), anal malignancy, abscess/fistula disease, cytomegalovirus, herpes, *Chlamydia,* syphilis, acquired immunodeficiency syndrome, and some blood dyscrasias may all mimic anal fissure/ulcer disease. Initial manifestations of Crohn's disease are limited to the anal canal in 10% of patients. Anal TB usually is associated with a prior or concomitant history of pulmonary TB. Anal cancer may present as a painless ulcer. Patients with nonhealing ulcers should undergo biopsy to rule out malignancy, infection, and inflammatory bowel disease.

Complications

Complications are related to persistence of the disease with associated pain, bleeding, and alteration in bowel habits. Fissures do not become malignant.

Treatment

A. MEDICAL

Stool softeners, bulk agents, and sitz baths are successful in healing 90% of anal fissures. Recurrent episodes also have a 60–80% chance of healing with conservative measures. Sitz baths after painful bowel movements soothe muscle spasm. While soaking in a hot bath, patients should contract the anal sphincter to identify the source of spasm and focus on sphincter relaxation. This serves to decrease the pain associated with the spasm and improve local blood flow promoting healing. Stool softeners and bulk agents soften the stool decreasing recurrent anal trauma. Patients with a chronic (more than 1 month) fissure or chronic recurrent fissures should be considered for definitive therapy.

Botulinum toxin (Botox) injection of 20–25 units into the internal anal sphincter appears effective in the treatment of anal fissures. Botox inhibits the release of acetylcholine from presynaptic nerve fibers affecting a reversible paralysis that last several months. This allows for improved perfusion of the disrupted anoderm and healing. Controlled and uncontrolled studies suggest that botulinum injection results in healing in 60–90% of patients with chronic fissures. Although botulinum toxin reduces resting anal sphincter pressure by 30%, it does not cause incontinence acutely or chronically.

Studies suggest 0.2% nitroglycerin is effective in the treatment of anal fissures in >60% of cases. In a recent controlled trial, nitroglycerin was significantly less effective than botulinum injection. Nitroglycerin ointment is a nitric oxide source. Nitric oxide is an inhibitory neurotransmitter that causes relaxation of the internal sphincter and improved blood flow to the anoderm. The major side effect, headache, occurs even at the lower therapeutic levels of nitoglycerin (0.2 or 0.3%), leading some to question the utility of this therapy.

B. Surgical

Lateral internal anal sphincterotomy is the procedure of choice for many surgeons after conservative measures have failed. This may be performed in "open" fashion, whereby an incision is made in the skin and the distal one-third of the internal sphincter is divided under direct vision. It may also be done in a "closed" manner, whereby a scalpel is passed in the intersphincteric plane and swept medially dividing the internal sphincter blindly. Both techniques are associated with similar results. Randomized trials of botulinum injection versus lateral sphincterotomy are needed.

Prognosis

Lateral internal anal sphincterotomy is successful in 90–95% of patients with chronic anal fissure/ulcer disease. Fewer than 10% of surgically treated patients are incontinent of mucous and gas. Fissure recurrence is less than 10%.

Altomare DF et al: Glyceryl trinitrate for chronic anal fissure—healing or headache? Results of a multicenter, randomized, placebo-controlled, double-blind trial. Dis Colon Rectum 2000;43(2):174; discussion 179.

Argov S, Levandovsky O: Open lateral sphincterotomy is still the best treatment for chronic anal fissure. Am J Surg 2000;179 (3):201.

Brisinda G et al: A comparison of injections of botulinum toxin and topical nitroglycerin ointment for the treatment of chronic anal fissure [see comments]. N Engl J Med 1999; 341(2):65.

Dorfman G et al: Treatment of chronic anal fissure with topical glyceryl trinitrate. Dis Colon Rectum 1999;42(8):1007.

Hananel N, Gordon PH: Re-examination of clinical manifestations and response to therapy of fissure-in-ano. Dis Colon Rectum 1997;40(2):229.

Lund JN, Scholefield JH: A randomised, prospective, double-blind, placebo-controlled trial of glyceryl trinitrate ointment in treatment of anal fissure [see comments] [published erratum appears in Lancet 1997;349(9052):656]. Lancet 1997;349 (9044):11.

Maria G et al: Influence of botulinum toxin site of injections on healing rate in patients with chronic anal fissure. Am J Surg 2000;179(1):46.

Nelson RL: Meta-analysis of operative techniques for fissure-in-ano. Dis Colon Rectum 1999;42(11):1424; discussion 1428.

Nyam DC, Pemberton JH: Long-term results of lateral internal sphincterotomy for chronic anal fissure with particular reference to incidence of fecal incontinence. Dis Colon Rectum 1999;42(10):1306.

Richard CS et al: Internal sphincterotomy is superior to topical nitroglycerin in the treatment of chronic anal fissure: results of a randomized, controlled trial by the Canadian Colorectal Surgical Trials Group. Dis Colon Rectum 2000;43(8):1048; discussion 1057.

■ INFECTIONS OF THE ANORECTUM

ANORECTAL ABSCESS & FISTULA

ESSENTIALS OF DIAGNOSIS

- *Severe anal pain.*
- *A palpable mass is usually present on perineal or digital rectal examination.*
- *Systemic evidence of sepsis.*

General Considerations

Perirectal abscess fistulous disease not associated with a specific systemic disease most commonly arises from the 6–14 anal glands that lie in or near the intersphincteric plane between the internal and external sphincters. Projections from the glands pass through the internal sphincters and drain into the crypts at the dentate line. Glands may become infected when a crypt is occluded by impaction of vegetable matter, edema from trauma (firm stool or foreign body), or from adjacent inflammatory process. If the crypt does not decompress into the anal canal, an abscess may develop in the intersphincteric plane. Abscesses are classified by the space they invade (Figure 28–5). The extent of disease is

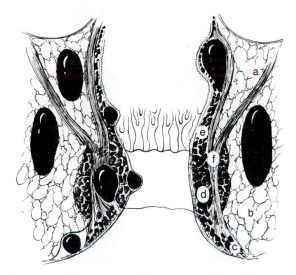

Figure 28–5. Composite diagram of acute anorectal abscesses (1–7) and spaces. **(a)** Pelvirectal (supralevator) space. **(b)** Ischiorectal space. **(c)** Perianal (subcutaneous) space. **(d)** Marginal (mucocutaneous) space. **(e)** Submucous space. **(f)** Intermuscular space. [Reproduced, with permission, from Welton ML: Anorectum. In: *Current Surgical Diagnosis & Treatment*, 11th ed. Way LW, Doherty GM (editors). McGraw-Hill, 2002.]

often difficult to determine without examination under anesthesia.

Early surgical consultation and operative drainage are the best measures to avoid the disastrous complications associated with undrained perineal sepsis. After the abscesses are drained to the skin, either surgically or spontaneously, 50% will have persistent communication with the crypt, creating a fistula from the anus to the perianal skin or "fistula-in-ano."

Clinical Findings

A. SYMPTOMS AND SIGNS

A perianal abscess typically causes severe continuous throbbing anal pain that worsens with ambulation and straining. Swelling and discharge are noted less frequently. Patients may develop fever, urinary retention, and life-threatening sepsis, especially patients who are diabetic or immunocompromised. A fistula-in-ano presents as chronic mucopurulent discharge that usually arises after a prior episode of severe pain followed by bloody purulent drainage associated with resolution of the pain.

Physical examination of the patient with an abscess reveals an exquisitely tender mass palpable externally in the perianal area or on digital examination of the anus or rectum. The size is often difficult to assess until the patient is provided adequate anesthesia. An apparently small abscess may extend high into the ischiorectal or supralevator space. A fistula is suggested by the presence of a small external opening outside the anal verge draining mucus, pus, or fecal matter. A fistula is confirmed by the demonstration of an internal opening within the anal canal. A firm fistulous tract is often palpable on digital examination.

B. LABORATORY AND IMAGING STUDIES

No imaging studies are necessary in uncomplicated abscesses or fistulous disease. Sinograms, transrectal ultrasound, computed tomography (CT), and magnetic resonance imaging (MRI) may be useful in the evaluation of complex and/or recurrent disease. Transrectal ultrasound can identify branching of fistulous tracts, the presence of persistent undrained abscesses, and the extent of sphincter involvement. Hydrogen peroxide injection of the tract may improve sensitivity of the ultrasound. CT scan may be helpful in identification of an undiagnosed supralevator abscess. MRI with endorectal coils may be of use in identifying and classifying fistulas.

Differential Diagnosis

Fistula disease of cryptoglandular origin must be differentiated from complications of Crohn's disease, pilonidal disease, hidradenitis suppurativa, tuberculosis, actinomycosis, trauma, fissures, carcinoma, radiation, chlamydia, local dermal processes, retrorectal tumors, diverticulitis, and urethral injuries.

About 10% of patients with Crohn's disease will present with anorectal abscesses or fistulous disease with no antecedent history of inflammatory bowel disease. TB may cause indolent, pale, granulomatous perianal disease but is usually associated with a known history of TB. Hidradenitis suppurativa is considered in the patient with multiple chronic, draining fistulas. Pilonidal disease may extend toward the perineum but may be distinguished from cryptoglandular disease by the presence of inspissated hairs, the direction of the tract, and the presence of other openings in the sacrococcygeal area. A colonic source may be suspected in a patient with known inflammatory bowel disease or diverticular disease. Other less common causes include tumors, radiation, infections, and urologic injuries.

Complications

Complications of an undrained anorectal abscess may be severe. In the absence of prompt drainage, infection may spread rapidly resulting in extensive tissue loss, sphincter injury, and even death. In contrast, the development of a fistula-in-ano, which may develop after abscess drainage, is not a surgical emergency. Chronic fistula may be associated with recurring perianal abscesses and, rarely, with cancer of the fistulous tract.

Treatment

Abscesses require surgical drainage. Drainage in the operating room with anesthesia allows for adequate evaluation of the extent of the disease. Abscesses thought in the office to be superficial may extend above the levators. Intersphincteric abscesses are treated by an internal sphincterotomy that drains the abscess and destroys the crypt. Perirectal and ischiorectal abscesses should be drained externally by catheter or with adequate excision of skin to prevent premature closure and reaccumulation of the abscess. If the internal opening of a fistula is identified and external sphincter involvement is minimal, a fistulotomy may be performed at the time of abscess drainage. However, the internal opening is often difficult to locate due to inflammation. In this instance, catheter drainage is preferred to skin excision (1) to establish drainage with a minimal disruption of normal perianal skin, (2) to facilitate later identification of the internal anal opening, and (3) to facilitate patient compliance and eliminate the need for packing the wound.

Patients with chronic or recurring abscesses after apparent adequate surgical drainage often have an undrained deep postanal space abscess that communicates with the ischiorectal fossa via a "horseshoe fistula." Treatment involves opening the deep postanal space and counterdraining the tract through the ischiorectal external opening. Once the postanal space heals, the counterdrain may be removed.

Immunocompromised patients are a particular challenge. In the moderately compromised host, such as the diabetic patient, urgent drainage in the operating room is required, as they are more prone to necrotizing anorectal infections. In the severely compromised host, such as patients receiving chemotherapy, an infection may be present without an "abscess" due to neutropenia. In these patients it is important to attempt to localize the process, establish "drainage," localize the internal opening, and obtain a biopsy for tissue examination and culture (to rule out leukemia and to select antibiotics).

The treatment of fistulas is dictated by the course of the fistula. Goodsall's rule is of assistance in identifying the direction of the tract (Figure 28–6). If the tract passes superficially and does not involve sphincter muscle, then a simple incision of the tract with ablation of the gland and "saucerization" of the skin at the external opening is all that is necessary. A fistula that involves a

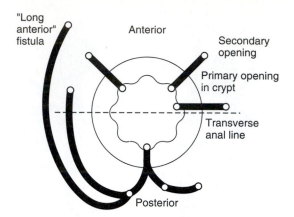

Figure 28–6. Goodsall's rule. The usual relation of the primary and secondary openings of fistulas. When there is an anterior and a posterior opening of the same fistula, the rule of the posterior opening applies; the "long anterior" fistula is an exception to the rule. [Reproduced, with permission, from Welton ML: Anorectum. In: *Current Surgical Diagnosis & Treatment,* 11th ed. Way LW, Doherty GM (editors). McGraw-Hill, 2002.]

small amount of sphincter may be treated similarly. A tract that passes deep, or that involves an undetermined amount of muscle, is best treated with a mucosal advancement flap (described in the section, "Rectovaginal Fistula"), because immediate or delayed (as with a Seton) muscle division is associated with a high rate of incontinence.

Prognosis

The prognosis for cryptoglandular abscess fistula disease is excellent, once the source of infection is identified. Fistulas persist when the source has not been identified or adequately drained, when the diagnosis is incorrect, or when postoperative care is insufficient.

Chapple KS et al: Prognostic value of magnetic resonance imaging in the management of fistula-in-ano. Dis Colon Rectum 2000;43(4):511.

Cintron JR et al: Repair of fistulas-in-ano using fibrin adhesive: long-term follow-up. Dis Colon Rectum 2000;43(7):944; discussion 949.

Garcia-Aguilar J et al: Anal fistula surgery. Factors associated with recurrence and incontinence. Dis Colon Rectum 1996;39(7):723.

García-Aguilar J et al: Patient satisfaction after surgical treatment for fistula-in-ano. Dis Colon Rectum 2000;43(9):1206.

Ho YH et al: Marsupialization of fistulotomy wounds improves healing: a randomized controlled trial. Br J Surg 1998;85(1):105.

Knoefel WT et al: The initial approach to anorectal abscesses: fistulotomy is safe and reduces the chance of recurrences. Dig Surg 2000;17(3):274.

Park JJ et al: Repair of chronic anorectal fistulae using commercial fibrin sealant. Arch Surg 2000;135(2):166.

Poen AC et al: Hydrogen peroxide-enhanced transanal ultrasound in the assessment of fistula-in-ano. Dis Colon Rectum 1998; 41(9):1147.

The Standards Practice Task Force. The American Society of Colon and Rectal Surgeons: Practice parameters for treatment of fistula-in-ano—supporting documentation. Dis Colon Rectum 1996;39(12):1363.

RECTOVAGINAL FISTULA

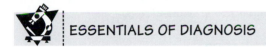 ESSENTIALS OF DIAGNOSIS

- *Passage of stool and flatus per vagina.*
- *Altered continence.*
- *Fistulous tract generally visible or palpable.*

General Considerations

Rectovaginal fistulas may result from obstetrical injuries, Crohn's disease, diverticulitis, radiation, undrained cryptoglandular disease, foreign body trauma, surgical extirpation of anterior rectal tumors, and malignancies of the rectum, cervix, or vagina. The fistulas are classified as low, middle, or high. Fistula location and etiology dictate the operative approach.

Clinical Findings

A. SYMPTOMS AND SIGNS

Patients with rectovaginal fistulas usually note passage of stool and flatus through the vagina and varying degrees of incontinence. These events are very disturbing and embarrassing to the patient. An opening in the vagina or rectum may be visualized or palpated on vaginal examination.

B. LABORATORY AND IMAGING STUDIES

A vaginogram or barium enema may identify the fistula. If the fistula is not demonstrated on radiographic study or physical examination, a dilute methylene blue rectal enema may be administered after insertion of a vaginal tampon. The presence of methylene blue stain on the tampon confirms the presence of a rectovaginal fistula.

Differential Diagnosis

The signs and symptoms of a rectovaginal fistula are unmistakable. Therefore, the focus of the differential diagnosis is the etiology of the fistula (discussed below), as this impacts on the management.

Complications

The major complication of a rectovaginal fistula is impaired hygiene and incontinence.

Treatment

The etiology and location of the rectovaginal fistula determine appropriate treatment. Involvement of tissue around the rectum and vagina by the underlying disease process may limit surgical options. Crohn's disease must be brought into remission before proceeding with fistula repair. In the surgical treatment of fistula caused by pelvic radiation, normal healthy tissues must be brought from outside the irradiated field.

Obstetric injuries, trauma from foreign bodies, Crohn's disease, and crypoglandular disease are associated with the development of low rectovaginal fistulas in which the rectal opening is near the dentate line and the vaginal opening is just above the fourchette. Obstetric injuries, traumatic fistulas, and complications of cryptoglandular disease may spontaneously close within 3 months. Waiting also allows inflammation to resolve, which facilitates surgical repair.

Fistulas secondary to Crohn's disease seldom heal spontaneously. Aggressive medical therapy and surgical control of perianal sepsis are necessary to preserve sphincteric function. Once the disease is in remission, local advancement flap procedures may be performed. Tissue uninvolved by Crohn's should be brought down over the fistulous tract and the rectal fistulous opening excised. Patients with severe Crohn's disease that does not respond to local measures may require temporary diverting colostomy. During fecal diversion, a single focus of Crohn's disease may be found and excised and an advancement procedure performed. Extensive destruction of the rectum or sphincters by Crohn's diseaes may mandate proctectomy without attempts at local preservation.

Mid-rectal fistulas from cryptoglandular disease, Crohn's disease, or obstetrical injury should be treated as outlined above. Mid-rectal fistulas caused by radiation usually are not amenable to local procedures because of radiation injury to the surrounding tissues, and transabdominal resection with coloanal anastomosis is preferred.

High rectal fistulas result from Crohn's disease, diverticular disease, operative injury, malignancy, and radiation. High rectovaginal fistulas are best treated with a transabdominal approach that allows for resection of the diseased bowel.

Prognosis

The prognosis is determined by the cause of the fistula.

Hull TL, Fazio VW: Surgical approaches to low anovaginal fistula in Crohn's disease. Am J Surg 1997;173(2):95.

Khanduja KS et al: Reconstruction of rectovaginal fistula with sphincter disruption by combining rectal mucosal advancement flap and anal sphincteroplasty. Dis Colon Rectum 1999;42(11):1432.

Marchesa P, Hull TL, Fazio VW: Advancement sleeve flaps for treatment of severe perianal Crohn's disease. Br J Surg 1998; 85(12):1695.

Tsang CB, Rothenberger DA: Rectovaginal fistulas. Therapeutic options. Surg Clin North Am 1997;77(1):95.

Tsang CB et al: Anal sphincter integrity and function influences outcome in rectovaginal fistula repair. Dis Colon Rectum 1998;41(9):1141.

Venkatesh KS, Ramanujam P: Fibrin glue application in the treatment of recurrent anorectal fistulas. Dis Colon Rectum 1999; 42(9):1136.

PILONIDAL DISEASE

 ESSENTIALS OF DIAGNOSIS

- *Acute chronic recurring abscess or chronic draining sinus over the sacrococcygeal or perianal region.*
- *Pain, tenderness, purulent drainage, inspissated hair, induration.*

General Considerations

The incidence of pilonidal disease is highest in white males (3:1 male/female ratio) between ages 15 and 40 with a peak incidence between 16 and 20 years of age. It was once widely accepted that pilonidal disease was a congenital condition that developed along an epithelialized tract of the natal cleft. However, it is now accepted that many of these cysts are acquired, particularly in hirsute individuals. It is hypothesized that a natal cleft hair follicle becomes obstructed, infected, and ruptures into the subcutaneous tissues forming a pilonidal abscess. Hair from the surrounding skin is pulled into the abscess cavity by the friction generated by the gluteal muscles during walking.

Clinical Findings

Patients with pilonidal disease may present with small midline pits or abscess(es) near the midline of the coccyx or sacrum. Patients are generally heavy, hirsute males. Physical examination may reveal acute suppuration with an undrained abscess or chronic draining sinuses with multiple mature tracts with hairs protruding from pit-like openings. Unless Crohn's disease is suspected, further evaluation beyond the physical examination is unnecessary.

Differential Diagnosis

The differential diagnosis includes cryptoglandular abscess/fistulous disease of the anus, hidradenitis suppurativa, furuncle, and actinomycosis.

Complications

Untreated pilonidal disease may result in multiple draining sinuses with chronic recurrent abscess, drainage, soiling of clothing, and rarely necrotizing wound infections or malignant degeneration.

Treatment

Pilonidal abscesses may be drained under local anesthesia. A probe is inserted into the primary opening and the abscess is unroofed. Granulation tissue and inspissated hair are removed by curettage but definitive therapy is not initially required. Cure rates of 60–80% are reported after primary unroofing. Nonoperative therapy with meticulous skin care (shaving of the natal cleft, perineal hygiene) and drainage of abscesses may significantly reduce the need for surgery.

For cysts that fail to heal after 3 months or that develop a chronic draining sinus, definitive therapy is recommended. Conservative excision of midline pits with removal of hair from lateral tracts and postoperative weekly shaving has almost a 90% success rate. Excision with open packing or marsupialization is proposed by some, however these leave the patient with painful, slowly healing wounds and have a reported recurrence rate of 6–10%. Our preference is to excise the pilonidal disease and close the defect primarily with rotational flaps over closed suction drainage. Simple primary closure often results in dehiscence because the midline skin has a poor blood supply, the wounds are closed under tension, and there is often dead space at the base of the defect that is susceptible to infection.

Prognosis

The prognosis after surgery is excellent. Recurrent or persistent disease may occur if there is inadequate excision with persistent external openings or occult tracts. Inadequate postoperative hygiene with ingrowth of hair into the wound also contributes to recurrence.

Abu Galala KH et al: Treatment of pilonidal sinus by primary closure with a transposed rhomboid flap compared with deep suturing: a prospective randomised clinical trial. Eur J Surg 1999;165(5):468.

Akinci OF, Coskun A, Uzunköy A: Simple and effective surgical treatment of pilonidal sinus: asymmetric excision and primary closure using suction drain and subcuticular skin closure. Dis Colon Rectum 2000;43(5):701; discussion 706.

Bozkurt MK, Tezel E: Management of pilonidal sinus with the Limberg flap. Dis Colon Rectum 1998;41(6):775.

Senapati A, Cripps NP, Thompson MR: Bascom's operation in the day-surgical management of symptomatic pilonidal sinus. Br J Surg 2000;87(8):1067.

Spivak H et al: Treatment of chronic pilonidal disease. Dis Colon Rectum 1996;39(10):1136.

PRURITUS ANI

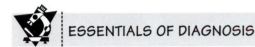

ESSENTIALS OF DIAGNOSIS

- Severe perianal itching, often at night.
- When chronic, skin is white, leathery, and thickened.

General Considerations

Pruritus ani is usually idiopathic. In some patients, poor hygiene of the perineum and/or local seepage may initiate irritation of the anoderm leading to pruritus. Conversely, some patients engage in frequent perineal washing with soap, detergents, and perfumes that dry the sensitive anoderm, leading to pruritus. Prior to seeking medical attention, most patients have tried over-the-counter preparations that have afforded no relief and may have exacerbated the problem by moistening and irritating the perineum, or by causing contact dermatitis. Pinworms (*Enterobius vermicularis*) are the most common cause of perianal itching in children.

Clinical Findings

A. SYMPTOMS AND SIGNS

The patient experiences severe perianal itching, often worse at night. In the acute stages, there may be acute dermatitis with erythema and weeping. In the chronic states, the skin becomes thickened, white, and lichenified. In children with pinworms, perianal itching is most severe at night when the pinworm deposits its eggs on the perianal skin.

B. LABORATORY AND IMAGING STUDIES

The diagnosis of pinworms is made by applying cellophane tape to the perianal skin, which collects the eggs and allows them to be viewed under a microscope. Scrapings of the perianal skin viewed microscopically may reveal fungal hyphae or yeast. Biopsy with histology may be necessary in refractory cases to rule out cutaneous malignancy.

Differential Diagnosis

Pruritus may be associated with other perianal lesions that distort normal anal anatomy, allowing friction of tissues or seepage of mucus or stool. These include hemorrhoids, fistulas, fissures, tumors of the anorectum, previous surgery, and radiation therapy. Primary dermatologic diseases such as lichen planus, atopic eczema, psoriasis, and seborrheic dermatitis may be confined initially to the perineum. Infections with fungae (dermatophytosis, candidiasis), parasites (*Enterobius vermicularis* scabies or pediculosis), and bacterial superinfection should be considered. Perianal yeast infection may be increased in patients with poorly controlled diabetes or chronic diarrhea. Other causes including contact dermatitis from local anesthetic creams or soaps, recent antibiotic usage, perianal neoplasms (Bowen's disease and extramammary Paget's disease), and dietary factors (see below). Pruritus may result from perspiration due to tight clothing, obesity, and climate. When all other causes are excluded it is considered idiopathic.

Complications

Complications include severe excoriation, ulceration, and secondary infection of the perineum.

Treatment

Identifiable causes of pruritus ani such as hemorrhoids, yeast infection, or parasites, should be treated. Patients should be educated about proper perineal care but should be advised to avoid excessive cleaning or scrubbing. Use of lanolin wipes ("baby wipes") may facilitate cleaning after bowel movements. Use of soaps and topical ointments should be discouraged. The perineum should be kept dry. Use of a blow dryer on the perineum after bathing may be helpful. Application of a loose cotton ball to the perineum may absorb seepage and perspiration. Coffee, tea, cola, beer, chocolate, and tomatoes cause perianal itching and should be removed from the diet for a minimum of 2 weeks. After resolution of symptoms, each food group may be added sequentially to identify the causative agent.

Prognosis

Relapse is common and reeducation is effective. In refractory cases, dermatologic and psychiatric consultation may be necessary.

■ PROCTITIS & ANUSITIS

General Considerations

Proctitis and anusitis are general, nonspecific terms that refer to inflammation of the anus or rectum due to infectious or inflammatory diseases. The causative agent or event determines the symptoms, signs, and appropriate management. In considering these diseases, particular attention should be paid to sexual practices and sexually transmitted diseases. The differential diagnoses and treatment of disorders causing proctitis are discussed.

HERPES PROCTITIS

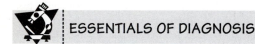

ESSENTIALS OF DIAGNOSIS

• *Painful perianal vesicles and ulcers.*

Clinical Findings

A. SYMPTOMS AND SIGNS

Patients present early with anal pain and discharge, rectal bleeding, tenesmus, and fear of defecation secondary to severe pain. External and anoscopic examination reveal vesicles, which may rupture to form ulcers. These ulcers may become secondarily infected. Fever and generalized malaise are often noted. Although patients often have a history of anoreceptive intercourse, disease may arise in women by extension from the vagina.

B. LABORATORY AND IMAGING STUDIES

Viral culture of the vesicle or biopsy of the ulcer is diagnostic. Herpes simplex type II is most common.

Treatment & Prognosis

Oral acyclovir is the treatment of choice but is not curative. It decreases the duration of outbreaks and viral shedding, and increases the interval between attacks. The first episode is associated with the most pain and longest duration of ulceration. Subsequent episodes are generally shorter and not as painful.

ANORECTAL SYPHILIS

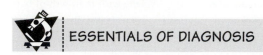

ESSENTIALS OF DIAGNOSIS

• *Asymptomatic perianal or anal ulcers (chancre).*

Clinical Findings

A. SYMPTOMS AND SIGNS

The chancre is an indurated, nontender perianal ulcer at the site of inoculation. Proctitis, pseudotumors, and condylomata lata may also be present. Condylomata lata are contiguous hypertrophic papules associated with secondary syphilis.

B. LABORATORY AND IMAGING STUDIES

Darkfield microscopy of exudate and serologic testing are the preferred methods of diagnosis. Serologic tests may initially be negative and should be repeated several months later.

Treatment & Prognosis

Penicillin is the treatment of choice. Prognosis is good. Contacts must be sought and treated.

GONOCOCCAL PROCTITIS

ESSENTIALS OF DIAGNOSIS

• *Cultures of anus, vagina, urethra, and pharynx.*

Clinical Findings

A. SYMPTOMS AND SIGNS

Patients may complain of rectal bleeding, discharge, perianal excoriation, or fistulas. However, patients may be asymptomatic. On anoscopic or proctoscopic examination, the mucosa appears friable and edematous with adherent mucopus.

B. LABORATORY AND IMAGING STUDIES

Swabs of the anus, vagina, urethra, and pharynx should be obtained and plated on a Thayer-Martin medium. The gram-negative diplococcus *Neisseria gonorrhoeae* is the causative agent.

Treatment & Prognosis

Intramuscular procaine penicillin G and oral probenecid is effective. Follow-up examination and cultures should be performed to confirm adequate therapy. The prognosis is excellent. Resistant strains should be treated with spectinomycin.

CHLAMYDIAL PROCTITIS & LYMPHOGRANULOMA VENEREUM

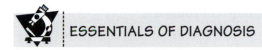

ESSENTIALS OF DIAGNOSIS

- *Inguinal adenopathy.*
- *Small, shallow ulcer.*

Clinical Findings

A. SYMPTOMS AND SIGNS

As in gonococcal proctitis, symptoms of chlamydial proctitis range from none to rectal pain, bleeding, and discharge. The small shallow ulcer of lymphogranuloma venereum (LGV) may be unnoticed but the inguinal adenopathy may become quite marked. Late findings include hemorrhagic proctitis and rectal stricture.

B. LABORATORY AND IMAGING STUDIES

The causative agent, *Chlamydia trachomatis,* is an intracellular parasite that is spread by anal intercourse or direct extension through the lymphatics of the rectovaginal septum. The diagnosis is made with the LGV complement fixation test. Tissue cultures are also used.

Treatment & Prognosis

Treatment with 21 days of tetracycline is recommended, but erythromycin is an acceptable alternative. Early strictures may be dilated. Although uncommon, strictures may cause bowel obstruction and require colostomy.

CONDYLOMATA ACUMINATA

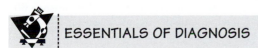

ESSENTIALS OF DIAGNOSIS

- *Characteristic perianal cauliflower-appearing warts.*

General Considerations

Human papilloma virus (HPV) is the cause of condylomata acuminatum. Multiple types have been identified. Types HPV-6 and HPV-11 are associated with the common "benign" genital wart, whereas HPV-16 and HPV-18 are associated with the development of high-grade anal dysplasia and anal cancer. In the United States, condylomata acuminatum is the most common sexually transmitted viral disease with 1 million new cases reported per year. It is the most common anorectal infection within homosexual men and is particularly prominent in human immunodeficiency virus (HIV)-positive patients. However the disease is not limited to men or women who practice anoreceptive intercourse. In women, the virus may track down from the vagina and in men, it may spread from the base of the scrotum. Patients with immunosuppression due to drugs (eg, posttransplantation) and HIV infection have a higher incidence of condylomatous disease with rates up to 4% and 86%, respectively.

Clinical Findings

A. SYMPTOMS AND SIGNS

The most frequent complaint is of a perianal growth. Pruritus, discharge, bleeding, odor, and anal pain are sometimes present. Physical examination reveals a cauliflower-like lesion, which may be isolated, clustered, or coalescent. The warts tend to spread in radial rows from the anus. The lesions may be quite large.

B. LABORATORY AND IMAGING STUDIES

Anoscopy and proctosigmoidoscopy are essential. The warts extend internally in more than three-fourths of patients and in >90% of affected homosexual men. Cultures and serologies for other veneral diseases may be taken from the penis, anus, mouth, and vagina.

Differential Diagnosis

Warts must be distinguished from condylomata lata and anal squamous cell carcinoma. Condylomata lata, the lesions of secondary syphilis, are flatter, paler, and smoother than condylomata acuminata. Anal squamous cell carcinoma is generally painful and may be tender and ulcerated, however condylomata is painless and nonulcerated.

Complications

Squamous cell carcinoma of the anal canal (discussed below) is the major complication.

Treatment & Prognosis

The extent of the disease and risk of malignancy (dysplasia treatment is discussed later) determine treatment. Minimal disease is treated in the office with topical agents such as bichloracetic acid or 25% podophyllin in tincture of benzoin. The former is preferred because of prompt response and few complications. Podophyllin must be washed off within 4–6 hours to limit pain and scarring. Patients are retreated at regular intervals until eradication is complete. More extensive disease may require initial treatment under anesthesia to allow excision of random lesions for pathologic evaluation to rule out dysplasia and extensive coagulation of remaining lesions. Electrocautery is useful to coagulate the lesions, taking care to spare the surrounding skin. Follow-up evaluation may reveal residual disease but this is often easily treated with topical agents in the office. Laser therapy is another method of condylomata destruction with acceptable recurrence rates. The main limitation is equipment cost.

Refractory disease may respond to surgical excision or fulgaration followed by intralesional interferon or autogenous vaccine created from excisional biopsies of the lesions. Recurrence rates of only 4.6% have been reported for destruction and vaccination combined, but the preparation of the vaccine is tedious and therefore has not gained wide acceptance.

Human papilloma viruses 16 and 18 are associated with a higher incidence of squamous cell carcinomas of the anal canal. This association has led to new screening techniques to screen high-risk patients (see section, "Anal Cancer"). Representative biopsies of clinically apparent condylomata should be sent to pathology to screen for unsuspected low- or high-grade dysplasia or squamous cell carcinoma of the anal canal may be found.

Buschke-Löwenstein tumors are giant condylomata acuminata that have benign histology but exhibit locally aggressive, malignant behavior. Radical excision is often the best therapeutic option for either palliation and cure, but wide local excision or combined surgery with adjuvant chemoradiation also have been used with success.

CHANCROID

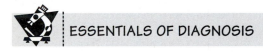

ESSENTIALS OF DIAGNOSIS

- *Multiple soft, painful lesions that bleed easily.*

Clinical Findings

A. SYMPTOMS AND SIGNS

Haemophilus ducreyi causes a soft perianal ulcer that is painful, often multiple, and bleeds easily. Autoinoculation is common. Inguinal lymph nodes become fluctuant, rupture, and drain.

B. LABORATORY AND IMAGING STUDIES

Cultures are diagnostic.

Treatment & Prognosis

Sulfonamides are the treatment of choice.

INFLAMMATORY PROCTITIS

General Considerations

Inflammatory proctitis is a mild form of ulcerative colitis that is limited to the rectum. The disease course is often self-limited. Only approximately 10% of the patients ever develop colonic manifestations of ulcerative colitis (see Chapter 7, Inflammatory Bowel Disease).

Clinical Findings

A. SYMPTOMS AND SIGNS

Rectal bleeding, discharge, diarrhea, and tenesmus are common. On sigmoidoscopy or colonoscopy, the rectal mucosa displays friability, granularity, erosions, or mucopus, but the colon proximal to the rectum appears normal on endoscopic and histologic examination.

B. LABORATORY AND IMAGING STUDIES

Rectal biopsies are taken at endoscopy to rule out infectious processes and Crohn's disease.

Differential Diagnosis

An infectious process must be ruled out before initiating steroid therapy. Distinguishing between Crohn's disease and inflammatory proctitis may be difficult. Lack of response to appropriate therapy is an indication to reassess the patient.

Treatment & Prognosis

Steroid foam or retention enemas (hydrocortisone 80–100 mg; prednisolone 20 mg) are given for 2–8 weeks. Alternatively, mesalamine (5-aminosalicylic acid; 5-ASA) may be given either orally (2.4 g/d) or rectally in an enema (4 g/d) or suppository (1 g/d). The choice of dosage forms (suppository, enema, or foam) is dependent upon the extent of proctitis and patient preference. Combination therapy with corticosteroids and mesalamine is superior to either agent alone and should be considered in refractory disease. Symptomatic improvement and endoscopic remission occur in >70% of patients with topical treatment. Refractory proctitis may require therapy with systemic corticosteroids. Judicious use of loperamide may decrease rectal urgency and incontinence.

RADIATION PROCTITIS

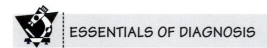

ESSENTIALS OF DIAGNOSIS

- *History of pelvic radiation.*

The rectum is subjected to radiation injury during radiation therapy for prostate, urinary bladder, testicular, and gynecologic cancers. It is particulary susceptible to injury due to its fixed position in the pelvis and proximity to the radiation field. Acute radiation injury occurs in up to 50–75% of patients but usually resolves with the discontinuation of therapy. Chronic radiation proctitis occurs in up to 30% of patients and is believe to be secondary to damage to the vascular endothelium.

Clinical Findings

A. SYMPTOMS AND SIGNS

Acute radiation proctitis develops during therapy and is characterized by diarrhea, rectal bleeding, discharge, tenesmus, pain, and incontinence. Chronic radiation proctitis may develop months to years after the injury. Symptoms of late disease are secondary to strictures, fistulas, and bleeding from ecstatic blood vessels in the anal and rectal mucosa. The most common symptom is bleeding that streaks or coats the stool, drips into the bowl, or stains the patient's undergarments. Patients with strictures or fistulas may report changes in bowel habits, urinary tract infections, and vaginal discharge.

B. LABORATORY AND IMAGING STUDIES

Endoscopy may reveal friable edematous mucosa with spontaneous or contact bleeding, myriad small telangiectasias, strictures, or internal fistulous openings.

Complications

The complications are those of late disease—strictures, fistulas, and telangiectasias.

Treatment & Prognosis

Initial therapy includes bulk-forming agents, antidiarrheal agents, and antispasmodics. Topical steroids, 5-ASA preparations, and misoprostol suppositories have been used in acute and chronic disease with only limited efficacy. Treatment of chronic recurrent bleeding from telangiectasias is effectively treated with laser or argon plasma coagulation. Alternatively, topical formaldehyde is effective and may be applied through a rigid sigmoidoscope. Fistulas to the bladder and vagina can be particularly challenging. Surgical success is optimized by interposition or transposition of healthy nonirradiated tissue into the radiated field. Seldom does the bladder require removal.

Centers for Disease Control and Prevention: 1998 guidelines for treatment of sexually transmitted diseases. MMWR 1998;47 (RR-1):1.

Counter SF, Froese DP, Hart MJ: Prospective evaluation of formalin therapy for radiation proctitis. Am J Surg 1999;177(5): 396.

El-Attar SM, Evans DV: Anal warts, sexually transmitted diseases, and anorectal conditions associated with human immunodeficiency virus. Primary Care; Clin Office Pract 1999;26(1): 81.

Fantin AC et al: Argon beam coagulation for treatment of symptomatic radiation-induced proctitis. Gastrointest Endosc 1999; 49(4 Pt 1):515.

Hemminki K, Dong C: Cancer in husbands of cervical cancer patients. Epidemiology 2000;11(3):347.

Khan AM et al: A prospective randomized placebo-controlled double-blinded pilot study of misoprostol rectal suppositories in the prevention of acute and chronic radiation proctitis symptoms in prostate cancer patients. Am J Gastroenterol 2000;95(8):1961.

Kobal B: Herpes simplex genitalis type 2: our experiences. Clin Exp Obstet Gynecol 1999;26(2):123.

Marshall J, Irvine EJ: Putting rectal 5-aminosalicylic acid in its place: the role in distal ulcerative colitis. Am J Gastroenterol 2000;95:1628.

Palefsky JM: Anal squamous intraepithelial lesions: relation to HIV and human papillomavirus infection. J Acquir Immune Defic Syndr 1999;21(Suppl 1):S42.

Palefsky JM: Anal squamous intraepithelial lesions in human immunodeficiency virus-positive men and women. Sem Oncol 2000;27(4):471.

Palefsky JM et al: Virologic, immunologic, and clinical parameters in the incidence and progression of anal squamous intraepithelial lesions in HIV-positive and HIV-negative homosexual men. J Acquir Immune Defic Syndr Human Retrovirol 1998;17(4):314.

Rompalo AM: Diagnosis and treatment of sexually acquired proctitis and proctocolitis: an update. Clin Infect Dis 1999;28 (Suppl 1):S84.

Taylor JG, Disario JA, Bjorkman DJ: KTP laser therapy for bleeding from chronic radiation proctopathy. Gastrointest Endosc 2000;52(3):353.

■ FECAL IMPACTION

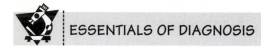

ESSENTIALS OF DIAGNOSIS

• *Rectal vault obstructed with hard, dry stool.*

General Considerations

Severe impaction of stool in the rectal vault may obstruct fecal flow leading to partial or complete large bowel obstruction. Predisposing causes include severe psychiatric disease, prolonged bed rest, chronic debilitation, neurogenic diseases of the colon, spinal cord disorders, constipating medications (narcotics, calcium channel blockers), and painful anorectal surgical procedures such as hemorrhoidectomy.

Clinical Findings

A. SYMPTOMS AND SIGNS

Patients with fecal impaction may present with "pseudodiarrhea" as only liquid stool is able to pass the obstructing fecal bolus. Some may complain of pelvic pain with episodic severe spasms from the pressure of the mass on the pelvic floor. Other symptoms include decreased appetite, nausea, vomiting, and abdominal distention. Abdominal examination may reveal a pelvic or abdominal mass much like a gravid uterus. Digital rectal examination reveals a hard, dry stool that obstructs the rectum.

Treatment

Initial treatment is directed at relieving the impaction with enemas or digitial disruption of the impacted material. Care must be taken not to injure the anal sphincter. Rarely, intervention in the operating room with local or regional anesthesia may be necessary to provide pelvic floor relaxation and pain control. At the completion of the disimpaction, sigmoidoscopy should be performed to exclude an obstructing inflammatory or malignant mass or rectal injury related to the disimpaction.

Long-term care is directed at maintaining soft stools and regular bowel movements with stool softeners (docussate, sorbitol, or milk of magnesia) and enemas, as needed.

Prather CM, Ortiz-Camacho CP: Evaluation and treatment of constipation and fecal impaction in adults. Mayo Clinic Proc 1998;73(9):881.

Tiongco FP, Tsang TK, Pollack J: Use of oral GoLytely solution in relief of refractory fecal impaction. Dig Dis Sci 1997;42(7): 1454.

■ ANAL/PERIANAL NEOPLASMS

General Considerations

It is important clinically to distinguish anal canal cancer from anal margin cancers, as these tumors have different epidemiology, risk factors, natural history, and treatment. Classification is based on anatomic landmarks, ie, the dentate line, the anal verge, and the anal sphincters. Efforts have been made by the World Health Organization and the American Joint Committee on Cancer (AJCC) to define these anatomic landmarks in order to distinguish anal margin and anal canal tumors. These organizations have established that the anal canal extends from the upper to the lower border of the internal anal sphincter (ie, from the pelvic floor to the anal verge). Anal margin tumors occur outside the anal verge but within a 5–6 cm radius of the anus.

Tumors of the **anal canal** account for 1.5% of gastrointestinal malignancies, with an estimated 3400 new cases per year. Chronic anal irritation may increase the risk of anal cancer, but more recent evidence implicates chronic infection with the human papilloma virus with anal cancer. Women infected with the papilloma virus are at increased risk for anal canal cancer (9/100,000). It is presumed that the virus pools in the vagina and tracks down to the anus. Anal infection may also be acquired through anoreceptive intercourse, the practice of which is reported to be increasing. Among men who have sex with men, the incidence of anal carcinoma is particularly high: 36/100,000 in those who are HIV negative and 70/100,000 in those who are HIV positive. Other factors associated with increased risk for anal cancer are anogenital warts, history of sexually transmitted disease, increased number of sexual partners, history of cervical, vulvar, or vaginal cancer (personal or partner), immunosuppression (HIV infection or organ transplantation), long-term use of corticosteroids, and cigarette smoking.

Although women are at increased risk for anal canal cancer, men have a four-fold increased risk of **anal margin carcinoma.** Tumors of the anal canal tend to be aggressive, nonkeratinizing, and associated with human papilloma virus infection. Tumors of the anal margin are generally well differentiated, keratinizing tumors that behave similarly to other squamous cell carcinomas of the skin and are treated accordingly.

Staging of anal and perianal malignancies is clinical. Physical examination includes bilateral inguinal nodal palpation and digital rectal examination. Anoscopy/sigmoidoscopy with biopsy are performed, under anesthesia if necessary, to confirm the diagnosis. Further staging is performed with endorectal ultrasound, CT, or MRI to assess tumor size and establish nodal and distant disease. The AJCC staging classification for both anal canal and anal margin tumors is presented in Table 28–1.

TUMORS OF THE ANAL MARGIN

1. Squamous Cell Carcinoma

ESSENTIALS OF DIAGNOSIS

- Rolled, everted edges, central ulceration.
- Arises in perianal skin.

Clinical Findings

A. SYMPTOMS AND SIGNS

Patients frequently complain of a mass, bleeding, pain, discharge, itching, or tenesmus. Typically the lesions are

Table 28–1. Staging for anal cancer.

Anal Cancer			
Tis	Carcinoma *in situ*		
T1	≤2 cm		
T2	>2 to 5 cm		
T3	>5 cm		
T4	Adjacent organ(s)		
N1	Perirectal		
N2	Unilateral internal iliac/inguinal		
N3	Perirectal and inguinal, bilateral internal iliac/inguinal		
Stage Grouping			
Stage 0	Tis	N0	M0
Stage I	T1	N0	M0
Stage II	T2	N0	M0
	T3	N0	M0
Stage IIIA	T1	N1	M0
	T2	N1	M0
	T3	N1	M0
	T4	N0	M0
Stage IIIB	T4	N1	M0
	Any T	N2, N3	M0
Stage IV	Any T	Any N	M1

Adapted, with the permission of the American Joint Committee on Cancer (AJCC), Chicago, Illinois. The original source of this material is the AJCC Cancer Staging Manual, 5th edition (1997) published by Lippincott-Raven Publishers, Philadelphia.

large, centrally ulcerated with rolled everted edges and have been present for over 2 years before detection. All chronic or nonhealing ulcers of the perineum should be biopsied to rule out squamous cell carcinoma.

Treatment & Prognosis

Small well-differentiated lesions (≤4 cm) are treated by wide local excision. Deep lesions that involve the sphincters require an abdominoperineal resection. Chemoradiation is used for less favorable lesions. Spread to the inguinal lymph nodes is included in the radiation fields. Excision of inguinal nodal disease is reserved for palpable and symptomatic disease. Recurrent cutaneous tumor may be treated with reexcision or abdominoperineal resection. Survival with T1 lesions approaches 100% at 5 and 10 years; however survival for T2 lesions is 60% and 40% at 5 and 10 years, respectively.

2. Basal Cell Carcinoma

ESSENTIALS OF DIAGNOSIS

- Raised, irregular edges and central ulceration.
- Superficial, mobile, rarely metastatic.

Clinical Findings

A. SYMPTOMS AND SIGNS

Bleeding, itching, and pain are presenting symptoms. The lesions appear with raised, irregular edges and central ulceration. They are more frequent in men.

Treatment & Prognosis

As with squamous cell carcinoma of the margin, treatment is wide local excision, where possible. Deeply invasive lesions may require abdominoperineal resection. Metastasis is rare. Local recurrence rates occur in up to 30% of patients and are treated with reexcision.

3. Bowen's Disease

ESSENTIALS OF DIAGNOSIS

- Intraepithelial squamous cell carcinoma.
- Associated with condylomata in young patients.

Clinical Findings

A. SYMPTOMS AND SIGNS

As with other perianal lesions, patients complain of perianal burning, itching, or pain. Lesions are sometimes found on routine histologic evaluation of specimens acquired at unrelated procedures. When grossly apparent, the lesions appear scaly, discrete, erythematous, and sometimes pigmented.

B. LABORATORY AND IMAGING STUDIES

In the immunocompromised patient (HIV positive, posttransplant), a Pap smear is a useful screening technique to detect evidence of dysplasia. If the Pap smear is positive, high-resolution anoscopy aided with acetic acid "painting" may reveal otherwise occult condylomata with dysplasia.

Treatment & Prognosis

Traditional treatment has been wide local excision with four quadrant biopsies to establish that no residual disease persists. Skin grafts may be necessary for larger lesions. However, radical skin excision does not address concomitant intraanal dysplastic lesions that may be even more aggressive than perianal disease. These intraanal dysplastic lesions have been successfully managed with local excision or destruction, even in the immunocompromised host. As fewer than 10% of the patients with Bowen's disease develop invasive squamous cell carcinoma of the anus, the need to perform radical excision and flap procedures is unclear.

4. Paget's Disease

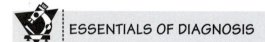

ESSENTIALS OF DIAGNOSIS

- Intraepithelial adenocarcinoma.
- Often associated with underlying gastrointestinal malignancy.

General Considerations

In contrast to the above three diseases, Paget's disease occurs predominantly in women. Patients are usually in the seventh or eighth decade. Up to 50% of patients have another coexistent carcinoma.

Clinical Findings

A. SYMPTOMS AND SIGNS

Severe intractable pruritus is characteristic. On physical examination an erythematous, eczematoid rash is apparent. Biopsy of nonhealing lesions should be taken to rule out this diagnosis. If Paget's disease is diagnosed, a thorough work-up for an occult malignancy is indicated.

Treatment & Prognosis

Wide local excision with multiple perianal biopsies is the treatment of choice. An abdominoperineal resection may be indicated for advanced disease. Lymph node dissection is performed if there is palpable adenopathy. The role for chemoradiotherapy is unclear. Prognosis is good unless there is metastatic disease or an underlying neoplasm, where patients do poorly.

Frisch M et al: Benign anal lesions, inflammatory bowel disease and risk for high-risk human papillomavirus-positive and -negative anal carcinoma. Br J Cancer 1998;78(11):1534.

Fuchshuber PR, Rodriguez-Bigas M: Anal canal and perianal epidermoid cancers. J Am Coll Surg 1997;185:494.

Marchesa P et al: Long-term outcome of patients with perianal Paget's disease. Ann Surg Oncol 1997;4(6):475.

Marchesa P et al: Perianal Bowen's disease: a clinicopathologic study of 47 patients. Dis Colon Rectum 1997;40(11):1286.

Nivatvongs S, Gordon PH: Surgical anatomy. In: *Principles and Practice of Surgery for the Colon, Rectum, and Anus.* Gordon PH, Nivatvongs S (editors). Quality Medical Publishing, 1999.

Peiffert D et al: Conservative treatment by irradiation of epidermoid carcinomas of the anal margin. Int J Radiat Oncol Biol Phys 1997;39(1):57.

Sarmiento JM et al: Paget's disease of the perianal region—an aggressive disease? Dis Colon Rectum 1997;40(10):1187.

TUMORS OF THE ANAL CANAL

Epidermoid (Squamous, Basoloid, Mucoepidermoid) Carcinoma

Clinical Findings

A. SYMPTOMS AND SIGNS

Prior to diagnosis, there is generally a long history of minor perianal complaints such as bleeding, itching, perianal discomfort, or a palpable, anal mass. At presentation, disease may be extensive with approximately half of lesions extending beyond the bowel wall or perianal skin. Inguinal nodal metastases are found initially in 15–20% of patients and develop in 10–15% over time.

Evaluation is reviewed under general considerations for perianal cancers

B. Laboratory and Imaging Studies

Endorectal ultrasound is the best test for determination of local invasion and identification of pararectal nodes. Abdominal CT and chest radiographs are performed to evaluate the liver and chest for distant disease.

Treatment

Early lesions that are small, mobile, confined to the submucosa, and well differentiated may be treated with local excision. Reported recurrence rates with local excision alone are high, with 5-year survivals of only 45–85%, although in highly selected patients recurrence rates after local excision are <10%.

Radiation therapy or chemoradiotherapy is the preferred treatment option for larger anal canal cancers. Chemoradiotherapy has now replaced surgery as the standard first line therapy for large lesions. Surgery is recommended only as a salvage procedure for persistent or recurrent disease. The established treatment regimen consists of 30 Gy radiation to the primary tumor and pelvic and inguinal nodes with mitomycin C (15 mg/m^2 intravenous bolus) on Day 1 of radiation therapy and 5-fluorouracil (1000 mg/m^2/24 h; 4 day infusion) on Days 1 and 28. Tumor response is excellent and 5-year disease-free survival is 67–90% after chemoradiotherapy. However there is significant morbidity associated with both the radiation and chemotherapy, leading some centers to modify the amount and type (cisplatin versus mitomycin) of chemotherapy and radiation dose (30–55 Gy) delivered.

Treatment failures occur most commonly at the primary site or in the locoregional lymph nodes. Disease occurs outside the pelvis in <17% of patients, most commonly in the liver. Salvage abdominoperineal resection for local recurrent or persistent tumor is associated with a 50% 5-year survival.

Prognosis

Metastatic disease is more likely with increasing depth of invasion, size, and worsening histologic grade. Tumor size is the most important prognostic factor. Mobile lesions ≤2 cm have cure rates of 80%, but tumors ≥5 cm have a 50% mortality. Long-term survival for node-negative disease (T1 to T3) is almost 90% and for node-positive disease is approximately 50%.

Allal AS et al: Effectiveness of surgical salvage therapy for patients with locally uncontrolled anal carcinoma after sphincter-conserving treatment. Cancer 1999;86(3):405.

Peiffert D et al: Preliminary results of a phase II study of high-dose radiation therapy and neoadjuvant plus concomitant 5-fluorouracil with CDDP chemotherapy for patients with anal canal cancer: a French cooperative study. Ann Oncol 1997;8 (6):575.

Pocard M et al: Results of salvage abdominoperineal resection for anal cancer after radiotherapy. Dis Colon Rectum 1998;41 (12):1488.

Ryan DP, Compton CC, Mayer RJ: Carcinoma of the anal canal. N Engl J Med 2000;342(11):792.

Miscellaneous Diseases of the Colon 29

Prashanthi N. Thota, MD & Bret A. Lashner, MD, MPH

This chapter comprises miscellaneous disorders of the colon and rectum that are characterized by obscure etiologies and diverse clinical presentations.

MICROSCOPIC COLITIS (Collagenous & Lymphocytic Colitis)

 ESSENTIALS OF DIAGNOSIS

- *Chronic secretory diarrhea.*
- *Normal endoscopic appearance of colon.*
- *Intraepithelial lymphocytosis.*
- *Subepithelial collagen deposition in collagenous colitis.*

General Considerations

Microscopic colitis is characterized by chronic, sometimes voluminous, watery, nonbloody diarrhea occurring in patients whose colons have normal endoscopic appearance but whose colonic biopsies have histologic evidence of inflammation. Two histologic types of microscopic colitis are seen: lymphocytic colitis and collagenous colitis. Both have lymphocytic infiltration of the colonic epithelium. Collagenous colitis, in addition, has subepithelial collagen deposition. It is unclear whether these are two diseases or variants of the same disorder. Because they both manifest and are treated similarly, they will be discussed together.

The mean age at presentation is in the sixth decade but ranges between the third and ninth decades. Among patients with collagenous colitis, women outnumber men by 10:1; however, among patients with lymphocytic colitis, the male-to-female ratio is nearly equal. Both entities are associated with autoimmune diseases in up to 20% of patients, including rheumatoid arthritis, scleroderma or sicca syndrome, pernicious anemia, chronic active hepatitis, primary biliary cirrhosis, idiopathic pulmonary fibrosis, idiopathic thrombocytopenic purpura, autoimmune thyroiditis, and diabetes mellitus. Seronegative peripheral arthritis may be seen in 10% of patients.

Pathophysiology

The etiology is unknown, but these colitic disorders may be due to autoimmunity or to mucosal injury from an unknown toxin. Some suggest that there is increased secretion of water and electrolytes due to an abnormal colonic immune response to a dietary toxin. In fact, the histologic appearance of microscopic colitis bears some resemblance to small intestinal celiac sprue. In sprue, there are inflammatory changes in the lamina propria and in one-third of patients there is submucosal collagen deposition. Furthermore, collagenous colitis may develop in patients with celiac sprue despite successful treatment with a gluten-free diet.

Drugs such as nonsteroidal antiinflammatory drugs (NSAIDs), H_2-receptor antagonists, simvastatin, ticlopidine, and flutamide have been implicated in some cases of microscopic colitis. Chronic use of NSAIDs has been implicated as a precipitating factor in up to half the patients with collagenous colitis.

Clinical Findings

A. SYMPTOMS AND SIGNS

The typical clinical presentation of patients with collagenous colitis is chronic watery diarrhea. Typically, patients have 5–10 stools per day and a stool volume greater than 500 mL/d. Nocturnal diarrhea may be present. The onset of the diarrhea may be acute in 40% of patients. Over 80% of patients complain of chronic, bothersome, intermittent symptoms, however the course is seldom severe. There may be mucus discharge or mild steatorrhea. Nausea, vomiting, abdominal pain, abdominal distention, flatulence, incontinence, and weight loss may also be presenting features of the disease. Physical examination and laboratory tests are normal. Mild elevation in the erythrocyte sedimentation rate (ESR) and fecal leukocytes may be present. Thyroid function tests should be obtained. In patients with severe collagenous colitis, serological tests [immunoglobulin A (IgA) antiendomysial antibody; IgG and IgA antigliadin antibodies] should be obtained to exclude celiac sprue.

B. HISTOLOGIC FINDINGS

In patients with watery diarrhea and a normal-appearing colonic mucosa at endoscopy, the diagnosis of microscopic colitis is confirmed by performing colonic biopsy for histologic assessment. In contrast to inflammatory bowel diseases (ulcerative colitis or Crohn's disease), there usually are no crypt abscesses, granulomas, alterations of crypt architecture, or immune complex deposits. In both entities, histologic abnormalities may be patchy, commonly sparing the rectum, and may be limited to the proximal colon. Flexible sigmoidoscopy with biopsy of the descending and sigmoid colon establishes the diagnosis in up to 90% of patients.

Collagenous colitis is characterized by a band of eosinophilic deposits under the surface epithelium that measures 7–100 μm in thickness. This is mainly composed of type III collagen and fibronectin, substances usually deposited following intestinal injury or inflammation. By contrast, normal basement membrane is less than 4 μm thick and is composed mostly of type IV collagen. Biopsy specimens also show inflammation in the lamina propria, characterized by lymphocytes or eosinophils.

Patients with lymphocytic colitis have an excess of intraepithelial lymphocytes as well as inflammation of the lamina propria characterized by plasma cells, eosinophils, and mast cells, but they do not have eosinophilic deposits.

Treatment & Prognosis

Diarrhea tends to be chronic and intermittent, but pursues a benign course. As there is no agent proven to be effective, initial treatment is directed toward control of symptoms. Medications (especially NSAIDs) associated with symptom onset should be discontinued, if possible. Symptomatic therapy with bulking agents and loperamide may provide effective control of diarrhea. Cholestyramine (believed to bind bile salts or bacterial toxins) may be of benefit in some patients. A course of empirical antibiotic therapy with metronidazole has also been recommended.

If symptoms persist, treatment with antiinflammatory medications should be considered. A 2-month course of treatment with bismuth subsalicylate may be beneficial. In an uncontrolled series of 13 patients with microscopic colitis (7 with collagenous colitis), eight tablets of 262 mg of bismuth subsalicylate for 8 weeks resulted in clinical response in 11 patients and histologic improvement in nine. If symptoms persist, treatment for 1–2 months with sulfasalazine or mesalamine should be tried, and continued for 2–3 months if symptoms improve. In case series, symptomatic improvement with these agents is reported in up to 60% of patients. Patients with severe or refractory symptoms may require treatment with corticosteroids (prednisone 40 mg/d; budesonide 3 mg three times a day). Although symptomatic improvement is common, symp-

tomatic relapse after discontinuation of steroids may occur. Histologic regression of collagen bands and inflammation have been reported with prednisone and sulfasalazine.

Resolution of symptoms occurs in approximately 60% of patients over time. Unlike ulcerative colitis and Crohn's disease, microscopic colitis is not associated with increased risk of colonic malignancy. There is no risk of development of inflammatory bowel disease.

PNEUMATOSIS CYSTOIDES INTESTINALIS

 ESSENTIALS OF DIAGNOSIS

- *Air-filled cysts in submucosa or serosa of small or large bowel.*
- *Often an incidental finding; cysts may produce cramping and bleeding.*
- *Rare fulminant form associated with other diseases, especially inflammatory or ischemic bowel disease.*

General Considerations

Pneumatosis cystoides intestinalis (PCI) is an uncommon condition characterized by air-filled cysts in the submucosa or the serosa of the large or small bowel. Cysts also may be found in the stomach, mesentery, or omentum. Two clinical syndromes have been described—a fulminant process and a benign, usually asymptomatic process, that have pathogenetic and therapeutic distinctions.

The uncommon fulminant form of PCI usually is associated with inflammatory or ischemic bowel disease in adults or necrotizing enterocolitis in children. Other associated diseases include graft-versus-host disease, complications from liver or kidney transplantation, cytomegalovirus colitis, and ulcerations from cancer chemotherapy. Cyst formation may arise from luminal gas entering the bowel wall through a disrupted mucosa or from migration of gas-forming organisms to the subepithelial layers.

The more common form of PCI is a chronic and often an incidental finding that is detected during the evaluation of unrelated complaints. It may be idiopathic in 15% of patients, but in most patients it is associated with predisposing conditions such as obstructive lung disease, scleroderma, intestinal obstruction, cystic fibrosis, nitrous oxide anesthesia, endoscopy, abdominal surgery, late stage human immunodeficiency virus (HIV) disease, or lactulose or steroid treatment.

Pathology

The cysts vary in size from a few millimeters to several centimeters and may be single or multiple. They are lined by endothelial cells that coalesce to form giant cells and do not communicate with the luminal surface. The gas in the cysts have an increased concentration of hydrogen and methane but a nitrogen:oxygen ratio similar to atmospheric air. Because the cysts are sterile in patients with chronic PCI, rupture results in pneumoperitoneum but does not cause peritonitis.

Clinical Findings

Pneumatosis can occur at any age but is more common in the sixth and seventh decades. It occurs equally among men and women. It usually is asymptomatic and is detected incidentally during radiographic imaging studies, endoscopy, or surgery. When symptomatic, larger cysts may produce cramping abdominal pain, rectal bleeding, mucus discharge, tenesmus, change in bowel habits, or obstruction caused by volvulus, cyst impaction, or intussusception.

Physical clues to the diagnosis include tympany throughout the abdomen and absence of dullness over the liver. Plain radiographs of the abdomen demonstrate linear or cystic lucencies in the bowel wall, and cyst rupture may result in pneumoperitoneum. Computed tomography (CT) is a more sensitive means of detecting intramural gas. The presence of air within the portal or mesenteric venous system may occur with benign PCI, but is worrisome for bowel ischemia and infection. On colonoscopy, the cysts appear as rounded pale or bluish masses protruding into the lumen and produce a popping sound when punctured with a needle.

Treatment

It is important to identify patients with fulminant PCI, for whom urgent surgery may be required to treat bowel ischemia, infarction, or infection. History, physical examination, abdominal CT scan, and laboratory data (leukocytosis, metabolic acidosis, and hyperamylasemia) should establish the diagnosis. For most patients with chronic or asymptomatic PCI, treatment is directed at the predisposing illness and no specfic therapy is necessary for the intestinal pneumatosis. Indeed, cysts may resolve spontaneously. When therapy is necessary for large or symptomatic cysts, increasing the partial pressure of oxygen in inspired air to achieve a pAO_2 of 200–250 mm Hg for 1–2 weeks allows diffusion of nitrogen from the cysts to the bloodstream, thereby reducing cyst size. Surgical resection may be necessary for refractory cases and for complicated disease.

COLITIS CYSTICA PROFUNDA

 ESSENTIALS OF DIAGNOSIS

- Hematochezia, mucus discharge, diarrhea, pain.
- Movable mass in anterior surface of rectum.

General Considerations

The presence of benign mucus-filled cysts in layers deeper than the muscularis mucosae defines **colitis cystica profunda (CCP).** A similar entity known as **colitis cystica superficialis** has asymptomatic cystic structures superficial to the muscularis mucosae; it is a rare condition usually associated with pellagra or celiac sprue, and resolves with treatment of the underlying disease.

CCP most likely represents an unusual reaction to colonic mucosal inflammation or trauma. Associated conditions include solitary rectal ulcers, rectal prolapse, and chronic ulcerative colitis. Epithelial-lined cysts often are large, are few in number, and can penetrate the muscularis propria. The overlying mucosa may be ulcerated or intact. There is a proliferation of muscularis layer in the lamina propria, similar to that found in the solitary rectal ulcer syndrome.

Clinical Findings

A. Symptoms and Signs

CCP typically affects men and women in their third or fourth decade. Presenting symptoms include hematochezia, mucus discharge, diarrhea, tenesmus, and abdominal and rectal pain. Digital examination may reveal a smooth, rubbery, movable mass in the anterior aspect of the rectum.

B. Endoscopy

Lesions are sessile and polypoid, and may be confused with adenomatous polyps. Biopsy is required for confirmation of diagnosis.

Differential Diagnosis

Differential diagnoses include juvenile polyps, adenomatous polyps, adenocarcinoma, intestinal lymphoma, lipoma, leiomyoma, pseudopolyps from inflammatory bowel disease, and cysts from PCI or endometriosis.

Treatment

Colonoscopic polypectomy usually is insufficient to control symptoms. Bulky symptomatic lesions require surgical resection. Rectal prolapse, a predisposing condition, may require surgical repair.

NONSPECIFIC OR "SOLITARY" ULCERATION OF THE COLON & RECTUM

Nonspecifc ulceration of the colon and rectum is a clinical entity characterized by ulceration in various segments of the large intestine and rectum. The common term "solitary ulceration" is a misnomer, as ulcers may be multiple. Rectal ulcers account for 5% of solitary ulcers, with the remainder occurring in the cecum (45%), ascending colon (20%), and sigmoid (16%). Three distinct syndromes are seen: nonspecific colonic ulcers, Dieulafoy-type ulcer, and solitary rectal ulcer syndrome.

1. Nonspecific Ulcer of the Colon

Ulcers are located along the antimesenteric border of the colon. They may be single or multiple and range in size from 5 mm to 6 cm. The etiology is unknown, although proposed mechanisms include ischemic injury, fecal stasis, peptic ulceration, foreign bodies, and focal diverticulitis. Patients may present with chronic abdominal pain and altered bowel habits, acute or recurrent colonic bleeding, or acute right lower quadrant abdominal pain that may be confused with appendicitis, Crohn's disease, or pelvic inflammatory disease. Spontaneous healing is common.

2. Dieulafoy-Type Ulcers

These are small mucosal ulcers thought to be caused by strong pulsations of an adjacent large-caliber submucosal artery. Patients present with profuse hematochezia and hypotension. If bleeding subsides or slows, colonoscopy may be performed, which may reveal a visible vessel or an adherent clot with normal mucosa or a minute mucosal defect. Endoscopic treatment coagulation or injection therapy may be applied. Patients with massive or recurrent bleeding require either mesenteric angiography with attempt at embolication of the bleeding vessel or colonic resection.

3. Solitary Rectal Ulcer Syndrome (SRUS)

 ESSENTIALS OF DIAGNOSIS

- Single or multiple rectal ulcers or mass lesion.
- Abdominal cramps, straining, hematochezia.
- Digital examination reveals indurated tissue, suggestive of malignancy.
- Associated with rectal prolapse and constipation.

General Considerations

SRUS is characterized by abdominal pain and hematochezia (especially in the setting of chronic constipation), straining at stool, and rectal prolapse. SRUS affects more women than men and the peak age range is 20–35 years old.

Pathophysiology

Rectal prolapse, seen in up to 95% of patients with SRUS, and self-induced trauma from manual disimpaction may lead to ulceration of the mucosa. More proximal ulcers are most likely caused by localized trauma from prolapse of the ileocecal valve, or even a short-lived intussusception. In the SRUS there may be histologic evidence of colitis cystica profunda, with glands buried in the adjacent mucosa, implying a common pathogenetic mechanism for these two disorders. Both entities are believed to be caused by a reaction to chronic constipation and prolonged straining at stool, with high intrarectal pressures.

Clinical Findings

Symptoms are dependent upon the location of the ulcer, with proximal ulcers causing cramping abdominal pain and more distal ulcers causing hematochezia. Digital examination may demonstrate firm tissue surrounding the ulceration, which may be confused with carcinoma. On endoscopic or proctoscopic examination, single or multiple ulcers may be seen, 5 mm to 5 cm in size, which usually are located on the rectal anterior wall, 6–12 cm above the anal verge. The lesions also may be raised and polypoid, resembling a neoplasm. Prolapse of the rectal mucosa may be demonstrated with abdominal straining. Histologically, there is excessive collagen deposition and muscular fibers of the lamina propria that extend to the deeper layers beyond the muscularis mucosae. Defecography may be useful to document rectal prolapse, intussusception, perineal descent, or other disorders of anorectal function. Rectal endosonorgraphy may be useful in differentiating SRUS from malignancy.

Differential Diagnosis

The differential diagnosis includes colonic ischemia, adenocarcinoma, Crohn's colitis, infectious colitis, colitis from NSAID use, and stercoral ulceration.

Treatment

Treatment options for solitary ulcers of the colon and rectum are of limited efficacy. The use of bulking agents and stool softeners as well as counseling to avoid straining and digital manipulation are the only medical options available. Sulfasalazine, 5-aminosalicylic acid agents, corticosteroids, and sucralfate enemas are ineffective. If rectal prolapse is present, surgical repair may result in symptom resolution. Severely symptomatic ulcers proximal to the rectum that do not respond to bulking agents require surgical resection.

FECAL IMPACTION & STERCORAL ULCERS

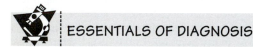

ESSENTIALS OF DIAGNOSIS

- *Vague abdominal pain, constipation, and sometimes passage of watery stool.*
- *Palpable firm fecal mass.*

General Considerations

Fecal impaction is defined as a large, firm, immovable fecal mass in the rectum or colon. Fecal impactions are usually rock-hard and often radiopaque. Most are in the rectum, but impactions may occur in the colon when the lumen is narrowed from a malignancy or fibrous stricture.

Pathophysiology

Predisposing conditions include chronic debility, pseudoobstruction, spinal cord injuries, diabetes, chronic renal failure, cystic fibrosis, immobility, painful anal disease (such as hemorrhoids, fissures, stricture, and cancer), chronic dehydration, and altered mental status, especially in institutionalized patients. Medications such as narcotics, anticholinergics, antihypertensives, aluminum-containing compounds such as sucralfate and antacids, and bulk-forming laxatives without sufficient hydration also may predispose to impaction. Barium examination without adequate evacuation may lead to barium impaction.

Clinical Findings

Clinically, patients may complain of vague abdominal pain, rectal fullness, tenesmus, anorexia, incontinence, and small amounts of watery stool, the so-called "diarrhea around a fecal impaction."

Complications

Left untreated, fecal impaction may lead to obstruction, stercoral ulceration, and possibly perforation. Ureteral obstruction from local compression, sigmoid volvulus, rectal prolapse, and perirectal fistulas are also reported.

Stercoral ulcerations arise from pressure necrosis of the rectal wall caused by fecal pressure. These ulcers have been dubbed the "decubitus ulcers" of the rectum and are usually irregular in appearance, conforming to the shape of the fecal mass. There is minimal inflammation surrounding this ulceration, but ischemic injury to the deeper layers makes localized perforation relatively common. Patients with stercoral ulceration present with hematochezia, fever, and localized tenderness. Because these ulcerations occur in the rectum (below the peritoneal reflection), free peritoneal air from perforation is rare. The diagnosis is suspected by clinical history and is confirmed by a digital examination and sigmoidoscopic examination.

Treatment

Fecal impaction and stercoral ulceration can be prevented by recognizing the predisposing conditions and intervening in high-risk patients. Preventive measures includes adequate hydration, bulk-forming agents, laxative use, and enemas, as needed. Chronic use of osmotic agents (sorbitol, lactulose, or polyethylene glycol) helps maintain soft, liquid stools. Once formed, fecal impactions usually require treatment with enemas (especially mineral oil or glycerin enemas to soften the fecal mass, or administration of gastrograffin enema under fluoroscopic visualization) and/or manual disimpaction followed by tap water enemas to assist expulsion. A local anesthetic may be required to assist with anal relaxation prior to disimpaction. More proximal impaction requires sigmoidoscopic removal.

DIVERSION COLITIS

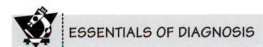

ESSENTIALS OF DIAGNOSIS

- *History of bowel bypass surgery.*
- *Blood and mucus discharge from rectum.*
- *Resolution with reanastomosis.*

Diversion colitis—also known as bypass colitis, exclusion colitis, or disuse colitis—is characterized by the occurrence of colitis in a previously normal segment of colon after it has been surgically diverted from the fecal stream. After surgical reanastomosis, the colitis completely resolves.

Pathophysiology

Colonocytes are nourished from the bloodstream as well as from luminal contents. Nonabsorbed carbohydrates are metabolized by colonic flora to synthesize, among other compounds, short-chain fatty acids (SCFAs). In vitro studies indicate that these SCFAs are preferred over glucose or ketone bodies as a metabolic substrate. The most favored nutrient source for colonocytes is butyrate, but propionate and acetate also are used efficiently. Blood concentrations of SCFAs are negligible. From a normal diet in an intact colon, 100–200 mmol/L of SCFAs are delivered into the colon; a diverted segment has less than 5 mmol/L. The preference of colonocytes for SCFAs increases aborally, making privations worse in diverted distal colonic segments. In laboratory animals, metabolic inhibition of the utilization of SCFAs induces a colitis similar to diversion colitis in humans.

Clinical Findings

A. SYMPTOMS AND SIGNS

Affected persons develop a bloody mucus discharge from the rectum or mucus fistula as early as 1 month after surgical diversion, but symptoms may develop up to 3 years after surgery. There may also be pelvic pain, fever, and anal irritation. However, many patients with evidence of diversion colitis on endoscopy are asymptomatic.

B. ENDOSCOPY AND HISTOLOGY

Among patients undergoing fecal diversion (eg, Hartman procedure with a rectal pouch) endoscopic or pathologic evidence of colitis almost always is present postoperatively in the diverted segment. Changes are more evident in the most distal segments. The endoscopic appearance may show narrowing, erythema, ulceration, friability, exudate, or a distorted mucosal vascular pattern. Histologic findings include mucin depletion, mucosal edema, decreased number and depth of crypts, superficial ulcerations, expansion of cellular elements of the lamina propria, granulocyte infiltration, and fibrosis of the lamina propria.

Treatment

The optimal and curative therapy for diversion colitis is reanastomosis of the diverted colonic segment to the colon or small bowel. Even in the face of mucosal inflammation in a patient with Crohn's colitis, surgery should proceed, when indicated. In a symptomatic patient who cannot undergo surgical anastomosis, twice-daily 60-mL enemas containing SCFA delivered into the diverted segment provide improvement within 6 weeks. This treatment resolves not only symptoms but also endoscopic and histologic inflammation. Response is not common with corticosteroid or 5-aminosalicylic acid enemas. SCFA enemas can be manufactured by a local pharmacy or laboratory. An effective formulation is 60 mmol acetate, 30 mmol propionate, and 40 mmol butyrate with sufficient sodium chloride and sodium hydroxide to bring the osmolality to 280 mOsm and the pH to 7.0. Success also has been achieved with 100 mmol butyrate enemas at the same osmolality and pH. Enemas given daily or every other day can be used to maintain remission until reanastomosis becomes feasible.

DRUG-INDUCED COLITIS

ESSENTIALS OF DIAGNOSIS

- *Colitis caused by oral contraceptives mimics Crohn's colitis: chronic diarrhea, aphthoid ulcers.*
- *NSAID colitis mimics ulcerative colitis: bleeding, diarrhea, and superficial ulcers.*
- *Resolution of symptoms when drugs are discontinued.*

General Considerations

Some medications, particulary oral contraceptives and NSAIDs, may cause mucosal inflammation of the colon resulting in symptoms and endoscopic findings that simulate inflammatory bowel disease. Even though the incidence is exceedingly low, the widespread use of these medications makes drug-induced colitis a potentially more important problem than inflammatory bowel disease. Other medications that may cause a drug-induced colitis include methyldopa, penicillamine, potassium supplements, 5-fluorouracil, oral gold, and isoretinoin.

Pathophysiology

The pathogenesis of colitis from oral contraceptives (OC) is unknown but is believed to result from an occlusive vascular phenomenon. NSAID-induced colitis is believed to arise from cyclooxygenase inhibition with loss of mucosal cytoprotective prostaglandins.

General Considerations

The distinction between drug-induced colitis and idiopathic inflammatory bowel disease is important, because drug-induced colitis may be treated effectively by withdrawal of the offending medication, whereas inflammatory bowel disease often requires the institution of potentially toxic medications.

Clinical Findings

A. OC PILL COLITIS

Colitis from oral contraceptives can be indistinguishable clinically and endoscopically from Crohn's colitis. Patients present with chronic diarrhea. On colonosocopy, aphthoid ulcers may be found scattered throughout the colon. Symptoms and signs of OC colitis completely resolve without sequelae upon discontinuation of the agents.

B. NSAID COLITIS

Colitis caused by NSAIDs mimics ulcerative colitis. Patients most often present with bleeding or bloody diarrhea. On colonoscopy, diffuse inflammation with superficial ulcers is seen. The distinction between inflammatory bowel disease and NSAID-induced colitis is further complicated by the fact that arthritis, a condition usually treated with NSAIDs, is common to both diseases. In an elderly patient with arthritis who develops symptoms and signs suggestive of ulcerative colitis, drug-induced colitis should be excluded before a diagnosis of inflammatory bowel disease is made. With discontinuation of medication, NSAID-induced colitis should completely resolve. NSAIDs also may induce a flare of ulcerative colitis in remission.

Complications

Besides bleeding and diarrhea, colonic complications of NSAIDS include diaphgragm-like strictures (especially in the small intestine and right colon) caused by submucosal fibrosis perforation from deep ulceration.

Treatment

Withdrawal of the offending agent is the only effective therapy.

RADIATION COLOPATHY

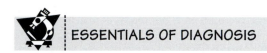

ESSENTIALS OF DIAGNOSIS

- Early disease: diarrhea, hematochezia occurring during or soon after radiation therapy.
- Late disease: abdominal pain, diarrhea, and rectal bleeding months to years after radiation.

General Considerations

One-half of patients diagnosed with cancer receive radiation therapy. Toxicity to the gastrointestinal tract is problematic and may limit the total dose that can be administered. Radiation colopathy occurs in approximately 5–10% of patients receiving therapy. Because of its proximity to other organs and its fixed pelvic location, the rectum is the most common organ affected. The malignancies most commonly associated with radiation colopathy are transitional cell carcinoma of the bladder, squamous cell carcinoma of the cervix, endometrial cancer, and adenocarcinoma of the prostate or rectum.

Pathophysiology

Radiation colopathy is dependent on the port, total dose, dose rate (fractionation), and type of energy (photon, neutron, or alpha particle). Cell death is exponentially related to the total dose, and rapid delivery is more lethal than slower delivery in fractions. Radiation causes molecules in the path of the beam to ionize and thereby damages living cells. Nuclear DNA is the prime target, resulting in either immediate cell death or loss of reproduction/division capacity. Most damage is done in the mitotic phase or late second rest phase (M or G_2 phase) of the cell cycle. Cell function may be altered by damage to cell membrane proteins. Early toxicity from radiation therapy is caused by injury to the crypt cells of the epithelium, whereas late injury is caused by damage to the vascular endothelium and connective tissue leading to vascular sclerosis and fibrosis. Delivery of 60 Gy to the region of the colon or 80 Gy to the region of the rectum will induce early or late radiation colopathy, or both, in approximately 50% of patients. There is a narrow margin of safety, since these doses are close to what is required for treatment of the tumor.

1. Early Radiation Colopathy

Clinical Findings

A. SYMPTOMS AND SIGNS

Early radiation colopathy usually occurs within the first month of therapy. Because the epithelium is disrupted, the most common symptoms are diarrhea and hematochezia. Tenesmus and mucus discharge also are common complaints.

B. ENDOSCOPY

The mucosa has edema, loss of mucosal vascular pattern, friability, and superficial ulcerations, similar to findings in ulcerative colitis. Involvement will be limited to the radiation port and therefore is not necessarily continuous.

C. HISTOLOGY

Histologic findings include mucosal cell loss, eosinophilic crypt abscesses, acute inflammatory infiltrate in the lamina propria, endothelial swelling of the arterioles, and rarely, ulceration. Thumbprinting, loss of haustrations, anterior rectal ulceration, and luminal narrowing are radiologic signs of early toxicity.

Treatment

Limiting total radiation dose significantly reduces the likelihood of symptoms. Symptoms of early toxicity may be treated with antispasmodics, antidiarrheals, bulking agents, and topical anesthetics. Steroid enemas and 5-aminosalicylic acid agents are of no benefit. Sucralfate enemas and short-chain fatty acid enemas have been tried with good initial results but the long-term effect benefit is unproven. A recent randomized clinical trial showed that misoprostol rectal suppositories prior to radiation reduce both acute and chronic symptoms.

2. Late Radiation Colopathy

Clinical Findings

A. SYMPTOMS AND SIGNS

Early symptoms may persist or new symptoms may arise 3 months or more after the conclusion of radiation. The peak symptom incidence is 9 months, but symptoms may occur up to several years after radiation. Symptoms are insidious and sometimes progressive. The most common presenting complaints are diarrhea, tenesmus, rectal pain, mucous discharge, change in stool caliber, and hematochezia. Stricture formation, fistulas, perforation, and impaired motility also may occur.

B. ENDOSCOPY

Telangiectasias, or "corkscrew" vessels, granularity, friability with mucosal oozing, discrete ulcers, or, uncommonly, strictures are found on endoscopy.

C. HISTOLOGY

In late radiation colopathy, histologic changes resemble ischemic colitis, with submucosal fibrosis, telangiectasias of small vessels, and hyalinized endothelium of larger blood vessels.

Treatment

Treatment of late complications of radiation therapy is difficult. Steroid and mesalamine enemas are of marginal benefit. Persistent rectal bleeding and discharge can be controlled by endoscopic cauterization of abnormal rectal vessels with a number of modalities, including argon plasma coagulation, argon or Nd:YAG laser, heater probe, or bipolar electrocoagulation. Patients may require repeated sessions. Topical application of formalin also has been shown to be effective for treatment of rectal bleeding. Symptomatic rectal strictures can be dilated with Savary-Gilliard or balloon dilators. Because of the compromised colonic vascular supply in the radiated bowel, dilation of colonic strictures has a higher risk of perforation. Rarely, surgery is indicated for high-grade obstruction, refractory bleeding, symptomatic fistulas, or perforation. Surgery should be considered as a last resort as it is often complicated by delayed healing, anastomotic leaks, local infections, strictures, obstruction, and fistulization.

FOREIGN BODIES IN THE RECTUM & COLON

Foreign bodies in the rectum and colon may occur from a variety of circumstances such as autoeroticism (most common), iatrogenic (eg, thermometer), inadvertent insertion (eg, enemas), sexual or criminal assault, accidental ingestion, or concealment (eg, body packing of cocaine). Both because of a narrower pelvis that more easily leads to impaction and more frequent practice of rectal eroticism, men more commonly present with foreign bodies than do women.

Clinical Findings

Patients most commonly report the presence of the rectal foreign body and their inability to remove it. Anal pain, pruritis, constipation, and bleeding may be other presenting symptoms. Findings are directly related to the size and type of the foreign body. Perforation, peritonitis, and obstruction rarely occur.

Diagnosis & Treatment

Based upon history, physical examination, and biplane pelvic x-ray, the clinician usually can identify the foreign body and assess the advisability of removal in the outpatient setting.

Low-lying rectal objects are palpable on digital examination and usually are situated in the ampulla. Extraction may be difficult because of the presence of spasm, blood, or edema caused by the object or prior attempts at removal. After sedation and local anesthesia, the object usually can be removed through an anoscope with a snare, forceps, or uterine tenaculum. Enemas should be avoided, since objects may be pushed out of reach, and blind removal should not be attempted. Anal dilation under general anesthesia with transanal removal usually is required for larger objects. After removal, proctosigmoidoscopy is recommended to evaluate for perforation, mucosal trauma, and bleeding.

High-lying objects are those that are located proximal to the rectosigmoid junction and hence not palpable on digital examination. High-lying objects in the colon that have been swallowed are thin enough to traverse proximal areas of physiologic narrowing and will usually pass within 48 hours on a high-fiber diet. Most others will descend within 24 hours with sedation. Otherwise, they are treated by moving them into a low-lying position. This can be done by sigmoidoscopic manipulation or bimanual manipulation under general anesthesia. If these methods are unsuccessful, surgical removal is required. The surgeon often may manipulate the object to the rectum and remove it transanally, thereby avoiding a colotomy on the unprepared colon. Sharp objects may become impacted and perforate or bleed, making laparotomy necessary.

REFERENCES

Babb R: Radiation proctitis: a review. Am J Gastroeneterol 1996; 91:1309.

Bjarnason I et al: Nonsteroidal antiinflammatory drug-induced intestinal inflammation in humans. Gastroenterology 1987;93: 480.

Davila M, McQuaid K: Management of rectal foreign bodies. In: *Consultations in Gastroenterology*. Snape W (editor). W.B. Saunders, 1994.

Fine D, Lee E: Efficacy of open label bismuth subsalicylate for the treatment of microscopic colitis. Gastroenterology 1998; 114:29.

Giardiello F, Lazenby A: The atypical colitides. Gastroenterol Clin 1999;28:479.

Harig JM et al: Treatment of diversion colitis with short-chain fatty acid irrigation. N Engl J Med 1989;320:23.

Khan A et al: A prospective randomized placebo-controlled double blinded pilot study of Misoprostol rectal suppositories in the prevention of acute and chronic radiation proctitis symptoms in prostate cancer patients. Am J Gastroenterol 2000;95: 1961.

SECTION V
Diseases of the Pancreas

Acute Pancreatitis

James H. Grendell, MD

Acute pancreatitis is an acute inflammatory process of the pancreas, with variable involvement of peripancreatic tissue or remote organ systems. It ranges in severity from a mild self-limited disease to a catastrophic one with multiple severe complications and the risk of death.

GENERAL CONSIDERATIONS

Gallstone disease and excessive alcohol use account for 70–80% of cases of acute pancreatitis in industrialized countries. Other important but less common causes include genetic hyperlipidemia (serum triglyceride levels typically >1000 mg/dL at the time of hospital admission for symptoms of pancreatitis), chronic hypercalcemia, surgery, abdominal trauma (blunt or penetrating), endoscopic retrograde cholangiopancreatography (ERCP), infection (eg, ascariasis, clonorchiasis, mumps, cytomegalovirus infection), and a variety of drugs (eg, azathioprine, mercaptopurine, didanosine, pentamidine, sulfonamides, 5-aminosalicylates). Pancreatic cancers and ampullary tumors can infrequently present as acute pancreatitis. Table 30–1 lists some of the causes of acute pancreatitis.

Patients with acquired immunodeficiency syndrome (AIDS) have an increased incidence of acute pancreatitis. In part, this is due to infections involving pancreatic tissue (eg, cryptosporidiosis, cryptococcosis, toxoplasmosis, or infection with cytomegalovirus, *Mycobacterium tuberculosis,* or *Mycobacterium avium* complex) and in part to use of medications (eg, didanosine, pentamidine, trimethoprim-sulfamethoxazole). In AIDS, serum amylase concentrations are also frequently elevated in the absence of evidence of pancreatitis; this may be due to abnormalities in renal tubular function

and increases in the salivary isoamylase fraction of total serum amylase or subclinical pancreatic inflammation below the threshold for detection by imaging studies.

Although most series classify 10–30% of patients as having idiopathic acute pancreatitis, recent reports suggest that occult gallstones (biliary microlithiasis or gallbladder sludge) can be demonstrated in 50–75% of these patients by microscopic examination of the bile or duodenal juice or by repeated abdominal ultrasound examinations. Treatments directed at gallstone disease (eg, cholecystectomy, endoscopic sphincterotomy, ursodeoxycholic acid therapy) appear to reduce the likelihood of recurrent pancreatitis for these patients.

Gallstone disease results in acute pancreatitis when a stone (usually only a few millimeters in diameter) migrates from the gallbladder into the common bile duct and reaches the duodenal papilla. This may lead to a sudden increase in pressure in the pancreatic duct, resulting in a "secretory block" of digestive enzymes at the level of the acinar (enzyme-secreting) cell, or may lead to reflux of bile or duodenal juice into the pancreatic duct.

The mechanism by which acute pancreatitis is induced by causative factors other than gallstone disease and direct trauma remains unknown. Experimental studies and some clinical observations suggest that development of a secretory block may be a common feature of acute pancreatitis, whatever the cause.

Identification of Occult Causes of Acute Pancreatitis

In most patients, the cause of acute pancreatitis will be identified by an initial evaluation consisting of history taking (looking for excessive alcohol use, medications, previous episodes of gallstone disease), physical exami-

Table 30–1. Major causes of acute pancreatitis.

Gallstone disease
Chronic excessive alcohol use
Drugs (eg, azathioprine, mercaptopurine, didanosine, pen-
    tamidine, sulfonamides, salicylates, valproic acid, furo-
    semide, methyldopa, angiotensin-converting enzyme
    inhibitors)
Infections (eg, ascariasis, clonorchiasis, mumps, toxoplasmo-
    sis, coxsackievirus, cytomegalovirus, tuberculosis, *M avium*
    complex)
Blunt or penetrating abdominal trauma
Surgery
ERCP[1]
Genetic hypertriglyceridemia
Chronic hypercalcemia
Pancreatic or ampullary tumors
Sphincter of Oddi dysfunction
Duodenal disease (eg, peptic ulcer, Crohn's disease, peri-
    ampullary diverticula)
Toxins (eg, organophosphate insecticides, scorpion venom)
Pancreas divisum
Vasculitis (eg, polyarteritis nodosum, systemic lupus eryth-
    ematosus, thrombotic thrombocytopenic purpura)
Cystic fibrosis
Hereditary disease
Idiopathic disease

---

[1]ERCP, endoscopic retrograde cholangiopancreatography.

nation, determination on admission of serum triglyceride and calcium concentrations, and abdominal ultrasound (or, previously, oral cholecystography). In most
series, however, 10–30% of patients have been considered to have "idiopathic" acute pancreatitis.

Several recent reports suggest that about one-half or
more of these patients have occult gallstone disease (eg,
microlithiasis, biliary sludge), which is best identified
by examination of bile for cholesterol and calcium
bilirubinate crystals or by repeated abdominal ultrasound examinations. Additionally, genetic hyperlipidemia is frequently missed because serum triglycerides
are not measured until after the patient has been fasting
for several days, by which time triglyceride levels may
have fallen substantially. Several studies have suggested
that sphincter of Oddi dysfunction may account for
15% of cases of acute pancreatitis otherwise considered
idiopathic. In addition, some less common mutations
of the cystic fibrosis transmembrane conductance regulator (CFTR) gene have been proposed to result in otherwise unexplained episodes of acute pancreatitis in
adults.

The more common identifiable causes of "idiopathic" acute pancreatitis and the means of diagnosing
them are given in Table 30–2.

PATHOPHYSIOLOGY

Acute pancreatitis is believed to begin as an autodiges-
tive process within the gland as a result of premature
activation of zymogens (digestive enzyme precursors)
within the pancreatic secretory (acinar) cells, duct system, or interstitial space. This results in acinar cell
damage and necrosis, edema, and inflammation. In addition to digestive enzyme activation, oxidative stress,
impaired microcirculation of blood in the pancreas, and
release of cytokines (in particular, interleukin-1, tumor
necrosis factor, platelet-activating factor, and nitric
oxide) also appear to contribute to both pancreatic injury and extrapancreatic complications.

Extension of this inflammatory process beyond the
pancreas frequently leads to localized complications
(Table 30–3) and can result in a variety of systemic
complications (Table 30–4).

In about 75–80% of patients, the inflammatory
process is self-limited, involving only the pancreas and
immediate peripancreatic tissue and resolving spontaneously in a few days to a week. In the other 20–25%, a
severe course ensues, with multiple local and systemic
complications, prolonged hospitalization, and risk of
death. The overall mortality rate for hospitalized patients with acute pancreatitis is 5–10%.

CLINICAL FINDINGS

Symptoms & Signs

Abdominal pain is the cardinal manifestation of acute
pancreatitis, present in about 95% of patients. Pain is
epigastric and radiates to the back in one-half to two-
thirds of patients. Nausea, vomiting, and abdominal
distention are also frequent symptoms.

On examination, abdominal tenderness is usually
present, along with guarding and rebound tenderness in
more severe cases. Depending on the severity of the disease, patients may also exhibit fever, tachycardia,
tachypnea, and hypotension.

Laboratory Findings

Because the history and physical findings are nonspecific,
confirmation by laboratory tests or abdominal imaging is
necessary. The serum amylase concentration is increased
in 80–85% of patients with acute pancreatitis but in only
65–70% with pancreatitis resulting from alcohol use;
serum amylase may also be normal in pancreatitis due to
hyperlipidemia. Amylase levels may also be elevated in a
variety of conditions that can mimic acute pancreatitis
(eg, cholangitis, gastrointestinal perforation or ischemia,
ruptured ectopic pregnancy), as well as in salivary gland
disease. Serum lipase determination, at least by some
methods, is as sensitive as amylase determinations but has

Table 30–2. Possible occult causes of acute pancreatitis.

Cause	Useful Diagnostic Tests
Occult gallstone disease (negative abdominal sonogram)	Biliary drainage for crystal analysis Repeated abdominal sonograms ERCP[1]
Undiagnosed hypertriglyceridemia	Previous serum triglyceride concentration, if available Serum triglyceride determination *after* patient is placed on regular diet and medications
Abnormalities of bile and pancreatic ducts	ERCP
Sphincter of Oddi dysfunction	ERCP Sphincter of Oddi manometry
Pancreatic cancer, ampullary and other tumors	CT scanning or endoscopic ultrasound and fine-needle aspiration biopsy of suspicious areas[1] ERCP Serial determination of CA 19-9 levels
Cystic fibrosis	Genetic testing

[1]ERCP, endoscopic retrograde cholangiopancreatography; CT, computed tomography.

greater specificity, and lipase levels may remain elevated longer than amylase levels. In acute or chronic renal failure, both lipase and amylase levels may be elevated up to five times the upper limits of normal, although typically they are elevated less than three times normal. A three-fold or greater increase above the upper limit of normal for serum alanine aminotransferase (ALT) is strongly suggestive of gallstones as the cause for acute pancreatitis. Measurement in serum or urine of other pancreatic enzymes (eg, trypsin, elastase) or amylase isoenzymes has not proved useful.

Imaging Studies

Abdominal imaging, particularly computed tomography (CT) scanning, has made the greatest contribution to the accurate diagnosis of acute pancreatitis and many of its complications. Abdominal ultrasound is useful in determining whether gallstone disease may be the cause of an episode of acute pancreatitis; however, the sensi-

Table 30–3. Local complications of acute pancreatitis.

Pancreatic complications
   Phlegmon (inflammatory mass)
   Peripancreatic effusions
   Infected necrosis or pancreatic abscess
Nonpancreatic complications
   Gastrointestinal ileus
   Pancreatic ascites and pleural effusions
   Bile duct obstruction

Table 30–4. Systemic complications of acute pancreatitis.

Cardiovascular complications
   Hypovolemia
   Hypotension or shock
Renal complications
   Oliguria
   Azotemia or renal failure
Hematologic complications
   Vascular thrombosis
   Disseminated intravascular coagulation
Pulmonary complications
   Hypoxemia
   Atelectasis or pleural effusion
   ARDS or respiratory failure[1]
Metabolic complications
   Hypocalcemia
   Hyperglycemia
   Hypertriglyceridemia
   Metabolic acidosis
Gastrointestinal bleeding
   Stress gastritis
   Pseudoaneurysm
   Gastric varices
Other complications
   Peripheral fat necrosis
   Encephalopathy

[1]ARDS, acute respiratory distress syndrome.

tivity of this modality in diagnosing acute pancreatitis is relatively low, and examinations are frequently technically inadequate in patients with significant ileus. CT scans may be normal in 15–30% of patients with mild acute pancreatitis but are virtually always abnormal in moderate to severe attacks (Figure 30–1). Thus, CT scanning is the most useful means of differentiating severe acute pancreatitis from other intraabdominal catastrophic processes that may mimic pancreatitis.

So far, magnetic resonance imaging (MRI) has not improved upon CT scanning as a diagnostic technique for pancreatic inflammatory disease, but it may be use-

ful in evaluating patients unable to receive intravenous contrast medium for CT scanning.

Criteria for Assessing the Severity of Acute Pancreatitis

Extensive efforts have been devoted to establishing a method for predicting the severity of acute pancreatitis, so that the 75–80% of patients who will have a relatively mild course can be differentiated from those possibly destined for serious illness and death (Table 30–5).

Ranson criteria have been the prognostic indicator most commonly used in the United States (Table 30–6). Patients with two or fewer risk factors have a low probability of serious illness or death; with three or more risk factors, both of these probabilities increase, and they continue to increase as the number of risk factors increases.

The modified Glasgow (Imrie) criteria are similar to Ranson criteria and have been used extensively in the United Kingdom. Neither the Ranson nor the Glasgow score can be computed until the patient has been hospitalized for 48 hours, and neither can be used to follow the patient's course after that point. The Acute Physiologic and Chronic Health Evaluation (APACHE) II system is a complex scoring system that can be calculated prior to 48 hours of hospitalization and then recalculated throughout the course of hospitalization to measure progress. The Ranson and Glasgow criteria and APACHE II scoring system are similar in their abilities to predict the severity of disease at 48 hours of hospitalization. Dynamic CT scanning to look for nonenhance-

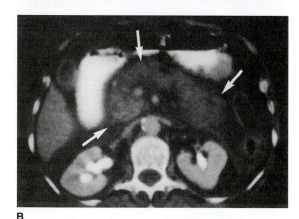

Figure 30–1. **A:** The normal pancreas on computed tomography. The gland *(arrows)* is homogeneous in appearance and, like the adjacent stomach (S) and left kidney (K), sharply demarcated. **B:** The pancreas on computed tomography in acute pancreatitis *(arrows)* is enlarged and inhomogeneous because of edema and inflammation. In addition, inflammatory changes have increased the density of the tissue surrounding loops of intestine (I) near the tail of the pancreas.

Table 30–5. Predictors of severity in acute pancreatitis.

Multiple clinical criteria
Ranson criteria
Glasgow (Imrie) criteria
APACHE II[1]
Multiple-organ failure score
CT scanning criteria[1]
Anatomic findings
Bolus contrast (dynamic pancreatography)
MRI[1]
Abdominal paracentesis
Individual laboratory tests
Methemalbumin
Phospholipase A_2
C-reactive protein
Granulocyte elastase
Interleukin-6
Trypsinogen activation peptide

[1]APACHE, Acute Physiologic and Chronic Health Evaluation; CT, computed tomography; MRI, magnetic resonance imaging.

Table 30–6. Ranson criteria of severity.

Gallstone pancreatitis
  On admission to hospital
    Age > 70 years
    WBC[1] > 18,000/μL
    Glucose > 200 mg/dL
    Lactate dehydrogenase > 400 U/L
    AST[1] > 250 U/L
  Within 48 hours of hospital admission
    Decrease in hematocrit > 10 points
    Increase in blood urea nitrogen > 2 mg/dL
    Serum calcium < 8 mg/dL
    Base deficit > 5 mmol/L
    Fluid deficit > 4 L
Pancreatitis due to causes other than gallstones
  On admission to hospital
    Age > 55 years
    WBC > 16,000/μL
    Glucose > 200 mg/dL
    Lactate dehydrogenase > 350 U/L
    AST > 250 U/L
  Within 48 hours of hospital admission
    Decrease in hematocrit > 10 points
    Increase in blood urea nitrogen > 5 mg/dL
    Calcium < 8 mg/dL
    Pa_{O_2} < 60 mm Hg
    Base deficit > 4 mmol/L
    Fluid deficit > 6 L

[1]WBC, white blood cells; AST, aspartate aminotransferase.

ment of pancreatic tissue following intravenous contrast is just as accurate but is costly (if done only to estimate prognosis) and associated with the risk of renal toxicity from intravenous contrast medium. The other predictors listed in Table 30–5 have not been as extensively validated as these three scoring methods or CT scanning.

Although several of these predictors function reasonably well (particularly APACHE II) in defining or stratifying patient populations for clinical research, none so far is clearly superior to close observation and careful clinical judgment as a basis for making therapeutic decisions for an individual patient.

TREATMENT

The goals of therapy of acute pancreatitis are to provide supportive care; decrease pancreatic inflammation and its results; and prevent, identify, and treat complications.

Mild Acute Pancreatitis

Most patients will have a mild, self-limited course requiring only bed rest, no oral intake, intravenous hydration and electrolytes, and analgesia. Traditionally,

meperidine has been the analgesic of choice because of reports that it is less likely than other opiates to raise the sphincter of Oddi pressure. The clinical importance of this is uncertain, however, and other narcotics can be substituted if needed. Nasogastric suction does not shorten the course of the disease but is useful in relieving symptoms of nausea, vomiting, or abdominal distention. Patients may be cautiously fed once abdominal pain has mostly abated, nausea (if present) has resolved, and serum amylase or lipase values have begun to return to normal.

Severe Acute Pancreatitis

A. EARLY MANAGEMENT

Care of the patient with severe pancreatitis poses a much greater challenge. In the earliest stages, vigorous resuscitation with intravenous hydration and electrolytes is critical. Volume requirements may be staggeringly large, and these patients will frequently require an intensive care unit setting, with careful attention to monitoring of hemodynamics, urine output, and renal and respiratory function. Acute renal failure may require dialysis, and respiratory failure (due to acute respiratory distress syndrome) may necessitate mechanical ventilation. The presence of renal or respiratory failure markedly increases mortality rates; however, both complications are reversible if the underlying pancreatic inflammation abates and other complications (eg, sepsis) do not supervene. Large amounts of intravenous analgesics are frequently needed for pain and nasogastric suction for severe ileus, nausea, and vomiting.

A number of pharmacologic agents have been tried to inactivate proteases (eg, aprotinin, gabexate), decrease pancreatic secretion (eg, atropine, somatostatin), or reduce inflammation (eg, indomethacin). None of these has been shown to be beneficial in good controlled studies, however. A potent platelet-activating factor antagonist (lexipafant) also failed to prove beneficial. Additionally, the efficacy of peritoneal lavage and early operative approaches (eg, "necrosectomy," debridement and drainage) in the absence of documented infection remains to be demonstrated.

B. MANAGEMENT OF GALLSTONES

Several recent randomized controlled studies have examined the value of ERCP with sphincterectomy and stone extraction, if indicated, in diminishing the severity of presumed gallstone pancreatitis. Gallstones should be suspected as the cause of acute pancreatitis in high-incidence areas (eg, Hong Kong) and in patients who abstain from alcohol or use it moderately, are of female gender, are over 60 years of age, have a greater than three-fold elevation in ALT levels, or have a history of gallstones or a dilated common bile duct visualized on abdominal ultrasound or CT scanning. ERCP for possible sphincterotomy and stone extraction should be performed for patients with likely gallstone acute pancreatitis and findings suggestive of cholangitis (right upper quadrant abdominal pain and tenderness, fever >39°C, leukocyte count >20,000/mL). However, in Western countries, cholangitis complicates gallstone pancreatitis in fewer than 10% of cases. Currently available studies yield conflicting results concerning whether ERCP performed within 24–72 hours of hospital admission reduces the severity of the disease for patients with presumed gallstone pancreatitis of moderate to severe degree who do not have cholangitis.

C. MANAGEMENT OF INFECTED NECROSIS OR ABSCESS

Patients with moderate to severe acute pancreatitis are at risk for lethal septic complications resulting from infected necrosis or abscess, usually presenting a week or more after admission to the hospital as clinical deterioration (eg, worsening pain or nausea and vomiting), fever (especially if >39.5°C), or leukocytosis (especially if >20,000/μL). The prophylactic use of antibiotics to try to prevent septic complications is now frequently employed in the treatment of patients predicted by multiple criteria scores or dynamic CT to have severe acute pancreatitis. The most commonly used regimens are imipenem or the combination of a quinolone and metronidazole administered intravenously for 10–14 days. These antibiotics reach therapeutic levels in pancreatic tissue and cover the organisms most commonly found in areas of infected necrosis (enteric gram-negative organisms, anaerobes, enterococci, and, less commonly, *Staphylococcus aureus*). Most recent studies have shown a benefit from prophylactic antibiotics, although the studies are generally small and differ in the type of benefit conferred. Patients receiving antibiotic prophylaxis, particularly those getting imipenem, are at risk for superinfection with fungi or multiresistant bacteria.

Although the value of prophylactic antibiotics is currently somewhat uncertain, over the past 20 years the earlier diagnosis and aggressive treatment of pancreatic infected necrosis and abscess have resulted in a reduction in mortality rates for this complication, from 70–80% to 10–20%. This has resulted from the widespread use of CT scanning in the early evaluation of patients with suspected infected necrosis or abscess. Suspicious (low-density) areas in the pancreas or fluid collections adjacent to it should be aspirated and material sent for culture and, most importantly, immediate preparation of gram-stained smears. The presence of both bacterial organisms and polymorphonuclear white blood cells (PMNs) on gram-stained smear is strongly indicative of infected necrosis or abscess, and patients with this finding should generally undergo emergency operation, with extensive debridement and drainage. A

few recent reports have proposed that some patients can be adequately treated with endoscopic or percutaneous catheter drainage or even antibiotics alone. However, selection criteria have yet to be defined to determine which patients may do well with nonoperative approaches because the viscous nature of the infected material and the frequent presence of loculations make catheter drainage difficult and antibiotic penetration uncertain. Patients who develop signs of recurrent sepsis after initial operative treatment for infected necrosis or abscess should be carefully evaluated for fungal (usually *Candida*) sepsis.

Needle aspiration in the evaluation of suspected infected necrosis or abscess is safe and highly reliable if adequate sampling has been achieved. The presence in aspirates of PMNs without bacterial organisms indicates a sterile necrotizing process. Operative debridement and drainage are sometimes performed in patients with sterile necrosis because of failure to improve (eg, persisting multiple-organ failure); however, the benefits of this approach have not been established.

D. NUTRITIONAL MANAGEMENT

Nutritional support should be considered for those patients who appear unlikely to resume oral intake within 7 days. Recent reports suggest that instituting enteral feeding of an elemental diet into the jejunum within 48 hours of admission is optimal. This has been shown for patients with acute pancreatitis to be well tolerated and to carry less risk and cost than total parenteral nutrition (TPN). In addition, enteral feeding may decrease septic complications by helping to maintain the integrity of the intestinal mucosa, thereby preventing bacterial translocation across the intestine. For those patients who cannot be fed enterally, lipid emulsions can be used as a component of TPN if the serum triglyceride level is maintained below 500 mg/dL. Oral feedings should not be restarted until (1) any major complications have been effectively treated; (2) the patient is free of pain and nausea; and (3) serum amylase or lipase concentrations have returned to normal. If an operation is necessary to treat a complication of acute pancreatitis, surgical placement of a tube jejunostomy greatly facilitates subsequent nutritional support by obviating the need for TPN.

Management of Pseudocysts & Hemorrhage

As many as two-thirds to three-fourths of patients with acute pancreatitis will have fluid collections (peripancreatic effusions) demonstrated early in their illness by abdominal ultrasound or CT scanning. Most of these will resolve spontaneously. Only about 15% of patients with acute pancreatitis develop an encapsulated collection of inflammatory fluid and pancreatic juice (**pseu-docyst**). If asymptomatic or mildly symptomatic (eg, mild pain), pseudocysts should be followed by ultrasound studies or CT scanning for at least 6 weeks to see if they will resolve or decrease in size without treatment. Asymptomatic pseudocysts less than 6 cm in diameter or those decreasing in size can be watched without treatment indefinitely.

Pseudocysts larger than 6 cm in diameter and persisting for more than 6 weeks after an episode of acute pancreatitis should be considered for therapy. The standard definitive treatment has been open internal surgical drainage of the cyst into the stomach, duodenum, or a Roux loop of jejunum. Newer alternative treatments include minimally invasive (laparoscopic) surgery, percutaneous catheter drainage, and endoscopic drainage. The treatment decision should be based on the specific circumstances for a given patient and the local expertise. For clinically infected pseudocysts (patients typically presenting with fever and leukocytosis who have pseudocyst aspirates demonstrating both polymorphonuclear leukocytes and bacterial organisms on gram-stained smear), percutaneous catheter drainage is as effective as the previous operative approach (open external drainage) with a lower rate of pseudocyst recurrence and fistula formation.

Significant hemorrhage (requiring transfusion) is only rarely seen as a complication of acute pancreatitis. Potential causes include stress gastritis, development of pseudoaneurysm in the peripancreatic arterial circulation, bleeding from small vessels in the wall of a pseudocyst into the cyst contents, or gastric varices due to splenic vein thrombosis. Stress gastritis and gastric varices usually present with hematemesis, melena, and a falling blood hemoglobin and are best diagnosed by upper gastrointestinal endoscopy. Bleeding from a pseudoaneurysm or into a pseudocyst may not communicate with the intestinal tract (best diagnosed by abdominal CT scanning) or may result in bleeding via the pancreatic duct (hemosuccus pancreaticus) with melena and blood or clots in the region of the duodenal papilla at endoscopy without the finding of any luminal lesion that could account for it.

Angiography is of great value in identifying the site of bleeding from a pseudoaneurysm. Some pseudoaneurysms can be definitively treated by angiographic embolization, whereas others require direct operative control.

REFERENCES

Banks PA: Practice guidelines in acute pancreatitis. Am J Gastroenterol 1997;92:377.

Baron TH, Morgan DE: Acute necrotizing pancreatitis. N Engl J Med 1999;340:1412.

Beger HG, Isenmann R: Surgical management of necrotizing pancreatitis. Surg Clin North Am 1999;79:783.

Fernandez-del Castillo C, Rattner DW, Warshaw AL: Acute pancreatitis. Lancet 1993;342:475.

Forsmark CE, Grendell JH: Complications of pancreatitis. Semin Gastrointest Dis 1991;2:165.

Grendell JH: Nonsurgical therapy of acute pseudocysts. In: *Acute Pancreatitis: Diagnosis and Therapy.* Bradley EL III (editor). Raven Press, 1994, pp 191–195.

Norman J: The role of cytokines in the pathogenesis of acute pancreatitis. Am J Surg 1998;175:76.

Runzi M, Layer, P: Nonsurgical management of acute pancreatitis. Use of antibiotics. Surg Clin North Am 1999;79:759.

Steinberg W, Tenner S: Acute pancreatitis. N Engl J Med 1994; 330:1198.

Whitcomb DC: Hereditary pancreatitis: new insights into acute and chronic pancreatitis. Gut 1999;45:317.

Wyncell DL: The management of severe acute necrotizing pancreatitis: an evidence-based review of the literature. Intensive Care Med 1999;25:146.

Chronic Pancreatitis & Pancreatic Insufficiency

31

Chris E. Forsmark, MD

Patients with chronic pancreatitis seek medical attention primarily because of chronic or episodic abdominal pain and less frequently for consequences of maldigestion (eg, steatorrhea, weight loss, or malnutrition) or diabetes mellitus. Although most patients develop pain, approximately 15% will develop steatorrhea or diabetes in the absence of pain, and a substantial number will suffer from pain alone and will never develop pancreatic exocrine or endocrine insufficiency. Chronic pancreatitis is defined histologically by irreversible damage to the pancreas with the development of inflammation, fibrosis, and eventually destruction of exocrine and endocrine tissue. The inability to obtain histologic confirmation of disease in most cases has made diagnosis and classification of chronic pancreatitis difficult. Although a series of international panels have attempted to draw up categories and definitions, these have often been based on histology and so have never become useful to clinicians. Other attempts to define and categorize chronic pancreatitis have focused on abnormalities of pancreatic morphology as visualized by computed tomography (CT), ultrasound (US), or endoscopic retrograde cholangiopancreatography (ERCP). Although more useful to clinicians, these are also inadequate as morphologic abnormalities (such as diffuse pancreatic calcifications or a dilated pancreatic duct) may take years to develop and may not even develop in some patients. More recent attempts to categorize chronic pancreatitis have focused more on etiology, but no single, widely accepted method for categorizing chronic pancreatitis exists. Given the rapid pace of our evolving knowledge of the genetic basis of pancreatic disease, it is likely this information will also need to be included in subsequent classification schemes.

Chronic pancreatitis is a progressive disease with variable tempo. Despite the fact that the damage due to the disease is usually irreversible, medical, endoscopic, and surgical therapy can often produce substantial improvement in the major complaints of abdominal pain, maldigestion, and diabetes mellitus.

DEMOGRAPHIC FINDINGS

The true incidence and prevalence of chronic pancreatitis are unknown. The fact that estimates of incidence and prevalence vary widely should not be surprising,

given the various presentations, definitions, causative factors, and diagnostic tests used in the disease. Autopsy studies suggest a prevalence of 0.04–5%. Retrospective clinical studies also vary widely, ranging from less than 1 to more than 10 new cases per 100,000 population. The only prospective study, a study essentially limited to patients with alcoholic chronic pancreatitis, found a prevalence of 27.4 cases per 100,000 population and an incidence of 8.2 new cases per 100,000 population. In the United States, approximately 20,000 admissions primarily for chronic pancreatitis occur yearly to non-Federal hospitals, with another 40,000 admissions in which chronic pancreatitis is one of the discharge diagnoses. These are underestimates of overall disease prevalence. All these data are based on populations primarily having alcohol-induced chronic pancreatitis. In the majority of these patients, substantial abnormalities of pancreatic morphology are usually readily apparent and the diagnosis of chronic pancreatitis is obvious based on CT, US, or ERCP. None of these studies reflects the incidence or prevalence of other forms of chronic pancreatitis. In particular, patients with idiopathic chronic pancreatitis often lack these changes of pancreatic morphology and hence can escape detection and may not be included in demographic data. The same can be said for less advanced cases of alcoholic chronic pancreatitis. Recent clinical studies have clearly demonstrated histologic findings of chronic pancreatitis in patients with severe chronic pain in the absence of abnormalities of the main pancreatic duct, as defined by CT scanning or ERCP. If these patients were included, the true incidence and prevalence of chronic pancreatitis would be higher than the figures suggested by the available epidemiologic studies.

The financial burden to society of chronic pancreatitis is not known. In a recent analysis of both acute and chronic pancreatitis, the total costs (direct costs for care and indirect costs such as loss of work productivity) total 2.5 billion dollars yearly. This would suggest that chronic pancreatitis accounts for substantial morbidity and health care costs. We have few data on quality of life in patients with chronic pancreatitis. Abdominal pain and continued alcohol abuse are the major negative influences on quality of life. Mortality is also strongly influenced by ongoing alcohol abuse. Overall,

496

10-year survival is about 70% and 20-year survival is about 45%. Death is usually not due to chronic pancreatitis itself but rather other medical conditions (emphysema, coronary artery disease, stroke, and malignancy), continued alcohol abuse, and postoperative complications.

PATHOPHYSIOLOGY & ETIOLOGY

The exact pathophysiologic mechanism producing pancreatic injury and chronic pancreatitis is unknown for all of the common underlying etiologies. We have begun to gain some new insights into pathophysiology based on rapidly evolving studies in genetic forms of pancreatitis. It is possible that different causes have different mechanisms of injury. Regardless of the cause, the ultimate effect is damage to the pancreatic acini, ducts, nerves, and islet cells. This damage is responsible for the cardinal manifestations of abdominal pain, maldigestion, and diabetes mellitus. The specific causes of chronic pancreatitis and their presumed pathophysiology are discussed below and are presented in Table 31–1.

Alcohol Consumption

Alcohol consumption is the major cause of chronic pancreatitis in Western societies. The incidence of chronic pancreatitis at autopsy is 50 times higher in alcoholics than in nondrinkers, and there appears to be a direct relationship between daily alcohol consumption and the risk of chronic pancreatitis. Prolonged alcohol intake is usually required before chronic pancreatitis develops (eg, four pints of beer or 800 mL of wine per day for 6–12 years). Only 15% of alcoholics with this level of intake ultimately develop chronic pancreatitis, and this suggests that other factors such as diet (particularly one high in fat), genetic predisposition (see below), or some other cofactor may also be important. In Western societies, 70% of cases of chronic pancreatitis are the result of alcohol consumption, with the remaining 30% due to other causes or idiopathic disease. The mechanism by which alcohol produces pancreatic injury and chronic pancreatitis is unknown. Alcohol appears to interfere with intracellular transport and secretion of digestive enzymes and augments the pancreatic response to cholecystokinin. In addition, alcohol promotes the formation of protein precipitates in the pancreatic duct. Whether these changes entirely explain the development of chronic pancreatitis remains to be elucidated.

Most patients with alcoholic chronic pancreatitis have an early phase of recurrent attacks of acute pancreatitis and later develop more chronic abdominal pain. Most patients (80%) who present with an acute attack of alcoholic chronic pancreatitis will ultimately progress to clear-cut chronic pancreatitis. Continued alcohol abuse after diagnosis hastens the pace of pancreatic damage, although, unfortunately, complete abstinence cannot prevent ongoing damage. The prognosis of alcoholic chronic pancreatitis is poor, with the frequent development of exocrine or endocrine insufficiency and increased mortality due to the consequence of continued alcohol abuse.

Tropical Pancreatitis

Chronic pancreatitis is commonly seen in certain areas within 30° of latitude from the equator, particularly in Indonesia, India, and Africa. Although rare in people born in the United States, this disease can be seen in immigrants to the United States. Patients typically present with abdominal pain beginning in childhood, with subsequent diabetes, malnutrition, and diffuse pancreatic calcifications. Most people ultimately die from complications of the disease. Although malnutrition is important in the development of chronic pancreatitis, toxic products contained in the diet (eg, cassava or sorghum) or the environment may also play a role in pancreatic injury.

Pancreatic Duct Obstruction

Obstruction of the main pancreatic duct by tumors, strictures or scarring, stents, or anatomic variants can lead to chronic pancreatitis. The pathologic hallmarks are acinar atrophy and fibrosis and dilatation of the pancreatic duct "upstream" of the obstruction. Long-standing obstruction can lead to irreversible chronic

Table 31–1. Causes of chronic pancreatitis.

Alcohol abuse
Obstruction of pancreatic duct
   Trauma to pancreatic duct
   Ductal stricture or stone
   Long-standing pancreatic duct stent
   Pancreas divisum, with associated accessory papillary
     stenosis
Genetic causes
   Cystic fibrosis
   Familial pancreatitis (trypsinogen gene mutations and
     others)
Tropical pancreatitis
Autoimmune chronic pancreatitis
Recurrent or severe acute pancreatitis
   Hyperlipidemia
   Severe necrotizing pancreatitis
Idiopathic pancreatitis
   Early onset
   Late onset

pancreatitis, but both functional and structural improvement can be seen if the obstruction is discovered and relieved. Obstruction may be due to posttraumatic strictures, ampullary stenosis or neoplasms, pancreatic tumors or pseudocysts, endoscopically placed pancreatic duct stents, or, rarely, inflammatory strictures resulting from a severe episode of acute pancreatitis.

Pancreas divisum, or failure of fusion of the embryologic dorsal and ventral pancreatic ducts, may also lead to obstruction to flow and chronic pancreatitis. In this condition, the small ventral pancreas drains through the major papilla and the larger dorsal pancreas drains through the accessory papilla. Pancreas divisum may occur in up to 7% of the population, and the vast majority of individuals with this congenital abnormality have no symptoms. In fact, two large studies of several thousand patients did not find pancreas divisum to be associated with either acute or chronic pancreatitis. There is a subset of patients, however, with both divisum and obstruction to flow at the accessory papilla in whom clinical pancreatic disease does occur. The clinical challenge arises in attempting to determine which patients have obstruction at the accessory papilla. Significant structural abnormalities limited to the upstream dorsal pancreatic duct (eg, dilatation) is the most specific finding and usually confirms that pancreas divisum is responsible for the clinical pancreatic disease. The finding of a normal dorsal duct does not exclude the possibility that pancreas divisum is responsible for chronic pain or chronic pancreatitis, but additional confirmatory evidence is required.

Autoimmune Chronic Pancreatitis

A rare form of chronic pancreatitis is associated with autoantibodies, elevated levels of immunoglobulins (particularly immunoglobulin G_4), and pathologic features of a dense lymphocytic infiltrate. In 60% of cases, it is associated with other autoimmune diseases including primary sclerosing cholangitis, primary biliary cirrhosis, autoimmune hepatitis, and Sjögren's syndrome. This disease may respond to steroid therapy.

Recurrent Acute Pancreatitis

Repeated attacks of acute pancreatitis or even one very severe single attack may produce enough damage to the gland to result in chronic pancreatitis. This is most likely in the setting of significant pancreatic necrosis with the development of strictures in the pancreatic duct that produce ongoing injury to the gland upstream of the stricture. Chronic pancreatitis may also occur as a consequence of repeated attacks of less severe acute pancreatitis, including hyperlipidemic pancreatitis and familial pancreatitis.

Hypertriglyceridemia may precipitate episodes of acute pancreatitis. Triglyceride levels above 1000 mg/dL are usually required to initiate acute pancreatitis, commonly as a result of familial hyperlipidemias (types IV and V) often exacerbated by estrogen use or poorly controlled diabetes. Recurrent attacks of hyperlipidemic pancreatitis may ultimately produce chronic pancreatitis. Although rare, this cause of both acute and chronic pancreatitis should not be forgotten, as effective therapy is available. The incidence of hyperlipidemic pancreatitis may be increasing because of the use of estrogens for prevention of postmenopausal osteoporosis.

Familial Pancreatitis

A number of kindreds have been described with the clinical features of recurrent acute pancreatitis beginning at an early age, which usually culminates in a markedly dilated pancreatic duct, diffuse calcifications, steatorrhea, and diabetes mellitus. Symptoms typically begin in childhood. The pattern of inheritance is autosomal dominant with incomplete penetrance. Pancreatic cancer is a common complication, occurring in up to 40% of these patients. There are a number of genetic defects that have been identified in kindreds with hereditary pancreatitis. The initial abnormality identified was a single point mutation in the cationic trypsinogen gene. Based on molecular modeling, this mutation was felt to convey a gain-of-function mutation, in which the mutated trypsinogen was resistant to inactivation once activated. Trypsin, the activated form of trypsinogen, can activate all of the other pancreatic digestive enzymes. This continual low-grade activation of digestive enzymes within the pancreas is felt to produce ongoing damage, which ultimately produces severe chronic pancreatitis. Since this initial discovery, several other gene mutations have been identified in both the cationic trypsinogen gene as well as within an enzyme meant to inactivate trypsin, the trypsin inhibitor protein (serine protease inhibitor). Initial studies have not identified these gene mutations frequently in patients with idiopathic and alcoholic chronic pancreatitis, but further studies are needed to determine whether these genetic defects can predispose to other forms of chronic pancreatitis.

Cystic Fibrosis

Cystic fibrosis is the most common cause of pancreatitis in children but can also be seen in young adults as improved overall medical care leads to more prolonged survival times in these patients. A defect in the chloride channel causes reduced flow of pancreatic secretions, the development of supersaturated pancreatic juice, and the precipitation of protein plugs within the duct. Recent studies have noted cystic fibrosis gene mutations in patients with "idiopathic" acute and chronic pancreatitis who have no clinical evidence of pulmonary or sinus conditions associated with cystic fibrosis. In preliminary studies 13–55% of patients with "idiopathic" chronic pancreatitis have at least one cystic fibrosis allelic mutation. Further studies are needed to define the role of these mutations in causing chronic pancreatitis in patients without classic sinopulmonary cystic fibrosis.

Idiopathic Pancreatitis

Despite careful evaluation, 10–30% of patients may not have a definable cause of chronic pancreatitis. Idiopathic chronic pancreatitis is the second most common cause of chronic pancreatitis in adults, the first being alcohol abuse. Some of these patients abuse alcohol surreptitiously, but a substantial number are not imbibers. Some may suffer from a *forme fruste* of cystic fibrosis, as noted above. There appear to be two forms of idiopathic chronic pancreatitis, a late-onset form and an early-onset form. The late-onset form has a mean age of onset of 56 years and commonly presents with steatorrhea or diabetes but only half have abdominal pain initially and only three-quarters develop it even with long-term follow-up. The early-onset form begins at about age 20 years and is characterized by severe pain in essentially all patients but very infrequently by steatorrhea or diabetes. Many of these patients with early-onset idiopathic chronic pancreatitis do not have easily identifiable abnormalities of the pancreatic duct and are commonly misdiagnosed.

CLINICAL FINDINGS

Symptoms & Signs

A. PAIN

For most patients with chronic pancreatitis, abdominal pain is the predominant symptom and the one that most affects quality of life. There are no characteristic features, and the pain varies tremendously in severity, pattern, quality, and frequency. An episode of acute pancreatitis superimposed on an already irreversibly damaged gland may produce the more abrupt abdominal pain associated with acute pancreatitis. In up to one-third of patients, these acute exacerbations are absent, and a more gradual onset of chronic pain is noted. The most commonly noted type of chronic pain is dull, constant, located in the epigastrium with associated back pain, and often made worse by eating or the supine position. Food may be avoided, leading to weight loss and malnutrition. Episodes of pain usually last from days to weeks, although some patients develop

continuous pain. The pain may be quite mild or severe, requiring narcotics for relief in up to 20% of patients. Pain never develops in up to 15% of patients with alcoholic chronic pancreatitis and in up to 25% or more of patients with late-onset idiopathic chronic pancreatitis.

The cause of pain in chronic pancreatitis is not well understood and is certainly multifactorial. Factors that may contribute include inflammation within the gland or affecting neural pain fibers supplying the pancreas through the celiac plexus; elevated pressures within the pancreatic ductal system or the parenchyma of the gland; associated extrapancreatic complications such as bile duct or duodenal obstruction; associated pancreatic pseudocysts; and hyperstimulation of the pancreas due to interruption of the normal negative-feedback control of the pancreas. The specific contribution of these (or other mechanisms) to pain in an individual patient is often impossible to determine. In many patients, the pain may "burn out" after many years of chronic pancreatitis, although this is unpredictable.

B. MALABSORPTION

Steatorrhea due to pancreatic exocrine insufficiency does not occur until the secretory capacity of the pancreas is reduced to less than 10% of normal. This degree of damage is not usually present until late in the clinical course of disease, so that steatorrhea is most often a marker of far advanced chronic pancreatitis. The ability of the pancreas to secrete proteases tends to be preserved longer than the ability to secrete lipase, so that protein malabsorption occurs later than fat malabsorption. In addition, carbohydrate malabsorption may rarely occur. Malabsorption is not only due to diminished secretion of pancreatic enzymes; reduced secretion of bicarbonate from the pancreatic ductal system also lowers the duodenal pH and further interferes with digestion. Weight loss occurs as a consequence of malabsorption, but may be worsened by avoidance of food due to pain or by inadequate dietary intake due to chronic alcoholism. Signs and symptoms of specific vitamin deficiencies are rare, although folate deficiency may be seen as a consequence of dietary deficiency in chronic alcoholics. In addition osteopenia and osteoporosis may develop as a consequence of vitamin D deficiency.

C. DIABETES MELLITUS

The pancreatic islet cells appear to be more resistant to damage than the acinar and ductal cells, so that diabetes occurs less frequently than steatorrhea. Diabetes mellitus ultimately develops in up to 30% of patients with chronic pancreatitis and in as many as 70% of patients when diffuse pancreatic calcifications (a marker of far advanced disease) are present. This secondary diabetes is characterized by frequent treatment-associated episodes of hypoglycemia (due to inadequate glucagon reserve) and infrequently by ketoacidosis. Complications such as diabetic retinopathy or neuropathy occur as frequently as in other diabetics if corrected for the duration of diabetes.

Diagnostic Studies

The diagnosis of chronic pancreatitis is usually suggested by clinical features such as abdominal pain, steatorrhea, or diabetes. A wide range of diagnostic tests for evaluation of pancreatic function and structure are available. Chronic pancreatitis is a slowly progressive disease. Exocrine or endocrine insufficiency or significant structural abnormalities may take years to develop. Most of the diagnostic tests currently in use rely on detecting these structural abnormalities. As the disease progresses, easily recognizable structural abnormalities may be seen, including a markedly dilated pancreatic duct, pancreatic atrophy, or diffuse pancreatic calcifications. This makes the diagnosis straightforward. In less advanced disease, however, the diagnosis can be quite challenging, particularly in early-onset idiopathic chronic pancreatitis in which characteristic structural changes develop very infrequently. This indicates that the etiology of disease and stage of disease may have a substantial impact on the overall sensitivity and specificity of diagnostic tests. This has led to a general clinical distinction: "big-duct disease" and "small-duct disease."

"Big-duct disease" is the presence of significant structural abnormalities of the pancreas and particularly dilation of the main pancreatic duct and is a marker of advanced chronic pancreatitis, particularly alcohol-induced. "Small-duct disease" implies the absence of these advanced structural abnormalities. This differentiation is useful in that those with "big-duct disease" are easiest to diagnose, are usually alcoholic, and are candidates primarily for endoscopic or surgical therapy. Those with "small-duct disease" are much more difficult to diagnose, are more likely idiopathic, and are candidates primarily for medical therapy. A few diagnostic tests are available that measure abnormalities of pancreatic function rather than abnormalities of pancreatic structure. With the exception of the direct hormonal stimulation test, all these tests of function are only abnormal in far-advanced disease when exocrine insufficiency has already developed. When evaluating patients with possible chronic pancreatitis, it is important for the physician to know the value of the various tests and to have a plan for using them. The true "gold standard" for diagnosis is pancreatic biopsy, which demonstrates pancreatic inflammation, fibrosis, destruction of acinar tissue, and intraductal concretions and plugs. Pancreatic tissue is rarely available, however, so another test usually must be substituted. Diagnostic tests used for chronic pancreatitis are listed in Table 31–2 and outlined in Figure 31–1.

A. IMAGING STUDIES

1. X-ray studies—Plain abdominal radiographs are inexpensive, simple, and noninvasive. The finding of diffuse pancreatic calcification is specific for chronic pancreatitis but is seen only in far-advanced disease. Focal pancreatic calcification is not specific for chronic pancreatitis and may be due to trauma, islet cell tumors, or hypercalcemia. The test is insensitive in less advanced disease; in addition, these calcifications may disappear in some patients.

2. Abdominal ultrasonography—Abdominal ultrasonography may demonstrate calcifications, pancreatic atrophy, or a markedly dilated pancreatic duct. The sensitivity of ultrasonography is greater than plain x-rays but less than CT. The procedure has a limited ability to visualize the pancreas because bowel gas may obstruct the view.

3. Computed tomography (CT)—CT findings that suggest chronic pancreatitis include atrophy of the gland, irregular contour of the pancreas, dilatation or irregularity of the pancreatic duct, and calcified pancreatic calculi (Figure 31–2). CT scanning is the most sensitive method for detecting pancreatic calcification and is also useful in screening for complications of chronic pancreatitis (eg, pancreatic pseudocyst). CT scanning is an accurate diagnostic test in advanced chronic pancreatitis, with reported sensitivities of 74–90%, but is substantially less sensitive in less advanced disease. The use of modern "spiral" CT scanning technology can more readily reveal small structures such as the pancreatic duct.

Table 31–2. Diagnostic tests and studies for chronic pancreatitis, listed in order of decreasing sensitivity.

Function	Structure
Secretin or secretin-cholecystokinin test	Endoscopic ultrasound[1]
Fecal elastase	Endoscopic retrograde cholangiopancratography
Serum trypsin	MRI/MRCP[2]
Fecal fat	Computed tomography
Blood glucose	Ultrasonography
	Plain abdominal radiograph

[1]The exact sensitivity of endoscopic ultrasound is unknown, but appears to be better than ERCP, MRI, and CT. The specificity of EUS is unknown and limits its overall accuracy.
[2]The sensitivity of MRI/MRCP is not known but is still less than ERCP with current imaging and image analysis technology.

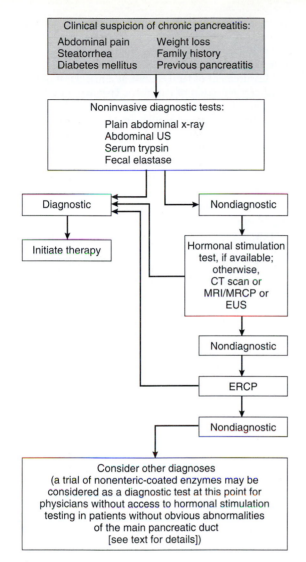

Figure 31–1. Diagnostic strategy for chronic pancreatitis.

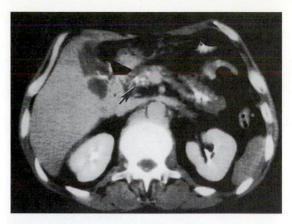

Figure 31–2. A CT scan demonstrating a dilated pancreatic duct and multiple pancreatic calcifications **(arrow).**

5. Endoscopic ultrasonography (EUS)—EUS utilizes a high-frequency ultrasound probe mounted on the end of a flexible endoscope. It allows finely detailed images of the pancreatic duct, parenchyma, and surrounding structures to be acquired. Studies of EUS suggest it may be more sensitive than CT scanning or MRCP, but further evaluation is required to confirm this. EUS is highly accurate in advanced chronic pancreatitis. The sensitivity and especially specificity of the test in patients without these obvious abnormalities are unknown.

6. Endoscopic retrograde cholangiopancreatography (ERCP)—ERCP is a commonly used imaging technique in the evaluation of patients with chronic pancreatitis or symptoms suggestive of that disease. ERCP remains the most sensitive method for defining pancreatic duct abnormalities but is associated with substantial cost and risk. The diagnosis of chronic pancreatitis by ERCP is based on changes in both the main pancreatic duct and the side branches. The most widely used criteria include duct dilatation, narrowing or stricture formation, irregular contour, associated filling of cavities or pseudocysts, and filling defects (ie, pancreatic ductal calculi) (Figure 31–3). At its most advanced stage, the "chain-of-lakes" appearance is quite characteristic of chronic pancreatitis. The reported sensitivity of ERCP is 67–90% and the specificity is 89–100%. The test is quite accurate in advanced disease but, like all tests of pancreatic structure, is less sensitive in less severe disease. It has not usually been appreciated that many patients with clear-cut chronic pancreatitis may have normal or only minimally abnormal ERCP findings. ERCP is also limited by a number of complicating factors including the following: (1) in up to 30% of pa-

4. Magnetic resonance imaging (MRI)—MRI has also not been extensively evaluated, but the use of new contrast agents and imaging technology has markedly improved image quality. Magnetic resonance cholangiopancreatography (MRCP) allows an anatomic reconstruction of the biliary and pancreatic ductal systems. MRCP is most useful in evaluating biliary tract diseases, but is also highly accurate in advanced chronic pancreatitis. The accuracy in patients with less advanced chronic pancreatitis is substantially less. The technology to perform MRCP is widely, although not universally, available.

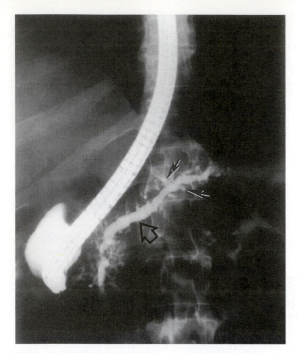

Figure 31–3. An endoscopic retrograde pancreatogram demonstrating moderate changes of chronic pancreatitis, with a dilated main pancreatic duct *(large arrow)* and dilated, clubbed side branches *(small arrows)*.

tients the pancreatogram is of inadequate quality to allow a definitive conclusion; (2) a variety of clinical conditions such as pancreatic carcinoma, acute pancreatitis, pancreatic duct stenting, and even normal aging may produce changes in the pancreatic duct that are indistinguishable from those of chronic pancreatitis; (3) the procedure requires substantial experience and skill to perform; (4) complications occur in up to 10% of patients undergoing ERCP; and (5) it is expensive. These factors make ERCP a late step in the evaluation of patients with suspected chronic pancreatitis. ERCP does, however, have certain advantages over all of the previously mentioned tests in that therapy can be accomplished in some patients. This therapeutic, rather than diagnostic, role of ERCP is discussed in the section on Therapy.

B. PANCREATIC FUNCTION TESTS

1. Laboratory tests—The measurement of serum glucose levels as a marker of diabetes mellitus is too insensitive to be of any clinical use in chronic pancreatitis, and serum amylase or lipase levels are often normal and also not of diagnostic importance. Serum trypsin levels

appear to be a reasonably accurate marker of advanced chronic pancreatitis (when steatorrhea is present); levels below 20 mg/dL appear to be quite specific for chronic pancreatitis.

Measurement of fecal elastase as a marker of intraluminal concentration of pancreatic enzymes and, hence, pancreatic function has also been evaluated. Overall, the sensitivity approaches 90% in advanced disease but is only about 50–60% in less advanced disease. This is equivalent to the accuracy of serum trypsin. Measurement of 72-hour fecal fat concentrations can document steatorrhea, but this is an overly cumbersome, insensitive test. With the exception of serum trypsin and fecal elastase, these simple laboratory evaluations are not helpful in diagnosis.

2. Indirect tests of pancreatic function—Indirect tests of pancreatic function are based on documentation of exocrine insufficiency. Because this does not occur until 90% of exocrine function has been lost, these tests will be accurate in advanced or end-stage disease but inaccurate in earlier disease. Many variations of this type of test have been developed, which involve giving an oral substrate and then measuring the presence of a metabolite. The metabolite requires pancreatic digestive enzymes to be released. These tests have included the bentiromide test, pancrealauryl test, Lundh test meal, amino acid consumption test, and dual-label Schilling test. None of these tests is accurate except in advanced disease, and none is available in the United States for clinical use.

3. Direct tests of pancreatic function—Direct tests of pancreatic function attempt to measure the stimulated secretory capacity of the pancreas (like a "stress test"). The secretin and secretin-cholecystokinin tests both require the collection of pancreatic secretions (with a tube placed in the duodenum) after stimulation of the pancreas with one or both of these hormonal secretagogues. These tests depend on the adequate collection of pancreatic secretions and on the technical ability to measure bicarbonate or proteases in the collected fluid. The sensitivity of these tests, like all diagnostic tests, depends on the severity of the disease (sensitivity is 74–90% and specificity is 80–90%). A number of studies have compared these direct tests of pancreatic function with other diagnostic tests, especially ERCP, EUS, CT, and even histology. All of these studies have reached similar conclusions: these hormonal stimulation tests are more sensitive, more accurate, and more able to diagnose chronic pancreatitis in its less severe stages compared with other tests. All of these studies have also documented patients who have normal pancreatic appearance on radiographic imaging (CT scanning or ERCP) but abnormal results of hormonal stimulation tests. Long-term follow-up of small numbers of these patients has confirmed that the majority develop clear-cut chronic pancreatitis. In addition, recent studies have been able to document histologic findings of chronic pancreatitis in patients with normal pancreatic duct anatomy. Direct hormonal stimulation tests therefore appear to diagnose chronic pancreatitis at a somewhat earlier stage than any other available test. Substantial expertise is required for these tests to be performed reliably, and they are used at only a few referral centers and are unavailable to most clinicians.

C. Diagnostic Strategy

The ideal diagnostic test, which is highly accurate in both early and advanced disease and is also inexpensive, safe, and widely available, does not yet exist. The strategy for evaluating patients should therefore initially focus on tests that are safe, simple, and inexpensive. More invasive, risky, or costly tests should be reserved for cases in which diagnostic uncertainty remains or in which therapeutic rather than diagnostic information is required. Simple tests that identify more advanced disease are used first. These could include a plain abdominal radiograph, abdominal ultrasound, serum trypsin measurement, or fecal elastase. Second-echelon tests include hormonal stimulation tests, CT scan, MRI MRCP, or EUS. Invasive or risky tests such as ERCP are used last and only in a subset of patients for whom diagnostic uncertainty exists. A general diagnostic algorithm is outlined in Figure 31–1.

D. Differential Diagnosis

The abdominal pain associated with chronic pancreatitis is not specific, and a variety of other abdominal conditions may mimic it. These include acid peptic disease, biliary tract disease, acute pancreatitis, mesenteric ischemia or infarction, aortic dissection, motility disorders, and a variety of others. Some of these conditions may also be associated with elevations in amylase or lipase levels, and they are more often confused with acute pancreatitis than chronic pancreatitis. The major diagnostic dilemma is, however, none of these conditions, but rather the differentiation of chronic pancreatitis from pancreatic cancer.

Pancreatic carcinoma may closely mimic the symptoms, signs, and radiographic appearance of chronic pancreatitis. Chronic pancreatitis is in fact a risk factor for pancreatic carcinoma, and the two often coexist. The overall risk for pancreatic cancer in patients with chronic pancreatitis is 4% but is up to 40% in those with hereditary pancreatitis. The use of CT scanning, ERCP with pancreatic duct cytology or biopsy, EUS with fine needle aspiration biopsy, percutaneous biopsy, tumor markers such as CA 19-9, and, possibly, positron emission tomography (PET) scanning can often allow carcinoma to be distinguished from chronic

pancreatitis. In a subset of patients, laparotomy is required to establish the diagnosis. This is discussed more fully in Chapter 32.

TREATMENT

Treatment of Direct Manifestations of Chronic Pancreatitis

A. Steatorrhea

Steatorrhea occurs primarily as a consequence of inadequate delivery of pancreatic digestive enzymes to the gut lumen, and only when 90% of pancreatic output has been lost. Deficient delivery of bicarbonate may also contribute to steatorrhea, because gastric acid may be inadequately neutralized, and this may cause inactivation of digestive enzymes and precipitation of bile salts. Therapy for steatorrhea is directed at delivering adequate amounts of exogenous pancreatic enzymes to the gut lumen. Appropriate use of these enzymes leads to resolution of diarrhea and weight loss despite the fact that steatorrhea cannot usually be totally corrected.

The lipase content of pancreatic enzyme preparations is the critical determinant of efficacy in treating steatorrhea. Most of the commercially available preparations are of low potency, although newer, more concentrated preparations have been developed. The enzymes are either packaged in a conventional form, which begins to dissolve in the stomach, or are contained in enteric-coated microspheres, which do not release their contents until the pH rises above 5.5. These preparations are listed in Table 31–3.

Effective treatment of steatorrhea usually requires the delivery of at least 30,000 IU of lipase to the duodenum during a 4-hour prandial and postprandial period. Patients using the lower-potency preparations must therefore take three to eight pills with each meal. Fewer pills must be taken with the more potent formulation. Formulation containing more than 25,000 IU of lipase per pill have been recalled by the manufacturers after colonic strictures were noted in young patients with cystic fibrosis taking high dosages of these preparations. No such complications have been reported in adults or patients with other forms of chronic pancreatitis.

The most common reason for failure of pancreatic enzymes to correct steatorrhea is the patient's unwillingness to take the number of pills required. The second most common reason is inactivation of lipase by gastric acid, which is only a problem in patients receiving conventional (nonenteric-coated) preparations. To prevent this, cotreatment to keep the gastric pH above 4.0 should be used (H_2-receptor antagonists or proton-pump inhibitors). If the reason for enzyme therapy is only treatment of steatorrhea, one of the enteric-coated preparations of lipase may be used as these do not re-

Table 31–3. Pancreatic enzymes for the treatment of steatorrhea[1] or pain.[2]

Brand Name	Units of Lipase per Pill
Conventional enzyme preparations	
Viokase, Viokase 16	8,000, 16,000
Ku-Zyme HP	8,000
Generic pancrelipase	8,000
Enteric-coated enzyme preparations	
Creon 5, 10, 20	5,000, 10,000, 20,000
Pancrease MT 4, 10, 16, 20	4,000, 10,000, 16,000, 20,000
Ultrase, Ultrase MT 12, 18, 20	4,500, 12,000, 18,000, 20,000

[1]For the treatment of steatorrhea, both conventional and enteric-coated preparations can be used. The dosage depends on the lipase content. 30,000 units of lipase should be delivered with each meal. Low-potency formulations (5000–8000 units of lipase per pill) require four to six pills with each meal. Higher potency formulations require two to three pills with each meal. Conventional enzymes require cotreatment with agents to suppress gastric acid.

[2]For the treatment of pain, conventional enzyme preparations are used, four to eight pills (depending on potency) before meals and at night. An adjuvant agent to reduce gastric acid is required, either H$_2$-receptor antagonists or a proton-pump inhibitor.

quire cotreatment with acid-suppressing medications and are of greater potency. Failure of a patient with pancreatic insufficiency to improve despite confirmed intake of adequate amounts of an enteric-coated enzyme supplement suggests the need for evaluation for possible concomitant small intestinal diseases such as bacterial overgrowth or celiac sprue.

Dietary manipulations may also be helpful in the management of malabsorption and malnutrition. The diet should usually contain a moderate amount of fat (30%), high amount of protein (24%), and low amount of carbohydrates (40%). Decreasing the amount of long-chain triglycerides in the diet or adding medium-chain triglyceride supplements, or both, may improve steatorrhea in selected patients who fail therapy with enzymes alone.

B. DIABETES MELLITUS

Diabetes is an independent predictor of mortality in patients with chronic pancreatitis. Morbidity and mortality can occur from progressive microangiopathic complications or from treatment-induced hypoglycemia. These patients often have inadequate glucagon as well as insulin reserves, and cannot respond to hypoglycemia with a glucagon surge and subsequent increase in blood glucose levels. Overly vigorous attempts to control blood sugar can be associated with disastrous complications of treatment-induced hypoglycemia.

Some patients will respond to oral hypoglycemics. If insulin is required, the goal is usually to control urinary losses of glucose rather than attempt tight control of blood sugar. Tight control of blood sugar is usually indicated in only one subgroup, those with hyperlipidemic pancreatitis. In this group, diabetes is a primary

disease and tight control of blood sugar is required to allow control of serum triglycerides.

C. PAIN

1. Medical treatment—The management of pain is often unsatisfactory, in large part because there are many causes of pain, so that one treatment will not be effective in all patients. Abstinence from alcohol should be strongly encouraged in those with alcoholic chronic pancreatitis, as this may produce some pain relief. Abstinence also reduces the risk of other alcohol-related complications (eg, cirrhosis), prolongs life, and slows the rate of progression of chronic pancreatitis. Analgesics are often required, and nonnarcotic analgesics should be used first. Narcotic agents are required in a subset of patients, and the least potent formulation should be tried initially (eg, Darvocet-N 100, tramadol). Narcotic addiction occurs in up to 20% of these patients. In patients who require narcotics, the addition of a tricyclic antidepressant can be helpful as these can potentiate the effect of narcotics. The use of other antidepressants (eg, selective serotonin reuptake inhibitors) can also be useful in some patients.

Several small controlled trials have demonstrated that conventional (nonenteric-coated) pancreatic enzymes can provide pain relief in some patients with chronic pancreatitis. These preparations are felt to reestablish normal negative feedback of pancreatic secretion, reducing hyperstimulation of the gland by cholecystokinin and thereby reducing pain. This feedback loop is operative only in the duodenum, so enteric-coated preparations that do not release enzymes until they reach the jejunum are ineffective. Patients who respond best to the use of conventional enzymes are those with mild to moderate chronic pancreatitis (without steatorrhea) and minimal abnormalities on ERCP (ie, "small-duct disease"). In some studies, up to 75% of these patients responded to the use of these enzymes. Conversely, patients with steatorrhea or marked abnormalities of the pancreatic duct ("big-duct disease") are unlikely to respond. This therapy is of moderate effectiveness in carefully selected patients and is risk free. If this therapy is used, it is necessary to choose the right patient ("small-duct disease"), use the right enzyme (nonenteric-coated) and the right dose (eg, 8 Viokase or 4 Viokase 16 with meals and at bedtime), and use an adjuvant agent to reduce gastric acid (H_2-receptor antagonist or proton-pump inhibitor).

A few studies of octreotide (Sandostatin) have suggested that the use of this agent may reduce the pain of chronic pancreatitis. A few small studies have also suggested that the use of antioxidants (mixtures of vitamins E and C, selenium, and methionine, and beta carotene) may reduce pain. Further studies of both are needed to define their potential effectiveness.

2. Celiac plexus block and other blocks—Ablation of the celiac plexus by radiographically guided or EUS-guided injection of anesthetics or alcohol can be effective for the pain of pancreatic cancer but provides only short-lived relief in patients with chronic pancreatitis. EUS-guided techniques appear to work better and for longer periods of time than CT-guided techniques. Use of percutaneous splanchnic nerve blocks or thoracoscopic splanchnicectomy has also been tried, but their efficacy remains to be established in chronic pancreatitis.

3. Endoscopic therapy of chronic pancreatitis—The endoscopic therapies of chronic pancreatitis include pancreatic duct stenting, pancreatic duct sphincterotomy of both the major and minor papilla, dilation of strictures, removal of pancreatic calculi, and treatment of complications such as pseudocyst or biliary obstruction. Like most forms of therapy in chronic pancreatitis, no randomized trials have been performed in patients with chronic pancreatitis for any of these endoscopic techniques. The goal of endoscopic therapy is to remove or bypass any obstruction within the pancreatic duct. Candidates for endoscopic therapy include those with a significant pancreatic ductal stricture in the head of the pancreas and those with a few obstructing stones in the head of the gland. Only a subset of patients with "big-duct disease" satisfies these criteria, hence endoscopic therapy is an option in only a highly selected subset of patients. In these highly selected groups, pain relief after endoscopic therapy can be seen in about 75% of patients.

Complications of endoscopic treatment of chronic pancreatitis occur in up to 15–20% of patients, including pancreatitis, bleeding, perforation, and sepsis. In addition, pancreatic stents in and of themselves can induce ductal changes resembling those of chronic pancreatitis in up to 50% of patients treated, and these changes may not resolve. Endoscopic therapy requires substantial expertise and is available only at larger, tertiary referral centers but is a reasonable alternative in appropriately selected patients.

4. Surgical treatment—Surgical therapy can be considered for complications of chronic pancreatitis (pseudocyst, bile duct obstruction, duodenal obstruction) or "big-duct disease" with refractory pain. Performance of a lateral pancreaticojejunostomy (Puestow procedure) leads to immediate pain relief in 70–90% of patients. Long-term pain control is achieved in 50% of patients after 1–3 years of follow-up. The pancreatic duct must usually be dilated to 7–8 mm or more for the technical performance of a Puestow procedure. This is usually defined by ERCP, EUS, CT, or MRCP preoperatively. The dilated pancreatic duct is widely filleted along its length and overlaid with a defunctionalized Roux limb. The procedure carries acceptable rates of complications (5%) and mortality (2%). In some centers, resection of all or part of the head of the pancreas is combined with a ductal drainage procedure. These operations have higher rates of long-term pain relief but at the cost of increased surgical morbidity and mortality. Subtotal or total pancreatic resections are rarely needed for pain control and are associated with significant rates of postoperative complications, particularly brittle diabetes mellitus. For selected patients with an inflammatory mass involving the head of the pancreas, pancreaticoduodenectomy (eg, modified Whipple procedure) or duodenum-sparing resection of the pancreatic head may be beneficial.

5. Choosing treatment for pain—The choice of a treatment for pain depends on the severity of symptoms, etiology of chronic pancreatitis, pancreatic ductal anatomy, presence of complications, and local expertise. The first step is to make sure the diagnosis is correct. It is then always worthwhile to search for specific complications that might have specific therapy, such as pancreatic pseudocyst, duodenal obstruction, common bile duct obstruction, peptic ulcer disease, or even gastroparesis. These are discussed below. Medical therapy is appropriate in all patients and should include abstinence from alcohol (if applicable), low-fat diet, and analgesics. The choice of subsequent therapy depends in large part on whether the patient has "small-duct" or "big-duct disease." In those with "small-duct disease," a trial of high-dose nonenteric-coated enzymes coupled with acid suppression is appropriate. Treatment options for those with "big-duct disease" are largely mechanical, with either endoscopic or surgical attempts to decompress the enlarged pancreatic duct. Patients who fail the above therapies may be considered for more experimental therapies such as celiac plexus block, splanchnicectomy, or octreotide. Significant pancreatic resections are considered an option of last resort in both groups of patients.

Treatment of Complications of Chronic Pancreatitis

A. EPISODES OF ACUTE PANCREATITIS

Patients with chronic pancreatitis may experience flareups of disease or episodes of acute pancreatitis superimposed on an already irreversibly damaged gland. These flare-ups tend to be mild and decrease in severity with evolution of the disease. A subset of patients will experience a more severe attack and may develop all of the complications associated with severe acute pancreatitis, such as renal failure or acute respiratory distress syndrome. These complications and their management are discussed fully in Chapter 30.

B. PANCREATIC PSEUDOCYST

Collections of pancreatic fluid in and around the pancreas may occur as a consequence of acute or chronic pancreatitis. Pseudocysts occurring in the setting of acute pancreatitis are usually due to ductal disruption and necrosis with the escape of pancreatic juice containing activated enzymes. Pseudocysts complicating chronic pancreatitis may also be due to downstream obstruction of the pancreatic duct, causing a "retention cyst" filled with inactive enzymes. These different pathophysiologic mechanisms are reflected in somewhat different clinical presentations and natural histories. Pseudocysts occurring in the setting of acute pancreatitis are more likely to produce complications than pseudocysts associated with chronic pancreatitis, but are also paradoxically more likely to resolve.

Patients with a pseudocyst complicating acute pancreatitis may remain asymptomatic or may present with complications such as pseudocyst rupture or infection. Although patients with pseudocysts complicating chronic pancreatitis may present in a similar fashion, they are also likely to notice worsening chronic pain, develop a wasting syndrome, or remain asymptomatic.

The diagnosis of pseudocyst is best made by CT scanning. Pseudocysts are characterized as rounded collections of fluid surrounded by a visible capsule (Figure 31–4). Other fluid collections that have not matured into this form are better termed acute pancreatic fluid collections. It appears to take at least 6 weeks for an acute pancreatic fluid collection to mature into a pseudocyst, although many will resolve without developing into pseudocysts.

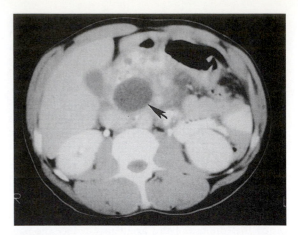

Figure 31–4. A CT scan demonstrating a pseudocyst ***(arrow)*** in the head of the gland, with areas of associated calcification.

The natural history of pseudocysts is variable. Initial studies suggested that complications developed in up to 40% of patients and that only 20% of pseudocysts spontaneously resolved. Resolution of pseudocysts usually happened within the first 6 weeks, and many of the complications occurred after this period. Six weeks was also approximately the amount of time it took for an acute pancreatic fluid collection to develop into a mature pseudocyst, and was considered the most appropriate time for surgical intervention. These early studies appear to have overestimated the severity of the natural history of pseudocysts. Several recent studies using CT scanning have noted resolution rates as high as 64%, with complications occurring in less than 10%. In addition, the long-term risk of pseudocysts less than 6 cm in diameter producing complications appears to be extremely small. The risk of complications has probably been overestimated and the chance of spontaneous resolution underestimated. In practice, relatively small (<6 cm) pseudocysts that are asymptomatic can be safely followed without therapy, especially if the patient can stop drinking alcohol.

Symptomatic pseudocysts that have not caused significant complications can be treated with surgical, endoscopic, or percutaneous drainage. Surgical therapies include decompression into an adjacent hollow viscus (eg, cystjejunostomy, cystgastrostomy) or resection of the pseudocyst along with a portion of the pancreas (typically for pseudocysts in the tail of the pancreas). Endoscopic therapy involves puncture of a pseudocyst through the gastric or duodenal wall with placement of one or more stents into the collection. Percutaneous aspiration of pseudocysts with catheter drainage is also effective and is usually the treatment of choice for infected pseudocysts. Endoscopic and percutaneous therapy are often effective in the short term (90% success rate), but the long-term success rates are not clearly known. In some patients, pseudocysts may recur when the stent or catheter is removed, although this may take months and the recurrent pseudocyst may remain asymptomatic. In addition, stent or catheter drainage does not allow differentiation of pseudocysts from cystic neoplasms of the pancreas. This differentiation generally requires biopsy of the cyst wall, which is usually possible only with surgical techniques. Cystic neoplasms should be particularly suspected when an asymptomatic or minimally symptomatic fluid collection is found in a middle-aged person (particularly female) without a history of pancreatitis and without risk factors for pancreatitis. Unlike what is seen in pseudocysts, CT scans of cystic neoplasms demonstrate a thick capsule around the collection with mural tumor nodules or internal septations. The therapy of these neoplasms is surgical resection, not drainage. Despite these drawbacks, endoscopic and percutaneous drainage is used widely due to their technical simplicity and low rate of complications.

1. Hemorrhage due to pseudocyst—Only 2–7% of patients with pancreatic pseudocysts bleed, but the development of bleeding is associated with a substantial rate of mortality (up to 35%). Bleeding from a pseudocyst can originate in small vessels in the pseudocyst capsule or in larger visceral arteries that are damaged and disrupted by the pseudocyst or associated pancreatitis, producing a pseudoaneurysm. Pseudoaneurysms most commonly form in the splenic artery, followed by the gastroduodenal and pancreaticoduodenal arteries. Blood may remain in the pseudocyst, enter the gut via the pancreatic duct (hemosuccus pancreaticus), or rupture into an adjacent hollow viscus. Rarely, the pseudocyst or pseudoaneurysm may rupture into the peritoneal cavity.

Pseudocyst-associated bleeding should be suspected when gastrointestinal bleeding develops in a patient with a known or suspected pseudocyst, when sudden abdominal pain develops in association with an enlarging abdominal mass, or when a patient with a pseudocyst develops sudden unexplained blood loss. Upper endoscopy is usually performed first, after fluid resuscitation, to search for other potential sources of bleeding. If no obvious abnormality is documented, radiographic evaluation is required. An initial ultrasound study may reveal the pseudocyst and even occasionally a pulsatile pseudoaneurysm, but CT scanning is usually more accurate and associated with fewer inadequate examinations. The finding of high-density fluid (blood) within a pseudocyst or an enhancing vascular structure within the pseudocyst should prompt emergent angiography.

Angiography can be used to confirm the presence of a pseudoaneurysm and also allows therapeutic embolization for stabilization or definitive therapy. In some patients, definitive therapy may require surgical ligation of the pseudoaneurysm and cystenterostomy or resection.

2. Infected pseudocyst—Pseudocysts may become infected in up to 15% of patients. Gram-negative enteric organisms are most commonly involved, but streptococci and anaerobes also may be causative organisms. In up to 40% of patients, more than one organism is responsible. Pseudocyst infection presents clinically with abdominal pain, fever, and leukocytosis. The presence of gas in a pseudocyst demonstrated by ultrasonography or CT scanning is strongly suggestive of pseudocyst infection, but most infected pseudocysts will not have gas present. The diagnosis can usually be established by puncture of the pseudocyst, with gram-stained smear and culture of the fluid.

Treatment requires the initiation of broad-spectrum antibiotics and drainage. Both percutaneous catheter drainage and surgical drainage are usually effective. Percutaneous drainage is preferred because of lower rates of pseudocyst recurrence and fistula formation. However, it should not be used if the infected material cannot be adequately removed through a small-bore tube, as is the case with infected pancreatic necrosis and fluid collections containing solid necrotic tissue or multiple septations.

3. Obstruction of surrounding organs by pseudocyst—Pseudocysts in the head of the pancreas may obstruct the common bile duct as it passes through the head of the pancreas. Bile duct obstruction due solely to pseudocysts is rare; usually, the bile duct is primarily obstructed from fibrosis due to chronic pancreatitis. Although common bile duct obstruction is common, clinically important obstruction is less common. Radiographic evidence of bile duct narrowing, seen on ERCP, in and of itself is not an indication for therapy. Conservative management is usually appropriate, unless clinical evidence (eg, cholangitis) or biochemical evidence (eg, markedly elevated alkaline phosphatase levels) of biliary obstruction develops; this is an indication for surgical biliary bypass along with cyst decompression (if present). The development of cholangitis usually requires emergent endoscopic treatment with ERCP and biliary stenting, followed by definitive surgical therapy. Duodenal obstruction may also occur as a result of an inflammatory mass in the head of the pancreas or large pseudocyst (1–7% of patients with pancreatic pseudocysts). Persistent symptomatic obstruction is an indication for gastrojejunostomy. Obstruction of the portal vein, ureters, and colon has also been rarely observed.

4. Rupture of pseudocyst—Pseudocyst rupture occurs in less than 10% of patients and is associated with a mortality rate of 14–40%. The rate is highest with abrupt rupture into the peritoneal cavity or rupture associated with bleeding. Rupture into a surrounding hollow viscus is often well tolerated, creating a spontaneous cystenterostomy, which obviates the need for further therapy. Rupture into the peritoneal cavity often produces a severe chemical peritonitis and usually requires surgical therapy, with external cyst drainage the treatment of choice.

C. PANCREATIC FISTULA

Disruption of the pancreatic duct or rupture of a pseudocyst may lead to a controlled leak of pancreatic secretions. This fluid may enter a number of spaces, including the peritoneal cavity and pleural spaces. The fluid may become walled off as a pseudocyst or remain connected to the pancreatic duct (internal pancreatic fistula) due to persistent leakage. Pancreatic ascites is usually associated with persistent leakage and a fistula on the anterior surface of the pancreas. Posterior fistulas usually reach the pleural space or mediastinum, producing pancreatic pleural effusions from a pancreaticopleural fistula. These persistent fistulas occur almost exclusively in patients with chronic pancreatitis. Surprisingly, signs and symptoms of pancreatitis are often absent, and patients may instead complain of abdominal distention or dyspnea. Abdominal pain is absent in up to 20% of these patients, and only 50% have a history compatible with previous attacks of pancreatitis. These fistulas should be suspected when an exudative pleural effusion or ascites with an elevated amylase level is found. The amylase value in the fluid is usually markedly elevated (median >18,000 IU/L). Radiographic studies, including CT scanning and ERCP, can often document chronic pancreatitis and localize the fistulous tract and any associated pseudocyst.

Medical therapy is effective in less than 40% of patients and includes allowing nothing by mouth, using hyperalimentation, repeatedly draining fluid that has collected, and giving octreotide to reduce pancreatic secretion. Endoscopic therapy can be quite useful in this setting, with either pancreatic duct sphincterotomy or placement of a pancreatic duct stent across the disrupted ductal system. Surgical therapy is effective for patients who fail endoscopic therapy and usually includes either resection of the pancreas upstream from the leak or capping of the fistulous tract with a small bowel Roux-en-Y limb.

D. GASTROINTESTINAL BLEEDING

In addition to the bleeding associated with pseudocysts, bleeding may occur in acute and chronic pancreatitis due to thrombosis of the splenic vein. This typically results in segmental portal hypertension. The endoscopic correlates of this left-sided portal hypertension are isolated gastric varices or large gastric varices with minor or trivial esophageal varices. Doppler ultrasound, CT, MRI/MRA, or angiography can usually confirm the diagnosis of splenic vein thrombosis. The treatment of this condition is splenectomy, which is usually curative.

E. PANCREATIC CARCINOMA

Chronic pancreatitis is a risk factor for the development of pancreatic carcinoma. The overall risk is about 4%. There is currently no effective screening method. Pancreatic carcinoma is usually suspected when a patient with known chronic pancreatitis develops worsening pain or weight loss.

F. OTHERS

Gastroparesis in not uncommon in patients with chronic pancreatitis and can mimic many of the symptoms of chronic pancreatitis including abdominal pain, nausea, and vomiting. In addition, it can interfere with the action of pancreatic enzyme therapy. It should be considered in patients who do not respond to initial therapies. In addition, small bowel bacterial overgrowth may occur in patients with chronic pancreatitis and should be considered in those with diarrhea not responsive to enzymes.

REFERENCES

AGA technical review: Treatment of pain in chronic pancreatitis. Gastroenterology 1998;115:763.

Ammann RW et al: Course of alcoholic chronic pancreatitis: a prospective clinicomorphological long-term study. Gastroenterology 1996;224:111.

Ammann RW et al: The natural history of pain in alcoholic chronic pancreatitis. Gastroenterology 1999;116:1132.

Beckingham IJ et al: Long-term outcome of endoscopic drainage of pancreatic pseudocysts. Am J Gastroenterol 1999;94:71.

Cohn JA et al: Cystic fibrosis mutations and genetic predispositions to idiopathic chronic pancreatitis. Med Clin North Am 2000; 84:621.

Criado E et al: Long term results of percutaneous catheter drainage of pancreatic pseudocysts. Surg Gynecol Obstet 1992;175:293.

Etemad B, Whitcomb DC: Chronic pancreatitis: diagnosis, classification, and new genetic developments. Gastroenterology 2001;120:682.

Forsmark CE: The diagnosis of chronic pancreatitis. Gastrointest Endosc 2000;52:293.

Forsmark CE, Grendell JH: Complications of pancreatitis. Semin Gastrointest Dis 1991;2:165.

Forsmark CE, Toskes PP: What does an abnormal pancreatogram mean? Gastrointest Endosc Clin North Am 1995;5:105.

Hayakawa T et al: Relationship between pancreatic function and histologic changes in chronic pancreatitis. Am J Gastroenterol 1992;87:1170.

Layer P et al: The different courses of early- and late-onset idiopathic and alcoholic chronic pancreatitis. Gastroenterology 1994;107:1481.

Lowenfels AB et al: Pancreatitis and the risk of pancreatic cancer. N Engl J Med 1993;328:1433.

Mishra G, Forsmark CE: Cystic neoplasms of the pancreas. Curr Treat Options Gastroenterol 2000;3:355.

Saforkas GH et al: Long-term results after surgery for chronic pancreatitis. Int J Pancreatol 2000;27:131.

Steinberg W: The clinical utility of the CA 19-9 tumor-associated antigen. Am J Gastroenterol 1990;85:350.

Toskes PP: Hyperlipidemic pancreatitis. Gastroenterol Clin North Am 1990;19:783.

Vitas GJ, Sarr MG: Selected management of pancreatic pseudocysts: operative versus expectant management. Surgery 1992; 111:123.

Wallace MB, Hawes RH: Endoscopic ultrasound in the evaluation and management of chronic pancreatitis. Pancreas 2001; 23:26.

Walsh TN et al: Minimal change chronic pancreatitis. Gut 1992; 33:1566.

Wong GY et al: Palliation of pain in chronic pancreatitis: use of neural blocks and neurotomy. Surg Clin North Am 1999; 79:873.

Yeo CJ et al: The natural history of pancreatic pseudocysts documented by computed tomography. Surg Gynecol Obstet 1990;170:411.

Tumors of the Pancreas

Randall E. Brand, MD

The vast majority of pancreatic neoplasms are adeno-carcinomas of ductal epithelial origin. A relatively small percentage of pancreatic tumors consist of islet-cell tumors, cystadenomas, adenoacanthomas, or pancreatic lymphomas. The clinician caring for patients with pancreatic neoplasms needs to be aware that most of these tumors grow rapidly and are fatal.

Incidence & Risk Factors

About 29,200 patients with pancreatic neoplasms are diagnosed annually in the United States, and there are 28,900 cancer-related deaths. The estimated annual incidence in the United States is nearly 10 per 100,000 persons over the age of 75, making carcinoma of the pancreas the fourth most common cause of death from cancer in men and women. The disease is somewhat more common in men than in women. Risk increases with age, and the mean age of onset occurs in the seventh and eighth decades of life. Certain ethnic and racial groups are noted to have an increased incidence: blacks, Polynesians, and native New Zealanders.

Genetic predisposition is the greatest risk factor for the development of pancreatic adenocarcinoma. It is estimated that up to 10% of patients will have one or more first- or second-degree relatives with pancreatic cancer. A very small percentage of cases of pancreatic cancer arise in families with hereditary chronic pancreatitis, an autosomal dominant condition. This disease is caused by a mutation in the trypsinogen gene that results in bouts of recurrent pancreatitis beginning early in life that may progress to chronic pancreatitis. Affected members have a 40% risk of developing cancer by age 70. The risk of pancreatic cancer is also increased in certain other family cancer syndromes, including Peutz-Jehgers syndrome, hereditary nonpolyposis colon cancer, von Hippel-Lindau syndrome, and ataxia telangiectasia. The most significant environmental risk factor is cigarette smoking with most studies reporting an increased relative risk of 1.5- to 5.5-fold.

Patients with chronic pancreatitis appear to have a 4% risk of developing pancreatic cancer within 20 years. Additional risk factors include alcohol consumption, gallbladder stones, diabetes mellitus, and high intake of animal fat. Other dietary factors associated with an increased risk of pancreatic cancer include high pro-tein consumption and the use of highly refined flour. Coffee consumption was once identified as a risk factor but recent studies do not confirm an association with pancreatic cancer. Certain environmental agents are associated with pancreatic cancer, including prolonged contact with petroleum products and wood pulp.

Pathophysiology

Pancreatic adenocarcinoma is believed to originate from ductal cells in which a series of genetic mutations have occurred in protooncogenes and tumor suppressor genes. Mutations in the K-*ras* oncogene are believed to be an early event in tumor development and are present in more than 90% of tumors. Loss of function of each of several tumor suppressor genes (*p16, p53, DCC, APC,* and *DPC4*) is found in 40–60% of tumors. Detection of K-*ras* mutations from pancreatic juice obtained at endoscopic retrograde cholangiopancreatography has been used in clinical research settings to diagnose pancreatic cancer.

The clinical manifestations, laboratory features, and abdominal imaging characteristics can be explained by the pathology of pancreatic neoplasms. Adenocarcinoma of the pancreas, the histologic type of over 90% of pancreatic neoplasms, is characterized by a dense, fibrotic reaction surrounding a compact mass of hard pancreatic tissue. Because the pancreas lacks a mesentery and is adjacent to the bile duct, duodenum, stomach, and colon, the most common clinical manifestations of pancreatic cancers are those related to invasion or compression of these adjacent structures. Neoplasms such as islet-cell tumors, lymphomas, and cystadenomas tend to be less fibrotic, thus distortion rather than compression or encasement of adjacent structures is more common with these neoplasms.

ESSENTIALS OF DIAGNOSIS

- *Vague, dull midepigastric abdominal discomfort.*
- *Weight loss.*
- *Anorexia.*
- *Dysgeusia.*

- *Diarrhea.*
- *Jaundice.*
- *Weakness.*
- *Vomiting.*

ADENOCARCINOMA

Clinical Findings

A. SYMPTOMS AND SIGNS

Most pancreatic neoplasms present late in the course of the disease, at which time diagnosis confirms a nonresectable neoplasm. Early in the course of pancreatic neoplasms, there are few characteristic signs or symptoms that suggest the diagnosis. As the tumor progresses, patients may complain of pain, which is described most commonly as a vague, dull midepigastric discomfort that may radiate to the back. Weight loss, anorexia, dysgeusia, diarrhea, weakness, and vomiting are also commonly seen in patients with pancreatic neoplasms, particularly adenocarcinoma. Jaundice is noted in over 50% of patients with pancreatic neoplasms, particularly those involving the head of the gland. Most tumors in this region are large and bulky, encasing the distal portion of the common bile duct. On occasion, a small (1–2 cm) focal pancreatic mass involving only the periampullary area obstructs the common bile duct and produces jaundice at a very early—and potentially curable—stage of the disease. For the unfortunate 30–40% of patients who develop a pancreatic malignancy in the body or tail of the gland, jaundice is a late manifestation of the disease, commonly associated with a large retroperitoneal mass or extensive hepatic metastases.

Obstruction of the distal common bile duct by a pancreatic neoplasm may be accompanied by a palpably distended nontender gallbladder, called **Courvoisier's sign.** This feature may also be noted in patients with bile duct obstruction from carcinoma of the ampulla of Vater, duodenal carcinoma, or cholangiocarcinoma. Uncommon manifestations of pancreatic neoplasms include severe back pain, thrombophlebitis, pruritus due to cholestasis, acute pancreatitis, psychiatric disturbances, or diabetes. Infrequently, patients present with signs and symptoms of upper gastrointestinal tract bleeding caused by erosion of the pancreatic neoplasm into the duodenal lumen.

B. LABORATORY FINDINGS

1. Abnormalities—The most common laboratory abnormalities include anemia, elevation of the erythrocyte sedimentation rate (ESR), and elevation of serum alkaline phosphatase, bilirubin, and transaminases. Because most patients with pancreatic neoplasms have adenocarcinoma arising in the head of the pancreas high-grade common bile duct obstruction is frequently encountered. Malignant obstruction of the distal common bile duct characteristically elevates the serum alkaline phosphatase four to five times above the upper limits of normal. Serum alkaline phosphatase levels increase out of proportion to bilirubin until late in the course of the disease, when alkaline phosphatase levels may exceed 1000 IU/L and serum bilirubin values rise >20 mg/dL. Despite biliary stasis, cholangitis (manifested by right upper quadrant pain, fever, leukocytosis, and modest elevations of the serum aminotransferases) is distinctly uncommon. Elevations of serum amylase may occasionally be seen, and, rarely, patients present with acute pancreatitis caused by pancreatic duct obstruction.

2. Tumor markers—A tumor marker may be defined as any substance that when measured in abnormal concentration in a body fluid or in tissue may indicate the presence of a malignancy or define its site of origin. Most studies have focused on the role of tumor markers in establishing a diagnosis of pancreatic cancer or in monitoring treatment response. To date, the clinical role of tumor markers has been limited. CA 19-9, a sialylated Lewis antigen associated with circulating mucins, is the most widely used marker for pancreatic malignancy. The sensitivity and specificity for the diagnosis of pancreatic adenocarcinoma are dependent on the cutoff level selected, and at the most commonly used cutoff level of 37 U/mL, ranges from 81 to 85% and 81 to 90%, respectively. Although CA 19-9 is most frequently elevated in pancreatic adenocarcinoma, it may also be expressed in other malignancies, particularly those of the bile duct, stomach, and colon. Levels can also be moderately elevated in benign conditions such as acute and chronic pancreatitis, hepatitis, and biliary obstruction; and marked elevations may be seen in patients with cirrhosis or acute cholangitis. The search for a reliable tumor marker for the diagnosis of pancreatic cancer has generated tremendous enthusiasm (Table 32–1). An elevated carcinoembryonic antigen (CEA) is noted in over 70% of patients with pancreatic neoplasm. Other tumor markers such as α-fetoprotein, RNase, galactosyltransferase II (GT-II), and oncofetal antigen are elevated in small numbers of patients with pancreatic neoplasms.

Serum trypsin levels and trypsin-creatinine clearance are also increased in some patients with pancreatic cancer. These and other biochemical and serologic markers for pancreatic cancer will need extensive evaluation in larger prospective trials before being used in the clinical setting.

Table 32–1. Investigational pancreatic tumor markers.

Category	Tumor Markers
Complex glycoconjugates	CA 19-9, CA 125, CA 242, TAG-72 (CA 72-4), MUC4, CAM17.1, CA 50, Span-1, DUPAN-2, TPA,[1] TPS[2]
Oncofetal proteins	CEA, AFP,[3] POA[4]
Tumor suppressor gene	*p53*
Oncogenes	K-*ras*
Enzymes	Elastase, ribonuclease, amylase, lipase, telomerase, GT-II[5]
Hormone and peptides	Amylin (IAPP), TATI,[6] insulin, gastrin, glucagon, TIMP-1[7]

[1]Tissue polypeptide antigen.
[2]Tissue polypeptide specific antigen.
[3]α-Fetoprotein.
[4]Pancreatic oncofetal antigen.
[5]Galactosyltransferase isoenzyme II.
[6]Tumor-associated trypsin inhibitor.
[7]Tissue prohibitor of metalloproteinase type I.

C. DIAGNOSTIC STUDIES

There are many imaging modalities available for the diagnosis and staging of a pancreatic adenocarcinoma. Optimal diagnostic algorithms for pancreatic cancer are dependent on clinical context including availability of imaging modalities and patient presentation. Transabdominal ultrasound and computed tomography (CT) (Figure 32–1) are the two most commonly utilized imaging techniques for the evaluation of suspected pancreatic carcinoma. Endoscopic retrograde cholangiopancreatography (ERCP) is considered the gold standard for the visualization of the pancreatic duct and biliary system (Figure 32–2). The clinical role of newer imaging modalities, such as endoscopic ultrasound (EUS), positron emission tomography (PET), and magnetic resonance imaging (MRI), is still evolving. All of these techniques base the diagnosis of cancer on at least one of the following imaging findings in the pancreas: morphologic changes (ie, focal deformity or enlargement), density changes, pancreatic and biliary duct changes (ie, dilatation or stricture), or signs of local extension into adjacent structures.

In most instances, a helical CT scan should be the initial radiologic study, since it provides staging information pertaining to the presence of local tumor invasion, metastasis, and vascular involvement superior to that obtained from abdominal ultrasonography. Helical CT allows for continuous imaging of a large volume of tissue using a single breath-hold period. Moreover, this technique permits retrospective reconstruction of images, which increases its diagnostic accuracy. If abdominal CT imaging suggests the presence of a pancreatic neoplasm that appears to be surgically resectable, EUS should be performed next. This study provides superior definition of tumor invasion of adjacent organs and vessels. EUS

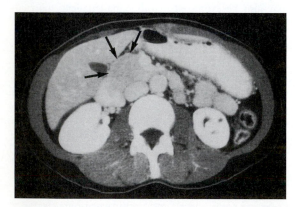

Figure 32–1. Computed tomography of the abdomen in a patient with carcinoma of the head of the pancreas. An irregular, low-density mass is noted in the head of the pancreas *(arrows)*. Pancreatic carcinoma was subsequently confirmed by fine-needle aspiration cytology.

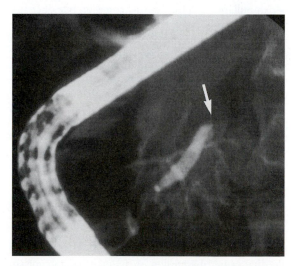

Figure 32–2. Endoscopic retrograde pancreatogram in a patient with carcinoma of the head of the pancreas. An abrupt cutoff of the pancreatic duct is noted, with filling of secondary pancreatic ductules in the head and uncinate process. Such an abrupt cutoff *(arrow)* is invariably due to pancreatic adenocarcinoma arising in the main pancreatic duct.

should also be performed in patients with suspected pancreatic neoplasm when CT fails to demonstrate a discrete pancreatic mass as it is superior to CT for resolution of small pancreatic tumors. Endoscopic retrograde cholangiopancreatography (ERCP) remains a useful diagnostic and therapeutic procedure in the management of patients with pancreatic neoplasms. It may aid in diagnosis by providing cytologic brushings of malignant pancreatic strictures. Biliary obstruction may be treated at ERCP in nonoperative candidates by placement of a stent. ERCP, PET, and MRI may also be useful in selected cases when the suspicion of cancer is high yet CT scan and EUS are not diagnostic. The ability to differentiate between an in-

flammatory mass and cancer remains a problem with all imaging modalities. After staging of the tumor, the disease is often categorized as resectable, locally advanced, or metastatic.

Cytology is the principal means for establishing the diagnosis of pancreatic cancer. Fine-needle aspiration (FNA), which can be performed percutaneously using CT or ultrasonographic guidance or across the stomach or duodenum using EUS guidance, has become the preferred method of obtaining a definitive tissue diagnosis and can in most instances differentiate adenocarcinomas from other malignant or benign pancreatic mass lesions (Figure 32–3). However, FNA of a pancre-

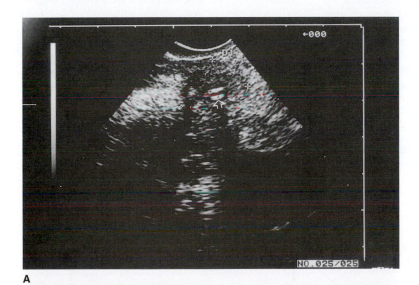

A

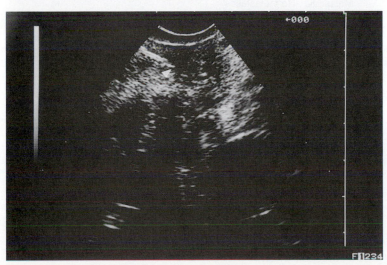

B

Figure 32–3. Endoscopic ultrasound (EUS) of a 2-cm mass in the head of the pancreas. **A:** Mass encompasses the common bile duct, which has a biliary stent *(arrow).* **B:** EUS-guided fine-needle aspiration of the mass. *Arrow* denotes tip of the needle.

atic mass should be performed only if it will affect patient management. Most patients present late in the course of the disease and are found on imaging with CT, transabdominal ultrasound, or EUS to have large mass lesions that are not surgically resectable. Those individuals can undergo FNA under CT or transabdominal ultrasound guidance to establish a definitive diagnosis of pancreatic cancer in order to guide medical decisions about nonoperative therapies. However, if probable liver metastases are evident on radiologic imaging, it usually is easier and safer to obtain FNA specimens from the hepatic lesions rather than the pancreatic mass. Similarly, FNA should be performed during staging with EUS if this study demonstrates features that indicate the tumor is not surgically resectable for cure. FNA should also be performed in pancreatic mass lesions of any size to confirm a diagnosis of malignancy when comorbid medical conditions increase the risk of safe surgical resection. At present, FNA should not be performed in patients with suspected pancreatic cancer when imaging studies suggest that the tumor may be resectable because of concerns that tumor cells may

spread outside the pancreas along the FNA needle track. However, this recommendation may change in the future if neoadjuvant (preoperative) therapy is shown to be useful in the treatment of pancreatic adenocarcinoma. If FNA is to be performed in patients with potentially resectable tumors, EUS-guided FNA is preferred to percutaneous methods due to a lower risk of tumor seeding. If an ERCP is performed, pancreatic ductal brushings or biopsy samples can be obtained and evaluated for malignant cytology (see Figure 32–4).

Differential Diagnosis

Because most pancreatic neoplasms present as solid masses in the pancreas, the primary differential diagnosis is with chronic pancreatitis, which may cause focal or generalized enlargement of the pancreatic head or body. In patients with enlargement of the pancreas suspicious for pancreatic neoplasm, the clinician must decide between pursuing fine-needle aspiration cytology, laparotomy with operative biopsy and/or excision, or a period of observation followed by repeated imaging.

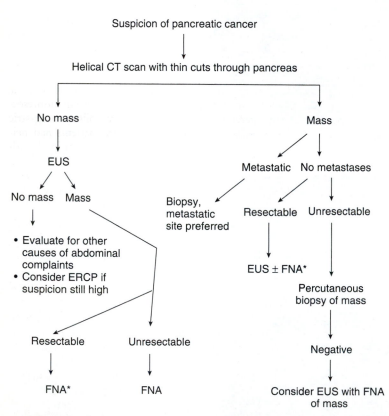

Figure 32–4. Diagnostic algorithm for pancreatic cancer. EUS, endoscopic ultrasound; ERCP, endoscopic retrograde cholangiopancreatography; FNA, fine-needle aspirate; CT, computed tomography.

* If neoadjuvant protocol, patient found to be unresectable by EUS or need to confirm diagnosis preoperatively.

Percutaneous radiologic or EUS-guided FNA usually confirms the histologic diagnosis of pancreatic neoplasm, when present; however negative or nondiagnostic results do not definitively exclude a diagnosis of malignancy (see Figure 32–2). For patients with negative or equivocal results on cytologic studies, an ERCP may differentiate between chronic pancreatitis and pancreatic neoplasms.

Cystic pancreatic neoplasms (mucinous or serous cystadenoma, cystadenocarcinoma) that must be differentiated from pancreatic pseudocysts are rare (see section, "Cystic Neoplasms").

In patients with jaundice, carcinoma of the ampulla of Vater must be differentiated from cancer of the pancreatic head that is obstructing the distal bile duct. The diagnosis of ampullary cancer usually is suggested on CT or ultrasonography by the presence of dilation of the extrahepatic bile ducts and the pancreatic duct without a detectable pancreatic mass lesion.

Endoscopic examination of the medial wall of the duodenum usually establishes the diagnosis of ampullary carcinoma, which results in enlargement of the duodenal papilla. Biopsy and pancreatography are confirmatory.

Treatment

Pancreatic adenocarcinoma can be cured only by surgical excision. Unfortunately, a potentially curative surgical resection is possible in less than 20% of patients at the time of diagnosis. The importance of preoperative staging cannot be overstated. Patients with tumors associated with vascular invasion (eg, superior mesenteric artery), peripancreatic or distal nodal involvement, or distant metastases have a median survival of less than 1 year, which is not improved with surgical resection. Table 32–2 shows the staging of carcinoma of the pancreas. However, this staging system is not commonly used for management decisions, and criteria for resection vary from institution to institution. Therapeutic approaches for pancreatic adenocarcinoma are outlined in Table 32–3.

Table 32–2. Staging of carcinoma of exocrine pancreas.

Stage 0	*In situ* carcinoma
Stage I	Tumor localized within pancreatic capsule
Stage II	Invasion of duodenum, bile duct, or peripancreatic tissues
Stage III	Involvement of lymph nodes
Stage IV	Tumor extends directly into stomach, spleen, colon, or adjacent large vessels; distant metastases

Table 32–3. Options for therapy.

Stage I (resectable) Good performance status	Surgery with adjuvant chemoradiation
Stage I (unresectable) Good performance status	Consider entry into experimental protocol to down-stage tumor Clinical trials Chemoradiation Gemcitabine
Stage I Poor performance status	Gemcitabine-based therapy Supportive care
Stages II and III Good performance status	Clinical trials Chemoradiation Gemcitabine-based therapy
Stage IV Good performance status	Clinical trials Gemcitabine-based therapy
Stages II, III, and IV Poor performance status	Gemcitabine-based therapy Supportive care

A. Surgery

The minority of patients with pancreatic neoplasms undergo curative surgical resection, primarily because less than 20% present with potentially curable disease. For example, of over 300 patients with pancreatic carcinoma who were referred to UCLA Medical Center over a 15-year period, only 15% underwent resection of the pancreatic tumor, whereas 50% underwent nonresective operative procedures to relieve biliary or gastric outlet obstruction. One-third of the patients had neither resection nor surgical bypass because of locally advanced or metastatic disease, advanced age, or debility.

For patients with confirmed carcinoma of the head of the pancreas, the Whipple resection (pancreaticoduodenectomy) is the procedure of choice. This involves resection of the pancreas to mid-body, the duodenum, the common bile duct, and the gallbladder, followed by anastomosis of a limb of jejunum to the stomach, proximal bile duct, and stomach. Due to improvements in operative technique, the mortality rate from this operation is less than 5% in patients with experienced surgeons. The main source of morbidity and mortality from the Whipple procedure arises from the pancreaticojejunostomy, through which anastomotic leaks and hemorrhage may occur. Despite its technical difficulty and associated morbidity, Whipple resection provides the only real hope of cure for patients with carcinoma of the head of the pancreas. Even when cure is not achieved, it may provide a long period of palliation with improved quality of life, particularly among good-risk patients who have small periampullary neoplasms. Despite improved rates of operative mortality and morbidity, the 5-year survival remains only 20% for the selected subset of patients who undergo potential curative surgical resection of tumor.

En bloc resection of the entire pancreas, duodenum, spleen, and greater omentum with subtotal gastrectomy has been suggested by some investigators to have advantages over the Whipple procedure for patients with carcinoma of the head of the pancreas. Total pancreatectomy obviates the need for the difficult and problematic pancreaticojejunal anastomosis. Furthermore, for many patients who have carcinoma of the pancreatic head, the body and tail of the pancreas may be quite fibrotic and unlikely to function normally postoperatively. Some studies have shown that among patients whose carcinoma seems confined to the head of the pancreas, microscopic or macroscopic tumor foci can often be found far from the margin of pancreatic resection. One study from the Mayo Clinic failed to demonstrate a significant difference in 5-year survival between patients undergoing Whipple procedure and those having total pancreatectomy.

Patients with advanced disease do not benefit from surgical excision—even if such excision is technically feasible. These include patients whose pancreatic neoplasm at the time of presentation is large and bulky with either metastases, retroperitoneal extension, high-grade common bile duct obstruction, invasion of vascular structures, or all these findings. Nonresective bypass surgery may be warranted in such patients for palliation of symptoms due to biliary obstruction or duodenal obstruction. For patients with symptoms of pruritus, jaundice, or cholangitis, palliative surgical decompression of the bile duct may be performed by transection of the bile duct above the tumor with creation of a choledochojejunostomy. Unfortunately, the mean survival following surgical bypass is about 6 months. Therefore, this procedure should be considered in otherwise good-risk patients with a reasonable life expectancy, particularly those who have coexistent obstruction of the pylorus or the second portion of the duodenum. Surgical biliary and gastric bypass usually can be performed rapidly and safely. However, endoscopic biliary stenting is the preferred initial therapeutic palliative procedure for obstruction of the distal common bile duct (Figure 32–5). Either small-caliber (3.3-mm) removable plastic stents or large-caliber (10-mm) permanent metal mesh stents may be placed at ERCP over guidewires into the bile duct. It is advantageous for the endoscopist to have already established a diagnosis of pancreatic carcinoma prior to ERCP, so that the permanent large metal stents may be placed. Problems may be encountered at ERCP with attempts at passage of a guidewire through a distal high-grade common bile duct obstruction, since there may be virtually no lumen available for cannulation. Problems may also occur in the patient whose tumor has

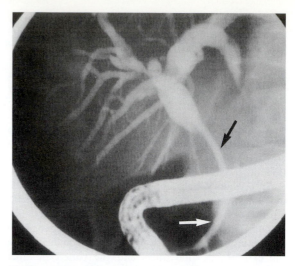

Figure 32–5. Endoscopic retrograde stenting of the common bile duct. A long polyethylene stent has been placed *(arrows)* with the proximal margin of the stent draining the dilated ductal system. The distal portion of the stent is left within the duodenum.

eroded into the duodenum since the papillary orifice may not be visible. In patients in whom endoscopic stent placement is not feasible, percutaneous transhepatic stenting can be performed by experienced interventional radiologists to palliatively decompress dilated bile ducts and relieve the symptoms of obstructive jaundice. Given the large array of surgical, radiologic, and endoscopic options for palliation of biliary obstruction, close cooperation and consultation among the primary care physician, surgeon, gastroenterologist, and interventional radiologist ensure that palliation is individualized to patient need and anatomy. Gastric outlet obstruction occurs in 15% of patients due to tumor compression or invasion of the stomach, pylorus, or duodenum. Patients may present with early satiety, postprandial vomiting, and weight loss. A surgical gastrojejunostomy is the optimal palliative treatment for this complication in patients who otherwise have a reasonable quality of life and short-term survival. Among poor operative candidates with gastroduodenal obstruction, large (18–20 mm) expandable metallic stents may be placed through to the obstructed region using endoscopic and fluoroscopic guidance and appear to provide reasonable short-term palliation.

B. CHEMOTHERAPY

Gemcitabine appears to be the most promising chemotherapeutic agent for the palliation of patients with nonresectable pancreatic cancer. Other single and combination-agent chemotherapies do not provide substantive palliation or improvement in survival. Gemcitabine produces only modest improvement in survival, but does appear to be effective in improving quality of life. However, overall response rates to gemcitabine are <15% and the 1-year survival rate for these patients is only 20%. Current studies with gemcitabine are focusing on optimal drug schedules designed to enhance the intracellular production of the active drug metabolite as well as combination therapy with other chemotherapeutic agents.

Prior to the widespread use of gemcitabine, 5-fluorouracil (5-FU) was the most commonly used chemotherapy agent for the palliative treatment of pancreatic cancer. However, the response rate to 5-FU administration is only 10–15% and the mean survival time is less than 20 weeks. Mitomycin, streptozotocin, ifosfamide, and doxorubicin likewise provide only a 10–25% response rate without improvement in long-term survival. Combination chemotherapy with streptomycin, mitomycin-C, and 5-FU may produce more objective tumor responses but do not prolong the median survival over that expected with single-agent treatment. These dismal results emphasize the necessity for new therapeutic approaches, using both novel and conventional agents, as well as the need for physicians to refer patients for participation in clinical trials.

C. RADIATION THERAPY

When used alone, external beam radiation therapy gives very disappointing results, with median survivals of only 6–12 months. Moreover, radiation can produce substantial injury to adjacent organs, such as the spinal cord, liver, and duodenum, although improvements in radiation equipment and delivery techniques have decreased the occurrence of these complications. The use of external beam radiation therapy combined with chemotherapy (5-FU) is widely used as adjuvant therapy following surgical resection of pancreatic adenocarcinoma. Newer approaches to the management of patients with potentially resectable disease include the use of neoadjuvant (ie, preoperative) therapy with chemotherapy and radiation therapy to reduce tumor bulk and improve local disease control with the hope of improving the chances for curative surgical resection. Many centers also use chemoradiation therapy as an initial treatment for patients with locally unresectable disease.

D. CELIAC PLEXUS BLOCK

For many patients, extensive retroperitoneal tumor infiltration produces disabling, intractable pain. Although narcotics and radiation therapy may be helpful, celiac plexus block can help patients who do not respond to standard narcotics or radiation therapy. These blocks may be performed by an experienced clinician using guidance by EUS, fluoroscopy, or CT. Although no prospective randomized trials have examined this therapy, complications are few and adequate palliation can be achieved with very low risk. For those patients who do not obtain adequate pain relief from a celiac plexus block, percutaneous splanchnic nerve blocks or thoracoscopic splanchnicectomy can be tried.

PANCREATIC ISLET-CELL TUMORS

Pancreatic islet-cell tumors constitute about 2% of all pancreatic neoplasms. Up to half of these tumors are "functional" and secrete one or more biologically active peptides (hormones), which result in the development of clinical symptoms. Five clinical types of tumors have been described: insulinoma, gastrinoma, glucagonoma, somatostatinoma, and vasoactive intestinal peptide-secreting tumors (VIPoma). Occasionally these tumors will secrete more than one peptide. A significant proportion of the tumors are not associated with hormone overproduction ("nonfunctional") and are diagnosed on the basis of symptoms caused by local or metastatic tumor growth.

Clinical Findings

Many of the patients with pancreatic islet-cell tumors present with signs and symptoms of excess hormone secretion. The most common tumor of islet-cell origin, namely the insulinoma, usually is manifested by profound hypoglycemia with diaphoresis, confusion, and syncope. Gastrinoma is the second most common tumor of islet-cell origin. Classically, these tumors present with peptic ulcer disease. Other common symptoms include diarrhea and esophagitis. About one-third of gastrinomas are associated with multiple endocrine neoplasia syndrome type 1 (MEN-1). VIPomas are associated with a syndrome of watery diarrhea, hypokalemia, and achlorhydria (WDHA). Glucagonomas can present with diabetes, deep-vein thrombosis, depression, and dermatitis (necrolytic migratory erythema). Somatostatinomas are quite rare and may present with symptoms including cholelithiasis, weight loss, abdominal pain, diabetes, steatorrhea, and diarrhea. Hormonally inactive (nonsecreting) islet-cell tumors of the pancreatic head may present with jaundice, pruritis, or abdominal pain. Islet tumors commonly metastasize to the liver, where they may cause hepatic enlargement, pain, or jaundice.

Diagnostic Studies

In most patients, elevated serum hormone levels (insulin, gastrin, vasoactive intestinal peptide, glucagons) or other serologic tests suggest the presence of a syndrome that may be caused by a pancreatic islet-cell tumor. Subsequent tests are directed at identification of the tumor source of the hormone and determination of whether the tumor is localized (and resectable) or metastatic. Previously, transhepatic portal venous sampling for these amine precursor uptake and decarboxylation (APUD) cell hormones was performed, but currently this test has only limited clinical use due to its invasiveness. The initial diagnostic procedure for localizing the tumor should be contrast-enhanced dynamic CT of the pancreas, employing sections through the liver and pancreas using a "pancreatic protocol." In most instances, pancreatic islet-cell tumors are hypervascular; using an optimal CT imaging technique, lesions less than 1 cm in size can be detected. The development of somatostatin receptor scintigraphy (SRS) has greatly improved the localization and staging of islet-cell tumors. Most APUD-derived islet-cell tumors have a large number of somatostatin receptors, which bind a radiolabeled somatostatin analogue (octreotide). SRS is extremely useful for the localization of tumors with overall sensitivity of 80–100% for all islet-cell tumors except for insulinomas, for which the sensitivity is <50%. Additional techniques for locating small APUD cell tumors not seen by CT or SRS include MRI, EUS, intraoperative surgical palpation of the gland, and intraoperative ultrasonography. EUS is especially helpful in localizing small islet-cell tumors and demonstrating resectability by showing normal tissue planes between the pancreas and adjacent great vessels. It is also useful for identification of tumors in the duodenal wall or adjacent peripancreatic lymph nodes, a common site of gastrinomas.

Treatment

The vast majority of pancreatic islet-cell neoplasms can be treated by segmental resection of the gland or enucleation of the tumor. Complete surgical resection is the only curative treatment of these tumors. Somatostatin analogues, such as octreotide, have been used to control hormonally related symptoms, and, in some cases, may cause inhibition of tumor growth.

CYSTIC NEOPLASMS

Pancreatic carcinomas other than adenocarcinoma of pancreatic ductal origin and islet-cell tumors are uncommon, representing only 5% of pancreatic cancers. Special mention is made of cystadenomas and cystadenocarcinomas because they are often mistaken for benign pancreatic pseudocysts and because they have a much more favorable natural history than noncystic pancreatic adenocarcinoma.

Clinical Findings

A. Symptoms and Signs

Cystic neoplasms are most commonly found in the body or tail of the pancreas of young to middle-aged adults, especially women. The tumors remain asymptomatic until they become quite large, when they may present with symptoms caused by local tumor growth with compression of adjacent abdominal structures. These include abdominal pain, a palpable mass, weight loss, nausea, and vomiting. Obstruction of the common bile duct resulting in jaundice, pruritis, and cholangitis is less common than with noncystic adenocarcinoma. Similarly, upper gastrointestinal tract bleeding caused by splenic vein thrombosis with formation of gastric varices or direct tumor invasion is a less common presentation.

B. Diagnostic Studies

The diagnosis usually is suggested by abdominal CT or ultrasonographic detection of a large, cystic pancreatic mass. These studies usually are obtained for evaluation of vague abdominal complaints. It may be difficult from these noninvasive imaging studies to differentiate cystic pancreatic neoplasms from nonneoplastic pancreatic pseudocysts. It is extremely important to consider the diagnosis of cystic neoplasms of the pancreas in patients who present with isolated cystic lesions who do not have risk factors for pancreatic pseudocysts. The absence of trauma, alcoholism, a history of acute or chronic pancreatitis, or biliary tract disease makes pancreatic pseudocysts unlikely and cystic neoplasm of the pancreas more likely in patients who are found to have an isolated cystic lesion of the gland. EUS is extremely useful in the evaluation of cystic lesions, often providing additional detail not seen by CT. It can clarify whether the lesion is a simple cyst (strongly suggesting pseudocyst) or a cystic mass. For cystic mass lesions, it can often distinguish serous cystic lesions (which are almost always benign) from mucinous cystic lesions (which have a high risk of malignancy). Serous ("microcystic") cystadenomas have a characteristic honeycomb appearance with central fibrosis or calcification. EUS can be used to sample cystic fluid, which can be examined for enzyme levels, viscosity, tumor marker levels, and cytology. Pancreatic pseudocysts have a high amylase content. Serous cystadenomas have a clear serous fluid, a low amylase content, and low CEA level. Mucinous cystadenomas have a fluid that is viscous, contains mucin, and has a low amylase level. Malignant cystadenocarcinomas may have a high CEA level and/or positive cytology. ERCP may also be performed to help clarify the diagnosis. Most patients with pancreatic pseudocysts have abnormal pancreatic ducts consistent with chronic pancreatitis; connection of the duct to the pseudocyst often can be demonstrated. Conversely, patients with cystic tumors usually have normal pancreatic ductal anatomy—which does not communicate with the cystic lesion.

Intraductal papillary mucinous tumors (IPMT) are rare mucinous tumors that arise in the main or segmental pancreatic ducts as papillary growths that produce a large amount of mucin. They may be benign or malignant. Approximately 80% occur in the pancreatic head and two-thirds of affected patients are men. Symptoms caused by pancreatic duct obstruction include acute or recurrent pancreatitis or pancreatic insufficiency.

Treatment

Most patients with either benign or malignant cystic neoplasms should be considered for surgical resection, even if the tumor is large or locally invasive. High-risk patients (especially those with a lesion in the pancreatic head, for which surgical excision is more complicated) whose preoperative studies suggest benign cystic neoplasms may be monitored closely with radiologic or EUS imaging. Although serous ("microcystic") adenomas have no malignant potential, resection is recommended in most patients whose operative risk is minimal because symptoms may arise from local tumor growth. It may be very difficult to distinguish benign mucinous ("macrocystic") cystadenomas from malignant cystadenomas by preoperative studies. Because of the high propensity of benign tumors to evolve into malignancy, resection is recommended. Long-term survival following resection of malignant pancreatic cystic neoplasms exceeds 70%. Treatment of IPMT usually involves distal pancreatectomy; if the tumor is confined to the pancreatic duct, surgery is curative.

PANCREATIC LYMPHOMAS

Pancreatic lymphomas are infrequent, probably representing 1–3% of all pancreatic neoplasms. An increase in pancreatic lymphomas is now being seen among patients with AIDS. These latter patients have B cell non-Hodgkin's lymphomas arising primarily in the pancreas, wall of the duodenum, or even common bile duct.

Clinical Findings

The differentiation of pancreatic lymphoma from pancreatic adenocarcinoma is important preoperatively because the primary form of therapy for lymphoma is chemotherapy rather than surgical resection. In general, patients with pancreatic lymphoma present with signs and symptoms identical to those with adenocarcinoma. However, patients with pancreatic lymphoma have lower levels of serum bilirubin and alkaline phosphatase than patients with comparably bulky pancreatic adenocarcinoma. Percutaneous transabdominal aspiration cytology usually establishes the diagnosis of lymphoma. However, an uncertain preoperative diagnosis may necessitate surgery.

Treatment

Surgery may also be warranted when there is clear-cut high-grade biliary or gastric outlet obstruction, or both. When patients with pancreatic lymphoma are diagnosed preoperatively, chemotherapy can be initiated with cyclophosphamide, prednisone, and doxorubicin.

REFERENCES

INCIDENCE & RISK FACTORS, PATHOPHYSIOLOGY

Gold EB, Goldin SB: Epidemiology of and risk factors for pancreatic cancer. Surg Oncol Clin North Am 1998;7;67.

Greenlee RT et al: Cancer statistics 2001. CA Cancer J Clin 2001; 51:15.

Hruban RH et al: Genetics of pancreatic cancer. From genes to families. Surg Oncol Clin North Am 1998;7:1.

Lillemoe KD, Yeo CJ, Cameron JL: Pancreatic cancer: state-of-the-art care. CA Cancer J Clin 2000;50:241.

Lowenfels AB et al: Hereditary pancreatitis is caused by a mutation in the cationic trypsinogen gene. J Natl Cancer Inst 1997; 89:442.

DIAGNOSTIC STUDIES

Ahmad N et al: Role of endoscopic ultrasound and magnetic resonance imaging in the preoperative staging of pancreatic adenocarcinoma. Am J Gastroenterol 2000;95:1926.

Brugge WR: The role of EUS in the diagnosis of cystic lesions of the pancreas. Gastrointest Endosc 2000 (Suppl):52:S18.

DiMagno EP, Reber HA, Tempero M: AGA technical review on the epidemiology, diagnosis, and treatment of pancreatic ductal adenocarcinoma. Gastroenterology 1999;117:1464.

Hawes RH et al: A multispecialty approach to the diagnosis and management of pancreatic cancer. Am J Gastroenterol 2000; 95:17.

Kim H et al: A new strategy for the application of CA 19-9 in the differentiation of pancreaticobiliary cancer: analysis using a receiver operating characteristic curve. Am J Gastroenterol 1999;94:1941.

Somogyi L, Mishra G: Diagnosis and staging of islet cell tumors of the pancreas. Current Gastroenterol Rep 2000;2:159.

TREATMENT

Burris HA et al: Improvements in survival and clinical benefit with gemcitabine as first-line therapy for patients with advanced pancreatic cancer: a randomized trial. J Clin Oncol 1997;15: 2403.

Carr J et al: Adenocarcinoma of the head of the pancreas: effects of surgical and nonsurgical therapy on survival—a ten year experience. Am Surg 1999;65:1143.

Castillo CF, Warshaw AL: Current management of cystic neoplasms of the pancreas. Adv Surg 2000;34:237.

Chamberlain AK: The surgical management of pancreatic neuroendocrine tumors. Surg Clin North Am 2001;81:511.

Heinemann V et al: Gemcitabine and cisplatin in the treatment of advanced or metastatic pancreatic cancer. Ann Oncol 2000; 11:1399.

Huibregtse K: The Wallstent for malignant biliary obstruction. Gastrointest Endosc Clin North Am 1999;9:491.

Karpoff H et al: Results of total pancreatectomy for adenocarcinoma of the pancreas. Arch Surg 2001;136:44.

Klinkenbijl J et al: Adjuvant radiotherapy and 5-fluorouracil after curative resection of cancer of the pancreas and periampullary region: phase III trial of the EORTC Gastrointestinal Tract Cancer Cooperative Group. Ann Surg 1999;230:776.

Millikan K et al: Prognostic factors associated with resectable adenocarcinoma of the head of the pancreas. Am Surg 1999;65: 618.

Nevitt A et al: Expandable metallic prostheses for malignant obstructions of gastric outlet and proximal small bowel. Gastrointest Endosc 1998;47:271.

Pedrazzoli S et al: Standard versus extended lymphadenectomy associated with pancreatoduodenectomy in the surgical treatment of adenocarcinoma of the head of the pancreas: a multicenter, prospective, randomized study. Ann Surg 1998;228: 508.

Prat F et al: A randomized trial of endoscopic drainage methods for inoperable malignant strictures of the common bile duct. Gastrointest Endosc 1998;47:1.

Saltz BR: Islet cell tumors of the pancreas: the medical oncologist's perspective. Surg Clin North Am 2001;81:527.

Sohn T et al: Surgical palliation of unresectable periampullary adenocarcinoma in the 1990s. J Am Coll Surg 1999;188:658.

Spitz F et al: Preoperative and postoperative chemoradiation strategies in patients treated with pancreaticoduodenectomy for adenocarcinoma of the pancreas. J Clin Oncol 1997;15:928.

Strasberg S, Drebin J, Soper N: Evolution and current status of the Whipple procedure. An update for gastroenterologists. Gastroenterology 1997;113:983.

Takao S et al: Comparison of relapse and long-term survival between pylorus-preserving and Whipple pancreaticoduodenectomy in periampullary cancer. Am J Surg 1998;176:467.

Tempero M: *Chemotherapy of Pancreatic Cancer.* Humana Press, 1998.

Yeo C et al: Pancreaticoduodenectomy for pancreatic adenocarcinoma: postoperative chemoradiation improves survival. Ann Surg 1997;225:621.

Yim H et al: Clinical outcome of the use of enteral stents for palliation of patients with malignant upper GI obstruction. Gastrointest Endosc 2001;53:329.

SECTION VI
Diseases of the Liver & Biliary System

Approach to the Patient with Suspected Liver Disease

33

J. Gregory Fitz, MD

The clinical manifestations of liver injury are diverse, ranging from isolated and clinically silent laboratory abnormalities to dramatic and rapidly progressive liver failure. This spectrum relates in part to the broad range of pathophysiologic processes that can damage the liver, and in part to the reserve capacity of the organ, which is large and can mask significant injury. It is estimated that approximately 40% of patients with cirrhosis are asymptomatic. Once symptoms develop, however, the prognosis is poor and the human and economic costs of liver disease are high. Cirrhosis accounts for over 40,000 deaths each year in the United States, and more than 228,145 years of potential life lost. The average patient with alcoholic liver disease loses 12 years of productive life, a much larger loss than that for heart disease (2 years) and cancer (4 years). The poor outcome and high cost of treatment of advanced liver disease reinforce the need for early diagnosis and intervention.

This chapter provides general guidelines for evaluating suspected liver disease. Clinical categories that reflect common patterns of liver injury are emphasized and include isolated aminotransferase elevation in the absence of symptoms, jaundice and cholestasis, and chronic liver disease. There is obvious overlap between these categories, but recognition of the dominant pattern of injury provides an important framework for subsequent diagnosis of the underlying causes of liver injury. Indeed, this accounts for much of the challenge of clinical practice in liver disorders. Specific disease processes are described in more detail in subsequent chapters.

CLINICAL EVALUATION OF SUSPECTED LIVER DISEASE

Liver disease is identified in most patients by suggestive laboratory abnormalities, or signs or symptoms that result from hepatocyte necrosis and fibrosis. These abnormalities are often nonspecific, initiating a more focused evaluation to establish the extent of liver damage, identify the underlying causes, and guide therapy. Points of the history, physical, and laboratory examinations that merit special emphasis are summarized here.

Clinical History: Risk Factors for Liver Disease

Evaluation of suspected liver disease begins first with a detailed assessment of risk factors. Initially, basic demographic factors (ie, age, gender, and race) are used to establish a hierarchy of possibilities. Usually, males and nonwhites represent high-risk groups for liver disease, as evidenced by an increased number of hospital admissions. Men younger than 20 years of age are at risk for acute viral hepatitis, but with increasing age, overuse of alcohol, biliary disease, and chronic hepatitis are more commonly identified. Men older than 55 years of age are at increased risk for cirrhosis, biliary disease, and hepatobiliary malignancies. Women are subject to the same general processes, but in addition are much more likely to develop autoimmune hepatitis in young and middle-aged cohorts, or primary biliary cirrhosis in those above age 40 years. Primary biliary cirrhosis is about nine times more common in women as compared with men.

Attention to the family history can also identify patients at risk. Classic genetic diseases such as hemochromatosis, α₁-antitrypsin deficiency, or Wilson's disease are the best defined. Hemochromatosis involves men more than women, and is associated with coexisting diabetes, heart disease, and pigmentation in many patients. Deficiency of α₁-antitrypsin is associated with pulmonary disease and younger age of onset. Wilson's disease is suggested by coincidence of neurologic abnormalities and an earlier age of onset. These familial disorders are relatively uncommon, however, and together account for less than 5% of visits to most hepatology practices. Instead, a positive family history of liver disease usually indicates either shared risks (eg, exposure to viral hepatitis) or more common inherited traits that have a much more complex genetic basis. Alcoholism, hyperlipidemia, and diabetes represent important risk factors that have unequivocal but poorly understood genetic links. These disorders are more common and likely to be associated with a family history of liver disease, and therefore may require the appropriate use of other diagnostic tests.

Personal habits and exposures also represent important risk factors (Table 33–1). As a rule, focused questions about high-risk behavior are required because of the temporal delay between the actions and the onset of clinical symptoms. Among these risk factors, alcohol abuse deserves special emphasis because of its prevalence. Alcohol-related liver disease accounts for 30% or more of hepatologic consultations. The precise mechanisms responsible for alcohol-related liver damage remain uncertain; there is evidence both for direct damage to liver cells by alcohol and its metabolites, and for indirect damage because of nutritional depletion (see Chapter 39). Most individuals have a history of substantial exposure. In men, it is estimated that consumption of 60–80 g of alcohol daily (approximately four beers, glasses of wine, or mixed drinks) establishes a clear risk for subsequent cirrhosis. In women, only 40–60 g/d establishes the same risk. Alcohol use must usually be continued for 10 years or more before cirrhosis develops. There is a broad range of susceptibility, however, and lower levels of consumption can be toxic in some individuals. In addition, binge drinking, with exposure to higher alcohol levels, can cause alcoholic hepatitis and fatty liver. Although these usually resolve with cessation of drinking, a history of alcoholic hepatitis identifies individuals at high risk for subsequent cirrhosis.

Attention to past medical events represents a final focus of the initial history. Male homosexuality, prior episodes of hepatitis, jaundice, or blood transfusions indicate increased risk for acute or chronic viral hepatitis, and a history of alcohol-related pancreatitis or hepatitis identifies a cohort with sufficient consumption to be at risk for cirrhosis. Prior cholecystectomy or biliary surgery represents a major risk for development of biliary strictures. Finally, many general medical conditions are accompanied by hepatic manifestations (see Table 33–1).

Physical Examination

Physical manifestations of liver disease can result from loss of hepatocyte mass, bile duct obstruction, or development of portal hypertension. Chronic hepatitis and cirrhosis are clinically silent in a significant portion of patients because of the large reserve capacity of the liver. Consequently, the absence of physical findings provides no guarantee that liver disease can be ruled out, thus emphasizing the importance of a systematic evaluation.

A. JAUNDICE

Jaundice results from an increase in serum bilirubin concentration (see following discussion) and is detected as a yellow-green coloration of skin, mucous membranes, and sclerae. The onset usually coincides with a rise in serum bilirubin to over 3.5 mg/dL, and is of sufficient concern to most patients that they seek medical

Table 33–1. Risk factors for liver disease.

Risk Factors	Associated Liver Diseases
Family history	Hemochromatosis, Wilson's disease, α₁-antitrypsin deficiency, cystic fibrosis, thalassemia
Alcohol consumption (usually ≥ 50 g/d)	Alcoholic fatty liver, alcoholic hepatitis, cirrhosis
Hyperlipidemia, diabetes, obesity	Fatty liver
Previous blood transfusion	Hepatitis B, C, non-A, non-B
Autoimmune diseases	Autoimmune hepatitis, primary biliary cirrhosis
Medications	Drug-induced liver injury
Parenteral exposures (intravenous drug use, health care workers)	Hepatitis B and C
Male homosexuality	Hepatitis B
Foreign travel	Hepatitis A and B
Ulcerative colitis	Primary sclerosing cholangitis
History of jaundice or hepatitis	Chronic viral hepatitis, autoimmune hepatitis, cirrhosis
Hepatobiliary surgery	Postoperative stricture of bile ducts, recurrent gallstones

attention quickly. Unfortunately, not all patients are careful observers, and the multiple potential causes of jaundice limit the specificity of this finding. Instead, the clinical interpretation depends on the duration of the hyperbilirubinemia as well as laboratory and radiographic testing to assess whether there is intra- or extrahepatic cholestasis.

Jaundice accompanying acute liver necrosis that results from acetaminophen overdose, viral hepatitis, or hypotension is due to the loss of hepatocellular mass and impaired bilirubin secretion. In the early stages, detection of right upper quadrant tenderness and an increase in liver size (span >12 cm) support active hepatocellular necrosis and inflammation. Appearance of asterixis, confusion, or coma mark further deterioration, and the onset of bleeding may indicate profound synthetic defects and coagulopathy. Liver size may decrease in the later stages, and decorticate or decerebrate posturing and neurogenic hyperventilation accompany irreversible damage.

The abrupt onset of jaundice accompanied by abdominal pain, fever, and right upper quadrant tenderness suggests acute cholangitis with or without cholecystitis. The liver is not usually enlarged, and a history of previous gallbladder stones or surgery is suggestive. A more indolent onset of jaundice in the absence of tenderness may indicate underlying transport abnormalities, cirrhosis, or duct obstruction.

B. MANIFESTATIONS RESULTING FROM LOSS OF HEPATOCELLULAR MASS AND PORTAL HYPERTENSION

Other physical manifestations of chronic liver disease result from sustained loss of hepatocellular mass and development of portal hypertension (see Chapter 42). A small liver (<8 cm) or a liver with a nodular contour suggests the presence of established cirrhosis, although interobserver variability limits the reproducibility of this finding. As the metabolic capacity of the liver deteriorates, the estrogen precursor androstenedione can accumulate and lead to gynecomastia, testicular atrophy, and palmar erythema. In addition, spider angiomas are common and most frequently involve the face, shoulders, and trunk. These may result from increased circulating levels of angiogenic factors.

Anatomic distortion of the liver caused by fibrosis and regeneration leads to distortion and loss of sinusoidal area and an increase in portal vein pressures. Portal hypertension may remain clinically silent but more commonly leads to predictable clinical sequelae, including renal Na^+ retention, which results in ascites and edema; hypersplenism with thrombocytopenia; portal-systemic shunting, resulting in hemorrhoids and distended superficial and periumbilical (caput medusa) abdominal veins; and esophageal varices. In chronic cirrhosis, hepatic encephalopathy correlates more closely with the degree of portal hypertension and shunting of blood away from the liver than with the loss of hepatocyte mass. Although any one of these features may predominate in an individual patient, they often coexist and may change over time.

C. MANIFESTATIONS MORE COMMON TO SPECIFIC DISORDERS

Some physical findings have more specificity in that they occur with greater frequency according to the underlying cause of cirrhosis. Chronic alcohol use is associated with fibrosis of the palmar fascia, leading to Dupuytren's contractures involving the fourth and fifth fingers, atrophy of proximal muscles, and peripheral neuropathy. Hemochromatosis is accompanied by a characteristic metallic-gray pigmentation related to melanin deposition on sun-exposed areas of the body; pigmentation can also be seen in the genital regions and in areas of scarring. Hemochromatosis is also accompanied by a characteristic arthropathy involving the small joints of the hands, particularly the second and third metacarpophalangeal joints. Wilson's disease can cause acute liver failure with hemolytic anemia, or chronic liver failure with associated neurologic findings due to involvement of basal ganglia; findings include movement disorders, tremors, spasticity, rigidity, chorea, and dysarthria. Kayser-Fleischer rings due to deposition of copper in Descemet's membrane are highly suggestive of Wilson's disease.

Laboratory Findings

Because many of the clinical features of liver injury are nonspecific, the history and physical examination are routinely supplemented by "liver function" tests, which are so widely available that they have become a standard and essential component of the evaluation. In this section, a brief overview of standard laboratory tests is provided to serve as a basis for later definition of specific clinical syndromes.

A. HEPATOCELLULAR INJURY: AMINOTRANSFERASES

Aspartate aminotransferase (AST) and alanine aminotransferase (ALT) are found in high concentrations inside hepatocytes, where they catalyze transfer of α-amino groups from their respective amino acids to ketoglutaric acid, resulting in the formation of oxaloacetic acid and pyruvate plus glutamate. The aminotransferases are detectable in serum in concentrations of less than 60 IU/L, as a result of normal cell turnover and regeneration. Any insult that leads to liver cell injury or necrosis releases intracellular enzymes and results in increases in serum AST and ALT concentrations. Consequently, the aminotransferases provide a sensitive but relatively nonspecific measure of liver inflammation. Aminotransferase levels may be elevated to the same degree in patients with benign conditions such as fatty liver, or more serious conditions, including chronic viral hepatitis and cancer. Thus, detection of elevated aminotransferases mandates more specific evaluation to identify the underlying cause.

Recognizing that there are exceptions to every rule, some useful generalizations regarding interpretation of aminotransferase elevations appear consistently and have enhanced their utility in the clinical setting. First, an AST to ALT ratio greater than 2 with AST levels of less than 300 IU/L is suggestive of alcohol-related liver disease. In contrast, viral hepatitis, ischemia, and other causes of injury result in more equivalent increases in AST and ALT and can produce higher serum concentrations. Second, increases in AST are not always related to liver injury, since this enzyme is also found in heart, muscle, kidney, brain, and pancreatic tissue and in erythrocytes. Because there are no tissue-specific isoenzymes of AST, it is important to suspect extrahepatic origins and confirm hepatic inflammation by measurement of ALT, which is found almost exclusively in the liver. Third, acute elevations of aminotransferases to values of more than 1000 IU/L usually reflect severe necrosis and necessitate rapid evaluation, with the aim of implementing specific therapy as soon as possible. Viral hepatitis, toxin-induced hepatitis (acetaminophen overdose, *Amanita phylloides* ingestion), and hepatic ischemia represent important causes of markedly elevated aminotransferases and should be considered according to the clinical presentation.

B. Alternative Markers for Hepatocellular Injury

Other hepatic enzymes have been used to supplement measurements of aminotransferase activity, with the aim of improving sensitivity or permitting early detection of alcohol-related injury. These include glutamate dehydrogenase, alcohol dehydrogenase, and lactate dehydrogenase. Their clinical utility has been limited by a lack of specificity, however, and they provide little information beyond that provided by AST and ALT.

C. Ductular Injury and Cholestasis: Alkaline Phosphatase and 5′-Nucleotidase

The alkaline phosphatases represent a family of enzymes that hydrolyzes organic phosphate esters in an alkaline environment. In the liver, they are localized to the canalicular region of hepatocytes and to bile duct cells. Ductular obstruction and cholestasis lead to increased production of alkaline phosphatase and to release of alkaline phosphatase from damaged cells. Consequently, elevation of serum alkaline phosphatase levels provides an important marker for duct cell injury, duct cell proliferation, and cholestasis.

Increases in alkaline phosphatase to levels four times normal or more are highly suggestive of ductular injury; representative causes include intrahepatic cholestasis, infiltrative processes, extrahepatic biliary obstruction, primary sclerosing cholangitis, primary biliary cirrhosis, malignant liver disease, and organ rejection after liver transplantation (Table 33–2). Lesser increases in alkaline phosphatase can accompany a broader range of injuries, including viral hepatitis, cirrhosis, and congestive hepatopathy.

Elevations of alkaline phosphatase also accompany diseases affecting bone, adrenal cortex, placenta, intestine, kidney, and lung. These diverse sources mandate that the hepatic origin of elevated alkaline phosphatase levels be confirmed by detection of associated evidence of liver disease and by evaluation for nonhepatic sources. Traditionally, this was done by fractionation of the alkaline phosphatase, since the hepatic and nonhepatic isoenzymes can be separated on the basis of different electrophoretic mobilities and susceptibility to urease and heat. This has largely been replaced by measurement of 5′-nucleotidase, which is a reliable and relatively specific marker of cholestasis and ductular injury. 5′-Nucleotidase activity is also abundant in the canalicular region, and usually increases in parallel with hepatic alkaline phosphatase levels.

Elevations of γ-glutamyl transpeptidase (GGT) also accompany the rise in alkaline phosphatase and 5′-nucleotidase levels. GGT is frequently elevated in patients ingesting alcohol, dilantin, barbiturates, and other drugs, and this has led to its use as a possible marker for occult alcohol use or liver disease. Isolated elevations of

Table 33–2. Common clinical findings in hepatic disease.

Test	Hepatocellular Injury	Cholestatic Disorders
Aminotransferases	> 8 times normal	< 3 times normal
Alkaline phosphatase	< 3 times normal	> 4 times normal
Bilirubin	Variably elevated	Elevated
5′-Nucleotidase	Variably elevated	Elevated
Prothrombin	Prolonged, poorly responsive to vitamin K	Prolonged, responsive to vitamin K
Abdominal pain	Uncommon	Common in extrahepatic obstruction
Fever, leukocytosis	Uncommon	Common in extrahepatic obstruction

GGT in the absence of other findings are nonspecific, however, and most cases are not associated with clinically significant liver disease. This represents an obvious limitation for the use of GGT as a screening test.

D. CHOLESTASIS: BILIRUBIN

Under normal conditions, serum bilirubin levels are maintained at less than 1.2 mg/dL, despite a continuous bilirubin load related to catabolism of heme molecules from senescent red blood cells. Maintenance of low serum levels requires three basic steps, which are illustrated in Figure 33–1. These steps include (1) hepatic uptake of bilirubin from the circulation, an efficient process mediated by specific carrier proteins in the basolateral membrane; (2) intracellular conjugation of bilirubin to glucuronic acid to improve water solubility; and (3) canalicular secretion of bilirubin into the canalicular space between cells. From there, bilirubin

conjugates are directed through the intrahepatic network of bile ducts and ultimately into the duodenum. Bilirubin is deconjugated in the intestinal lumen by bacteria. This secretory cycle can be interrupted at many levels, resulting in accumulation of bilirubin in the serum and clinical jaundice.

The subtleties of bilirubin metabolism and the susceptibility of the metabolic pathways to nonspecific injury complicate the interpretation of individual tests. Canalicular secretion is usually the rate-limiting step in the bilirubin cycle. Consequently, most jaundice encountered in adults is caused by conjugated hyperbilirubinemia resulting from defective canalicular transport and export of conjugated bilirubin out of the hepatocyte and back into the circulation. Unconjugated hyperbilirubinemia is encountered less commonly, and relevant causes include Gilbert syndrome and hemolysis. Bilirubin elevations in the hospitalized patient with

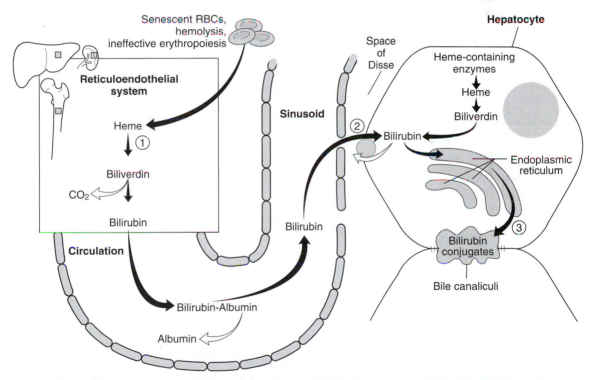

Figure 33–1. Bilirubin metabolism. Senescent red blood cells (RBCs) are removed from the circulation by reticuloendothelial cells in the liver, spleen, and bone marrow. Heme oxygenase (1) catalyzes cleavage of the tetrapyrrole ring to the linear tetrapyrrole biliverdin. Biliverdin is subsequently reduced to bilirubin. After production in the reticuloendothelial system, bilirubin is released into the circulation, where it is bound primarily to albumin. Fenestrations in the endothelial cells lining the hepatic sinusoids allow proteins access to Disse's space, where free bilirubin is transported into the hepatocyte (2). Bilirubin is poorly soluble in water and requires conjugation with glucuronide for excretion into the bile canaliculi (3). Conjugated bilirubin is actively transported into the bile canaliculi, where it is carried to the biliary tree and, ultimately, the duodenum.

other medical or surgical problems are most often multifactorial, with contributions from increased bilirubin production and impaired secretion. Systemic bacteremia, for example, causes a selective defect in secretion of conjugated bilirubin. In the absence of specific diagnostic tests, this syndrome is suggested by elevations of bilirubin out of proportion to alkaline phosphatase levels, without evidence of biliary obstruction.

Most clinical laboratories use the van den Bergh reaction to measure serum bilirubin levels. This colorimetric approach detects conjugated bilirubin as a "direct" fraction, and unconjugated bilirubin as an "indirect" fraction. Conjugation of bilirubin to glucuronide greatly increases its water solubility. Because conjugated bilirubin is then freely excreted by the kidneys, it has a short half-life in the circulation. The van den Bergh approach tends to overestimate the direct fraction as compared with high-resolution chromatography methods, which indicate that almost all circulating bilirubin in normal individuals is unconjugated. With intra- or extrahepatic cholestasis, there are increases in both the conjugated and unconjugated forms, but conjugated bilirubin usually predominates, since uptake and conjugation continue despite limited canalicular secretion. Over time, a third form of bilirubin appears that is covalently bound to albumin. This is often referred to as a delta fraction, which increases with the degree and duration of the bilirubin elevation. Protein-bound bilirubin is detected as part of the "direct" fraction by colorimetric assays, but protein-bound bilirubin is not secreted by the kidneys and has a much longer half-life in the circulation. Consequently, hyperbilirubinemia may persist for weeks after resolution of cholestasis if there is an appreciable amount of protein-bound (delta) bilirubin present.

E. SYNTHETIC FUNCTIONS OF THE LIVER

Loss of hepatocyte mass results in impairment of the biosynthetic functions of the liver and is reflected in common symptoms, including fatigue and loss of muscle mass. Measurement of the serum albumin concentration and the prothrombin time provides a more quantitative assessment of functional impairment. Decreases in serum albumin result primarily from decreased production, and sustained values of less than 3 mg/dL indicate substantial impairment. Because albumin has a half-life in the circulation of approximately 28 days, several weeks or months of impaired synthesis are required before there are detectable decreases in serum concentrations. Nonhepatic causes of hypoalbuminemia include protein-losing enteropathies, nephrosis, and malnutrition.

Prolongation of the prothrombin time is a more reliable indicator of defective synthetic function. Maintenance of normal values requires synthesis of multiple vitamin K–dependent factors in the coagulation cascade. With loss of hepatocyte mass, the decrease in factor levels leads to incremental defects in coagulation. A decrease in factor VII levels to less than 30% of normal or an increase in the prothrombin time of more than 3 seconds correlates with marked impairment. Because cholestasis, malabsorption, and nutritional deprivation can all contribute to vitamin K deficiency, it is important to replete vitamin K stores to ensure that the prothrombin time accurately reflects synthetic capacity rather than vitamin K depletion.

Clinical Assessment & Prognosis

Although individual laboratory findings lack specificity, the use of a panel of laboratory and clinical findings has been shown to provide important insights into the severity of the underlying disease and the long-term prognosis. This approach helps to quantitate functional reserve and is becoming increasingly important with the advent of newer therapies. The appropriate timing of transplantation, for example, is critical to successful and cost-effective outcomes (see Chapter 54). Transplantation too early in the clinical course would improve surgical outcomes at the expense of some unnecessary operations, while transplantation late in the clinical course at a time when hepatic reserve is exhausted predicts poorer outcomes and increased costs.

Several methods for evaluating functional hepatic reserve have been developed. One of the best validated and easiest to use is the *Child-Pugh score,* which is based on the original observations of Child and Turcotte. This approach uses a graded system to assign a numerical risk on the basis of serum albumin and serum bilirubin measurements, the presence of ascites and encephalopathy, and nutritional status, as shown in Table 33–3. The sum of these clinical and laboratory parameters, on a scale of 0–15, provides an important overall assessment of the severity of cirrhosis. A total score of less than 6 is considered grade A (well-compensated) disease; 7–9 grade B (sig-

Table 33–3. Modified Child-Pugh classification of the severity of liver disease.[1]

Parameter	Points Assigned		
	1	2	3
Ascites	Absent	Slight	Moderate
Bilirubin (mg/dL)	≤ 2	2–3	> 3
Albumin (g/dL)	> 3.5	2.8–3.5	< 2.8
Prothrombin time (seconds over control)	1–3	4–6	> 6
Encephalopathy	None	Grade 1–2	Grade 3–4

[1]Total score of 1–6, grade A; 7–9, grade B; 10–15, grade C.

nificant functional compromise) disease; and 10–15 grade C (decompensated) disease, which has the highest risk for subsequent complications. The ease and prognostic utility of this scoring system provide important advantages for routine assessment of most patients with cirrhosis. Separate disease-specific measures may be more reliable in primary biliary cirrhosis, where alkaline phosphatase and bilirubin are specifically influenced by the illness. Recently the Model for End-Stage Liver Disease (MELD) score has been proposed as an alternative to the Child-Pugh score. The score consists of serum bilirubin and creatinine levels, international normalized ratio for prothrombin time, and etiology of liver disease. Efforts are underway to use the MELD score to determine organ allocation rather than the Child-Pugh score (see Chapter 54).

CLINICAL PRESENTATIONS OF LIVER INJURY

The following sections delineate several of the more common clinical presentations that account for most consultations to liver specialists. Because the hepatic response to diverse injuries may be similar, emphasis is placed on pattern recognition and categorization into basic pathophysiologic syndromes. It is important to emphasize that this is not an end unto itself but is useful as a guide to management and provides a framework for the efficient evaluation of the underlying cause of liver damage. Specific etiologic diagnoses, as described in subsequent chapters, are always preferred, since they allow better definition of the natural history and potential complications.

Isolated Aminotransferase Elevation in the Asymptomatic Patient

A. CLINICAL PRESENTATION

Most patients with liver disease are asymptomatic during much of the course of the disease due to the large reserve capacity of the organ. They come to medical attention only when abnormal blood tests suggest underlying liver damage, usually in the form of modest AST or ALT elevations (or both). Unfortunately, lack of symptoms is no assurance of a benign cause, since chronic active hepatitis, cirrhosis, and other threatening disorders are not distinguished from transient and clinically insignificant processes without further assessment. A systematic evaluation such as the one shown in Figure 33–2 is warranted, to identify patients with significant disease and initiate treatment to prevent progression to cirrhosis.

B. PATHOPHYSIOLOGIC FINDINGS

AST and ALT are widely used as screening tests because they provide a sensitive index of active liver inflammation. In the absence of symptoms, values are usually less than 400 IU/L; higher values more often reflect an acute process such as viral or ischemic hepatitis with accompanying clinical manifestations. The increase in aminotransferases alone provides little insight into the underlying cause; and the degree of transaminase elevation has only a weak correlation with the degree of inflammation as assessed histologically. Consequently, even modest transaminase elevations should not be dismissed without further consideration.

It is helpful to consider some of the more common causes of increased aminotransferase elevation in asymptomatic populations as a guide to designing an appropriate evaluation. Alcohol overuse, fatty liver, chronic viral and autoimmune hepatitis, and drug toxicity account for two-thirds of cases. Unsuspected cirrhosis, liver tumors, and genetic diseases such as hemochromatosis are less common.

C. DIAGNOSTIC EVALUATION

Evaluation of increased aminotransferase values is challenging for both the patient and the physician. Although many of the causes are benign and self-limited, the recognition that a potentially serious disease could be present necessitates a systematic approach in order to identify the underlying cause and establish the severity. The approach summarized in Figure 33–2 is predicated upon the lack of symptoms and no evidence for cholestasis; coexisting increases in alkaline phosphatase and bilirubin levels mandate concomitant evaluation for ductular diseases (eg, primary biliary cirrhosis), cirrhosis, and bile duct obstruction.

1. Initial evaluation—The initial evaluation of these patients begins with a careful history to identify risk factors and a physical examination to identify features of unrecognized chronic liver disease. Use of alcohol or potential hepatotoxic medications should be prohibited, and in the absence of symptoms, there is usually a window of opportunity for observation to determine whether test abnormalities will improve without further intervention. More commonly, persistent or intermittent elevations require more focused testing. Initially, this should include testing for viral hepatitis, with emphasis on hepatitis B surface antigen and hepatitis C viral antibodies to identify those at risk for chronic viral disease (see Chapter 36). Positive tests for autoimmune markers, including antinuclear antibodies, might suggest an autoimmune basis for the disease. The evaluation of persistent aminotransferase elevations in the setting of positive viral or autoimmune markers usually requires a liver biopsy for confirmation of the diagnosis, assessment of disease activity, and guidance of therapy.

2. Fatty liver—If viral and autoimmune markers are unrevealing, the possibility of fatty liver, which is found in up to 20–60% of these patients, should be considered.

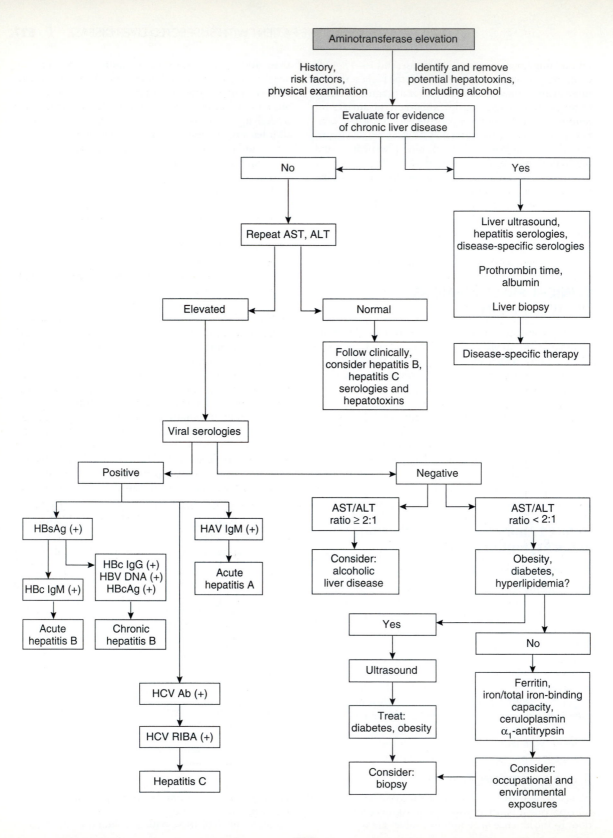

Obesity, hyperlipidemia, and glucose intolerance represent important risk factors for fatty liver, which is characterized histologically by accumulation of lipids inside hepatocytes. The clinical course of fatty liver is usually benign. Because the abnormalities reflect a systemic metabolic abnormality, treatment is aimed at correction of the underlying risk factors. Even when fatty liver is suspected on clinical grounds, an ultrasound examination is warranted to address the possibility of an unsuspected mass lesion. In more severe cases, ultrasound may reveal a diffuse increase in echogenicity because of increased fat accumulation. A more worrisome entity referred to as nonalcoholic steatohepatitis occurs with greater frequency in overweight women and can mimic simple fatty liver or autoimmune liver disease (see Chapter 45). Unlike fatty liver, nonalcoholic steatohepatitis can progress to hepatic fibrosis and cirrhosis. Consequently, if there is uncertainty about the diagnosis, or if the test abnormalities do not respond to treatment of the underlying risk factors, a liver biopsy is warranted.

3. Drug-induced liver disease—A common clinical quandary is that many of the drugs used to treat hyperlipidemia or hyperglycemia can themselves cause elevation of aminotransferases. Although this is limited to less than 5% of patients, drug-induced liver disease can have serious sequelae. As a general rule, the benefits of these medications in controlling the risk factors outweigh their potential for liver toxicity. Careful surveillance for an increase in AST or ALT is warranted. Control of risk factors through diet and exercise is important but not always successful.

4. Other diseases—In patients without a clear working diagnosis, or in whom a conservative course of observation and risk-factor reduction fails, additional studies should be performed. These include ultrasound examination of the liver to minimize the possibility of an unsuspected anatomic abnormality or mass lesion, and screening for genetic diseases, including hemochromatosis, Wilson's disease, and α_1-antitrypsin deficiency. Suspicion of these disorders usually requires liver biopsy for definitive diagnosis.

Jaundice & Cholestasis

A. CLINICAL PRESENTATION

Cholestasis is detected clinically by the onset of jaundice and an increase in serum bilirubin concentrations.

Due to the central role of the liver in bilirubin metabolism, the onset of jaundice localizes the abnormality to the hepatobiliary system in most patients. An efficient diagnostic approach helps to minimize unnecessary tests in those with benign causes, focuses the work-up in those with extrahepatic causes, and provides a clear therapeutic rationale for those with significant underlying pathologic changes.

When cholestasis develops acutely, impaired bile flow is often associated with jaundice, pruritis, and anorexia. Nausea and vomiting are nonspecific but frequently present. With sustained cholestasis, the decrease in bile flow has more far-reaching metabolic effects. Weight loss and fat malabsorption are related to impaired intestinal micelle formation, coagulopathy and bleeding to impaired absorption of dietary vitamin K, and osteomalacia to malabsorption and impaired metabolism of vitamin D.

A central focus of the diagnostic evaluation is to determine whether jaundice results from "medical" causes, including increased bilirubin load and intrahepatic cholestasis, or from "surgical" causes, such as obstruction of the bile ducts. Clinical judgment based on a careful history, physical examination, and routine laboratory studies is a powerful tool in differentiating between intrahepatic and extrahepatic jaundice. Clinical judgment is more sensitive but less specific than duct visualization by ultrasonography. Clinical features that suggest extrahepatic obstruction include fever, leukocytosis, right upper quadrant pain, elevated alkaline phosphatase values, or previous biliary surgery; features that suggest intrahepatic cholestasis include a history of chronic hepatitis, cirrhosis, portal hypertension, or exposure to hepatocellular toxins.

B. PATHOPHYSIOLOGIC FINDINGS

Cholestasis in the strictest sense refers to impaired bile formation. Although this is usually associated with a rise in bilirubin, it is important to emphasize that the formation of bile does not depend upon bilirubin but is driven by the transport of other organic and inorganic solutes, including bile salts, glutathione, and HCO_3^-. The increase in bilirubin itself is not harmful, but in the presence of cholestasis, it is a marker for underlying changes in bile flow. Indeed, parallel increases in the serum concentrations of bile salts and other solutes may contribute more importantly to the clinical symptoms of cholestasis.

Figure 33–2. An approach to the patient with elevated aminotransferases (see text for details). HBsAg, hepatitis B surface antigen; HBc, hepatitis B core; IgM, IgG, immunoglobulin M, G; HBcAg, hepatitis B core antigen; HCV Ab, hepatitis C virus antibody; RIBA, recombinant immunoblot assay; HAV, hepatitis A virus.

Figure 33–1 shows an outline of bilirubin production, metabolism, and secretion. A working knowledge of these pathways provides an important framework for clinical evaluation, since disorders at any of these steps can lead to an increase in bilirubin concentrations. Unconjugated (indirect) hyperbilirubinemia suggests increased bilirubin production or defective conjugation, whereas conjugated (direct) hyperbilirubinemia suggests impaired secretion or obstruction. Because secretion of conjugated bilirubin across the canalicular membrane is rate limiting, most patients with hepatitis or cirrhosis have an increase in conjugated bilirubin levels.

C. DIAGNOSTIC EVALUATION

Evaluation of jaundice or hyperbilirubinemia begins with a careful history to determine whether risk factors of liver disease are present, a review of routine liver function tests, and a physical examination focusing on liver size, tenderness, and evidence of chronic liver disease. In addition, conjugated and unconjugated bilirubin fractions should be measured. One algorithm for evaluation of jaundice is shown in Figure 33–3.

1. Intravascular hemolysis and Gilbert syndrome—
In the absence of other liver function test abnormalities, the differential diagnosis of unconjugated hyperbilirubinemia centers either on increased bilirubin production resulting from intravascular hemolysis or impaired conjugation as in Gilbert syndrome. A large number of other possibilities exist but are rarely encountered clinically. As a general rule, hemolysis sufficient to elevate serum bilirubin levels is not subtle and is readily detected by routine studies. Note that AST but not ALT can be released from damaged red blood cells, and that a large hematoma can have similar effects on bilirubin production. In the absence of hemolysis, Gilbert syndrome is suggested when peak bilirubin values are less than 3–5 mg/dL, an appreciable portion is unconjugated, and other liver function tests are normal. Gilbert syndrome is not a disease but a genetic variant characterized by diminished bilirubin UDPglucuronyltransferase, the enzyme that catalyzes the conjugation of bilirubin to glucuronide. This benign variant is important to keep in mind because it is common, occurring in 4–7% of the population, and does not have known clinical sequelae. Consequently, recognition of Gilbert syndrome may limit unnecessary testing and concern in the future. Typically, episodes of jaundice are mild and occur intermittently. An increase in serum bilirubin levels is brought out by fasting, exercise, or stress. Values usually return to normal with resumption of normal activities. If the diagnosis is in doubt, patients should be subjected to supervised fasting for 1–2 days to determine if there is an increase in unconjugated bilirubin concentrations. Assurance and counseling about the benign course and familial basis for the disease are the only treatments needed.

2. Conjugated hyperbilirubinemia—Conjugated hyperbilirubinemia with otherwise normal liver tests is relatively uncommon. Attention to medication exposure, including antibiotics, sulfa derivatives, and azathioprine, may suggest drug-induced cholestasis. Potential offending agents should be discontinued and tests followed over time to ensure resolution. Occasionally, conjugated hyperbilirubinemia is the only manifestation of well-compensated cirrhosis; the normal aminotransferase and alkaline phosphatase values indicate the lack of clinically active hepatocellular necrosis and duct obstruction, respectively. Sustained hyperbilirubinemia following acute hepatitis or other events may persist for many weeks due to the persistence of protein-bound bilirubin, which forms slowly over time in the setting of prolonged cholestasis. Genetic disorders such as Rotor's disease and Dubin-Johnson syndrome result in conjugated hyperbilirubinemia but are distinctly uncommon.

3. Bile duct obstruction or proliferation—Concomitant elevations of alkaline phosphatase, 5′-nucleotidase, or GGT mandate a careful evaluation of the bile ducts to rule out obstruction or duct proliferation. Chronic cholestasis with elevated alkaline phosphatase values presents indolently with pruritis and malabsorption. Acute presentations with associated pain, fever, and leukocytosis increase the index of suspicion for cholangitis. Common duct stones with or without cholecystitis are encountered frequently. Increases in bilirubin levels above 5 mg/dL are uncommon in uncomplicated stone disease, and suggest a more complete obstruction resulting from duct strictures or cancer. Again, direct visualization of the ducts is required, along with consideration of chronic duct-oriented diseases such as primary biliary cirrhosis and sclerosing cholangitis.

Ultrasonography is the preferred initial screening test for duct obstruction, and offers the advantages of relatively low cost, high sensitivity for gallstones and duct dilatation, and wide availability. False-negative

---

Figure 33–3. An approach to the patient with hyperbilirubinemia. ERCP, endoscopic retrograde cholangiopancreatography.

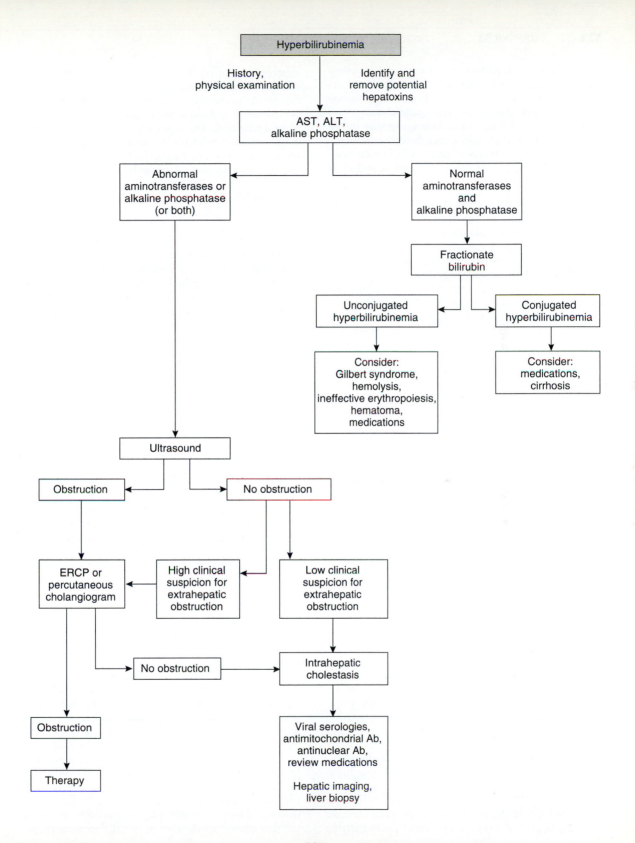

studies can occur in patients with cirrhosis and previous biliary tract surgery. Consequently, if the index of suspicion for an obstructive lesion is high, it is reasonable to proceed with endoscopic retrograde cholangiopancreatography or percutaneous cholangiography for definitive diagnosis. Similarly, direct duct visualization is required for the diagnosis of primary biliary cirrhosis, sclerosing cholangitis, duct strictures, and most duct tumors.

4. Intrahepatic disorders—If jaundice is accompanied by significant elevation of aminotransferases out of proportion to alkaline phosphatase concentrations, the origin is more likely to be intrahepatic. Evaluation focusing on acute or chronic hepatitis, cirrhosis, and primary hepatocellular disorders as described below is indicated. There is obviously overlap between these presentations. When in doubt, visualize the biliary tree. If there is no obstruction, consider a liver biopsy for definitive diagnosis of the underlying disease process.

Chronic Hepatocellular Injury & Cirrhosis

A. CLINICAL PRESENTATION

Chronic hepatocellular injury is suspected when there are clinical or laboratory findings suggesting poorly compensated liver function. These may be subtle, such as sustained fatigue or decreased albumin concentrations, or life threatening, such as variceal hemorrhage or prolongation of the prothrombin time. Evidence of decompensation imparts a sense of urgency because of the potential benefits of treatment and the poor prognosis of established cirrhosis. Consequently, efforts to treat the manifestations of liver injury and establish the diagnosis should proceed in parallel (eg, treatment of ascites should not await an etiologic diagnosis). This is particularly true as no definitive cause can be ascertained in more than 30% of cirrhotic patients.

Clinical symptoms related to loss of hepatocyte mass are nonspecific outside of the setting of fulminant liver failure (see Chapter 43). Fatigue, weight loss, poor memory, and inability to concentrate are common. Menstrual irregularities or a decrease in libido also develop relatively early; direct questioning may be required to elicit the history. Hepatic origin of the symptoms is suspected when there are suggestive physical features such as jaundice, gynecomastia, or cutaneous angiomas or associated liver test abnormalities.

Development of portal hypertension contributes importantly to the clinical manifestations of chronic hepatocellular injury (see Chapter 43). The increase in portal pressure leads directly to engorged varices or hemorrhoids, and the probability of bleeding increases with the degree of pressure elevation. Accompanying abnormalities of renal function lead to Na^+ and water retention and, if uncorrected, to ascites and edema. Although the pathophysiologic basis is complex, defective Na^+ secretion is thought to initiate the cascade leading to fluid retention. The hepatorenal syndrome marks the most extreme manifestation and is characterized by severe Na^+ retention (urine Na^+ concentrations <10 meq/L), oliguria, and a decrease in creatinine clearance. This is reversible with correction of liver function, but untreated disease can result in uremia.

Hepatic encephalopathy deserves special emphasis as a clinical manifestation of chronic liver injury because it is often unrecognized in the early stages, when it responds best to therapy. Indeed, most patients with cirrhosis will have subtle impairment of fine motor skills and memory that can be improved with moderate protein restriction, lactulose intake, and a decrease in portal pressures. Attention to subtle symptoms, measurement of serum ammonia levels, and cognitive testing are helpful when the diagnosis is suspected. More often, a therapeutic trial will be instrumental in establishing the diagnosis. Usually, overt encephalopathy with asterixis, mental confusion, and disturbed sleep patterns is readily detectable.

B. PATHOPHYSIOLOGIC FINDINGS

The pathophysiologic processes that result in the clinical manifestations of chronic liver injury are directly related to loss of liver cell mass or development of portal hypertension (or both), as described above. Clinically, it is important to establish a time course or rate of change of symptoms as an aid to understanding the pathophysiologic changes. Chronic liver injury due to viral hepatitis, autoimmune diseases, and sometimes alcohol abuse is most often indolent, with a clinical course developing over many months or years. More acute presentations suggest either acute injury (ie, toxic, infectious, or vascular cause) or decompensation of previously unrecognized chronic disease. The latter is surprisingly common.

Chronic liver injury also predisposes patients to predictable complications that can cause rapid clinical deterioration. Portal vein thrombosis deserves special mention as an important but underrecognized complication of chronic liver disease. Liver function depends upon portal flow for maintaining the cellular supply of nutrients and oxygen, so even small decreases in portal flow can result in significant functional deterioration, particularly when there is preexisting hepatocellular disease. Portal vein thrombosis can occur in the absence of preexisting liver disease (eg, as a manifestation of hypercoagulability or portal bacteremia), but it is more often observed as a complication of chronic liver disease and cirrhosis. Doppler sonography is a reliable screening test that allows visualization of portal flow to assess patients at risk. The relative risk for hepatocellular carcinoma is markedly increased in the setting of preexisting cirrhosis, particularly if cirrhosis is related to chronic hepatitis B or C infection or hemochromatosis. Again, an ultrasound study of the liver is a reasonable screening test for identification of a liver mass. The utility of α-fetoprotein for screening and early diagnosis in high-risk patients has not been firmly established, but its use is widespread (see Chapter 46). Finally, an increased rate of infection is associated with cirrhosis and portal hypertension. This is due in part to increased seeding of the portal vein with enteric pathogens, and in part to defective clearance of circulating microorganisms by the reticuloendothelial system. Attention to these complications of chronic liver disease may account for unexplained deterioration in liver function or worsening of ascites and encephalopathy.

C. DIAGNOSTIC EVALUATION

When chronic liver disease or cirrhosis is suspected on clinical grounds, the first goals are to establish the degree of functional impairment and look for reversible causes of deterioration. The history focuses on assessment of risk factors (see Table 33–1) and the physical examination on detection of portal hypertension, encephalopathy, liver size, and cutaneous manifestations of cirrhosis. The clinical findings are used in association with laboratory studies to calculate a Child-Pugh score,

which should be followed routinely to assess changes in functional hepatic reserve (see Table 33–3).

Laboratory studies also provide some insight into the causes of liver damage by suggesting whether the underlying pathologic basis is primarily obstructive ductular disease or hepatocellular damage (Figure 33–4). Patients with alkaline phosphatase or bilirubin levels elevated out of proportion to aminotransferase levels are more likely to have duct-centered pathologic causes such as sclerosing cholangitis, primary biliary cirrhosis, infiltrative liver diseases, or biliary obstruction. Accordingly, an evaluation focusing on imaging of the biliary system and screening for antimitochondrial antibodies is appropriate. Patients with sustained aminotransferase elevation usually have ongoing cell necrosis such as that caused by toxic injury (due to alcohol, medications, or occupational exposures), chronic viral hepatitis, or autoimmune hepatitis. An evaluation focusing on viral and autoimmune markers, alcoholism, and medications is appropriate. In each case, the laboratory findings are rarely definitive, so liver biopsy is required for staging and diagnosis.

Although such an approach is orderly and logical, most findings are nonspecific. Consequently, the authors' impressions are that every patient with chronic or poorly compensated liver disease suspected of having underlying cirrhosis should undergo a detailed evaluation, which includes abdominal ultrasound examina-

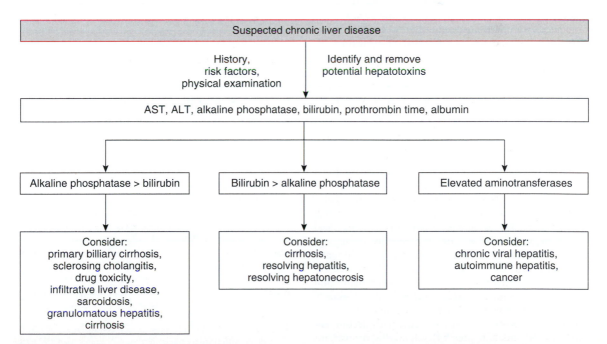

Figure 33–4. An approach to the patient with chronic hepatocellular injury or suspected cirrhosis.

tion with Doppler flow studies, screening tests for chronic hepatitis, and definitive assessment of ductular anatomy. This approach is based on the premise that early investigation offers the best chance of definitive diagnosis and correction, but it may or may not be cost effective.

Ultrasound study is readily justified, as it is noninvasive, widely available, and provides information about the liver parenchyma, biliary tree, and vasculature. Findings suggestive of cirrhosis, including a diffuse increase in echogenicity and a nodular contour, provide presumptive evidence of chronic disease with established fibrosis. More importantly, findings of duct dilatation, gallstones, mass lesions, or portal vein thrombosis rapidly alter the diagnostic and therapeutic approaches.

Screening for unsuspected hepatitis B and C is also justified because of the prevalence of these viruses and the potential for treatment with α-interferon. Because serologic testing for hepatitis B surface antigen and hepatitis C antibodies is relatively inexpensive, even patients with alternative diagnoses such as alcoholic liver disease or primary biliary cirrhosis should be tested. Moreover, identification of unsuspected viral hepatitis has important long-term ramifications, including a risk for viral transmission and effects of immunosuppressive drugs if liver transplantation is considered.

Guidelines for appropriate screening for genetic diseases in patients with established liver disease are not clear. Liver disease related to Wilson's disease and α_1-antitrypsin deficiency has an earlier age of onset, whereas that related to hemochromatosis typically appears later and affects men more than women. Be pragmatic. Because patients at this stage of evaluation already have active liver disease, they represent a high-risk group. In the absence of another clear cause, ferritin, ceruloplasmin, and α_1-antitrypsin levels are obtained, as these tests are relatively inexpensive and positive results have clear implications for treatment and family counseling. Among these, serum ferritin levels are particularly important due to the higher prevalence of hemochromatosis and the beneficial effects of phlebotomy. Suggestive or equivocal results are evaluated by liver biopsy for definitive diagnosis.

Two final caveats in the evaluation of chronic hepatocellular injury merit emphasis. First, always have a high index of suspicion for biliary obstruction, as it may lead to cirrhosis, and endoscopic or percutaneous cholangiography allows definitive diagnosis and treatment in many situations. If the sonogram is unrevealing but other features suggest obstruction, proceed to direct visualization of ductular anatomy with a cholangiogram. Second, rapid advances in liver transplantation have made this the treatment of choice for many patients with decompensated cirrhosis (see Chapter 54). Operating on patients with minimal functional reserve and multiple medical complications leads to higher costs and poorer outcomes. Because the timing of transplantation is so important, early referral to a transplant center is warranted for appropriate candidates.

REFERENCES

EPIDEMIOLOGY

Dufour MC: Chronic liver disease and cirrhosis. In: *Digestive Diseases in the United States: Epidemiology and Impact.* Everhart JE (editor). US Department of Health and Human Services, Public Health Service, National Institutes of Health, National Institute of Diabetes and Digestive and Kidney Diseases, Washington, DC. US Government Printing Office, 1994. NIH Publication no. 94-1447.

PHYSICAL EXAMINATION

Naylor CD: Physical examination of the liver. JAMA 1994;271: 1859.

HEPATOCELLULAR INJURY

Cohen JA, Kaplan MM: The SGOT/SGPT ratio: an indicator of alcoholic liver disease. Dig Dis Sci 1979;24:835.

Goddard CJR, Warnes TW: Raised liver enzymes in asymptomatic patients: investigation and outcome. Dig Dis Sci 1992;10: 218.

Katkov WN et al: Elevated serum alanine aminotransferase levels in blood donors: the contribution of hepatitis C virus. Ann Intern Med 1991;115:882.

Reichling JJ, Kaplan MM: Clinical use of serum enzymes in liver disease. Dig Dis Sci 1988;33:1601.

Sherman KE: Alanine aminotransferase in clinical practice. Arch Intern Med 1991;151:260.

Simko V: Alkaline phosphatase in biology and medicine. Dig Dis Sci 1991;9:189.

HYPERBILIRUBINEMIA & JAUNDICE

Anciaux ML et al: Prospective study of clinical and biochemical features of symptomatic choledocholithiasis. Dig Dis Sci 1986;31:449.

Borsch G et al: Clinical evaluation, ultrasound, cholescintigraphy, and endoscopic retrograde cholangiography in cholestasis: a prospective comparative clinical study. J Clin Gastroenterol 1988;10:185.

Frank BB: Clinical evaluation of jaundice: a guideline of the patient care committee of the American Gastroenterological Association. JAMA 1989;262:3031.

Matzen P et al: Ultrasonography, computed tomography, and cholescintigraphy in suspected obstructive jaundice: a prospective comparative study. Gastroenterology 1983;64:1492.

Richter JM, Silverstein MD, Schapiro R: Suspected obstructive jaundice: a decision analysis of diagnostic strategies. Ann Intern Med 1983;99:46.

Sherlock S, Scheuer PJ: The presentation and diagnosis of 100 patients with primary biliary cirrhosis. N Engl J Med 1973;289: 674.

CHRONIC LIVER DISEASE

Child CG, Turcotte JG: Surgery in portal hypertension. In: *Major Problems in Clinical Surgery: The Liver and Portal Hypertension.* Child CG (editor). Saunders, 1964.

Kamath PS et al: A model to predict survival in patients with end-stage liver disease. Hepatology 2001;33:464.

Pugh RNH et al: Transection of the oesophagus for bleeding oesophageal varices. Br J Surg 1973;60: 646.

Saunders JB et al: A 20-year prospective study of cirrhosis. Br Med J 1981;282:263.

Van Ness MM, Diehl A: Is liver biopsy useful in the evaluation of patients with chronically elevated liver enzymes? Ann Intern Med 1989;111:473.

Acute Liver Failure

Emmet B. Keeffe, MD

ESSENTIALS OF DIAGNOSIS

- An acute liver disease that evolves rapidly and is complicated by coagulopathy and hepatic encephalopathy.
- Most common underlying causes include drug-induced liver injury, particularly acetaminophen-related, and acute viral hepatitis.
- Nonspecific symptoms are followed rapidly by jaundice and altered mental status, with or without coma.
- Laboratory findings include markedly elevated serum aminotransferases, hyperbilirubinemia, hypoprothrombinemia, and, in advanced cases, hypoglycemia and metabolic acidosis.

General Considerations

Acute liver failure is an uncommon but catastrophic illness resulting from sudden marked impairment of liver cell function. In most cases, acute liver failure evolves from a severe, rapidly progressive course of an acute liver disease such as drug-induced or viral hepatitis. In a few cases, acute liver failure is the first manifestation of an underlying chronic liver disease, eg, Wilson's disease, autoimmune hepatitis, or reactivation of chronic hepatitis B. Multiorgan failure often accompanies acute liver failure, and the mortality rate with supportive care only ranges from 50% to 90%.

A. TERMINOLOGY

Acute liver failure is a term reserved for the presence of acute liver disease associated with significant coagulopathy, which has been arbitrarily defined by a prothrombin time or factor V level of less than 50% of normal (Table 34–1). The term **fulminant hepatic failure** was introduced by Trey and Davidson in 1970 to designate acute liver failure associated with hepatic encephalopathy developing within 8 weeks of the onset of illness. The term is now widely used, although changes in the time interval between the onset of symptoms and encephalopathy have been proposed. In addition, some investigators use the time interval between the onset of jaundice, rather than symptoms, and the development of hepatic encephalopathy to define acute liver failure. Alternative terminology has been introduced to characterize a group of patients with a more delayed onset of encephalopathy.

Bernuau and colleagues at the Hôpital Beaujon base their classification of acute liver failure on the interval between the first detection of jaundice and the appearance of encephalopathy (Table 34–1). They define fulminant hepatic failure as the development of hepatic encephalopathy within 2 weeks of the onset of jaundice. The term **subfulminant hepatic failure** is used to designate another subgroup of disorders causing acute liver failure characterized by the development of encephalopathy 2 weeks to 3 months after the appearance of jaundice. By contrast, Gimson and colleagues at King's College Hospital in London define fulminant hepatic failure as originally proposed by Trey and Davidson. They use the term late-onset hepatic failure as synonymous with subfulminant hepatic failure, but the interval between the onset of illness and encephalopathy is defined as 8 weeks to 6 months.

O'Grady and colleagues, also from King's College Hospital, proposed a new terminology based on the interval between the onset of jaundice and subsequent encephalopathy: (1) hyperacute liver failure, with an interval of less than 7 days; (2) acute liver failure, with an interval of between 8 and 28 days; and (3) subacute liver failure, with an interval of between 5 and 12 weeks. The classifications of Bernuau and colleagues and O'Grady and associates allow the inclusion of patients with chronic liver disease who have previously been asymptomatic and then exacerbate under the designation of acute liver failure.

The distinction between fulminant (hyperacute or acute) and subfulminant (late-onset or subacute) hepatic failure is important clinically, because patients with the shortest interval between jaundice and the onset of encephalopathy have the best prognosis. Moreover, the causes of acute liver failure are usually different in patients experiencing fulminant and subfulminant hepatic failure. The management of patients with acute liver failure must be individualized according to the pace and tempo of the illness, which can often be predicted by the cause of liver failure. The overall goal of treatment is to

Table 34–1. Definitions of acute liver failure.

Acute liver failure	Acute liver disease, with prothrombin time or factor V less than 50% of normal
Fulminant hepatic failure	Acute liver failure with hepatic encephalopathy, developing less than 2 weeks[1] (or 8 weeks[2]) after onset of jaundice[1] (or illness[2])
Subfulminant hepatic failure[3]	Acute liver failure with hepatic encephalopathy, developing from 2 weeks[1] (or 8 weeks[2]) to 3 months[1] (or 6 months[2]) after onset of jaundice[1] (or illness[2])

[1]Criteria from Bernuau J, Rueff B, Benhamou J-P: Fulminant and subfulminant liver failure: definitions and causes. Semin Liv Dis 1986;6:97.
[2]Criteria from Trey C, Davidson LS: The management of fulminant hepatic failure. In: *Progress in Liver Diseases*, Vol 3. Popper H, Schaffner F (editors). Grune & Stratton, 1970; and Gimson AES et al: Clinical and prognostic differences in fulminant hepatitis type A, B, and non-A, non-B. Gut 1983;24:1194.
[3]Also called late-onset hepatic failure.

provide supportive care and buy time to allow hepatic regeneration, while at the same time assessing for prognostic indices that suggest a poor outcome and the need to proceed rapidly to liver transplantation.

As noted above, a small subset of patients with acute liver failure will, in reality, have a previously unrecognized chronic liver disease. For example, Wilson's disease may initially present with the symptoms and signs of acute hepatitis or, if severe, acute liver failure, usually subfulminant hepatic failure. Wilson's disease, however, more commonly presents as a chronic illness with a clinical picture of chronic hepatitis or cirrhosis. Another example of a chronic liver disease that may present acutely is autoimmune hepatitis, which occasionally is first recognized in a rapidly progressive form that meets the criteria of acute liver failure.

The true incidence of acute liver failure is unknown, but approximately 2000 individuals are affected annually in the United States. Because it is an uncommon condition, patients tend to be referred to tertiary centers that are able to provide aggressive supportive intensive care and liver transplantation, which is performed in 200–300 patients with acute liver failure per year in the United States. Thus, referral bias certainly influences the published information regarding the causes and outcome of acute liver failure.

B. ETIOLOGY

The causes of acute liver failure are diverse, but drug-induced liver injury and viral hepatitis account for 80–85% of all cases for which a cause can be determined (Table 34–2). Toxins, metabolic diseases, vascular events, and a few miscellaneous conditions explain the remaining causes. The distribution of causes varies in different geographic regions. In the United States and Europe, drug-induced liver injury, particularly acetaminophen related, is the dominant cause, while acute viral hepatitis is the most common etiology in developing countries. In a a large series from King's College Hospital, 431 of 763 patients (56%) had acetaminophen overdose as the cause of fulminant hepatic failure. A recent study showed that 38% of acute liver failure in the United States is acetaminophen related. There also is emerging evidence that the use of excessive therapeutic doses of acetaminophen by heavy drinkers of alcohol accounts for an increasing percentage of acute liver failure in the United States, with one center reporting that two-thirds of cases could be explained by this combination of events.

Acute viral hepatitis is a common cause of acute liver failure. Most cases of fulminant hepatic failure secondary to hepatitis A and hepatitis B follow the hyperacute course (ie, encephalopathy within 1 week of jaundice). In the large referral experience with this disorder

Table 34–2. Known causes of acute liver failure.

Viral hepatitis
Hepatitis A, B, C, D, and E viruses
Hepatitis due to other viruses
Herpesviruses 1, 2, and 6
Adenovirus
Epstein–Barr virus
Cytomegalovirus
Drug-induced liver injury
Acetaminophen overdose
Idiosyncratic drug reaction
Toxins
Amanita phalloides
Organic solvents
Phosphorus
Metabolic disorders
Acute fatty liver of pregnancy
Reye's syndrome
Vascular events
Acute circulatory failure
Budd-Chiari syndrome
Venoocclusive disease
Heat stroke
Miscellaneous disorders
Wilson's disease
Autoimmune hepatitis
Massive infiltration with tumor
Liver transplantation with primary graft nonfunction

at Hôpital Beaujon, 72% of 330 cases in adults could be attributed to viral hepatitis. All five hepatotropic viruses have been implicated as a cause of acute liver failure, although the contribution of hepatitis C virus is doubtful. According to compilations of the causes of acute liver failure at referral centers, non-A, non-B hepatitis, a designation based on the exclusion of hepatitis A, hepatitis B, and other causes of acute liver failure and presumed to represent an unidentified specific viral agent, was typically the most common etiology, followed by hepatitis B and then hepatitis A. The currently preferred terminology for a patient with an unknown cause of acute liver failure is "cryptogenic" rather than "non-A, non-B." Finally, one must keep in mind that viral hepatitis is complicated by the development of acute liver failure in less than 1% of cases.

Hepatitis A virus is only rarely complicated by the development of fulminant hepatic failure (0.1–0.5% of cases). In addition, patients who experience fulminant hepatitis A have a relatively good prognosis, with a survival rate of 50–60% and a less frequent need for liver transplantation. Fulminant hepatitis A is common in intravenous drug users, and is more severe in older patients and individuals with preexisting chronic liver disease, including chronic hepatitis C.

Hepatitis B virus is the most common known viral cause of fulminant hepatic failure, and is the most prevalent cause in many southern European countries, France, and the Far East. Most patients who experience fulminant hepatitis B are young adults. Immunosuppressed patients who are acutely infected with hepatitis B virus are less likely to experience fulminant hepatic failure. Massive hepatic necrosis with fulminant hepatic failure has also been reported in asymptomatic chronic hepatitis B surface antigen (HBsAg) carriers after withdrawal of immunosuppressive or chemotherapeutic drugs. Patients with acute liver failure secondary to acute hepatitis B may have rapid clearance of hepatitis B virus in one-third to one-half of cases, most likely related to a major immunologic attack on infected hepatocytes; these individuals will not have detectable HBsAg several days after the onset of illness. For this reason, occult hepatitis B virus infection may explain some cases of fulminant hepatic failure classified in the past as non-A, non-B hepatitis. This hypothesis is supported by the finding of serum or hepatic (or both) hepatitis B virus DNA in some patients undergoing liver transplantation for cryptogenic acute liver failure. Mutants of hepatitis B virus, as well as the more common wild type of this virus, have been shown to cause fulminant hepatic failure. The most common hepatitis B virus mutant has a stop codon inserted in the precore region of the C gene, such that hepatitis B e antigen is not released from hepatocytes.

Hepatitis D virus is also associated with the development of acute liver failure, particularly in intravenous drug users, who are often infected with this virus. Markers of delta hepatitis are more prevalent among patients with fulminant hepatitis B than in patients with typical acute hepatitis B. Patients with fulminant hepatic failure may be acutely coinfected with hepatitis B and hepatitis D viruses simultaneously; alternatively, patients with chronic hepatitis B may develop fulminant hepatic failure secondary to later superinfection with hepatitis D virus. Some data suggest that the risk of fulminant hepatic failure is higher in patients coinfected with hepatitis B and hepatitis D viruses than in patients having acute hepatitis B alone.

The recently identified enteric hepatitis E virus often causes infection in the setting of epidemics and is characterized by an unusually high incidence of fulminant hepatic failure in pregnant women, who experience a case fatality rate approaching 40%. Overall, however, fulminant hepatic failure appears to be an infrequent complication of hepatitis E, and hepatitis E virus infection is not commonly found in patients with acute liver failure of indeterminate cause. To date, hepatitis E has only rarely been identified in the United States.

As noted above, the designation non-A, non-B hepatitis had in the past been applied to patients with fulminant hepatic failure and no viral markers or other recognized cause of acute liver failure. This terminology had implied that hepatitis C virus, or some other viral agent, was the likely causative factor. In fact, hepatitis C virus RNA or antibody (or both) to hepatitis C virus has rarely been identified in patients designated as having cryptogenic fulminant hepatic failure. It thus seems unlikely that hepatitis C virus plays an important role in the development of acute liver failure. In cases of fulminant hepatic failure of indeterminate cause, there may be one or more novel viral agents causing this syndrome. In some studies, virus-like particles have been identified in the cytoplasm of infected liver cells in patients with fulminant hepatic failure of uncertain cause. Other cases of cryptogenic fulminant hepatic failure may be explained by occult hepatitis B virus infection, including mutant forms of hepatitis B.

Acute liver failure has rarely been attributed to hepatitis caused by other viruses, including herpes viruses 1, 2, and 6, adenovirus, Epstein–Barr virus, and cytomegalovirus.

Drug-induced liver injury is the most common cause of acute liver failure, accounting for more than 50% of all cases in the United States and United Kingdom. Acute liver failure complicates drug-induced hepatitis (≤20% of cases), which is a relatively more frequent incidence than after acute viral hepatitis (<1% of cases). Drug-induced liver injury occurs most often in individuals older than 40 years of age, and is more common in women. It has classically been divided into two categories: predictable and idiosyncratic. Predictable hepatotoxicity occurs in a dose-dependent fashion, whereas idiosyncratic liver injury occurs in less than 1% of users of an individual drug; the latter is therefore unpredictable, and is unrelated to the administered dose (see Chapter 44).

Acetaminophen hepatotoxicity is an example of dose-dependent, predictable liver injury, but its effect can be exaggerated by drugs, including alcohol, which induce its cytochrome P-450 isoenzyme, or by starvation, which depletes glutathione. Neither acetaminophen nor its major sulfate or glucuronide metabolites are toxic. A small percentage of acetaminophen, however, is metabolized via its P-450 isoenzyme to a reactive metabolite that is conjugated to a nontoxic product by glutathione. Acetaminophen is generally safe within the recommended dosage of 3–4 g/d. Acetaminophen hepatotoxicity uniformly follows a hyperacute course. It may occur as the result of a suicidal overdose following the ingestion of more than 10 g of a drug or by excessive therapeutic doses used by alcoholics who have induced cytochrome P-450 enzymes. From either the ingestion of a large dose of acetaminophen that overwhelms available glutathione, or from the excessive therapeutic use of acetaminophen by alcoholic patients with induced P-450 isoenzymes or reduced glutathione stores, or both, the toxic intermediate of acetaminophen accumulates, binds to liver cytoplasmic proteins, and causes liver cell necrosis. Whereas the fatality rate for untreated acetaminophen overdose approximates 50%, excessive ingestion of acetaminophen by the alcoholic is associated with as much as a 20% fatality rate. Markedly elevated serum aminotransferase levels are a characteristic diagnostic feature of acetaminophen hepatotoxicity, with values typically exceeding 3000–4000 IU/L.

A number of drugs are associated with the rare development of idiosyncratic drug-induced liver injury, which is not uncommonly associated with progression to acute liver failure. In some cases, eosinophilia or the presence of a rash, or both, suggests that hypersensitivity plays a role; however, in most cases, presumed idiosyncratic abnormalities in hepatic drug metabolism are likely the key pathophysiologic factors. Examples of drugs that have been implicated in idiosyncratic drug-induced liver injury resulting in acute liver failure include halothane, isoniazid, disulfiram, valproate, phenytoin, sulfonamides, methyldopa, propylthiouracil, nonsteroidal antiinflammatory drugs, bromfenac, and troglitazone.

A small number of toxins have been associated with the development of acute hepatic failure, which in this setting is frequently accompanied by concomitant renal failure. Organic solvents, including the fluorinated hydrocarbons trichloroethylene and tetrachloroethane,

have been associated with the development of acute liver failure. *Amanita phalloides,* the death cap mushroom, has been associated with the development of acute liver failure in association with renal failure, particularly in central Europe, where mushroom collecting and consumption are common. Liver transplantation has been used to successfully treat a handful of patients fortunate enough to be promptly referred to liver transplant centers.

Metabolic causes of acute liver failure include acute fatty liver of pregnancy and Reye's syndrome. Both of these syndromes are associated with microvascular fatty change rather than the more typical massive hepatic necrosis characteristic of other causes of fulminant hepatic failure. Acute fatty liver of pregnancy usually occurs in the third trimester and is characterized by the rapid onset of jaundice and encephalopathy, frequently accompanied by hypoglycemia. Even though the prothrombin time is markedly prolonged, the serum aminotransferase levels are usually not elevated more than 1000 IU/L. Treatment consists of rapid delivery of the fetus (see Chapter 47).

A number of vascular events have also been associated with the development of acute liver failure (see Table 34–2). Cardiac causes include myocardial infarction or cardiomyopathy associated with acute circulatory failure. In some cases, the underlying cardiac disease is not immediately apparent, and, thus, careful cardiovascular evaluation is appropriate in patients who initially have acute liver failure of uncertain cause. Hepatic venous outflow obstruction secondary to an acute form of Budd-Chiari syndrome or venoocclusive disease has also rarely been associated with acute liver failure. Heat stroke with liver failure has been noted in miners as well as long-distance runners and is typically reversible.

Miscellaneous causes of acute liver failure include the aforementioned Wilson's disease and autoimmune hepatitis. Massive infiltration of the liver with metastatic tumor that spreads in an intrasinusoidal pattern has also rarely been associated with acute liver failure. The onset of fulminant hepatic failure may be the first clinical manifestation of hepatic metastasis, and hepatic imaging with ultrasonography or computed tomography (CT) scanning may show only homogeneous hepatomegaly. Finally, liver transplantation may be complicated by primary graft nonfunction and the rapid onset of acute liver failure, requiring retransplantation in the first few days after orthotopic liver transplantation.

The multiple causes of acute liver failure may follow a course characteristic of fulminant or subfulminant hepatic failure (Table 34–3). In 75% or more of cases, hepatitis A, B, D, and E, *Amanita phalloides* poisoning, acetaminophen overdose, and acute fatty liver of pregnancy are associated with a relatively short interval from

Table 34–3. Course of acute liver failure according to cause.

Predominantly fulminant (hyperacute > acute[1]) hepatic failure
   Hepatitis A, B, D, and E
   Amanita phalloides
   Acetaminophen overdose
   Acute fatty liver of pregnancy
Predominantly subfulminant (or subacute[1]) hepatic failure
   Indeterminate or sporadic
   Drug-induced liver injury
   Budd-Chiari syndrome
   Venoocclusive disease
   Wilson's disease
   Autoimmune hepatitis

---

[1]Acute liver failure terminology (hyperacute vs acute vs subacute) of O'Grady et al: Acute liver failure: redefining the syndromes. Lancet 1993;342:373.

the onset of jaundice to the development of hepatic encephalopathy (ie, fulminant hepatic failure). By contrast, patients with an indeterminate cause of acute liver failure, drug-induced liver injury, hepatic venous outflow obstruction, Wilson's disease, and autoimmune hepatitis more often have a subfulminant course. The other important distinction between fulminant and subfulminant hepatic failure is the better survival rates of patients affected by fulminant as opposed to subfulminant hepatic failure (Table 34–4).

Clinical Findings

The essential clinical findings of acute liver failure include jaundice, hepatic encephalopathy, and coagulopathy. When severe, acute liver failure is also characterized by multiorgan failure, particularly cardiovascular

Table 34–4. Examples of survival rates of fulminant and subfulminant hepatic failure according to cause.[1]

Cause	Survival Rate (%)
Fulminant hepatic failure	
Acute hepatitis A	50–60
Acetaminophen overdose	50–55
Acute hepatitis B	40–50
Subfulminant hepatic failure	
Indeterminate or sporadic	25–30
Drug-induced liver injury	10–25

[1]In the absence of liver transplantation.

and renal changes, multiple metabolic abnormalities, and an increased incidence of infection.

A. SYMPTOMS AND SIGNS

Acute liver failure often begins with nonspecific symptoms such as malaise or nausea, which are rapidly followed by jaundice, and, over a variable period of time, changes in mental status. Hepatic encephalopathy is traditionally divided into four stages based on the mental state and the presence or absence of neurologic signs (Table 34–5). Stage 1 hepatic encephalopathy is characterized by mild confusion and mental slowness, with only subtle neurologic abnormalities. In stage 2, drowsiness is prominent and accompanied by personality changes and inappropriate behavior; asterixis and dysarthria are typically present. In stage 3, the patient sleeps most of the time. Although arousable, the patient is unable to perform mental tasks and is disoriented with respect to time or place. In stage 4, the patient is in coma and may or may not respond to painful stimuli. Hepatic encephalopathy itself is an important predictor of outcome; in patients with stage 4 coma, the survival rate is less than 20%.

On physical examination, characteristic abnormalities include changes in mental status, jaundice, and decreased or absent hepatic dullness on hepatic percussion.

B. LABORATORY FINDINGS

Laboratory findings that support the presence of acute liver failure include markedly elevated serum aminotransferases, hyperbilirubinemia, hypoprothrombinemia, and, when liver failure is particularly severe, hypoglycemia and metabolic acidosis. Other laboratory abnormalities that may be present include hyponatremia and respiratory alkalosis early in the course of illness. The hallmark laboratory abnormality is coagulopathy, which by definition in acute liver failure is associated with a prothrombin time or factor V level of less than 50% of normal.

Differential Diagnosis

The diagnosis of acute liver failure is typically straightforward, but the disease or disorder may be initially mistaken for gram-negative septicemia or a drug overdose. Once coagulopathy and hepatic encephalopathy supervene in the patient with markedly elevated serum aminotransferases, acute liver failure can be diagnosed with confidence.

The most important aspect of diagnosis in the setting of acute liver failure is the determination of the specific cause, since the pace of the illness and prognosis can be estimated based on the underlying condition (see Table 34–4). In addition, the approach to supportive therapy may vary according to the underlying etiologic diagnosis

Table 34–5. Clinical stages of hepatic encephalopathy.

Stage	Mental State	Neurologic Signs
1	Mild confusion, euphoria, or depression; decreased attention; mental slowness; irritability; inverted sleep pattern	Incoordination; slight tremor; poor handwriting
2	Drowsiness; lethargy; deficits in analytic ability; personality changes; inappropriate behavior; intermittent disorientation	Asterixis; ataxia; dysarthria
3	Somnolent but arousable; unable to perform mental tasks; disorientation with respect to time or place; marked confusion; amnesia; fits of rage; incoherent speech	Hyperreflexia; muscle rigidity; fasciculations; Babinski's sign
4	Coma	Oculovestibular responses lost; response to painful stimuli lost; decerebrate posture

(eg, acetylcysteine for acetaminophen overdose), and determination of the cause of liver failure can predict the likelihood that liver transplantation will be needed.

Complications

Life-threatening complications are common in patients with acute liver failure. Meticulous attention to detail in the management and anticipation of possible complications is critical to a successful outcome.

A. GENERAL MEASURES

All patients with acute liver failure should be managed in an intensive care unit to carefully watch for the unpredictable development of multiorgan failure. Because it is often difficult to predict which patients will recover and which will require liver transplantation, patients should be transferred to a hospital with the capability of performing transplantation. Once at a transplant center, the patient is usually evaluated urgently by hepatologists and liver transplant surgeons, with the goal of promptly assessing the patient's suitability for urgent transplantation. Once contraindications to urgent transplantation are excluded (Table 34–6), patients are often placed on the United Network for Organ Sharing (UNOS) transplant waiting list (see also Chapter 54). Intensive neurologic monitoring, usually including the direct measurement of intracerebral pressure and early treatment of cerebral edema, is critical to a successful outcome without permanent neurologic damage. If stage 3 or stage 4 hepatic encephalopathy develops, the patient is intubated for mechanical ventilation and UNOS status is upgraded to the highest priority. Additional monitoring includes the placement of Swan-Ganz and intraarterial catheters, a urinary catheter, and a nasogastric tube, with frequent gastric pH monitoring.

B. HEPATIC ENCEPHALOPATHY AND CEREBRAL EDEMA

Hepatic encephalopathy and cerebral edema, although both having the similar clinical manifestation of changes in mental status, are likely caused by different pathogenic events. Accumulation of toxic substances in the central nervous system, particularly ammonia and endogenous benzodiazepine agonists, is postulated to mediate hepatic encephalopathy. Although hepatic encephalopathy is typically reversible and seldom fatal, cerebral edema is frequently lethal secondary to uncal herniation. In spite of a number of theories to explain

Table 34–6. Contraindications to orthotopic liver transplantation for acute liver failure.[1]

Seropositivity for human immunodeficiency virus
Active alcohol or drug abuse
Advanced cardioplumonary disease
Uncontrolled sepsis
Widespread thrombosis of portal and mesenteric veins
Irreversible brain damage
Sustained elevation of intracerebral pressure to > 50 mm Hg
Cerebral perfusion pressure < 40 mm Hg for > 2 hours
Improving hepatic function

[1]Modified, with permission, from Muñoz SJ: Difficult management problems in fulminant hepatic failure. Semin Liv Dis 1993;13:395
© Thieme Medical Publishers, Inc.

the development of cerebral edema, its precise pathogenesis in acute liver failure remains poorly understood. Swelling of brain cells and disruption of the blood–brain barrier likely play contributory roles, however. Neurologic complications account for approximately 30% of the conditions that preclude liver transplantation (see Table 34–6). The overall prognosis for patients with grade 1 or grade 2 encephalopathy is usually good, although that for grade 3, and particularly grade 4, hepatic encephalopathy is much poorer. Cerebral edema is the leading cause of death in patients with grade 4 encephalopathy and is estimated to occur in approximately three-quarters of patients reaching this stage of cerebral dysfunction. Cerebral ischemia will occur if cerebral perfusion pressure (the difference between mean arterial pressure and intracerebral pressure) is not maintained at above 40 mm Hg.

The treatment of hepatic encephalopathy in the setting of fulminant hepatic failure is challenging. Patients should be placed in the intensive care unit, with the head elevated at 20–30%. Although lactulose is the cornerstone of treatment for chronic hepatic encephalopathy in patients with cirrhosis, it is less effective in patients with fulminant hepatic failure. In general, however, a trial of lactulose either orally (or by nasogastric tube, if necessary) or by rectal enemas is worthwhile. Lactulose is titrated to achieve two to four loose bowel movements daily. The effectiveness of antibiotics, such as neomycin or metronidazole, for hepatic encephalopathy secondary to fulminant hepatic failure is even less certain. Factors known to worsen hepatic encephalopathy such as gastrointestinal bleeding, hypokalemia, or sepsis should be identified and treated.

Cerebral edema is frequently manifested by hypertension, bradycardia, decerebrate rigidity and posturing, abnormal pupillary reflexes, and brainstem respiratory patterns and apnea. These clinical signs may occur late; therefore, the general preference is to monitor intracerebral pressure and institute therapy to maintain a pressure of less than 20 mm Hg at all times. CT scanning of the head is not a reliable way to estimate intracerebral pressure in fulminant hepatic failure, but CT scanning is often used to exclude other intracerebral problems, such as hemorrhage or other structural lesions, before proceeding with orthotopic liver transplantation.

In patients with fulminant hepatic failure, intracranial pressure is usually monitored with either subdural or epidural transducers. The risk of placement of intracerebral pressure transducers is hemorrhage, but the benefit appears to outweigh this risk. Epidural monitors are safer to place than subdural transducers, although their sensitivity may be lower. The goal of intracerebral pressure monitoring is to maintain the pressure at less than 20 mm Hg; a persistent pressure greater than 40 mm Hg

and refractory to treatment precludes orthotopic liver transplantation. In addition, the cerebral perfusion pressure should be maintained above 50 mm Hg.

When cerebral edema develops on the basis of intracerebral pressure recordings or clinical signs, treatment with mannitol at a dosage of 0.5–1 g/kg is given by intravenous infusion over 5 minutes. Repeated doses of mannitol may be required to treat recurrent increases of intracerebral pressure. Mannitol should be given only if serum osmolality is less than 320 mOsm/L. In patients who have renal failure, mannitol can be given only in combination with hemodialysis or continuous arteriovenous hemofiltration. Pentobarbital boluses of 100–150 mg intravenously every 15 minutes for 1 hour followed by a continuous infusion of 1–3 mg/kg/h can be given if mannitol fails to lower the intracerebral pressure.

Other useful therapies for the prevention or management of increases in intracerebral pressure include disturbing the patient as little as possible, controlling agitation, elevating the head 20–30 degrees above the horizontal, providing moderate hyperventilation to a partial carbon dioxide pressure of 25–30 mm Hg, and administering phenytoin therapy for subclinical seizures detectable by electroencephalography.

C. COAGULOPATHY

In acute liver failure, there may be a number of abnormalities of coagulation. Decreased levels of factors II, V, VII, IX, and X account for prolongation of the prothrombin time and partial thromboplastin time. The patient's clinical condition and prognosis are best determined by serial measurements of prothrombin time and factor V levels; thus, infusion of fresh frozen plasma is indicated only for bleeding or at the time of invasive procedures. In fulminant hepatic failure, coagulopathy predisposes patients to bleeding from the gastrointestinal tract, venous access sites, and arterial lines.

Thrombocytopenia is also common in fulminant hepatic failure, with platelet counts frequently less than 100,000/μL. The thrombocytopenia may be related to bone marrow suppression and low-grade disseminated intravascular coagulation. Clinical evidence of bleeding may necessitate the use of platelet transfusions if the platelet count is <50,000/μL.

D. RENAL FAILURE

Renal failure develops in approximately half of patients with fulminant hepatic failure and worsens the prognosis. The renal failure is oliguric and typically functional (ie, the hepatorenal syndrome), but acute tubular necrosis may also be found. Drug-induced nephrotoxicity should also be excluded. Any potentially nephrotoxic agent, such as aminoglycosides or contrast agents, should be avoided. Hypovolemia and hypotension should be corrected with intravenous colloids, such as fresh-frozen plasma or albumin, to achieve adequate cardiac filling pressures. Hemodialysis is frequently necessary for severe metabolic acidosis, hyperkalemia, or fluid overload, although most transplant centers prefer to use continuous arteriovenous hemofiltration. Other electrolyte abnormalities that are common and may require correction include hyponatremia, hypophosphatemia, hypocalcemia, or hypomagnesemia. Hepatorenal syndrome in the setting of fulminant hepatic failure can be reversed by orthotopic liver transplantation, and, thus, the development of renal failure should not exclude proceeding with transplantation.

E. Cardiovascular Abnormalities

Increased cardiac output and low systemic vascular resistance characterize the usual cardiovascular derangements in fulminant hepatic failure. Hypotension with poor organ perfusion may exacerbate hepatic failure, and lactic acidosis resulting from tissue hypoxia may also occur. Adequate replacement of volume to maintain blood pressure and infusion of dopamine may be required. It is important that sepsis be excluded as a potential contributing cause of cardiovascular instability.

F. Hypoglycemia

Hypoglycemia is a common complication of severe fulminant hepatic failure. Hence, blood glucose levels should be monitored at least every 4 hours during all stages of hepatic encephalopathy. The pathophysiology of hypoglycemia is multifactorial, including impaired hepatic glucose release, impaired hepatic gluconeogenesis, and elevated serum insulin levels. All patients with fulminant hepatic failure should receive a continuous intravenous infusion of 10% dextrose. Treatment of hypoglycemia may occasionally require infusion of hypertonic glucose by central venous lines, with a reasonable goal of maintaining blood glucose levels at 60–200 mg/dL. Caloric requirements of 35–50 kcal/kg are required to meet resting metabolic demand.

G. Infection

Patients with fulminant hepatic failure are at increased risk for a number of bacterial and fungal infections. Such infections will compromise a patient's eligibility for liver transplantation; sepsis accounts for approximately 20% of conditions that contraindicate transplantation (see Table 34–6). Bacteremia is a frequent problem because patients are often comatose and have numerous indwelling catheters, which increases the chance for infection. A number of recent prospective studies have shown that 80% or more of patients with fulminant hepatic failure have infection based on clinical assessment or culturing, with the respiratory and urinary tracts being the primary sites involved. The predominant infectious organisms are gram-positive strep-

tococci, *Staphylococcus aureus,* and gram-negative organisms. As many as one-third of patients with fulminant hepatic failure develop fungal infections, primarily *Candida albicans.* These patients often have coexistent renal failure and have received antibiotics. Regular surveillance cultures and aggressive treatment of presumed or documented infection are critical to management. An alternative approach is prophylactic, empiric antibiotic therapy, including parenteral, broad-spectrum antibiotics combined with enteral amphotericin B and clotrimazole, which may reduce the incidence of infection to 20%. Prophylactic antifungal agents are more commonly used for patients with advanced hepatic encephalopathy, because of the relatively high incidence and level of morbidity of fungal infection.

Treatment

A number of proposed treatments, including corticosteroids, insulin, glucagon, and prostaglandin analogs, have no benefit in patients with fulminant hepatic failure. In particular, several controlled trials have failed to confirm any favorable effect from the use of corticosteroids. Historically, a number of aggressive therapies, such as repeated exchange transfusions, plasmapheresis, total body washout, and hemoperfusion through isolated primate livers, have either shown no benefit or been associated with a worse outcome. Charcoal hemoperfusion initially demonstrated promise in an uncontrolled trial, but a subsequent controlled trial in over 100 patients showed no improvement in survival rates with this therapy.

Because specific therapies have been ineffective, the two primary goals of therapy are (1) to provide good supportive care in an intensive care unit and (2) to assess whether liver transplantation is indicated. An important approach to therapy is also to determine the cause of fulminant hepatic failure, because specific antidote therapy for certain conditions, such as acetaminophen and possibly mushroom poisoning, may be beneficial. *N*-Acetylcysteine is particularly effective in the suicidal patients who present early after ingestion of a large quantity of acetaminophen. H_2-receptor blockers are routinely given to prevent stress-induced ulceration and gastrointestinal hemorrhage. Pulmonary artery monitoring is helpful in the management of intravascular volume and optimal oxygenation. If the patient progresses to grade 3 or grade 4 hepatic encephalopathy, intubation with mechanical ventilation is begun, and consideration should be given to intracerebral pressure monitoring.

The only proven therapy for fulminant hepatic failure is liver transplantation (see Chapter 54). For this reason, all patients should be transferred to a liver transplant center that is able to promptly assess patients and proceed with transplantation if indicated. In a retrospective, 2-year study in the United States of 295 patients with acute liver failure, 41% had transplantation, 25% recovered with supportive care, and 34% died. In this series, the 1-year survival rate after liver transplantation was 76%. The factor that has improved the results of liver transplantation for fulminant hepatic failure, other than the general improvements in surgical techniques and development of more effective immunosuppressive drugs, is a multidisciplinary approach to the intensive care management of these patients with anticipation and treatment of complications such as cerebral edema, bleeding, and infection. It is important to note that this 1-year survival rate is approximately 10% less than the survival rate of patients undergoing liver transplantation for end-stage liver disease. Before proceeding with transplantation, the patient must be promptly assessed for potential contraindications to transplantation (see Table 34–6). Some of the obstacles to successful transplantation include safe transportation of a patient with cerebral edema to a transplant center, obtaining a reliable psychosocial assessment, securing funding on an urgent basis, and obtaining a suitable organ. In the setting of fulminant hepatic failure, marginal donors may be used and orthotopic liver transplantation may also be performed across ABO blood groups.

Alternative approaches to the treatment of hepatic encephalopathy remain experimental. Auxiliary heterotopic liver transplantation has been performed in emergency situations with good results. If the native liver recovers function, immunosuppression can be withdrawn and the heterotopic graft will undergo rejection and atrophy. Living donor liver transplantation, providing a donor right lobe to an adult and donor left lobe or left lateral segment to a child, has also been used in patients with fulminant hepatic failure, if a suitable donor can be identified and evaluated in a timely fashion. An extracorporeal human donor graft has even been used for temporary support for a few days if the organ is otherwise deemed not suitable for implantation at orthotopic liver transplantation.

Other methods of temporary liver support include various hepatic assist or support devices. The original approach was to transplant isolated hepatocytes, either alone or with pancreatic islets, into the spleen. The most common approach is to perfuse blood or plasma through cultured, immortalized human hepatocellular cancer lines or fresh, isolated porcine hepatocytes placed in cartridges. Other clinicians have attached hepatocytes to various microcarriers and injected them into the peritoneal cavity. These approaches remain experimental and may or may not reach the level of clinical application. There is also efforts to develop transgenic pig livers that might provide an extracorporeal organ as a bridge to liver transplantation.

Prognosis

The decision whether to proceed with liver transplantation to treat/counter fulminant hepatic failure is difficult. The underlying cause of fulminant and subfulminant hepatic failure, as displayed in Table 34–4, is a major determinant of the likelihood of recovery and survival without transplantation. Perhaps the single most reliable guide to outcome is the stage of hepatic encephalopathy, with poor survival rates being expected in stage 3, and particularly stage 4, encephalopathy. The most comprehensive experience with fulminant hepatic failure has been reported from King's College Hospital in London. Ongoing studies at this center have demonstrated an improvement in survival rates over the past 20 years due to better supportive care of patients with acute liver failure in intensive care units. A multivariate analysis of 588 patients seen at King's College Hospital over a 12-year period was used to develop criteria predicting death from fulminant hepatic failure and the need for orthotopic liver transplantation (Table 34–7). The cause of acute liver failure was important, with patients having acetaminophen overdose experiencing the best survival rates and patients with non-A, non-B hepatitis or idiosyncratic drug reactions having the worst survival rates. Other laboratory thres-

Table 34–7. Criteria for liver transplantation in fulminant hepatic failure.

Criteria of King's College, London[1]
Acetaminophen patients
pH < 7.30, or
Prothrombin time 6.5 (INR)[2] and serum creatinine
> 3.4 mg/dL
Nonacetaminophin patients
Prothrombin time 6.5 (INR), or
Any three of the following variables
Etiology: non-A, non-B hepatitis or drug reaction
Age < 10 and > 40 years
Duration of jaundice before encephalopathy > 7 days
Serum bilirubin > 17.6 mg/dL
Prothrombin time > 3.5 (INR)
Criteria of Hôpital Paul-Brousse, Villejuif[3]
Hepatic encephalopathy, and
Factor V level < 20% in patient younger than 30 years
of age, or
Factor V level < 30% in patients 30 years of age or older

[1]Data from O'Grady JG et al: Early indicators of prognosis in fulminant hepatic failure. Gastroenterology 1989;97:439.
[2]INR, international normalized ratio.
[3]Data from Bernuau J et al: Criteria for emergency liver transplantation in patients with acute viral hepatitis and factor V below 50% of normal: a prospective study (Abstract). Hepatology 1991; 14:49A.

hold values, particularly prothrombin times, were useful in predicting outcome. In this series, nearly all patients ultimately developed advanced stages of hepatic encephalopathy, which was not an independent prognostic variable. Thus, irrespective of the grade of encephalopathy, the presence of the adverse prognostic indicators shown in Table 34–7 should lead to the placement of a patient with fulminant hepatic failure on the list for orthotopic liver transplantation, if there are no contraindications. In addition, Bernuau and colleagues have shown that factor V levels of less than 20% in patients younger than 30 years of age or less than 30% in older patients are an indication that failure to survive is likely when viral hepatitis is the cause of fulminant hepatic failure. Use of these prognostic criteria and daily assessment of patients usually allow early determination of the need for liver transplantation prior to the onset of grade 4 encephalopathy with its risks of cerebral edema and death.

Assessment of prognosis is critically important, so that liver transplantation, with its lifelong requirement for immunosuppression and continuous care, can be avoided in patients who would otherwise recover from fulminant hepatic failure, while transplantation can expeditiously be carried out in patients who would otherwise die of acute liver failure. Proper application of transplantation has favorably altered the outcome of acute liver failure, which was dismal before the widespread availability of this procedure.

REFERENCES

Lee WM: Acute liver failure. N Engl J Med 1993;329:1862.

Lee WM, Schiødt FV: Fulminant hepatic failure. In: *Schiff's Diseases of the Liver,* 8th ed. Schiff ER, Sorrell MF, Maddrey WC (editors). Lippincott-Raven, 1999.

Lidofsky SD: Liver transplantation for fulminant hepatic failure. Gastroenterol Clin North Am 1993;22:257.

Riordan SM, Williams R: Fulminant hepatic failure. Clin Liver Dis 2000;4:25.

Shakil AO et al: Acute liver failure: clinical features, outcome analysis, and applicability of prognostic criteria. Liver Transpl 2000;6:163.

Schiødt FV et al. Etiology and outcome for 295 patients with acute liver failure in the United States. Liver Transpl Surg 1999;5:29.

Viral Hepatitis

35

Rena Kramer Fox, MD & Teresa L. Wright, MD

The first cause of viral hepatitis was identified more than 20 years ago when hepatitis B virus (HBV) was shown to be the pathogen responsible for "serum hepatitis." Since then, there has been extensive characterization of properties of HBV and the host immune response to infection. Advances in molecular biology have resulted in the identification and sequence analysis of two viruses acquired by the fecal–oral route of transmission (hepatitis A virus, HAV, and hepatitis E virus, HEV) and two viruses acquired parenterally (hepatitis C virus, HCV, and hepatitis D virus, HDV). Other viruses that cause hepatitis (including cytomegalovirus, CMV) are discussed elsewhere (see Chapter 38). The pathogenesis, diagnosis, and treatment of chronic viral hepatitis continue to be the focus of research. Sensitive and specific assays are available for all five forms (A to E) of viral hepatitis. Nevertheless, at least 5–20% of cases of acute and chronic hepatitis are cryptogenic in that they cannot be attributed to any of the known forms of viral hepatitis and do not appear to result from toxic, metabolic, or genetic conditions. These include 5–20% of cases of acute viral hepatitis, 10–20% of cases of chronic hepatitis, and approximately 50% of cases of fulminant hepatitis and hepatitis-associated aplastic anemia. Whether additional unidentified viruses cause acute or chronic liver disease is under intense investigation. This chapter will focus on clinical features of the five main viruses that cause acute and chronic hepatitis (Table 35–1).

GENERAL CONSIDERATIONS

Essentials of Diagnosis

Diagnostic tests for different clinical situations are summarized in Table 35–2. Antibodies or antigen in serum are usually detected by enzyme-linked immunosorbent assay (ELISA) or radioimmunoassays.

Clinical Findings

A. ACUTE VIRAL HEPATITIS

Symptoms of acute viral hepatitis are usually nonspecific with malaise, fatigue, nausea, anorexia, and arthralgias. Fever, if present, is usually low grade. With disease progression, pruritus, dark urine, scleral icterus, and jaundice may occur. In any acute viral hepatitis, serum transaminases are typically greater than 500 U/L

and often greater than 1000 U/L, with the alanine aminotransferase (ALT) characteristically higher than the aspartate aminotransferase (AST). Transaminase elevation starts in the prodromal phase and precedes the rise in bilirubin level. Serum alkaline phosphatase may be normal or only mildly elevated. Serum bilirubin is variably elevated, but albumin and prothrombin time should be normal unless there is significant impairment of hepatic synthetic function. In most instances bilirubin is equally divided between conjugated and unconjugated fractions; values above 20 mg/dL that persist late into the course of viral hepatitis are more likely to be associated with severe disease. Prolongation of the prothrombin time (greater than 3 seconds above control value) should raise concern and prompt close monitoring of the patient for worsening hepatic failure. Neutropenia and lymphopenia are transient and followed by a relative lymphocytosis. Hypoglycemia occurs occasionally in severe acute hepatitis. A mild and diffuse elevation of the γ-globulin fraction is common. Liver biopsy is rarely necessary in acute viral hepatitis except when the diagnosis is questionable or when chronic hepatitis is suspected. Radiologic studies are rarely necessary unless biliary tract disease is suspected. In patients with profound intrahepatic cholestasis (such as occurs with hepatitis A infection), ultrasonography may be helpful in eliminating extrahepatic biliary tract obstruction.

B. CHRONIC VIRAL HEPATITIS

Chronic viral hepatitis is typically asymptomatic, with patients frequently unaware of their diagnosis until incidental findings or symptoms of advanced liver disease develop in later stages. Laboratory values may reflect normal liver function tests or fluctuations in transaminases, specifically ALT. For these reasons, liver biopsy can be most useful for staging the extent of disease. Ultrasound or computed tomography (CT) scan can also be useful to assess liver parenchyma, spleen size, existence of varicies, and possibilities of focal mass lesions.

Differential Diagnosis

A. ACUTE VIRAL HEPATITIS

Infections with other viruses such as CMV, infectious mononucleosis, herpes simplex, and coxsackieviruses

Table 35–1. Properties and clinical characteristics of viruses.

	Hepatitis A	Hepatitis B	Hepatitis C	Hepatitis D	Hepatitis E
Size	27 nm	42 nm	32 nm	36 nm	27–34 nm
Length	7.5 kb	3.2 kb	10 kb	1.7 kb	7.6 kb
Genome	RNA	DNA	RNA	RNA	RNA
Incubation	14–49 days	14–84 days	14–160 days	21–42 days	21–63 days
Transmission	Fecal/oral (98%) Transfusion (2%)	IVDA (35%) Sexual (19%) Vertical (<5%) Transfusion (<5%) Needlestick (1%) Unknown (49%)	IVDA (35%) Sexual (10%) Vertical (5–6%) Transfusion (<5%) High-risk occupation (7%) Unknown (49%)	Parenteral	Fecal/oral
Vaccine	Available	Available	None	None	None
Severity of acute illness	Usually mild, particularly in children	70% subclinical, 30% clinical, <1% severe	Usually subclinical <1% severe	Can be severe	May be severe— 30% mortality in pregnancy
Chronic infection	None	90% neonatal 50% infants 20% children <5% adults	>85%	5% with HBV coinfection, 70–80% with HBV superinfection	None

can result in an acute viral hepatitis syndrome and elevated serum transaminases. Toxoplasmosis may also share clinical features with acute hepatitis. If HBsAg, anti-HBc, and immunoglobulin M (IgM) anti-HAV are negative, serological tests for these agents should be considered. Several drugs and anesthetic agents can produce a picture similar to acute hepatitis with cholestasis, and thus it is important to take a careful drug history. A past history of unexplained and repeated episodes of hepatitis raises the possibility of underlying chronic hepatitis. Alcoholic hepatitis is associated with a history of ethanol abuse, as well as with stigmata of alcoholism (see Chapter 39). In patients with alcoholic liver disease, serum transaminase levels rarely rise above

Table 35–2. Serologic diagnosis of viral hepatitis.

Significance	Anti-HAV IgM	HBsAg	HBeAg	Anti-HBc IgG	Anti-HBc IgM	Anti-HBs IgG	Anti-HCV IgM/IgG	Anti-HDV IgM	Anti-HEV IgM
Acute HAV	+	–	–	–	–	–	–	–	–
Acute HBV	–	+	+	–	+	–	–	–	–
Chronic HBV, active replication	–	+	+	+	–	–	–	–	–
Chronic HBV, quiescent	–	+	–	+	–	–	–	–	–
Resolved HBV	–	–	–	–	+	+	–	–	–
Postvaccine immune HBV	–	–	–	–	–	+	–	–	–
Chronic or recent HCV	–	–	–	–	–	–	+	–	–
Acute or chronic HDV	–	+	–	–	–	–	–	+	–
Acute HEV	–	–	–	–	–	–	–	–	+

500 U/L, and typically, serum AST levels are greater than serum ALT levels. When abdominal pain is prominent, acute viral hepatitis may be confused with acute cholecystitis, common duct stone, or ascending cholangitis. Careful clinical and radiologic evaluation will assist in making the correct diagnosis and therefore avoiding unnecessary surgery. Cholestatic viral hepatitis may be confused with obstructive jaundice due to pancreatic carcinoma or a common bile duct stone. Clinical features help to distinguish acute hepatitis from congestive hepatopathy and acute ischemic injury. Uncommonly, inherited metabolic disorders, such Wilson's disease, mimic acute viral hepatitis.

B. CHRONIC VIRAL HEPATITIS

When diagnosing chronic viral hepatitis, consideration should be given to autoimmune chronic active hepatitis, connective tissue disorders such as systemic lupus erythematosis and rheumatoid arthritis, Wilson's disease, and primary biliary cirrhosis. Serology, biochemical testing, and liver histopathology help in arriving at the correct diagnosis in most instances.

HEPATITIS A

Pathophysiology

Hepatitis A virus is an RNA virus that is transmitted by fecal–oral mode through ingestion of contaminated food (eg, shellfish) or water. The incubation period is 2–6 weeks and the phase when virus is present in serum is short (5–7 days); hence, parenteral transmission is rare. Infection is sporadic and is associated with poor socioeconomic conditions, which can lead to epidemics. In several developing countries hepatitis A is endemic, with infection occurring in the majority of children before the age of 5 years. Improved socioeconomic conditions and sanitation have led to an increase in the mean age of infection in southern Europe. The liver cell damage probably results from cell-mediated cytotoxicity. Serum neutralizing antibodies protect against HAV infection. The necroinflammatory changes are prominent in periportal areas and are accompanied by many plasma cells. In some cases, centrilobular cholestasis may be severe, particularly in adults. HAV antigen can be demonstrated by immunohistochemical staining as fine granules in the cytoplasm of hepatocytes and Kupffer cells.

Essentials of Diagnosis

Diagnosis of HAV infection depends on detection of antibodies [immunoglobulin G (IgG) for prior infection, IgM for recent infection]. A positive anti-HAV result usually reflects total antibodies (both IgG and IgM) and cannot be used to distinguish between acute or prior exposure unless IgM is specified. Anti-HAV IgM may persist for 6–12 months after acute infection. Hence, in a patient with acute transaminase elevation, presence of anti-HAV IgM, does not always signify acute hepatitis A infection but may represent hepatitis A infection within the prior year, with a superimposed, unrelated hepatitis.

Clinical Findings

Most cases of acute hepatitis A are asymptomatic (particularly in children) or have nonspecific symptoms. When clinically apparent, patients present with jaundice, fatigue, and malaise. Uncommonly, HAV infection may result in a cholestatic picture.

Natural History

Hepatitis A is rarely fulminant and never chronic. Systemic manifestations are uncommon and include cryoglobulinemia, nephritis, and leucytoclastic vasculitis. Concomitant meningoencephalitis has been reported in some patients. Cholestatic hepatitis with protracted cholestatic jaundice and pruritus can occur as a variant of acute hepatitis A. It has been suggested that in genetically susceptible individuals, HAV infection may trigger an autoimmune hepatitis. Hepatitis A may have a relapsing course, symptomatic for 6 months or more. The relapses are generally benign, with eventual complete resolution. Chronic infection never ensues, and complete recovery is the rule. Rarely (less than 1% of cases), fulminant hepatic failure with encephalopathy and coagulopathy results from acute infection. Such patients should be referred for consideration of liver transplantation. Once profound encephalopathy develops in elderly patients, mortality is high (up to 80%). In younger patients, the prognosis is better than in patients with fulminant liver failure of other causes. The overall case fatality rate with HAV infection is very low (about 0.1%), although in patients with chronic underlying liver disease, the morbidity and mortality are increased in the presence of a hepatitis A superinfection.

Treatment

Treatment is largely supportive and consists of bed rest until jaundice subsides, a high caloric diet, discontinuation of potentially hepatotoxic medication, and restriction of alcohol intake. Most cases do not require hospitalization, which is recommended for patients with advanced age, serious underlying medical conditions, or chronic liver disease, malnutrition, pregnancy, immunosuppressive therapy, hepatotoxic medication, severe vomiting that excludes adequate oral intake, and clinical and laboratory findings that suggest fulminant hepatitis.

The occasional patient with fulminant hepatic failure, defined as the onset of encephalopathy within 8 weeks of the onset of symptoms, should be referred for consideration of liver transplantation (see Chapters 34 and 54).

Prevention

Prevention of hepatitis A is justified for public health reasons. General measures to prevent the spread of HAV include careful handwashing, safe water supply, and proper sewage disposal. Human trials with inactivated whole HAV vaccines have shown a protective efficacy of 94–100% after two or three doses and only minor side effects. Such a vaccine is licensed in several countries, including the United States, and is widely available. Indications for HAV vaccination are listed in Table 35–3. Immunoglobulin has also been shown to be safe and effective in preventing HAV infection in both pre- and postexposure situations. If immediate protection is required, travelers should receive passive immunization with immunoglobulin as well as vaccine to confer protection. Passive immunization is by a single intramuscular dose of immune serum globulin of 0.02–0.06 mL/kg. In postexposure setting, immune serum globulin, if given within 10–14 days of exposure, has an efficacy of about 85%, and usually aborts or reduces the severity of the HAV infection. The protection offered by immune serum globulin lasts only a few months.

Lednar WM, Lemon SM, Kirkpatrick JW: Frequency of illness associated with epidemic hepatitis A virus infection in adults. Am J Epidemiol 1985;122:226.

Lemon SM: Type A viral hepatitis: new developments in an old disease. N Engl J Med 1985;313:1059.

Prevention of hepatitis A through active or passive immunization: recommendations of the Advisory Committee on Immunization Practices (ACIP). MMWR 1999;48:1.

Stapleton JT: Host immune response to hepatitis A virus. J Infect Dis 1995;171(Suppl 1):S9.

Vento S, Garofano R, Renzini C: Fulminant hepatitis associated with hepatitis A virus superinfection in patients with chronic hepatitis C. N Engl J Med 1998;338:286.

HEPATITIS B

Pathophysiology

Hepatitis B virus is a DNA virus transmitted by blood, or by sexual or needle contact. In the United States, the most common modes of transmission are sexual and parenteral (horizontal spread), whereas in Asia, the most common mode is from mother to child (vertical spread). Injecting drug users are at high risk of also acquiring hepatitis C and D (see the following sections). HBV is a partially double-stranded DNA virus, which replicates through an RNA intermediate. Although HBV is strongly hepatotrophic, viral sequences, including HBV replicative intermediates, are present in

Table 35–3. Indications for vaccination.

Indications for HAV Vaccination in Adults	Indications for HBV Vaccination in Adults
Persons traveling to or working in countries with high or intermediate endemicity of infection	Health care workers
Men who have sex with men	Public safety workers with exposure to blood in the workplace
Illegal drug users (injection and noninjection)	Clients and staff of institutions for the developmentally disabled, day care centers, schools
Persons who have occupational risk for infection	Hemodialysis patients
Persons who have clotting factor disorders/receive clotting factor concentrates	Persons who have clotting factor disorders/receive clotting factor concentrates
Persons who have chronic liver disease	Household contacts and sex partners of HBV carriers
Persons who either are awaiting or have received liver transplantation	Adoptees from countries where HBV infection is endemic
Persons who work as food handlers in areas where such vaccination is cost effective	International travelers who plan to spend more than 6 months in endemic area, who will have close contact with the local population, or who are likely to have contact with blood or sexual contact with residents
	Men who have sex with men
	HIV-infected persons
	Sexually active heterosexual men and women who recently acquired other sexually transmitted diseases, who are sex workers, or who have a history of sexual activity with more than one partner in the previous 6 months.
	Inmates of long-term correctional facilities

extrahepatic tissues (lymph nodes, peripheral blood mononuclear cells). There are four open reading frames in HBV that encode four major proteins: (1) surface gene for hepatitis B surface antigen (HBsAg); (2) core gene for hepatitis B core antigen (HBcAg); (3) pol gene for the DNA polymerase, which catalyzes several steps in viral replication and assembly; and (4) the hepatitis B X gene for the X protein, which appears to up-regulate the replication of other viruses such as human immunodeficiency virus (HIV). HBsAg, the envelope protein of the virus that is excreted in excess as 20-nm particles in serum, indicates ongoing infection. HBcAg, the protein found in the inner core of HBV, is not secreted into serum but is expressed on the hepatocyte surface. As such, it is the target of the host immune response to infection, playing an important role in the pathogenesis of HBV-induced liver damage. HBcAg can also be detected in the nuclei of hepatocytes. HBeAg is the secretory form of HBcAg, whose presence indicates active viral replication and increased infectivity. The C region has two initiation codons, and therefore two gene transcripts (precore and core), which result in two protein products (HBcAg and HBeAg). These polypeptides have considerable amino acid homology and immune cross-reactivity at the T cell level. Anti-HBc appears at the onset of clinical hepatitis and may be the only marker detectable between the disappearance of HBsAg and appearance of anti-HBs. Anti-HBe usually appears at the time of peak clinical symptoms and in combination with HBsAg implies low viral replication and infectivity. Four antigenic subtypes of HBV exist (adw, ayw, adr, ayr), and there is geographic variation in the distribution of these subtypes.

HBV enters and mainly survives in hepatocytes as a noncytopathogenic virus. The viral components responsible for attachment to host cells are not fully characterized. Viral replication takes place in the cytoplasm. The host immune mechanisms of defense include the production of antibodies, such as anti-HBs. However, HbsAb is effective at neutralizing virus only when HBV is extracellular. Once HBV has entered the cell, these antibodies offer no protection. Most damage from HBV infection is caused by host immune response. Cell-mediated response directed against cellular HBcAg is the primary cause of cell injury, with immune lysis of infected hepatocytes by HBV-specific and activated cytotoxic T-lymphocytes (CTL) resulting in hepatitis.

The clinical outcome of HBV infection depends on the balance between the viral behavior and the host defense. In the case of acute HBV infection, if the immune response begins when only a small number of hepatocytes are infected, the infection may resolve without symptoms. If the immune response begins to be effective once a large number of hepatocytes are infected, the reaction may lead to symptomatic hepatitis.

Even if the immune response ultimately overcomes the infection, the HBV-specific CTL response is maintained for years, despite loss of serum markers of HBV infection.

In vertically acquired infection, the neonate has an immature immune system and is unable to mount an adequate immune response. This leads to a state of viral "tolerance" characterizing the asymptomatic carrier state.

In the case of chronic HBV infection, if the humoral immune response is insufficient to overcome infection, then a chronic infection results, as occurs in 3–8% of adults. Hepatocytes with ground glass cytoplasm are seen, particularly in patients with little or no necroinflammatory activity. HBcAg can be demonstrated in the hepatocyte nuclei and also the cytoplasm and cell membrane. HLA-restricted cytotoxic T lymphocytes directed against the molecular complex of viral and histocompatibility antigens on the liver cell surface are the effector cells that mediate cell damage. Cytokine-mediated cell injury and other mechanisms may also be involved in cell damage. HBeAg negative variants result from mutations in the precore region with failure of HBeAg synthesis, yet with continued viral replication. These mutant viruses have been associated with fulminant hepatitis and aggressive chronic disease.

Chronic HBV infection is strongly linked epidemiologically to the development of hepatocellular carcinoma (in up to 50% of patients with HBV-induced cirrhosis) (see Chapter 46). The mechanism of viral oncogenesis has been extensively studied. Viral integration into the host genome is required but no consistent sites of integration have been shown (eg, adjacent to a host tumor promotor or suppressor gene). Cell turnover associated with chronic inflammation likely contributes to the pathogenesis of hepatocellular carcinoma, as do environmental cofactors such as aflatoxins and alcohol.

HBV Variants

A. PRECORE MUTANTS

A precore nucleotide mutation leads to premature termination of the precore protein, preventing production of HbeAg. This mutation is seen in both chronic infections and asymptomatic carriers. The basis for selection of this mutation is unclear, but HBV DNA levels are not higher in precore mutants compared with wild-type HBV. The prevalence of this mutation is unclear but appears to be increasing.

B. S MUTANTS

A mutation in the S gene has been reported in infants who are born to carrier mothers but develop HBV despite vaccination and in liver transplant recipients who develop HBV reinfection despite hepatitis B immunoglobulin.

C. P Mutants

Mutations in the polymerase gene are associated with resistance to HBV antivirals such as lamivudine and famciclovir.

Prevalence & Epidemiology

More than 50% of the world's population has been infected with hepatitis B. HBV is endemic in areas containing 45% of the world's population. However, prevalence is difficult to estimate. In endemic areas, carrier rates range from 8 to 25% and exposure rates (measured by anti-HBs) range from 60 to 85%. In low prevalence areas such as the United States, chronic carrier prevalence is less than 2%. The Centers for Disease Control (CDC) estimates that 200,000–300,000 new infections occur per year and there are 1.25 million chronic carriers in the United States.

Essentials of Diagnosis

Diagnosis of HBV infection largely relies on the presence of HBsAg. Acute and chronic infections are distinguished by the presence of IgM versus IgG antibodies to the inner hepatitis B core protein (anti-HBc). Acute HBV infection in the absence of HBsAg positivity but anti-HBc IgM positive is theoretically possible but rare and is referred to as the "window period." The presence of IgM anti-HBc indicates recent infection, although this marker may occasionally be present during acute reactivation of chronic infection. Hepatitis B e antigen (HBeAg) is a cleaved protein product of the hepatitis B core gene, which is indicative of active HBV replication. Antibodies to HBeAg (anti-HBe) are present in inactive or nonreplicative HBV infection. Precore mutants, described above, are actively replicating with detectable HBV DNA in serum, but have absent HBeAg. Isolated antibodies to hepatitis B surface antigen (anti-HBs) indicate vaccine-induced immunity. Antibodies to both core and surface proteins (anti-HBc and anti-HBs) indicate prior HBV infection. Interpretation of isolated anti-HBc (IgG) positivity is problematic since this may represent ongoing, low-level HBV infection, prior HBV infection, or a false-positive test. Typically anti-HBc IgM is indicative of acute HBV infection and anti-HBc IgG is indicative of prior or resolving HBV infection. On occasion, acute flares of chronic HBV are associated with anti-HBc IgM positivity.

Clinical Findings

A. Acute Hepatitis B

The patient with acute HBV infection is infective for many weeks before clinical presentation. The incubation period is between 6 weeks and 6 months. In 5–10% of acute hepatitis B patients, a serum sickness-like syndrome with arthralgias, rash, angioedema, and rarely proteinuria and hematuria may develop in the prodromal phase. In children, hepatitis B may rarely present as anicteric hepatitis associated with a nonpruritic papular rash on the face, buttocks, and limbs. Fatigue, anorexia, icterus, and alanine transaminase elevation correlate with anti-HBc appearance.

B. Chronic Hepatitis B

Progression to chronic active hepatitis is suggested by ongoing anorexia, weight loss, and fatigue, although most patients with chronic replication are asymptomatic. Physical findings may include persistent hepatomegaly. Other findings may include the persistence of HbsAg, elevations of the aminotransferase, bilirubin, and globulin levels, and the presence of bridging or multilobular hepatic necrosis on liver biopsy for at least 6 months after clinically acute hepatitis. However, most patients with chronic infection are "healthy carriers" and have normal liver enzymes, no symptoms, are anti-HBe positive, and have normal or near normal liver histology. Extrahepatic manifestations, when they occur, may include arthralgias, arthritis, Henoch-Schönlein purpura, angioneurotic edema, polyarteritis nodosa, glomerulonephritis, pleural effusions, pericarditis, and aplastic anemia. Uncommon complications of HBV infection include pancreatitis, myocarditis, atypical pneumonia, transverse myelitis, and peripheral neuropathy.

Natural History

Ninety percent of adult patients with acute HBV infection have a favorable course and recover completely. Case fatality rate is low (0.1%), but increases with age and associated systemic illnesses. Older persons and patients with diabetes mellitus and congestive heart failure may have a severe hepatitis with a prolonged course. Less than 5% of normal, immunocompetent young adults remain chronically positive after acute infection. Overall, the risk of chronicity is related to the age of acquisition: more than 90% in newborns, about 50% in early childhood, less than 5% in immunocompetent adults, and greater than 50% in immunocompromised adults such as transplant recipients, HIV-positive individuals, and patients with leukemia or leprosy. Chronically infected patients may be asymptomatic carriers or may have chronic hepatitis with or without cirrhosis.

Hepatitis B does account for about 50% of cases of fulminant hepatitis of viral cause (see Chapter 34). The diagnosis is suggested by decreasing liver size, rising bilirubin, an increasing prothrombin time, and signs of encephalopathy. Cerebral edema is common, and brainstem compression, gastrointestinal (GI) bleeding, sepsis, respiratory failure, cardiovascular collapse, and renal failure are terminal events in this condition, which has a very high mortality. Survivors may have complete biochemical and histologic recovery.

Chronic carriers seem to be immunologically tolerant to this virus and have an excellent prognosis. When there is a loss of tolerance with emergence of reactive T cell clones, hepatic inflammation and T cell-mediated liver damage may follow.

Chronic replicative hepatitis B patients mostly have active liver disease and active viral replication demonstrated by the presence of HBeAg and HBV DNA. HBV DNA has been found integrated into chromosomal DNA of hepatocytes. Predominantly episomal HBV DNA is detectable in carriers with high levels of viral replication, with integrated HBV DNA detectable in those with less active viral replication. These patients are at a greater risk of death from liver disease or hepatocellular carcinoma than those with inactive disease. The proportion of patients with integrated HBV DNA and anti-HBe positivity increases with the increasing age of the cohort. The outcome in HBsAg-positive patients is also influenced by histologic stage. Five-year survival rates in patients with early histologic changes (chronic persistent hepatitis) are higher (97%) than in patients with chronic active hepatitis (85%). Development of cirrhosis is associated with a reduction in 5-year survival to about 50%.

Hepatitis B is a major risk factor for the development of hepatocellular carcinoma (HCC). In regions where this viral infection is endemic, HCC is the leading cause of cancer-related death. Cirrhosis is present in more than 90% of HBV-related HCC, and the chronic inflammation and regenerative cellular proliferation associated with cirrhosis may predispose to cellular transformation and frank malignancy. However, the risk of HCC is still significantly elevated even in the absence of cirrhosis, which is unlike HCV patients. In otherwise healthy HBV carriers, the HCC incidence is 0.06–0.3% per year. In those with chronic hepatitis, the annual incidence is 0.5–0.8% and in those with cirrhosis, the rate of developing HCC is 1.5–6.6% per year. Furthermore, the risk of HCC is also significantly higher among men than women and is higher in patients with HBV–HCV coinfection than in those with HBV alone. Population- and clinic-based screening programs using serum α-fetoprotein and liver ultrasound have led to identification of patients with small and potentially resectable tumors. Despite earlier detection, it is not clear that the mortality due to HCC carcinoma is reduced by screening programs (see Chapter 46).

Treatment

A. Treatment of Fulminant Hepatitis B

In fulminant hepatitis, intensive care in a specialized unit likely reduces mortality, which otherwise approaches 80% (see Chapter 34). Protein intake should be restricted and oral lactulose or neomycin administered. Patients should be supported by maintaining fluid and electrolyte balance and cardiorespiratory function, controlling bleeding, and managing other complications. Large corticosteroid doses, exchange transfusions, plasma perfusion, human cross-circulation, and porcine liver cross-perfusion have not proven effective. Orthotopic liver transplantation is being performed with increasing frequency, with good results. Thus, patients should be supported maximally until spontaneous recovery or until prognostic factors indicate worsening outcome necessitating transplantation. Measures should be taken to prevent HBV infection of the graft (see below).

B. Treatment of Chronic Hepatitis B

The treatment of chronic hepatitis B aims at suppressing HBV replication and reducing liver injury. This is manifest by three major end points: (1) HBeAg seroconversion to anti-HBe, (2) loss of HBV DNA in the serum, and (3) normalization of ALT levels. It is hoped that with sustained effects, histologic progression to cirrhosis and HCC is delayed or halted. Two main therapies are currently available for treatment of chronic HBV.

1. Interferon-α-2b—The first therapy, interferon-α-2b, has been approved by the Food and Drug Administration (FDA) for treatment of hepatitis B since 1992. Interferon-α-2b is a glycoprotein that has direct antiviral mechanisms and also has mechanisms of enhancing immune responses to viruses. Interferon is indicated for patients with detectable HBsAg, HBeAg, HBV DNA, and compensated disease. It is acceptable to use in early cirrhosis. The usual dose is 10 MU three times per week or 5 MU daily for 4 months, although a prolonged course may also have additional benefits. Approximately 30–40% of patients with the 4-month course will clear HBV DNA and lose HBeAg. Seroconversion to anti-HBe occurs in approximately 20%. Approximately 10% of patients will clear HBsAg after their initial course. Approximately 10–25% of initial responders will relapse within the first 2 years of follow-up. The main predictors of response to interferon in terms of the short-term end points are HBV DNA level of <100 pg/mL and high ALT of >200 U/L. Other predictors include an active hepatitis on liver biopsy and short duration of infection. Compensated cirrhotic patients do have a 20–30% sustained response to interferon. However, in decompensated cirrhosis, interferon may precipitate hepatic failure and infection and therefore is not recommended. Retreatment of nonresponders can be considered. Pretreatment with prednisone has been studied as a method of increasing response to interferon. However, improved response has not been clearly found and some serious hepatitis flares have occurred. Side effects of interferon are the major limitation to its use and include (1) flu-like symptoms of fever, myalgias, and headache, (2) leukopenia, neutropenia, and thrombocytopenia, (3) fatigue, and (4) depression. Contraindications include (1) immune suppression or autoimmune disease and (2) significant psychiatric disease or depression. Interferon should be considered in a young person with mild liver disease, low levels of replication, and high serum transaminase levels.

2. Lamivudine—The second major therapy, lamivudine (3TC), has been approved by the FDA for treatment of hepatitis B since 1998. Lamivudine is a nucleoside analog that inhibits viral DNA synthesis by blocking reverse transcriptase. It was originally approved for use in human immunodeficiency virus (HIV) in 1995. It is dosed orally, once daily at 100 mg, and is renally cleared. Randomized controlled clinical trials of patients treated for 1 year have demonstrated effects in seroconversion of HBeAg in 17–33% of patients compared with 4–6% spontaneous seroconversion in control subjects. Furthermore, lamivudine-treated patients showed a loss of detectable HBV DNA in the majority of patients, normalization of ALT in 50% of patients, and improvement in inflammatory histology in 56% of patients compared with 25% in control subjects. Reductions in the progression of fibrosis and progression to cirrhosis have also been demonstrated. It is notable that the HBeAg seroconversion rate rises with extended courses of therapy, yet the optimal duration of treatment with lamivudine is unclear. Determination of the optimal duration of treatment is further complicated since mutant strains of HBV with resistance to lamivudine appear in approximately 13% of patients treated for 1 year and 30–50% of patients treated for 3 years. Mutations are found in the YMDD motif of the HBV polymerase. Unfortunately, other than duration of treatment, there are no known markers for predicting the appearance of these resistant variants before treatment. Lamivudine is safe to use in patients with cirrhosis and, unlike interferon, can be used for patients with decompensated disease. Furthermore, it is used in patients with end-stage liver disease awaiting transplantation and is a mainstay of therapy in postrenal and postliver transplantation. However, there are many questions regarding the benefits of early lamivudine treatment versus the risk of development of resistance. Combination therapy with lamivudine and interferon is safe, but has not been shown to have greater efficacy than either drug alone. The side effect profile of combination therapy is similar to interferon alone.

3. Special groups—There are several subgroups of chronic HBV disease that should be discussed. In **HBV–HIV coinfection,** interferon therapy is ineffec-tive, although lamivudine resistance is common since many patients have received long-term lamivudine as part of their HIV treatment regimen. In **HBV–HDV coinfection,** neither lamivudine nor interferon has been extensively studied. In **HBV–HCV coinfection,** interferon is not effective and results with lamivudine are unclear. In **precore mutants,** both interferon and lamivudine appear to have transient benefits only and optimal duration of treatment is even less clear than in the treatment of wild-type cases. In **postliver transplantation patients,** lamivudine prophylaxis with hepatitis B immunoglobulin has been shown to decrease HBV reinfection as measured by HBsAg, HBeAg, and HBV DNA. In **interferon nonresponders,** lamivudine is superior to either combination therapy or placebo.

C. POSTEXPOSURE PROPHYALXIS

For neonates born to infected mothers and any patient with a clear exposure, hepatitis B immunoglobulin is available. Active vaccination should also be offered.

D. LIVER TRANSPLANTATION

Liver transplantation has been employed as therapy for end-stage chronic HBV-associated liver disease (see Chapter 54). HBV is the sixth most common indication for liver transplantation in the United States. Until recently, transplantation resulted in an 80% rate of reinfection in the absence of prophylaxis, and the resulting hepatitis could be severe and was almost invariably chronic. The risk was higher in patients with chronic liver disease versus fulminant disease and lower in those with HBD–HDV coinfection than in HBV alone. Interferon-α treatment in the peritransplant period has been ineffective in preventing reinfection. The most effective approach to delaying and preventing recurrent HBV infection has been high-dose hepatitis B immunoglobulin (HBIG) perioperatively and postoperatively. The use of high-dose prophylactic HBIG has resulted in prolonged survival following liver transplantation in those with and without active pretransplantation viral replication. Short-term HBIG use still resulted in high recurrence rates but with indefinite therapy, recurrence decreased significantly. Lamivudine has recently had a major impact on decreasing posttransplant reinfection. However, lamivudine alone, without HBIG, leads to the development of reinfection and resistant mutations in 25% of patients. A combined posttransplant regimen of HBIG and lamivudine is highly effective in preventing recurrence with fewer HBIG mutations and fewer polymerase variants as well. The optimal dose of lamivudine and HBIG combination is still unclear. Disadvantages of prolonged HBIG include cost, patient inconvenience, tolerability, and limited availability. One study compared HBIG monotherapy as long-term prophylaxis with short-term HBIG for 6 months posttransplantation combined with long-term lamivudine. Results showed that the combination regimen was as effective as long-term HBIG in preventing reinfection; clearly this regimen would be a less costly and inconvenient regimen. Recurrent HBV post-transplantation now occurs in less than 5% of patients treated with HBIG plus lamivudine. Additional antivirals are in development for the treatment of lamivudine-resistant variants as well.

Prevention

Hepatitis B vaccine is protective in over 90% of normal individuals. Recombinant vaccines have largely supplanted the original plasma-derived vaccine in most parts of the world. Common adverse effects are local reactions at the injection site (soreness, tenderness, pruritus, and swelling); serious adverse effects have not been reported. For reasons that are unclear, approximately 9% of healthy patients receiving HBV vaccine do not develop protective antibodies. Vaccination of those at high risk has been of only limited success, since compliance in even highly educated groups such as health care workers has been poor. Despite the availability of an effective vaccine for more than a decade, targeted vaccination programs for those at highest risk of infection have failed. The United States Public Health Service currently recommends universal vaccination of all neonates and prepubertal teenagers. In addition, HBV vaccination is currently recommended for immunocompromised patients, hemodialysis patients, patients with existing chronic liver disease including chronic hepatitis C, health care workers, injection drug users, and those with high-risk sexual exposures (see Table 35–3). Protection is afforded against HBV surface antigenemia, clinically apparent hepatitis B, and chronic infection. Currently, booster immunization is not recommended routinely, although booster immunization may be useful in immunosuppressed persons who have lost detectable anti-HBs or immunocompetent persons who sustain HBsAg inoculation after losing detectable antibody.

Colquhoun SD, Belle SH, Samuel D: Transplantation in the hepatitis B patient and current therapies to prevent recurrence. Sem Liver Dis 2000;20:7.

Deres K, Rubasmen-Waigmann H: Development of resistance and perspectives for future therapies against hepatitis B infections: lessons to be learned from HIV. Infection 1999;27:S45.

Dienstag JL, Schiff ER, Wright TL: Lamivudine as initial treatment for chronic hepatitis B in the United States. N Engl J Med 1999;341:1256.

Farrell G: Hepatitis B e antigen seroconversion: effects of lamivudine alone or in combination with interferon-α. J Med Virol 2000;61:374.

Lau DT, Khokhar MF, Doo E: Long-term therapy of chronic hepatitis B with lamivudine. Hepatology 2000;32:828.

Lin OS, Keeffe EB: Current treatment strategies for chronic hepatitis B and C. Annu Rev Med 2001;52:29.

Lok AS: Hepatitis B infection: pathogenesis and management. J Hepatol 2000;32:89.

Peters MG, Shouval D, Bonhan A: Posttransplantation: future therapies. Sem Liver Dis 2000;20:19.

HEPATITIS C

Pathophysiology

Hepatitis C virus is a single-stranded RNA virus. Its genome is fully characterized, encoding two structural proteins (core and envelope) and five nonstructural proteins (including a helicase, protease, and RNA polymerase) that are important in viral replication). Six major HCV genotypes have been described and designated 1–6; these are further divided into subtypes (1a, 1b, 2a, etc) of which over 50 have been described. There is considerable variation in geographic distribution of HCV genotypes. In the United States, 75% of patients are genotype 1. This genotypic variation has significant clinical implications. First, genotypes 1 and 4 have increased resistance to interferon therapy compared with genotypes 2 and 3. Second, hypervariability of regions of the HCV envelope proteins may be important in persistence of HCV infection, facilitating evasion of the host immune response. Third, vaccine development may be more difficult due to variation in immune responses to different genotypes.

Levels of HCV in serum are lower than levels of HBV, and HCV antigens are not detectable in blood. Liver biopsies from patients with chronic HCV infection demonstrate micro- or macrovesicular steatosis (in 50%), bile duct damage (in 60%), and lymphocyte aggregates or follicles (in 60%). Immune-mediated damage is thought to produce hepatitis in HCV infection, although the mechanism of cell injury is not fully understood. A direct cytopathic effect of HCV may also contribute to the damage in some situations.

Prevalence & Epidemiology

The NHANES III study found that 3.9 million people in the United States, 1.8% of the population, have been exposed to HCV. Approximately 2.7 million have chronic infection. Worldwide, it is estimated that 3% of the population, 170 million people, have chronic HCV. In the United States, HCV is the most common blood-borne infection, the leading cause of chronic liver disease, and the most common indication for liver transplantation. The annual incidence of new HCV infection is decreasing, but the overall number of chronically infected patients is likely to remain high.

Groups at risk for HCV include, but are not limited to, transfusion recipients, injection drug users, hemodialysis patients, Vietnam-era veterans, and health care workers. HCV accounts for most posttransfusion hepatitis prior to 1992. However, risk from transfusion is now greatly decreased with proper donor screening. Hemophiliacs have a 74–90% prevalence of infection. In intravenous drug users, prevalence is 72–90%. Needlestick spread in health care workers innoculated with blood-contaminated needles has been confirmed by anti-HCV testing, but the seroconversion rate is low (approximately 4%), and this accounts for a very small proportion of HCV infections (<1%). Sporadic HCV infection, in which the mode of transmission is unknown, is responsible for 12% of cases. Vertical transmission occurs but is inefficient and only 5–6% of infected mothers have chronically infected neonates, regardless of the route of delivery.

Sexual transmission is a highly debated issue. It is clear that HCV is much less efficiently transmitted sexually as compared with HBV. Stable partners of HCV patients are rarely infected, with prevalence of anti-HCV ranging from 0.4 to 3%. In those partners with infection, other risk factors were commonly identified. However, a 2–12% prevalence of anti-HCV is seen in sexually promiscuous individuals (homosexual or heterosexual) who deny other HCV risk factors. The U.S. Public Health Service currently does not recommend a change in sexual practices in stable sexual partners.

The NHANES III survey analyzed which factors are independently associated with HCV infection. The strongest include illegal drug use and high-risk sexual behavior. Other factors include poverty, low education, and having been divorced or separated. However, neither sex nor racial–ethnic group was independently associated with infection.

Essentials of Diagnosis

A. ANTIBODY TESTING

The first step in diagnosis of HCV infection is the enzyme-linked immunosorbent assay (ELISA) for anti-HCV, detecting past exposure or ongoing infection. Three generations of the ELISA have been developed, all of which have high sensitivity and specificity. The ELISA III is >99% sensitive and specific. The window for serologic conversion after initial exposure varies with a range of 20–150 days with a mean of approximately 50 days. Eighty percent of patients have measurable antibody at 15 weeks. No HCV IgM assays are available. False-positive tests are most often seen in low-risk populations, such as blood donors. False-negative tests are most often seen in immunocompromised patients, including dialysis patients and transplant recipients. When a false-positive test is suspected, such as in the blood donor population, recombinant immunoblot

assays (RIBA) are confirmatory tests for HCV Ab, reported as positive/indeterminate/negative. However, RIBA should not be employed as routine testing in clinical practice when HCV infection is suspected based on risk factors.

B. VIROLOGIC DETECTION

The second main step in diagnosis of chronic HCV infection is detection of HCV RNA in serum. Virus is generally detectable 7–21 days following exposure. There are three main assays available. Qualitative HCV RNA by polymerase chain reaction (PCR) is the most sensitive technique, detecting as few as 50 copies/mL but does not quantitate the viral titer. Quantitative HCV RNA by PCR is less sensitive, but still able to detect as few as 1000 copies/mL and is able to provide an absolute viral titer. It is currently reported in both copies/mL and in international units/mL (IU/mL). Finally, the branched-DNA technique is the least sensitive, able to detect only as few as 200,000 copies/mL, but is the most reproducible for quantitative measures. After a World Health Organization (WHO) consensus meeting, a standarized international unit (IU) was developed. The WHO concluded that 800,000 IU/mL was the clinically relevant threshold whereas greater than 800,000 IU/mL was considered a high viral titer and less than 800,000 IU/mL was considered a low viral titer. The distinction is clinically relevant in regard to the likelihood of treatment response.

C. GENOTYPE

The HCV genotype is not necessary for the diagnosis of HCV but is extremely important and useful information in making treatment decisions (discussed below) given that it is a major predictor of response. Genotype testing is not necessary in patients without detectable RNA.

D. LIVER FUNCTION TESTS

An elevation of aminotransferases is not required for diagnosis. Up to 30% of patients with chronic HCV have persistently normal ALT. Patients with normal ALT are significantly younger and weigh less compared with those with elevated ALT, but there is no correlation to gender, race, baseline viral titer or HCV genotype. On pretreatment biopsy, 50% of patients with normal ALT had histologic activity index (HAI) scores of 7 or higher and 11% had fibrosis scores of 3–4, compared with 73% and 25%, respectively, in patients with elevated ALT.

E. LIVER BIOPSY

Because the severity of liver damage cannot be determined noninvasively, a liver biopsy is necessary for accurately assessing the degree of inflammation and fibrosis. Biopsy is useful in guiding decisions for therapy initiation and therapy duration. The NIH Consensus Development Conference on Hepatitis C recommended a biopsy in all patients prior to treatment. However, in some cases where results will not alter management, it is acceptable to treat without biopsy.

Clinical Findings

A. ACUTE HCV INFECTION

Acute HCV is asymptomatic in approximately 84% of cases and is usually not recognized clinically. Jaundice, fatigue, fever, nausea, vomiting, and right upper quadrant discomfort can occur, usually within 2–12 weeks of exposure and lasting from 2 to 12 weeks. Diagnosis requires PCR for RNA since acute infections may be seronegative for anti-HCV.

B. CHRONIC HCV INFECTION

Chronic HCV is also asymptomatic in the majority of patients. However, compared with nonhepatitis C control subjects, patients more often report fatigue and right upper quadrant pain, have hepatomegaly, tender liver, and thrombocytopenia, as well as elevated transaminases and bilirubin. ALT values fluctuate in most patients. Extrahepatic manifestations develop in approximately 15% of patients with chronic infection, and may include membranoproliferative glomerulonephritis, thyroiditis, leukocytoclastic vasculitis, porphyria cutanea tarda, and essential mixed cryoglobulinemia.

Natural History

Approximately 85% of those infected with HCV will develop chronic infection and 15% will spontaneously clear virus, although the rate of viral clearance appears to be less common in blacks and those coinfected with HIV. With chronic viremia, the progression of liver damage appears to average approximately one activity grade or fibrosis stage every 7–10 years. Approximately 20–30% of chronic HCV patients develop cirrhosis over 10–20 years of infection. Once cirrhosis develops, however, patients are at increased risk of gastrointestinal bleeding, encephalopathy, life-threatening bacterial infections, and hepatorenal failure. Finally, HCV cirrhosis increases the risk of HCC dramatically. It is estimated that between 2 and 6.7% of all patients with HCV cirrhosis will develop HCC over 10 years and the annual risk is 1–4%. It is rare that HCC will develop in patients without cirrhosis or advanced fibrosis.

The actual rate at which patients with hepatitis C develop serious complications is unclear. The above estimates are based primarily on retrospective analyses, which are often flawed in that they are usually based on patients seen in referral centers. A few prospective studies have gathered outcome data on hepatitis C cohorts, but given the relatively recent discovery of hepatitis C, at this point, these studies have follow-up time only on the order of 5–8 years. Other prospective studies have focused on acute transfusion-associated hepatitis with 4–16 years of follow-up. Although these studies have a defined date of infection, they were not originally designed to examine the clinical outcomes of hepatitis C and do not control for alcohol, do not have biopsy data, and do not have control groups. Cohort studies using stored sera from prior transfusion-associated hepatitis events with renewed prospective follow-up have also been performed, using matched transfused nonhepatitis control subjects from the same studies. One large study of 222 HCV cases and 377 control subjects from three studies with stored sera revealed cirrhosis in 35% of those biopsied and clinical complications of liver disease in 86% of those with cirrhosis and 23% of those with chronic hepatitis alone.

Special Groups

A. CHILDREN

Children who are infected with hepatitis C appear to have a more benign course than adults. In a study of children who contracted hepatitis C genotype 1 through infant cardiac surgery in Germany, 45% of children cleared the virus spontaneously. At a mean of 21 years after infection, only 3 of 17 children had evidence of progressive liver disease on biopsy. These results suggest that viral elimination is more frequent in children and that the interval between infection and development of chronic liver disease seems to be longer than for adults.

B. HCV–HIV

Coinfection with HCV and HIV is common. In one European cohort of over 3000 HIV patients, 33% were anti-HCV positive and in those who were injection drug users, 75% were anti-HCV positive. HIV appears to accelerate the course of disease in HCV infection. In one series, 25% of coinfected patients developed cirrhosis within 15 years, compared with 6.5% in those with only HCV.

C. HCV–HBV

As discussed above, coinfection with HCV and HBV increases the rate of development of cirrhosis and the risk for HCC compared with infection with either virus alone.

Treatment

A. INTERFERON-α AND RIBAVIRIN

Interferon-α is the backbone of treatment for chronic HCV. As discussed in regards to hepatitis B, interferon-α is a glycoprotein that has direct antiviral mechanisms and also has mechanisms of enhancing immune responses to viruses. However, monotherapy with interferon at 3 million units 3 times weekly for 48 weeks produces low sustained virologic response rates of 10–19%. Ribavirin, a synthetic guanosine analogue, has direct action against RNA and DNA viruses and is thought to inhibit a viral-dependent RNA polymerase. Ribavirin given alone has no effects on hepatitis C. However, the combination of ribavirin with the standard interferon regimen improves sustained virologic responses to 38–43%. Recent use of pegylated formulations of interferon-α with ribavirin suggests a somewhat higher response rate (see below). In patients who do develop a sustained virologic response on either monotherapy or combination therapy, histologic improvements also occur. Studies have found that in 86–89% of sustained responders, inflammation decreased on serial liver biopsy. Although some studies have failed to demonstrate an effect on fibrosis, others do demonstrate regression of fibrosis after treatment in 59% of responders compared with 5% of untreated controls. In a pooled analysis of 1509 paired biopsies from subjects in the three major combination therapy trials, 55% of responders had significant regression of fibrosis versus 22% of treated nonresponders after a 3-year follow-up. Reduced morbidity and mortality rates from hepatitis C should parallel these improved rates of virologic and histologic response, but this hypothesis will need to be confirmed in long-term follow up studies with clinical outcome measurements.

Combination therapy is currently indicated for initial therapy in HCV patients. Furthermore, 47% of patients who had an initial response but relapsed after monotherapy have been found to have a sustained response to combination therapy. For those who were nonresponders to monotherapy, response to combination therapy is usually poor (14%) but combination therapy may be offered. Therapy also might be indicated in those with serious extrahepatic manifestations. The typical regimen is interferon-α-2b at 3 million units subcutaneously three times weekly and ribavirin 1000 mg orally daily for patients 75 kg or less and 1200 mg orally daily for patients over 75 kg.

Several variables are associated with increased likelihood of achieving a sustained virologic response: HCV genotype other than 1, low serum HCV RNA levels, and the absence of fibrosis or cirrhosis at baseline. Baseline ALT levels do not predict response to therapy. However, the absence of these characteristics should not be a reason to deny a patient therapy, but may be reason to treat a patient for 48 weeks duration as opposed to 24 weeks. In controlled, multicenter, randomized trials, patients with genotype 1a or 1b had sustained virologic response rates of 16% with a 24-week course of therapy but 28% with a 48-week course. In patients with non-genotype 1, response rates are 66–69% and do not vary significantly with a 24- or 48-week course of therapy. Across all genotypes, patients with baseline cirrhosis or bridging fibrosis, 29% respond to a 24-week course and 38% respond to a 48-week course. In those with minimal or no fibrosis, there is no significant difference in response according to the duration of therapy.

B. SIDE EFFECTS AND MONITORING

Side effects to interferon may include influenza-like symptoms, gastrointestinal symptoms, psychiatric symptoms, leukopenia, neutropenia, thrombocytopenia, thyroid dysfunction, and occasionally respiratory and dermatologic symptoms (Table 35–4). Furthermore, all patients on interferon must be counseled on the possible side effect of birth defects and all female patients should be required to use effective birth control while on treatment. Additional side effects are associated with combination therapy, specifically a hemolytic anemia due to ribavirin. In 8% of patients, a decrease in hemoglobin to less than 10 g/dL necessitated a dose reduction of ribavirin. The frequency of anemia is not associated with duration of therapy and this effect cannot be predicted. Counts recover typically within 4 weeks after treatment is stopped. However, patients with unstable coronary artery or pulmonary disease or those with baseline cell count depression may not be able to tolerate these side effects safely.

Once a patient is started on therapy, close follow-up is essential. Monitoring complete blood counts and platelets is necessary every 1–2 weeks during the first 2 months and then typically every 4–8 weeks during treatment. Periodic thyroid tests are also recommended. In terms of monitoring HCV RNA, in up to 50% of patients who ultimately have a sustained virologic response,

Table 35–4. Side effects of interferon-α and ribavirin in hepatitis C.

Side effects of interferon-α and ribavirin
Leukopenia
Neutropenia
Thrombocytopenia
Hemolytic anemia
Fatigue
Depression and other psychiatric symptoms
Flu-like symptoms: fever, myalgias
Gastrointestinal symptoms: nausea, anorexia
Respiratory symptoms: dyspnea, cough
Diabetes management: irregular glucose control
Thyroid dysfunction: hyperthyroidism, hypothyroidism
Dermatologic symptoms: rash, alopecia

clearance will not occur until after week 12 or 24 of therapy. Therefore, virologic response should not be used to guide duration of therapy until 24 weeks of treatment. Generally, earlier monitoring is unnecessary and may only be discouraging to patient and provider. If HCV RNA is still present at 24 weeks, therapy can be stopped.

C. PEGYLATED INTERFERON-α

Most recently, pegylated interferon-α has been developed and was approved by the FDA in 2001. Pegylated interferons have a covalently attached polyethylene glycol moiety that results in a more sustained absorption and reduced clearance. This has allowed a once-weekly dosing, as compared with the three times weekly dosing required for standard interferon. Results of pegylated interferon-α-2b monotherapy and pegylated α-2a monotherapy are superior to interferon monotherapy. Sustained virologic response was seen in 39% on peginterferon-α-2a versus 19% on interferon. In patients with HCV cirrhosis, 30% achieved a sustained virologic response versus 8% on standard interferon. The safety profile is similar to standard interferon. Pegylated interferon has recently been approved by the FDA in conjunction with ribavirin (Table 35–5).

D. ONGOING ISSUES IN TREATMENT

In addition to the above therapies, amantadine has been studied in combination with interferon but does not have proven additional benefits. Finally, patients frequently inquire about and use herbal medicines. Currently, these have not been systematically evaluated and no guidelines exist for incorporating these into the management of hepatitis C.

Finally, despite the very important and significant improvements in drug treatments, the majority of patients are still not benefited by these therapies, for sev-

eral reasons. First, for many patients, treatment is contraindicated—such as those with major depression or risk for suicide, autoimmune disorders, significantly depressed cell lines, or active cardiopulmonary disease. HIV is not a contraindication to therapy and sustained response rates are approximately equal in HCV with and without HIV. Second, many patients decline treatment due to concern for side effects or do not tolerate treatment. Third, approximately 60% of patients overall do not have a sustained response despite successful completion of therapy. Finally, the effectiveness of current regimens is seen in highly select patients in clinical trials and may not be duplicated in routine practice.

E. OTHER ASPECTS OF DISEASE MANAGEMENT

Although most patients with hepatitis C are asymptomatic, there are many aspects of disease management outside of the treatment possibilities described above. Education and counseling are major aspects to caring for patients with hepatitis C. Due to the risk of increased morbidity and mortality from hepatitis A superinfection, patients who lack hepatitis A IgG antibody should be vaccinated against hepatitis A. Due to the increased risk of cirrhosis and hepatocellular carcinoma, patients who lack hepatitis B surface antibody and have no hepatitis B surface antigen should be vaccinated against hepatitis B. If a patient has isolated positive hepatitis B core antibody, but negative surface antibody, vaccination guidelines are unclear. Alcohol consumption promotes progression of HCV and therefore avoidance of alcohol is recommended. However, it is not known whether small amounts of alcohol are safe. Many patients inquire about diet but none has been shown to be beneficial. Finally, screening for hepatocellular carcinoma in patients is recommended for patients

Table 35–5. Peginterferon-α-2b (12 kDa) plus ribavirin versus interferon-α-2b plus ribavirin, as reported in the product insert[1] and by Manns et al.[2]

	PEG 1.5 µg/kg per Week Plus Ribavirin 800 mg/d		Interferon 3 mU Three Times a Week Plus Ribavirin 1000/1200 mg/d	
	Product Insert	Manns et al	Product Insert	Manns et al
SVR[3] (overall)	52% (264/511)	54% (274/511)	46% (231/505)	47% (235/505)
SVR Genotype 1	41% (141/348)	42% (145/348)	33% (112/343)	33% (114/343)
SVR Genotypes 2–6	75% (123/163)	2/3: 82% (121/147) 4/5/6: 50% (8/16)	73% (119/162)	2/3: 79% (115/146) 4/5/6: 38% (6/16)

[1]Peg-Intron (peginterferon-α-2b) product insert.
[2]Manns MP et al and the International Hepatitis Interventional Therapy Group: Peginterferon α-2b plus ribavirin compared with interferon α-2b plus ribavirin for initial treatment of chronic hepatitis C: a randomized trial. Lancet 2001;358:958.
[3]SVR, sustained virologic response.

with cirrhosis or advanced fibrosis. Although evidence-based guidelines for screening are not available, current recommendations are for α-fetoprotein and radiologic imaging (ultrasound or CT scan) every 6–12 months.

Prevention

Hepatitis C incidence can be reduced by blood donor screening. However, because transfusions account for only 5% of all cases of HCV infection in the United States, reduction in the incidence of posttransfusion HCV infection is unlikely to have an impact on the overall prevalence of disease. Prevention of high-risk drug-related behaviors is the best way to prevent the majority of new infections in the United States since the injection drug using population represents a large reservoir that transmits the virus. Although case studies report success with postexposure interferon therapy, this has not been systematically studied and is not recommended until the diagnosis of infection is established. Efficacy of standard immunoglobulin after needlestick, sexual, or perinatal exposure to HCV has not been determined and is not recommended. Currently there is no vaccine available.

Alter MJ, Kruszon-Moran D, Nainan OV: The prevalence of hepatitis C virus infection in the United states, 1988 through 1994. N Engl J Med 1999;341:556.

McHutchinson J, Gordon SC, Schiff ER: Interferon-α 2-b alone or in combination with ribavirin as initial treatment for chronic hepatitis C. N Engl J Med 1998;339:1485.

National Institutes of Health Consensus Development Conference Panel Statement: management of hepatitis C. Hepatology 1997;26:2S.

Poynard T, Marcellin P, Lee SS: Randomised trial of interferon-α-2b plus ribavirin for 48 weeks or for 24 weeks versus interferon-α-2b plus placebo for 48 weeks for treatment of chronic infection with hepatitis C virus. Lancet 1998;352: 1426.

Reddy KR, Wright TL, Pockros PJ: Efficacy and safety of pegylated (40-kd) interferon-α-2a compared with interferon-α-2a in noncirrhotic patients with chronic hepatitis C. Hepatology 2001;33:433.

Seeff LB, Hollinger FB, Alter HJ: Long-term mortality and morbidity of transfusion-associated non-A, non-B and type C hepatitis: a National Heart, Lung, and Blood Institute collaborative study. Hepatology 2001;33:455.

Shiratori Y, Imazeki F, Moriyama M: Histologic improvement of fibrosis in patients with hepatitis C who have sustained response to interferon therapy. Ann Intern Med 2000;132:517.

Thomas DL, Astemborski J, Rai RM: The natural history of hepatitis C virus infection. JAMA 2000;284:450.

HEPATITIS D

Pathophysiology

Hepatitis D virus (HDV) is a unique hepatitis virus. It is the smallest known animal RNA virus (1.7 kb), approximately 36 nm in size. It contains the HDV RNA genome, two forms of hepatitis delta antigen (HDAg), and a protein envelope. It is replication defective, though, in that it is incapable of making its own envelope protein; rather its envelope consists of the hepatitis B surface antigen (HbsAg). Therefore, envelope production requires HBV and HDV transmission and entry into hepatocytes requires HBV. Overall, HDV infection and replication can occur only in a host with HBV infection. However, HDV inhibits HBV replication, and thus, patients with both HBV and HDV infection are usually HbsAg positive, HBeAg negative, anti-HBe positive, and HBV DNA negative.

In contrast to HBV, the virus is believed to be directly cytopathic. Also unlike HBV, HDV infects only hepatocytes and no extrahepatic sites of viral replication are yet identified. In acute HDV infection, microvesicular steatosis and granular eosinophilic necrosis are often seen. In chronic hepatitis D, necroinflammatory activity is often severe but no specific histologic features are noted, and HDAg is readily demonstrated in nuclei and, to a lesser extent, cytoplasm of hepatocytes.

HDV is classified into three genotypes that appear to have clinical significance. Genotype II is relatively less pathogenic than genotype I. Genotype III is frequently associated with fulminant hepatitis.

Prevalence & Epidemiology

HDV infection occurs worldwide but incidence and prevalence data are limited due to inaccurate reporting and delayed detection. Worldwide, HDV is present in less than 5% of chronic HBV carriers. The number of new cases appears to be steadily decreasing in all parts of the world as well, although in the 1970s an epidemic of HDV was occurring. Higher prevalence also exists in older populations, reflecting an earlier cohort effect.

HDV is transmitted primarily by parenteral or inapparent parenteral routes. HDV is most commonly found in patients with prior or ongoing parenteral drug use, or in their sexual contacts. In parts of the Mediterranean and other endemic areas, HDV is transmitted without known parenteral contact.

HDV has significant geographic distribution by genotype. Genotype I is predominant in most areas, specifically North America, North Africa, the Middle East, Italy, and East Asia. Genotype II is isolated only from Japan and Taiwan. Genotype III is found exclusively in northern South America.

Essentials of Diagnosis

HDV infection occurs only in the presence of HBV infection (HBsAg positive) and is detected by anti-HDV (IgM for acute or IgG for chronic infection). There are no commercial assays for detection of HDAg. As described above, given that HBV replication is usually suppressed by HDV, HBV markers may resemble a carrier state with HbsAg positive, HBeAg negative, anti-HBe positive, and HBV DNA negative. Assessing the severity of liver disease would require a work-up similar to that described for chronic hepatitis B.

Clinical Findings

A. ACUTE HBV–HDV COINFECTION

Acute coinfection is characterized by a severe hepatitis with hepatocellular necrosis and inflammation. The majority of cases, however, are self-limiting, with clearance of HBV and therefore HDV. Fulminant hepatitis is infrequent overall, but is still 10 times more common than in acute hepatitis B alone. Labrea fever is an unusual form of delta hepatitis described from the Amazon basin in which fulminant hepatitis results in jaundice, fever, and black vomit.

B. ACUTE HDV SUPERINFECTION

Acute superinfection of HDV on a chronic HBV patient is often clinically distinguishable. Typically a severe marked hepatitis is seen, with high levels of HDV virus. The majority of cases do not resolve but rather lead to chronic coinfection.

C. CHRONIC HBV–HDV INFECTION

HDV viremia continues, although at lower levels than is seen during acute HDV superinfection. On biopsy, necroinflammatory lesions are notable and are typically more severe than that seen in chronic HBV. Episodes of acute hepatitis can also mark the course in chronic coinfection.

Natural History

A. ACUTE HBV–HDV COINFECTION

Acute coinfection resolves in 80–95% of cases, with elimination of HBV through humoral immune mechanisms. The immune response to HDV is usually limited to IgM but with HbsAg clearance, HDV infection is also cleared. However, 2–20% develop fulminant hepatitis and in 30% of cases of fulminant hepatitis due to acute hepatitis B, a simultaneous acute hepatitis D infection is detected. In addition, 2–5% of acute coinfection cases result in chronic infection. Finally, in acute simultaneous HBV and HDV infection among drug addicts, the case fatality rate approaches 5%.

B. ACUTE HDV SUPERINFECTION

Unlike acute coinfection, HDV superinfection results in chronic HDV–HBV in more than 70–80% of cases.

Similar to acute coinfection, acute HDV superinfection results in fulminant hepatitis in 2–20% of cases. In 30% of cases of fulminant hepatitis in chronic hepatitis B patients, acute hepatitis D infection can be demonstrated. Superinfection resolves in approximately 20%. In some outbreaks of severe delta superinfection in populations with a high HBV carrier rate, mortality is in excess of 20%.

C. CHRONIC HBV–HDV INFECTION

Initial associations of chronic HDV were that of severe liver disease, but there also may be a chronic healthy carrier state for HDV, similar to that noted with HBV. Chronic HDV does progress to cirrhosis frequently. In Italy, 50% of chronic hepatitis B carriers with cirrhosis had HDV infection, although only 3% of chronic hepatitis B carriers are infected with HDV. The development of cirrhosis is also more rapid than for chronic HBV or chronic HCV, and there is a predominance of coinfected patients with cirrhosis who are young. Also in Italy, 10–15% of patients progress to cirrhosis and clinical liver failure within a few years after superinfection of HDV while the remainder progress to cirrhosis slowly and similarly to an isolated HBV infection. Although chronic HBV infection is a well-recognized risk factor for the development of hepatocellular carcinoma, a similar association has not been clearly demonstrated for chronic HDV infection. Overall, the pattern of disease progression appears to vary with geography, genotype, and mode of transmission. Slowly progressive, mild disease is more common in endemic areas. On the other hand, HDV disease appears to be more severe in nonendemic areas where injection drug use is the main form of transmission.

Treatment

Therapy for chronic hepatitis D is problematic. Interferon-α results in initial biochemical and virologic responses but relapses are common unless the HbsAg is cleared. Long-term interferon has been tried but the side effects, inconvenience and cost, make this a difficult option. A pilot study of lamivudine monotherapy has been reported, but although HBV DNA suppression occurred, HDV RNA was not cleared. A pilot study of lamivudine and interferon-α combination therapy has also recently been reported, but neither aminotransferase nor HDV RNA levels normalized. Patients with decompensated cirrhosis resulting from chronic delta hepatitis are good candidates for liver transplantation, as risk of recurrent hepatitis is lower than that in patients with chronic HBV cirrhosis without HDV.

Prevention

Because of its requirement for chronic HBV infection, HDV infection can be prevented by vaccinating susceptible persons with hepatitis B vaccine. No effective vaccine is available for preventing delta superinfection in HBsAg carriers.

Casey JL: Hepatitis delta virus: genetics and pathogenesis. Clin Lab Med 1996;16:451.

Hadziyannis SJ: Delta hepatitis. J Gastroenterol Hepatol 1997;12:289.

Huang YH, Wu JC, Sheng WY: Diagnostic value of anti-hepatitis D virus (HDV) antibodies revisited: a study of total and IgM anti-HDV compared with detection of HDV-RNA by polymerase chain reaction. J Gastroenterol Hepatol 1998;13:57.

Huo TI, Wu JC, Chung-Ru L: Comparison of clinico-pathological features in hepatitis B virus-associated hepatocellular carcinoma with or without hepatitis D virus superinfection. J Hepatol 1996;25:439.

Lau DT, Doo E, Park Y: Lamivudine for chronic delta hepatitis. Hepatology 1999;30:546.

London WT, Evans AA: The epidemiology of hepatitis viruses B, C, and D. Clin Lab Med 1996;16:251.

Taylor JM: Hepatitis delta virus. Intervirology 1999;42:173.

Wolters LM, Van Nunen AB, Honkoop P: Lamivudine—high dose interferon combination therapy for chronic hepatitis B patients co-infected with the hepatitis D virus. J Viral Hepatitis 2000;7:428.

HEPATITIS E

Pathophysiology

Hepatitis E virus (HEV) is a small, 32–34 nm, nonenveloped spherical RNA virus. Its genome has been cloned. Transmission is through the fecal–oral route and the main target cells are hepatocytes. There are two main strains, Burmese (or Asian) and Mexican. However, new isolates of HEV have recently been identified in the United States, Italy, Greece, and China. The new United States isolates appear to be near identical to a swine HEV, ubiquitous in pigs in the United States.

Prevalence & Epidemiology

HEV is endemic in India and Southeast and Central Asia. It is responsible for common source outbreaks in these and other developing countries. Outbreaks can be marked with either an increase in the number of sporadic cases or an attack in thousands of people. These outbreaks develop most frequently after rainy seasons, as ingestion of fecally contaminated water is a common route for transmission. The largest group affected is young adults, aged 15–40 years, with relatively low attack rates in children.

HEV infection is rare in the United States except when imported by visitors from endemic areas.

Essentials of Diagnosis

HEV infection is diagnosed by the presence of anti-HEV. Assays are available for either IgM or IgG class. The IgM anti-HEV is nondetectable after a few months whereas IgG persists for several years. PCR for the detection of HEV RNA in the stool or serum is also now available.

Clinical Findings

The incubation period for hepatitis E ranges from 2 to 10 weeks. The clinical course is similar to hepatitis A, but generally the infection is more severe. Acute hepatitis E has an insidious onset, most commonly beginning with a prodromal phase of a few days with flu-like symptoms, fever, abdominal pain, nausea and vomiting, dark urine and clay-colored stools, diarrhea, and a transient macular skin rash. This leads to development of jaundice, resolution of the prodromal symptoms, and a severe hepatitis with bilirubinemia, transaminitis, and mild alkaline phosphatase elevations. Histologicly, cholestasis with rosette formation of hepatocytes and polymorphonuclear leukocytes may be prominent, but the degree of transaminitis does not correlate with the degree of liver injury.

Natural History

Acute hepatitis E is self-limiting and the illness usually lasts 1–4 weeks although some patients have a prolonged cholestatic hepatitis lasting 2–6 months. There are no reports of persistent viremia, chronic hepatitis E, or cirrhosis resulting from acute infection. The case fatality rate is 1–2% although there is a much higher mortality (10–30%) in pregnant women, particularly if they are in the third trimester. Children appear to have a milder course than adults.

Treatment

Treatment is largely supportive, and no effective vaccine is yet available.

Prevention

The only prophylactic measures against HEV infection that can be currently recommended are improved sanitation and sanitary handling of food and water. Boiling water appears to reduce the risk of contraction. There is no indication for isolation of affected persons, as person-to-person transmission is rare. The efficacy of passive immunization with immunoglobulin for prevention of HEV infection is under evaluation. Currently, vaccines for pregnant women and travelers are under development.

Aggarwak R, Krawczynski K: Hepatitis E: an overview and recent advances in clinical and laboratory research. J Gastroenterol Hepatol 2000;15:9.

Chadha MS, Walimbe AM, Arankalle VA: Retrospective serological analysis of hepatitis E patients: a long-term follow-up study. J Viral Hepatitis 1999;6:457.

Harris TJ: Hepatitis E virus—an update. Liver 1999;19:171.

Krawczynski K, Aggarwak R, Kamili S: Hepatitis E. Infect Dis Clin North Am 2000;14:669.

Reichler MR, Valway SE, Onorato IM: Acute hepatitis E infection acquired in California. Clin Infect Dis 2000;30:618.

Schwartz E, Jenks NP, Van Damme P: Hepatitis E virus infection in travelers. Clin Infect Dis 1999;29:1312.

Wu JC, Sheen IJ, Chiang TY: The impact of traveling to endemic areas on the spread of hepatitis E virus infection: epidemiological and molecular analyses. Hepatology 1998;27:1415.

Chronic Nonviral Hepatitis

36

Albert J. Czaja, MD

Chronic nonviral hepatitis is an unresolving inflammation of the liver of unknown cause. Autoimmune hepatitis, cryptogenic chronic hepatitis, autoimmune cholangitis, and autoimmune hepatitis with variant features ("overlap syndromes") warrant the designation. Each entity lacks pathognomonic features, and diagnosis is based on the exclusion of other similar conditions. A careful clinical history, a battery of laboratory tests, and expert examination of liver tissue can confidently secure the diagnosis in most instances. Granulomatous hepatitis is not a true hepatitis, but it can be included within the category.

By definition, patients lack serological evidence of active infection with viruses that can produce chronic hepatitis (hepatitis B and C viruses) or syndromes that can resemble chronic hepatitis (Epstein–Barr virus and cytomegalovirus) (Table 36–1). Disease activity can usually be documented for at least 6 months, but an abrupt and rarely fulminant presentation is also recognized. Hereditary diseases (Wilson disease, genetic hemochromatosis, and α₁-antitrypsin deficiency), alcoholic and nonalcoholic steatohepatitis, bile duct diseases (primary biliary cirrhosis and primary sclerosing cholangitis), and drug-induced liver disease (especially those associated with minocycline, nitrofurantoin, isoniazid, propylthiouracil, or α-methyldopa) may at times resemble chronic nonviral hepatitis. Each has pathogenic mechanisms, pertinent historic features, clinical and histologic findings, and/or behaviors that distinguish them (see Table 36–1).

AUTOIMMUNE HEPATITIS

Autoimmune hepatitis is an inflammatory process involving mainly hepatocytes that is self-perpetuated by a presumed immune reaction against normal liver cell membrane protein or antigens expressed on that membrane. The disease implies the existence of a triggering factor, impairment of host immune modulation, membrane expression of a target autoantigen, and expansion of cytotoxic T lymphocytes that infiltrate and destroy liver tissue. The bases for the loss of self-tolerance are unclear, but a genetic propensity for autoimmune expression is an important requisite.

CD4 T helper cells are the key effectors, and they can differentiate into cytotoxic T lymphocytes or au-

toantibody-producing cells depending on the cytokine milieu. Polymorphisms of the *tumor necrosis factor-α* gene can favor a type 1 cytokine response, and antigen-sensitized cytotoxic T lymphocytes can be present within liver tissue. These findings have supported hypotheses of pathogenesis based on a cell-mediated form of cytotoxicity. Overexpression of interleukin 10 can favor a type 2 cytokine response in some patients, and antigen–antibody complexes on the hepatocyte membrane can be targeted by natural killer cells. These findings have supported hypotheses of pathogenesis based on an antibody-dependent, cell-mediated form of cytotoxicity. Cytokines are cross-regulatory and interactive, and there may be different cytokine responses at different stages of the disease. Cell-mediated and antibody-dependent mechanisms of liver cell injury may coexist and variably dominate during the illness.

Diagnosis

Autoimmune hepatitis is characterized by autoantibodies directed against nuclear, cytosolic and/or microsomal components of the hepatocyte (Table 36–2), hypergammaglobulinemia with predominant elevation of the immunoglobulin G fraction, and the presence of at least interface hepatitis ("piecemeal necrosis" or "periportal hepatitis") on histologic examination (Figure 36–1). The disease typically responds to corticosteroid therapy, but this response is not a requisite for the diagnosis. Acute, even fulminant, presentations are possible, and the diagnosis can be made at presentation without establishing 6 months of disease duration.

The definite diagnosis of autoimmune hepatitis requires negative serologic markers of active viral infection; denial of parenteral exposure to blood or blood products; absence of other etiologic factors such as excess alcohol consumption and drug use; seropositivity for antinuclear antibodies (ANA), smooth muscle antibodies (SMA), or antibodies to liver/kidney microsome type 1 (anti-LKM1) at titers of at least 1:80; total serum globulin, γ-globulin or immunoglobulin G levels of greater than 1.5 times the upper limit of normal; predominant serum aminotransferase elevations; interface hepatitis with or without lobular hepatitis; and no biliary lesions, granulomas, siderosis, copper deposits, or other histologic changes suggestive of a different etiol-

Table 36–1. Differential diagnosis of chronic nonviral hepatitis and features of alternative diagnoses.[1]

Differential Diagnosis	Features Suggestive of Alternative Diagnosis
Chronic hepatitis B	HBsAg, HBV DNA
Chronic hepatitis C	Anti-HCV, RIBA reactivity, HCV RNA
Wilson disease	Low ceruloplasmin level, Kayser-Fleischer rings
α_1-Antitrypsin deficiency	Low α_1-antitrypsin level, MZ or ZZ phenotype
Genetic hemochromatosis	Elevated serum ferritin level, high transferrin saturation, hepatic iron index > 1.9, homozygosity for C282Y or H63D mutations
Alcoholic steatohepatitis	Fatty liver, Mallory bodies, regular alcohol excess
Nonalcoholic steatohepatitis	Fatty liver, Mallory bodies, alcohol abstinence, obesity, diabetes, and/or hyperlipidemia
Primary biliary cirrhosis	Antimitochondrial antibodies, florid duct lesions, interlobular duct damage
Autoimmune cholangitis	High titer ANA, absent AMA, no inflammatory bowel disease, florid duct lesion, or interlobular duct damage and/or loss
Primary sclerosing cholangitis	Inflammatory bowel disease, abnormal cholangiogram, fibrous obliterative cholangitis, or interlobular bile duct damage and/or loss
Drug-induced liver disease	Active exposure to minocycline, nitrofurantoin, isoniazid, propylthiouracil, or α-methyldopa

[1]HBsAg, hepatitis B surface antigen; HBV DNA, hepatitis B virus DNA in serum; anti-HCV, antibodies to hepatitis C virus; RIBA, recombinant immunoblot assay; HCV RNA, hepatitis C virus RNA in serum; ANA, antinuclear antibodies; AMA, antimitochondrial antibodies.

Table 36–2. Autoantibodies associated with autoimmune hepatitis.

Autoantibodies[1]	Autoantigen(s)	Clinical Implication(s)
Antinuclear	Histones, centromere, ribonucleoproteins	Type 1 autoimmune hepatitis
Smooth muscle	Actin and nonactin components (tubulin, vimentin, desmin, and skeletin)	Type 1 autoimmune hepatitis
Liver/kidney microsome type 1	P450 IID6 (CYP2D6)	Type 2 autoimmune hepatitis Autoimmune polyglandular syndrome type 1
Soluble liver antigen/liver pancreas	Transfer ribonucleoprotein complex (tRNP(ser)sec)	Type 1 autoimmune hepatitis "Type 3" autoimmune hepatitis Cryptogenic chronic hepatitis
Perinuclear antineutrophil cytoplasmic antibodies	Unknown; reacts to neutrophils and monocytes; possible nuclear membrane lamina	Type 1 autoimmune hepatitis Cryptogenic chronic hepatitis
Asialoglycoprotein receptor	Transmembrane hepatocytic glycoprotein	Common marker for all types Reflects disease activity Indicates relapse tendency
Actin	Polymerized F actin	Type 1 autoimmune hepatitis Early age onset disease Lower frequency of remission
Liver cytosol type 1	Formiminotransferase cyclodeaminase Argininosuccinate lyase	Type 2 autoimmune hepatitis Early age onset Aggressive disease

[1]Italics indicated limited availability and/or investigational use only.

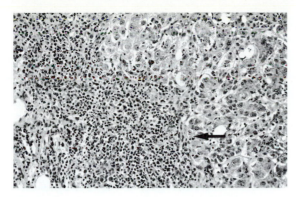

Figure 36–1. Interface hepatitis. Interface hepatitis ("piecemeal necrosis" or periportal hepatitis) is the histologic hallmark of autoimmune hepatitis, but it is not pathognomonic of the disease. It connotes disruption of the limiting plate of the portal tract by a mononuclear inflammatory infiltrate (H&E; original magnification ×200).

ogy. Portal plasma cell infiltration is characteristic of the disease but not a requirement for diagnosis. A cholestatic form of autoimmune hepatitis is not recognized.

A probable diagnosis of autoimmune hepatitis is justified if serum γ-globulin levels are abnormal but not high; autoantibody titers are less than 1:80; other than conventional liver-related autoantibodies are present such as antibodies to soluble liver antigen/liver pancreas (anti-SLA/LP) or antibodies to asialoglycoprotein receptor (anti-ASGPR); and risk factors such as previous alcohol use or exposure to hepatotoxic medications are present but not associated with current inflammatory activity.

A scoring system has been proposed to accommodate all manifestations of the disorder and grade the net strength of the diagnosis (Table 36–3). Inconsistent findings, such as the presence of antimitochondrial antibodies (AMA), absence of immunoserologic markers, evidence of concurrent viral infection, or histologic features

Table 36–3. Scoring system for the diagnosis of autoimmune hepatitis.[1]

Category	Factor	Score	Category	Factor	Score
Gender	Female	+2	Other associated antibodies	Anti-SLA/LP Anti-ASGPR pANCA	+2
Alk Phos: AST (or ALT) ratio	>3 <1.5	−2 +2	Immune disease	Patient or relative	+2
γ-Globulin or IgG levels above normal	>2.0 1.5–2.0 1.0–1.5 <1.0	+3 +2 +1 0	Histologic features	Interface hepatitis Rosettes Plasma cells None of above Biliary changes Other changes	+3 +1 +1 −5 −3 −3
ANA, SMA, or LKM1 titers	>1:80 1:80 1:40 <1:40	+3 +2 +1 0	Responses to steroid therapy	Complete Relapse	+2 +3
AMA	Positive	−4			
Viral markers	Positive Negative	−4 +1			
Drugs	Yes No	−4 +1	Pretreatment score Definite diagnosis Probable diagnosis		>15 10–15
Alcohol intake	<25 g daily >60 g daily	+2 −2	Posttreatment score Definite diagnosis Probable diagnosis		>17 12–17
HLA	DR3 or DR4	+1			

[1]Alk phos, serum alkaline phosphatase level; AST, serum aspartate aminotransferase level; ALT, serum alanine aminotransferase level; IgG, serum immunoglobulin G level; ANA, antinuclear antibodies; SMA, smooth muscle antibodies; LKM1, antibodies to liver/kidney microsome type 1; AMA, antimitochondrial antibodies; HLA, human leukocyte antigens; anti-SLA/LP, antibodies to soluble liver antigen/liver pancreas; anti-ASGPR, antibodies to asialoglycoprotein receptor; pANCA, perinuclear antineutrophil cytoplasmic antibodies.

of bile duct damage, do not preclude the diagnosis if other more characteristic features outweigh these isolated occurrences. Responsiveness to corticosteroid therapy can upgrade the diagnosis in those patients with probable or indefinite diagnoses at presentation. The scoring system is useful in evaluating patients with variant or overlap syndromes to determine the predominant manifestations of the disease. It can also be used to establish the strength of a clinical trial and the comparability of different clinical trials. In most instances, the scoring system is unnecessary for routine clinical practice. Prospective application is required to confirm its validity.

Liver biopsy examination is essential for the definite diagnosis. Interface hepatitis with or without acinar (lobular) hepatitis can occur in acute and chronic viral and drug-related liver disease, but it is the *sine qua non* for the diagnosis of autoimmune hepatitis. Individual histologic findings, such as moderate to severe interface hepatitis (see Figure 36–1), acinar (lobular) hepatitis (Figure 36–2), and plasma cell infiltration of the portal tracts (Figure 36–3) in the absence of portal lymphoid aggregates, steatosis, and bile duct injury (Figure 36–4), can distinguish autoimmune hepatitis from chronic hepatitis C. These patterns have a specificity of 81% and overall predictability of 62% for autoimmune hepatitis. Their sensitivity, however, is only 40%, and many patients with autoimmune hepatitis lack these characteristic histologic features. In these patients with compatible but not distinctive histologic features, diagnosis depends on the strength of the other findings.

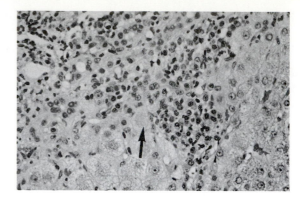

Figure 36–3. Plasma cell infiltration. Numerous plasma cells in groups or sheets in the portal tracts or as groups in the sinusoids characterize autoimmune hepatitis, but they are not requisites for the diagnosis (H&E; original magnification ×400).

Subclassifications

Three types of autoimmune hepatitis have been proposed based on immunoserologic markers, and a jargon has evolved to accommodate this proposal (Table 36–4). None of the types has been officially endorsed, and treatment strategies are similar for each. Confident subclassifications await the identification of distinctive etiologic factors and pathogenic mechanisms.

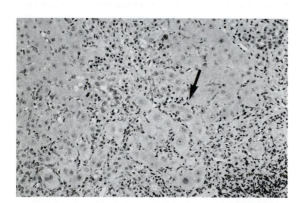

Figure 36–2. Acinar hepatitis. Prominent cellular infiltrates lining sinusoidal spaces in association with liver cell degenerative or regenerative changes connote acinar (lobular) hepatitis. Moderate to severe acinar hepatitis can be present in autoimmune hepatitis, especially during relapse after corticosteroid withdrawal (H&E; original magnification ×200).

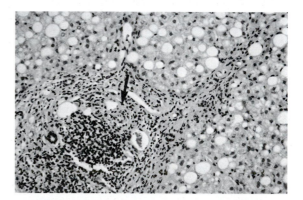

Figure 36–4. Portal lymphoid aggregate and steatosis. Densely packed small lymphocytes within a portal tract or a germinal center with surrounding small lymphocytes support the diagnosis of chronic hepatitis C. Small, large, or mixed-size vacuoles of lipid within the cytoplasm of hepatocytes also typify chronic hepatitis C (H&E; original magnification ×400).

Table 36–4. Subclassification of autoimmune hepatitis based on immunoserologic markers.[1]

Features	Type 1	Type 2	Type 3
Signature autoantibodies	SMA, ANA	LKM1	SLA/LP
Associated autoantibodies	Actin, pANCA	Liver cytosol 1	SMA, ANA
Autoantigen	Unknown	P450 IID6 (CYP2D6)	tRNP [(ser) sec]
Associated syndromes	None	Autoimmune polyglandular syndrome type 1	Type 1 autoimmune hepatitis
Populations at risk	Adult	Children	Adult
Common associated immune diseases	Autoimmune thyroiditis, Graves' disease, synovitis, ulcerative colitis	Type 1 diabetes, vitiligo, autoimmune thyroiditis	Same as type 1
Acute onset	Common	Common	Common
HLA associations	HLA DR 3 HLA DR4	HLA B14 HLA DR3	HLA DR3
Susceptibility alleles	DRB1*0301 DRB1*0401	C4A-QO DRB1*07	Uncertain
Treatment	Prednisone alone or with azathioprine	Prednisone alone or with azathioprine	Prednisone alone or with azathioprine

[1]SMA, smooth muscle antibodies; ANA, antinuclear antibodies; LKM1, antibodies to liver/kidney microsome type 1; SLA/LP, antibodies to soluble liver antigen/liver pancreas; pANCA, perinuclear antineutrophil cytoplasmic antibodies; tRNP[(ser)sec], transfer ribonucleoprotein complex; HLA, human leukocyte antigen.

A. TYPE 1 AUTOIMMUNE HEPATITIS

Type 1 autoimmune hepatitis is characterized by the presence of SMA and/or ANA, and it constitutes the vast majority (80%) of patients with autoimmune hepatitis in the United States (see Table 36–4). Seventy percent are women who are typically less than 40 years old. Thirty-four percent have concurrent immune diseases, especially autoimmune thyroiditis, Graves' disease, and/or ulcerative colitis. The presence of ulcerative colitis is compatible with the diagnosis, but it compels cholangiography and expert histologic examination to exclude primary sclerosing cholangitis. Forty-two percent of patients with ulcerative colitis have cholangiographic changes of primary sclerosing cholangitis and recalcitrance to corticosteroid therapy. In contrast, most patients with ulcerative colitis have normal cholangiograms and a good response to corticosteroid treatment. Ulcerative colitis per se is not a determinant of treatment response.

Twenty-five percent of patients with type 1 autoimmune hepatitis have cirrhosis at the time of presentation, indicating that the disease has an indolent but aggressive subclinical stage. Forty percent have an acute onset of symptoms that can be mistaken for an acute self-limited

viral infection or toxic injury. Failure to recognize this presentation may needlessly delay institution of potentially life-saving therapy. Patients with an acute onset commonly have features that suggest chronicity, such as hypoalbuminemia, hypergammaglobulinemia, ascites, or cytopenia. In these cases, the "acute" onset of illness may represent an exacerbation of longstanding, preexistent, subclinical disease. Signs of chronicity, including histologic features of fibrosis, are not required for the diagnosis, and autoimmune hepatitis should be considered in all individuals with acute liver disease of undetermined cause.

The target autoantigen of type 1 autoimmune hepatitis remains uncertain, and none of the autoantibodies that characterize the disorder is pathogenic. Viruses have been proposed as triggering agents, and isolated case reports have linked the disease to infections with hepatitis A virus, hepatitis B virus, hepatitis C virus, measles virus, and the human immunodeficiency virus. Multiple drugs, especially minocycline and nitrofurantoin, have also been incriminated. The diversity of putative inciting agents suggests that molecular mimicry between foreign antigens and self antigens triggers a common pathogenic pathway. The critical epitope may be short and shared by multiple antigens. The cause of autoimmune hepatitis may not be necessary for its perpetuation, and a long lag time between the trigger and the clinical disease may prevent discovery of the etiology.

Hepatitis C virus (HCV) has been the most thoroughly studied of the candidate agents. Initial studies using first-generation immunoassays for the detection of antibodies to HCV (anti-HCV) indicated seropositivity in over 40% of patients with autoimmune hepatitis. Subsequent studies recognized a high frequency of false positivity associated with the confounding effects of hypergammaglobulinemia on the assay system. Second- and third-generation immunoassays and assessments by polymerase chain reaction for HCV RNA in serum now indicate that HCV infection is uncommon in type 1 autoimmune hepatitis (6–11%) and either an unimportant etiologic factor or a coincidental finding.

B. TYPE 2 AUTOIMMUNE HEPATITIS

Type 2 autoimmune hepatitis is characterized by anti-LKM1 (Table 36–4). These antibodies infrequently coexist with SMA and/or ANA (4% concurrence in adult patients). Detection by indirect immunofluorescence requires reactivity against the proximal tubules of the murine kidney and the cytoplasm of murine hepatocytes. An exuberant reaction can obscure the distinction between proximal and distal renal tubules and suggest the presence of AMA. Retrospective analyses have indicated that 27% of patients with autoimmune hepatitis and AMA are seropositive for anti-LKM1.

Type 2 autoimmune hepatitis affects mainly children (ages 2 to 14 years) (see Table 36–4). It is most prevalent in France and Germany and rare among children and adults with autoimmune hepatitis in the United States. Patients with type 2 autoimmune hepatitis can have low serum levels of immunoglobulin A; absence of ANA and SMA; frequent concurrent immune diseases, including vitiligo, insulin-dependent diabetes, and autoimmune thyroiditis; and diverse organ-specific autoantibodies, including antibodies to parietal cells, islets of Langerhans, and thyroid. Corticosteroid therapy is effective, and outcomes are similar to patients with type 1 disease.

The cytochrome monooxygenase, P-450 IID6 (CYP2D6), is the target autoantigen. This drug-metabolizing enzyme is expressed on the hepatocyte membrane of humans with the disease, and its expression can be modulated by tumor necrosis factor and interleukins. P-450 IID6 (CYP2D6) exhibits genetic polymorphism, and it is absent in 10% of individuals. Genetic variability in the expression of the autoantigen may explain in part regional differences in the prevalence of type 2 disease.

Antibodies to LKM1 recognize a short linear amino acid sequence of the recombinant P-450 IID6 (CYP2D6) antigen, and they inhibit enzyme function

in vitro. Recombinant P-450 IID6 (CYP2D6) has been mapped for T and B cell epitopes, and it has been used as the basis for a diagnostic enzyme immunoassay to detect antibodies to the antigen (anti-P-450 IID6). Serum from patients with type 2 autoimmune hepatitis reacts with amino acid sequence 254–271 in the recombinant antigen, and reactivity against this "core motif" distinguishes patients with type 2 autoimmune hepatitis from patients with nonspecific reactivity to other epitopes on the same antigen.

Homologies exist between the recombinant P-450 IID6 (CYP2D6) antigen and the genome of the hepatitis C virus. This molecular mimicry can result in cross-reacting antibodies, and as many as 10% of patients with true HCV infection have anti-LKM1. This association is more common in western Europe than in the United States where surveys have failed to detect anti-LKM1 in any patients with chronic hepatitis C. Genomic sequencing has not indicated differences in the viral genome of patients with and without anti-LKM1, and the basis for expression of anti-LKM1 in some patients with chronic hepatitis C may reflect host susceptibility factors that remain undefined. Homologies also exist between the recombinant P-450 IID6 (CYP2D6) antigen and the herpes simplex type 2 virus, and there may be yet undescribed mimicries with other viruses. Antibodies to LKM1 associated with chronic hepatitis C react to diverse epitopes of the recombinant P-450 IID6 (CYP2D6) antigen, and they can usually be distinguished from the anti-LKM1 of type 2 autoimmune hepatitis, which react only to the amino acid sequence 254–272.

Fifteen percent of patients with the autoimmune polyglandular syndrome type 1 (APS1) have anti-LKM1 and type 2 autoimmune hepatitis (see Table 36–4). This syndrome must be distinguished from patients with classic type 2 autoimmune hepatitis since patients with APS1 have an aggressive liver disease that may be recalcitrant to corticosteroid treatment. APS1 is characterized by ectodermal dystrophy, mucocutaneous candidiasis, multiple endocrine gland failure (parathyroids, adrenal, and/or ovaries), autoantibody production, and autoimmune hepatitis in various syndromatic combinations. APS1 has a mendelian pattern of inheritance, complete penetrance of the gene, no HLA associations, and no female predominance. The susceptibility gene is located on chromosome 21q22.3, and it encodes a transcription factor, designated the autoimmune regulator (AIRE), which modulates clonal deletion of autoreactive T cells in the thymus and affects self-tolerance. The autoantigens of APS1 are P-450 IA2 and P-450 IA6.

C. TYPE 3 AUTOIMMUNE HEPATITIS

Type 3 autoimmune hepatitis is the least established form of the disease (see Table 36–4). It is characterized by the presence of antibodies to anti-SLA/LP. These antibodies have high specificity for autoimmune hepatitis, and a transfer ribonucleoprotein complex responsible for incorporating selenocysteine into peptide chains (tRNP$^{(ser)sec}$) is the probable autoantigen. Patients with type 3 autoimmune hepatitis are young and predominantly women (90%). They typically lack anti-LKM1, but 74% have other autoantibodies, including SMA or AMA. Eleven percent of patients with type 1 autoimmune hepatitis have anti-SLA/LP, and these patients are indistinguishable from seronegative counterparts by clinical and laboratory findings. Preliminary studies have suggested that patients with anti-SLA/LP have more severe disease and/or a higher frequency of relapse after corticosteroid withdrawal than their seronegative counterparts, but these distinctions have not yet justified their separate classification. The greatest clinical value of testing for anti-SLA/LP may be in assessing patients with cryptogenic chronic hepatitis. Eighteen percent of these patients have anti-SLA/LP, and they can be redesignated as autoimmune hepatitis.

Other Autoantibodies

Other autoantibodies have been associated with autoimmune hepatitis, but clinically distinct subgroups have not been identified or been generally available. New antibodies continue to be characterized in the hope of improving diagnostic and prognostic tools or discovering pathogenic mechanisms.

A. ANTIBODIES TO ASIALOGLYCOPROTEIN RECEPTOR

Antibodies to asialoglycoprotein receptor (anti-ASGR) are present in all types of autoimmune hepatitis, and they are generic markers of the disease (see Table 36–2). The autoantibodies are directed against a transmembrane hepatocytic glycoprotein that can capture, display, and internalize potential antigens, induce T cell proliferation, and activate cytotoxic T cells. The function and location of the asialoglycoprotein receptor are ideal for processing self-antigens or foreign antigens that resemble self-antigens, and the receptor may be important in triggering the autoimmune response. Antibody reactivity correlates with inflammatory activity and the antibodies disappear during successful therapy. Loss of these antibodies prior to drug withdrawal may identify patients who are less likely to relapse.

B. ANTIBODIES TO ACTIN

Antibodies to actin (antiactin) have greater specificity for autoimmune hepatitis than SMA, but they are frequently absent in patients with definite disease (see Table 36–2). Consequently, screening for antiactin has limited value, and testing for SMA is the preferred diagnostic tool. Preliminary studies using multiple assays for antiactin have indicated their occurrence in patients with early age onset disease and poor response to corticosteroid therapy. They may evolve as indices of prognosis, but their clinical utility depends on the emergence of a confident assay. Currently, there are four assays for antiactin and controversy about the importance of a thermolabile F-actin depolymerizing factor on assay performance.

C. ANTIBODIES TO LIVER CYTOSOL TYPE 1

Antibodies to liver cytosol type 1 (anti-LC1) are specific markers of autoimmune hepatitis, and they may have prognostic implications (see Table 36–2). Seropositivity is rare in patients older than 40 years, and it increases in populations younger than 20 years. Antibodies to LC1 commonly are associated with anti-LKM1 and type 2 autoimmune hepatitis, concurrent immune diseases, severe inflammation, and progression to cirrhosis. Formiminotransferase cyclodeaminase and argininosuccinate lyase have been proposed as the target autoantigens. Failure to detect anti-LC1 in children with fulminant autoimmune hepatitis and the occurrence of these antibodies in patients with chronic hepatitis C or primary sclerosing cholangitis have raised questions about their clinical utility. Serum levels of anti-LC1 fluctuate with inflammatory activity, and the assay may prove useful as a barometer of disease severity or a probe of pathogenic mechanisms.

D. PERINUCLEAR ANTINEUTROPHIL CYTOPLASMIC ANTIBODIES

Perinuclear antineutrophil cytoplasmic antibodies (pANCA) are found in high titer in 50–90% of patients with type 1 autoimmune hepatitis, and they have been useful in reclassifying patients with cryptogenic chronic hepatitis (see Table 36–2). Their absence in type 2 autoimmune hepatitis suggests that they have specificity for certain clinical syndromes, but their occurrence in ulcerative colitis and primary sclerosing cholangitis indicates that this specificity is limited. The pANCA of type 1 autoimune hepatitis react against neutrophils and monocytes, and they are mainly of the immunoglobulin G_1 isotype. The autoantigen is unknown, and the nomination of actin as the target has not been confirmed. Reactivity has not been associated with a prognostic significance, and recent studies have suggested that the antibodies are better designated as "antineutrophil nuclear antibodies" ("ANNA") since reactivity is against nuclear lamina.

Genetic Predispositions

Human leukocyte antigens (HLA) DR3 and DR4 are independent risk factors for type 1 autoimmune hepatitis in white North Americans and northern Europeans (see

Table 36–4). Fifty-two percent of white patients with type 1 autoimmune hepatitis have HLA DR3 and 42% have HLA DR4. Human leukocyte antigen B8 is in strong linkage disequilibrium with HLA DR3 (94% co-occurrence), and it is present in 47% of patients. The HLA phenotype, A1-B8-DR3, is found in 37% of individuals and 11% are heterozygous for HLA DR3 and HLA DR4. High resolution DNA-based techniques have indicated that the *DRB1* gene influences susceptibility to type 1 autoimmune hepatitis, and the principal susceptibility alleles are *DRB1*0301* and *DRB1*0401*. The predominant HLA phenotype of type 2 autoimmune hepatitis remains uncertain, but HLA B14, DR3, and *C4A-QO* have been implicated. Recent studies have indicated that *DRB1*07* is a risk factor in Brazilian and white German patients (see Table 36–4).

The HLA phenotype may also affect the clinical expression of type 1 autoimmune hepatitis and its response to corticosteroid treatment (Table 36–5). Individuals with HLA B8 are younger, and they have more active disease, as assessed by serum aminotransferase levels and histologic findings of confluent necrosis and cirrhosis, than patients without HLA B8. Similarly, patients who are HLA A1 negative and B8 positive relapse more frequently after corticosteroid withdrawal than patients with other phenotypes.

Patients with HLA DR3 (*DRB1*0301*) enter remission less frequently and deteriorate more commonly during corticosteroid therapy than counterparts with other phenotypes, and they require liver transplantation more often (see Table 36–5). In contrast, patients with HLA DR4 (*DRB1*0401*) are older and more commonly women than those with HLA DR3 (*DRB1*0301*). They also have higher serum levels of γ-globulin, a greater frequency of concurrent immune diseases, a higher frequency of remission during therapy, and a lower occurrence of treatment failure than patients with HLA DR3 (*DRB1*0301*). The presence

of HLA DR3 (*DRB1*0301*) does not preclude responsiveness to corticosteroid therapy, and all patients should be treated similarly.

The genetic bases for susceptibility and disease expression are unclear, but they probably relate to the amino acid sequences encoded by the susceptibility alleles in the antigen binding groove of the class II molecules of the major histocompatibility complex (MHC). Analyses of amino acid sequence variations encoded by the susceptibility alleles indicate that the risk of type 1 autoimmune hepatitis is associated with a six amino acid motif at positions 67–72 in the DRβ polypeptide chain of the HLA DR molecule. *DRB1*0301* and *DRB1*0401* each encodes this motif, and a lysine residue at position DRβ71 is critical for antigen presentation and immunocyte activation. DRβ71 is at the lip of the antigen binding groove and at a contact point between the class II MHC molecule, autoantigen, and T cell antigen receptor of CD4 T helper cells. Lysine at this location may facilitate orientation of the antigen and recognition of the antigen-presenting complex. Class II MHC molecules containing lysine at DRβ71 may also form dimers on the surface of antigen-presenting cells and increase the intensity of antigen display and vigor of immunocyte activation.

According to the "shared motif hypothesis," disease susceptibility relates to a short amino acid sequence within the antigen binding groove and multiple alleles can encode this sequence. This hypothesis accommodates observations that not all patients with type 1 autoimmune hepatitis have *DRB1*0301* and/or *DRB1*0401*. The susceptibility allele for type 1 autoimmune hepatitis in Mestizo Mexicans is *DRB1*0404*. In Japanese patients and in Argentine adults, it is *DRB1*0405*. In Brazilian patients and Argentine children, it is *DRB1*1301*. Most susceptibility alleles are subtypes of HLA DR4, and they encode a similar amino acid sequence at DRβ67–72. In these patients, an arginine re-

Table 36–5. Clinical associations with HLA phenotype and susceptibility alleles.[1]

HLA DR3/*DRB1*0301*	HLA DR4/*DRB1*0401*
Early age onset (median age, 37 years)	Late age onset (median age, 52 years)
Commonly men (32%)	Mainly women (89%)
Relapse common after drug withdrawal	Frequent immune diseases (59%)
High frequency of treatment failure (32%)	High serum γ-globulin levels
Liver transplantation more common	High frequency of remission (85%)
Associated with disease-nonspecific autoimmune promoters (*TNF-α* and *CTLA-4* polymorphisms)	

[1]*TNF-α*, tumor necrosis factor-α-promoter gene; *CTLA-4*, cytotoxic T lymphocyte antigen-4 gene; HLA, human leukocyte antigen.

places a lysine at DRβ71. The arginine residue is a polar, positively charged, molecule that is sufficiently similar to lysine to not greatly affect autoantigen presentation. In contrast, *DRB1*1501* is protective against type 1 autoimmune hepatitis in white northern Europeans, and it encodes an isoleucine for leucine at DRβ67 and more importantly, an alanine for lysine at DRβ71. Alanine is a nonpolar, negatively charged residue that is structurally different from lysine, and its substitution could alter immunocyte recognition of the class II MHC-peptide complex. The association of *DRB1*1301* with type 1 autoimmune hepatitis in South America is inconsistent with the "shared motif hypothesis," and it suggests a different disease in this population or a selection of patients susceptible to a common etiologic trigger, such as hepatitis A virus.

The "autoimmune promoter hypothesis" accommodates observations that not all patients with the same susceptibility alleles behave similarly and not all patients with the same disease have the same susceptibility alleles. According to this hypothesis, multiple factors other than the principal susceptibility alleles can synergize with each other or the main risk factors and affect disease expression. Ten alleles other than *DRB1*0301* and *DRB1*0401* are known to encode lysine at DRβ71, and patients with one or more of these lysine-encoding alleles may have an increased risk of type 1 autoimmune hepatitis despite the absence of the principal risk factors. These same alleles may also enhance the vigor of the immune response in patients with the principal risk factors by increasing the "dose effect" of the lysine substitution at DRβ71.

Other factors outside the MHC may also contribute to disease risk and behavior. Polymorphisms of the tumor necrosis factor-α promoter gene (*TNF*-α) and the cytotoxic T lymphocyte antigen-4 gene (*CTLA-4*) have been recognized in patients with type 1 autoimmune hepatitis. The polymorphism of *TNF*-α may enhance a type 1 cytokine response that promotes clonal expansion of liver-infiltrating cytotoxic T cells, and the polymorphism of *CTLA-4* may impair modulation of immunocyte activation. In each instance, disease risk and severity may be increased. The occurrence of these promoters in other autoimmune liver diseases indicates that they are not disease specific but rather constitutive aspects of the host that promote autoimmune expression. In this fashion, they may have an impact on susceptibility akin to the female gender. Other disease-nonspecific autoimmune promoters undoubtedly exist, and their recognition will be critical in understanding the pathogenesis of the disease, identifying populations at risk, and developing site-specific therapies. A strong dependence on genetic predispositions may explain differences in disease frequency and severity in different geographic regions and ethnic groups.

Treatment

Prednisone alone or in combination with azathioprine induces clinical, biochemical, and histologic remission in 65% of patients with severe autoimmune hepatitis within 2 years. The benefit–risk ratio strongly favors therapy in these patients regardless of their autoantibody profile. The 10- and 20-year life expectancies after therapy exceed 80%, and they are similar to those of an age- and sex-matched normal population from the same geographic region. Untreated disease of similar severity is associated with a 3-year mortality of 50% and 10-year mortality of 90%.

The benefit–risk ratio of corticosteroid therapy in patients with mild disease is less clear. Cirrhosis develops in 49% within 15 years, and the 10-year mortality is 10%. Interface hepatitis progresses to cirrhosis in 17% within 5 years, and spontaneous resolution occurs in 13–20%. This low potential for shortened immediate survival must be balanced against the risk for treatment-related side effects. Cosmetic changes occur in 80% of patients after 1 year of continuous therapy, and the risk of extrahepatic malignancy in patients on long-term treatment is 1.4-fold normal (95% confidence interval, 0.6- to 2.9-fold normal). Thus, the treatment decision must be highly individualized and tempered by the realization that in some patients the treatment may create more complications than the disease. Controlled clinical trials have not been performed in patients with mild autoimmune hepatitis, and there are no evidence-based guidelines that have justified corticosteroid therapy.

The absolute indications for corticosteroid treatment are incapacitating symptoms, sustained extreme elevations of serum aspartate aminotranferase and γ-globulin levels, and/or the presence of bridging necrosis or multilobular necrosis on histologic examination (Table 36–6). Relative indications for therapy are moderate symptoms, laboratory changes, and/or evidence of disease progression. Corticosteroid treatment is not indicated in patients with inactive cirrhosis with or without features of hepatic decompensation. Patients with less severe disease should be monitored closely for disease progression and exacerbation of inflammatory activity. The decision to treat these patients must be individualized and based largely on symptoms such as severe fatigue, myalgia, and/or arthralgia.

Prednisone (20 mg daily) alone and prednisone (10 mg daily) in combination with azathioprine (50 mg daily) are maintenance regimens of comparable efficacy (Table 36–7). The combination regimen is preferred since it is associated with fewer side effects than the higher dose regimen of prednisone alone (10% versus 44%). Postmenopausal women and patients with exogenous obesity, cushingoid features, labile hyperten-

Table 36–6. Indications for treatment of autoimmune hepatitis.

Absolute	Relative	None
Sustained serum AST[1] level greater than 10-fold normal	Moderate serum AST and γ-globulin levels	Mild or minimal serum AST and γ-globulin levels
Sustained serum AST level greater than 5-fold normal and serum γ-globulin level more than twice normal	Interface hepatitis	Cirrhosis with little or no inflammation
	Moderate symptoms	Minimal or no symptoms
	Disease progression	Ascites, encephalopathy, or variceal bleeding and little or no inflammatory activity
Bridging necrosis		
Multilobular necrosis		
Incapacitating symptoms		

[1]AST, serum aspartate aminotransferase level.

sion, and brittle diabetes are ideal candidates for the combination schedule if azathioprine is not contraindicated by severe cytopenia. Active malignancy, pregnancy, or the contemplation of pregnancy are relative contraindications for the use of azathioprine. Prednisone alone is preferred in patients with severe cytopenia associated with hypersplenism, those who are pregnant or contemplating pregnancy, or individuals with neoplastic disease. It is also appropriate for patients in whom a short treatment trial is proposed (3 to 6 months) since the advantages of combination treatment in reducing side effects are evident only after long-term use. Demonstration of a normal thiopurine methyltransferase level is reassuring before institution of azathioprine therapy in patients with cytopenia.

Treatment is continued until clinical, biochemical, and histologic remission, drug toxicity, deterioration or death (treatment failure), or inability to resolve abnormalities after protracted (≥3 years) therapy (incomplete response). Histologic improvements lag behind clinical and biochemical resolution by 3 to 6 months, and liver biopsy assessment is necessary to establish histologic remission and prevent premature withdrawal of medication. Medication should always be withdrawn in a gradual tapered fashion over a 6-week period whenever a treatment end point is reached.

Hepatocellular cancer occurs in patients with cirrhosis of at least 5 years duration, and it should be sought in those individuals with clinical deterioration. The availability of sensitive and specific markers for viral in-

Table 36–7. Treatment regimens for autoimmune hepatitis.

Prednisone (Daily Dose)	Combination Therapy (Daily Dose)	
	Prednisone	Azathioprine
60 mg for 1 week	30 mg for 1 week	50 mg until end point
40 mg for 1 week	20 mg for 1 week	
30 mg for 2 weeks	15 mg for 2 weeks	
20 mg until end point	10 mg until end point	
Relative Contraindications		
Postmenopausal	Cytopenia	
Osteopenia	Active neoplasm	
Emotional lability	Pregnancy or desire for pregnancy	
Acne or cushingoid features	Azothioprine intolerance	
Obesity	Low thiopurine methyltransferase activity	
Labile hypertension	Short (≤6 months) treatment trial	
Brittle diabetes		

fection has identified patients with autoimmune hepatitis who have concurrent viral infection and an increased risk of hepatocellular cancer. The frequency of a neoplasm in uninfected patients with cirrhosis of at least 5 years duration is 1 per 965 patient-years of observation.

Management of Suboptimal Responses

A. RELAPSE

Relapse occurs in 49% of patients within 6 months after drug withdrawal, and it eventuates in 74% within 3 years. Reinstitution of the original treatment regimen usually induces another remission, but the probability of another relapse after drug withdrawal exceeds 80%. Patients who relapse appear to progress to cirrhosis (38% versus 10%) and die from liver failure (14% versus 4%) more commonly than counterparts who sustain their remission after treatment. The only statistically significant consequence of relapse, however, is a higher frequency of corticosteroid-induced side effects (70% versus 21%).

Because relapse and retreatment are associated with a diminishing benefit–risk ratio, alternative therapies are appropriate for patients who relapse multiply (Table 36–8). Low-dose indefinite therapy with prednisone or azathioprine is a treatment option. In the former strategy, the dose of prednisone is reduced each month by decrements of 2.5 mg until the lowest dose is achieved that will control symptoms and maintain serum aminotransferase levels below five-fold normal. In this fashion, 87% of patients can be managed satisfactorily on less than 10 mg of prednisone daily (median dose, 7.5 mg daily). Side effects that had accrued during conventional treatment improve during low-dose maintenance therapy, new side effects do not develop, and survival is unaffected. In the latter strategy, azathioprine (2 mg/kg daily) is administered indefinitely after corticosteroid withdrawal. Withdrawal myalgias and arthralgias can persist for up to 12 months, but biochemical and histologic features of inflammatory activity are usually controlled. The regimen does have the theoretical risks of teratogenicity and oncogenicity. Individual treatment schedules have not been directly compared, and there is no objective basis for preference.

B. TREATMENT FAILURE

Treatment failure connotes clinical, laboratory, and/or histologic deterioration despite compliance with the conventional treatment schedule. Progression to cirrhosis is not a treatment failure if the histologic features of in-

Table 36–8. Management after a suboptimal response to conventional corticosteroid therapy.

Suboptimal Response	Treatment Options
First relapse after drug withdrawal	Retreatment with original schedule
Multiple relapses after drug withdrawal	Low-dose prednisone titrated to prevent symptoms and maintain serum AST[1] ≤5-fold normal
	Indefinite azathioprine (2 mg/kg daily) after corticosteroid withdrawal
Treatment failure	High-dose prednisone (60 mg daily) for 1 month or prednisone (30 mg daily) and azathioprine (150 mg daily) for 1 month followed by dose reductions each month of laboratory improvement until conventional doses achieved
	Empiric therapies, including 6-mercaptopurine (1.5 mg/kg daily), mycophenolate mofetil (2 g daily), or cyclosporine (5–6 mg/kg daily)
	Liver transplantation if decompensation despite therapy
Incomplete response after 3 years of continuous therapy	Low-dose prednisone or indefinite azathioprine therapy
	Liver transplantation at first sign of decompensation (ascites)
Drug toxicity	Dose reduction or drug withdrawal depending on severity
	Maintenance with tolerated drug (prednisone or azathioprine)
	Empiric therapies with alternative drugs (6-mercaptopurine, mycophenolate mofetil, cyclosporine)

[1]AST, serum aspartate aminotransferase level.

flammatory activity are improved. High doses of prednisone alone (60 mg daily) or prednisone (30 mg daily) in combination with azathioprine (150 mg daily) are able to induce clinical and biochemical improvement in 75% of patients within 2 years, but histologic remission occurs in only 20% (see Table 36–8). Patients who fail conventional therapy commonly become corticosteroid dependent, and they are at risk for drug-related side effects and death from liver failure. 6-Mercaptopurine (1.5 mg/kg daily) has been used empirically in small numbers of patients with recalcitrant disease and is reported to be useful in suppressing inflammatory activity. Cyclosporine (5–6 mg/kg daily) has also been used successfully in selected patients. Relapse after drug withdrawal is typical, and patients become dependent on cyclosporine and at risk for its complications (hypertension, renal injury, and malignancy). Other treatments with anecdotal success have been tacrolimus (3 mg twice daily) and mycophelonate mofetil (2 g daily). Ursodeoxycholic acid (13–15 mg/kg daily) and budesonide (3 mg three times a day) have been ineffective in the problematic patient.

Liver transplantation is the preferred treatment for patients who deteriorate during therapy (see Table 36–8). The 5-year survival of patient and graft after transplantation is 80%, and autoantibodies and hypergammaglobulinemia disappear in all individuals within 2 years. Seventeen percent of patients have recurrent disease, and rarely recurrence can result in cirrhosis and graft failure. Typically, recurrence is mild and is managed successfully by adjustments in the immunosuppressive regimen. HLA DR3 mismatching between donor and recipient does not affect recurrence, but recipients who have recurrent disease are usually HLA DR3 positive. The decision to transplant must be based on failure to respond to corticosteroid therapy as there are no findings at presentation that confidently predict survival before treatment. Patients with multilobular necrosis at presentation whose hyperbilirubinemia does not improve after 2 weeks of corticosteroid treatment invariably die, and they are candidates for expeditious transplantation. Patients who have required continuous corticosteroid therapy for at least 4 years become candidates for liver transplantation at the first sign of decompensation (usually ascites formation). Autoimmune hepatitis can develop *de novo* after liver transplantation for nonautoimmune liver disease, and it has been described in a patient transplanted for primary biliary cirrhosis. Autoimmune hepatitis should be included in the differential diagnosis of all individuals who develop liver dysfunction after transplantation.

C. PROTRACTED TREATMENT OR INCOMPLETE RESPONSE

Protracted treatment or incomplete response connotes failure to induce remission after 3 years of continuous therapy. Treatment extended beyond 3 years is associated with only a 7% probability of remission per annum, and the risk of drug-related side effects equals this likelihood. Empiric low-dose prednisone or indefinite azathioprine therapy is an option in these patients as efforts are best directed at preserving well-being rather than inducing a sustained remission (see Table 36–8).

D. DRUG TOXICITY

Drug toxicity necessitates premature discontinuation of medication in 13% of patients. The major reasons for termination of therapy are intolerable obesity or cosmetic changes (47%), osteoporosis with vertebral compression (27%), brittle diabetes (20%), and peptic ulceration (6%). The offending medication must be reduced in dose or discontinued if the complication is severe. Usually, treatment can be continued with the one tolerated agent (prednisone or azathioprine) in adjusted dose. Therapy must be individualized to control manifestations of the liver disease and prevent worsening of the side effects (see Table 36–8).

Promising Treatments

A. CYCLOSPORINE

Cyclosporine (5–6 mg/kg daily) inhibits the release of soluble lymphokines and suppresses clonal expansion of activated T helper cells (Table 36–9). It offers greater blanket immunosuppression than either prednisone or azathioprine, and it has been used in anecdotal reports to rescue patients with treatment failure or corticosteroid intolerance. Recent studies have also advocated its use as initial therapy in treatment-naive pediatric and adult patients. Controlled treatment trials are needed to establish its role as first line and rescue therapy.

B. TACROLIMUS

Tacrolimus is an immunosuppressive agent that has been used mainly to rescue patients with graft rejection after liver transplantation (see Table 36–9). Preliminary results from an open-labeled trial in a small group of patients with autoimmune hepatitis indicate that the drug can decrease serum aminotransferase and bilirubin levels after 3 months at an oral dose of 4 mg twice daily. Patients were not treated to clinical and biochemical remission; liver biopsy assessments were not performed to document histologic response; and most patients developed abnormalities of the serum creatinine and blood urea nitrogen levels. The role of tacrolimus in the therapeutic armamentarium has not been established, but the early experiences justify controlled clinical trials.

C. MYCOPHENOLATE MOFETIL

Mycophenolate mofetil inhibits inosine monophosphate dehydrogenase, which in turn restricts DNA syn-

Table 36–9. Promising new treatments.

Blanket Immunosuppressive Agents	Site-Specific Interventions
Cyclosporine (5–6 mg/kg daily)	Competing peptides for antigen binding groove of class II MHC[1] molecule
Tacrolimus (4 mg twice daily)	
Mycophenolate mofetil (1 g twice daily)	Soluble cytotoxic T lymphocyte antigen-4
Ursodeoxycholic acid (13–15 mg/kg daily in selected patients)	T cell vaccination
	Cytokine antibodies or supplements
Budesonide (3 mg three times a day in selected patients)	Oral tolerance
	Gene therapy
Rapamycin (untested)	
Brequinar (untested)	

[1]MHC, major histocompatibility complex.

thesis and lymphocyte proliferation (see Table 36–9). It has actions similar to those of azathioprine, but they are more lymphocyte specific. In a small treatment trial of seven patients in whom conventional therapies had failed or been poorly tolerated, biochemical remission and histologic improvement was achieved in five patients after treatment with 1 g twice daily for 7 months. The only side effect was a single episode of leukopenia that required dose adjustment. Mycophenolate mofetil has been identified by the International Autoimmune Hepatitis Group as a drug of sufficient promise to warrant further vigorous investigation.

D. Ursodeoxycholic Acid

Ursodeoxycholic acid, administered daily for 2 months in doses of 250 mg, 500 mg, and 750 mg, has reduced serum aminotransferase and γ-glutamyltransferase levels in some patients with chronic hepatitis (see Table 36–9). It has also been used in small pilot studies to improve treatment-naive Japanese patients with mild autoimmune hepatitis. The putative actions of ursodeoxycholic acid, including displacement of hydrophobic (highly detergent) bile acids from the liver, prevention of their ileal absorption, protection of the hepatocyte membrane from noxious insults, alteration of class I HLA expression on hepatocyte membranes, and modulation of apoptosis, make it an appealing agent for further study in autoimmune hepatitis. Controlled trials have not demonstrated efficacy in patients with suboptimal responses to corticosteroids, and its therapeutic role may be restricted to the treatment-naive patient with mild disease.

E. Budesonide

Budesonide is a second-generation corticosteroid that has a high first-pass clearance by the liver and metabolites that are devoid of glucocorticoid activity (see Table 36–9). Theoretically, budesonide can be delivered to the injured organ at a low risk of side effects. A small pilot study has justified this expectation by demonstrating a reduction in serum aminotransferase and γ-globulin levels and good drug tolerance. Similar efficacy and safety have not been shown in corticosteroid-dependent patients with problematic disease who received budesonide, 3 mg three times a day for 6 months. These patients were unable to be removed long term from prednisone, and they commonly developed corticosteroid-related side effects. The promise of budesonide may also be restricted to treatment-naive patients with mild disease.

F. Brequinar and Rapamycin

Brequinar, which inhibits B and T cell function, and rapamycin, which suppresses interleukin 2 production, are other drugs that have putative actions of theoretical advantage to patients with autoimmune hepatitis. Neither has been sufficiently studied to allow incorporation into a management algorithm (see Table 36–9).

G. Site-Specific Interventions

Future treatments promise to be site specific and based on pathogenic mechanisms (see Table 36–9). Peptides that competitively inhibit the display of autoantigen within the class II MHC molecule and soluble CTLA-4 that can interfere with the second signal of immunocyte activation are interventions that promise to dampen the CD4 T helper cell response. T cell vaccination can limit clonal expansion of liver infiltrating cytotoxic T cells and prevent the disease or attenuate it in the animal model. Treatment with interleukin 10 or antibodies to tumor necrosis factor-α can alter the cytokine milieu, and oral tolerance therapy may induce systemic nonresponsiveness to the autoantigen. Lastly, gene therapy has the potential to deliver immunoregulatory or regenerative growth factors that can correct or counterbalance disturbances promoting autoreactivity. Site-specific interventions are already being assessed in rheumatoid arthritis and type 1 diabetes mellitus, and they await the development of a reliable animal model before testing in autoimmune hepatitis.

CRYPTOGENIC CHRONIC HEPATITIS

Cryptogenic chronic hepatitis is an active inflammatory process that lacks epidemiologic risk factors for viral hepatitis, evidence of drug or toxin-induced liver injury, viral markers, and autoantibodies. The designation does not include end-stage, inactive cirrhosis that has lost all distinguishing features. Cryptogenic chronic hepatitis is second only to type 1 autoimmune hepatitis as the most common diagnosis in adults with chronic nonviral hepatitis (13% versus 80%).

Typically, patients with cryptogenic chronic hepatitis are indistinguishable from patients with autoimmune hepatitis by age, gender, duration of illness, serum immunoglobulin levels, frequency of concurrent immune disorders, and histologic findings. Human leukocyte antigens B8, DR3, and DR4 occur as commonly in these patients as in autoimmune hepatitis and at a higher frequency than in counterparts with chronic viral hepatitis. Most importantly, these patients respond to corticosteroids as well as patients with autoimmune hepatitis. They enter remission (83% versus 78%) and fail treatment (9% versus 11%) as commonly. Patients with cryptogenic chronic hepatitis may have "autoantibody-negative autoimmune hepatitis," and they should be selected for treatment by the same criteria and treated with the same regimens as patients with classic disease.

Twenty percent of individuals with cryptogenic chronic hepatitis ultimately express SMA and/or ANA, and they can be reclassified as type 1 autoimmune hepatitis. Antibody–antigen binding at presentation may have prevented detection of the diagnostic autoantibodies. Other patients may be reclassified as autoimmune hepatitis because they express anti-SLA/LP or pANCA, whereas others remain seronegative by the currently available battery of markers. These latter patients may have autoimmune hepatitis with a novel yet undiscovered autoantibody, a sporadic form of viral hepatitis that has eluded detection by second-generation immunoassays, or a hepatitis due to a virus not yet identified. Future investigations will undoubtedly diminish the significance of this category. Currently, symptomatic patients with severe disease should be treated with corticosteroids and monitored closely. Failure to improve within 3 months justifies corticosteroid withdrawal.

AUTOIMMUNE CHOLANGITIS

Autoimmune cholangitis is a cholestatic hepatitis with autoimmune features. Antinuclear antibodies (typically in high titer) and/or SMA are commonly present, and AMA (including antibodies against the M2 mitochondrial autoantigens) and inflammatory bowel disease are absent. Destructive cholangitis (including florid duct lesions), ductopenia, ductular proliferation, portal fibrosis, and/or cholestasis may be present on histologic examination, and these patterns can resemble primary biliary cirrhosis or primary sclerosing cholangitis. In the latter instance, cholangiography is an important component of the evaluation. Autoimmune cholangitis is probably a heterogeneous disorder that encompasses AMA-negative primary biliary cirrhosis, small duct primary sclerosing cholangitis, idiopathic adulthood ductopenia, and transition states between syndromes with overlapping features.

Corticosteroid therapy has been of limited or no value in the treatment of this condition. Clinical and biochemical indices of inflammation may improve, but the histologic features are typically unchanged. Similarly, anecdotal experiences with ursodeoxycholic acid have indicated an inconsistent and incomplete response. Therapies are empiric and based on the predominant manifestations of the disease (hepatitic versus cholestatic findings). Combination therapy with prednisone and ursodeoxycholic acid can be used in symptomatic patients with equally mixed features. Liver transplantation is an option for advanced and/or decompensated disease.

AUTOIMMUNE HEPATITIS WITH VARIANT FEATURES

Patients with autoimmune hepatitis can have concurrent features of viral infection, primary biliary cirrhosis, or primary sclerosing cholangitis ("overlap syndromes"). These mixed findings generate speculation about etiologic relationships, and they complicate treatment strategies. Recombinant interferon-α enhances display of HLA antigens on the hepatocyte membrane and reduces suppression of T cell function. Its administration to patients with autoimmune features can exacerbate those manifestations and increase the expression of nonpathogenic autoantibodies. Similarly, corticosteroids may fail to reduce disease activity in patients with predominant viral features or those with primary sclerosing cholangitis. Indeed, corticosteroids in patients with active viral infection may enhance the virus burden and make long-term management more difficult. To successfully manage the variant syndromes, the predominant disorder must be identified and then treated with the most appropriate regimen. Variant syndromes have been described in 18% of patients with autoimmune liver disease, and they should be considered in all patients who are recalcitrant to conventional corticosteroid regimens (Table 36–10).

Autoimmune Hepatitis with Viral Markers

Patients with autoimmune hepatitis may have serologic markers of an earlier viral infection, false-positive tests for a current viral infection, or a coexistent true viral infection. Hepatitis B surface antigen (HBsAg)-negative patients with autoimmune hepatitis who have antibodies to HBsAg (anti-HBs) and hepatitis B core antigen (anti-HBc) have had previous viral infection, and they should be treated in a standard fashion as autoimmune hepatitis. Similarly, patients with isolated seropositivity for anti-HBc or antibodies to HCV whose specificity

against HCV-encoded antigens cannot be confirmed by recombinant immunoblot assay (RIBA) and/or who lack HCV RNA in serum have false-positive viral markers, and they should be treated as autoimmune hepatitis (see Table 36–10).

Difficulties arise in the diagnosis and management of patients with active viremia and autoimmune manifestations. Thirty-eight percent of individuals with chronic hepatitis B or C have ANA or SMA. Typically, the autoantibodies are low titer background reactivities, and they are not coexpressed. These patients do not have compelling features of autoimmune hepatitis, and they can be classified as "chronic viral hepatitis with autoimmune features" and treated with antiviral regimens. In one study, there were no patients with ANA titers of greater than 1:100 who were anti-HCV positive, whereas 64% with ANA titers of less than 1:100 were anti-HCV positive. In another series, patients

Table 36–10. Management of autoimmune hepatitis with variant features.[1]

Variant Features	Treatment
Previous viral infection (HBsAg negative, anti-HBs and anti-HBc positive)	Prednisone alone or with azathioprine
False-positive viral markers (anti-HBc only; anti-HCV positive, RIBA negative, or HCV RNA negative)	Prednisone alone or with azathioprine
Concurrent true viral infection	Antiviral therapy if anti-LKM1, low-titer autoantibodies, histologic features of steatosis, portal lymphoid aggregates, and/or bile duct damage
	Prednisone alone or with azathioprine if high-titer autoantibodies and histologic changes of moderate to severe interface hepatitis (especially portal plasma cell infiltration) in absence of steatosis, portal lymphoid aggregates, and bile duct changes
Concurrent primary biliary cirrhosis	Prednisone alone or with azathioprine if serum alkaline phosphatase level less than 2-fold normal
	Prednisone (20 mg daily) and ursodeoxycholic acid (13–15 mg/kg daily) if serum alkaline phosphatase level more than 2-fold normal and/or florid bile duct lesions
Concurrent primary sclerosing cholangitis	Empiric treatment with prednisone (20 mg daily) and ursodeoxycholic acid (13–15 mg/kg daily)
	Investigational protocols

[1]HBsAg, hepatitis B virus surface antigen; anti-HBs, antibodies to hepatitis B surface antigen; anti-HBc, antibodies to hepatitis B core antigen; anti-HCV, antibodies to hepatitis C virus; RIBA, recombinant immunoblot assay; HCV RNA, hepatitis C virus RNA in serum; anti-LKM1, antibodies to liver/kidney microsome type 1.

with chronic viral hepatitis more commonly had serum titers of SMA or ANA of 1:80 or less compared with those with autoimmune hepatitis (89% versus 16%). Moreover, only 23% of patients with chronic viral hepatitis and autoantibodies had titers of 1:320 or higher, and no patients had concurrent SMA and ANA.

In contrast, patients with classical autoimmune hepatitis have a median SMA titer of 1:160 and ANA titer of 1:320. The range of seropositivity may be as low as 1:40, but other immune features are typically present to support the diagnosis. Only 6% of patients with autoimmune hepatitis have just one autoantibody of low titer (less than 1:80). These observations facilitate the categorization of most patients with mixed viral and autoimmune features. Patients with true viral infection who have low titers of autoantibodies (<1:320) or anti-LKM1 have viral predominant disease, and they are candidates for antiviral therapy. Patients with high titer autoantibodies (≥1:320) and/or multiple autoantibodies must be evaluated further for autoimmune disease (see Table 36–10).

Liver tissue examination is essential in the evaluation of patients with viremia and high titer autoantibodies. Moderate to severe interface hepatitis, especially with portal plasma cell infiltration, suggests autoimmune hepatitis. Patients with true HCV infection and these histologic features in the absence of portal lymphoid aggregates, steatosis, and bile duct injury have more aggressive disease than patients without these features, a higher frequency of HLA DR3, and responsiveness to corticosteroid therapy. Patients with autoimmune hepatitis and coincidental or background true viral infection are rare, but several case reports have indicated that corticosteroids are a treatment option in these highly selected cases. Individuals in whom a confident diagnosis of autoimmune hepatitis would have been made if viral markers had not been present are candidates for a 3–6 month course of prednisone. Improvement during this period justifies continuation of the corticosteroid regimen, whereas lack of improvement justifies drug withdrawal and treatment with antiviral agents (see Table 36–10).

Autoimmune Hepatitis & Primary Biliary Cirrhosis

Patients with autoimmune hepatitis may have features of primary biliary cirrhosis (see Table 36–10). Twenty percent of patients with autoimmune hepatitis have AMA, and 8% have antibodies to the E2 subunits of pyruvate dehydrogenase and/or branched-chain ketoacid dehydrogenase. AMA titers are typically low (≤1:40), but 12% have titers that exceed 1:160. Serum alkaline phosphatase levels are increased in 81% of patients with autoimmune hepatitis, but they are greater than two-fold normal in 33% and more than four-fold normal in 10%. Serum immunoglobulin M levels may exceed 6.0 mg/mL; histologic examination can indicate bile duct damage in 12%; and rhodanine stains of liver tissue can rarely demonstrate the presence of hepatic copper. Patients with autoimmune hepatitis and AMA who have one or more of these cholestatic features constitute an overlap syndrome with primary biliary cirrhosis.

The treatment of patients with autoimmune hepatitis and primary biliary cirrhosis depends on the cholestatic component of the disease (see Table 36–10). Patients with serum alkaline phosphatase levels of less than two-fold normal at presentation respond to corticosteroid therapy as well as patients with classic autoimmune hepatitis. These patients should be treated with conventional regimens for autoimmune hepatitis. Patients with serum alkaline phosphatase levels greater than two-fold normal and/or florid duct lesions on liver tissue examination are candidates for therapy with prednisone in combination with ursodeoxycholic acid. Treatments are empiric, and they must be individualized according to the response.

Autoimmune Hepatitis & Primary Sclerosing Cholangitis

Clinical, biochemical, and histologic features of autoimmune hepatitis are present in 6% of patients with primary sclerosing cholangitis, and lymphoid, fibrous, and pleomorphic cholangitis suggestive of primary sclerosing cholangitis are found in 20% of patients with autoimmune hepatitis. Both diseases have similar frequencies of HLA DR3, and they may share pathogenic pathways that account for their concurrence. AMA-negative patients with autoimmune hepatitis and cholestatic features constitute an overlap syndrome with primary sclerosing cholangitis if characteristic cholangiographic changes are present. Patients with autoimmune hepatitis and inflammatory bowel disease should undergo cholangiography to exclude this diagnosis since the presence of primary sclerosing cholangitis diminishes the likelihood of a response to corticosteroids. A normal cholangiogram does not exclude primary sclerosing cholangitis since a small duct variety is recognized. Under such circumstances, the diagnosis of an overlap syndrome requires the presence of inflammatory bowel disease since patients would otherwise be classified as autoimmune cholangitis.

Only 20% of patients with autoimmune hepatitis and primary sclerosing cholangitis achieve remission with corticosteroid therapy, and responsiveness relates to the cholestatic component. Serum alkaline phosphatase levels less than two-fold normal identify patients who may respond. Most patients have high serum alkaline phosphatase concentrations, and they are candidates for empiric therapy with prednisone in

CHRONIC NONVIRAL HEPATITIS / **579**

combination with ursodeoxycholic acid. This strategy has not been shown to be effective, but it may ameliorate symptoms in some patients.

Children with autoimmune hepatitis may have cholangiographic changes that justify the diagnosis of "autoimmune sclerosing cholangitis." These children typically do not have inflammatory bowel disease, and they respond well to conventional corticosteroid regimens. The place of "autoimmune sclerosing cholangitis" within the spectrum of variant syndromes is uncertain, and it is best regarded as a separate entity among children. Its occurrence has not been substantiated on a global basis, and its manifestations and outcome differ from adult patients with autoimmune hepatitis and primary sclerosing cholangitis.

GRANULOMATOUS HEPATITIS

Hepatic granulomas are focal collections of epithelioid cells with surrounding lymphocytes that can occur anywhere within the liver (Figure 36–5). Most commonly, they are in or near portal tracts. Caseation necrosis and multinucleated giant cells may be components of the lesion, and clinical and biochemical manifestations may or may not be present. In some instances, the granulomas are isolated, unsuspected, serendipitous findings of uncertain clinical significance; in other instances, they may explain laboratory changes that reflect a focal infiltrative disorder of the liver characterized by prominent elevations of serum alkaline phosphatase and γ-glutamyltransferase levels. When the granulomas are the predominant histologic findings, the designation of granulomatous hepatitis is justified. Granulomatous hepatitis is not a true hepatitis, and its classification as such reflects convention rather than conviction.

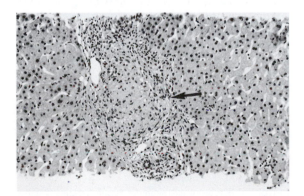

Figure 36–5. Noncaseating granuloma in idiopathic granulomatous hepatitis. The focal collection of epithelioid cells and surrounding lymphocytes is adjacent to a portal tract (H&E; original magnification ×100).

There are many causes of hepatic granulomas, including infectious agents of a bacterial, fungal, parasitic, and viral nature (tuberculosis, histoplasmosis, coccidioidomycosis, blastomycosis, brucellosis, Q fever, syphilis, schistosomiasis, tularensis, ascariasis, leprosy, Epstein–Barr virus, and cytomegalovirus), drugs (methyldopa, allopurinol, quinidine, phenytoin, hydrochlorothiazide, benzodiazapines, sulfonamides, and phenylbutazone), foreign bodies (beryllium, talc), immunologic reactions (primary biliary cirrhosis, inflammatory bowel disease, polymyalgia rheumatica, rheumatoid arthritis, Wegener's granulomatosis), sarcoidosis, and neoplasms (hairy-cell leukemia, Hodgkin's disease, melanoma, non-Hodgkin's lymphoma) (Table 36–11). The most common causes of granulomatous hepatitis are tuberculosis (10–53% of cases) and sarcoidosis (12–55% of cases). Because granulomas are common (2–35% of liver biopsy examinations), the frequency of idiopathic granulomatous hepatitis is high (30–50% of cases). Most likely, granulomas reflect a cell-mediated immunologic reaction against a variety of different antigens that are frequently undefined.

Fever is present in up to 75% of patients with granulomatous hepatitis, and it may be relapsing or continuous in nature. In patients with idiopathic granulomatous hepatitis, activated mononuclear phagocytes within the granulomas probably release endogenous pyrogens, including interleukin 1, which affect hypothalamic thermoregulation. Nonspecific symptoms, such as anorexia, fatigue, and malaise, may also accompany the syndrome. Typically, liver biopsy examination is performed to evaluate the cause of fever rather than the basis of liver test abnormalities. Multiple sections of the liver tissue sample are necessary to discover the lesions. Acid-fast and fungal stains are essential components of the tissue examination, although diagnostic findings are unusual and their absence is not exclusionary. Cultures of the liver tissue have a low yield for mycobacteria (<10%), but results are better for fungi such as *Histoplasma capsulatum* (50% yield), and they should be performed. Portal hypertension may occur with extensive granulomatous infiltration of the liver, but this occurrence is rare. Cirrhosis is not an expected consequence of granulomatous hepatitis, and it may reflect a coincidence rather than a consequence.

The cause of granulomatous hepatitis must be sought in a thoughtful cost-effective fashion. The long list of etiologic possibilities (see Table 36–11) can be shortened considerably by clinical assessment and a careful travel, drug, and occupational history. Specific etiologic factors can then assessed by order of likelihood. Cultures of sputum, urine, gastric washings, and liver tissue for mycobacteria; serological tests for fungi, Q fever, Epstein–Barr virus, cytomegalovirus, and toxoplasmosis; examination of stools for parasites; culture of liver tissue

Table 36–11. Common causes of granulomatous hepatitis.

Bacterial agents	Parasitic agents	Foreign bodies
Brucellosis	Amebiasis	Beryllium
Borreliosis	Ascariasis	Silica
Mycobacteria	Giardiasis	Talc
Salmonellosis	Toxoplasmosis	Thorium dioxide
Secondary syphilis	**Rickettsial agents**	**Immune diseases**
Whipple's disease	Q fever	Polymyalgia rheumatica
Fungal agents	**Drugs**	Primary biliary cirrhosis
Actinomycosis	Allopurinol	Rheumatoid arthritis
Aspergillosis	Cephalexin	Sarcoidosis
Blastomycosis	Chlorothiazide	Ulcerative colitis
Candidiasis	Chlorpromazine	Wegener's granulomatosis
Coccidioidomycosis	Dapsone	**Malignancies**
Cryptococcosis	Diazepam	Hairy-cell leukemia
Histoplasmosis	Diltiazem	Hodgkin's
Nocardiosis	Isoniazid	Melanoma
Viral agents	Methyldopa	Non-Hodgkin's lymphoma
Cytomegalovirus	Nitrofurantoin	Crohn's disease
Epstein–Barr virus	Oxacillin	
Human immunodeficiency virus type 1	Phenylbutazone	
	Phenytoin	
	Sulfasalazine	
	Sulfonamides	
	Quinidine	

Adapted, with permission, from Bonkovsky H: Granulomatous hepatitis and hepatic granulomas. In: *Medicine: For the Practicing Physician.* Hurst JW (editor). Butterworths-Heinemann, 1992.

for fungi; blood cultures for bacteria; chest x-rays; and imaging studies can then be tailored to the clinical situation.

Management is based on the cause of the condition and the severity of symptoms. Discontinuation of all medication and elimination of an infectious agent are obvious strategies. Patients with idiopathic disease can be observed or treated symptomatically. Such patients commonly have a benign prognosis and rarely manifest changes of tuberculosis, histoplasmosis, or sarcoidosis later in their course. Forty-one percent of patients with idiopathic granulomatous hepatitis may improve spontaneously within 1 to 12 months.

Febrile symptomatic patients warrant empiric therapy. Individuals with risk factors for tuberculosis or caseating hepatic granulomas should be treated with isoniazid (8 mg/kg daily) and ethambutol (15–25 mg/kg daily) for 8 weeks. If there has been no improvement on antituberculosis therapy, the medication can be discontinued and therapy with either indomethacin or prednisone (0.75–1.0 mg/kg daily) instituted. A response to antituberculosis treatment warrants the addition of pyridoxine (100 mg daily) to the regimen and continuation of therapy for 18 months. Symptomatic patients without risk factors for tuberculosis, negative

cultures for mycobacteria, and no evidence of caseation can be treated directly with indomethacin or prednisone. Prompt defervescence and symptomatic improvement should be expected in all such patients, and the dose of medication can be withdrawn as tolerated in a gradual fashion. The duration of treatment is variable, and it may range from 3 to 79 months. Close surveillance is indicated for emergence of the rare occult infection. Isoniazid (300 mg daily) and pyridoxine should be administered in conjunction with prednisone in those patients with positive tuberculin skin tests or a past history of tuberculosis.

REFERENCES

Alvarez F et al: International Autoimmune Hepatitis Group report: review of criteria for diagnosis of autoimmune hepatitis. J Hepatol 1999;31:929.

Bach N et al: The histologic features of chronic hepatitis C and autoimmune chronic hepatitis: a comparative analysis. Hepatology 1992;15:572.

Ben-Ari Z et al: Autoimmune cholangiopathy: part of the spectrum of autoimmune chronic active hepatitis. Hepatology 1993; 18:10.

Bonkovsky H: Granulomatous hepatitis and hepatic granulomas. In: *Medicine: For the Practicing Physician.* Hurst JW (editor). Butterworths-Heinemann, 1992.

Costa M et al: Isolation and characterization of cDNA encoding the antigenic protein of the human tRNP$^{(Ser)Sec}$ complex recognized by autoantibodies from patients with type 1 autoimmune hepatitis. Clin Exp Immunol 2000;121:364.

Czaja AJ: Low dose corticosteroid therapy after multiple relapses of severe HBsAg-negative chronic active hepatitis. Hepatology 1990;11:1044.

Czaja AJ: Chronic active hepatitis: the challenge for a new nomenclature. Ann Intern Med 1993;119:510.

Czaja AJ: Autoimmune hepatitis and viral infection. Gastroenterol Clin North Am 1994;23:547.

Czaja AJ: Autoimmune hepatitis: current therapeutic concepts. Clin Immunother 1994;1:413.

Czaja AJ: Autoimmune hepatitis: evolving concepts and treatment strategies. Dig Dis Sci 1995;40:435.

Czaja AJ: The variant forms of autoimmune hepatitis. Ann Intern Med 1996;125:588.

Czaja AJ: Frequency and nature of the variant syndromes of autoimmune liver disease. Hepatology 1998;28:360.

Czaja AJ: Behavior and significance of autoantibodies in type 1 autoimmune hepatitis. J Hepatol 1999;30:394.

Czaja AJ: Drug therapy in the management of type 1 autoimmune hepatitis. Drugs 1999;57:49.

Czaja AJ: Understanding the pathogenesis of autoimmune hepatitis. Am J Gastroenterol 2001;96:1224.

Czaja AJ et al: Clinical and prognostic implications of human leukocyte antigen B8 in corticosteroid-treated severe autoimmune chronic active hepatitis. Gastroenterology 1990;98:1587.

Czaja AJ et al: Frequency and significance of antibodies to liver/kidney microsome type 1 in adults with chronic active hepatitis. Gastroenterology 1992;103:1290.

Czaja AJ et al: Evidence against hepatitis viruses as important causes of severe autoimmune hepatitis in the United States. J Hepatol 1993;18:342.

Czaja AJ et al: Genetic predispositions for the immunological features of chronic active hepatitis. Hepatology 1993;18:816.

Czaja AJ et al: Significance of HLA DR4 in type 1 autoimmune hepatitis. Gastroenterology 1993;105:1502.

Czaja AJ et al: The nature and prognosis of severe cryptogenic chronic active hepatitis. Gastroenterology 1993;104:1755.

Czaja AJ et al: Antibodies to soluble liver antigen, P-450IID6, and mitochondrial complexes in chronic hepatitis. Gastroenterology 1993;105:1522.

Czaja AJ et al: Sensitivity, specificity and predictability of biopsy interpretations in chronic hepatitis. Gastroenterology 1993;105:1824.

Czaja AJ et al: Hepatitis C virus infection as a determinant of behavior in type 1 autoimmune hepatitis. Dig Dis Sci 1995;40:33.

Czaja AJ et al: The validity and importance of subtypes of autoimmune hepatitis: a point of view. Am J Gastroenterol 1995;90:1206.

Czaja AJ et al: Validation of a scoring system for the diagnosis of autoimmune hepatitis. Dig Dis Sci 1996;41:305.

Czaja AJ et al: Histologic findings in chronic hepatitis C with autoimmune features. Hepatology 1997;26:459.

Czaja AJ et al: Genetic distinctions between types 1 and 2 autoimmune hepatitis. Am J Gastroenterol 1997;92:2197.

Czaja AJ et al: Associations between alleles of the major histocompatibility complex and type 1 autoimmune hepatitis. Hepatology 1997;25:317.

Czaja AJ et al: Immune phenotype of chronic liver disease. Dig Dis Sci 1998;43:2149.

Czaja AJ et al: Cytokine polymorphisms associated with clinical features and treatment outcome in type 1 autoimmune hepatitis. Gastroenterology 1999;117:645.

Czaja AJ et al: Ursodeoxycholic acid as adjunctive therapy for problematic type 1 autoimmune hepatitis: a randomized placebo-controlled treatment trial. Hepatology 1999;30:1381.

Czaja AJ et al: Autoimmune cholangitis within the spectrum of autoimmune liver disease. Hepatology 2000;31:1231.

Czaja AJ et al: Autoimmune hepatitis: the investigational and clinical challenges. Hepatology 2000;31:1194.

Czaja AJ et al: Failure of budesonide in a pilot study of treatment-dependent autoimmune hepatitis. Gastroenterology 2000;119:1312.

Czaja AJ et al: Nature and behavior of serum cytokines in type 1 autoimmune hepatitis. Dig Dis Sci 2000;45:1028.

Czaja AJ et al: Autoantibodies in liver disease. Gastroenterology 2001;120:239.

Czaja AJ et al: Shared genetic risk factors in autoimmune liver disease. Dig Dis Sci 2001;46:140.

Desmet VJ et al: Classification of chronic hepatitis: diagnosis, grading and staging. Hepatology 1994;19:1513.

Doherty DG et al: Allelic sequence variation in the HLA class II genes and proteins in patients with autoimmune hepatitis. Hepatology 1994;19:609.

Donaldson PT et al: Susceptibility to autoimmune chronic active hepatitis: human leukocyte antigens DR4 and A1-B8-DR3 are independent risk factors. Hepatology 1990;13:701.

Homberg J-C et al: Chronic active hepatitis associated with antiliver/kidney microsome antibody type 1: a second type of "autoimmune" hepatitis. Hepatology 1987;7:1333.

Lunel F et al: Liver/kidney microsome antibody type 1 and hepatitis C virus infection. Hepatology 1992;16:630.

Manns M et al: Characterization of a new subgroup of autoimmune chronic active hepatitis by autoantibodies against a soluble liver antigen. Lancet 1987;1:292.

Manns MP et al: LKM-1 autoantibodies recognize a short linear sequence in P-450IID6, a cytochrome P-450 monooxygenase. J Clin Invest 1991;88:1370.

Poralla T et al: The asialoglycoprotein receptor as target structure in autoimmune liver diseases. Semin Liver Dis 1991;11:215.

Sartin JS, Walker RC: Granulomatous hepatitis: a retrospective review of 88 cases at the Mayo Clinic. Mayo Clin Proc 1991;66:914.

Wies I et al: Identification of target antigen for SLA/LP autoantibodies in autoimmune hepatitis. Lancet 2000;355:1510.

Yamamoto AM et al: Characterization of the anti-liver-kidney microsome antibody (anti-LKM1) from hepatitis C virus-positive and -negative sera. Gastroenterology 1993;104:1762.

Zoutman DE et al: Granulomatous hepatitis and fever of unknown origin: an 11-year experience of 23 cases with three years' follow-up. J Clin Gastroenterol 1991;13:69.

■ BACTERIAL INFECTIONS

PYOGENIC LIVER ABSCESS

Pathophysiology

Pyogenic bacteria gain access to the liver by a variety of routes. Biliary tract disease currently accounts for the greatest percentage of cases, and may occur from either benign or malignant obstruction of the biliary tree with resultant cholangitis. Before antibiotics became available, seeding through the portal venous system occurred most frequently with appendicitis or diverticulitis. In childhood or infancy, pyogenic liver abscesses occur most frequently with umbilical vein infections. Infection via the hepatic artery may occur during bacteremia secondary to endocarditis, osteomyelitis, or other sources. Direct extension of infection from contiguous organs may permit bacteria to gain entry to the liver such as in pneumonia or subphrenic abscess. Penetrating injuries to the liver may directly seed bacteria into the organ. In almost one-half of the cases of pyogenic liver abscess, no clear cause is ever found.

Pyogenic liver abscesses may be single or multiple; most single abscesses are located in the right lobe. Most abscesses of portal vein origin are single, whereas those of biliary tract origin are often multiple. The organisms recovered from pyogenic liver abscesses vary considerably. Approximately one-half are found to be due to infection with anaerobic organisms or mixed cultures of anaerobic and aerobic organisms. The most common organisms isolated include gram-negative enteric bacilli, anaerobic gram-negative bacilli, and microaerophilic streptococci (Table 37–1). *Escherichia coli* has been the organism most commonly isolated.

ESSENTIALS OF DIAGNOSIS

- *Fever, malaise, hepatomegaly, right upper quadrant tenderness.*
- *Leukocytosis, elevated alkaline phosphatase, and γ-glutamyl transpeptidase (GGTP).*
- *Round or oval defects seen on ultrasound, computed tomography (CT) scan, or magnetic resonance imaging (MRI).*

Clinical Findings

A. SYMPTOMS AND SIGNS

The clinical features of pyogenic liver abscess are often nonspecific and variable, but most often include fever, malaise, weight loss, and right upper quadrant abdominal pain. Hepatomegaly and right upper quadrant abdominal tenderness are the most common findings on physical examination. Jaundice is seen in approximately 25% of cases.

B. LABORATORY FINDINGS

Laboratory findings can be nonspecific and most often include leukocytosis and anemia, elevations of the alkaline phosphatase and GGTP, and hyperbilirubinemia in about 25% of cases. Aerobic and anaerobic culture of the abscess yields specific results in over three-quarters of pyogenic liver abscesses. Blood culture results are positive for the responsible bacteria in about one-half of cases.

C. IMAGING

Routine chest x-rays are abnormal in almost 50% of patients with pyogenic liver abscess. Findings can include elevation of the diaphragm, air–fluid levels within a liver mass, or both. Ultrasonography detects pyogenic liver abscesses in 80–100% of cases. The characteristic appearance is a round or oval area within the liver that is less echogenic than the surrounding hepatic parenchyma. It may be difficult to image either abscesses that are high in the dome of the liver or multiple microabscesses. CT scanning reveals lesions that are less dense (lower attenuation values) than surrounding normal liver. Using intravenous contrast improves detection because an abscess does not enhance like surrounding normal liver parenchyma (Figure 37–1). Contrast-enhanced MRI has been used to demonstrate pyogenic abscesses, but CT scanning remains the imaging test of choice.

Table 37–1. Organisms cultured from pyogenic liver abscesses.

Aerobic	Anaerobic
Escherichia coli	Anaerobic streptococci
Klebsiella	Microaerophillic streptococci
Streptococcus viridans group	Bacteroides species
	Fusobacterium species
Staphylococcus aureus	Clostridium species
Enterococcus	Actinomyces
Proteus species	Eubacterium
Pseudomonas species	Propionibacterium
Enterobacter	
Listeria	
Yersinia	

Adapted, with permission, from Goldman IS, Farber BF, Brandborg LL: Bacterial and miscellaneous infections of the liver. In: *Hepatology: A Textbook of Liver Disease,* 3rd ed. Zakim D, Boyer TD (editors). Saunders, 1995.

Complications

Most complications of pyogenic liver abscess result from rupture or extension of the abscess into adjacent structures. In early series, pleuropulmonary involvement occurred in 15% of patients, while subphrenic abscess developed in about 3% of cases.

Treatment

If possible, a diagnostic aspiration under ultrasound or CT guidance should be performed before starting antibiotic therapy. Pyogenic liver abscesses can be effectively treated with antibiotics, alone or used in conjunction with percutaneous drainage. Significant coagulopathy or ascites are relative contraindications to percutaneous drainage, but in most other cases a percutaneous drainage should be attempted. When culture results from percutaneous aspiration are available, antibiotic choice can be specifically tailored to the sensitivities of the organism. Because growth in anaerobic cultures may take several days, however, it is advisable to continue antianaerobic coverage until all culture results are final. A large number of antibiotics can be used either singly or in combination as initial empiric therapy (Table 37–2). Antibiotic treatment before culture results are available should include coverage against gram-negative bacilli, microaerophilic streptococci, and anaerobic bacteria. The duration of antibiotic therapy varies, but should be given for at least 10–14 days intravenously, followed by a longer course of oral therapy lasting 6 or more weeks. The total duration of antimicrobial therapy may be guided by imaging studies. Open surgical drainage is reserved for those who do not respond to antibiotics and percutaneous drainage.

Prognosis

The mortality associated with untreated pyogenic liver abscess is extremely high. Multiple abscesses and polymicrobial infections are adverse risk factors. The recognition and diagnosis of pyogenic liver abscess are often delayed because the symptoms are nonspecific, adding to morbidity and mortality. Liver abscesses must be considered in patients with fever of unknown

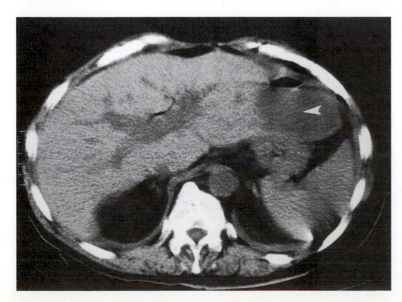

Figure 37–1. CT scan showing a large low-density (attenuation) mass in the left lobe of the liver **(arrow).** Aspiration documented an *E coli* pyogenic liver abscess.

Table 37–2. Antibiotics used as empiric therapy for hepatic abscess.

Second-generation cephalosporin (cefotetan), with or with-
out aminoglycoside
Broad-spectrum penicillin (Timentin, ampicillin-sulbactam)
with or without aminoglycoside
Imipenem
Third-generation cephalosporin plus metronidazole or clin-
damycin
Clindamycin plus aminoglycoside

Adapted, with permission, from Goldman IS, Farber BF, Brandborg LL: Bacterial and miscellaneous infections of the liver. In:
Hepatology: A Textbook of Liver Disease, 3rd ed. Zakim D, Boyer TD
(editors). Saunders, 1995.

origin. Early use of ultrasound or CT imaging will detect abscesses that might otherwise go unrecognized.
Even with prompt recognition and treatment, the mortality rate may be as high as 50%.

Barnes PF et al: A comparison of amebic and pyogenic abscess of
the liver. Medicine 1987;66:472.

Barreda R, Roso P: Diagnostic imaging of liver abscess. Crit Rev
Diagn Imaging 1992;33:29.

Johannsen EC et al: Pyogenic liver abscess. Infect Dis Clin North
Am 2000;14:547.

Stain SC et al: Pyogenic liver abscess: modern treatment. Arch Surg
1991;126:991.

LEPTOSPIROSIS

Leptospirosis in humans is caused by infection with a
spirochete of the *Leptospira interrogans* complex, of
which there are approximately 240 serotypes. The
milder form of leptospirosis is usually anicteric, whereas
the more severe and less common presentation, known
as Weil's disease, is characterized by jaundice and severe
systemic illness.

Pathophysiology

Leptospires are found in a number of both domestic
and wild animals and are excreted in the urine. Humans are incidental hosts and are most often infected
through contact with the urine of rodents, the most important vector for human exposure. Sewer workers, vet-
erinarians, and slaughterhouse workers have occupational exposure, but disease may occur in patients in
urban and suburban areas without such occupational
risk. The organisms enter humans through a cut in the
skin or via mucous membranes, and incubate for 5–20
days before clinical illness begins. Some patients have
a biphasic illness. During the first, or leptospiremic

phase, organisms can be isolated from the blood or
cerebrospinal fluid. The first phase usually lasts 4–9
days, followed by a few days of symptomatic improvement. The second, or immune phase, is caused by the
patient's immune response to the leptospiral infection.
Any of the signs and symptoms of the first phase of illness may recur. In the immune phase, leptospires can
no longer be isolated from the blood. In an usually severe form of leptospirosis, known as Weil's disease,
there is profound hepatic, renal, and central nervous
system dysfunction.

 ESSENTIALS OF DIAGNOSIS

- *Exposure history to infected animal tissue or
  urine.*
- *Abrupt onset of high fever, headache, myalgias,
  nausea, abdominal pain.*
- *Conjunctival suffusions may be present.*
- *May have biphasic illness; first phase lasts 4–9
  days, followed by 1–3 days of defervescence, then
  recurrence of symptoms.*
- *Microscopic agglutination test and enzyme-
  linked immunosorbent assay (ELISA) used to confirm the diagnosis.*
- *Weil's disease: jaundice, renal impairment, central nervous system dysfunction.*

Clinical Findings

A. SYMPTOMS AND SIGNS

The first phase of illness is characterized by the abrupt
onset of rapidly rising high fever, chills, severe myalgias,
nausea, abdominal pain, headache, and malaise. The
headache is often severe and constant. Conjunctival
suffusions, arthralgias, rashes, cough, and evidence of
hemorrhage may also be present. These symptoms usually last 4–9 days, after which there are a few days of
clinical improvement with return of the temperature to
normal. After another 1–3 days, fever recurs although
not as high as initially. Headache is the most common
symptom of this phase, though any of the symptoms
may recur, especially myalgias and abdominal pain.

In Weil's disease, a severe form of leptospirosis occurring in 5–10% of cases, the illness is also biphasic,
although the severity of illness may make this less evident. Jaundice and evidence of renal insufficiency may
be seen as early as 2–3 days into the illness, and reach a

peak during the second week of illness. Hypotension, bleeding, and confusion may be seen in Weil's disease.

B. LABORATORY FINDINGS

Leukocytosis is common. Mild forms of leptospirosis are characterized by minor elevations of the aminotransferases, alkaline phosphatase, GGTP, and a normal bilirubin. Weil's disease is characterized by hyperbilirubinemia that may reach 30 mg/dL or higher, and moderate elevations in the aminotransferases and alkaline phosphatase. The blood urea nitrogen and creatinine are high and renal insufficiency may become severe enough to cause anuria and require renal dialysis. The prothrombin time may be elevated. During the first phase of illness, diagnosis may occasionally be made by direct culture of the leptospires from blood or cerebrospinal fluid (CSF). Serologic tests, including an immunoglobulin M (IgM) ELISA and the microscopic agglutination test, are the most reliable ways to make the diagnosis. There should be a significant rise between the acute and convalescent antibody titers. Leptospira organisms may be isolated from the blood, urine, or CFS.

Treatment

Antibiotic treatment is most effective only when given within the first phase of illness, a time when the diagnosis is difficult to make. Doxycycline and penicillin G have both been shown to decrease the severity of infection when given early, but are ineffective once significant hepatorenal dysfunction has occurred. The treatment of Weil's disease is largely supportive, including renal dialysis.

Gollop JH et al: Rat-bite leptospirosis. West J Med 1993;159:76.

Jacobs R: Leptospirosis. West J Med 1980;132:440.

Lomar AV et al: Leptospirosis in Latin America. Infect Dis Clin North Am 2000;14:23.

McClain JB et al: Doxycycline therapy for leptospirosis. Ann Intern Med 1984;100:696.

Shpilberg O et al: Long-term follow-up after leptospirosis. South Med J 1990;83:405.

■ HEPATIC CANDIDIASIS

ESSENTIALS OF DIAGNOSIS

- *Immunocompromised patient; especially after bone marrow transplantation, with prolonged periods of neutropenia, broad-spectrum antibiotic treatment.*
- *Fever, may have right upper quadrant abdominal pain.*
- *Elevated alkaline phosphatase and GGTP.*
- *Multiple low-attenuation areas in liver on CT scan, may have "halo" sign.*

General Considerations

Involvement of the liver and spleen with *Candida* is an increasingly frequent complication of disseminated candidiasis. Infection usually occurs in patients with hematologic malignant tumors who have postchemotherapy neutropenia, and who have had prolonged treatment with broad-spectrum antibiotics. In some patients, empiric amphotericin treatment may have been given for prolonged fever. Spread is hematogenous from mucocutaneous sites throughout the body. Damage to the mucosa lining the gastrointestinal tract from chemotherapy may allow colonization with *Candida,* then dissemination via the portal vein to the liver.

Clinical Findings

A. SYMPTOMS AND SIGNS

Persistent fever is the hallmark of hepatic candidiasis, with fever spikes occurring in a random pattern. Right upper quadrant abdominal pain and tenderness are often found.

B. LABORATORY FINDINGS

Leukocytosis, after resolution of prior neutropenia, may be seen. Although the liver tests may be entirely normal, the alkaline phosphatase and GGTP are usually elevated. Mild elevations in the aminotransferases may be seen.

C. IMAGING

Multiple, small 1- to 2-cm lesions may be seen throughout the liver and have been demonstrated with ultrasonography, CT scanning, and MRI. CT scanning may show enhancing rings of increased attenuation surrounding low-attenuation abscesses ("halo" sign). Lesions are often also seen in the spleen (Figure 37–2).

Diagnosis

Definitive diagnosis is difficult because cultures from percutaneously obtained aspirates are often negative, especially in patients who have received amphotericin. Laparoscopically directed biopsy, with culture and stain of aspirated material, may increase the diagnostic yield.

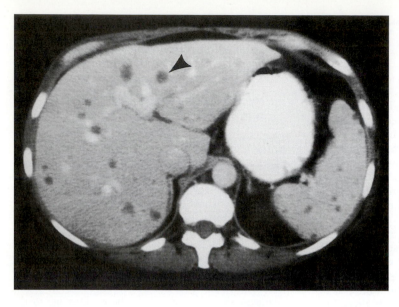

Figure 37–2. CT scan showing numerous low-density (attenuation) abscesses in the liver and spleen due to *Candida*. The arrow points to an abscess with an enhancing rim or "halo" sign, characteristic of hepatic candidiasis.

Treatment

Successful treatment of hepatic candidiasis is difficult and requires long periods of therapy with amphotericin B. Cumulative doses of greater than 4 g have been required. Fluconazole may be effective in some patients with chronic hepatic candidiasis who have not previously responded to amphotericin.

Flannery MT et al: Fluconazole in the treatment of hepatosplenic candidiasis. Arch Int Med 1992;152:406.

Gordon SC et al: Focal hepatic candidiasis with perihepatic adhesions; laparoscopic and immunohistologic diagnosis. Gastroenterology 1990;98:214.

Thaler M et al: Hepatic candidiasis in cancer patients: the evolving picture of the syndrome. Ann Intern Med 1988;108:88.

■ PARASITIC INFECTIONS OF THE LIVER

PROTOZOAN INFECTIONS

1. Amebic Liver Abscess

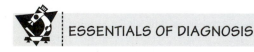

ESSENTIALS OF DIAGNOSIS

- *Right upper quadrant abdominal pain and tenderness, hepatomegaly, and fever are common.*

- *Leukocytosis and anemia are common. Liver tests may be normal or minimally elevated (especially the GGTP).*

- *Serologic tests positive in over 90% of cases; IgM ELISA available.*

- *Right hemidiaphragm often elevated on chest x-ray. Ultrasound, CT, or MRI demonstrates abscess.*

General Considerations

Entamoeba histolytica is the only ameba responsible for liver abscesses, because of its ability to cause tissue invasion. The parasite exists as either a trophozoite or a cyst, the infective form. Up to 5% of the population of the United States may at some time be asymptomatic carriers of *E histolytica* cysts. Transmission occurs via the fecal–oral route.

Risk factors for amebic liver abscess include travel to or origin from an endemic area as well as being an immunocompromised host (such as HIV infection).

Clinical Findings

A. SYMPTOMS AND SIGNS

Right upper quadrant abdominal pain is the most common symptom of an amebic liver abscess. Ten to 20 percent of patients either have had diarrhea prior to or at the time of diagnosis. Patients with pleuropulmonary complications may complain of a cough. Tender hepatomegaly and fever are the most common presenting signs on physical examination. About one-half of patients will have dullness or decreased breath sounds at the right lung base or right intercostal tenderness.

B. LABORATORY FINDINGS

Leukocytosis and anemia are the most consistent laboratory abnormalities. The aminotransferases, alkaline phosphatase, and GGTP may be normal or minimally elevated. Fewer than 10% of patients have an elevated bilirubin. Over 90% of patients have positive serologic tests. There are a number of currently available tests including ELISA, gel diffusion, indirect hemagglutination, and others. DNA probes for *E histolytica* are being developed as diagnostic tools. Due to variation in the sensitivity of serologic tests, using two of them in combination is helpful to confirm a diagnosis. When amebic abscesses are aspirated, the aspirate is usually reddish brown in color. The material is usually culture negative and may demonstrate amebic forms as well as necrotic material.

C. IMAGING

Plain chest x-ray demonstrates elevation of the right hemidiaphragm in 50% of patients. Amebic abscesses appear similar to pyogenic abscesses by ultrasonography, but are more commonly single than multiple. They are usually round or oval, located at the periphery of the right lobe, and may have enhancement of the rim. CT scanning is a more sensitive method for detecting hepatic amebic abscesses as well as extrahepatic extension. They appear as hypodense, round or oval lesions, and may have an enhancing wall or internal trabeculae. The diagnostic yield of MRI is similar to that of CT.

Complications

Pleuropulmonary complications are most common. Rupture of an abscess high in the dome of the right lobe through the diaphragm and pleura may lead to amebic empyema or consolidation of the right lung. Pleuritic chest pain, cough, and dyspnea are the most frequent symptoms of this complication. Left-sided perforations are less common. Rupture of an abscess into the peritoneum results in peritonitis and formation of an intraabdominal abscess. Amebic abscesses of the left hepatic lobe may rarely perforate into the pericardium, which is associated with pericarditis, hypotension, and a high mortality rate.

Treatment

Metronidazole, 750 mg, given orally three times a day for 10 days, is the drug of choice. Following this, iodoquinol, an intestinal amebicide, is given at a dose of 650 mg orally, three times a day for 20 days. Elimination of amebae from the intestine decreases the risk of recurrent liver abscess. Therapeutic aspiration should be performed if the abscess is large and in danger of rupture, or there is no clinical response to medical therapy within a few days. Pleural effusions, if present, should be aspirated. Surgery is rarely needed except in cases with rupture of abscesses into the chest or peritoneum.

Prognosis

The mortality rate of an uncomplicated liver abscess is less than 1%. Pleuropulmonary complications raise the mortality rate to about 6%, and pericardial involvement to close to 50%.

Barreda R, Ross PR: Diagnostic imaging of liver abscess. Crit Rev Diagn Imag 1992;33:29.

Hoffner RJ et al: Common presentations of amebic liver abscess. Ann Emerg Med 1999;34:351.

Maltz G et al: Amebic liver abscess: a 15 year experience. Am J Gastroenterol 1991;86:704.

Reed SL: Amebiasis: an update. Clin Infect Dis 1992;14:385.

Seeto RK, Rockey DC: Amebic liver abscess: epidemiology, clinical features, and outcome. West J Med 1999;170:104.

2. Malaria

 ESSENTIALS OF DIAGNOSIS

- *High spiking fever, chills, headache, nausea.*
- *Tender hepatosplenomegaly.*
- *Mild elevations in the aminotransferases, alkaline phosphatase, and GGTP may be seen. Indirect bilirubin may be elevated in* Plasmodium falciparum *infection.*
- *Thick smear of blood shows parasites frequently; parasitized red blood cells (RBCs) are rarely seen on liver biopsy.*

General Considerations

There are four species of *Plasmodium* that cause malaria in humans; *P falciparum, P vivax, P ovale, and P malariae.* When infected mosquitoes bite humans, saliva containing infectious sporozoites enter the bloodstream and are cleared by the liver. The sporozoites enter hepatocytes where asexual reproduction may occur. Periportal mononuclear infiltrates, Kupffer cell hyperplasia, iron deposition, and, rarely, parasitized red blood cells may be seen on liver biopsy.

Clinical Findings

A. SYMPTOMS AND SIGNS

High fever, with temperatures at times over 40°C, chills, headaches, and nausea are quite common presenting symptoms. The physical findings are nonspecific but may include tender hepatomegaly or splenomegaly. In severe forms of *P falciparum* malaria, signs of hepatic decompensation including encephalopathy and jaundice may be seen.

B. LABORATORY FINDINGS

Mild leukocytosis as well as elevations of the aminotransferases, alkaline phosphatase, and GGTP are common. About 5% of those with *P falciparum* malaria have elevations of the serum bilirubin greater than 2 mg/dL. The liver tests return to normal after treatment. Thick blood smears typically demonstrate parasitized red blood cells. Liver biopsy findings are nonspecific other than occasional parasitized red blood cells in hepatic sinusoids.

Treatment

Preventive treatment is recommended for all those traveling to endemic areas. There has been an increase in chloroquine-resistant *P falciparum* malaria, making both prophylactic and treatment regimens more complex. The Centers for Disease Control and Prevention (CDC), in Atlanta, Georgia, have telephone advice on current treatment programs available 24 hours a day. In rare cases of liver or other organ failure due to severe *P falciparum* malaria, exchange transfusion has been used with good results.

Ayyub M et al: Usefulness of exchange transfusion in acute liver failure due to severe falciparum malaria. Am J Gastroenterol 2000;95:802.

Hollingdale M: Malaria and the liver. Hepatology 1985;5:327.

Mishra SK et al: Hepatic changes in *P falciparum* malaria. Ind J Malariol 1992;29:167.

HELMINTHIC INFECTIONS

1. Echinococcosis

Echinococcus in humans is caused by *E granulosus* and *E multilocularis*. These tapeworms live in the intestine of carnivores, which are definitive hosts, including dogs, cats, foxes, wolves, and other animals. Humans are the intermediate hosts of the larval stage (hydatid cyst) of the parasite, as are sheep, cattle, pigs, and other herbivores. *E granulosus* is found worldwide, but is most commonly seen in sheep-raising areas. In the United States, the disease is most commonly found in the western states, Alaska, and the lower Mississippi valley. *E multilocularis* infection is different from *E granulosus* in that herbivores are not involved in the life cycle of infection. The definitive hosts are foxes, and rarely dogs or cats. The intermediate hosts are a number of rodent species. The definitive host becomes infected with tapeworms after eating the intermediate host. Humans become infected accidentally by ingesting *Echinococcus* eggs excreted in the feces of the definitive host. The disease is most common in parts of Alaska, Canada, Russia, and Europe.

ESSENTIALS OF DIAGNOSIS

- *Exposure to dogs or foxes in sheep- and cattle-raising regions.*
- *Nonspecific symptoms, which may include right upper quadrant abdominal pain.*
- *Cystic mass in the liver, or rarely other organs on ultrasound, CT, or MRI.*
- *Positive echinococcal serology.*

Pathophysiology

Echinococcus granulosus eggs are passed in the stool of definitive hosts and are accidentally swallowed by humans or other animals (intermediate hosts). The outer shell of the egg is digested in the duodenum and the embryo is released. The embryo moves into the intestinal mucosa, enters small blood vessels, and is transported by the portal circulation until trapped in the microcirculation of the liver. Whereas most of the embryos are trapped by the liver, some larvae reach the lungs, spleen, brain, kidney, bone, and other organs. Although most of the embryos are destroyed by host defenses, surviving ones develop into the hydatid stage within several days while trapped in the microcirculation. The hydatid cysts have three layers and generally grow slowly, approximately 1 cm/year. The germinal layer, from which scoleces develop, is surrounded by the two outer layers. The life cycle is completed when a definitive host (dog) ingests infected tissue from the intermediate host (sheep). The adult worm develops in the intestine of the definitive host, where it sheds eggs in the intestinal lumen, to be then passed in the stool.

In *E multilocularis* infection, the germinal membrane is not surrounded by a cyst wall. Scoleces develop in an uncontrolled manner, invading adjacent tissue, much like a neoplasm. This continuous budding of the germinal membrane produces multiple small cavities, 2–5 mm, causing alveolar hydatid disease.

Clinical Findings

A. SYMPTOMS AND SIGNS

Echinococcal infection is generally asymptomatic until growth of the hydatid cyst enlarges to the point that it impinges on some other structure or becomes visible as an abdominal mass. Since the growth rate is only about 1 cm/year, clinical symptoms and signs may take 10 or more years to develop. Right upper quadrant abdominal pain and nausea may occur when the cyst is large. Abdominal masses, at times tender, may be found. Enlarging cysts may obstruct blood flow within the liver causing portal hypertension, or cause biliary obstruction with resultant jaundice or cholangitis. Cysts enlarging toward the abdomen may rupture into the peritoneal cavity, colon, or small intestine. Because the fluid in the cysts is highly antigenic, sudden rupture into the peritoneum may cause anaphylaxis and death.

B. LABORATORY FINDINGS

Routine laboratory tests are rather nonspecific. The liver tests are usually normal until the cyst has enlarged enough to cause jaundice from biliary obstruction. There may be a mild leukocytosis and eosinophilia, especially if a cyst has ruptured or is slowly leaking. Serologic tests are available including ELISA and indirect hemagglutination. However, false-positive reactions may occur with other parasitic infections. Tests to distinguish *E granulosus* from *E multilocularis* infection are being developed.

C. IMAGING

Routine chest and abdominal x-rays may reveal cystic masses that occasionally are calcified around the rim. Ultrasonography, CT, MRI, or radionuclide scanning may also demonstrate echinococcal cysts. CT findings are those of a sharply delineated, low-attenuation mass, with a rim that may enhance. The presence of daughter cysts within a cyst with a calcified rim is virtually pathognomonic of echinococcal disease. MRI may be more sensitive than CT in distinguishing echinococcal from epithelial cysts. Endoscopic retrograde cholangiopancreatography (ERCP) has been useful in demonstrating involvement of the common bile duct with hydatid disease.

E multilocularis infection resembles polycystic disease on ultrasound, CT, or MRI. There may be myriad small, 2- to 5-mm cystic areas, at times with calcified rims.

Complications

Continued growth of hydatid cysts cause problems because of their size and location. Biliary obstruction may cause cholangitis, especially with secondary bacterial infection. Rupture of a hepatic cyst into the biliary tree has been reported in various series to occur in 5–17% of cases with liver involvement. Portal hypertension may result in esophageal varices, bleeding, and cirrhosis. Cyst rupture into the peritoneum may result in anaphylactic shock. Cysts may also rupture into the pleura, pulmonary parenchyma, or bronchi.

Treatment

Treatment of hepatic hydatid disease is primarily surgical, with considerable controversy as to the best type of surgical approach. The major objectives are to (1) remove all parasitic material including the germinal membrane lining the cyst, (2) avoid spilling cyst contents, (3) close connections between cysts and other structures such as the biliary tree, and (4) manage the residual space remaining after cyst removal. The conservative surgical approach involves evacuating the cyst followed by cyst enucleation. Scolicidal agents such as hypertonic saline may cause sclerosing cholangitis resulting from their diffusion from the cyst into the biliary tree. Although the morbidity of this approach is low, recurrence rates may be as high as 10–30%. Those who favor the more aggressive approach of pericystectomy and partial hepatectomy argue that only the removal of the pericyst lining will result in complete cure. A pedicle of greater omentum (omentoplasty) is favored as the technique to close the cyst cavity. Albendazole is given preoperatively as prophylaxis against cyst spillage. A recent report of laparoscopic treatment of hepatic hydatid cysts shows short-term mortality, morbidity, and recurrence rates comparable to open surgical series.

Selected cases in which cysts are primarily fluid filled, anechoic on ultrasonography, and do not communicate with the biliary tree can be treated with percutaneous ultrasound-guided drainage plus albendazole treatment. This has been referred to as the PAIR method, for percutaneous puncture of cysts, aspiration of fluid, infusion of scolicidal agent, and reaspiration. ERCP has been used to extract daughter cysts from the common bile duct in both *E granulosis* and *E multilocularis* disease. When surgery is contraindicated or if patients have alveolar hydatid disease caused by *E multilocularis,* drug therapy is the primary treatment. Albendazole, 400 mg orally twice a day for 28-day cycles, is the drug of choice since it achieves higher tissue and cyst levels than mebendazole. The drug is repeated in 28-day cycles as needed, with a 1–2 week break between cycles, with treatment lasting up to 6 months. Albendazole causes elevation of the aminotransferases in up to two-thirds of treated patients. The liver tests should be monitored frequently.

Liver transplantation has been used successfully in otherwise unresectable alveolar hydatid disease caused by *E multilocularis*.

Akoglu M, Davidson BR: A rational approach to the terminology of hydatid disease of the liver. J Infect 1992;24:1.

Ammann RW, Eckert J: Cestodes: Echinococcus. Gastroenterol Clin North Am 1996;25:655.

Behrns KE, Van Heerden JA: Surgical management of hepatic hydatid disease. Mayo Clin Proc 1991;66:1193.

Gschwantler M et al: Combined endoscopic and pharmaceutical treatment of alveolar echinococcosis with rupture into the biliary tree. Gastrointest Endosc 1994;40:238.

Khuroo MS et al: Percutaneous drainage versus albendazole therapy in hepatic hydatidosis: a prospective, randomized study. Gastroenterology 1993;104:1452.

Steven R et al: Laparoscopic treatment of hepatic hydatid cysts. Surgery 2000;128:36.

2. Schistosomiasis

Pathophysiology

Human hepatic schistosomiasis is due to infection with the flukes *Schistosoma mansoni* or *S japonicum*. Humans are the definitive hosts and snails serve as intermediate hosts. *S mansoni* is found throughout the Middle East and Africa as well as parts of South America and the Caribbean. *S japonicum* has a more limited geographic distribution within Asia. There are differences between the two parasites in their patterns of egg laying in humans with resultant variation in disease responses to the parasites.

The schistosomal life cycle involving humans begins with the infective larvae (cercariae) from snails penetrating the skin or mucous membranes. They lose their tails and become schistosomulae, which then migrate into the circulation. After many cercariae are destroyed by host defense mechanisms, those remaining mature to adult worms in various branches of the portal venous system. Within a month, these worms begin to lay eggs in the small terminal venules within the intestines. *S mansoni* lay eggs primarily in branches of the inferior mesenteric vein within the colon, whereas *S japonicum* deposit their eggs in the superior mesenteric vessels of the colon and small intestine. A pair of *S mansoni* worms can release 1000 eggs per day; *S japonicum* worms can release up to three times that number. Some eggs develop to miracidia, which may live in tissue for up to a month. Other eggs reach the bowel lumen and may appear in feces as early as 40 days after cercarial infection. Under proper conditions, these eggs hatch into miracidia, which may find a snail host. Within the snail, a mother sporocyst develops giving rise to daughter sporocysts and cercariae. The life cycle is completed when the cercariae leave the snail, in water, where they survive for only a few hours unless they find an acceptable definitive host.

Adult worms are well tolerated within humans, perhaps by incorporating human antigens into their lumens. Dead worms produce local inflammatory responses within terminal venules in the lung and liver resulting in necrosis and progressive fibrosis of these vessels. Most of the clinical manifestations of schistosomal disease result from the host's response to eggs trapped in tissues. This involves both circulating immune complexes and cell-mediated immune responses that are responsible for liver injury. These become more intense with repeated exposures to schistosomal antigens. Lymphocytes sensitized by cercarial antigens may stimulate collagen synthesis in areas such as the liver, where eggs are trapped. This has recently been shown to be a dynamic process under the control of fibrogenic cytokines. With increasing fibrosis, presinusoidal portal hypertension develops. Schistosomiasis-induced acquired lymphangiectasia and weakness in the portosystemic venous system may also promote the formation of gastric and esophageal varices.

Worm load influences the severity of the disease in conjunction with the host's response to the foreign antigens from these worms and eggs. *S japonicum* infection may be more severe than *S mansoni* infection because of the larger number of eggs trapped in the host's tissues.

 ESSENTIALS OF DIAGNOSIS

- *History of travel to an endemic area.*
- *Acute disease: fever, chills, nausea, diarrhea, myalgias, cough, hepatomegaly, mild splenomegaly, and mild leukocytosis with eosinophilia.*
- *Chronic disease: may be asymptomatic until late in disease. Diarrhea, hepatomegaly with significant splenomegaly, ascites, esophageal varices.*
- *Species specific ova found in stool.*

Clinical Findings

A. SYMPTOMS AND SIGNS

1. Acute schistosomiasis—Many patients infected with schistosomiasis remain asymptomatic. The initial symptom may be a pruritic, maculopapular rash caused by cercariae penetrating the skin. After a variable period of a few weeks to 2 months, patients develop anorexia, fatigue, headache, intermittent fevers, chills, myalgias, nausea, diarrhea, and cough. Both fevers and diarrhea may persist for 1–2 months. Hepatosplenomegaly along with generalized lymphadenopathy may be present. Red, edematous rectosigmoid mucosa associated with small ulcerations and petechiae may be seen on sigmoidoscopic examination. An acute toxic reaction associated with severe abdominal pain, distention, jaundice, and even coma has been seen rarely in endemic areas.

2. Chronic schistosomiasis—Chronic schistosomiasis is asymptomatic in the majority of patients, and it may take many months to years to develop the initial symptoms of abdominal pain, hepatosplenomegaly, and progressive weight loss and fatigue. Hepatosplenic schistosomiasis develops in about 10% of patients in endemic areas and may not occur until 5–15 years or longer after infection. Variceal bleeding and ascites may complicate the development of portal hypertension. Other stigmata of chronic liver disease are usually not present, or occur with terminal disease. Pulmonary hypertension and right-sided congestive heart failure may complicate late stages of the disease. Large confluent schistosomal granulomas within the intestine or mesentery may be mistaken for colonic polyps or tumors. Central nervous system disease such as transverse myelitis, immune complex glomerulonephritis, and prolonged *Salmonella* infection are other complications of chronic schistosomiasis.

B. LABORATORY FINDINGS

In acute disease, eosinophilia is the most common laboratory abnormality seen. Routine liver tests are usually normal. With the development of chronic schistosomiasis, anemia and thrombocytopenia are seen, but eosinophilia is not a common feature. Low serum albumin and hyperγglobulinemia are common. The aminotransferases are normal or minimally elevated.

The definitive diagnosis is generally made by finding ova in the stool. There are characteristic findings to distinguish between *S mansoni* and *S japonicum* eggs. Rectal biopsy with immediate examination of fresh tissue between two glass slides (crush prep) is a sensitive technique to demonstrate eggs or miracidia in tissue. Among the serologic tests available, ELISA is the screening test of choice. Immunoblot tests are used to confirm the diagnosis and distinguish between schistosome species.

C. IMAGING

Ultrasonography of the liver may demonstrate characteristic findings of scarred portal tracts that appear as thick echogenic bands with central lucency. In ad-

vanced disease, with increasing fibrosis, this central lucency may disappear. There is a good correlation between ultrasonographic grading of hepatic fibrosis and clinical stage or endoscopic grading of size of esophageal varices. Characteristic CT and MRI findings have also been described, but these techniques are less useful for large-scale screening in endemic areas. Endoscopy and upper gastrointestinal series may be useful in demonstrating esophageal varices.

Treatment

Praziquantel is the drug of choice for both *S mansoni* and *S japonicum.* It is given at a dose of 20 mg/kg, three times a day for 1 day for *S japonicum,* and 20 mg/kg, twice a day for 1 day for *S mansoni.* Some reversal of fibrosis is possible with antihelminthic drugs provided the lesion is not advanced. Dizziness and headache are frequent, but transient side effects. Oxamniquine, 15 mg/kg as a single oral dose, is an alternative treatment for *S mansoni.* Injection sclerotherapy or variceal banding has been the treatment of choice for managing esophageal varices. Propranalol may decrease portal pressure and reduce the risk of hemorrhage. Splenectomy is necessary in some patients to control thrombocytopenia and other effects of hypersplenism. Esophagogastric devascularization (EGDS) or distal splenorenal shunt is the surgical treatment of choice for bleeding esophageal varices that have not responded to sclerotherapy.

Abdel-Wahab MF et al: Grading of hepatic schistosomiasis by the use of ultrasonography. Am J Trop Med Hyg 1992;46:403.

Aboul-Enein A, Arafa S, Sakr M: Pathogenesis of varices in schistosomal portal hypertension. Dig Dis Sci 1994;39:39.

DaSilva LC, Carrilho FJ: Hepatosplenic schistosomiasis. Pathophysiology and treatment. Gastroenterol Clin N Am 1992;21:163.

Elliot DE: Schistosomiasis: pathophysiology, diagnosis, and treatment. Gastroenterol Clin North Am 1996;25:599.

Tsang VCW, Wilkins PP: Immunodiagnosis of schistosomiasis. Clin Lab Med 1991;11:1029.

3. Clonorchiasis & Opisthorchiasis

Clonorchiasis and opisthorchiasis are liver fluke infections with similar clinical, pathologic, and epidemiologic features. These diseases are found throughout Asia and Southeast Asia, where in some areas up to 90% of the population might be infected, but some studies have shown that up to 25% of Asian immigrants to the United States have active liver fluke infection.

Pathophysiology

Clonorchis sinensis, Opisthorchis felineus, and *Opisthorchis viverrini* are the three species of liver flukes that most commonly cause disease in humans. Humans, as well as other animals such as cats and dogs, are the definitive hosts. There are two intermediate hosts in the life cycle of these species, snails and freshwater fish. The adult liver flukes inhabit the bile ducts, gallbladder, and pancreatic ducts of humans or other animals where the eggs are shed, pass into the duodenum, and out into the stool. Snails ingest these eggs, miracidia develop into cercariae, and the free-swimming cercariae are shed into the water where they may penetrate the skin of freshwater fish. The parasite encysts in the muscles of fish where it becomes a metacercaria. Humans and other fish-eating animals acquire infection by eating raw or incompletely cooked fish. The parasites excyst in the definitive host's duodenum after action of digestive enzymes, migrate to the ampulla of Vater, and complete their life cycle in the bile ducts, pancreatic duct, and gallbladder. The worms may live for up to 30 years in the bile ducts of the definitive host. Adult worms begin to lay eggs within 3–4 weeks after initial infection of the definitive host.

Mechanical obstruction from worm burden, as well as potential injury from toxic metabolites of the worms, cause inflammation, thickening, and dilatation of the bile ducts. There may be secondary bacterial infection due to obstruction and bile stasis. Clonorchiasis predisposes patients to form intrahepatic gallstones, an uncommon finding in opisthorchiasis. Occasionally, ova, granulomas, and eosinophilic infiltrates are found within the hepatic parenchyma. Intrahepatic abscesses may form. Late disease may be complicated by secondary biliary cirrhosis and portal hypertension. There is an increased incidence of cholangiocarcinoma in these patients, although some authors have ascribed this to the high prevalence of hepatitis B in the same group of patients.

ESSENTIALS OF DIAGNOSIS

- *Travel to an endemic area; history of eating raw or undercooked fish.*
- *Acute disease: asymptomatic with mild infection. Moderate disease causes fever, tender hepatomegaly, eosinophilia.*
- *Chronic disease: jaundice, tender hepatomegaly, enlarged gallbladder, eosinophilia. Dilated common or intrahepatic bile ducts on imaging studies.*
- *Definitive diagnosis based on finding ova in stool or duodenal aspirate.*

Clinical Findings

A. SYMPTOMS AND SIGNS

Clinical presentation is dependent on the worm burden and duration of infection. Patients with light infection (under 100 worms) are usually asymptomatic, whereas moderate infection (up to 1000 worms) causes mild fever, nausea, anorexia, and occasionally tender hepatomegaly. In severe infection symptoms are due to the mass of worms present. Upward of 10,000–20,000 flukes may be found in rare cases. Anorexia, right upper quadrant abdominal pain, hepatomegaly, enlargement of the gallbladder, and jaundice are common. If there is associated cholangitis, high fever, chills, and worsening jaundice are usually present. In late disease, secondary biliary cirrhosis may occur with portal hypertension and subsequent variceal bleeding. Cholangiocarcinoma is a late complication that may develop in up to 50% of those infected.

B. LABORATORY FINDINGS

In early, mild disease the liver tests are usually normal. There is mild leukocytosis with eosinophilia. In moderate to severe cases, the alkaline phosphatase, GGTP, bilirubin, and aminotransferases are elevated. Low albumin and hyperγglobulinemia may be found. Definitive diagnosis is made by finding characteristic ova in the stool or duodenal aspirate. Serologic testing has not been useful in diagnosis, since many parasites share similar group antigens, and the false-positive rate of detection is quite high. DNA probes for diagnosis are being developed.

C. IMAGING

Dilatation of the common bile duct, intrahepatic bile ducts, and gallbladder are best seen on ultrasonography. CT and MRI may also demonstrate bile duct or gallbladder dilatation, as well as cystic defects and abscesses. ERCP may be useful in demonstrating biliary strictures, cysts, or the flukes themselves.

Treatment

Praziquantel, 25 mg/kg three times a day for 1 day, is the drug of choice. Albendazole, 400 mg two times a day for 7 days, is an alternative.

Chan CW, Lam SK: Diseases caused by liver flukes and cholangiocarcinoma. Baillieres Clin Gastroenterol 1987;1:297.

Chin A et al: Late complications of infection with *Opisthorcis viverrini.* West J Med 1996:164:174.

Harinasuta T, Pungpak S, Keystone JS: Trematode infections. Opisthorchiasis, clonorchiasis, fascioliasis, and paragonimiasis. Infect Dis Clin North Am 1993;7:699.

Liu LX, Harinasuta KT: Liver and intestinal flukes. Gastroenterol Clin North Am 1996;25:627.

Ona FV, Dytoc JN: Clonorchis-associated cholangiocarcinoma: a report of two cases with unusual manifestations. Gastroenterology 1991;101:831.

OTHER PARASITES

A number of other parasites are known to cause liver disease. American (Chagas' disease) and South American trypanosomiais, visceral leishmaniasis (Kala-Azar), strongyloidiasis, fascioliasis, capillariasis, ascariasis, toxocariasis, and toxoplasmosis are fairly uncommon and discussion of these illnesses is outside the scope of this chapter.

■ OTHER INFECTIONS

Liver involvement in syphilis had been described as occurring in 1–10% of cases, although an increased incidence of *T pallidum* has been seen in association with human immunodeficiency virus (HIV) infection. Hepatic manifestations occur in the stage of secondary syphilis, often in association with other systemic manifestations such as rash, lymphadenopathy, and arthritis. The symptoms may mimic those seen in acute viral hepatitis. Elevations in the alkaline phosphatase and GGTP are common and persist longer than the elevations in the aspartate aminotransferase (AST) and alanine aminotransferase (ALT). Liver biopsy findings include Kupffer cell hyperplasia, focal necrosis of hepatocytes, and periportal inflammatory cell infiltrates. Spirochetes may be demonstrated with silver stains.

Lyme disease, caused by the spirochete *Borrelia burgdorferi,* is occurring with increasing incidence in a number of regions in the United States, particularly the northeast and western states. Diagnosis is often made when the characteristic rash, erythema migrans, is seen in association with arthritis and a history of tick exposure. Acute hepatitis may rarely occur in early Lyme disease, with demonstration of *B burgdorferi* on liver biopsy. Liver test abnormalities, however, are fairly common, with elevations seen in up to 40% of cases. Elevation in the GGTP is the most common finding, with ALT elevations almost as common. Liver test abnormalities usually resolve within 3 weeks after antibiotic treatment.

Liver test abnormalities may also rarely be seen in association with other infections such as in typhoid fever, shigellosis, brucellosis, Legionnaire's disease, Q fever, or tuberculosis but will not be reviewed in detail in this chapter. Opportunistic infections seen in association with HIV infection are covered in Chapter 38.

Goellner MH et al: Hepatitis due to recurrent Lyme disease. Ann Intern Med 1988;108:707.

Horowitz HW et al: Liver function in early Lyme disease. Gastroenterology 1996;23:1412.

Kazakoff MA et al: Liver function test abnormalities in early Lyme disease. Arch Fam Med 1993;2:409.

Parcek SS: Liver involvement in secondary syphilis. Dig Dis Sci 1979;24:41.

■ LIVER DYSFUNCTION ASSOCIATED WITH SEPSIS

Liver test abnormalities and jaundice in association with bacteremia constitute an entity distinguishable from primary infection of the liver. Although initially described in infants and young children, cholestasis associated with sepsis is now recognized in both gram-negative and gram-positive infections. Elevations in the AST, ALT, and alkaline phosphatase are found in approximately 50% of patients who are bacteremic. These elevations are usually less than twice the upper limit of normal. Elevation of the bilirubin occurs less frequently, but may cause profound, and at times prolonged, jaundice. Liver biopsy is characterized by cholestasis without liver cell necrosis. Mild periportal inflammatory cell infiltration and Kupffer cell hyperplasia have been described. Dilation of the bile canaliculi has been demonstrated on transmission electron microscopy.

The mechanism of cholestasis associated with sepsis is not clear, but is probably multifactorial. Fever, hepatic hypoxia, bacterial endotoxins, and sepsis-induced cytokines may all play a role in causing hepatic dysfunction.

Oka Y et al: The mechanism of hepatic cellular injury in sepsis: an in vitro study of the implications of cytokines and neutrophils in its pathogenesis. J Surg Res 1993;55:1.

Sikuler E et al: Abnormalities in bilirubin and liver enzyme levels in adult patients with bacteremia. A prospective study. Arch Intern Med 1989;149:2246.

Liver & Biliary Disease in Patients with Human Immunodeficiency Virus Infection

38

Lorna Dove, MD, MPH & Scott L. Friedman, MD

There is a broad spectrum of liver disease described in those with human immunodeficiency virus (HIV) infection. In some cases, a diagnosis of hepatic or biliary disease establishes the diagnosis of acquired immunodeficiency syndrome (AIDS) (Table 38–1). In HIV-infected patients, liver diseases can be classified into four groups: (1) those that are associated with HIV-related immune compromise and are rarely encountered in nonimmune suppressed individuals [eg, AIDS cholangiopathy, *Mycobacterium avium*, and cytomegalovirus (CMV) hepatitis]; (2) those that occur in both immune-compromised and immune-competent individuals, but that are more prevalent in those who are HIV positive than those who are HIV negative [hepatitis B virus (HBV) and hepatitis C virus (HCV) infection, which, because of overlapping risk factors with HIV for infection, can occur in up to 90% of subpopulations with HIV]; (3) drug-induced hepatotoxicity, which results from the multiple HIV-specific antiretroviral drugs and antimicrobials used in HIV-infected individuals to prevent and control HIV-related infectious complications; and (4) all the common hepatobiliary diseases that afflict those who are HIV negative (eg, gallstone-associated cholecystitis and alcoholic liver disease). Given that liver test abnormalities are common in HIV-infected individuals, the clinician must be aware of the broad differential diagnosis for hepatobiliary disease when evaluating a patient with HIV infection and right upper quadrant symptoms or abnormal liver tests, or both.

ESSENTIALS OF DIAGNOSIS

- *Symptoms and signs alone are unreliable; further evaluation is required for specific diagnosis.*
- *Diagnosis often depends on the level of immuno-compromise.*

- *Multiple infections are common, especially in late-stage disease.*

General Considerations

The first year in which a decrease in both AIDS deaths and AIDS-defining opportunistic infections was documented was 1996. Over the past 5 years, this decline has continued with the greatest decrease noted in the incidence of *Mycobacterium avium* complex (MAC). Now that patients are remaining healthy for longer periods of time, a change might be predicted in the spectrum of liver disease seen in those who are HIV seropositive. In the past, the majority of patients with HIV infection who presented to a health care provider with an abnormal liver test had advanced immune compromise (defined as a CD4 count less than 100 cells/μL). In this population, biliary tract disorders such as AIDS cholangiopathy or infiltrative disorders such as disseminated *Mycobacterium avium-intracellulare* complex (MAC) were frequently encountered. Today, most of these patients evaluated by a practitioner have well-controlled HIV infection and chronic viral hepatitis, particularly HCV.

Clinical signs and symptoms alone rarely suggest a specific diagnosis. Some additional evaluation is almost always required in both symptomatic patients and asymptomatic patients with an elevated liver function test. Likely diagnoses may be stratified based on the extent of immunocompromise (Table 38–2). For example, patients with well-controlled HIV infection and preserved immune function, as manifested by normal or near-normal CD4 lymphocyte counts, are prone to bacterial infection, neoplasia, or drug-induced liver disease. In contrast, those with CD4 counts of less than 200/μL are additionally at risk for opportunistic infections with CMV, fungi, atypical mycobacteria, and esoteric protozoa. In late-stage HIV disease, hepatobiliary

Table 38–1. Hepatobiliary diseases that establish a diagnosis of AIDS.[1]

A diagnosis of AIDS can be made	
1. *Without* laboratory evidence of HIV infection (and assuming there are no other causes of immuno-suppression)	And with *definite* evidence of cryptosporidiosis > 1 month; cytomegalovirus infection > 1 month; herpesvirus infection > 1 month; disseminated *M avium* or *M kansasii* infection
2. *With* laboratory evidence of HIV infection	And with *definite* evidence of disseminated nontubercular mycobacterial infection; extrapulmonary tuberculosis; recurrent *Salmonella* bacteremia; Kaposi's sarcoma; disseminated coccidioidomycosis; disseminated histoplasmosis; non-Hodgkin's lymphoma
3. *With* laboratory evidence of HIV infection	And with *presumptive* evidence of disseminated mycobacterial disease

[1]From 1987 revised CDC criteria.

pathogens (eg, CMV and MAC) are almost always part of systemic infection.

The evaluation should proceed from less to more invasive. Multiple infections are not unusual, especially in late-stage immunocompromise. The main goal is identification of treatable infections or neoplasia. However, failure to establish a specific cause for abnormal tests or persistent symptoms is not unusual in HIV disease. Clinicians must always individualize the need for invasive evaluation based on the overall clinical status.

Clinical Findings

A. SYMPTOMS AND SIGNS

Patients may present with right upper quadrant discomfort, jaundice, or nonspecific symptoms such as malaise and anorexia. Another common scenario is an asymptomatic patient with rising levels of transaminases or alkaline phosphatase; the next step is to decide how extensive further evaluation should be.

Table 38–2. Hepatic disease in HIV based on CD4 lymphocyte count.

CD4 Lymphocyte Count	Predominantly Cholestatic	Predominantly Hepatocellular
500 or less	Drug toxicity	Drug toxicity
	Mycobacterium tuberculosis	Steatosis
	Kaposi's sarcoma	Viral hepatitis
	Lymphoma	Herpes simplex
	Cholelithiasis	
	Acalculous cholecystitis	
	Bacterial abscess	
250 or less	Fungal infection	*Pneumocystis carinii*
	Candidiasis	
	Histoplasmosis	
	Cryptococcosis	
	Blastomycosis	
	Cryptosporidium	
	AIDS cholangiopathy	
	Bartonella/bacillary angiomatosis and peliosis	
100 or less	Cytomegalovirus	Cytomegalovirus
	Mycobacterium avium (MAC)	
	Microsporidia	

B. LABORATORY FINDINGS

1. ALT, AST, alkaline phosphatase—The clinical presentation alone is rarely enough to distinguish between hepatic parenchymal disease and biliary disease. Specific patterns of liver tests may provide useful clues. For example, disproportionate elevation of alkaline phosphatase compared with alanine aminotransferase (ALT) or aspartate aminotransferase (AST) suggests either biliary tract disease or an infiltrative process such as lymphoma, mycobacterium, or fungal infection. In contrast, marked elevation of transaminases more commonly reflects primary parenchymal disease, such as that due to viral hepatitis or drug toxicity.

2. Serology and virology—All patients with HIV should be screened for markers of previous and/or current infection with hepatitis A, B, and C. These tests should include hepatitis B surface antigen (HBsAg), hepatitis B surface antibody (HBsAb), HCV antibody, and hepatitis A virus (HAV) antibody (total). The HAV and HBsAb are included to determine if vaccination is needed. In patients who are HBsAg positive, further evaluation should include HBV DNA and hepatitus B e antigen (HBeAg) to evaluate for active viral replication. In patients with a positive HCV antibody, a qualitative HCV RNA may be needed to establish chronic infection if there is no other evidence of liver disease, eg, a patient with normal liver enzymes. A quantitative HCV RNA is needed only if the patient is to receive treatment and wants prognostic information about the likelihood of response.

3. Liver histology—Liver biopsy should be pursued if it is believed that the findings will change clinical management. In patients in whom a treatable hepatic complication is suspected and other less invasive measures (including imaging studies, blood and bone marrow cultures, lymph node biopsy, and a trial of medication withdrawal) are not diagnostic, it should be considered. In patients with chronic viral hepatitis, a liver biopsy may be necessary to determine the stage of disease, especially if treatment is an option.

Directed find needle liver biopsy is a more appropriate test for patients with identified focal hepatic lesions. Abnormalities uncovered through abdominal imaging (see section, "Imaging Studies"), such as focal hepatic or intraabdominal masses, must be sampled by directed aspiration and are suitable for cytology studies, gram-stained smears, and cultures for acid-fast bacteria, viruses, and fungi.

Although there are some anecdotal reports of an increased incidence of postbiopsy bleeding in HIV-infected patients, biopsy is generally believed to be safe. Normal contraindications to biopsy including thrombocytopenia, coagulopathy, or other bleeding disorders continue to apply to this population. If a contraindica-

tion to percutaneous biopsy is present but histology would help with patient care, a transjugular liver biopsy can be performed by an interventional radiologist.

In any situation in which liver biopsy is contemplated in this population, the clinician must determine that the liver disease is a more proximate cause of illness or death than other concurrent extrahepatic diseases.

C. IMAGING STUDIES

Abdominal imaging plays a critical role in the early evaluation of hepatobiliary disease. Any patient who is symptomatic and has elevated liver tests or right upper quadrant pain, or both, requires early imaging with abdominal ultrasound or computed tomography (CT) scanning to identify regions of pathologic change. Findings of interest include focal or mass lesions of the liver, lymph node enlargement, intra- or extrahepatic bile duct dilatation, and gallbladder wall abnormalities. Imaging studies can also reveal findings consistent with chronic liver disease, including varices and ascites, as well as other intraabdominal disorders such as pancreatic or peritoneal disease.

Patients with evidence of bile duct abnormalities typically require a contrast study of the biliary tree, either via endoscopic retrograde cholangiopancreatography (ERCP) or percutaneous transhepatic cholangiography (PTC). In patients in whom the clinical suspicion for AIDS cholangiopathy (see discussion below) is high, a contrast study is appropriate even in the absence of dilated ducts on initial imaging. One study noted normal initial imaging studies in 25% of patients later demonstrated to have disease by cholangiogram.

The role of magnetic resonance imaging (MRI) and magnetic resonance cholangiopancreatography (MRCP) has not been defined in the setting of HIV infection. MRI is an important imaging study to identify several causes of liver abnormalities including hepatocellular carcinoma, cholangiocarcinoma, fatty infiltration, and metastatic disease. MRCP has become accepted as a valuable, noninvasive tool for evaluation of the biliary system. No HIV-specific data have been published on these modalities. Therefore, at this time, the indications for these studies should be no different for HIV-infected patients than for patients without HIV.

Differential Diagnosis

A. HEPATIC PARENCHYMA DISEASE

The differential diagnosis of hepatic parenchymal disease in patients with HIV infection is broad, and includes viral infection, adverse drug reaction, neoplasm, and opportunistic infections (see Table 38–2). Virtually any opportunistic infection can involve the liver; those more commonly seen are included below.

1. Infections

a. Hepatitis C virus infection—HCV and HIV coinfection are common, particularly in those who have a history of injection drug use. The clinical course of HCV infection is often more aggressive in the setting of HIV. Multiple studies have demonstrated an increased rate of fibrosis and prevalence of cirrhosis in this population compared with patients without HIV. In addition, HIV increases the cotransmissibility of HCV virus by sexual or perinatal transmission, although not because of an increase in HCV RNA levels.

b. Hepatitis B virus infection—HBV coinfection is also common in HIV disease. Patients with coinfection by HBV and HIV have high levels of HBV DNA polymerase and surface antigen, making their body fluids highly infectious. Some patients with previous evidence of serologic clearance, manifested by positive HBsAb, have converted from surface antigen negative to positive following HIV infection. In HIV-positive patients without serologic evidence of past or present HBV infection, vaccination is largely ineffective.

c. *Mycobacterium avium intracellulare* infection—Typically, this is a late-stage infection, and the liver involvement is part of a systemic infection. The pathologic hallmark is the presence of poorly formed granulomas associated with large numbers of acid-fast bacilli within foamy histiocytes (Figure 38–1). Acid-fast smear of infected tissue usually reveals organisms, although distinction from *Mycobacterium tuberculosis* is not possible by smear alone. Patients typically have systemic symptoms, including fever, lymphadenopathy, diarrhea, and night sweats. Associated bone marrow infiltration is common. The diagnosis can often be established by blood culture, bone marrow, or lymph node examination prior to consideration of liver biopsy. Imaging studies may reveal diffuse intraabdominal adenopathy. As noted in the preceding section, liver abnormalities typically include disproportionate elevation of serum alkaline phosphatase, with only modest elevations of bilirubin, AST, and ALT.

d. *Mycobacterium tuberculosis* infection—*M tuberculosis* infection may occur before patients are markedly immunocompromised. Symptoms are those associated with tuberculous infection in immunocompetent individuals and include fever, cough, night sweats, and, occasionally, lymphadenopathy. Extrapulmonary tuberculosis, including liver disease, is more common in HIV-infected patients, and may be manifested by abdominal pain, jaundice, or hepatosplenomegaly.

e. Bacillary peliosis hepatis—Bacillary peliosis hepatis is a systemic infection caused by *Bartonella quintana* or *Bartonella henselae* (previously called *Rochalimaea* sp.), two organisms closely related to other *Bartonella* species. In this lesion, bacilli are seen within dilated vascular (peliotic) spaces. Patients typically present with fever and elevated liver enzymes, often in association with cutaneous or bony involvement. The causative organism appears within amorphous clusters near dilated vascular spaces in the liver. These peliotic spaces may be micro- or macroscopic. Diagnosis is established by Warthin-Starry silver staining of infected tissue, chocolate agar culture, or polymerase chain reaction using specific primers.

f. Cytomegalovirus infection—CMV infection of the liver has been documented in many patients with

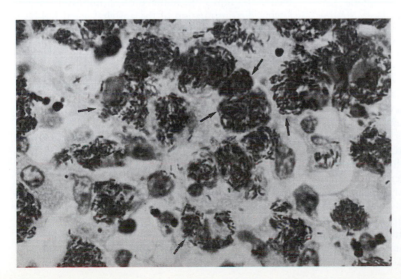

Figure 38–1. *Mycobacterium avium* complex in the liver. High-power photomicrograph of a liver biopsy specimen from a patient with late-stage HIV disease, in which tissue has been stained with an acid-fast stain, revealing large numbers of organisms within macrophages **(arrows)**. (Courtesy of B Herndier, MD.)

late-stage HIV infection, although luminal tract infection by CMV is more common. As with other opportunistic infections, CMV hepatitis is always part of systemic infection. Clinical findings with liver infection may include fevers and right upper quadrant pain in association with nonspecific elevations of transaminases. Infected tissue reveals typical viral inclusions, creating an owl's eye appearance within endothelial cells, macrophages, or hepatocytes. Mononuclear cell infiltration or neutrophils may be present.

g. Cryptococcal, coccidioidal, or histoplasmal infection—Cryptococcal, coccidioidal, and histoplasmal infections are usually seen in association with systemic disease. Liver involvement may be macro- or microscopic. *Candida* rarely infects the liver, despite its high prevalence in mucocutaneous sites. Hepatic *Candida* infections are confined to patients who are neutropenic, typically in response to systemic chemotherapy used to treat non-Hodgkin's lymphoma.

h. *Pneumocystis carinii* infection—Rare cases of *Pneumocystis carinii* or microsporidial infection in the liver have been reported. The presence of *P carinii* in extrapulmonary sites typically is seen in patients who have had inhalation therapy with a drug such as pentamidine, which fails to protect sites outside the airways.

i. HIV infection—Typically, HIV is found within hepatic macrophages and occasionally sinusoidal endothelial cells. Infection of macrophages is not surprising given the propensity of the virus to infect the cell type in other organs. Nonetheless, infection of hepatic macrophages by HIV suggests that the liver may be a large reservoir of virus. Additionally, HIV infection of Kupffer's cells could result in impaired cell function, leading to the increased incidence of enteric bacteremias in this population. Despite the demonstration of HIV in liver, there is no discrete clinical syndrome of liver disease that has been ascribed to HIV alone.

j. Drug reaction—Potentially hepatotoxic drugs frequently used in the management of HIV-positive patients are summarized in Table 38–3. Liver abnormalities associated with most of these drugs are typically indicative of hepatocellular injury, although certain drugs are associated with a predominantly "cholestatic" pattern of liver injury. The use of highly active antiretroviral therapy (HAART) against HIV has become the standard of care. Hepatotoxicity has been noted with all of the protease inhibitors as well as many of the nucleoside and nonnucleoside analog drugs. A recent study compared the incidence of hepatotoxicity in patients receiving several different regimens with and without protease inhibitors and found that ritonavir was associated with a higher incidence of hepatotoxicity when

Table 38–3. Drugs commonly associated with liver abnormalities used in the treatment of HIV and its complications.

Predominantly Hepatocellular Disease	Predominantly Cholestatic Disease
Clarithromycin	Rifampin
Delaviridine	Ketoconazole
Didanosine (ddI)	Trimethoprim-sulfamethoxazole
Dideoxycytidine (ddC)	Dapsone
Efavirenz	
Indinavir	
Isoniazid	
Ketoconazole	
Nelfinavir	
Nevirapine	
Pentamidine	
Ritonavir	
Saquinavir	
Stavudine (d4T)	
Trimethoprim-sulfamethoxazole	
Zidovudine	

compared with indinavir, nelfinavir, saquinavir, and nucleoside analog regimens.

Hepatic steatosis is another pattern of injury noted as a complication of HIV medications. Hepatic steatosis in the setting of lactic acidosis has been described for zidovudine, didanosine, and now stavudine. Some patients have developed progressive, fatal hepatic steatosis. Typically, the syndrome has occurred in patients who appear to be relatively well and has been ascribed to mitochondria injury. In nonfatal cases, improvement following discontinuation of the antiviral agent has been observed, with no documented progression to chronic liver injury. Two other frequently noted problems are sulfa allergy with associated liver toxicity and hyperbilirubinemia in the setting of indinavir. This is primarily an elevation in unconjugated bilirubin and is not related to liver injury.

2. Neoplasms

a. Non-Hodgkin's lymphoma—Non-Hodgkin's lymphoma (now referred to as either large cell lymphoma or Burkitt's lymphoma, depending on the histologic findings) typically presents in extranodal sites, and occurs at all stages of HIV infection with equal frequency. The liver is among the more common extranodal sites; there may be focal hepatic lesions associated with pain, weight loss, night sweats, and a progressive rise in both alkaline phosphatase and transaminase levels. The lesion is typically identified by noninvasive imaging, and diagnosis can be established by an experienced pathologist using fine-needle aspiration and cytologic or conventional liver biopsy (Figure 38–2). The prognosis of non-Hodgkin's lymphoma is largely correlated with the stage of HIV infection and extent of immunocompromise (see section, "Prognosis"). Although not strictly an AIDS-defining diagnosis, advanced-stage Hodgkin's lymphoma, often with visceral involvement, is also seen with increased prevalence in all risk groups.

b. Kaposi's sarcoma—Kaposi's sarcoma is a neoplasm that is largely confined to skin and mucous membranes but can involve the liver. Recent evidence has revealed that greater than 85% of tumors are associated with a virus that has been named Kaposi's sarcoma-associated herpes virus (KSHV) or human herpesvirus 8 (HHV-8). Hepatic lesions are usually asymptomatic; however, there have been reports of bleeding from lesions following liver biopsy.

B. BILIARY TRACT DISEASE

The differential diagnosis of biliary tract disease is dominated by a syndrome called AIDS cholangiopathy but also includes other opportunistic infections and neoplasms (Table 38–4).

1. AIDS cholangiopathy—AIDS cholangiopathy is a syndrome characterized by marked abnormalities of biliary ducts in patients with HIV disease (Figure 38–3). These abnormalities may include papillary stenosis, sclerosing cholangitis, or long extrahepatic strictures. The cause of this syndrome is uncertain, but in many cases it is associated with the presence of one or more organisms in the biliary epithelium, including microsporidium, cryptosporidium, or CMV. Typical

Table 38–4. Differential diagnosis of biliary tract disease in HIV infection.

AIDS cholangiopathy
Lymphoma
Kaposi's sarcoma
Acalculous cholecystitis (often due to cytomegalovirus)
Non-AIDS disorders, including gallstone disease

symptoms include right upper quadrant pain and fever, although the patients may sometimes be asymptomatic. Laboratory abnormalities include marked elevation of alkaline phosphatase and modest elevation of AST and ALT. Jaundice is extremely unusual in this syndrome and should raise the possibility of an alternative or additional hepatobiliary disorder. Imaging studies are useful in evaluating AIDS cholangiopathy, as 75% of patients will have abnormal CT scans or ultrasound studies revealing ductal dilatation (see section, "Imaging Studies").

2. Non-Hodgkin's lymphoma; Kaposi's sarcoma—Rare cases of non-Hodgkin's lymphoma or Kaposi's sarcoma have been reported in the biliary tree, reflecting the aggressive nature and unusual presentations of these neoplasms in this setting.

3. Cytomegalovirus cholecystitis—Acalculous cholecystitis due to gallbladder involvement by CMV has been described. Patients present with severe abdominal pain with or without peritonitis. CMV cholecystitis is not part of the AIDS cholangiopathy syndrome but should be suspected in any patient with clinical evidence of cholecystitis. Prolonged fasting (eg, in patients

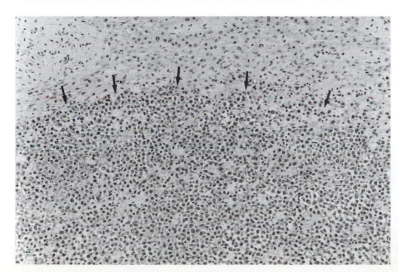

Figure 38–2. Non-Hodgkin's (large cell) lymphoma of liver. Low-power photomicrograph of lymphoma invading hepatic tissue. A monomorphic population of lymphocytes is evident *(arrows)* (hematoxylin & eosin stain). (Courtesy of B Herndier, MD.)

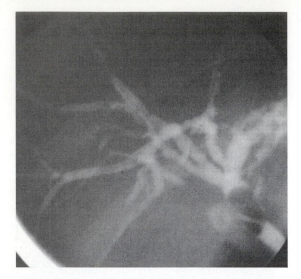

Figure 38–3. AIDS cholangiopathy. A cholangiogram of papillary stenosis with a secondary dilated common bile duct. (Courtesy of J Cello, MD.)

receiving total parenteral nutrition) may also lead to gallbladder distention and pain, although fasting has not been directly linked to acalculous cholecystitis in this population.

Treatment

Treatment of hepatobiliary abnormalities in patients with HIV infection is dictated by the specific findings uncovered during evaluation, the severity of immuno-compromise, and the presence of concurrent underlying infections or neoplasms.

A. HEPATIC DISEASE

1. Drug reaction—Any medication should be seen as potentially hepatotoxic and its discontinuation or substitution considered. Particularly culpable agents include sulfonamides and antiretrovirals. Development of drug resistance in HIV is not rare; therefore, any withdrawal of antiretrovirals should be done judiciously under the advice of a practitioner experienced in HIV care.

2. *M avium complex* infection—For documented *M avium* infection, the goal is reduction in bacterial burden and relief of symptoms rather than complete eradication of the organism. Because of its prevalence, current recommendations for management of HIV disease include prophylactic use of antibiotics in patients with profound immunocompromise (CD4 count < 100/μL). In those with documented disease, multidrug regimens

are required. Macrolide-based therapy is associated with improved survival and decreased relapse. Treatment is with azithromycin 500 mg/d or clarithromycin 500 mg two times a day plus ethambutol 25 mg/kg/d or rifabutin 300 mg/d. Life-long therapy for supresion is required.

3. *M tuberculosis* infection—The treatment of *M tuberculosis* can be very complex in patients with HIV infection. Protease inhibitors (PI) and nonnucleoside reverse transcriptase inhibitors (NNRTI) may inhibit or induce cytochrome P-450 isoenzymes (CYP450). Rifamycins used for the treatment of tuberculosis may induce CYP450; therefore, drug–drug interactions can be expected. Patients who are taking PIs and/or NNRTIs and undergoing treatment for active tuberculosis (TB) with rifabutin or rifampin should be monitored closely for the possibility of TB treatment failure, antiretroviral treatment failure, and drug toxicities associated with increased serum concentrations of rifamycins. In patients on no antiretrovirals or taking only nucleoside reverse transcriptase inhibitors (NRTIs) adjustments in therapy are not required. Initial treatment of *M tuberculosis* in this population should include four drugs initially for 2 months while awaiting the results of sensitivity testing: isoniazid, 300 mg orally or intramuscularly; rifampin, 600 mg orally or intramuscularly; pyrazinamide, 15 mg/kg intramuscularly up to 1 g; and ethambutol, 15–25 mg/kg orally. This regimen is followed by 6 months of isoniazid and rifampin for susceptible strains. Treatment of patients on PIs or NNRTIs should be individualized based on their antiretroviral regime and in conjunction with the published guidelines.

4. Bacillary peliosis hepatis—Bacillary peliosis hepatis responds to erythromycin, 500–1000 mg, four times per day, which is the drug of choice for 8–12 weeks; parenteral administration may be required in severe cases. Responses to tetracycline, minocycline, or cephalosporin have also been documented; sulfonamides are ineffective. Long-term (ie, more than 2 months) or chronic therapy is recommended in patients with HIV infection. Resolution of peliosis has been documented in several cases following antibiotic therapy.

5. Non-Hodgkin's lymphoma; Kaposi's sarcoma—Treatment options for Kaposi's sarcoma and non-Hodgkin's lymphoma include chemotherapy or radiation therapy. Any patient treated should be treated with the consultation of an oncologist. Although no improved survival rates have been documented following such regimens, some treatment is usually required because of the rapid growth of these tumors, particularly lymphomas. Chemotherapy is especially difficult to use in these immunocompromised patients, because most agents can further increase the susceptibility to infection, and also suppress the bone marrow. In patients with lymphoma and CD4 counts of less than 200/μL, chemotherapy is given in standard dosages combined with granulocyte–macrophage colony-stimulating factor (GM-CSF); more immunosuppressed patients require lower dosage regimens. Novel immunologic and anticytokine therapies are currently under investigation but are not yet available for general use. Visceral symptomatic Kaposi's sarcoma is often treated with combination chemotherapy, including doxorubicin, bleomycin, or vincristine.

6. Cytomegalovirus infection—CMV infection is rarely localized only to the liver; patients with systemic CMV disease involving the liver are treated with ganciclovir, 5 mg/kg intravenously every 12 hours for 14–21 days (induction), followed by 5–6 mg/kg for 5–7 days per week (maintenance). Alternatives to ganciclovir in patients who do not respond are (1) foscarnet, 90 mg/kg intravenously every 8 hours for 14–21 days, infused over 1 hour (induction), followed by 90–120 mg/kg/d intravenously as a 2-hour infusion (maintenance); dosages must be reduced in patients with impaired creatinine clearance. Vigorous hydration and careful monitoring of serum calcium levels are essential when using foscarnet, as life-threatening renal failure with hypocalcemia is a potential adverse reaction; the drug should not be used simultaneously with pentamidine. (2) Cidofovir, 5 mg/kg intravenously every week followed by 5 mg/kg every 2 weeks for maintenance. Probenecid should be coadministered with cidofovir to minimize renal toxicity. Patients with concurrent ocular CMV infection must be treated chronically with either ganciclovir or foscarnet, whereas those with only visceral disease may be treated for 4–8 weeks. For recurrence, chronic maintenance therapy is appropriate. Chronic parenteral therapy usually requires placement of an indwelling venous catheter to permit outpatient administration.

7. Fungal infections—Visceral fungal infections involving the liver, including histoplasmosis, coccidiomycosis, candidiasis, and cryptococcosis, require aggressive therapy as outlined below.

    a. Disseminated histoplasmosis—Amphotericin B, 1 mg/kg for a mininum of 15 mg/kg total dose followed by consolidation therapy with itraconazole 200 mg twice a day for 12 weeks, followed by itraconozole 200–400 mg daily for life.

    b. Coccidiomycosis—Amphotericin B, 1.0–1.5 mg/kg/d for a cumulative dose of 1.0–2.5 g. Life-long suppressive therapy with ketoconazole (400 mg/d orally) or fluconazole (400–600 mg/d orally) must be instituted to prevent relapses.

    c. Candidiasis—Disseminated candidiasis is exceedingly rare. Treatment decisions should be made on a case by case basis with the guidance of an infectious disease specialist.

    d. Cryptococcosis—Amphotericin B, 0.6–0.8 mg/kg/d intravenously plus flucytosine 25 mg/kg orally four times a day for 2 weeks followed by fluconazole 400 mg daily for 8 weeks followed by fluconazole 200 mg orally daily for life.

8. Hepatitis C infection—Treatment of chronic HCV infection is indicated if the provider feels that the patient's life expectancy is more likely to be determined by liver disease than HIV. There are limited data on the efficacy of HCV treatment in the setting of HIV. Current data indicate that interferon at 3 million units three times per week and ribavirin 800–1200 mg/d are well tolerated and are associated with similar initial response rates. Pegylated interferon has recently been approved by the Food and Drug Administration (FDA) and several studies are underway evaluating the efficacy of this drug in the setting of HIV.

9. Hepatitis B infection—The current FDA-approved therapies for hepatitis B are interferon and lamivudine. Data suggest that there is limited benefit of interferon alone in the setting of HIV. However, there are good response rates to lamivudine in coinfected patients. Therefore, patients with evidence of actively replicating virus and liver disease should be considered for treatment. Lamivudine administered at 100 mg/d is sufficient to control HBV, but HIV patients are often on higher doses given that lamivudine is also used as a treatment for HIV at a dose of 300 mg/d. Unfortunately, mutation of the HBV virus and subsequent resistance to lamivudine is common. Currently,there are no additional drugs approved for the treatment of lamivudine-resistant HBV.

10. *P carinii* infection—Those rare cases of *P carinii* infection involving the liver will respond to oral therapy with dapsone and trimethoprim in mild cases. Severely ill patients require parenteral therapy for 14–21 days with pentamidine, 3–4 mg/kg/d intravenously, or trimethoprim, 15 mg/kg/d, and sulfamethoxazole, 100 mg/kg/d.

B. BILIARY TRACT DISEASE

1. AIDS cholangiopathy—Effective therapy of AIDS cholangiopathy is confined to patients with papillary stenosis, whose pain is improved in at least 50% of cases by endoscopic sphincterotomy. In all patients, the syndrome is associated with progressive elevation of alkaline phosphatase, possibly reflecting progressive intrahepatic biliary lesions.

2. Acalculous cholecystitis—Acalculous cholecystitis is usually a surgical emergency. In otherwise stable patients, cholecystectomy is indicated, but patients are often too ill to tolerate laparotomy. In this circumstance, cholecystotomy by a percutaneous catheter or minilaparotomy may be feasible. Evidence or strong suspicion of CMV infection as an underlying cause may necessitate use of ganciclovir or foscarnet.

Prognosis

The prognosis in the patient with HIV infection is dictated almost entirely by the extent of immunocompromise and control of HIV replication. Indicators of long-term disease progression (several months to years) in HIV infection include HIV viral load, serum CD4 lymphocyte counts, and CD4:CD8 lymphocyte ratios. Severe wasting also portends a reduced survival time. In one study, patients with serum albumin of less than 2 g/dL had a dramatically reduced mean survival rate, compared with those whose albumin was greater than 3 g/dL. Now that morbidity and mortality have improved in HIV, we anticipate that health care providers will see potential complications of liver disease increase, in particular viral hepatitis.

REFERENCES

Adal KA, Cockerell CJ, Petri WA: Cat scratch disease, bacillary angiomatosis, and other infections due to *Rochalimaea*. N Engl J Med 1994;330:1509.

Benhamou Y et al: Liver fibrosis progression in human immunodeficiency virus and hepatitis C virus coinfected patients. Hepatology 1999;30:1054.

Benhamou Y et al: Long-term incidence of hepatitis B virus resistance to lamivudine in human immunodeficiency virus-infected patients. Hepatology 1999;30:1302.

Bica I et al: Increasing mortality due to end-stage liver disease in patients with human immunodeficieny virus infection. Clin Infect Dis 2001;32:492.

Cello J: AIDS-related biliary tract disease. Gastrointest Endosc Clin North Am 1998;8:963.

Centers for Disease Control: Prevention and treatment of tuberculosis among patients infected with human immunodeficiency virus: principles of therapy and revised recommendations. MMWR 1998;47(no. RR-20).

Centers for Disease Control: Notice for readers: updated guidelines for the use of rifabutin or rifampin for the treatment and prevention of tuberculosis among HIV-infected patients taking protease inhibitors or nonnucleoside reverse transcriptase inhibitors. MMWR 2001;49:185.

Centers for Disease Control. Guidelines for national human immunodeficiency virus case surveillance, including monitoring for human immunodeficiency virus infection and acquired immunodeficiency syndrome. MMWR 1999;48(RR-13):1, 29.

Chalasani N, Wilcox N: Etiology, evaluation, and outcome of jaundice in patients with acquired immunodeficiency syndrome. Hepatology 1996;23(4):728.

Freiman JP et al: Hepatomegaly with severe steatosis in HIV-seropositive patients. AIDS 1993;7:379.

Friedman SL (guest editor): AIDS: a review for the hepatologist. Semin Liver Dis 1993;12:103.

Greub G et al: Clinical progression, survival, and immune recovery during antiretroviral therapy in parties with HIV-1 and hepatitis C virus coinfection: the Swiss HIV Cohort Study. Lancet 2000;356:1800.

Herndier BG, Kaplan KD, McGrath MS: Pathogenesis of AIDS lymphomas. AIDS 1994;8:1025.

Housset C et al: Immunohistochemical evidence for human immunodeficiency virus-1 infection of liver Kupffer cells. Human Pathol 1990;21:404.

Landau A et al: Efficacy and safety of combination therapy with interferon-alfa 2b and ribavirin for chronic hepatitis C in HIV-infected patients. AIDS 2000;14(14):839.

McDonald JA et al: Effect of human immunodeficiency virus (HIV) infection on chronic hepatitis B hepatic viral antigen display. J Hepatol 1987;4:337.

Miller KD et al: Lactic acidosis and hepatic steatosis associated with use of stavudine: report of four cases. Ann Intern Med 2000; 133(3):192.

Perkocha L et al: Clinical and pathological features of bacillary peliosis hepatis in association with human immunodeficiency virus infection. N Engl J Med 1990;323:1581.

Poles N et al: Liver biopsy findings in 501 patients infected with human immunodeficiency virus (HIV). J Acquir Immune Defic Syndr Human Retrovirol 1996;11: 170.

Schmitt MP, Steffan AM, Gendrault JL: Multiplication of human immunodeficiency virus in primary cultures of human Kupffer cells: possible role of liver macrophages infection in the physiopathology of AIDS. Res Virol 1990;141:143.

Sulkowski M et al: Hepatotoxicity associated with antiretroviral therapy in adults infected with human immunodeficiency virus and the role of hepatitis C or B virus infection. JAMA 2000;283:74.

Thomas D et al: Effect of human immunodeficiency virus on hepatitis C virus infection among injection drug users. J Infect Dis 1996;174:690.

Volberding PA, Aberg JA (editors): *The San Francisco General Hospital Handbook of HIV Management.* The Parthenon Publishing Group, 1999.

Wong D et al: Interferon alfa treatment of chronic hepatitis B: randomized trial in a predominantly homosexual male population. Gastroenterology 1996;108:165.

Alcoholic Liver Disease

39

Jacquelyn J. Maher, MD

ESSENTIALS OF DIAGNOSIS

- *History or strong suspicion of heavy ethanol use (at least 20 g, but typically 40–80 g ethanol/d).*
- *Mild to moderate elevation of hepatic transaminases [<500 IU/L, with aspartate aminotransferase:alanine aminotransferase (AST:ALT) ratio >2].*
- *Liver biopsy with steatosis; Mallory bodies; ballooning degeneration of hepatocytes; neutrophilic infiltrate; with or without pericellular fibrosis.*

General Considerations

Excessive alcohol consumption can lead to several abnormalities in the liver, ranging from steatosis, to alcoholic hepatitis, to hepatic fibrosis and cirrhosis. These terms are based largely on histologic status; they infer a spectrum of increasing disease severity, although clinically there can be significant overlapping among these disorders. Steatosis represents a purely biochemical disturbance in hepatocytes. It does not connote true liver injury, and is completely reversible with abstinence. Hepatitis and fibrosis, by contrast, are serious disorders characterized by hepatic inflammation, necrosis, and scarring. In many patients, alcoholic hepatitis precedes fibrosis, although the two lesions often occur together and may arise from different pathophysiologic mechanisms. Hepatic fibrosis, if unchecked, ultimately leads to irreversible cirrhosis.

There is little doubt that chronic ethanol ingestion plays a key role in the development of liver disease. Countries from around the world report a direct correlation between cirrhosis-related mortality rates and per capita ethanol consumption; in the United States, cirrhosis represents the tenth leading cause of death, with most patients suffering from alcoholic liver disease. Over 900,000 persons in the United States are estimated to have cirrhosis; at least 40% and perhaps as many as 90% of these individuals consume ethanol chronically.

Figure 39–1 provides proof of a cause-and-effect relationship between alcohol consumption and mortality rates from cirrhosis. This graph, which depicts the age-adjusted death rates from cirrhosis in the United States from 1910 to 1997, demonstrates a sharp decline in cirrhosis-related mortality rates after the enactment of Prohibition in 1916 and a gradual increase following its repeal in 1932. Cirrhosis mortality rose until the mid-1970s, coincident with the peak in per capita ethanol consumption. Over the past two decades, ethanol consumption and cirrhosis mortality have both been steadily declining.

Alcoholic liver disease was once believed to require prolonged periods of heavy ethanol use. Recent data, however, indicate that more modest levels of alcohol consumption can also place individuals at risk. Population-based studies show that the relative risk of liver disease begins to rise at daily doses of ethanol as low as 30 g (three drinks), which has led to a recommendation that the maximum safe dose of ethanol is 20 g (two drinks) daily. It is important to note that although the *relative* risk of liver disease is substantially increased by ethanol consumption, the *absolute* risk is low. Indeed, even among individuals who drink more than 60 g/d of ethanol, the incidence of cirrhosis is only 15%. This suggests that other factors, perhaps hereditary, environmental, or both, interact with ethanol to produce liver disease.

Bellentani S et al: Drinking habits as cofactors of risk for alcohol induced liver damage. The Dionysos Study Group. Gut 1997;41:845.

Pathophysiology

Ethanol has been described as an idiosyncratic hepatotoxin in humans because it does not reproducibly cause liver damage even in heavy drinkers. A number of different mechanisms have been proposed by which ethanol induces liver disease; to date, no single theory is considered predominant. The following section describes how chronic ethanol ingestion (in the absence of hereditary or environmental cofactors) might produce liver damage.

A. ETHANOL METABOLISM IN THE LIVER

Ethanol metabolism is essential to the development of alcoholic liver injury. In the liver, ethanol is oxidized

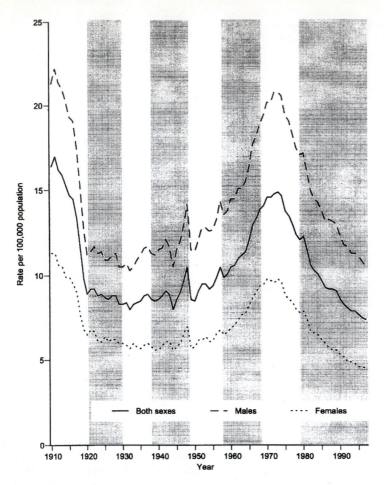

Figure 39–1. Age-adjusted death rates of liver cirrhosis: Death Registration States, 1910–1932, and United States, 1933–1997. (Death rates per 100,000 population.) (Reprinted from Saadatmand F et al: Surveillance Report #54—Liver Cirrhosis Mortality in the United States, 1970–97. Division of Biometry and Epidemiology, National Institute on Alcohol Abuse and Alcoholism, December 2000.)

primarily by the cytosolic enzyme alcohol dehydrogenase (ADH). ADH converts ethanol to acetaldehyde, which is then oxidized to acetate (primarily in mitochondria) by aldehyde dehydrogenase (ALDH). Both ADH-mediated ethanol oxidation and ALDH-mediated acetaldehyde oxidation are coupled to the reduction of NAD⁺ to NADH (Figure 39–2).

Alternate pathways of ethanol metabolism also exist in the liver. In alcoholics, ethanol can be oxidized in microsomes by the cytochrome P-4502E1(CYP2E1); this mixed-function oxidase is greatly induced by chronic ethanol consumption. In both alcoholics and nonalcoholics, ethanol can also be metabolized in peroxisomes by catalase, although this is considered a minor pathway in relation to ADH and CYP2E1. CYP2E1-mediated ethanol metabolism in alcoholics is particularly relevant to liver injury because it leads to formation of reactive oxygen intermediates (see following discussion). CYP2E1 has a much higher K_m for ethanol than does ADH; thus, even in alcoholics, ADH

metabolizes much of the ethanol reaching the liver, with CYP2E1 contributing to its metabolism only when blood levels are high. Both ADH and CYP2E1 are present in highest concentration near terminal hepatic venules; this may account in part for the centrizonal distribution of alcoholic liver injury.

Recent studies indicate that ADH is present in the stomach and intestine as well as the liver. A portion of ingested ethanol is metabolized by the gastric enzyme (referred to as the "first-pass" metabolism of ethanol). Metabolism of ethanol in the stomach limits the amount available for absorption and ultimate delivery to the liver. Gastric ADH activity is lower in women than in men; consequently, equivalent doses of ingested ethanol tend to cause higher blood ethanol levels in women than in men.

B. DIRECT TOXIC EFFECTS OF ETHANOL (TABLE 39–1)

1. Alteration of lipid and carbohydrate metabolism—The reduction of NAD⁺ to NADH that accom-

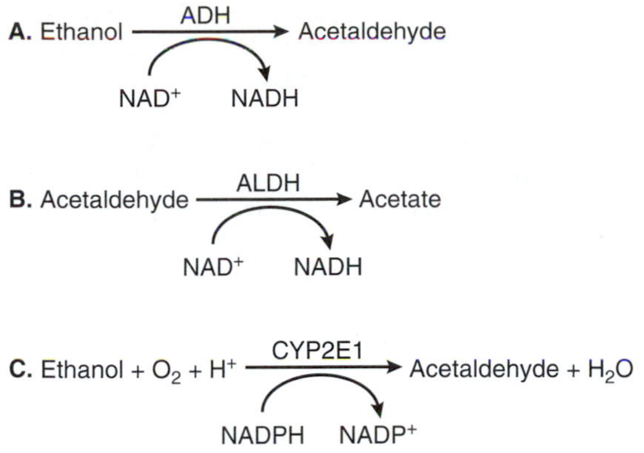

A. Ethanol $\xrightarrow{\text{ADH}}$ Acetaldehyde

$\text{NAD}^+ \quad \text{NADH}$

B. Acetaldehyde $\xrightarrow{\text{ALDH}}$ Acetate

$\text{NAD}^+ \quad \text{NADH}$

C. Ethanol + O_2 + H^+ $\xrightarrow{\text{CYP2E1}}$ Acetaldehyde + H_2O

$\text{NADPH} \quad \text{NADP}^+$

Figure 39–2. **A:** Oxidative metabolism of ethanol. Ethanol is oxidized to acetaldehyde by alcohol dehydrogenase (ADH). **B:** Acetaldehyde is then metabolized to acetate by aldehyde dehydrogenase (ALDH). Both reactions are accompanied by the conversion of NAD^+ to NADH. **C:** In alcoholics, CYP2E1 can also contribute to ethanol metabolism. This reaction uses oxygen and NADPH, producing NADP^+ and H_2O.

panies ethanol oxidation shifts the redox state of hepatocytes. The excess NADH alters several NAD^+-dependent processes, particularly those involved in intermediary metabolism. The redox shift enhances triacylglycerol synthesis in hepatocytes; at the same time, it inhibits β-oxidation of fatty acids, resulting in esterification and storage as triglyceride. Ethanol also alters the expression of several enzymes involved in fat metabolism. Those that oxidize fatty acids tend to be inhibited, whereas those that promote lipid synthesis are enhanced. The net result of these processes is hepatic steatosis.

A high NADH:NAD^+ ratio also causes disturbances in gluconeogenesis by limiting the availability of several intermediates in the gluconeogenic pathway (oxaloacetate, pyruvate, and dihydroxyacetone-phosphate) and by inhibiting the activity of key enzymes involved in glucose production. Together, these alterations can result in profound hypoglycemia, particularly in alcoholics with underlying carbohydrate malnutrition.

2. Oxidative stress—Metabolism of ethanol by CYP2E1 gives rise to oxygen-derived free radicals, including the superoxide ion radical (O_2^-) and the hydroxyl radical ($^\bullet$OH). These reactive oxygen species, particularly the hydroxyl radical, can interact with cellular proteins, lipids, or DNA to begin a chain reaction of peroxidation that results in cell injury or death. ADH-mediated ethanol oxidation may also promote free radical production in liver cells by a different mechanism. In this case, the high NADH:NAD^+ ratio resulting from ethanol oxidation promotes mobilization of iron from ferritin, which can then react with H_2O_2 to produce hydroxyl and superoxide radicals. The resultant oxidative stress can lead to hepatocellular injury.

Other metabolic processes linked to ethanol metabolism may also promote oxidative stress in the liver. Acetaldehyde oxidation, for example, yields acetate; in high concentrations, acetate promotes conversion of pyridine nucleotides to purines in liver cells, which are then catabolized by xanthine oxidase in a reaction that generates oxygen radicals. Acetaldehyde oxidation itself can potentially lead to free radical production, if catalyzed by alternate pathways from ALDH (such as aldehyde oxidase or xanthine oxidase). Neutrophils and Kupffer cells, which produce superoxide upon activation, can be stimulated by chronic ethanol ingestion and provide an additional source of oxygen radicals. The traditional view was that Kupffer cells and neutrophils played a supporting role in

Table 39–1. Putative mechanisms of alcoholic liver injury.

Direct toxic effects of ethanol

Oxyradical formation	→ Peroxidation of membrane lipids
Acetaldehyde–protein adduct formation	→ Altered enzyme function; altered protein trafficking
Disturbance of intermediary metabolism	→ Fatty liver; hypoglycemia

Immune responses to ethanol

Cytokine production	→ Hepatocellular necrosis; neutrophil infiltration
Autoimmune responses to hepatocellular proteins	→ Hepatocellular necrosis; ? fibrosis

Mechanisms of fibrosis

Oxyradical formation	
Lipid peroxidation	
Local production of transforming growth factor-β	→ Stellate cell activation
Extracellular deposition of acetaldehyde–protein adducts	

ethanol-induced oxidant stress, subordinate to CYP2E1-mediated oxidant stress in hepatocytes. Recent data from experimental animals, however, suggest that the opposite is true. Studies in genetically engineered mice indicate that elimination of CYP2E1 has no impact on the development of early alcoholic liver injury, whereas elimination of NADPH oxidase from Kupffer cells ameliorates ethanol-induced steatosis and inflammation. Thus, Kupffer cells may play a central role in the pathogenesis of alcoholic liver injury.

The oxidative stress induced in the liver by ethanol metabolism can be exacerbated by a concomitant decrease in the liver's ability to defend against free radical attack. Chronic ethanol ingestion leads to a reduction in hepatic glutathione, a nonprotein thiol that plays a key role in protection against oxidative injury. Ethanol affects mitochondrial levels of glutathione preferentially; this renders cells particularly susceptible to oxidative injury because mitochondria represent a major site of H_2O_2 production and because these organelles lack alternative mechanisms of antioxidant defense. This combination of enhanced oxidant stress and impaired antioxidant defense in alcoholics may contribute importantly to alcoholic liver injury.

3. Acetaldehyde effects—Acetaldehyde is a highly reactive compound that may directly promote hepatocellular injury and necrosis. One means by which acetaldehyde can provoke cellular damage is by reacting with lysine residues on cellular proteins to form acetaldehyde–protein adducts. Adduct formation may interfere with the catalytic activity of lysine-dependent enzymes; it may also have profound effects on protein transport processes in hepatocytes, such as glycoprotein secretion and receptor-mediated endocytosis. The latter may result from interactions between acetaldehyde and tubulin. *In vitro,* acetaldehyde reacts readily with lysine residues on tubulin; acetaldehyde-modified tubulin does not assemble properly into microtubules, and *in vivo,* this could slow microtubule-dependent processes such as protein trafficking. Acetaldehyde has been linked to protein secretory abnormalities in hepatocytes, which represent the major event underlying hepatocellular swelling ("ballooning"). Whether the effect of acetaldehyde is mediated through adduct formation with tubulin remains unproved. Finally, some evidence suggests that acetaldehyde–protein adducts serve as "neoantigens," provoking an immune response that may contribute to hepatocellular injury (see following discussion).

C. IMMUNE AND INFLAMMATORY MECHANISMS OF ALCOHOLIC LIVER INJURY (TABLE 39–1)

1. Cytokine production—Several cytokines are upregulated in individuals with alcoholic liver disease. Interleukin-1, interleukin-6, interleukin-8, and tumor necrosis factor-α along with other members of these cytokine families, are increased in the liver and plasma of patients with alcoholic hepatitis. Many of these compounds are known for their proinflammatory effects; they are believed to contribute to the leukocytosis and tissue inflammation characteristic of alcoholic hepatitis. Tumor necrosis factor-α may play an independent role in alcoholic liver disease by promoting apoptosis of hepatocytes. Studies show that alcohol sensitizes hepatocytes to the cytotoxic effects of this cytokine.

Among all the cytokines identified in alcoholic liver disease, tumor necrosis factor and interleukin-8 correlate best with disease severity. In patients with alcoholic hepatitis who undergo hospitalization, clinical improvement coincides with a reduction in these circulating cytokines. In addition, drugs that inhibit tumor necrosis factor-α show some efficacy in the treatment of alcoholic hepatitis (see below).

2. Immune responses to altered hepatocellular proteins—Chronic ethanol ingestion may lead to autoimmune liver injury by inducing cellular or humoral responses to various proteins. The targets of these immune responses are hepatocellular proteins altered *in vivo* by ethanol, such as acetaldehyde–protein adducts or Mallory bodies (see section, "Histology"). Antibodies directed against these compounds can be found in the serum of alcoholic patients, and in some cases are used as markers of alcohol consumption. It remains controversial, however, whether autoantibodies actually contribute to alcoholic liver injury. One problem related to the immune theory of alcoholic liver injury is that most of the autoantibodies identified to date in alcoholics are directed against *intracellular* proteins. This makes it difficult to envision how the antibodies reach their target antigens and lead to cytotoxicity. Antibodies directed against plasma membrane antigens may more readily provoke liver injury; studies have identified antibodies against membrane antigens, including liver membrane antibody (LMA) and CYP2E1. Ongoing studies are searching for other acetaldehyde–protein adducts that could lead to liver injury by an autoimmune mechanism.

Cell-mediated immune responses to acetaldehyde–protein adducts or Mallory bodies may also lead to alcoholic liver injury. *In vitro,* acetaldehyde-modified liver membranes stimulate neutrophils to degranulate and produce superoxide; likewise, Mallory bodies, when incubated with lymphocytes in culture, induce activation and cytokine production. Whether the same cell-mediated responses occur in alcoholics *in vivo* is unknown.

D. MECHANISMS OF FIBROSIS (TABLE 39–1)

The deposition of excess connective tissue in the liver may be mediated by some of the same compounds that induce hepatocellular injury in alcoholics. The main effectors of fibrosis are hepatic stellate cells, which are mesenchymal liver cells that reside in the space of Disse. Acetaldehyde and lipid aldehydes both promote collagen synthesis by stellate cells; these compounds may either be produced by stellate cells (which have a modest capacity to oxidize ethanol) or released from hepatocytes during ethanol metabolism. Transforming growth factor-β may also be an important stimulus to hepatic fibrosis in alcoholics; this fibrogenic cytokine is produced by Kupffer cells in response to chronic ethanol ingestion, and is a potent inducer of stellate cell collagen synthesis. Oxyradicals are toxic to stellate cells; in low concentrations they may stimulate collagen production.

Friedman SL: Stellate cell activation in alcoholic fibrosis—an overview. Alcohol Clin Exp Res 1999;23(5):904.

Lieber CS: Alcoholic liver disease: new insights in pathogenesis lead to new treatments. J Hepatol 2000;32(1 Suppl):113.

McClain CJ et al: Cytokines in alcoholic liver disease. Semin Liver Dis 1999;19(2):205.

Thurman RG II: Alcoholic liver injury involves activation of Kupffer cells by endotoxin. Am J Physiol 1998;275(4 Pt 1):G605.

Tuma DJ, Klassen LW: Immune responses to acetaldehyde-protein adducts: role in alcoholic liver disease. Gastroenterology 1992;103(6):1969.

Cofactors Implicated in Alcoholic Liver Disease

In an effort to explain why only a small proportion of alcoholics develop serious liver disease, confounding variables have been sought that might contribute to end-organ damage in the large population at risk. Numerous cofactors have been implicated in the pathogenesis of alcoholic liver disease, including inherited differences in ethanol metabolism, nutritional abnormalities (eg, protein–calorie malnutrition, antioxidant depletion, and iron overload), and concomitant infection with hepatitis viruses. One or more of these variables is often present in alcoholics with liver disease (Table 39–2).

A. HEREDITARY FACTORS

A number of investigators have attempted to identify subpopulations of alcoholics at high risk for liver disease by examining their histocompatibility antigen profiles. Although several antigens of the A and B classes are more common in patients with liver injury than in those without injury, none has proved to be a reliable predictor of disease risk. More recently, investigators have focused on inherited differences in ethanol and acetaldehyde *metabolism* as potential contributors to alcoholic liver injury. Variations in ethanol metabolism may be caused by genetic polymorphisms of ADH, ALDH, or CYP2E1. ADH is a homodimeric enzyme with at least three alleles encoding the hepatic enzyme. Studies suggest that varia-

Table 39–2. Cofactors implicated in the pathogenesis of alcoholic liver disease.

Cofactor	Means of Enhancing Liver Injury
Inherited variations in ADH, ALDH	Rapid ethanol oxidation Slow acetaldehyde elimination
Female gender	Diminished gastric ethanol metabolism
Nutrition	Enhanced lipid peroxidation via (1) Antioxidant depletion (2) Increased iron stores (3) Increased polyunsaturated fat
Viral hepatitis	Enhanced viral replication
Cigarette smoking	Unknown

tions in ADH phenotype among individuals can result in 3- to 10-fold differences in the ethanol elimination rate. Interestingly, it appears that individuals with the most rapid elimination rates may be at higher risk of alcoholic liver disease. ALDH polymorphisms have also been linked to alcoholic liver injury, but in this case, the allele that results in slow acetaldehyde elimination appears to be responsible. The *ALDH2*2* allele, which is present in about 50% of Chinese and Japanese persons, is completely inactive toward acetaldehyde. Patients homozygous for *ALDH2*2* experience a severe flushing reaction after drinking ethanol and generally avoid ethanol completely. Patients heterozygous for *ALDH2*2*, however, occasionally abuse ethanol, and these individuals develop liver injury more frequently and with lower alcohol intake than patients with a normal ALDH phenotype.

B. GENDER

Women are more susceptible to alcoholic liver injury than men. Studies suggest that women who consume 80 g/d of ethanol begin to display signs of liver disease after as short a time as 10 years; women consuming smaller quantities of ethanol can also develop liver injury over longer periods of time (eg, 40 g/d of ethanol for 20 years). This predisposition to alcoholic liver disease is unexplained. Some have attempted to connect the increased risk to gastric ethanol metabolism, which is slower in women than in men; this means that in women, a larger proportion of ingested ethanol escapes gastric metabolism and enters the portal circulation. The relative paucity of gastric ADH in women may explain why they display higher blood ethanol levels than men after drinking similar quantities of ethanol. It does not fully explain their predisposition to alcoholic liver injury. Behavioral scientists argue that the higher blood ethanol levels achieved in women should act as a negative stimulus to further ethanol consumption, and thus limit the total amount of ethanol consumed.

C. NUTRITION

The role of nutrition in the pathogenesis of alcoholic liver injury is quite controversial. Studies in baboons indicate that ethanol can induce liver injury despite adequate protein–calorie and vitamin nutrition; clinical studies, however, suggest that alcoholic liver injury correlates strongly and inversely with nutritional status. Despite the fact that malnutrition portends a poor prognosis in alcoholic hepatitis, it remains to be determined whether it is a precipitating factor in the development of alcoholic liver disease. Malnutrition could facilitate alcoholic liver injury by several mechanisms. Depletion of antioxidant vitamins could lead to enhanced oxidative stress in the livers of alcoholics; vitamins A and E in particular are known to be depleted by chronic ethanol consumption. A diet high in polyunsaturated fat may also enhance the risk of alcoholic liver injury by permitting the accumulation in the liver of substrates for ethanol-induced lipid peroxidation. Chronic ethanol ingestion enhances absorption of iron from the gut and increases hepatic iron stores. Given the importance of iron in free radical production during the metabolism of ethanol and acetaldehyde, it too provides a means of enhancing ethanol-induced oxidative liver injury.

D. VIRAL HEPATITIS

There is general agreement among all investigators that hepatitis C virus infection contributes importantly to liver injury in alcoholics. Roughly 18–25% of alcoholics are infected with this virus. Infection has been reported to correlate strongly with the presence of advanced liver disease; 40% of cirrhotic patients are positive for hepatitis C virus as compared with 25% with nonfibrotic liver injury.

Hepatitis B virus infection also increases the incidence of chronic liver injury in alcoholics. Epidemiologic data suggest that hepatitis B poses an additive, rather than synergistic, risk of liver injury in combination with alcohol. Hepatitis C and alcohol may be a more serious combination; laboratory studies indicate that alcohol enhances hepatitis C virus replication, and some clinical studies confirm this by showing increased viral loads in alcoholics.

E. EXCESS HEPATIC IRON

Alcoholics with liver disease frequently exhibit increased serum iron saturation, and liver biopsy may reveal quantitative iron levels as high as 5000 μg/g of dry liver weight. These abnormalities are likely due to increased intestinal absorption of dietary iron or increased hepatic uptake of transferrin-bound iron, or both. In the setting of ethanol oxidation, iron catalyzes several reactions that lead to free radical production (see section, "Pathophysiology"); excess iron can enhance these processes and lead

to oxidative liver injury. It is interesting to note that patients with hereditary hemochromatosis, who progressively accumulate hepatic iron with age, develop cirrhosis earlier if they also abuse alcohol.

F. CIGARETTE SMOKING; COFFEE DRINKING

Alcoholics who smoke more than one pack of cigarettes per day have three times the risk of cirrhosis as those who do not smoke. By contrast, alcoholics who consume four or more cups of coffee daily have a 5-fold lower incidence of cirrhosis than those who do not drink coffee. The reason for the synergistic effect of smoking and the protective effect of coffee is uncertain; the effect of coffee appears unrelated to caffeine, as tea drinking does not afford the same benefit.

Adams PC: Iron overload in viral and alcoholic liver disease. J Hepatol 1998;28(Suppl 1):19.

Bosron WF, Ehrig T, Li TK: Genetic factors in alcohol metabolism and alcoholism. Semin Liver Dis 1993;13:126.

Corrao G, Arico S: Independent and combined action of hepatitis C virus infection and alcohol consumption on the risk of symptomatic liver cirrhosis. Hepatology 1998;27:914.

Frezza M et al: High blood alcohol levels in women: the role of decreased gastric alcohol dehydrogenase activity and first-pass metabolism. N Engl J Med 1990;322:95.

Klatsky AL, Armstrong MA: Alcohol, smoking, coffee, and cirrhosis. Am J Epidemiol 1992;136:1248.

Mendenhall CL et al: Protein-calorie malnutrition associated with alcoholic hepatitis. Veterans Administration Cooperative Study Group on Alcoholic Hepatitis. Am J Med 1984;76: 211.

Mezey E: Dietary fat and alcoholic liver disease. Hepatology 1998; 28(4):901.

Naveau S et al: Excess weight risk factor for alcoholic liver disease. Hepatology 1997;25:108.

Clinical Findings

The term alcoholic hepatitis is used to describe the acute clinical manifestations of alcoholic liver disease. For this diagnosis to be made, patients should have a significant history of ethanol consumption (approximately 80 g/d of ethanol, preferably for 1 year or more), along with signs or symptoms of active liver injury. Because alcoholics frequently underestimate or deny active alcohol consumption, the only accurate estimation of recent drinking habits may come from family members or acquaintances, who should be interviewed whenever possible. Patients who meet diagnostic criteria for alcoholic hepatitis can exhibit a wide range of disease severity. As shown below, features such as encephalopathy, hyperbilirubinemia, and hypoprothrombinemia are good predictors of advanced injury. Stratification of patients according to the severity of illness is useful for predicting prognosis and planning therapy. The clinical use of the term alcoholic hepatitis is more broad than the histologic use; in fact, patients with clinical alcoholic hepatitis may have a combination of steatosis, inflammation, and fibrosis on biopsy. In contrast to histologic findings in the liver, the clinical features of alcoholic hepatitis correlate reliably with patient outcome.

A. Symptoms and Signs

The most common clinical manifestation of alcoholic liver disease is hepatomegaly. Liver enlargement can be detected in more than 75% of patients who are actively drinking, and is observed consistently at all stages of liver injury. Hepatomegaly is related in part to the accumulation of fat within liver cells; this may explain its presence even in patients with mild disease. Hepatocyte swelling, rather than steatosis, is believed to be the major cause of liver enlargement in moderately or severely ill patients.

1. Mild disease—The symptoms of mild alcoholic liver disease are vague, with anorexia and weight loss predominating (Table 39–3). These symptoms are present in only one-third of patients, making a history of heavy ethanol consumption important for establishing a diagnosis. Ascites is detectable in 30% of patients; this may be due to hepatomegaly and resultant "acute" portal hypertension, even in the absence of cirrhosis. Altered mentation may be indicative of hepatic encephalopathy. Fewer than one-fourth of patients with mild alcoholic liver injury complain of abdominal pain.

2. Moderate to severe disease—Patients with moderate to severe alcoholic liver disease exhibit different signs and symptoms, with jaundice, ascites, and encephalopathy predominating (see Table 39–3). Jaundice is a good predictor of disease severity, as it is present in 100% of patients with mild to moderate disease but only 17% of patients with mild disease. Ascites is detectable in over three-fourths of patients, and encephalopathy in over half. Another important feature of alcoholic hepatitis is fever, which is present in roughly 25% of patients and does not necessarily predict infec-

tion. Diffuse abdominal pain is distinctly uncommon, and should raise concern about concurrent peritonitis.

B. Laboratory Findings

Derangements can be found in both the hematologic and biochemical profiles of alcoholics (Table 39–4). Patients with alcoholic hepatitis are often anemic (average hematocrit 36%); over three-fourths exhibit macrocytosis (mean corpuscular volume 102 mm^3). Leukocytosis is also common in alcoholic hepatitis, particularly in patients with moderate to severe disease.

Hepatic transaminases are only modestly elevated in alcoholic hepatitis; regardless of disease severity, aspartate aminotransferase (AST) and alanine aminotransferase (ALT) rarely exceed 500 IU/L. Elevations significantly greater than 500 IU/L should raise concern about other or concurrent causes of liver injury (eg, drug toxicity or ischemia).

The ratio of AST to ALT is helpful in distinguishing alcoholic from nonalcoholic liver disease. Patients with alcoholic hepatitis often have an AST:ALT ratio of more than 2; this is in contrast to patients with viral hepatitis or nonalcoholic steatohepatitis, in which the ratio is commonly less than 1 (Figure 39–3). An AST:ALT ratio between 1 and 2 is not diagnostic of alcoholic liver disease; such ratios can be seen in patients with nonalcoholic liver disease and postnecrotic cirrhosis. A ratio of more than 3 is very suggestive of alcoholic liver injury.

It is important to note that active drinkers who develop acute nonalcoholic liver injury will often display elevated AST:ALT ratios in serum. A classic example of this phenomenon is acetaminophen poisoning, which in alcoholics causes AST elevation in marked disproportion to ALT. The reason for the discrepancy is that

Table 39–3. Clinical manifestations of alcoholic liver disease.

Sign or Symptom	Mild Disease (%)	Moderate to Severe Disease (%)
Hepatomegaly	84	80–95
Jaundice	17	100
Ascites	30	79–86
Anorexia	39	57–60
Encephalopathy	27	55–70
Alcohol withdrawal	36	15–30
Weight loss	37	8–28

Excerpted, with permission, from Mendenhall CL: Alcoholic hepatitis. Clin Gastroenterol 1981;10:420.

Table 39–4. Laboratory abnormalities in alcoholic liver disease.

Laboratory Test[1]	Mild Disease	Moderate Disease	Severe Disease
Hematocrit	38	36	33
WBC (thousand)	8	11	12
AST (mU/mL)	84	124	99
ALT (mU/mL)	56	56	57
Alkaline phosphatase (mU/mL)	166	276	225
Bilirubin (mg/dL)	1.6	13.5	8.7
Prothrombin time (sec over control)	0.9	2.4	6.4
Albumin (g/dL)	3.7	2.7	2.4

Excerpted, with permission, from Mendenhall CL: Alcoholic hepatitis. Clin Gastroenterol 1981;10:422.
[1]WBC, white blood cells; AST, aspartate aminotransferase; ALT, alanine aminotransferase.

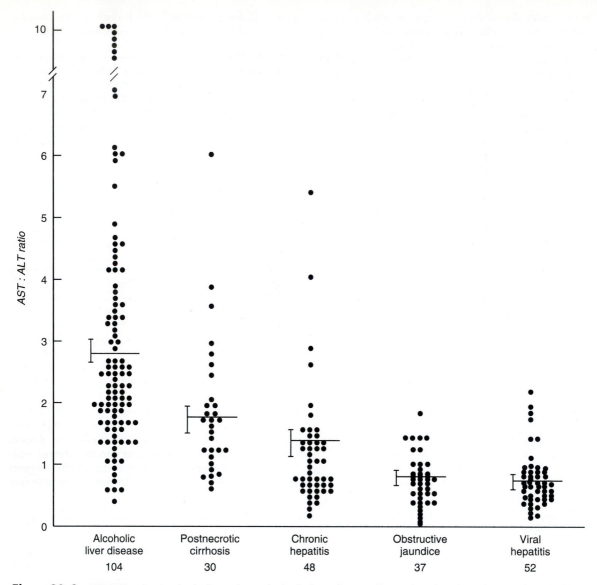

Figure 39–3. AST:ALT ratios in alcoholic and nonalcoholic liver disease. (Reproduced, with permission, from Cohen JA, Kaplan MM: The SGOT/SGPT ratio: an indicator of alcoholic liver disease. Dig Dis Sci 1979;24:835.)

chronic alcohol consumption, even in the absence of liver disease, alters the proportion of AST to ALT in hepatocytes. Consequently, when active drinkers contract acute liver disease, they are prone to release more AST than ALT into the circulation. This tendency is present regardless of the cause of the acute liver injury.

The laboratory parameters that are most useful in predicting the severity of alcoholic liver injury are bilirubin levels, prothrombin time, and perhaps albumin levels. The first two have been used to formulate a "discrimi-

nant function" (defined as (4.6 × [prothrombin time – control]) + bilirubin); when the result is greater than 32, a mortality rate of 50% can be predicted within 1 month. Similar criteria were used to subdivide alcoholic patients into the mild, moderate, and severe disease categories displayed in Tables 39–3 and 39–4. Of note is that the level of serum bilirubin, once a value of 5 mg/dL has been reached, does not correlate with disease severity. The prothrombin time increases progressively with worsening illness.

Other laboratory tests have been evaluated as markers of alcohol consumption or alcoholic liver injury but are not yet used in clinical practice. These include mitochondrial AST, carbohydrate-deficient transferrin, and serum markers of connective tissue metabolism such as collagen propeptides and tissue inhibitor of metalloproteinase. Carbohydrate-deficient transferrin appears to be useful for detecting recent ethanol consumption; the collagen propeptides, despite their relationship to collagen metabolism, distinguish patients with alcoholic hepatitis more reliably than those with alcoholic fibrosis. The overall objective in searching for new parameters is to develop reliable noninvasive methods for diagnosing alcoholism and alcoholic liver injury.

C. Imaging Studies

There are no characteristic radiographic features of alcoholic liver disease. The most common finding is hepatic steatosis, detectable by increased echogenicity on sonography or by extremely low attenuation of the liver on unenhanced computed tomography (CT) scan.

Histology

Ideally, a diagnosis of alcoholic liver disease should be based on histologic findings. In practice, many physicians dispense with liver biopsy when clinical clues strongly suggest alcohol-related illness. If alcoholic liver disease is suspected on the basis of clinical and laboratory information, the diagnosis is correct in approximately 90% of cases. Liver biopsy is still quite useful, however, in distinguishing other types of liver injury that often coexist in alcoholics (eg, chronic hepatitis in patients coinfected with hepatitis C virus). Liver biopsy is helpful in determining the extent of fibrosis in patients with good synthetic function. In the early stages of alcoholic liver injury, perivenular fibrosis can portend progression to hepatic fibrosis and ultimately cirrhosis. Cardinal features of alcoholic liver injury that can be recognized with light microscopic studies include steatosis, ballooning of hepatocytes, Mallory bodies, an inflammatory infiltrate in which neutrophils are prominent, and fibrosis. The first four features are frequently observed together, while fibrosis may be absent, mild, or extensive.

Steatosis, which connotes the presence of fat droplets in hepatocytes, is present in almost 100% of patients with alcoholic liver injury. Alcoholic steatosis is most prominent in pericentral zones, but in severe cases exhibits a panlobular distribution. The classic pattern of alcoholic steatosis is macrovesicular, with the large fat droplets pushing hepatocyte nuclei into an eccentric position. Despite this, a recent survey showed that alcoholic steatosis often is both macrovesicular and microvesicular. In microvesicular steatosis, small fat droplets fill the hepatocyte cytoplasm but leave the nucleus in a central position. This pattern of steatosis has also been termed "alcoholic foamy degeneration."

Ballooning degeneration of hepatocytes describes marked cell swelling, with a pale, often granular appearance of the cytoplasm. This pattern is not unique to alcoholic liver disease but can also be observed in many conditions that result in hepatocellular necrosis. Like steatosis, ballooning degeneration in alcoholic liver injury is most prominent pericentrally. In association with ballooned hepatocytes, one may see acidophil bodies, which are small, densely eosinophilic structures that represent apoptotic hepatocytes. Hepatocyte ballooning can be detected in over 75% of patients with clinical alcoholic liver injury.

Mallory bodies are crescent-shaped, eosinophilic structures that often wrap around the nucleus of hepatocytes. They represent a condensation of intermediate filaments, particularly cytokeratins, within the cytoplasm of hepatocytes. Mallory bodies are found in 76% of patients undergoing biopsy for alcoholic liver disease; they can be distinguished by periodic acid–Schiff (PAS) staining from enlarged mitochondria, which can also be present in alcoholics (mitochondria stain positive; Mallory bodies stain negative). Because Mallory bodies are seen in patients with primary biliary cirrhosis and Wilson's disease as well as alcoholic liver disease, and can be induced by drugs such as griseofulvin or amiodarone, their presence is not diagnostic of alcoholic liver injury.

Neutrophils are often present in the livers of alcoholics and are commonly found in the pericentral zones, adjacent to fatty or ballooned hepatocytes. Neutrophils are rarely found in nonalcoholic liver disease. Mononuclear cell infiltrates can also be observed pericentrally in alcoholics; at times, the pattern suggests chronic active hepatitis, which may reflect infection with hepatitis C or B virus.

Fibrosis in alcoholic liver injury begins with deposition of connective tissue around the terminal hepatic venule. As the lesion progresses, connective tissue extends into the hepatic parenchyma, surrounding hepatocytes in a "chicken-wire" fashion. Pericellular fibrosis is quite delicate and may be detectable only with special stains such as the Masson trichrome stain. In advanced fibrosis, bridging is common, involving central or portal veins, or both. Cirrhosis connotes distortion of the parenchyma into nodules, usually less than 1 cm in size, that are completely surrounded by bands of connective tissue. Moderate to severe fibrosis can be detected in roughly half of patients with alcoholic liver injury.

For diagnostic and investigational purposes, liver histologic findings in alcoholics can be arranged in categories such as fatty liver, alcoholic hepatitis, cirrhosis, and cirrhosis with alcoholic hepatitis. Histologic classification of patients with alcoholic hepatitis, however, does not always correlate well with the severity of clinical disease.

Differential Diagnosis

A. Nonalcoholic Steatohepatitis

Patients who do not abuse ethanol can develop liver disease that is clinically and histologically indistinguishable from alcoholic hepatitis. This entity is termed nonalcoholic steatohepatitis, and occurs in patients who are obese, diabetic, or taking medications such as estrogens, diethylstilbestrol, glucocorticoids, or amiodarone (see Chapter 45). It has also been reported after jejunoileal bypass surgery and in patients receiving total parenteral nutrition. Nonalcoholic steatohepatitis affects women predominantly; it is often asymptomatic and is discovered only by elevation of hepatic transaminases. Patients do not commonly have an exaggerated AST:ALT ratio. Cirrhosis is found in 7–16% of patients on initial liver biopsy; whether the natural history of the disease parallels that of alcoholic liver disease is yet unknown.

B. Hemochromatosis

In patients who display high serum iron saturations and have siderosis on liver biopsy, there may be some difficulty in distinguishing alcoholic liver disease from hereditary hemochromatosis. Differentiation can be made by performing genetic testing for hemochromatosis gene mutations and by measuring hepatic iron levels and calculating a "hepatic iron index" [(micrograms hepatic iron divided by 58) divided by age in years]. An index of greater than 2 indicates hereditary hemochromatosis (see Chapter 40).

Cohen JA, Kaplan MM: The SGOT/SGPT ratio: an indicator of alcoholic liver disease. Dig Dis Sci 1979;24:835.

Diehl AM et al: Relationship between pyridoxal 5′-phosphate deficiency and aminotransferase levels in alcoholic hepatitis. Gastroenterology 1984;86:632.

French SW et al: Pathology of alcoholic liver disease. Veterans Administration Cooperative Study Group 119. Semin Liver Dis 1993;13:154.

Mendenhall CL: Alcoholic hepatitis. Clin Gastroenterol 1981;10:417.

Reid A: Nonalcoholic steatohepatitis. Gastroenterology 2001;121:710.

Complications

The complications of alcoholic liver disease are similar to those encountered in nonalcoholic chronic liver disease. Ascites, gastrointestinal hemorrhage, and encephalopathy are related to portal hypertension; coagulopathy and hypoalbuminemia arise from hepatocellular dysfunction. Hypoglycemia can occur in malnourished patients who are actively drinking; it may also be a sign of overt liver failure.

There is some uncertainty whether alcoholic cirrhosis predisposes patients to hepatocellular carcinoma. Although 80% of all patients with hepatocellular carcinoma have underlying cirrhosis, some studies suggest that the risk is borne primarily by patients with postnecrotic cirrhosis and those with hereditary diseases such as hemochromatosis. Others suggest that alcohol is a risk factor for hepatocellular carcinoma, even when it is separated from cofactors such as viral hepatitis. At present, screening for hepatocellular carcinoma is prudent in males over 50 years old with alcoholic cirrhosis, particularly if they also have hepatitis C infection.

Treatment

The mainstay of treatment for alcoholic liver disease is abstinence. Abstinence substantially improves the survival time of patients, even those with cirrhosis and portal hypertension at the time of diagnosis (see section, "Prognosis"). For patients with severe alcoholic hepatitis, whose short-term mortality rate is high, pharmacologic therapy has been tried as an adjunct to abstinence and general supportive care. The utility of certain drugs in the treatment of alcoholic hepatitis is discussed below.

A. Corticosteroids

Patients with severe alcoholic hepatitis, judged either by a discriminant function of more than 32 (see section, "Laboratory Findings") or by the presence of encephalopathy, benefit from methylprednisolone (32 mg intravenously) or prednisolone (40 mg orally) administered daily for 28 days. Short-term survival rates in treated patients increase from 63% to over 90%. The salutary effect of corticosteroids has been confirmed in numerous clinical trials. Finding adequate candidates for treatment can be difficult; corticosteroids are not recommended for patients with active gastrointestinal hemorrhage, infection, or renal insufficiency. The long-term effect of corticosteroids on liver injury and survival rates beyond 1 year is unknown.

B. Nutrition

Nutritional supplements, provided either by the enteral or parenteral route, have been studied as adjuncts to the care of patients with severe alcoholic hepatitis. For the most part, these treatments consist of conventional amino acids, with some protocols substituting branched-chain amino acids and others adding lipid. Alcoholic patients treated with nutritional supplements often display more rapid normalization of biochemical liver tests (AST, bilirubin, albumin) than those receiving standard hospital diets. Such therapy has little or no effect on survival rates. Conventional amino acid preparations are tolerated well by most patients, even those with advanced cirrhosis. They should be the first choice for therapy, with branched-chain amino acids being reserved for patients who develop encephalopathy in response to routine formulas. Diets supplemented with medium-chain triglycerides may also be of benefit, and are under study in clinical trials.

C. PENTOXIFYLLINE

Pentoxifylline is a drug with many mechanisms of action, one being inhibition of tumor necrosis factor-α. It was recently studied as treatment for acute alcoholic hepatitis, in a placebo-controlled trial involving 101 patients. All patients had severe alcoholic hepatitis as judged by a discriminant function >32. Pentoxifylline (400 mg orally three times a day) increased 4-week survival from 53.9% to 75.5%. This is true despite the lack of any demonstrable difference in plasma tumor necrosis factor-α between the two treatment groups. Of note, pentoxifylline reduced the incidence of hepatorenal syndrome from 34.6% to 8.2%. This may be ultimately responsible for the beneficial effects of the drug. The pronounced effect of pentoxifylline on renal function is unexplained, but may be related to a direct influence of the drug on the renal microcirculation.

D. S-ADENOSYLMETHIONINE

This drug has the potential to reduce alcoholic liver injury by replenishing mitochondrial glutathione and diminishing oxidative stress. A controlled trial of 123 patients was recently completed to determine the effects of S-adenosylmethionine (400 mg orally three times a day) over a 2-year interval. The drug failed to show a significant survival benefit over placebo in the entire study group. However, when Child class C patients were excluded, a modest benefit emerged (88% survival with S-adenosylmethionine, 71% with placebo). Life-table analysis confirmed a benefit, but only at $P = .046$. Additional studies are required for confirmation of the effect.

E. SILYMARIN

This antioxidant compound extracted from milk thistle has been studied as a long-term treatment for alcoholic cirrhosis. Two controlled trials have been reported, with conflicting results. In the study that showed a survival benefit with silymarin (140 mg orally three times a day for 2 years), the improved outcome was restricted to patients in Child class A. In the study that showed no benefit of the drug, overall survival was good even in the placebo group and was attributed to rigorous attempts to reinforce abstinence from ethanol. Thus, the existing data suggest that silymarin can improve survival in select patients with alcoholic cirrhosis, but that the outcome may not exceed that achievable by abstinence alone.

F. POLYUNSATURATED LECITHIN

This compound, extracted from soybeans, has been shown to prevent hepatic fibrosis in alcohol-fed baboons. It supposedly acts by stimulating collagenase ac-

tivity in hepatic stellate cells, thus down-regulating the net amount of collagen deposited by these same cells in alcoholic liver injury. A trial of polyunsaturated lecithin in human alcoholics is currently under way, with published results awaited.

G. PROPYLTHIOURACIL

This drug is advocated for alcoholic hepatitis based on evidence that liver injury is related to a "hypermetabolic state," with increased hepatic oxygen consumption. Controlled trials of propylthiouracil suggest that it significantly increases the survival rates of patients with alcoholic liver injury (87% as compared with 75% at 2 years). Despite this, clinical use of this drug has not expanded, perhaps because of concerns about hypothyroidism or speculation that differences between experimental and control patients were not attributable to the drug (they occurred early, before the expected antithyroid effect of propylthiouracil in euthyroid patients). Clinical trials of this drug in alcoholic liver disease are ongoing.

H. COLCHICINE

Colchicine (1 mg/d orally for 30 days) is of no benefit in the treatment of acute alcoholic hepatitis. Long-term treatment of cirrhotic patients with colchicine (1 mg/d for up to 14 years), on the other hand, has been reported to significantly improve patient survival rates. To date, the benefit of colchicine has been demonstrated in only one clinical trial. This study has been criticized on several counts, including a high dropout rate, poor documentation of compliance, and uncertainty as to whether deaths in the placebo group were attributable to liver disease. For these reasons, colchicine is not widely used in the treatment of alcoholic liver disease.

I. LIVER TRANSPLANTATION

Transplantation is an option for some patients with end-stage alcoholic liver disease, provided that a defined period of abstinence (preferably 6 months or longer) precedes the surgery (see Chapter 54). In spite of concerted efforts at careful patient selection, the rate of recidivism is as high as 20–50%. The 5-year survival rate for alcoholic patients undergoing transplantation is comparable to that for nonalcoholic patients (about 70%).

Akriviadis E et al: Pentoxifylline improves short-term survival in severe acute alcoholic hepatitis: a double-blind, placebo-controlled trial. Gastroenterology 2000;119(6):1637.

Imperiale TF, McCullough AJ: Do corticosteroids reduce mortality from alcoholic hepatitis? A meta-analysis of the randomized trials. Ann Intern Med 1990;113:299.

Jain A et al: Long-term follow-up after liver transplantation for alcoholic liver disease under tacrolimus. Transplantation 2000;70(9):1335.

Lieber CS et al: Phosphatidylcholine protects against fibrosis and cirrhosis in the baboon. Gastroenterology 1994;106:152.

Mato JM et al: S-Adenosylmethionine in alcoholic liver cirrhosis: a randomized, placebo-controlled, double-blind, multicenter clinical trial. J Hepatol 1999;30:1081.

McCullough AJ, O'Connor JF: Alcoholic liver disease: proposed recommendations for the American College of Gastroenterology. Am J Gastroenterol 1998;93:2022.

Orrego H et al: Long-term treatment of alcoholic liver disease with propylthiouracil. Part 2. Influence of drop-out rates and of continued alcohol consumption in a clinical trial. J Hepatol 1994;20:343.

Pares A et al: Effects of silymarin in alcoholic patients with cirrhosis of the liver: results of a controlled, double-blind, randomized and multicenter trial. J Hepatol. 1998;28:615.

Schenker S, Halff GA: Nutritional therapy in alcoholic liver disease. Semin Liver Dis 1993;13:196.

Prognosis

The outcome of patients with alcoholic liver disease is dependent upon several variables, including (1) the clinical severity of liver injury at diagnosis, (2) the ex-

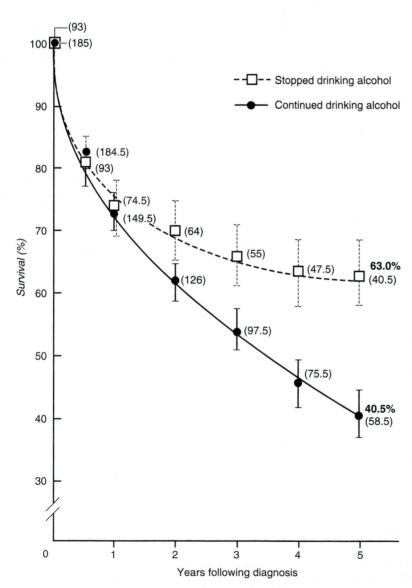

Figure 39–4. Five-year survival rates in patients with alcoholic cirrhosis as a function of ethanol intake. Even in the setting of irreversible hepatic fibrosis, patients who abstain from ethanol *(open squares)* have a significantly better prognosis than those who continue to drink *(closed circles).* (Reprinted from Powell WJ, Klatskin G: Duration of survival in patients with Laennec's cirrhosis: influence of alcohol withdrawal, and possible effects of recent changes in general management of the disease. Am J Med 1968;44:406 Copyright 1968, with permission from Excerpta Medica Inc.).

tent of irreversible liver damage (ie, cirrhosis) at diagnosis, and (3) subsequent drinking behavior. Patients with severe alcoholic hepatitis (determined clinically by indices such as the discriminant function) have an estimated mortality rate of 50%; the overall mortality rate of alcoholic hepatitis is roughly 17%. Even in the absence of acute alcoholic hepatitis, alcoholic cirrhosis alone has a negative effect on survival rates (30% mortality rate within 3–5 years, as opposed to an 18% mortality rate in those without cirrhosis). When clinical and histologic parameters are monitored together, cirrhosis with alcoholic hepatitis clearly emerges as the most ominous combination. Patients with both cirrhosis and alcoholic hepatitis have a 5-year mortality rate of approximately 60%.

Abstinence dramatically improves the survival rates of patients with alcoholic liver disease, even if cirrhosis is present at the time of diagnosis. Figure 39–4 demonstrates that patients with alcoholic cirrhosis have a

5-year survival rate approaching 65% with abstinence; if drinking continues, the survival rate drops to 40.5%.

Chedid A et al: Prognostic factors in alcoholic liver disease. Veterans Administration Cooperative Study Group. Am J Gastroenterol 1991;86:210.

Goldberg S et al: Veterans Administration Cooperative Study on Alcoholic Hepatitis. IV. The significance of clinically mild alcoholic hepatitis: Describing the population with minimal hyperbilirubinemia. Am J Gastroenterol 1986;81:1029.

Niemela O et al: Markers of fibrogenesis and basement membrane formation in alcoholic liver disease: relation to severity, presence of hepatitis, and alcohol intake. Gastroenterology 1990; 98:1612.

Orrego H et al: Prognosis of alcoholic cirrhosis in the presence and absence of alcoholic hepatitis. Gastroenterology 1987;92:208.

Powell WJ, Klatskin G: Duration of survival in patients with Laennec's cirrhosis: influence of alcohol withdrawal, and possible effects of recent changes in general management of the disease. Am J Med 1968;44:406.

Iron Overload Diseases

40

Paul C. Adams, MD

HEMOCHROMATOSIS

Pathophysiology

Hemochromatosis is now recognized as one of the most common autosomal recessive diseases, occurring in 1 in 200 persons with northern European ancestors. The hemochromatosis gene (*HFE*) has been localized to an area of chromosome 6, linked to the HLA complex (6p21.3). The HFE protein is localized to the crypts of the duodenum. In hemochromatosis, the mutated HFE protein results in a relatively iron-deficient crypt cell that migrates to the tip of the duodenal villus. This results in the expression of another iron transport gene (DMT1) and increased intestinal iron absorption occurs. Newer iron transport genes and proteins have been described (DcytB, IREG1, SFT, hephaestin) and their role in hemochromatosis remains to be determined. It is likely that a cascade of events leads to the increased iron absorption similar to the series of events that has been described for blood coagulation or complement activation. The progressive accumulation of iron probably results in oxidative damage to parenchymal organs.

Clinical Findings

A. SYMPTOMS AND SIGNS

Because the signs and symptoms of hemochromatosis are nonspecific and occur at a late stage of the disease, patients that would benefit the most from early therapeutic intervention are often undetected. The classic description of "bronze diabetes" is a late and uncommon presentation of the disease that is seen in less than 10% of patients. Hemochromatosis is most commonly diagnosed as an incidental finding. A common presentation is that the physician orders serum ferritin in a patient with fatigue. The physician was anticipating a low serum ferritin and is surprised to have found iron overload. As more patients are screened for hemochromatosis, the percentage of asymptomatic patients is increasing. Attribution of a symptom to hemochromatosis is difficult because of the nonspecific nature of symptoms, such as fatigue and arthralgias. A referral bias is present in most clinical series of patients. When only family members of the proband cases were reviewed in a series of 214 relatives, 38% had a hemochromatosis-related symptom (52% of men, 10% of women). In these unselected relatives, cirrhosis was present in 7% of men and 1% of women.

1. Hepatic disease—Hepatomegaly is one of the most common physical signs in this condition. The extent of liver damage depends on the age and gender of the patient. Signs of chronic liver disease can insidiously develop over many years.

2. Articular disease—Arthritis is one of the most common symptoms associated with hemochromatosis. Although chondrocalcinosis is also associated with the disease, a degenerative osteoarthritis involving the metacarpophalangeal joints is the most common articular manifestation. Nonspecific antiinflammatory therapy is the treatment of choice.

3. Endocrine disease—Diabetes is a late complication of the disease. Early studies implied that iron deposits damaged the pancreatic islet cells, but more detailed studies on insulin metabolism have shown that many patients with hemochromatosis have high insulin levels, with insulin resistance similar to that of most patients with type II diabetes. Insulin resistance has also been associated with iron overload in patients without the HFE genetic mutations. Iron-depletion therapy does not usually affect the diabetes.

Endocrine dysfunction is usually manifested as impotence, which is related to pituitary hypofunction, although testicular atrophy can also occur. Hypothyroidism is a less common endocrine manifestation. Testosterone therapy is often ineffective in the treatment of impotence but may prevent osteoporosis.

4. Cardiac disease—Cardiac disease is one of the less common presenting features, although some young males may present with life-threatening cardiomyopathy. This can be seen in juvenile hemochromatosis, which may be a different genetic disease localized to chromosome 1. Cardiac biopsy of patients in transplantation centers has also led to inadvertent discovery of the disease. Iron depletion can lead to marked improvement in cardiac function. Cardiac arrhythmias have also been described, particularly during major surgery.

5. Asymptomatic cases—As more cases are detected through genetic screening and at an earlier age, many asymptomatic cases have been discovered. Progression to symptomatic disease is not inevitable and the natural history in these cases has not been well defined.

B. LABORATORY FINDINGS

1. Genetic testing—A major advance has been the use of genetic testing for the diagnosis of hemochromatosis. Typical patients with hemochromatosis are homozygous for the C282Y mutation of the *HFE* gene in greater than 90% of cases. Compound heterozygotes (C282Y mutation and H63D mutation) and H63D homozygotes have a much lower risk of significant iron overload and have normal iron studies in most population screening studies. Familial iron overload is rare in the absence of HFE mutations. Several pedigrees have been described in Italy including cases with a mutation in the transferrin receptor 2 gene. A new iron overload syndrome has been described in a Dutch family with a mutation in the IREG1 gene. A typical genetic profile (C282Y homozygote) may alleviate the need for diagnostic liver biopsy. A "negative" genetic test in the setting of iron overload requires further investigations including liver biopsy. C282Y homozygotes without iron overload are not uncommon, particularly in young women. An interpretation of genetic testing is shown in Table 40–1.

2. Serum ferritin and transferrin saturation—Patients can be readily screened for hemochromatosis with serum ferritin and transferrin saturation (serum iron/total iron-binding capacity) (Figure 40–1). Serum iron alone is an unreliable marker for the disease. The transferrin saturation is usually abnormal at a young age, and the ferritin saturation rises progressively with age. Females will have a lower serum ferritin level because of menstruation. To discuss the sensitivity and specificity of the iron tests for the diagnosis of hemochromatosis, a "gold standard" must be established. Prior to genetic testing the iron tests were often used as part of the diagnostic criteria so the sensitivity was overestimated. If genetic testing is used as the gold standard (C282Y homozygosity), the sensitivity of transferrin saturation has been reported to be as low as 52% at a threshold of 50%. This is a reflection of the increasing number of nonexpressing homozygotes that have been described.

Serum ferritin can be elevated in both acute and chronic inflammation as well as in certain tumors

Table 40–1. Interpretation of genetic testing for hemochromatosis.

C282Y homozygote

This is the classic genetic pattern that is seen in > 90% of typical cases. Expression of disease ranges from no evidence of iron overload to massive iron overload with organ dysfunction. Siblings have approximately a one in four chance of being affected and should have genetic testing. For children to be affected, the other parent must be at least a heterozygote. If iron studies are normal, false-positive genetic testing or a nonexpressing homozygote should be considered.

C282Y/H63D—Compound heterozygote

This patient carries one copy of the major mutation and one copy of the minor mutation. Most patients with this genetic pattern have normal iron studies. A small percentage of compound heterozygotes have been found to have mild to moderate iron overload. Severe iron overload is usually seen in the setting of another concomitant risk factor (alcoholism, viral hepatitis).

C282Y heterozygote

This patient carries one copy of the major mutation. This pattern is seen in about 10% of the white population and is usually associated with normal iron studies. In rare cases, the iron studies are high in the range expected in a homozygote rather than a heterozygote. These cases may carry an unknown hemochromatosis mutation and liver biopsy is helpful to determine the need for venesection therapy.

H63D homozyote

This patient carries two copies of the minor mutation. Most patients with this genetic pattern have normal iron studies. A small percentage of these cases have been found to have mild to moderate iron overload. Severe iron overload is usually seen in the setting of another concomitant risk factor (alcoholism, viral hepatitis).

H63D heterozygote

This patient carries one copy of the minor mutation. This pattern is seen in about 20% of the white population and is usually associated with normal iron studies. This pattern is so common in the general population that the presence of iron overload may be related to another risk factor. Liver biopsy may be required to determine the cause of the iron overload and the need for treatment in these cases.

No HFE mutations

Iron overload has been described in families with mutations in other iron-related genes (transferrin receptor 2 and IREG1). Other hemochromatosis mutations will likely be discovered in the future. If iron overload is present without any HFE mutations, a careful history for other risk factors must be reviewed and liver biopsy may be useful to determine the cause of the iron overload and the need for treatment. Most of these are isolated, nonfamilial cases.

A

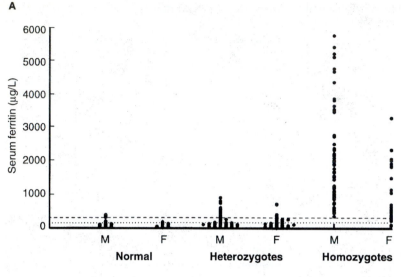

B

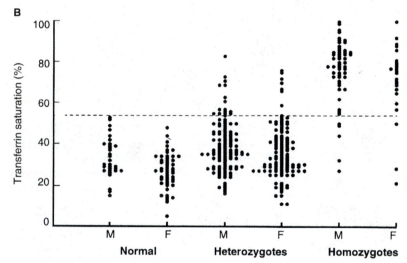

Figure 40–1. **A:** Serum ferritin in C282Y homozygotes, C282Y heterozygotes, and normal (wild type) for hemochromatosis. The reference range was 15–200 μg/L for females and 30–300 μg/L for males. The dashed line represents the upper limit of normal in males and the dotted line in females. **B:** Transferrin saturation (%)in C282Y homozygotes, C282Y heterozygotes, and normal (wild type) for hemochromatosis. The reference range was 20–55%. The dashed line represents the upper limit of the reference range. (Reproduced, with permission, from Adams PC: Prevalence of abnormal iron studies in heterozygotes for hereditary hemochromatosis: an analysis of 255 heterozygotes. Am J Hematol 1994;45:147–148. © 1994, reprinted with permission of Wiley-Liss, a division of John Wiley & Sons, Inc.)

(Table 40–2). Extreme elevations (>100,000 μg/L) can be seen in malignant histiocytosis, and this has led to speculation that macrophages are the source of serum ferritin. Heterozygous patients do not develop progressive iron overload. Most heterozygotes with minor elevations in serum ferritin or transferrin saturations have now been shown with genetic testing to be compound heterozygotes (C282Y/H63D).

3. AST and ALT—Mild abnormalities in aspartate aminotransferase (AST) and alanine aminotransferase (ALT) have been described in 65% of referred patients. The mean elevation in AST is typically less than 100 IU/L in both cirrhotic and noncirrhotic patients, however. Hemochromatosis is not associated with extensive liver inflammation and hepatocyte necrosis. Thus, the patient with marked elevations in AST and ALT in association with increased serum ferritin or transferrin saturations (or both) is unlikely to have hemochromatosis alone but rather some other inflammatory disease.

4. Liver biopsy—The liver biopsy had previously been the "gold standard" for the diagnosis of hemochromatosis, however with genetic testing, the role of liver biopsy has shifted from a diagnostic test to a prognostic test in typical patients with hemochromatosis. Iron staining shows excess parenchymal iron deposition. At

Table 40–2. Causes of elevated serum ferritin levels.

Hereditary hemochromatosis
Chronic hepatitis
Alcoholic liver disease
Histiocytosis
Hepatocellular carcinoma
Hyperthyroidism
Adult Still's disease
Chronic inflammation

advanced stages of the disease, there may be portal fibrosis, cirrhosis, bile duct iron deposition, and hepatocellular carcinoma. Iron-free foci may represent a premalignant lesion. The hepatic iron concentration can be measured from the paraffin block by means of atomic absorption spectrophotometry; this is a more accurate method of assessing the degree of iron loading than iron staining. Patients with hemochromatosis will have at least twice as much iron as patients with alcoholic siderosis of the same age. This has been expressed as the hepatic iron index [(µmol/g)/age] and is usually greater than 2 in homozygotes. This index assumes less clinical relevance in the era of genetic testing.

C. POPULATION SCREENING FOR HEMOCHROMATOSIS

Because hemochromatosis is a common disease that can be detected by simple blood tests, some have advocated screening of the general population for this disease. Widespread screening has been studied in blood donors and in inpatient and outpatient clinics using serum ferritin and transferrin saturations and genetic testing. Selective screening strategies in arthritis and diabetes clinics have also been studied. Because patients who are diagnosed in the precirrhotic stage of the disease have survival rates similar to those of the general population, early diagnosis and therapy based on these relatively inexpensive screening tests can be highly advantageous to the individual patient. The study of 65,238 Norwegian patients in primary care resulted in a high prevalence of 1 in 220 but a low morbidity with many asymptomatic C282Y homozygotes. In studies in which genetic testing has been done in all cases, there are many C282Y homozygotes without iron overload. This has been estimated to represent as many as 50% of C282Y homozygotes. There has been concern about genetic discrimination with widespread genetic testing, but the benefits of early treatment are likely greater than potential discrimination (insurance, labeling, stigmatization). For the primary care physician, it would be reasonable to screen all patients with any symptoms, abnormal liver enzymes, or a family history of the disease using serum ferritin and transferrin saturation and follow up abnormal iron tests with genetic testing.

Patients with cirrhosis of the liver are at risk for hepatocellular carcinoma. In a collected series of 649 cirrhotic patients with hemochromatosis, hepatocellular carcinoma was described in 18.5%. This is similar to the prevalence in other types of cirrhosis, such as that of hepatitis B and C, and suggests that cirrhosis is the major risk factor rather than iron overload. Although screening studies for hepatocellular carcinoma in patients with hemochromatosis with α-fetoprotein measurements and ultrasound have led to earlier detection, the therapeutic options of resection, chemoembolization, and transplantation are often not curative.

D. IMAGING STUDIES

Abdominal imaging [computed tomography (CT) and magnetic resonance imaging (MRI) scanning] can detect moderate to severe iron overload. The current lack of sensitivity of available imaging methods limits their usefulness in the detection of early disease. Genetic testing has been a more significant clinical advance than imaging for iron overload.

Differential Diagnosis

Confusion persists about the differential diagnosis of iron overload, particularly in a patient who consumes alcohol heavily. In an era of intensive diagnostic evaluations, it is alarming to note that in many major centers in the United States, hemochromatosis is diagnosed initially at the time of liver transplantation.

As previously noted, hemochromatosis is strongly suggested by a marked elevation in the serum ferritin and transferrin saturation. The two major problems associated with these tests are the failure to order them in the first place and the misinterpretation of mild abnormalities. A typical clinical presentation that often creates confusion is a middle-aged patient with a mild elevation in serum ferritin (<1000 µg/L), a borderline elevation in serum transferrin saturation, significant alcohol consumption, and no family history of hemochromatosis. The clinical diagnosis is alcoholic liver disease, but the elevated iron levels raise the possibility of hemochromatosis. A concomitant rise in the erythrocyte sedimentation rate or C-reactive protein level suggests that the ferritin elevation may be secondary to inflammation rather than iron overload (Figure 40–2). Although alcoholic liver disease can coexist with hemochromatosis, in my experience, the relationship between alcoholism and hemochromatosis has been overemphasized, and the literature on hemochromatosis historically has erroneously included patients who actually have alcoholic siderosis rather than hemochromatosis. An increasing number of patients with chronic

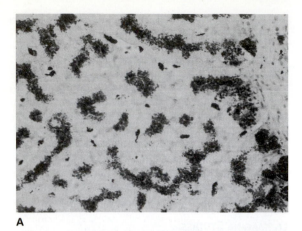

A

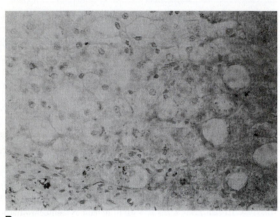

B

Figure 40–2. Comparative liver biopsies from a patient with **(A)** hereditary hemochromatosis and **(B)** alcoholic siderosis. The degree of iron overload is much greater in the patient with hemochromatosis. The alcoholic patient of a similar age has much less stainable iron, iron in Kupffer cells and hepatocytes, polymorphonuclear infiltrates, and fat. (Photomicrographs courtesy of J Frei.)

hepatitis (hepatitis B or C or idiopathic hepatitis) have been found to have elevated ferritin and transferrin saturation with mild elevations in hepatic iron concentration. Genetic testing has been a major advance in the assessment of patients with multiple risk factors such as alcohol abuse or chronic viral hepatitis.

Treatment

A. VENESECTION

The goal of therapy is to deplete iron stores to prevent any further tissue damage. Patients begin a program of

weekly venesections of approximately 500 mL. The author determines the hemoglobin at the time of each venesection and proceed with the next venesection if the hemoglobin is greater than 10 g/dL. A mild anemia (10–12 g/dL) is common throughout therapy and stimulates erythropoiesis and iron mobilization. Serum ferritin levels are monitored every 3 months, and venesections are continued until the level is approximately 50 µg/L. Young patients can often tolerate two venesections per week, whereas elderly patients may tolerate only one venesection every 2 weeks. The duration of therapy depends on the age of the patient and the iron burden at the time of diagnosis. Weekly venesection therapy can last for as long as 3 years in an older male proband or as little as a few months in a young female.

Following depletion of iron stores, patients can begin a maintenance program of three or four venesections per year on a lifelong basis. The interval between venesections can be adjusted based on an annual serum ferritin measurement. An alternative approach is to follow the serum ferritin level annually and restart weekly venesections when it becomes abnormal.

B. CHELATION THERAPY

Chelation therapy with deferoxamine is reserved for the patient with iron overload secondary to iron-loading anemia. Hepatotoxicity is a concern with the oral iron chelator, deferiprone, that has been studied in thalassemia. Despite iron depletion, many of the symptoms such as arthritis, impotence, and diabetes do not improve.

C. LIVER TRANSPLANTATION

Liver transplantation is indicated for patients with end-stage liver disease (see Chapter 54). Preliminary data suggest that patients with hemochromatosis have a higher mortality rate following transplantation than other cirrhotic patients because of concomitant cardiac disease and a higher incidence of infection. Initial studies also suggest gradual reaccumulation of iron in the transplanted liver. The inadvertent transplantation of a hemochromatosis liver into a normal recipient resulted in complete mobilization of the excess hepatic iron within the first year following transplantation. This is compelling evidence against an intrahepatic defect being the primary metabolic abnormality in hemochromatosis. Transplantation of a hemochromatosis intestine and liver simultaneously resulted in progressive iron overload in the recipient.

Prognosis

Cirrhosis is the major clinical factor influencing long-term survival rates, and patients with cirrhosis at the time of diagnosis are 5.5 times more likely to die than

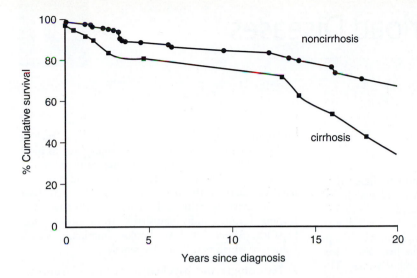

Figure 40–3. Cumulative survival (%) in 277 C282Y homozygotes for the *HFE* gene. Survival rates were significantly reduced in cirrhotic patients as compared with noncirrhotic patients (*P* < .004; log-rank test).

noncirrhotic patients. Diagnosis and venesections prior to the development of cirrhosis will prevent this complication. Patients that are noncirrhotic at the time of diagnosis have an estimated survival rate that does not differ from age- and sex-matched members of the normal population (Figure 40–3).

REFERENCES

Adams PC: Population screening for haemochromatosis. Gut 2000; 46:301.

Asberg A et al: Screening for hemochromatosis—high prevalence and low morbidity in an unselected population of 65,238 persons. Scand J Gastroenterol 2001;36:1108.

Bacon BR: Diagnosis and management of hemochromatosis. Gastroenterology 2001;120:718.

Bulaj Z et al: Disease-related conditions in relatives of patients with hemochromatosis. N Engl J Med 2000;343:1529.

Feder A et al: A novel MHC class I-like gene is mutated in patients with hereditary hemochromatosis. Nature Genet 1996; 13:399.

Griffiths W, Cox T: Haemochromatosis: novel gene discovery and the molecular pathophysiology of iron metabolism. Human Genet 2000;9:2377.

Niederau C et al: Long term survival in hereditary hemochromatosis. Gastroenterology 1996;110:1107.

Tavill A: Diagnosis and management of hemochromatosis. Hepatology 2001;33:1321.

Copper Overload Diseases

Michael L. Schilsky, MD

WILSON'S DISEASE

Pathophysiology

Copper is an essential metal that must be ingested in our diets, absorbed by the intestine, and distributed and eliminated by the liver in accordance with our overall metabolic needs (Figure 41–1). Wilson's disease (WD) is an autosomal recessive disorder in which copper accumulates to toxic levels in the liver and thereafter in the neurologic system and other tissues. The prevalence of this disease is about 1:30,000 in almost all populations. The genetic basis for WD is the mutation of both alleles on chromosome 13 encoding the ATP7B protein, a copper-transporting ATPase expressed mainly in hepatocytes. Individuals homozygous for a single *ATP7B* mutation, or more commonly with two different mutations of this gene (compound heterozygotes), have reduced or failed copper transport activity of the ATP7B protein. Loss of this physiologic copper transport function leads to reduced biliary copper excretion and subsequent copper accumulation in the liver, and to reduced copper incorporation into ceruloplasmin. Untreated, the accumulated copper results in hepatocellular injury by oxidative damage to membranes, organelles such as mitochondria, and nucleic acids, and to altered protein synthesis, among other ill effects. Liver injury ranges from mild steatosis and inflammation at first, to cirrhosis and liver failure. Excess copper that increases in the circulation following hepatic copper accumulation and injury leads to toxic accumulation in the central nervous system with resultant neurologic or psychiatric manifestations of this disease. Other organs that may also be affected by copper accumulation include the kidneys, heart, and bone.

Clinical Findings

A. SYMPTOMS AND SIGNS

1. Hepatic disease—The clinical presentation of Wilson's disease varies widely. Liver disease may be present without apparent clinical signs, or patients may experience fatigue, jaundice, or other complications of liver disease and portal hypertension such as ascites and variceal bleeding. Some patients may present with acute fulminant hepatic failure. Typically, patients under the age of 5 years will not present with signs of their illness unless there is concurrent injury to the liver, such as viral or other infectious hepatitis or injury due to medications. The majority of patients presenting with liver disease are in their second decade of life and most will have cirrhosis of the liver. Some patients may have chronic active hepatitis and a few may also have overlapping features indistinguishable from autoimmune hepatitis. About 5% may develop fulminant hepatic failure, of which two-thirds are female.

2. Neurologic and psychiatric disease—Neurologic manifestations of WD typically present later than the liver disease, most often in the third decade of life. However, earlier and sometimes subtle findings in pediatric patients can include changes in behavior, deterioration in schoolwork, or the inability to perform activities requiring motor coordination such as dance, gymnastics, or other athletics. Handwriting may deteriorate and micrographia may develop. Other common findings in older patients presenting with neurologic disease include tremor, motor discoordination, drooling, dysarthria and dystonia, and spasticity. Some patients experience migraine headaches and insomnia. It is unclear whether seizures are more common in WD. Transfer dysphagia may also occur, with a risk of aspiration in some. Along with behavioral changes, other psychiatric manifestations include depression, anxiety and even psychosis.

3. Ophthalmologic—Kayser-Fleischer rings are deposits of copper in Descemet's membrane in the cornea of the eye. It is a pathognomonic finding almost invariably present in patients with neuropsychiatric manifestations of WD, but in only ~50% of patients with hepatic presentations. This finding, best detected by slit-lamp examination, disappears with treatment of the disease. An example of the findings seen on slit-lamp examination are shown in Figure 41–2. Very rarely, Kayser-Fleischer rings may be present in patients with chronic cholestasis such as primary biliary cirrhosis or primary sclerosing cholangitis. Sunflower cataracts are another rare finding associated with WD. These typically do not affect visual acuity, and as with Kayser-Fleischer rings, disappear with treatment.

4. Systemic manifestations—A Coombs-negative hemolytic anemia may be present in patients presenting with acute fulminant hepatic failure. In other patients,

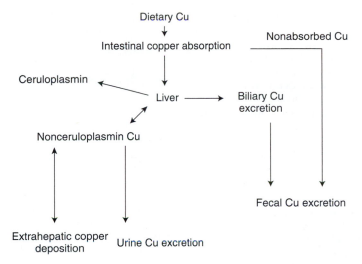

Figure 41–1. Copper metabolism. Copper absorbed by the small intestine is delivered by the portal circulation to the liver where it is avidly extracted. The liver utilizes some copper for metabolic needs, exports copper synthetically incorporated into ceruloplasmin, and eliminates excess copper into bile for excretion in the feces. The normal amount of nonceruloplasmin copper in the circulation is ~10 μg/dL or about 10% of the total serum copper. In Wilson's disease, there is reduced incorporation of copper into ceruloplasmin and reduced excretion of copper into bile, with a subsequent increase in hepatic copper and nonceruloplasmin copper in the circulation. It is from the nonceruloplasmin pool of copper that the extrahepatic deposition of copper occurs, and from which the kidney extracts copper for excretion (normally a minor component of daily loss). Medical therapy for this disorder aims at reducing copper absorption (zinc salts) or eliminating excess copper by increasing urinary excretion (chelating agents). Liver transplant with a normal donor organ restores physiologic copper metabolism.

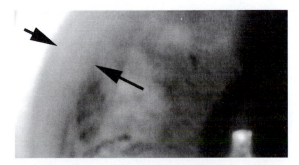

Figure 41–2. A picture of a Kayser-Fleischer ring in a patient with Wilson's disease presenting with neurologic symptoms. Note the gradation of the copper rings in Descemet's membrane of the cornea outward to the periphery *(arrows)*. These rings are typically largest at the superior and inferior poles, but may be circumferential in some untreated patients such as the one shown here. (Courtesy of SL Guillory, MD.)

abnormalities of the bones, joints, kidneys, heart, and other endocrine systems can occur. Bone and joint abnormalities include osteoporosis and osteomalacia, osteoarthritis, and chondrocalcinosis. Cardiomyopathy and arrhythmia have been reported, however these findings are rarely clinically evident. Renal abnormalities include a renal tubular acidosis, aminoaciduria, and in the acute fulminant setting, acute tubular damage. Amennorhea and irregular menstrual cycles are frequently noted in women, and often resolve with treatment.

B. LABORATORY FINDINGS

1. Biochemical findings—Reduced levels of serum ceruloplasmin are found in 90–95% of patients with WD, but may also be present in 20% of heterozygous carriers. Ceruloplasmin may also be reduced in some patients with severe hepatic insufficiency, in severe protein-losing enteropathy or nephropathy, and in other rare genetic disorders such as Menkes disease and aceruloplasminemia. As ceruloplasmin is also an acute phase reactant and responsive to estrogens, some individuals with WD and active liver injury and others who are pregnant or on hormonal supplementation who would otherwise have diagnostically reduced levels of this protein may have ceruloplasmin levels above the lower limit of the normal range (typically >20 mg/dL, the level varying somewhat with the laboratory).

Due to the reduction in serum ceruloplasmin, levels of serum copper are most often reduced as ceruloplasmin-copper normally comprises ~90% of the copper in the circulation. The exception is the patient with fulminant liver failure who has a marked increase in the circulating level of non-ceruloplasmin-bound copper. Because the copper that is excreted in the urine is derived from the non-ceruloplasmin bound copper in the circulation, symptomatic patients have an elevated urinary copper excretion above 100 μg per 24-hour period. This elevated level of urine copper may also be found in patients with acute liver failure due to other etiologies and in those individuals taking chelating agents.

Hepatic copper content ≥250 μg/g dry weight remains the best biochemical evidence for Wilson's disease. In long-standing cholestatic disorders, hepatic copper content may also be increased to this level. Markedly elevated levels of hepatic copper may also be found in idiopathic copper toxicosis.

Patients with fulminant hepatic failure due to WD almost always have a relatively low alkaline phophatase, and the ratio of alkaline phosphatase (U/L) to bilirubin (mg/dL) is ≤2.0. These patients may also have relative low levels of transaminase elevations despite the massive hepatic injury.

Low serum uric acid levels are found in many patients, and ammoaciduria and electrolyte changes due to renal tubular acidosis may be present.

2. Liver biopsy findings: histology and ultrastructure

—The liver biopsy may yield several characteristic histologic features. Steatosis is the most common early finding, which is microvesicular and macrovesicular, with glycogenated nuclei in some hepatocytes (Figure 41–3). Varying degrees of fibrosis and inflammatory infiltrates may be present with time, and cirrhosis is frequently found in most patients by the second decade. There are some older individuals who do not appear to have cirrhosis even after this time although they have neurologic disease; however, their hepatic histology is not normal.

Histochemical analysis of liver biopsy specimens may reveal the presence of copper-binding protein in some nodules and its absence in others (Figure 41–4). The absence of histochemically identifiable copper does not exclude WD.

Ultrastructural analysis of liver specimens at the time steatosis is present reveals specific mitochondrial abnormalities that include dilated cristae and crystalline inclusions (Figure 41–5). At later stages of the disease, dense deposits within lysosomes are present. Although

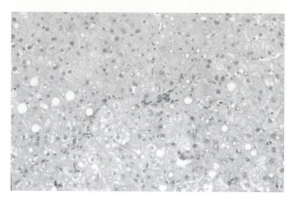

Figure 41–3. A light microscopic image of a liver biopsy specimen from a patient with Wilson's disease. Micro- and macrovesicular steatosis shown in this image is a common finding early in the course of the disease.

electron microscopic analysis of liver biopsy specimens is not routine, ultrastuctural analysis may be a useful adjunct for diagnosis in helping to distinguish between heterozygous carriers and patients.

Molecular genetic studies are becoming available for clinical use, but only pedigree analysis using haplotypes or polymorphisms surrounding the WD gene are commercially available. This analysis requires the identification of a patient within the family (the proband) by clinical and biochemical studies as above, and then analysis of first-degree relatives using haplotyping is

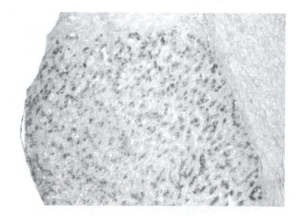

Figure 41–4. Histochemical staining for copper in Wilson's disease. A light microscopic image of a liver biopsy specimen from a patient with Wilson's disease demonstrates the presence of copper-binding protein identified by Rhodanine staining. Note the presence of brown pigmented granules within cells.

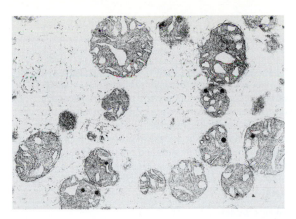

Figure 41–5. Ultrastructural findings in Wilson's disease. Abnormal mitochondria with dilated cristae and crystalline deposits are evident in this specimen from a patient with Wilson's disease. (Ultrastructural analysis and photograph courtesy of I Sternlieb, MD.)

possible. *De novo* diagnosis by molecular studies remains difficult at present as over 200 mutations of ATP7B have been found to be disease specific, and only rare populations have a single dominant mutation. In these populations with a single dominant mutation, direct mutation analysis is useful.

C. IMAGING STUDIES

In patients symptomatic with neuropsychiatric disease and in some without symptoms, computed tomography (CT) or magnetic resonance imaging (MRI) of the brain reveals significant abnormalities. Most frequently found are increased density on CT and hyperintensity on T2 MRI in the region of the basal ganglia. Abnormal findings are not limited to this region, and other abnormalities have been described.

Imaging of the liver by sonography, CT, or MRI may show evidence of cirrhosis, splenomegaly, and other signs of portal hypertension.

Differential Diagnosis

WD must be considered in any patient with unexplained liver disease or cirrhosis. Although the vast majority of individuals with WD present before 40 years of age, rarely this disorder has been identified in patients in their seventh and eighth decades. In patients with neurologic and psychiatric symptoms and evidence of liver disease, this diagnosis must always be considered. Individuals with hepatic histology suspicious for WD, with radiologic imaging of the brain with compatible findings, and those in whom Kayser-

Fleischer rings were identified spuriously should be evaluated further to establish or exclude this disorder.

Difficulty arises in establishing the diagnosis noninvasively most frequently in patients presenting with liver disease, however, quantitative copper analysis on an adequate specimen is almost always diagnostic. Quantitative analysis for copper can be performed on fresh specimens handled properly, or may be performed on liver biopsy specimens extracted from the paraffin block when the diagnosis is considered retrospectively.

Combinations of signs and laboratory findings that establish the diagnosis of WD include the presence of Kayser-Fleischer rings and a low ceruloplasmin, Kayser-Fleischer rings and neurologic or psychiatric symptoms, and an elevated hepatic copper with appropriate histology. Molecular studies using haplotype analysis can be used to identify affected siblings, however, the diagnosis must be firmly identified in the proband. For those in whom specific *ATP7B* mutations are identified, direct sequence analysis can be utilized.

Treatment

Treatment for WD includes lifelong pharmacologic therapy and liver transplant. Medical therapy of WD aims to prevent further copper accumulation and reverse the toxic effects of this metal by promoting its excretion or blocking its intestinal absorption. Chelating agents such as penicillamine, trientine, or British antilewisite (BAL) promote copper excretion in the urine. Zinc salts act by reducing copper absorption from the intestine. Currently recommended treatment dosages are shown in Table 41–1. Liver transplant corrects the underlying hepatic defect and changes the phenotype to that of the donor liver.

The approach to treatment is dependent upon whether there is active disease or symptoms, whether neurologic or hepatic, or whether the patient is identified prior to the onset of disease. Patients with symptomatic disease should initially be treated with chelating agents, or more recently with trials of chelating agents and zinc salts temporally separated. Although the most extensive experience for treatment has been with penicillamine, trientine as initial therapy is gaining favor given that this drug has a better safety profile than penicillamine. Tetrathiomolybdate is another chelating agent that is being tested for initial treatment of neurologically affected patients as 10–50% of individuals treated with penicillamine develop worsening neurologic symptoms during this phase of treatment that may not reverse. For asymptomatic individuals identified with WD or for those in whom treatment has stabilized their disease, treatment with a lower dose of chelating agent or with zinc is effective as maintenance therapy. For those asymptomatic or presymptomatic

Table 41–1. Treatment of Wilson's disease.

Medication	Dosage	Comment
D-Penicillamine	25–30 mg/kg in divided doses,[1] 15 mg/kg for maintenance therapy	Initial therapy with lower dosage increased to full dosage over 1–2 weeks time; monitoring for side effects is essential; dosage reduction for surgery and pregnancy necessary
Trientine	~20 mg/kg in divided doses,[1] 15 mg/kg for maintenance therapy	Initial therapy with lower dosage increased to full dosage over 1–2 weeks time; initial hypersensitivity is rare, however a reversible sideroblastic anemia may occur with long-term use; dosage reduction for surgery and pregnancy necessary
Zinc salts	25 mg two or three times a day for pediatric patients, 50 mg three times a day for adults	Used as maintenance therapy or for initial therapy for asymptomatic patients, may be used adjunctively with chelating agent as initial therapy

[1]Rounded to the nearest 250 mg as these medications are supplied in 250-mg capsules.

patients, treatment with a chelating agent or with zinc is effective in preventing disease symptoms or progression. Patients with fulminant hepatic failure due to Wilson's disease and those with severe liver disease unresponsive to medical therapy require liver transplant, which is life-saving. Some patients with cirrhosis and portal hypertension have suffered variceal bleeding despite stabilization of their hepatic function by medical therapy, and have been treated successfully with surgical or portacaval shunts or transjugular intrahepatic portosystemic shunts, or by liver transplant. Some individuals that are transplanted for indications related to their liver disease also have had psychiatric or neurologic symptoms, and these can improve in some. Because severe neurologic impairment prior to liver transplant may not improve posttransplant, liver transplant is not recommended as a primary treatment for neurologic WD as the liver disease is stabilized by medical therapy in most of these individuals.

In pregnant women, treatment must be maintained throughout the course of pregnancy for all patients with WD. The dosage of zinc salts is maintained throughout without change, however dosages of chelating agents should be reduced for the last trimester and if caesarian section is performed, until wound healing is achieved. The chelating agents penicillamine and trientine and zinc salts have been shown to be effective and safe for use during pregnancy, and have been associated with good outcomes for the mother and fetus.

Prognosis

The prognosis for long-term survival in successfully treated and compliant patients with WD is excellent. Complications of cirrhosis and portal hypertension, although infrequent, can occur and may require other interventions. There does not appear to be an increased risk for the development of hepatocellular carcinoma in

treated patients with WD. One-year survival post-liver transplant is now ~80–87% for patients with WD, and long-term survival for these individuals is excellent.

IDIOPATHIC COPPER TOXICOSIS

The development of cirrhosis due to copper overload in Indian and non-Indian children is now referred to as idiopathic copper toxicosis, reflecting our lack of understanding of the etiology of this disorder. This disorder of hepatic copper overload typically occurs in infancy, ranging in age from 1 to 3 years of age, and is severe and progressive. Patients typically present with jaundice, ascites, and hepatosplenomegaly. Although liver content is massively increased, serum ceruloplasmin is normal and neurologic copper deposition is not reported. The current hypothesis regarding the pathogenesis of this rare disorder is that these individuals possess an underlying genetic predisposition to the development of copper overload, but that without alimental exposure to increased copper, the disease does not develop. Recent data from Germany suggest a possible autosomal inheritance in patients with this disorder. Idiopathic copper toxicosis is not genetically linked to any abnormality in the *ATP7B* gene. The histologic appearance of the liver is characterized by micronodular cirrhosis most commonly, or massive necrosis. A distinctive feature is the large number of Mallory bodies typically present, a finding that may be seen in WD, but in fewer numbers and not as a prominent feature. The elimination of further dietary copper intake and the use of chelating agents have been reported to modify the clinical course of the disease in some patients. In others, the development of significant hyperbilirubinemia heralded liver failure and death. The copper chelator penicillamine, along with dietary restriction, may alter the course of the disease by preventing progression and reversing the pathologic changes if recognized in the early stages of the illness.

REFERENCES

Bavdekar AR et al: Long term survival in Indian childhood cirrhosis treated with D-penicillamine. Arch Dis Child 1996;74:32.

Brewer GJ et al: Worsening of neurologic syndrome in patients with Wilson's disease with metal penicillamine therapy. Arch Neurol 1987;44:490.

Brewer GJ et al: Treatment of Wilson disease with ammonium tetrathiomolybdate. II: Initial therapy in 33 neurologically affected patients and follow-up with zinc therapy. Arch Neurol 1996;53:1017.

Brewer GJ et al: Treatment of Wilson's disease with zinc. XV: Long-term follow-up studies. J Lab Clin Med 1998;132:264.

Brewer GJ et al: Treatment of Wilson's disease with zinc. XVI: Treatment during the pediatric years. J Lab Clin Med 2001; 137:191.

Brewer GJ et al: Treatment of Wilson's disease with zinc. XVII: Treatment during pregnancy. Hepatology 2000;31:364.

Eghtesad B et al: Liver transplantation for Wilson's disease: a single-center experience. Liver Transplant Surg 1999;5:467.

Muller T et al: Non-Indian childhood cirrhosis. Eur J Med Res 1999;4:293.

Pandit A, Bhave S: Present interpretation of the role of copper in Indian childhood cirrhosis. Am J Clin Nutr 1996;63:830S.

Santos-Silva EE et al: Successful medical treatment of severely decompensated Wilson disease. J Pediatr 1996;128:285.

Scheinberg IH, Sternlieb I: *Wilson's Disease,* Volume XXIII. WB Saunders, 1984.

Scheinberg IH, Jaffe ME, Sternlieb I: The use of trientine in preventing the effects of interrupting penicillamine therapy in Wilson's disease. N Engl J Med 1987;317:209.

Schilsky ML: Treatment of Wilson disease: what are the relative roles of penicillamine, trientine and zinc supplementation? Curr Gastroenterol Rep 2001;3:54.

Schilsky ML, Tavill AS: Wilson's disease. In: *Diseases of the Liver.* Schiff ER et al (editors). Lippincott-Raven, 1999; 1091.

Schilsky ML, Scheinberg IH, Sternlieb I: Prognosis of Wilsonian chronic active hepatitis. Gastroenterology 1991;100:762.

Schilsky ML, Scheinberg IH, and Sternlieb I: Hepatic transplantation for Wilson's disease: indication and outcome. Hepatology 1994;19:583.

Sternlieb I: Wilson's disease and pregnancy. Hepatology 2000;31: 531.

Tanner MS: Indian childhood cirrhosis and Tyrolean childhood cirrhosis. Disorders of a copper transport gene? Adv Exp Med Biol 1999;448:127.

Hepatic Porphyrias

42

D. Montgomery Bissell, MD

GENERAL CONSIDERATIONS

Pathophysiology

The porphyrias comprise a group of diseases that is subdivided into acute (neurologic) and chronic (cutaneous) forms. The types most commonly encountered clinically in North America and Europe are acute intermittent porphryia (AIP) and porphyria cutanea tarda (PCT). AIP is one of the acute, neurologic forms, in which attacks are induced classically by medications. PCT is a purely cutaneous form, occurring most often on a background of liver disease and iron overload. Although genetically distinct, all types of porphyria represent disturbances in the formation of heme, an essential component of hemoglobin and cellular cytochromes. Because the pathway of heme formation is well understood, it serves as a logical framework for viewing the porphyrias. Porphyrins are darkly colored compounds (Greek *porphyos,* purple) that are either intermediates or side products of heme formation. They are detectable in urine or feces, but excretion normally represents less than 1% of the daily flux through the pathway. Porphyria denotes markedly increased excretion of porphyrins or porphyrin precursors, in association with symptoms.

A. THE PATHWAY OF HEME FORMATION

The formation of heme, investigated in the 1940s, was one of the first biosynthetic pathways elucidated through the use of radioisotopic tracers. It was proved that all of the carbons in heme are supplied by the amino acid glycine and by succinic acid, a Krebs cycle intermediate (Figure 42–1). These simple precursors combine to form δ-aminolevulinic acid (ALA), the first intermediate committed to heme synthesis. The reaction is catalyzed by ALA synthase and is normally rate limiting for the pathway as a whole. ALA synthase is subject to negative regulation by heme, which ensures that the flow of precursors into the pathway matches the need of the cell for new heme formation. In the second reaction, two molecules of ALA condense to form porphobilinogen (PBG), a five-membered ring with acetic and propionic side chains. Both ALA and PBG are colorless and water soluble. In the next reaction, four molecules of PBG are linked to create a linear tetrapyrrole in a reaction catalyzed by PBG deaminase.

The first porphyrin of the pathway (uroporphyrinogen) uses another enzyme, uroporphyrinogen synthase, which cyclizes the linear tetrapyrrole. As indicated in Figure 42–1, the true intermediates of the pathway, up to protoporphyrin, are porphyrinogens, which are reduced porphyrins. The corresponding porphyrins are side products of the pathway and are irreversibly oxidized: They cannot reenter the pathway and must be excreted into either bile (and then to feces) or urine. Such leakage from the pathway normally is minimal, although porphyrins are detectable in the urine and feces of healthy individuals. A marked increase in porphyrin excretion suggests a disturbance in the flow of heme precursors along the pathway.

The conversion of uroporphyrinogen, first into coproporphyrinogen and then into protoporphyrinogen, requires two enzymes (see Figure 42–1), which mediate a progressive decarboxylation of the original acetic and propionic side chains of uroporphyrinogen. As shown, this gives rise to a series of intermediates, named according to the number of carboxyl side chains on the porphyrin nucleus. Of these, the most important, quantitatively, are octacarboxyporphyrin, otherwise known as uroporphyrin, and tetracarboxyporphyrin, known as coproporphyrin. The hepta-, hexa-, and pentacarboxyporphyrins are minor.

The progressive decarboxylation of uroporphyrinogen leads to compounds with reduced water solubility and a change in their principal route of excretion: Uroporphyrin is excreted almost entirely in urine (as its name implies), coproporphyrin in both urine and feces, and protoporphyrin entirely in feces. In the final step of the pathway, iron is inserted into protoporphyrin forming heme; the reaction is catalyzed by heme synthase (ferrochelatase).

The pathway traverses both the mitochondrial and cytosolic compartments of the cell. It starts in the mitochondrion, with ALA synthase, then moves to the cytosol, where the next three enzymes are located (PBG synthase, PBG deaminase, and uroporphyrinogen synthase), returning to the mitochondrion, where coproporphyrinogen oxidase and heme synthase are located. Most of the newly synthesized heme is then exported to the cytosol for combination with globin (in erythropoietic cells) or apocytochromes (in other nucleated cells) (see Figure 42–1). A small fraction is degraded to bile pigment.

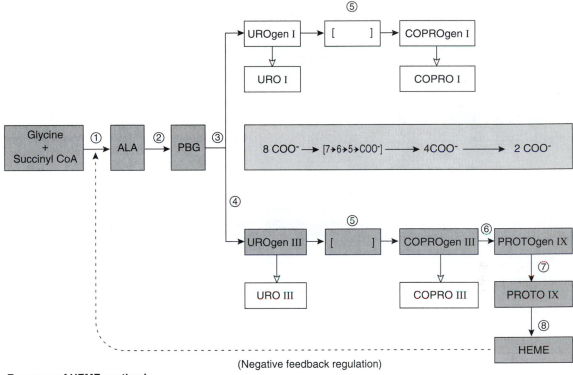

Enzymes of HEME synthesis

① ALA synthase
② PBG synthase
③ PBG deaminase
④ UROgen III synthase
⑤ UROgen decarboxylase
⑥ COPROgen oxidase
⑦ PROTOgen oxidase
⑧ HEME synthase (ferrochelatase)

Figure 42–1. The pathway of heme synthesis. The ***solid arrows*** indicate the flow of metabolites in the normal situation. The ***dashed arrows*** indicate side pathways, which normally are minor but increase in porphyria. [Reproduced, with permission, from Bissell DM: The porphyrias. In: *The Molecular and Genetic Basis of Neurological Disease.* Rosenberg R et al (editors). Butterworth Heinemann, 1992.]

B. ENZYME DEFECTS IN PORPHYRIA

The porphyrias represent hereditary or acquired defects in one of the enzymes of heme synthesis. The most important result from genetic deficiencies. The enzyme defect appears to create a partial block to the flow of heme precursors, with spillover of intermediates to excretory routes. The pattern of metabolic intermediates reflects the site of the block and is diagnostic for each type of porphyria (Figure 42–2).

C. CLASSIFICATION OF THE PORPHYRIAS

Porphyrias are usually classified as erythropoietic or hepatic, according to the principal source of excess porphyrin or porphyrin precursors. In genetic porphyria, the enzyme defect is present in all tissues. Heme synthesis, however, occurs principally in the bone marrow, where it serves hemoglobin production, and in the liver, where it is required for synthesis of microsomal heme proteins. Among the latter, the cytochrome P-450 family is pre-

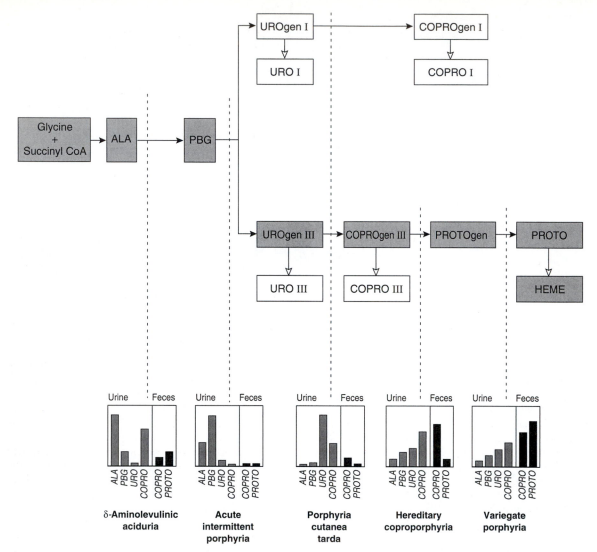

Figure 42–2. Urinary and fecal excretion of heme precursors associated with genetic hepatic porphyria. The **vertical dashed lines** indicate the point in the pathway at which an enzyme deficiency exists (see Figure 42–1 for a list of enzymes). Each defect gives rise to a unique excretory pattern of heme precursors. The "I" and "III" refer to isomers of porphyrin: only the III series are intermediates in heme formation. For the patterns associated with the individual acquired or erythropoietic porphyrias, see text. [Reproduced, with permission, from Bissell DM: The porphyrias. In: *The Molecular and Genetic Basis of Neurological Disease*. Rosenberg R et al (editors). Butterworth Heinemann, 1992.]

sent in high concentration and turns over rapidly, requiring a substantial level of ongoing heme synthesis. This classification is presented in Table 42–1. Clinically, the porphyrias can be grouped according to their presentation: acute (neuropsychiatric) or chronic (cutaneous). There is overlap, however, with some types being cutaneous and chronic but on occasion also acute.

D. PATHOGENESIS OF SYMPTOMS IN ACUTE PORPHYRIA

Most attacks are induced by drugs (see below). The inducers usually are compounds that elicit new synthesis of hepatic cytochrome P-450. Induction of cytochrome P-450 entails a demand for heme synthesis, to which the liver reacts with an increase in ALA synthase, the

Table 42–1. Classification of the prophyrias.[1]

Type	Enzyme Defect	Inheritance	Clinical Type
Hepatic porphyria			
Acute intermittent porphyria	PBG deaminase	Dominant	Acute, neurologic
Hereditary coproporphyria	COPROgen oxidase	Dominant	Acute, neurologic (+ cutaneous)
Variegate porphyria	PROTOgen oxidase	Dominant	Acute, neurologic (+ cutaneous)
δ-ALAuria	PBG synthase	Recessive	Acute, neurologic
Cutanea tarda	UROgen decarboxylase	Dominant (+ acquired?)	Chronic, cutaneous
Lead intoxication	PBG synthase + COPRO oxidase	(Acquired)	Neurologic
"Toxic" porphyria	UROgen decarboxylase	(Acquired)	Cutaneous
Erythropoietic porphyria			
Congenital erythropoietic porphyria	UROgen synthase	Recessive	Cutaneous
Protoporphyria	Heme synthase	Dominant	Cutaneous (+ hepatic)

[1]PBG, porphobilinogen; COPROgen, coproporphyrinogen; PROTOgen, protoporphyrinogen; UROgen, uroporphyrinogen; δ-ALA, δ-aminolevulinic acid.

rate-limiting enzyme of the pathway. In porphyria, where an inherited or acquired enzyme deficiency exists distal to ALA synthase, the affected enzyme limits the flow of precursors, resulting in heme production failing to meet the demand. As precursors prior to the block accumulate, an acute attack ensues.

All of the acute-attack porphyrias have overproduction of ALA and PBG in common, although it remains unclear whether such overproduction directly underlies symptoms. It has been noted that ALA bears a structural resemblance to the inhibitory neurotransmitter γ-aminobutyric acid (GABA), suggesting that it may act as a GABA analog *in vivo*. However, plasma ALA does not correlate well with symptoms in patients with AIP.

E. PATHOGENESIS OF SYMPTOMS IN CUTANEOUS PORPHYRIA

Although the precursors ALA and PBG are colorless, porphyrins are purple and fluorescent and, at a sufficient concentration in skin, photosensitizing. This effect has been proved by the finding that the "action spectrum" of photocutaneous injury (with a peak at about 400 nm) corresponds exactly to the wavelength at which a porphyrin is excited to its reactive form. In variegate porphyria and protoporphyria, the inherited deficiency appears to be both necessary and sufficient for porphyrin overproduction. On the other hand, the clinical expression of porphyria cutanea tarda clearly requires environmental factors as well as a deficiency in uroporphyrinogen decarboxylase (Table 42–2). Estrogens and a small number of other drugs play a role in some patients. Inducers of heme synthesis (such as barbiturates), however, do *not*. A moderate level of iron overload is present in virtually all patients, as indicated by transferrin saturation

in excess of 50% and stainable iron on liver biopsy. The basis for the excess iron is controversial. Genetic markers for hemochromatosis (mutations in the HFE gene) are present in some patients, but this varies widely by region. In North America and western Europe, the prevalence of HFE mutations in patients with PCT is significantly higher than in control populations (73% in one U.S. study), but in eastern Europe and Japan, few mutations have been found. This has led to the recommendation that depending on the geographic area, PCT patients should be screened for HFE mutations.

In addition to moderately increased iron stores, liver disease is common in porphyria cutanea tarda. In the past, this was viewed as alcoholic injury, postviral liver disease, or a porphyric hepatopathy. More recently, studies from North America have found that ~60% of PCT patients are infected with the hepatitis C virus (HCV). Most of the HCV-positive males also consume alcohol to excess, while a substantial proportion of the female patients take estrogen, confirming that multiple environmental factors contribute to the pathogenesis of PCT. Anecdotal reports of HCV-positive patients given antiviral therapy describe resolution of the cutaneous disease

Table 42–2. Environmental factors in porphyria cutanea tarda.

Iron overload; dietary iron supplements
Alcohol
Estrogens
Chronic liver disease
Acquired immunodeficiency syndrome

with loss of virus. However, in at least one reported case, PCT resolved (with normalization of urine porphyrin excretion) despite a failure to clear HCV. This case suggests that interferon was acting on PCT by mechanisms independent of its antiviral effect, perhaps through immunomodulation. Pointing also to an altered immune state in PCT is its higher than expected prevalence in patients infected with the human immunodeficiency virus. Although the immunologic hypothesis remains to be explored in detail, it is currently recommended that all patients with PCT be screened for HCV.

Diagnostic Screening Tests

Cutaneous lesions, in porphyrias displaying them (see Table 42–1), are characteristic and should immediately suggest the diagnosis. The "neurologic" syndrome, on the other hand, often takes the form of complaints (nausea, abdominal pain, constipation) that occur commonly in the general population. As in other unusual diseases, the "classic" clinical presentation of abdominal pain, psychosis, and dark urine in a young female is seldom seen. More often, porphyria comes under consideration only after other diagnostic possibilities have been exhausted. In such patients, accurate laboratory evaluation is the key to diagnosis. Various "screening" tests are available, but have important limitations.

A. Urinary ALA and PBG; Watson-Schwartz Test

For the evaluation of pain and neurologic symptoms, the appropriate tests are for urinary ALA and PBG, the porphyrin precursors. In all of the acute porphyrias, these are elevated, although in ALAuria and lead poisoning, only the ALA is increased. The Watson-Schwartz test, in which urine is mixed with Ehrlich's reagent (dimethylaminobenzaldehyde in hydrochloric acid), is a rapid qualitative test for PBG and suitable for emergency room use provided it is performed correctly. If no pink color forms, the test is negative. Importantly, however, formation of a pink color is positive *only* if the color proves resistant to extraction with *n*-butanol (ie, remains in the aqueous phase). Thus, the extraction step is critical to a correct interpretation of the test. Color that is present initially but extractable is due to urobilinogen or certain medications and is unrelated to porphyria.

B. Porphyrin Screening

Cutaneous symptoms are evaluated with measurement of porphyrins (not porphyrin precursors) in urine, stool, or blood. The choice of sample depends on the pattern of porphyrin overproduction in the disease under consideration. In porphyria cutanea tarda, for example, the salient change is increased uroporphyrin, and urine analysis is performed. In variegate porphyria, protoporphyrin is increased, and a stool analysis is appropriate (see Figure 42–2).

A "porphyrin screen" is useful for rapid assessment of cutaneous disease. Because it reflects total porphyrins irrespective of type, quantitative analysis of individual porphyrins is needed to ascertain the type of porphyria. With a complete profile of heme precursors in urine and feces (and, occasionally, in blood), virtually all porphyrias can be typed (see Figure 42–2). A point of emphasis is that persons with symptoms exhibit markedly abnormal porphyrin excretion. For example, in acute neurologic attacks, the amount of PBG in urine exceeds 30 mg/d (normal < 2 mg/d) and ranges up to 200 mg/d. For porphyria cutanea tarda with cutaneous symptoms, urine uroporphyrin exceeds 500 µg/d (normal < 50 µg/d). In short, the laboratory abnormalities associated with symptoms are not subtle.

A pattern of porphyrin excretion frequently encountered in clinical practice is an isolated, usually minor increase in urine coproporphyrin. As a rule, rather than signifying a hereditary porphyria, this is nonspecific, associated with a variety of acute and chronic illnesses, including acquired liver disease. The only specific diagnostic considerations are lead poisoning and asymptomatic hereditary coproporphyria. Diagnosis of the latter requires analysis of fecal coproporphyrin, which is elevated only in the hereditary condition.

Genetic Diagnosis

The acute-attack (neurologic) porphyrias are inherited in an autosomal dominant manner, except for δ-ALAuria, in which a double defect in the gene for PBG synthase is required for the expression of clinical disease. All porphyrias are viewed as rare, although their prevalence is relatively high in certain inbred populations. Acute intermittent porphyria is found in 1 in 1000 persons in northern Scandinavia; variegate porphyria is present in as many as 1 in 300 South Africans of Dutch ancestry. In the latter case, the gene has been traced back to the original group of Dutch settlers who emigrated to the Cape area in the late seventeenth century; the story is recounted by Dean (see references). Investigation of the molecular defect in acute intermittent porphyria has revealed more than 130 distinct mutations in the gene for PBG deaminase, all leading to an inactive or unstable enzyme. Because there is no predominant mutation, molecular diagnosis is not currently in use except for screening individual large kindreds.

With regard to the cutaneous porphyrias, two types of porphyria cutanea tarda are postulated. The first is clearly genetic, involving a partial deficiency of uroporphyrinogen decarboxylase. In a second type, the deficiency is expressed only in the liver and appears to be detectable only prior to treatment. The latter defect may be acquired, but because a genetic lesion has not been excluded, this form is termed "sporadic" porphyria cutanea tarda. For clinical purposes, the distinction is unimportant. All porphyria cutanea tarda is eminently treatable, and for this reason genetic analysis usually is not pursued. A third condition that can be grouped with porphyria cutanea tarda is hepatoerythropoietic porphyria, in which uroporphyrinogen decarboxylase is profoundly decreased. Although this is suggestive of homozygous porphyria cutanea tarda, the molecular defects identified to date have not been found in familial porphyria cutanea tarda.

Protoporphyria is autosomal dominant but with more than one subtype. Many carriers appear to be asymptomatic. The affected enzyme is heme synthase (ferrochelatase).

ACUTE INTERMITTENT PORPHYRIA

Acute intermittent porphyria is an acute hepatic porphyria with no cutaneous manifestations.

Clinical Findings

A. SYMPTOMS AND SIGNS

The principal symptoms are shown in Table 42–3. Pain is almost always present, often in the abdominal region but sometimes involving the back or extremities. It may be diffuse, deep, and achy or may be localized, mimicking a surgical abdomen. Nausea is frequent. Indeed, a history of recurrent abdominal pain with negative laparotomy should suggest the diagnosis. Porphyric symptoms have a characteristic course, increasing over a period of days rather than hours. Many patients will report chronic constipation that worsens at the onset of an attack. A family history should be sought but is often lacking because of the frequently silent state of most genetic carriers. Many attacks occur in the setting of an inducing drug; thus, a review of medications is particularly important. Attacks can occur also as a result of decreased caloric intake, either because of intercurrent illness, such as influenza, or an attempt at rapid weight reduction. Elective surgery can be the setting for an acute attack because of the routinely imposed preoperative fasting. Barbiturate induction of anesthesia is a particular hazard.

Attacks are more frequent in women than in men and have a peak incidence between age 20 and 40 years. Although reported, attacks are rare prior to puberty. Female sex hormones may predispose women to acute attacks and account also for the virtual absence of symptoms prior to puberty; oral contraceptives have been implicated in some cases. Cyclical premenstrual exacerbations can occur that resolve with the onset of menses. The effect of pregnancy is unpredictable.

The physical findings of acute porphyria are, for the most part, consistent with a neuropathic process (see Table 42–3). None is diagnostic, however. A clue to the examining physician may be the impression that symptoms are out of proportion to the physical findings. Psychosis is part of the classic description but usually is not overt. More commonly, patients exhibit an "hysterical" affect, which can be misconstrued as drug-seeking behavior. Weakness, when present, is initially proximal and, in a patient with abdominal pain, should suggest the diagnosis. Seizures can occur early and represent a particular risk in that use of phenytoin and related drugs may aggravate the attack and cause rapid progression of porphyria. Fever suggests a coexisting infection, a setting in which acute attacks may occur in the absence of an inducing drug.

B. LABORATORY FINDINGS

Minor abnormalities in blood urea, liver transaminases, and thyroxine have been reported. The most important finding, when present, is hyponatremia. It appears to be due in at least some patients to inappropriate secretion of antidiuretic hormone, and it can develop rapidly, particularly with aggressive administration of dextrose-in-water as initial therapy (see below). The diagnostic finding in acute porphyria is marked elevation of urinary (or serum) PBG. The Watson-Schwartz test is a rapid qualitative test for PBG; as noted above, the butanol extraction is critical for avoiding false positives. It should be confirmed by quantitative assay of PBG, which is available in many commercial laboratories. Quantitative urine porphyrins are needed for establishing the type of porphyria. In addition to the major porphyrins (uroporphyrin and coproporphyrin), many laboratories report the intermediate forms (hepta-, hexa-, and pentacarboxyporphyrins). The latter provide no

Table 42–3. Presentation of acute porphyria: percentage of patients with symptom or sign.[1]

Symptom	%	Sign	%
Abdominal pain	90	Tachycardia	83
Vomiting	80	Hypertension	55
Constipation	80	Motor neuropathy	53
Pain in limbs	51	Pyrexia	38
Pain in back	50	Leukocytosis (> 12,000)	20
Confused state	32	Bulbar involvement	18
Seizures	12	Sensory loss	15
Diarrhea	8	Cranial nerve involvement	9

[1]Modified from Eales M: Porphyria as seen in Cape Town: a survey of 250 patients and some recent studies. S Afr J Lab Chem Med 1963;9:151.

additional diagnostic information and are best ignored, being usually present in such low concentrations that accurate measurement is difficult.

C. GENETIC DIAGNOSIS

Because prevention of attacks plays a large role in management, identification of asymptomatic carriers (eg, first-degree relatives of an index case) is important. Although quantitative assay of urine PBG is appropriate as the initial screening test, there is a significant false-negative rate (estimated at 50% of the healthy carrier population). Therefore, the urine test is supplemented by assay of erythrocyte PBG deaminase, which is less than normal in most affected individuals regardless of symptoms. In some carriers, however, values are in the low-normal range, and in one genetic variant, the enzyme in erythrocytes is normal but in liver is deficient. Nonetheless, the combination of urinary PBG and erythrocyte PBG deaminase identifies at least 90% of carriers. Molecular diagnosis is a research procedure (discussed above).

D. PRENATAL TESTING

Although this is feasible by analysis of amniotic cells, it is not pursued because of the low probability of acute attacks, particularly if carriers are identified prospectively. This assumes, of course, that parents will have their offspring evaluated at the appropriate time and will ensure that those who are carriers understand how to avoid attacks (see below). Such testing can be deferred until well beyond infancy, in that symptoms of any sort are exceedingly rare prior to puberty.

Differential Diagnosis

Cholestasis, appendicitis, or other acute abdominal process can resemble porphyria. Such conditions should be excluded rigorously in patients manifesting fever and leukocytosis, which are not regularly part of a porphyric attack. Hereditary tyrosinemia has many features of acute porphyria, including increased urinary ALA, but it presents in childhood. Finally, the symptoms of lead intoxication may mimic those of acute porphyria, including abdominal pain and altered mental status. Urinary excretion of ALA and coproporphyrin is increased, presumably reflecting an inhibitory effect of lead on PBG synthase and coproporphyrinogen oxidase, respectively. Unlike acute porphyria, PBG is normal; erythrocyte protoporphyrin may be elevated. The diagnosis is confirmed by blood lead determination; assay of PBG synthase also has been used.

Treatment

The approach to an acute attack is outlined in Table 42–4. Carbohydrate reverses the fasting state, which ac-

Table 42–4. Initial management of acute prophyric attacks.

1. Suppress seizures, if present, with intravenous diazepam
2. Ensure that patient is receiving no porphyria-inducing drugs
3. Provide pain relief
4. Monitor electrolytes, particularly hyponatremia
5. Initiate a 24-hour urine collection for porphobilinogen
6. Administer carbohydrate
   If neurologic signs are present, or if the above regimen fails to produce a symptomatic response within 48 hours, then:
7. Administer intravenous hematin

cording to experimental evidence sensitizes the liver to porphyria-inducing chemicals. The goal is to give 400–500 g/d, orally if possible. If intravenous administration is necessary, careful monitoring of serum electrolytes, particularly sodium, is essential. Pain relief usually requires opiates such as meperidine. There is little risk of addiction for a patient with a bona fide acute porphyric attack, although caution is indicated where the diagnosis is in doubt. Chlorpromazine has been used, but sedation may be its principal effect.

For women who experience premenstrual exacerbations of porphyria, suppression of the ovulatory cycle may provide relief. Peptide analogs of luteinizing hormone-releasing hormone (LHRH) are the preferred agents; unlike estrogen-based drugs, these have no demonstrable porphyria-inducing activity. Known genetic carriers of acute porphyria may experience intermittent somatic complaints but without the expected elevation of urinary PBG. Such patients often do not respond to hematin and most likely have an unrelated condition. In the absence of a specific diagnosis, empiric therapy should be tried (with due regard for hazardous drugs); opiates are inappropriate.

When seizures occur in acute porphyria, their management poses a problem in that virtually all first-line anticonvulsants are contraindicated (Table 42–5). Diazepam will provide short-term suppression while the attack is brought under control with hematin (see below); intravenous magnesium sulfate also has been used. For chronic seizures in patients with porphyria, bromide is the only treatment that clearly is safe and also effective. Although this therapy was eclipsed 50 years ago by the discovery of phenytoins (Dilantin and others), it has been reintroduced for problems such as refractory childhood epilepsy. Close monitoring of serum bromide levels is essential, and side effects are frequent.

Hematin represents the only specific therapy for acute porphyria. In theory, it corrects heme deficiency,

Table 42–5. Unsafe and safe drugs in porphyria.[1]

	Unsafe	Believed to Be Safe
Anticonvulsants	**Barbiturates**	Bromides
	Carbamazepine	Diazepam
	Clonazepam	Magnesium
	Ethosuximide	sulfate
	Hydantoins	
	Phenytoin	
	Primidone	
	Valproic acid	
Hypnotics or	**Barbiturates**	Chloral hydrate
sedatives	Chlordiazepoxide	Chlorpromazine
	Ethchlorvynol	Diphenhydramine
	Gluthethimide	Lithium
	Meprobamate	Lorazepam
	Methyprylon	Meclizine
		Trifluoperazine
Other drugs	α-Methyldopa	ACTH
	Danazol	Allopurinol
	Diclofenac	Aminoglycosides
	Ergot preparations	Aspirin
	Estrogens	Atropine
	Griseofulvin	Codeine
	Imipramine	Colchicine
	Pentazocine	Dexamethasone
	Pyrazinamide	Furosemide
	Sulfonamides	Ibuprofen
	Sulfonylureas	Insulin
		Meperidine
		Morphine
		Naproxen
		Penicillins
		Warfarin

[1]The agents in **bold print** have been implicated repeatedly in acute attacks. For the other "unsafe" compounds, the clinical information is anecdotal but supported by tests in experimental animals or *in vitro*.

which is the fundamental metabolic defect in the disease ("hematin" refers to heme in aqueous solution). Although not evaluated in controlled trials, its efficacy is supported by substantial clinical experience. Hematin should be given early to all patients presenting with neurologic signs and otherwise to those whose symptoms fail to respond within 48 hours to the measures outlined in Table 42–4. It is provided as a dry powder (Panhematin, Abbott Laboratories, Chicago, IL), to be reconstituted immediately prior to infusion. In general, 1.5 mg/kg (or 100 mg) every 24 hours is effective. This can be given every 12 hours in urgent circumstances. Urinary excretion of PBG is monitored to ensure that the patient has received an effective dose; a decrease to

approximately 10% of prehematin levels should occur after 48 hours. A symptomatic response follows that is often dramatic, with the requirement for pain medication decreasing rapidly and disappearing on the fourth or fifth day of treatment. Side effects of hematin are minor. The solution is slightly alkaline and, if infused too rapidly or into a small vein, causes a local chemical phlebitis. It also causes transient anticoagulation and should be given cautiously, if at all, to patients at risk of bleeding or receiving anticoagulant therapy.

Prevention of Attacks

Once an index diagnosis is established, screening of first-degree relatives is performed to identify latent carriers by the procedures outlined above (see section, "Genetic Diagnosis"). Because the gene is inherited as an autosomal dominant, those family members not identified as carriers (50%, on average) are normal and will not pass on the condition to their children. The vast majority of carriers will remain asymptomatic if they avoid drugs that precipitate acute attacks (see Table 42–5). They are advised also to avoid fasting and fad diets. On the other hand, there is no convincing evidence that a diet rich in carbohydrates prevents attacks, and obesity is an unwanted side effect.

Prognosis

The most ominous development in acute porphyria is a motor neuropathy, which can progress to respiratory paralysis. Prior to the advent of modern intensive care and the use of hematin, the mortality rate in such attacks approached 50%. The outlook is much improved now. Neurologic deficits resolve slowly but, as a rule, completely. Although psychosis is a component of the acute presentation, it resolves promptly as the attack subsides. There is no evidence of long-term or progressive psychiatric disease. The incidence of hepatocellular carcinoma is increased in patients with acute hepatic porphyria, as in children with hereditary tyrosinemia, independent of other known risk factors (hepatitis viruses, alcohol, iron overload). Moreover, lesions may arise in a noncirrhotic liver. The appropriate surveillance strategy has not been defined. An atypical excretion pattern of heme precursors should trigger a search for liver cancer.

HEREDITARY COPROPORPHYRIA

Hereditary coproporphyria is an acute hepatic porphyria; because circulating porphyrins are increased, cutaneous manifestations occur in about 30% of cases. This type appears to be expressed clinically less frequently than is acute intermittent porphyria. Population surveys have not been done, and the prevalence of the carrier state is unknown.

Clinical Findings

A. SYMPTOMS AND SIGNS

The acute attack is indistinguishable from that of acute intermittent porphyria (see Table 42–4). The cutaneous manifestations, when present, may be chronic and resemble those of porphyria cutanea tarda (see below).

B. LABORATORY FINDINGS

In acute attacks, urinary PBG is elevated as in acute intermittent porphyria. The diagnostic finding in carriers is elevation of fecal coproporphyrin as well as urine coproporphyrin.

C. GENETIC DIAGNOSIS

Carriers usually are identified by analysis of urine and feces. Although a blood test for coproporphyrinogen oxidase is available commercially, the results should be confirmed with conventional analysis.

Treatment & Prognosis

Treatment and prognosis are the same as for acute intermittent porphyria.

VARIEGATE PORPHYRIA

Variegate porphyria is an acute hepatic porphyria, with chronic cutaneous manifestations in most genetic carriers.

Clinical Findings

A. SYMPTOMS AND SIGNS

Acute attacks are identical to those in acute intermittent porphyria. The cutaneous manifestations are chronic in many affected persons and are similar to those in porphyria cutanea tarda (see below).

B. LABORATORY FINDINGS

Urinary PBG is elevated in attacks, as in acute intermittent porphyria, but may be normal otherwise. In persons with cutaneous disease only or in asymptomatic individuals, the diagnosis relies on an elevation of fecal protoporphyrin, which identifies about 75% of genetic carriers.

C. GENETIC DIAGNOSIS

The affected gene is protoporphyrinogen oxidase, which encodes a mitochondrial enzyme. As with the other porphyrias, the specific mutation varies among

individuals, and none is predominant. Thus, DNA analysis, although highly accurate, has been applied only to large kindreds and is not commercially available. Testing for enzyme activity also is a research procedure only.

Treatment & Prognosis

Acute attacks are handled as in acute intermittent porphyria and have a similar prognosis. There is no satisfactory treatment for the cutaneous manifestations other than protective clothing. Topical sunscreens are ineffective.

δ-AMINOLEVULINIC ACIDURIA

This type of porphyria involves deficiency of the second enzyme in heme synthesis, PBG synthase. It is recessively inherited and is rare. Acute attacks are similar to those in acute intermittent porphyria, and there is no cutaneous component. The pattern on urinalysis is increased urinary ALA, with normal PBG and increased coproporphyrin. The findings are similar to those of lead intoxication (see below), which must be excluded.

PORPHYRIA CUTANEA TARDA

Porphyria cutanea tarda is a chronic hepatic type, with cutaneous manifestations only; acute attacks do not occur.

Clinical Findings

A. SYMPTOMS AND SIGNS

Patients typically fail to relate their cutaneous problem to sun exposure, complaining mainly of "fragile skin." Seemingly trivial contact to the back of the hand produces an ulcer or sloughing of skin. The problem can be disabling for mechanics and others who require heavy use of the hands. They may report dark-colored (usually brownish) urine, which is due to porphyrins. The photosensitizing effects of porphyrins in the skin are manifest initially as blisters that range in size from milia to 1–2 cm, typically on the dorsa of the hands or on the face. These eventually open, leaving shallow ulcerations. With chronic injury, pigmented or depigmented scars are present as well as increased hair growth, which is noticeable mainly on the face. Sclerodermatous plaques can occur.

B. LABORATORY FINDINGS

The hallmark of the disease is markedly increased urine uroporphyrin. The presence of skin disease implies uroporphyrin excretion of at least 500 μg/24 hours, and values in the range of 1500–3000 μg/24 hours are not unusual. Urine PBG is normal or minimally elevated; fecal coproporphyrin and protoporphyrin are normal, and this distinguishes porphyria cutanea tarda from hereditary coproporphyria and variegate porphyria. Assay of uroporphyrinogen decarboxylase is not usually available.

Pathologic changes in the liver in porphyria cutanea tarda are those of the associated liver disease (commonly due to alcohol abuse). In addition, a uroporphyrin hepatopathy has been described. The accumulation of uroporphyrin renders the tissue fluorescent under long-wave ultraviolet excitation.

Differential Diagnosis

A. Tumor-Associated Porphyria

Hepatic tumors may overproduce porphyrins in quantities sufficient to cause manifestations similar to those of porphyria cutanea tarda. The pattern in urine differs from that of porphyria cutanea tarda and should suggest the diagnosis. In patients with HCV (see above) and significant fibrosis or cirrhosis, surveillance with a semiannual serum α-fetoprotein and abdominal ultrasound is indicated.

B. Bullous Dermatosis of Hemodialysis

Patients with chronic renal failure on hemodialysis may have bullous lesions indistinguishable from those of porphyria cutanea tarda. Plasma porphyrins are minimally elevated in most cases, even though uroporphyrin is not effectively dialyzed. In a minority of patients, the condition improves after discontinuation of medications, particularly nonsteroidal antiinflammatory drugs (NSAIDs), hormones, tetracycline, furosemide, and antihistamines.

C. Toxic Porphyria

In the late 1950s, an outbreak of cutaneous porphyria occurred in Turkey after several thousand people consumed seed grain that had been treated with hexachlorobenzene, a fungicide. This prompted experimental studies of halogenated aromatic hydrocarbons, several of which caused a uroporphyria in animals. Dioxin was among the most potent and, moreover, was of interest as a known contaminant of herbicides such as Agent Orange, which had been used in Vietnam. Detailed evaluation of Vietnam veterans and other groups exposed to dioxin or hexachlorobenzene, however, has failed to produce convincing evidence of either porphyria or a subclinical state consistent with chemical porphyria. It would appear that environmental exposure to polychlorinated hydrocarbons (with mainly cutaneous absorption) is less risky to humans than was suggested by studies of humans or animals with systemic exposure.

Treatment

Alcohol, estrogen, and dietary iron supplements should be discontinued (see Table 42–2). Patients should be screened for HCV infection (see above) and considered for antiviral treatment. Whereas these steps alone may lead to improvement, iron-depletion therapy hastens recovery in virtually all patients. This is best accomplished by venesection at the rate of 500 mL weekly or biweekly, with monitoring of the hemoglobin level until transferrin saturation drops below 40%. Follow-up consists of an annual check of urine uroporphyrin and iron status, with resumption of phlebotomy as indicated. For patients unable to tolerate phlebotomy, continuous subcutaneous infusion of desferrioxamine is effective, albeit expensive. Chloroquine is an alternative, causing depletion of uroporphyrin apparently by complexing with it in the liver. It should be used at low doses (eg, 125 mg chloroquine base, twice weekly), however, to minimize the risk of adverse hepatic reactions.

Topical transparent sunscreens offer little or no protection from light-induced damage.

Prognosis

Virtually all patients respond to iron depletion, although the period of treatment required to produce a response can vary from a few weeks to 6 months or more. Provided the responsible environmental factors (notably alcohol) have been eliminated, the remission may be long lasting. In women who need replacement estrogen, transdermal patches may be tolerated better than oral medication.

CONGENITAL ERYTHROPOIETIC PORPHYRIA

This is a rare, recessively inherited disease in which levels of blood and urine uroporphyrin are massively elevated. Photocutaneous lesions are evident from an early age, beginning usually in infancy. The relevance to gastroenterology is that some cases are relatively mild and may present in adulthood with cutaneous disease resembling that of porphyria cutanea tarda. Activated charcoal by mouth is an experimental therapy that has proved beneficial in a few patients. It presumably binds porphyrin in the intestine, preventing its enterohepatic recirculation and thus decreasing the total body burden. Iron-depletion therapy is of no value.

PROTOPORPHYRIA

Protoporphyria is a chronic cutaneous porphyria; in most cases, the excess porphyrin originates from the bone marrow, but in some it comes at least in part from the liver.

Clinical Findings

A. SYMPTOMS AND SIGNS

The cutaneous disease involves an immediate edematous, urticarial reaction to sunlight, which is quite distinct from the blistering that occurs in porphyria cutanea tarda. Repeated exposure produces cutaneous thickening and fibrosis. Typically these patients appear in the dermatologist's office but, rarely, may present with cholestatic liver disease. Because circulating protoporphyrin is excreted essentially entirely into bile, relatively high levels may accumulate in the liver. Such deposition appears to be the basis for a hepatopathy that may progress rapidly to portal hypertension and a fatal outcome. Jaundice heralds hepatic decompensation. About 10% of patients have protoporphyrin-containing gallstones.

B. LABORATORY FINDINGS

The characteristic abnormality is elevation of erythrocyte and fecal protoporphyrin, with little, if any, change in the other heme precursors. Circulating erythrocytes may be fluorescent. Anemia usually is not present. The finding on liver biopsy of birefringent inclusions in hepatocytes under polarizing light is diagnostic. The best predictor of liver disease appears to be a plasma protoporphyrin level in excess of 100 µg/dL.

C. GENETIC DIAGNOSIS

Direct assay of the deficient enzyme, heme synthase (ferrochelatase), is not available except in research laboratories. In some families, carriers can be identified by their fluorescing erythrocytes.

Treatment & Prognosis

Individuals with worrisome levels of plasma protoporphyrin should have tests of liver function and needle biopsy, if necessary, to assess the activity of the liver disease. Cholestyramine or activated charcoal has been used to trap protoporphyrin in the intestine and facilitate its excretion. Anecdotal reports suggest some benefit of this approach. Red cell transfusion reduces protoporphyrin production by way of suppressing erythropoiesis but is cumbersome. β-Carotene (Lumitene) alleviates the cutaneous symptoms in many patients, apparently by quenching active oxygen, which mediates the light-induced damage. The recommended dosage for children is 100–200 mg/d and for adults 200–300 mg/d. At therapeutic levels, it causes a noticeable yellowing of the skin. Other antioxidants, such as vitamin C, may be helpful also. For patients with hepatic failure, liver transplantation has been performed, although its long-term benefit is uncertain. Operating room lights need to be equipped with special filters for avoiding phototoxic injury to exposed tissues during the procedure. A goal of current research is transfer of the normal heme synthase gene into erythropoietic stem cells followed by bone marrow transplantation. Experimental studies support the feasibility of this approach.

SUMMARY

The porphyrias are a group of diseases involving disturbances in heme synthesis. The most important are genetic and represent deficiency of a specific enzyme of the pathway. The "acute-attack" (neurologic) types have clinical features in common, including increased urinary excretion of ALA and PBG. Cutaneous porphyria results from overproduction of porphyrins, which are photosensitizing. The specific diagnosis is determined from the pattern of porphyrin intermediates in blood or excreta.

Management is tailored to the type of porphyria. The only specific treatment for acute attacks is hematin, which should be considered for any patient with objective neurologic signs and for those whose symptoms fail to respond to conservative measures. The most prevalent of the cutaneous porphyrias, porphyria cutanea tarda, is effectively treated by iron depletion, while the cutaneous symptoms in protoporphyria respond to administration of β-carotene. Toxic (acquired) porphyria occurs following intensive exposure to some halogenated hydrocarbons and resembles porphyria cutanea tarda. It appears, however, to be a rarity in Western Europe and North America under current standards of environmental safety.

REFERENCES

Andant C et al: Hepatocellular carcinoma in patients with acute hepatic porphyria: frequency of occurrence and related factors. J Hepatol 2000;32:933.

Anderson KE: LHRH analogues for hormonal manipulation in acute intermittent porphyria. Semin Hematol 1989;26:10.

Bissell DM: Treatment of acute hepatic porphyria with hematin. J Hepatol 1988;6:1.

Bonkovsky HL et al: Porphyria cutanea tarda, hepatitis C and HFE gene mutations in North America. Hepatology 1998;27:1661.

Cox TM et al: Protoporphyria. Sem Liver Dis 1998;18:85.

Daniell WE et al: Environmental chemical exposures and disturbances of heme synthesis. Environ Health Perspect 1997;105 (Suppl 1):37.

Dean G: Pursuit of a disease. Sci Am 1957;196:133.

McDonagh AF, Bissell DM: Porphyria and porphyrinology—the past fifteen years. Sem Liver Dis 1998;18:3.

Complications of Chronic Liver Disease

43

Thomas D. Schiano, MD & Henry C. Bodenheimer, Jr., MD

The complications of chronic liver disease are multiple and highly variable in presentation. Patients may be asymptomatic, with only incidentally detected laboratory test abnormalities, or may have obvious features of hepatic parenchymal failure and portal hypertension. Cirrhosis results when any chronic liver disease or insult leads to the diffuse destruction of hepatic parenchymal cells and the formation of nodules, which result in disorganization of the liver's lobular and vascular architecture, further compromising hepatocyte survival and function. A cirrhotic liver with a grossly normal liver for comparison is shown in Figure 43–1.

Cirrhosis and its complications (eg, hepatocellular carcinoma) constitute one of the greatest causes of mortality worldwide. Table 43–1 lists the most common causes of cirrhosis. It is estimated that there are over 3 million Americans with cirrhosis. In addition, cirrhosis is by far the most frequent indication for liver transplantation. Alcoholic liver disease alone is responsible for more than 100,000 hospitalizations annually, close to 14,000 deaths, and $1.8 billion in medical expenditures. Because of the increasing incidence of cirrhosis related to chronic hepatitis C virus (HCV) infection, similar estimates are predicted for patients with HCV over the next decade. Much of the morbidity and mortality occurring in cirrhosis is a direct consequence of hepatic synthetic failure, portal hypertension, or both.

HEPATIC SYNTHETIC FAILURE

Consequences

With hepatocellular damage and destruction, residual hepatic parenchyma may maintain production of liver-derived proteins such as albumin and clotting factors due to the large reserve capacity of the healthy liver. Additionally, the injured liver may regenerate lost hepatocyte mass. Extensive liver damage usually must occur before the hepatic reserve and regenerative capacity are overwhelmed; therefore, clinical evidence of inadequate liver protein synthesis indicates extreme damage. When severe hepatic synthetic failure complicates chronic liver disease and is clinically apparent, current therapies other than liver transplantation have little impact on

mortality rates. Management is most effectively directed toward the prevention and treatment of the complications of portal hypertension.

A. SYMPTOMS AND SIGNS

Fatigue is a hallmark of advanced chronic liver disease. Other symptoms are typically vague and nonspecific, such as malaise, anorexia, epistaxis, weight loss, skin fragility and bruisability, muscle cramps, and decreased libido and sexual function. In addition, patients with cirrhosis have anemia, are at risk for developing cholelithiasis and osteoporosis, have gonadal failure and subtle autonomic nervous system dysfunction, and may have QT prolongation on their electrocardiogram (ECG). Typical physical findings found in cirrhosis are shown in Figure 43–2.

Several signs of parenchymal failure (eg, edema and bleeding) result from reduced plasma concentrations of proteins that are synthesized by the liver (eg, albumin, fibrinogen, and coagulation factors), and the severity of these deficits is commonly used to estimate the severity of liver dysfunction. However, acute illness may transiently worsen the levels of hypoalbuminemia, coagulopathy, and hyperbilirubinemia, so these parameters are imprecise at best. The Child–Pugh–Turcotte classification and more recently the Model for End-stage Liver Disease (MELD) scoring system use parameters of hepatic synthetic dysfunction to help measure mortality risk in patients with end-stage liver disease and to determine liver allograft allocation priority. To date, no dynamic tests of hepatic functional reserve have been validated and widely adopted.

B. HYPOALBUMINEMIA/COAGULOPATHY

Low serum albumin levels are generally found in patients with cirrhosis. Albumin, however, is an imperfect indicator of liver function because the plasma concentration of albumin is also affected by nutritional and fluid status. Additionally, albumin production may decrease during acute illness as part of the acute phase response to stress. Albumin loss through proteinuria may be a consequence of several renal diseases (eg, diabetic nephropathy, HCV glomerulonephritis) associated with cirrhosis. Hypoalbuminemia out of proportion to

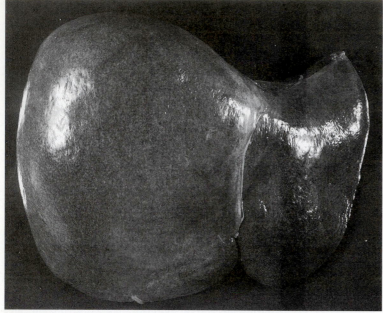

A

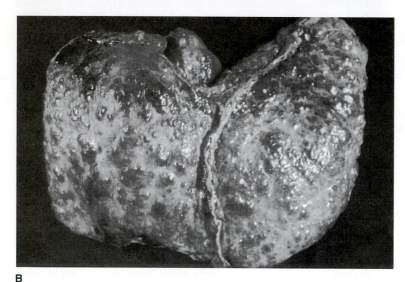

B

Figure 43–1. **A:** Autopsy photograph of a normal human liver. **B:** Photograph of an explanted cirrhotic liver. (Courtesy of M Isabel Fiel, MD and R Saxena, MD.)

other parameters of hepatic synthetic dysfunction should prompt an evaluation for renal protein loss. At times, gastrointestinal protein loss may contribute to low serum albumin levels in patients with portal hypertension. Hypoalbuminemia results in reduced plasma oncotic pressure, which permits the leakage of fluid from the vascular space and promotes tissue edema.

Another clinically important consequence of impaired hepatic protein synthesis is coagulopathy, be-

cause all protein-clotting factors except factor VIII are synthesized by hepatocytes. Bleeding risk is further increased in persons with cirrhosis because of concurrent thrombocytopenia, typically the result of hypersplenism. In the absence of vitamin K deficiency, the magnitude of prolongation of the prothrombin time is a better marker of the severity of the hepatic parenchymal dysfunction than measurement of serum albumin. Vitamin K deficiency, seen more commonly in cholestatic

Table 43–1. Causes of cirrhosis.

Autoimmune hepatitis
Alcohol-induced liver injury
Drug- or toxin-induced liver injury (ie, methotrexate)
Viral hepatitis B, C, or D
Metabolic diseases
    α_1-Antitrypsin deficiency
    Wilson's disease
    Hemochromatosis and other copper disorders
    Tyrosinemia
Nonalcoholic steatohepatitis or fatty liver
Vascular derangements
    Chronic right heart failure
    Budd–Chiari syndrome
    Long-standing portal vein thrombosis
Biliary disorders
    Primary biliary cirrhosis
    Cystic fibrosis
    Sarcoidosis
    Biliary cirrhosis secondary to chronic large bile duct
        obstruction
    Primary sclerosing cholangitis
    Biliary atresia
    Congenital paucity of intrahepatic ducts
    Progressive familial intrahepatic cholestasis
Malnutrition and postjejunoileal bypass surgery
Cryptogenic disease

liver diseases, can be adequately corrected with 10 mg vitamin K administered subcutaneously daily over 3 days. It should not be administered intramuscularly because of the risk of formation of hematoma. Consumptive coagulopathy associated with sepsis can be distinguished from the coagulopathy of cirrhosis by assaying factor VIII levels, which are decreased in sepsis but not in liver failure. Efforts to emergently correct coagulopathy with administration of preformed clotting factors should be reserved for patients who are actively bleeding or who are about to undergo procedures associated with a high risk of significant bleeding. In such circumstances, transfusion with fresh frozen plasma is effective, but typically large amounts are required and may exacerbate fluid overload.

C. JAUNDICE

Jaundice is an additional sign of hepatic parenchymal failure, with the extent of hyperbilirubinemia often paralleling the severity of liver disease. Jaundice occurs in parenchymal failure because the ability of liver cells to excrete conjugated bilirubin into bile becomes impaired. This results in elevation of both direct and indirect serum bilirubin. The magnitude of bilirubin elevation is not specific to worsening liver disease alone. Any

condition that causes overproduction of bilirubin (eg, hemolysis, blood transfusion), concurrent hepatocyte destruction (eg, drug hepatotoxicity, alcoholic hepatitis), decreased hepatic uptake or conjugation of bilirubin (eg, Gilbert's syndrome), or decreased bile excretion (intrahepatic or extrahepatic mechanical obstruction of the bile duct) can worsen the degree of jaundice in cirrhosis. Noninvasive imaging studies [eg, ultrasound, computed tomography (CT) scan, magnetic resonance (MR) cholangiogram] are useful in excluding bile duct obstruction that may be treated by mechanical decompression. Sepsis causes unconjugated hyperbilirubinemia because bacterial endotoxin impedes bilirubin transport across the canalicular membrane. Both the ability of the cirrhotic liver to conjugate bilirubin and the efficiency of other hepatic enzyme systems are impaired, including those responsible for detoxification and metabolism of hormones, cytokines, and drugs. Thus, the patient with cirrhosis is more susceptible to drug toxicity or overdose.

D. SUSCEPTIBILITY TO INFECTION

The incidence of bacterial infections in patients with cirrhosis admitted to the hospital is very high, and the incidence of nosocomial bacterial infection in this population is much higher than in the general hospital population. Facultative gram-negative bacilli appear to be increased in the jejunal flora of many patients with cirrhosis, some of whom have decreased gastric motility. This change in intestinal flora may increase the risk of gram-negative bacteremia, via translocation through the gut wall and a disruption of the normal intestinal permeability barrier. Hypoalbuminemia and ascites contribute to gut wall edema, predisposing to bacterial translocation.

The activity of the reticuloendothelial system is reduced in cirrhosis. Impairment may result, in part, from intrahepatic shunting of blood, which escapes the phagocytic action of the Kupffer cells located in the hepatic sinusoids. Additionally, circulating immune complexes associated with several liver diseases such as primary biliary cirrhosis and sclerosing cholangitis may directly affect macrophage function. Serum opsonic activity is reduced in cirrhosis, probably as a consequence of decreased serum concentration of complement and fibronectin. Decreased opsonic activity in ascites may predispose to bacterial peritonitis. Altered neutrophil function at different stages of cell maturation has been demonstrated in cirrhosis. The most frequent disturbance is a marked reduction of chemotaxis, probably caused by the presence of serum substances that inhibit granulocyte migration. Furthermore, the phagocytic and bactericidal capacity of neutrophils may also be reduced.

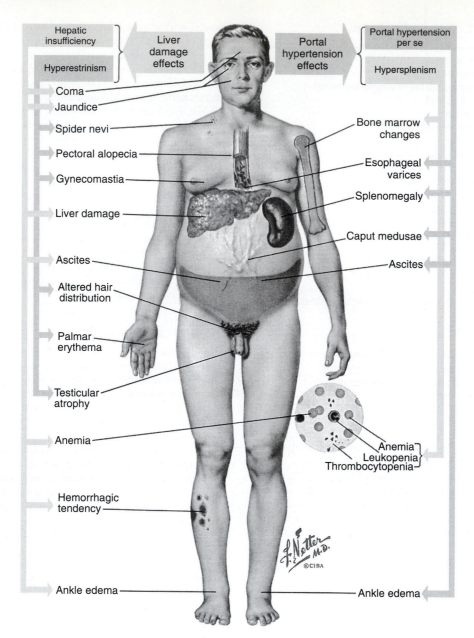

Figure 43–2. The clinical manifestations found in cirrhosis. A compilation of paintings on the normal and pathologic anatomy of the digestive system. (From the Netter Collection of Medical Illustrations, Vol. 3, Part 3: *Digestive System.* Copyright © 1957 Icon Learning Systems, LLC, a subsidiary of MediMedia USA Inc. Reprinted with permission from ICON Learning Systems LLC, illustrated by Frank H. Netter, MD. All rights reserved.)

Patients with cirrhosis, overall, are at increased risk for developing infectious complications as a result of the sequelae of portal hypertension. There is an increased risk of bacterial infection during acute variceal bleeding. Patients are at risk for aspiration pneumonia and atelectasis during bouts of hepatic encephalopathy, and anasarca and malnutrition predispose to poor wound healing and soft tissue infections. Because patients with cirrhosis may be hypothermic, and their peripheral white blood cell counts are frequently depressed due to hypersplenism, infection may not present with fever and leukocytosis. An abrupt rise in prothrombin time or in the degree of hyperbilirubinemia is an indicator of infection and should trigger more extensive evaluation. Infection may precipitate hepatorenal syndrome (HRS) or hepatic encephalopathy. Frequent cultures and at times prophylactic antibiotic use are beneficial in patients with cirrhosis. In spite of a decreased immune response to vaccines, patients with cirrhosis should be administered the pneumococcal and hepatitis A and B vaccinations.

E. Protein–Calorie Malnutrition

Cachexia and clinical evidence of protein–calorie malnutrition are seen in a majority of patients with cirrhosis. Many factors contribute to the development of malnutrition in these individuals, including malabsorption of nutrients because of intestinal edema, diarrhea, and decreased bile flow, and reduced hepatic stores of many water-soluble vitamins and trace elements. Anorexia and decreased oral intake result from fatigue, dysgeusia, nausea, early satiety due to ascites and decreased gastric emptying, and frequent hospitalizations. In addition, patients with cirrhosis have impaired hepatic and muscle intermediary metabolism as a result of increased circulatory levels of proinflammatory cytokines and altered balance of many hormones that maintain metabolic homeostasis (ie, insulin, insulin-like growth factor, glucagon). Glucose intolerance and diabetes are seen commonly in cirrhosis, in part related to decreased glycogen synthesis and reduced skeletal muscle glucose uptake and transport.

Patients with advanced liver disease have higher mean protein requirements (0.8–1.2 g/protein/kg/d) necessary to maintain nitrogen balance, but appear to have efficient utilization of dietary protein. The increased protein requirement may be due to an increased use of amino acids for energy expenditure via gluconeogenesis during postabsorptive periods, because of reduced postprandial glycogen stores and decreased protein accretion during feeding periods. Patients with cirrhosis have increased urinary nitrogen losses and elevated rates of whole-body protein degradation. Spontaneous protein intake in clinically stable malnourished patients is close to the requirements for balance, so patients with cirrhosis are therefore prone to rapid protein wasting during periods of decreased oral intake (ie, hospitalization). Prolonged fasting should be avoided and frequent feeding, including an evening supplement, may improve nutritional balance. Low-grade encephalopathy should not be considered a contraindication to otherwise indicated nutritional intervention.

Malnutrition is a definite risk factor that increases morbidity and mortality in patients with cirrhosis and in individuals undergoing liver transplantation. These patients need to maintain an adequate dietary intake. A high meal frequency or nocturnal nutritional supplementation can often meet dietary goals. In hospitalized patients, caloric intake should be frequently monitored and supplemental nutrition should be provided in the form of oral supplements or enteral feeding, when appropriate.

F. Renal Dysfunction

In the early stages of cirrhosis when ascites is not present, systemic circulatory dysfunction is subtle and renal function is normal. With time, however, diminished renal ability to excrete a sodium load develops. As cirrhosis and portal hypertension progress, renal sodium excretional capacity decreases, so patients can no longer excrete normal daily sodium intake, which results in fluid retention and formation of ascites. Patients may still have a normal glomerular filtration rate (GFR) and are able to dilute their urine after a water load. At this point patients with cirrhosis have a slight decrease in arterial blood pressure and, if sodium retention is intense, compensatory activity of the renin-angiotensin–aldosterone axis and sympathetic nervous system occurs. Patients with more severe liver disease develop greater impairment in their ability to excrete free water, resulting in delusional hyponatremia. Delusional hyponatremia indicates a severe derangement in systemic hemodynamics and a very high risk for developing HRS. Renal perfusion and GFR ultimately become impaired, related in part to compensatory increases that occur in plasma levels of antidiuretic hormones, renin and norepinephrine.

These pathophysiologic changes thus predispose patients with advanced liver disease to developing renal failure. Usual methods for measuring creatinine clearance generally overestimate renal functional capacity in patients with cirrhosis, in part because of the protein malnutrition, muscle wasting, and thus decreased urea and creatinine production observed in patients with cirrhosis. Therefore, patients with cirrhosis generally have reduced levels of blood urea nitrogen (BUN) and creatinine at baseline. Risks for developing renal impairment are further increased because of a greater susceptibility to infection, gastrointestinal bleeding, volume and electrolyte derangements due to ascites and the use of diuretics, decreased oral intake, and the nausea, vomiting, and diarrhea that many patients with cirrhosis experience. Occult infection is a frequent cause of renal decompensation in cirrhosis. Worsening renal function should prompt a work-up for infection including blood cultures and diagnostic paracentesis. It is often difficult to ascertain the effective arterial blood volume in patients with cirrhosis, which can be decreased even in the presence of significant peripheral edema. Thus, diuretics are usually discontinued in patients with cirrhosis having ascites in the setting of other potential precipitants of renal dysfunction, such as infection.

Patients with cirrhosis are exquisitely sensitive to the renal effects of aminoglycosides and nonsteroidal anti-inflammatory agents (NSAIDs), both of which can precipitate acute tubular necrosis (ATN) and, ultimately, HRS. These medications should not be used in patients with cirrhosis. The recently introduced cyclooxygenase 2 inhibitors share the renal effects of NSAIDs and should be similarly prescribed. Avoiding NSAIDs makes analgesic use somewhat problematic in patients with cirrhosis because opiates often can precipitate hepatic encephalopathy and aspirin can worsen chronic gastrointestinal tract blood loss. Acetaminophen, in a daily dose of less than 2 g, is a safe alternative to NSAIDs.

G. Pruritus

Pruritus may occur in any patient with cirrhosis, but occurs more commonly in patients with cholestasis, such as in primary biliary cirrhosis or sclerosing cholangitis. In some patients with cirrhosis, generalized itching limits normal activities, causes sleep deprivation, and has a major impact on the quality of life. Severe pruritus may lead to skin excoriations that can become superinfected. The pathogenesis of pruritus is unknown but may be related to increased central opioidergic tone. Evidence for this is suggested by the findings that opiate agonists induce pruritus of central (brain) origin, opioidergic tone in the central nervous system is increased in cirrhosis, and opiate antagonists reduce scratching activity in patients with the pruritus of cholestasis. The sites of synthesis of endogenous opioids mediating the pruritus of cholestasis are currently unknown, but one source may be the cholestatic or failing liver itself.

Pruritus can be a disabling symptom of advanced liver disease and is often difficult to palliate. Nails should be trimmed short and smooth to prevent excoriations. Xerosis will exacerbate pruritus so skin should be kept moist. Cholestyramine is often used as an initial medical treatment. Caution should be exercised that ample time is given between the administration of cholestyramine and other medications to prevent their malabsorption. Ursodeoxycholic acid and rifampicin may also have beneficial effects. Phenobarbital may be

helpful in some patients but can cause sedation, as will diphenhydramine. Opioid receptor antagonists (ie, naloxone) and serotoninergic antagonists (ie, ondansetron) have been effective in refractory cases, as has plasmapheresis.

Jones EA, Bergasa NV: The pruritus of cholestasis. Hepatology 1999;29:1003.

Kamath PS et al: A model to predict survival in patients with end-stage liver disease. Hepatology 2001;33:464.

Keeffe EB: Liver transplantation: current status and novel approaches to liver replacement. Gastroenterology 2001;120: 749.

Kim WR et al: Outcome of hospital care of liver disease associated with hepatitis C in the United States. Hepatology 2001;33: 201.

Kondrup J, Müller MJ: Energy and protein requirements of patients with chronic liver disease. J Hepatol 1997;27:239.

Marchesini G et al: Factors associated with poor-health-related quality of life of patients with cirrhosis. Gastroenterology 2001;120:170.

Moseley RH: Sepsis-associated cholestasis. Gastroenterology 1997; 112:302.

Navasa M, Rimola A, Rodes J: Bacterial infections in liver disease. Semin Liver Dis 1997;17:323.

CONSEQUENCES OF PORTAL HYPERTENSION

As shown in Figure 43–3, the portal vein is derived from the splenic and superior mesenteric veins, and drains the splanchnic circulation through the liver. As such, it provides the liver with over 60% of its blood supply, with the remainder supplied by the hepatic artery. The liver is the main site of resistance to portal blood flow and acts as a distensible vascular network of low resistance. Although portal hypertension can occur in the absence of cirrhosis due to extrahepatic vascular obstruction, cirrhosis is by far the most common cause.

Changes in pressure in the portal vein are regulated by Ohm's law, which states that changes in pressure $(P_1 - P_2)$ along a blood vessel are a function of the interaction of blood flow (Q) and vascular resistance (R), where $(P_1 - P_2) = Q \times R$. Increased resistance to portal blood flow can develop anywhere along the venous system, eg, in the portal vein or its tributaries before blood reaches the liver (prehepatic portal hypertension), in the vascular spaces within the liver (intrahepatic), or in the veins or vascular compartments that receive portal blood flow as it exits the liver (posthepatic). Intrahepatic obstruction to portal blood flow can occur at multiple sites within the liver. Occlusion of small portal vein branches within portal triads (presinusoidal portal hypertension) may complicate liver diseases in which there is extensive portal and periportal inflammation or fibrosis, such as in schistosomiasis. Alternatively, portal

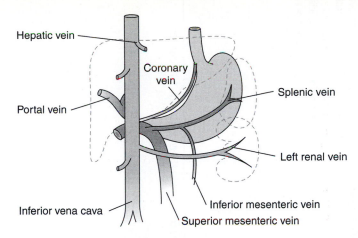

Figure 43–3. Normal venous anatomy of the liver and mesenteric axis.

blood flow may be impeded by narrowing of the hepatic sinusoids via collagen deposition and contractile sinusoidal occlusion by stellate cells, or blood flow may be obstructed at the level of the terminal hepatic venules (postsinusoidal) as in Budd–Chiari syndrome. Table 43–2 includes known causes of portal hypertension, and the sites at which portal blood flow is affected.

Portal vein pressure is indirectly estimated by "wedging" a catheter into a small branch of the hepatic vein, which measures hepatic sinusoidal pressure and thus indirectly pressure of the portal vein. Portal pressure is estimated by the difference between the wedged hepatic venous pressure and the free hepatic venous pressure. Cirrhosis leads to both an increase in hepatic sinusoidal pressure and an increase in portal pressure gradient (the pressure difference between the portal vein and posthepatic systemic veins). Pressure increases initially as a consequence of an increased resistance to portal flow at all levels of the intrahepatic vascular bed. This obstruction to flow is mostly caused by an architectural distortion of the liver secondary to fibrous tissue and regenerative nodules, but there is also a primary increase in intrahepatic vascular tone. This reversible component accounts for about 20–30% of increased intrahepatic resistance.

An elevated portal pressure gradient results in the formation of portosystemic collaterals (varices). Esophageal and gastric varices are connections between the coronary and short gastric veins, respectively, and the azygous vein. These collaterals are insufficient to decompress the portal venous system because their vascular resistance, although lower than that of the intrahepatic vasculature, is higher than normal portal resistance. In the early stages of cirrhosis, patients have a normal portal vein–inferior vena cava (IVC) pressure gradient but as disease progresses the gradient increases. Varices form when the por-

tal vein–IVC gradient reaches 10–12 mm Hg. Even when 100% of portal blood is shunted away from the portal venous system through collaterals, portal pressure remains elevated. This is due not only to the resistance that collaterals themselves offer to portal flow, but also to an increase in portal venous inflow. This increased inflow is the result of arteriolar vasodilation that occurs both in the splanchnic and systemic circulations. Esophageal varices are shown in Figure 43–4. Portal hypertension also leads to blood pooling in vascular beds that normally empty into the portal vein. Sequestration of blood in the spleen causes splenomegaly and hypersplenism, with secondary thrombocytopenia, neutropenia, and anemia.

CLINICAL COMPLICATIONS OF PORTAL HYPERTENSION

1. Gastrointestinal Bleeding

Portal hypertension leads to the development of portosystemic collaterals of which the most clinically significant are esophagogastric varices, because of their tendency to hemorrhage. Bleeding from these varices accounts for one-third of all deaths in patients with cirrhosis and portal hypertension. Esophageal varices develop at a rate of 5% per year, and up to 90% of all patients with cirrhosis will develop varices. The risk of bleeding from esophagogastric varices is 25–35% for both alcoholic and nonalcoholic cirrhosis, with the majority of sentinel bleeding occurring within the first year of diagnosis. For those patients who survive the initial episode of bleeding the risk of recurrent bleeding approaches 70%, with most episodes occurring within 6 months of the index bleed. The mortality for each episode of variceal bleeding is 30–50%, with infection being a major cause of death. The risk of dying from

Table 43-2. Classification of the types of portal hypertension.

Prehepatic	Presinusoidal	Presinusoidal Mixed	Sinusoidal Mixed	Sinusoidal	Postsinusoidal Mixed	Postsinusoidal	Posthepatic
Portal vein thrombosis	Schistosomiasis	Idiopathic portal hypertension	Alcoholic cirrhosis	Idiopathic portal hypertension	Alcoholic hepatitis	Budd–Chiari	Inferior vena cava web
Splenic arteriovenous fistula	Sarcoidosis	Primary biliary cirrhosis	Primary biliary cirrhosis		Hypervitaminosis A	Veno-occlusive disease	Constrictive pericarditis
Idiopathic tropical splenomegaly	Myeloproliferative diseases	Congenital hepatic fibrosis	Peliosis hepatis			Partial nodular transformation	Tricuspid insufficiency
Splenic capillary hemangiomatosis	Metastatic malignancy	Schistosomiasis	Fulminant hepatitis				Severe heart failure
	Intrahepatic arteriovenous fistula	Chronic active hepatitis	Methotrexate				
	Congenital hepatic fibrosis	Vinyl chloride toxicity	Idiopathic portal hypertension				
	Idiopathic portal hypertension	Vineyard sprayers in Portugal					
		Azathioprine					

Adapted, with permission, from Groszmann RJ, Jensen JE: Pathophysiology of portal hypertension. In: *Liver and Biliary Diseases*, 2nd ed. Kaplowitz N (editor). Williams & Wilkins, 1996.

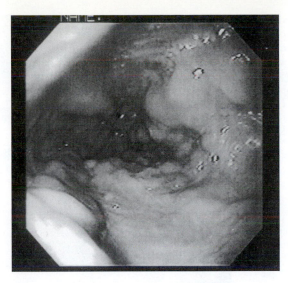

Figure 43–4. Endoscopic photograph of esophageal varices, which are the serpiginous structures lining all four walls of the esophagus. (Courtesy of D Jaffe, MD.)

variceal bleeding is directly related to the severity of the underlying liver condition.

Three risk factors for variceal hemorrhage have been established: size of varices, presence of red signs on varices (ie, blood blisters called hematocystic spots), and the severity of liver disease. There is a threshold portal vein–IVC pressure gradient of 10–12 mm Hg, below which varices do not develop. However, varices may not form even when this gradient is exceeded. The risk of variceal hemorrhage appears to be dependent more directly on the wall tension of the varix than on the portal pressure. Wall tension is determined by the diameter of the varix and its wall thickness, as well as the pressure within its lumen. Hence, large, thin-walled veins within the esophagus are at greatest risk of rupture. Patients who are actively drinking alcohol or who have large hepatocellular carcinomas appear to be at high risk for bleeding. Although varices of the esophagus and stomach occur most commonly, ectopic varices can infrequently occur in the duodenum, jejunum, colon, rectum, and peristomally in patients with ostomies following bowel surgery.

Prevention of Initial Variceal Hemorrhage

Once varices are demonstrated on screening endoscopy, medical therapy should be undertaken to prevent hemorrhage because of the high probability of eventual bleeding. The nonselective β-adrenegic blockers propranolol and nadolol have been extensively evaluated in randomized, controlled trials. They decrease both cardiac output and splanchnic blood flow, which decreases the hyperdynamic circulation and portal pressure. There is also a decrease in collateral blood flow and di-

ameter, which explains the efficacy of β-blockers in clinical trials despite only modest portal pressure reduction. There is a significant benefit of β-adrenegic blockers in preventing initial variceal hemorrhage. The benefit persists regardless of ascites or liver function, and is associated with a significant reduction in bleeding-related deaths. There is a 15% frequency of side effects from β-blockade when used prophylactically. The most common adverse effects are depression, light-headedness, fatigue, and cold extremities. Congestive heart failure, severe asthma, chronic obstructive lung disease, and insulin-dependent diabetes mellitus are relative contraindications to the use of β-blockers. Their dose should be adjusted to achieve a 25% reduction in resting heart rate, a maximal tolerable decrease in heart rate to a minimum of 55 beats/min, or until the appearance of symptoms. Some centers utilize serial measurements of portal pressure to gauge dosing of medical therapy. Therapy with β-blockade should be continued indefinitely, as cessation of treatment after 2 years has been associated with a recurrence of the risk of bleeding.

Carvedilol is a new nonselective β-blocker with additional anti-α-adrenegic activity that reduces portal pressure gradient, arterial blood pressure, and peripheral resistance. Isosorbide mononitrate may be as effective as propranolol in preventing initial variceal hemorrhage, but long-term follow-up of treated patients has been associated with a higher mortality. The use of nitrate monotherapy is not advocated. Although the combination of a β-blocker and mononitrate has a synergistic portal pressure-reducing effect, it does not improve or prevent a sentinel variceal hemorrhage and may be associated with more side effects and a higher incidence of ascites.

Prophylactic sclerotherapy is not recommended because of unproven efficacy and a high rate of complications. In contrast, prophylactic band ligation reduces the risks of variceal hemorrhage and mortality compared with untreated controls. Moreover, band ligation reduces the risk for sentinel variceal bleed compared with β-blockade, but has no effect on mortality. Thus, prophylactic ligation should be considered for patients with large esophageal varices who cannot tolerate β-blockers.

Management of Acute Variceal Hemorrhage

Patients with cirrhosis should thus be screened endoscopically for the presence of varices. The prevalence of varices in cirrhosis is proportional to the severity of portal hypertension and liver disease. Therefore, those patients who are Child's class A should be screened when there is clinical evidence of portal hypertension, eg, platelet count <100,000 or an enlarged portal vein diameter (>13 mm) on ultrasound. Patients who are Child's class B or C at the time of diagnosis of cirrhosis should always be screened for varices. The rate of growth of varices in patients with cirrhosis is proportional to the severity of liver disease. Therefore, patients who have no varices on screening endoscopy should be rescreened periodically, about every 2 years. The progression from small to large varices occurs in 10–20% of cases each year. Because the development of large varices is greater in patients with small varices on initial endoscopy compared with patients having no varices, patients who have small varices on screening endoscopy should be reassessed regularly.

Hemorrhage from varices is a dramatic event with painless hematemesis, melena, or hematochezia; bleeding is rarely insidious or chronic. The coagulopathy and thrombocytopenia typical of cirrhosis compound hemorrhage. Patients should be hemodynamically resuscitated and their coagulopathy corrected, with caution not to overhydrate the individual (the baseline systolic blood pressure of some patients with cirrhosis is 85–95 mm Hg), which could further acutely raise portal pressure. Optimal resuscitation requires careful monitoring of the patient's blood loss and observation in an intensive care unit. Femoral vein catheters may carry appreciable morbidity in patients with cirrhosis and should be avoided if possible. During acute bleeding, endoscopy is essential because nonvariceal sources of gastrointestinal bleeding are common in patients with cirrhosis. An actively bleeding esophageal varix is shown in Figure 43–5. Orotracheal intubation may be necessary prior to endoscopy because of the risks of aspiration and the potential toxicity of sedation in these pa-

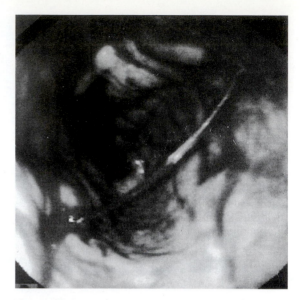

Figure 43–5. Endoscopic photograph of an actively bleeding esophageal varix. Another variceal column is noted on the superior wall. (Courtesy of T Lissoos, MD.)

tients. Figure 43–6 shows a treatment algorithm for the management of acute variceal hemorrhage.

A. ENDOSCOPIC SCLEROTHERAPY AND BAND LIGATION

Endoscopic control of variceal hemorrhage by sclerotherapy or band ligation is successful in approximately 90% of cases, especially when used in conjunction with intravenous somatostatin analogs (ie, octreotide). Sclerotherapy consists of the injection of a sclerosant agent (ie, ethanolamine oleate, sodium tetradecyl) into or next to a varix with the objective of producing thrombosis of the varix and/or inflammation of the surrounding tissue (Figure 43–7). Band ligation consists of the placement of rubber rings on variceal columns with the objective of interrupting blood flow and subsequently developing necrosis of mucosa and submucosa with replacement of varices by scar tissue (Figure 43–8). Endoscopic therapy is a local treatment that has no effect on the pathophysiologic mechanisms that underlie portal hypertension and variceal rupture. Even though endoscopic treatment can ultimately achieve variceal obliteration, varices will eventually recur.

Rebleeding after initial endoscopic control of variceal hemorrhage may occur in a majority of patients. Approximately 20–40% of patients undergoing sclerotherapy experience complications and side affects, including chest pain, fever, bacteremia, mediastinitis, acute esophageal ulceration with or without bleeding,

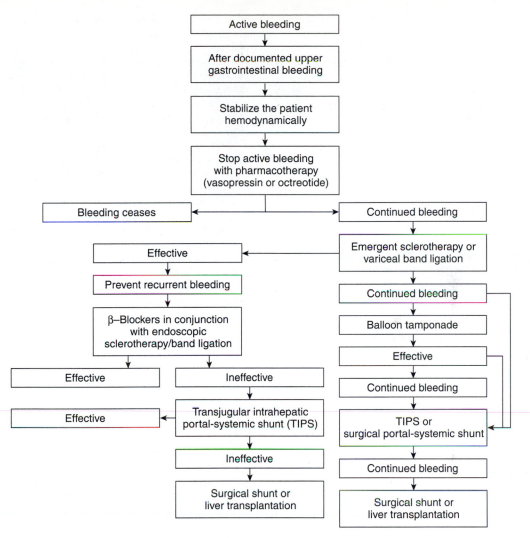

Figure 43–6. Management algorithm for active gastrointestinal bleeding resulting from portal hypertension.

and delayed development of esophageal strictures. Band ligation carries a much lower complication rate (although esophageal ulceration remains a problem) and because of its ease of use, has supplanted injection sclerotherapy as the preferred endoscopic treatment of variceal hemorrhage.

B. PHARMACOLOGIC THERAPY

Pharmacologic therapy can be initiated as soon as variceal hemorrhage is suspected, even before diagnostic endoscopy is performed since its safety profile is good. Terlipressin and somatostatin (neither available in the United States) are the most effective and safe pharmacologic agents, controlling acute variceal hemorrhage in 75–80% of cases. In the United States, vasopressin and octreotide are most commonly used. Vasopressin is limited by the frequency of side effects; its efficacy and safety are significantly improved by the addition of nitrates. Continuous infusion of vasopressin cannot be recommended for more than 24 hours because of these adverse effects (eg, cardiac ischemia). A recent meta-analysis suggests that octreotide had little or no effect on acute variceal hemorrhage when used alone. However, when used as an adjunct to endoscopic therapy, octreotide may decrease the failure rate for controlling acute variceal hemorrhage and may decrease the risk of early rebleeding. This, however, remains controversial as there may be rapid tachyphylaxis to octreotide's ef-

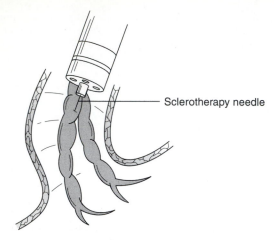

Figure 43–7. Diagram of endoscopic sclerotherapy. Note the sclerotherapy needle extending from the endoscope into the varix.

fects. Given the lack of side effects, use of intravenous octreotide is generally extended to 5 days, the period during which the risk of rebleeding is highest. The optimal dose of octreotide for controlling esophageal variceal hemorrhage is unknown.

C. TIPS

Despite urgent sclerotherapy/band ligation and pharmacologic therapy, variceal bleeding cannot be controlled or has an early recurrence in about 10–20%

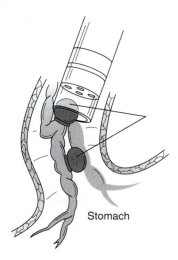

Figure 43–8. Diagram of endoscopic band ligation of esophageal varices. Note how the varix is suctioned into the device that is positioned at the tip of the endoscope, where the band is deployed.

of patients. Transjugular intrahepatic portosystemic shunting (TIPS) is an additional treatment option supplanting emergent surgical portal decompression and variceal balloon tamporade. TIPS is an angiographically placed shunt in which the portal vein is cannulated via the transjugular route through the liver, and then an expandable stent is inserted to construct an intrahepatic shunt between the portal circulation and a hepatic vein (Figure 43–9).

TIPS can effectively control acute variceal hemorrhage nonresponsive to endoscopic and pharmacologic therapy by acutely lowering the portal vein–IVC pressure gradient to <10 mm Hg. TIPS placement is technically successful in almost 100% of cases at experienced centers. Portal vein thrombosis may occur in the setting of cirrhosis or noncirrhotic portal hypertension or secondary to hepatocellular carcinoma, and generally precludes TIPS placement. Early complications of TIPS include fever, infection, renal dysfunction, intrahepatic or intraperitoneal hemorrhage, and, rarely, liver failure. Hyperbilirubinemia may occur due to hemolytic anemia related to the TIPS stent itself, until epithelialization occurs.

Long-standing problems associated with TIPS are hepatic encephalopathy and stent occlusion. *De novo* encephalopathy occurs in approximately 20% of patients with cirrhosis undergoing TIPS. Older age, presence of subclinical encephalopathy, and larger stent diameter are all risk factors for developing encephalopathy post-TIPS. Significant preexisting hepatic encephalopathy is a relative contraindication to TIPS placement in the nonemergent setting. TIPS stent occlusion occurs in more than 50% of patients within a year, mainly related to vascular endothelial ingrowth. Angioplasty or placement of a tandem stent is then undertaken. Regular surveillance of TIPS patency with Doppler ultrasound is essential.

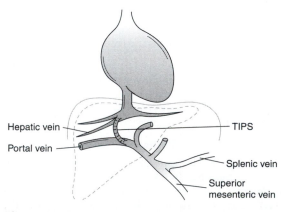

Figure 43–9. Diagram of a TIPS stent positioned between the hepatic and portal veins.

Doppler ultrasonography is very operator dependent and should be performed by experienced ultrasonographers, as less experienced operators frequently overlook TIPS malfunction. If there is any concern regarding the sensitivity of Doppler, venography should be performed. TIPS occlusion can lead to recurrent variceal bleeding.

D. Other Treatments

Prior to the advent of TIPS, portal decompression was typically accomplished by creating surgical shunts directing portal blood flow from the portal vein or its tributaries (the splenic vein or inferior mesenteric vein) into the inferior vena cava or its tributaries (the renal vein). Surgically created portosystemic shunts (eg, portacaval, mesocaval, and splenorenal shunts) are effective at decompressing the portal vein and controlling variceal hemorrhage, but have generally been supplanted by TIPS. Surgical decompression in the acute setting is avoided because of high perioperative morbidity and mortality rates, especially in patients with Child's class B or C cirrhosis. There are differing long-term patency rates for the different surgical procedures, which may also be utilized in cases of portal hypertension due to prehepatic vascular occlusion. Mesocaval and distal splenorenal shunts divert only a portion of portal blood flow away from the liver and thus achieve adequate portal decompression without excessive risk of hepatic encephalopathy. Surgical portal decompression is usually undertaken in patients with Child's class A cirrhosis who are not expected to have progressive hepatic synthetic dysfunction over the short term. Patients should be referred to specialized centers that are experienced in these procedures and in the care of patients with portal hypertension. Shunt surgery does not prevent death from other complications of advanced liver disease, and may make subsequent transplant surgery more difficult.

Mechanical balloon tamponade of persistent and uncontrolled esophageal or gastric variceal hemorrhage using specially designed nasogastric tubes (eg, Minnesota or Sengstaken-Blakemore tubes) is sometimes necessary. Only experienced individuals should place these tubes as malpositioning or overinflation can result in esophageal or gastric rupture. Endotracheal intubation protects the airway thereby reducing the risk of aspiration. Balloon tamponade is a temporizing and dangerous maneuver that stems hemorrhage but should be followed by more definitive decompression of the portal system as via TIPS or surgical shunt.

Prevention of Recurrent Variceal Hemorrhage

Both pharmacologic therapy with nonselective β-blockers and sclerotherapy reduce variceal rebleeding and death rates compared with untreated controls. Propra-

nolol and sclerotherapy are comparable in the prevention of variceal rebleeding and survival, but sclerotherapy is associated with a significantly higher rate of side effects. Band ligation is thus the endoscopic treatment of choice in the prevention of variceal rebleeding. Sessions are repeated at 14–21 day intervals until variceal obliteration, which usually requires two to four sessions. Long-term control of variceal hemorrhage by sclerotherapy requires regular endoscopy (every 2–3 weeks initially, then periodically) to detect and obliterate recurrent varices. The effectiveness of sclerotherapy appears to diminish over time, as esophageal varices are obliterated and replaced by gastric and intestinal collaterals that are less readily eradicated. Compared with sclerotherapy, band ligation is associated with lower rebleeding rates, a lower frequency of esophageal strictures, and the need for fewer sessions to achieve variceal obliteration.

Combining endoscopic therapy with pharmacologic therapy is rational because β-blockers will theoretically protect against rebleeding in the period before variceal obliteration would prevent variceal recurrence. The combination of variceal band ligation plus nadolol plus sucralfate is more effective in preventing variceal rebleeding than banding alone. Patients who rebled during pharmacologic/endoscopic therapy should be considered for shunt surgery, either surgical or TIPS, and in addition should be considered for urgent transplantation.

Gastric Varices and Portal Hypertensive Gastropathy

Gastric varices occur in the cardia and fundus of patients with portal hypertension (Figure 43–10), either isolated or in conjunction with esophageal varices. Endoscopic treatment of esophageal varices may increase the size and bleeding risk of gastric varices. Gastric varices account for about 10% of upper gastrointestinal bleeds in patients with portal hypertension. Because splenic vein thrombosis may cause gastric varices in the absence of liver disease, splenic vein patency should be documented in cases in which gastric varices are the predominant abnormality. Gastric varices tend to bleed more frequently and more severely than esophageal varices (requiring greater amounts of blood transfusions and having a greater mortality rate). Management of acute gastric variceal bleeding should be the same as the management of esophageal variceal hemorrhage, except that endoscopic treatment is difficult or impossible because the actual bleeding site is easily obscured by the hemorrhage. Band ligation or sclerotherapy with butylcyanoacrylate has shown some promise. Generally, however, patients with gastric varices will require surgical portosystemic shunting or TIPS.

Portal hypertensive gastropathy (PHG) is a gastric mucosal condition occurring in patients with cirrhosis.

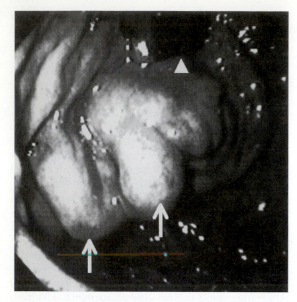

Figure 43–10. Endoscopic photograph of gastric varices (as denoted by ***arrows***) in the cardia of the stomach. The endoscope is seen on a retroflexion view (as denoted by the ***arrowhead***).

Histologically, dilatation of the capillaries and venules of the gastric mucosa with very little mucosal inflammation characterizes this condition. The gastric mucosa is edematous, erythematous, and associated with submucosal hemorrhage, and typically results in chronic blood loss. PHG is frequently noted during endoscopy in patients with cirrhosis, usually in the presence of esophagogastric varices, with its prevalence paralleling the severity of portal hypertension. Acute bleeding from PHG is relatively infrequent and rarely severe. β-Blockade is the treatment of choice for PHG although good clinical trials showing benefit are lacking. If β-blockade is unsuccessful in limiting the transfusion requirement in chronic bleeding, TIPS should be considered.

2. Ascites

The accumulation of ascites is often among the first signs of decompensated chronic liver disease. Both portal hypertension and parenchymal failure contribute to the pathogenesis of ascites, because clinically significant ascites is relatively unusual in patients with either acute liver failure or noncirrhotic portal hypertension. Approximately 50% of patients with cirrhosis will develop ascites within 10 years. The development of ascites in the setting of cirrhosis is an important landmark in the natural history of chronic liver disease, as approximately 50% of patients will die within 2 years. Thus, the de-velopment of ascites in a patient with cirrhosis should prompt referral for liver transplantation.

Pathophysiology

Portal hypertension and consequent hypoperfusion of hepatocytes with portal blood lead to enhanced renal reabsorption of sodium and water. This, in turn, expands the plasma volume and increases portal inflow. When resistance to that inflow is relatively fixed because of hepatic fibrosis, portal hypertension increases without further improvement in hepatocyte perfusion. Renal salt and water retention persist, leading to marked overexpansion of intravascular volume. Increased hydrostatic pressure forces fluid out of the vascular spaces and leads to tissue edema. This is exacerbated by hypoalbuminemia, which decreases oncotic pressure. At first, most of the extravasated fluid is returned to the vascular space by increased lymphatic flow. Eventually, however, the lymphatic capacity is overwhelmed, and excess fluid in the extracellular tissue space begins to "weep" into the peritoneal cavity, forming ascites. Splanchnic vasodilation triggers the release of sympathetic neurotransmitters and activation of the renin–angiotensin–aldosterone axis. This further stimulates retention of sodium and free water. Renal function in cirrhosis is disturbed long before ascites begins to form, and the mechanisms that drive ascites formation change as portal hypertension and parenchymal failure progress.

Clinical Findings

In the United States approximately 80% of patients having ascites will have cirrhosis (Figure 43–11). In 5% of patients, ascites may have two or more etiologies, eg, cirrhosis and another cause (peritoneal carcinomatosis or tuberculosis). Many patients with unexplained ascites have two or more causes for ascites formation, such as heart failure and diabetic nephropathy. In this setting the sum of predisposing factors leads to sodium and water retention although each individual factor itself might not be severe enough to cause fluid overload. Successful treatment of ascites depends on an accurate diagnosis of the etiology, eg, carcinomatous ascites does not respond to diuretic therapy. On physical examination in the setting of ascites, there is flank and shifting dullness in the presence of a bulging abdomen. Approximately 1500 mL of fluid must be present to detect flank dullness. Ultrasonography can detect as little as 100 mL of ascites.

The most useful parameter to classify ascites is the serum-ascites albumin gradient (SAAG), which is calculated by subtracting the ascites albumin concentration from the serum value. With approximately 97% accu-

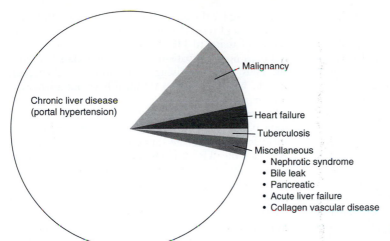

Figure 43–11. The different etiologies of ascites.

racy, a difference of 1.1 g/dL or greater is consistent with ascites secondary to portal hypertension. Gradients of <1.1 g/dL are associated with ascites due to pancreatitis, bile peritonitis, malignancy, or tuberculosis. Patients with portal hypertension undergoing serial outpatient therapeutic paracentesis need be tested only for cell count and differential once the SAAG has been determined on their initial tap. New-onset ascites should always be evaluated with diagnostic paracentesis to help determine its cause.

In patients with cirrhosis, umbilical hernias occur when long-standing ascites is present. Hernias persist and increase in size if ascites itself persists. Conversely, they decrease in size when ascites is controlled. Umbilical hernias expose patients with cirrhosis to potentially life-threatening complications, such as strangulation (which can be precipitated by rapid removal of ascites) and rupture (which is usually preceded by the formation of cutaneous ulcerations on the surface of the hernia). Rupture carries a high risk for infection of the ascites along with difficulty in wound healing. Abundant ascites frequently restricts the possibility of surgical treatment and increases operative risks. Therefore, surgical repair should not be recommended in patients with uncontrolled ascites and poor liver function. In patients with cirrhosis with incisional hernias and ascites, prosthetic meshes should be avoided because of the high risk of bacterial infection. Prevention of umbilical hernias is based on adequate control of ascites.

Treatment

A. SODIUM RESTRICTION

Treatment of ascites does not significantly improve survival. However, treating ascites is important not only because it improves the quality of life of patients with cirrhosis but because spontaneous bacterial peritonitis (SBP) cannot occur in the absence of ascites. Because sodium retention is one of the main mechanisms in the development of ascites, a central goal of therapy is the attainment of a negative sodium balance. To achieve this, sodium output must exceed sodium input. Patient education regarding stringent dietary sodium restriction (<2000 mg/d) is essential; sodium restriction can speed the loss of weight and edema. It is sodium restriction, not fluid restriction, that results in weight loss as fluid passively follows sodium. The latter is not necessary unless serum sodium is <120 mEq/L. Patients with cirrhosis typically do not have symptoms from hyponatremia until sodium levels fall below 110 mmol/L.

B. DIURETICS

Diuretics are required in most patients with ascites, particularly in those with moderate-to-tense ascites who retain sodium avidly and in whom sodium restriction will not be sufficient to obtain negative sodium balance. Sodium retention in cirrhosis is mainly the result of increased renal distal tubular reabsorption, so aldosterone antagonists, such as spironolactone, are the initial diuretics of choice. Spironolactone has a long duration of action and potassium-sparing effects, and is often used in combination with furosemide. Furosemide is less effective when used alone because the sodium that is not reabsorbed in the loop of Henle is taken up avidly in the distal and collecting tubules of the kidney because of the hyperaldosteronism seen in cirrhosis. A typical diuretic regimen consists of single morning doses of oral spironolactone and furosemide, 100 mg and 40 mg, respectively. The good oral bioavailability of furosemide together with acute reductions in GFR associated with its intravenous administration favor oral administration. The dose of both diuretics can be increased simultaneously to a maximum of 400 mg/d spironolactone and 160 mg/d furosemide. Patients with parenchymal renal disease may tolerate less spironolactone because of hyperkalemia. Single morning dosing maximizes compliance. Treatment with diuretics is associated with a high incidence of complications such as dehydration, severe muscle cramping, hyponatremia, and hepatic encephalopathy. Spironolactone may cause painful gynecomastia and can be replaced with amiloride, a potassium-sparing diuretic that has a less natriuretic effect.

A reasonable daily goal for weight reduction in patients with ascites is 0.5 kg. Diuretics should be discontinued if one of the following develop: encephalopathy, severe hyponatremia despite fluid restriction, or serum creatinine ≥2.0 mg/dL. In patients with extreme fluid overload, large volume paracentesis (LVP) may remove fluid more rapidly than careful diuresis, which may take up to weeks. Patients who fail to respond to diuretics after an aggressive regimen of dietary sodium restriction are considered refractory. Refractory ascites occurs in only 5–10% of patients with cirrhosis. LVP with albumin administration is standard treatment for refractory ascites.

C. Large Volume Paracentesis

Serial LVP is effective in controlling ascites. Concomitant plasma volume expansion with albumin has been used with LVP to correct decreased effective arterial volume that leads to sodium retention. Intravenous albumin infusion reduces the incidence of hyponatremia and renal impairment that occurs due to further decrease in effective arterial volume. LVP is a temporizing treatment that does not alter any of the mechanisms leading to ascites, and thus albumin infusion has only a temporary effect. Although the acute risks of LVP are low, repeated LVP is inconvenient for the patient and can result in significant depletion of total body protein stores.

D. Portal Decompression and Peritoneovenous Shunts

TIPS improves survival in patients with refractory or recurrent ascites, compared with LVP. In addition, TIPS is more effective than LVP in controlling ascites, with rates of complete or partial response of 83% and 84%, respectively. TIPS in the setting of ascites is associated with a marked and rapid improvement of sodium handling. It may take several weeks for the humoral and hemodynamic changes to occur post-TIPS, for ascites to optimally respond. During this time, diuretics should be used, probably utilizing smaller doses than pre-TIPS. Removal of as much ascites via LVP prior to TIPS may make the procedure less technically challenging for the interventional radiologist. Older patient age and renal dysfunction adversely affect the response of ascites to TIPS. A higher mortality with TIPS has been noted in patients with Child's class C cirrhosis. Thus, refractory ascites in Child's class C cirrhosis may be best treated by LVP until liver transplantation can be performed.

Peritoneovenous shunts (eg, LeVeen or Denver) were popularized in the 1970s as a physiologic treatment for ascites. These shunts are tubes burrowed underneath the skin, leading from the peritoneal cavity into the jugular vein. Shunt placement decreases the duration of hospitalization for ascites, the number of hospitalizations, and the dose of diuretics required to control ascites. However, use of these shunts is now limited because of poor long-term patency, excessive complications (eg, DIC, infection), and no survival advantage compared with medical therapy in controlled trials. TIPS has supplanted peritoneovenous shunting in treating patients with refractory ascites. The use of peritoneovenous shunts appears limited to those patients who are not candidates for liver transplantation.

3. Hepatic Encephalopathy

Portosystemic or hepatic encephalopathy is defined as a disturbance in central nervous system function due to hepatic insufficiency. It is a neuropsychiatric disorder characterized by changes in personality, cognition, motor function, or level of consciousness. Hepatic encephalopathy is usually reversible and is due to hepatic parenchymal failure, but may also occur in individuals with normal livers having spontaneous or surgically constructed portosystemic shunts. The development of overt hepatic encephalopathy portends a poor prognosis with a 1-year survival of 40%. Patients with cirrhosis should be referred for liver transplantation after their first episode of hepatic encephalopathy.

Pathophysiology

Although the precise pathogenesis of hepatic encephalopathy is unknown, the accumulation of nitrogenous substances derived from the gut, which produces adverse effects on brain function, plays a major role. These compounds gain access to the systemic circulation as a result of decreased hepatic function or portosystemic shunts (ie, TIPS). Once in brain tissue, they produce alterations of neurotransmission that affect consciousness and behavior. Abnormalities in glutamatergic, catecholamine, serotoninergic, and GABAergic pathways have all been described in experimental hepatic encephalopathy.

Ammonia appears to play a key role in the pathogenesis of hepatic encephalopathy. Portal vein ammonia is derived from both urease activity of colonic bacteria and the deamidization of glutamine in the small intestine, and is a key substrate for the synthesis of urea and glutamine in the liver. In chronic liver disease, increased arterial levels of ammonia are commonly seen, but there is little correlation between blood levels and severity of neuropsychiatric impairment. As blood–brain barrier permeability to ammonia is increased in patients having hepatic encephalopathy, blood levels correlate weakly with brain levels of ammonia. Furthermore, the alterations in neurotransmission induced by ammonia also occur after its metabolism within astrocytes, resulting in a series of neurochemical events caused by functional alteration of the astrocyte. Thus, the magnitude of ammonia level cannot be used to diagnose hepatic encephalopathy.

Other putative gut-derived mediators have also been studied. Endogenous ligands of the benzodiazepine receptor may arise from specific colonic bacteria and activate the GABAergic pathway, and along with neurotoxic short- and medium-chain fatty acids, phenols, and false neurotransmitters derived from amino acid imbalance, may variably contribute to the pathogenesis of hepatic encephalopathy. In some patients manganese may deposit in basal ganglia and induce extrapyramidal symptoms.

Clinical Findings

Hepatic encephalopathy may manifest with mild cognitive abnormalities recognizable only with psychometric testing or present as recurrent or chronic cognitive or motor disorders. This may significantly affect the quality of life in patients with cirrhosis. Altered mentation or level of consciousness can range from subtle personality changes to lethargy to coma. The spectrum of motor disorders is also quite broad, ranging from asterixis or ankle clonus to spastic paralysis. The gradation of severity and stages of hepatic encephalopathy are shown in Table 43–3. Subclinical hepatic encephalopathy may occur in 50–80% of patients with cirrhosis. The most common symptom is insomnia with reversal of the day/night sleep cycle. There are subtle deficits in visual and motor coordination that contribute to falls and traffic accidents. Recurrent attacks of clinically overt changes in mental status are the next most common presentation of hepatic encephalopathy; these attacks are usually precipitated by identifiable factors (Table 43–4). Medications used to treat hepatic encephalopathy may not be well tolerated, so noncompliance is a major cause of worsening neuropsychiatric symptoms. Correction of the precipitating factors typically permits patients with recurrent bouts of overt encephalopathy to return to subclinical states of the disorder. Chronic hepatic encephalopathy is much more difficult to manage because variable degrees of alteration in mental status occur in the absence of any identifiable precipitants.

Because the manifestations of hepatic encephalopathy are so variable, encephalopathy should be suspected in any patient with cirrhosis with a neuropsychiatric abnormality. For instance, patients with cirrhosis with encephalopathy have been arrested for alcohol or drug intoxication, or have been misdiagnosed with strokes because of unsteadiness of gait and slurring of speech. Other conditions to be considered in the differential diagnosis of hepatic encephalopathy are shown in Table 43–5. The detection of asterixis, ankle clonus, or psychomotor retardation may be clues to the diagnosis of hepatic encephalopathy, but are nonspecific. The absence of these clinical signs does not exclude the diagnosis of hepatic encephalopathy. Documentation of

Table 43–3. Stages of hepatic encephalopathy.

Stage	Consciousness	Cognition	Behavior	Motor Function	Psychometric Tests
0–1	Normal	Normal	Normal	Normal	Slow
1	Abnormal sleep	Attention	Moody	Dyscoordination	Very slow
2	Lethargy Ataxia Dysarthria	Memory	Dysinhibition	Asterixis	Poor
3	Confusion Delirium Semistupor Incontinence	Disoriented Incoherent Amnesic Rigidity	Bizarre Anger Paranoia Seizures	Abnormal reflexes Nystagmus Babinski reflex	
4	Coma	None	Absent	Oculocephalic or oculo-vestibular response, decorticate or decerebrate posture, dilated pupils	

Table 43–4. Precipitating factors for recurrent hepatic encephalopathy.

Gastrointestinal bleeding
Infection (especially spontaneous bacterial peritonitis)
Excessive dietary protein intake
Constipation
Overdiuresis
Electrolyte abnormalities (decreased potassium, increased or
    decreased sodium)
Azotemia and dehydration
Sedative and opiate analgesic use
Noncompliance with Lactulose and neomycin
Hepatic injury (viral infection, toxic damage, surgery, hepato-
    cellular carcinoma)
Portosystemic shunts (eg, TIPS)

---

normal blood ammonia levels may be helpful in a patient's initial evaluation when nonhepatic causes of encephalopathy are being considered. Serial levels are unnecessary and do not replace the evaluation of the patient's mental status. Alterations of the EEG are not specific in hepatic encephalopathy. Wilson's disease should be excluded in young patients who present with neuropsychiatric symptoms associated with liver disease (see Chapter 41).

Table 43–5. Differential diagnosis of hepatic encephalopathy.

Intracranial lesions
    Hemorrhage
    Infarct
    Tumor
    Abscess
Infections
    Meningitis
    Encephalitis
    Sepsis
Metabolic encephalopathies
    Dehydration
    Hyperglycemia or hypoglycemia
    Uremia
    Acidosis (including hypercarbia, ketoacidosis)
    Electrolyte imbalances
Alcohol-related disorders
    Intoxication
    Withdrawal
    Wernicke's encephalopathy
    Korsakoff's syndrome
Drug toxicity (sedatives, heavy metals, or other psychoactive
    drugs)
Postictal encephalopathy
Primary neuropsychiatric disorders

Treatment

A comprehensive search to identify and eliminate any precipitating factor(s) is a key initial step in treating encephalopathy. Supportive care must be provided to all patients when at home or while hospitalized. The mental state can change rapidly and disorientation can result in bodily harm. Prevention of falls is an important measure. In deeper stages of hepatic encephalopathy, prophylactic tracheal intubation to prevent aspiration may be required. Adequate nutrition should be provided during the period of altered mental status. Sedative-hypnotic medication must always be avoided. Constipation can precipitate hepatic encephalopathy. The use of opiate analgesics and calcium and iron supplements may constipate a patient; therefore, Lactulose or stool softeners should be instituted.

Medical treatment of hepatic encephalopathy is based on efforts to control the generation of putative neuroactive toxins. Nonabsorbable disaccharides such as Lactulose serve as laxatives, decreasing ammoniagenesis and reducing ammonia absorption from the gastrointestinal tract. Lactulose is not degraded by intestinal disaccharidases and thus reaches the colon where bacteria metabolize it into acetic and lactic acids. The acidification of the colon traps ammonia in the lumen. An excessively sweet taste, flatulence, and abdominal cramping are the most frequent complaints with use of Lactulose. It is dosed to produce two to three soft bowel movements a day. If diarrhea develops, Lactulose should be stopped and reinstituted at a lower dose, as diarrhea may lead to hypertonic dehydration, actually worsening the encephalopathy. Lactulose administered by enema is not as effective as oral administration. Antibiotics such as neomycin or metronidazole may be alternatives or adjuncts to Lactulose. Benefits from neomycin are attributed to effects on colonic bacteria. Associated toxicities may hamper the use of antibiotics for a prolonged period of time. In spite of its poor absorption, neomycin can cause auditory loss and renal failure, especially in patients with renal dysfunction. Patients require regular auditory testing if maintained on chronic neomycin. Dysgeusia and peripheral neuropathy may complicate metronidazole therapy.

Bowel cleansing may complement standard treatment of hepatic encephalopathy, especially in the presence of gastrointestinal hemorrhage. Protein intake should not be restricted in patients with chronic encephalopathy but can be limited during an acute episode. Flumazenil may be used to reverse selected cases of benzodiazepine-induced oversedation.

4. Hepatorenal Syndrome

HRS is a clinical condition developing in individuals with advanced chronic liver disease that is characterized by impaired renal function and marked abnormalities in arterial circulation resulting in marked renal vasoconstriction and decreased GFR. HRS is functional in nature, as no pathognomonic renal pathologic changes have been demonstrated. Kidneys of patients with HRS may recover their function when transplanted into patients with end-stage renal disease and a healthy liver, or when the diseased liver is replaced by transplantation. HRS can develop in the absence of any precipitating factors or can occur following events that reduce effective arterial blood volume (eg, dehydration or gastrointestinal bleeding). The development of HRS in patients with cirrhosis is associated with a poor prognosis, with more than 95% of patients dying within a few weeks of the onset of azotemia. Spontaneous recovery of renal function is rare. Thus, it is imperative to carefully monitor the renal function in patients with advanced cirrhosis, to avoid as much as possible all potential precipitants of HRS, and to aggressively intervene at the earliest evidence of renal decompensation.

Pathophysiology

HRS represents the extreme expression of circulatory dysfunction associated with portal hypertension, occurring in the setting of increased plasma volume and cardiac output and very low systemic vascular resistance. There is increased resistance in all major arterial vascular beds (ie, the afferent renal arteriole), except in the splanchnic circulation, in which vasodilation is responsible for homeostatic activation of endogenous vasoconstriction and further impairment of circulatory function. Renal hypoperfusion represents the extreme consequence of the underfilling of the arterial circulation secondary to this splanchnic vasodilation. With stimulation of endogenous vasoconstricting factors, there is also activation of renal vasodilation (ie, prostaglandins) to maintain renal perfusion and GFR. Renal failure may thus be induced in these patients through the inhibition of prostaglandin synthesis (ie, NSAIDs). HRS therefore develops when the activation of vasoconstrictor systems overcomes these renal vasodilatory mechanisms, or as a result of extreme progression of decreased effective arterial blood volume. Once renal vasoconstriction develops, intrarenal mechanisms may contribute to the perpetuation of HRS. This may explain why HRS can follow a rapidly worsening course despite the removal of the event that triggered the renal dysfunction.

Clinical Features

The reported incidence of HRS in hospitalized patients with cirrhosis is 7–15%. Criteria for establishing the diagnosis of HRS are shown in Table 43–6. It is important to differentiate HRS from other etiologies of renal failure common in cirrhosis, particularly prerenal azotemia secondary to volume depletion, glomerulonephritis, ATN, or drug-induced nephrotoxicity. As with HRS, prerenal azotemia is characterized by reduced renal perfusion and GFR. Prerenal azotemia can be reversed with intravenous hydration, whereas no significant changes in GFR are observed in HRS. To avoid a possible role of an unrecognized reduction in plasma volume, renal function should be evaluated in HRS after diuretic withdrawal and expansion of plasma volume. Hemodynamic monitoring is indicated if doubt persists about intravascular volume status. Table 43–7 shows other features that distinguish HRS from other causes of acute renal failure.

Table 43–6. Diagnostic criteria of hepatorenal syndrome (HRS) according to the International Ascites Club.[1]

Major criteria

Low glomerular filtration rate, indicated by serum creatinine > 1.5 mg/dL or 24-hour creatinine clearance < 40 mL/min

Absence of shock, ongoing bacterial infection, and fluid losses and current treatment with nephrotoxic drugs

No sustained improvement in renal function (decrease in serum creatinine to $\leq$ 1.5 mg/dL or increase in creatinine clearance to $\geq$ 40 mL/min) after diuretic withdrawal and expansion of plasma volume with 1.5 L of plasma expander

Proteinuria < 500 mg/d and no ultrasonographic evidence of obstructive uropathy or parenchymal renal disease

Additional criteria

Urine volume < 500 mL/d

Urine sodium < 10 mEq/L

Urine osmolality greater than plasma osmolality

Urine red blood cells < 50/high-power field

Serum sodium concentration < 130 mEq/L

[1]Only major criteria are necessary for the diagnosis of HRS.
Reproduced, with permission, from Arroyo V et al: Definition and diagnostic criteria of refractory ascites and hepatorenal syndrome in cirrhosis. Hepatology 1996;23:164.

Table 43–7. Differential characteristics of azotemia in patients with liver disease.

	Hepatorenal Syndrome	Prerenal Azotemia	Acute Tubular Necrosis
Urine sodium (mEq/L)	< 10	< 10	> 30
Urine/plasma creatinine	> 30	> 30	< 30
Urine/plasma osmolality	> 1	> 1	1
Urine sediment	Normal	Normal	Casts, cellular debris
Response to plasma expansion	Absent	Good	Absent

Two different types of HRS, which probably represent distinct expressions of the same pathogenic mechanism, have been defined. Type I HRS is characterized by rapid and progressive renal impairment. In most instances it occurs in association with other medical complications (ie, alcoholic hepatitis) or therapeutic intervention (ie, large volume paracentesis without plasma volume expansion). SBP has been recognized as the most common precipitant of type I HRS. Intravenous albumin administration in conjunction with antibiotic therapy may lessen the likelihood of HRS occurring in SBP. Type II HRS is characterized by a moderate and stable reduction in GFR, and may occur in patients with relatively preserved hepatic function. Survival is longer than in type I HRS, but is still poor without liver transplantation.

Treatment

Liver transplantation is the most effective treatment for patients with HRS because it provides a cure for both the diseased liver and the circulatory and renal dysfunction (see Chapter 54). The long-term outcome of patients for HRS post-liver transplantation is usually good, although there is increased morbidity and early mortality. More than 30% of patients require short-term hemodialysis, with only 5% progressing to end-stage renal disease and need for long-term dialysis. However, many patients with type I HRS die before transplantation.

Medical therapies are minimally effective for HRS. Vasodilator drugs have been used in an attempt to reverse the renal vasoconstriction of HRS. Dopamine has little or no benefit on GFR in small case series. Prostaglandin analogs (ie, misoprostol) have been used with the rationale of increasing intrarenal synthesis of prostaglandin, but also without significant success. Vasoconstrictors have also been administered, in an attempt to reverse intense splanchnic arterial vasodilation. Although their use in a condition characterized by marked renal vasoconstriction appears paradoxical, the rationale is that the initial event in the pathogenesis of HRS is arterial vasodilation causing homeostatic activation of endogenous vasoconstriction. Short-term infu-

sions of agonists of vasopressin receptors, such as ornipressin and terlipressin, have significantly improved creatinine clearance in HRS by decreasing cardiac output, increasing total peripheral vascular resistance, and markedly suppressing the renin–angiotensin–aldosterone axis and sympathetic nervous system. Terlipressin has a lower incidence of side effects than ornipressin. It has been used in combination with intravenous albumin over 5–15 days resulting in complete reversal of HRS. In studies of patients in whom normalization of serum creatinine was achieved, HRS did not recur after discontinuation of therapy.

Other modestly successful combination treatments for HRS include midrodine (an α-adrenergic agonist), octreotide, and albumin, and continuous intravenous infusion of ornipressin with renal dose dopamine. These studies indicate that a relatively long delay can occur between improvement in circulatory function and reversal of HRS. In small, uncontrolled studies TIPS has improved renal perfusion and GFR in patients with type I HRS. Typically, improvement in renal function requires a month or longer at times after some transient worsening in renal function. In patients with type II HRS, improvement in renal perfusion is associated with an increase in urinary sodium excretion and improved renal response to diuretics. It is unclear if TIPS in this setting improves patient survival and should be used in combination with medical therapy.

5. Spontaneous Bacterial Peritonitis

SBP is an infection of ascites fluid occurring in the absence of a contiguous source of infection (eg, intestinal perforation, intraabdominal abscess). The prevalence of SBP in hospitalized patients with cirrhosis ranges between 10 and 30%. In-hospital mortality of an episode of SBP is approximately 20% with a 1-year recurrence rate of 70%. For these reasons, the occurrence of SBP raises the priority for transplantation in the current UNOS liver allograft allocation system. All patients recovering from an episode of SBP should be evaluated for liver transplantation.

Pathophysiology

The gut is the main source of bacteria that cause SBP. Bacterial translocation, that is, the passage of viable microorganisms from the intestinal lumen to the mesenteric lymph nodes and other extraintestinal sites, plays a major role in causing SBP. An alternative mechanism may be peritoneal seeding after bacteremic episodes, as many patients developing SBP also have positive blood cultures. Impaired reticuloendothelial cell clearance of portal blood bacteremia also contributes to its development. Patients with low levels of total protein in their ascitic fluid (<1.5 g/dL) are at increased risk for SBP because of reduced ascitic fluid complement levels and opsonic activity. One of the most important predictors of death in patients with cirrhosis with SBP is the development of renal impairment, which occurs in patients with the highest concentration of cytokines in plasma and ascites, and is associated with marked activation of the renin–angiotensin system. Thus, SBP appears to further decrease effective arterial blood volume, which results from a cytokine-mediated increase in splanchnic vasodilation.

Clinical Findings

Fever, worsening jaundice or renal dysfunction, alterations in gastrointestinal motility (eg, vomiting), abdominal pain (occurring only in 50% of patients), and encephalopathy are the most common clinical findings in SBP. However, the patient is frequently asymptomatic. Patients with cirrhosis with gastrointestinal bleeding are at high risk for SBP. There must always be a high index of suspicion for SBP and a low threshold for the performance of a diagnostic paracentesis in the hospitalized patient with cirrhosis. A diagnostic tap should be performed on hospital admission in all patients with cirrhosis with ascites, even when they are admitted for other reasons. Coagulopathy is almost never a contraindication to diagnostic paracentesis.

Peritoneal infection causes an inflammatory reaction that results in an increased number of neutrophils in ascitic fluid. Because culture of ascites fluid is negative in a large number of patients with SBP, diagnosis should be based on the presence of >250 neutrophils/mm^3. The most common causative organisms of SBP are *Escherichia coli* and other coliforms such as *Klebsiella*, and streptococcal and enterococcal species. In patients with bloody ascites, a correction factor of one neutrophil per 250 red blood cells is used. The insensitivity of ascitic fluid cultures is probably due to the relatively low concentration of bacteria in the fluid. Bedside inoculation of aerobic and anaerobic blood culture bottles with 10 mL of ascitic fluid can increase this yield. Gram stains are typically negative in SBP. Bacterascites refers to the colo-

nization of ascitic fluid by bacteria, in the absence of an inflammatory reaction in the peritoneal fluid; there are positive ascites cultures in the setting of a neutrophil count <250/mm^3. This may represent a transient and spontaneously reversible colonization of ascites, but may also be the first evidence of the development of SBP. Thus, initiation of antibiotic therapy is advised.

The vast majority of patients with cirrhosis with ascites and peritoneal inflammation have SBP, but some may have secondary peritonitis due to an abdominal abscess, perforated viscus, etc. Secondary peritonitis should be suspected (1) in the presence of extremely high ascites fluid neutrophil counts, (2) when more than one organism is isolated from the fluid (particularly anaerobic bacteria or fungi), (3) when at least two of the following are found in the ascites fluid: glucose levels <50 mg/dL, protein concentration >10 g/dL, and lactic dehydrogenase concentration greater than normal serum levels, or (4) when there has been no response to antibiotic therapy as evidenced by no significant decrease in ascites neutrophil count on follow-up diagnostic paracentesis. If secondary peritonitis is suspected, CT scan or MRI should be performed to exclude an abdominal collection or perforated viscus, and antibiotic coverage broadened against anaerobic organisms and enterococci.

Treatment

If ascites neutrophil count is >250/mm^3, antibiotic therapy should be initiated, usually with 2–4 g daily of intravenous cefotaxime. Use of intravenous albumin as an adjunct to antibiotic therapy may lower the incidence of renal failure and improve survival, particularly in patients with poor baseline liver and renal function. Interventions that decrease effective blood volume should be avoided, such as diuretics and LVP. Antibiotic treatment can be safely discontinued after 5 days once the neutrophil count decreases below 250/mm^3. Follow-up diagnostic paracentesis performed 48 hours after starting therapy allows assessment of response to treatment and the need to modify antibiotic coverage.

Patients who have recovered from an episode of SBP are at a high risk of developing SBP recurrence. Long-term prophylaxis with oral norfloxacin 400 mg daily should be initiated as soon as intravenous antibiotics are discontinued. Prophylaxis is also indicated in those patients with ascites who have never had SBP, but who have ascitic fluid protein concentration <1.0 g/dL. Ciprofloxacin and trimethoprim-sulfamethoxazole are also effective prophylactic antibiotics that prevent SBP recurrence. Patients with cirrhosis with gastrointestinal hemorrhage are predisposed to develop bacterial infections. Approximately 20% of these patients are already infected at admission, and 50% develop an infection during hospitalization. Short-term (over a minimum of 7 days) antibiotic prophylaxis in these patients can significantly decrease the incidence of infection, including SBP, and improve survival.

6. Hydrothorax

Pleural effusions are an infrequent complication of portal hypertension occurring in approximately 5% of patients. The term hepatic hydrothorax is applied to the presence of a pleural effusion in a patient with cirrhosis in which the source of the pleural fluid is the abdominal cavity (ie, ascites). Patients with hepatic hydrothorax usually have advanced liver disease and are potential candidates for liver transplantation. Typical characteristics of the pleural fluid in hepatic hydrothorax are shown in Table 43–8.

Pathophysiology

Hydrothorax results from direct passage of ascites fluid into the pleural space via defects in the diaphragm. This has been demonstrated by the injection of radiolabeled materials into the peritoneal cavity of patients with hepatic hydrothorax and their relatively rapid movement from the abdominal cavity into the pleural space. Defects in the diaphragm have been identified (holes or blebs on the tendinous portion) that allow free access of ascites to the pleural cavity. These defects may close, which would account for the spontaneous resolution of the effusion, which may rarely occur in some patients. Hepatic hydrothorax may develop in patients without demonstrable ascites. Ascites may be drawn into the chest preferentially because of the negative intrathoracic

Table 43–8. Usual clinical and laboratory features of hepatic hydrothorax.

Clinical features
Right sided (85%)
Left sided (13%)
Bilateral (2%)
Laboratory features
Cell count <1000 cells/mm^3
Total protein concentration <2.5 g/dL
Total protein pleural fluid-to-serum ratio < 0.5
Lactate dehydrogenase pleural fluid-to-serum ratio <2:3
Serum-to-pleural fluid albumin gradient > 1.1 g/dL
Pleural fluid amylase concentration less than serum amylase concentration
pH 7.40–7.55

Reproduced, with permission, from Lazaridis KN: et al: Hepatic hydrothorax: pathogenesis, diagnosis and management. Am J Med 1999;107:262.

pressure, which also prevents the movement of the fluid back into the abdomen.

Clinical Findings

Symptoms may be quite variable with some patients being asymptomatic and others have significant pulmonary complaints of dyspnea on exertion, cough, and hypoxemia (initially ascribable to the presence of ascites). These symptoms in the absence of ascites may lead to an extensive evaluation for causes of the effusion without considering cirrhosis as the primary etiology. Hepatic hydrothorax most commonly occurs on the right side and is transudative. CT scan of the chest should be obtained to exclude other mediastinal, pulmonary, or pleural disease. If the effusion is left sided or if there is evidence of infection, thoracentesis should be performed. Akin to SBP, spontaneous bacterial empyema may develop when the polymorphonuclear count exceeds 250 mm^3 and can occur in the absence of SBP.

Treatment

In most patients with cirrhosis the size of the effusion is limited and symptoms are controlled effectively with sodium restriction and diuretics. However, in a few individuals the fluid accumulates to such a degree that quality of life is severely compromised. Thoracentesis is indicated for the rapid relief of symptoms. As many patients have underlying coagulopathy, this procedure carries increased risk for bleeding. Infusion of fresh frozen plasma can correct the coagulopathy, but also ultimately adds to the fluid excess. Loculated effusions greatly decrease the effectiveness of thoracentesis. In patients with both hepatic hydrothorax and appreciable ascites, the ascites is removed prior to the thoracentesis. As ascitic fluid is preferentially drawn into the pleural space, reducing the ascitic fluid volume, however, is unlikely to affect the rate at which the pleural effusion reaccumulates.

Chest tube placement in hepatic hydrothorax is contraindicated, as it is associated with significant complications due in large part to the continuous loss of large volumes of ascites via the chest tube. Chest tube removal is problematic because leakage of ascites along the chest tube tract can persist following its removal. Pleurodesis is ineffective in preventing recurrence of hepatic hydrothorax because of dilution of the sclerosant by the rapid movement of ascites into the pleural space. TIPS may be successful in decreasing the need for repeated thoracentesis in some patients with hepatic hydrothorax. Generally, however, prognosis remains poor despite symptomatic improvement, and patients should be considered candidates for liver transplantation.

7. *Hepatopulmonary Syndrome*

Hepatopulmonary syndrome is defined as hypoxemia occurring in the setting of advanced liver disease (cirrhosis or noncirrhotic portal hypertension) related to intrapulmonary vascular dilatation in the absence of intrinsic cardiopulmonary disease. Portal hypertension appears to be centrally involved in the pathophysiology of the hepatopulmonary syndrome. There is no clear relationship between biochemical measures of hepatic function and the presence or severity of the hepatopulmonary syndrome.

Pathophysiology

The cause of the vascular pathophysiology of hepatopulmonary syndrome is speculative. An imbalance between potential pulmonary vasodilators and vasoconstrictors is likely. It is unclear whether a particular vasodilatory substance is not cleared by a diseased liver, or whether there is an abnormal sensitivity by the pulmonary vascular bed to a substance (ie, endothelin) in patients with cirrhosis.

Clinical Findings

The majority of patients with hepatopulmonary syndrome have no respiratory symptoms and will be diagnosed by an increased alveolar–arterial gradient on arterial blood gas measurement when breathing room air. Patients with more severe disease will have dyspnea on exertion and may have clubbing of the digits, cyanosis, and substantial hypoxemia. Physical examination of the chest is usually unremarkable. Dyspnea may be worse with exercise or when the patient assumes the standing position (platypnea). Hypoxemia typically is worse when changing from the supine to the standing position (orthodeoxia), reflecting pulmonary vascular dilatation that occurs predominately in the lung bases. Hypoxemia may become profound with $PaO_2 \leq 50$ mm Hg with patients requiring continuous oxygen supplementation. Quality of life may be significantly impaired as patients may become bed or home bound due to severe dyspnea.

The initial diagnostic test for hepatopulmonary syndrome is contrast-enhanced transthoracic echocardiography, which establishes the presence of intrapulmonary shunting. Pulmonary angiography allows discrete intrapulmonary vascular dilatations pathognomonic of hepatopulmonary syndrome to be identified, and may also allow for therapeutic intervention. It is vital to exclude pulmonary hypertension as a cause of the oxygenation defects and symptoms. In hepatopulmonary syndrome, the pulmonary arterial pressures are generally not elevated above the mild increases typically observed in the high cardiac output state of cirrhosis. Shunt quantification can be performed using nuclear scanning with technetium-99m-labeled macroaggregated albumin.

The diagnosis of chronic liver disease usually occurs years prior to the onset of respiratory symptoms of hepatopulmonary syndrome. Worsening hypoxemia may portend poor survival and occur in the setting of clinically stable liver disease. Many medical treatments including methylene blue, nitric oxide, prostaglandin inhibitors, octreotide, angiographic embolization, and TIPS have had very limited success in improving hypoxemia and the quality of life of these patients. The gas exchange abnormalities associated with hepatopulmonary syndrome may be reversible after liver transplantation in most patients. In fact, severe hepatopulmonary syndrome is itself an indication for liver transplantation. However, the reversibility of hepatopulmonary syndrome after liver transplantation is unpredictable, and some patients may have persistent problems with oxygenation.

8. *Portopulmonary Hypertension*

Rarely, patients with cirrhosis and portal hypertension may develop pulmonary hypertension. Portopulmonary hypertension and hepatopulmonary syndrome are distinct entities. Individuals may have respiratory symptoms, digital clubbing, or evidence of pulmonary hypertension on chest radiography. More frequently, the diagnosis is made by demonstrating high right-sided cardiac pressures on transthoracic echocardiography, which is routinely performed in patients undergoing candidate evaluation for liver transplantation. It is imperative to diagnose portopulmonary hypertension prior to proceeding with liver transplantation, as its presence is a strict preoperative contraindication because of high intra- and postoperative mortality secondary to cardiopulmonary failure. In the absence of pharmacologic intervention, the prognosis is poor with a 6-month mortality of 50%.

The pulmonary pathophysiology of portopulmonary hypertension is similar to that of primary pulmonary hypertension, without evidence for venoocclusive disease or recurrent thromboembolism. The inciting factor(s) for the development of portopulmonary hypertension are unknown. Patients typically exhibit hemodynamic features of both primary pulmonary hypertension (elevated mean pulmonary artery pressure and pulmonary vascular resistance) and cirrhosis (elevated cardiac index and depressed systemic vascular resistance).

When portopulmonary hypertension is suspected, right heart catheterization is undertaken to assess the magnitude of the pulmonary pressures and response to vasodilator trials (ie, inhaled nitric oxide, calcium channel blockers). Recently, epoprostenol (a prostaglandin analog) has been successfully used to lower pulmonary arterial pressures sufficient to allow liver transplantation in some patients. Unlike hepatopulmonary syndrome for which liver transplantation may be curative, portopulmonary hypertension may not be reversible with transplantation, and patients may require continuous treatment of their elevated pulmonary pressures. Because of the complexities of diagnosis, treatment, and perioperative management of patients with portopulmonary hypertension, these individuals should be referred to a large liver transplant center with experience in this entity.

The Risk of Surgery in Patients with Cirrhosis

Because of impaired hepatic synthetic function, patients with cirrhosis are at increased risk for morbidity and mortality when undergoing any type of surgery. This is due in part to the following factors: (1) the pharmacokinetic of many drugs, particularly anesthetics, muscle relaxants, analgesics, and sedatives, can be affected by changes in plasma protein binding, detoxification, and excretion; (2) bleeding risk is increased because of coagulopathy and portal hypertension; (3) the incidence of renal failure is increased due to the presence of ascites and decreased creatinine clearance, and abnormal renal physiology results in marked fluid retention; (4) malnutrition impedes optimal wound healing; and (5) susceptibility to infection is increased because of altered functioning of hepatic reticuloendothelial cells and other changes in the immune system. Anesthesia generally reduces hepatic arterial blood flow and hepatic oxygen uptake, which typically do not affect the normal liver, but can lead to hepatic decompensation in cirrhosis.

The type of surgery is an important determinant of postoperative hepatic dysfunction in patients with cirrhosis. For example, abdominal surgery leads to a greater reduction in hepatic arterial blood flow than does extraabdominal surgery, in part because traction on abdominal viscera may cause reflex systemic hypotension as a result of dilation of capacitance vessels. Abdominal adhesions due to prior surgery can be highly vascular, leading to increased intraoperative bleeding. Cardiac surgery may also be associated with a high operative mortality in the setting of cirrhosis. Cardiopulmonary bypass may aggravate the coagulopathy of liver disease by inducing platelet dysfunction and fibrinolysis. Perioperative morbidity and mortality correlate well with the Child's class of cirrhosis. In 92 patients with cirrhosis undergoing abdominal surgery, Mansour et al described mortality rates of 10%, 30%, and 82% in persons classified as Child's class A, B, and C, respectively. Increased surgical risk is noted in emergent as opposed to elective surgery, in biliary tract operations, and with hepatic resection. Although hepatic resection is often considered in Child's class A patients with cirrhosis with hepatocellular carcinoma, patients with appreciable portal hypertension (measured by hepatic venous pressure gradient or indirectly by magnitude of thrombocytopenia) may still frequently experience hepatic decompensation. Only surgeons experienced in dealing with patients having portal hypertension should undertake this surgery.

Evaluation of any patient undergoing surgery should include careful history and physical examination. Risk factors for liver disease, such as previous blood transfusion, tattoos, illicit drug use, a family history of jaundice or liver disease, and alcohol use, should be elicited along with a complete review of all current prescription and nonprescription medications. Physical findings suggestive of occult cirrhosis should trigger additional evaluation. Coagulopathy and ascites require specific treatment before surgery; β-blockade may be instituted perioperatively if large varices are identified. The role of perioperative TIPS in lowering portal hypertension has not yet been studied. It is important to recognize hepatic encephalopathy prior to surgery, because of the high frequency of conditions that can precipitate or exacerbate encephalopathy in the postoperative period, including constipation, alkalosis, use of central nervous system depressants, hypoxia, sepsis, azotemia, and gastrointestinal bleeding.

REFERENCES

Angeli P et al: Reversal of type 1 hepatorenal syndrome with the administration of midodrine and octreotide. Hepatology 1999;29:1690.

Banares R et al: Carvedilol, a new nonselective beta-blocker with intrinsic anti-alpha-adrenergic activity, has a greater portal hypotensive effect than propranolol in patients with cirrhosis. Hepatology 1999;30:79.

Belghiti J, Durand F: Abdominal wall hernias in the setting of cirrhosis. Semin Liver Dis 1997;17:219.

Blei AT, Cordoba J, and The Practice Parameters Committee of the American College of Gastroenterology: Practice guidelines. Hepatic encephalopathy. Am J Gastroenterol 2001;96: 1968.

Butterworth RF: The neurobiology of hepatic encephalopathy. Semin Liver Dis 1996;16:235.

Cardenas A et al: Hepatorenal syndrome. Liver Transplant 2000;6: S63.

Chalasani N et al: Determinants of mortality in patients with advanced cirrhosis after transjugular intrahepatic portosystemic shunting. Gastroenterology 2000;118:138.

Corley DA et al: Octreotide for acute esophageal varical bleeding; a meta-analysis. Gastroenterology 2001;120:946.

DeFranchis R, Primignani M: Endoscopic treatments for portal hypertension. Semin Liver Dis 1999;19:439.

Friedman LS: The risk of surgery in patients with liver disease. Hepatology 1999;29:1617.

Garcia-Tsao G: Current management of the complications of cirrhosis and portal hypertension: variceal hemorrhage, ascites and spontaneous bacterial peritonitis. Gastroenterology 2001; 120:726.

Grace ND et al: Portal hypertension and variceal bleeding: an AASLD single topic symposium. Hepatology 1998;28:868.

Guevara M et al: Reversibility of hepatorenal syndrome by prolonged administration of ornipressin and plasma volume expansion. Hepatology 1998;27:35.

Imperiale TF, Chalasani N: A meta-analysis of endoscopic variceal ligation for primary prophylaxis of esophageal variceal bleeding. Hepatology 2001;33:802.

Krowka M: Hepatopulmonary syndrome and liver transplantation. Liver Transplant 2000;6:113.

Kuo PC et al: Portopulmonary hypertension and the liver transplant candidate. Transplantation 1999;67:1087.

Lazaridis KN et al: Hepatic hydrothorax: pathogenesis, diagnosis and management. Am J Med 1999;107:262.

Lo GH et al: Endoscopic variceal ligation plus nadolol and sucralfate compared with ligation alone for the prevention of variceal rebleeding: a prospective, randomized trial. Hepatology 2000;32:461.

Lo GH et al: A prospective randomized trial of butyl cyanoacrylate injection versus band ligation in the management of bleeding gastric varices. Hepatology 2001;33:1060.

Mansour A et al: Abdominal operations in patients with cirrhosis: still a major surgical challenge. Surgery 1997;122:730.

Merkel C et al: Long-term results of a clinical trial of nadolol with or without isosorbide mononitrate for primary prophylaxis of variceal bleeding in cirrhosis. Hepatology 2000;31:324.

Papatheodoridis GV et al: Transjugular intrahepatic portosystemic shunt compared with endoscopic treatment for prevention of variceal rebleeding. A meta-analysis. Hepatology 1999;30: 612.

Primignani M et al: Natural history of portal hypertensive gastropathy in patients with liver cirrhosis. The New Italian Endoscopic Club for the study and treatment of esophageal varices (NIEC). Gastroenterology 2000;7:181.

Rimola A et al: Diagnosis, treatment and prophylaxis of spontaneous bacterial peritonitis: a consensus document. International Ascites Club. J Hepatol 2000;32:142.

Riordan SM, Williams R: Treatment of hepatic encephalopathy. N Engl J Med 1997;337:473.

Rössle M et al: The first decade of the transjugular intrahepatic portosystemic shunt (TIPS): state of the art. Liver 1998;78: 73.

Rössle M et al: A comparison of paracentesis and transjugular intrahepatic portosystemic shunting in patients with ascites. N Engl J Med 2000;342:1701.

Runyon BA: AASLD Practice Guidelines. Management of adult patients with ascites caused by cirrhosis. Hepatology 1998;27; 264.

Sanyal AJ et al: The natural history of portal hypertension after transjugular intrahepatic portosystemic shunts. Gastroenterology 1997;112:889.

Schepis F et al: Which patients with cirrhosis should undergo endoscopic screening for esophageal varices detection? Hepatology 2001;33:333.

Sort P et al: Effect of intravenous albumin on renal impairment and mortality in patients with cirrhosis and spontaneous bacterial peritonitis. N Engl J Med 1999;341:403.

Strauss RM, Boyer TD: Hepatic hydrothorax. Semin Liver Dis 1997;17:227.

Drug-Induced Liver Disease

Nathan M. Bass, MD, PhD

Liver injury may be produced by a large variety of chemical substances, including medicinal agents, industrial toxins, and natural products. More than 900 different drugs have been implicated. Drugs are estimated to be responsible for up to 5% of hospital admissions for jaundice and as many as 10% of all cases investigated for liver disease. The problem of drug-induced liver disease assumes an even greater significance in patients over 50 years of age, in whom the combination of increased susceptibility to adverse drug reactions and greater exposure to therapeutic drugs plays a role. The type of injury produced is extremely varied, and may mimic the entire spectrum of hepatobiliary disorders. The degree of severity of liver disease produced is also highly varied. Many drugs cause subclinical liver injury manifested only as abnormal serum liver enzyme tests, which rapidly reverse upon withdrawal of the drug. At the other extreme, drugs can initiate progressive, chronic liver disease and are the single leading cause of acute, liver failure. A relatively small proportion of drugs causes predictable, dosage-dependent toxic injury to the liver; the vast majority of injuries occur as unexpected reactions to a therapeutic dosage of a drug. The understanding of the molecular mechanisms involved in drug-induced liver disease as well as the determinants of individual susceptibility that underlie the idiosyncratic nature of most cases has increased greatly over the past three decades, but much remains unknown.

MECHANISMS OF DRUG-INDUCED LIVER DISEASE

The central role played by the liver in the clearance and biotransformation of chemicals is fundamental to its susceptibility to drug-induced injury. A key concept in this type of injury is that the parent drug or chemical is rarely responsible for producing the injury. Rather, a metabolite derived from the parent drug as a result of biotransformation by the hepatic drug-metabolizing enzymes is usually more directly responsible for producing an injurious effect upon liver structure and function.

Role of Hepatic Drug Metabolism

Most drugs are lipophilic in nature (ie, they are readily soluble in lipids, such as body fat and cell membranes, but poorly soluble in water). The hepatic drug-metabolizing enzymes are responsible for rendering these agents more water soluble, thus permitting their efflux into the plasma and excretion in the urine, or elimination via the canalicular secretory apparatus into the bile. Hepatic metabolism of drugs and toxins is catalyzed by three classes of enzymes: oxidoreductases, hydrolases, and transferases. The oxidation–reduction and hydrolytic reactions, usually referred to as phase 1 reactions, tend to increase the polarity or water solubility of a molecule, often through the generation of metabolically active moieties, such as hydroxyl groups, in the parent compound. By contrast, the transferases catalyze synthetic reactions, referred to as phase 2 (ie, conjugation) reactions, in which polar compounds including acetate, amino acids, sulfate, glucuronic acid, and glutathione are covalently attached to the drug (Figure 44–1). Phase 2 reactions often employ as substrates drugs that have been metabolized via phase 1 reactions, and this further increases the water solubility of the drug. Many compounds, however, can be metabolized by phase 2 reactions without first having undergone phase 1 metabolism. As discussed below, phase 1 reactions may result in the generation of metabolites that are far more chemically reactive and hence potentially damaging to the cell. The importance of phase 2 reactions in such instances is in rendering these reactive phase 1 metabolic products relatively inert, commonly via the attachment of a polar compound (eg, glutathione) to the reactive chemical group generated by the phase 1 reaction on the parent drug.

The superfamily of cytochrome P-450 enzymes, which are located in the endoplasmic reticulum, is the most important family of hepatic phase 1 drug-metabolizing enzymes. There is a tremendous diversity of individual P-450 gene products. These comprise several structurally related subfamilies that are contained in about 10 distinct gene families in mammals. The P-450 isoenzymes that are important in drug metabolism belong largely to families 1, 2, and 3 (Table 44–1). It is the presence of multiple distinct, yet related, P-450 enzymes in the hepatocyte that allows the liver to perform oxidative metabolism on a vast array of xenobiotics and natural substances. Three important properties of the P-450 system have a direct bearing on the mechanisms of drug-induced liver disease:

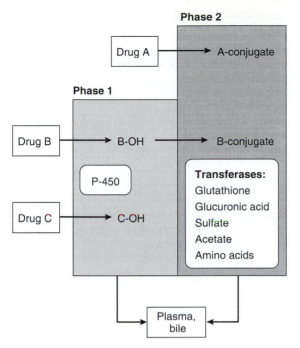

Figure 44–1. Pathways of hepatic drug metabolism. A, B, and C represent three different drugs. Drugs may undergo primary phase 2 biotransformation (A) or initial phase 1 and subsequent phase 2 metabolism (B). Drug C is secreted from the hepatocyte following phase 1 metabolism only.

A. GENETIC HETEROGENEITY

Each of the P-450 proteins identified to date appears to be a unique gene product, with genetic heterogeneity or polymorphism in its expression. This accounts, in part, for the wide range of individual human differences in the ability to perform P-450 metabolism on some drugs, the study of which has given rise to the new field of pharmacogenomics. Genetic variations in enzymes of phase 2 reactions are also emerging as important in individual susceptibility to drug-induced hepatotoxicity. For example, genetic deficiency in glutathione synthetase may increase the susceptibility to several drugs including acetaminophen.

B. VARIATIONS IN SPECIFIC P-450 ENZYME ACTIVITY

These variations occur in a given individual largely as a result of enzyme induction. Many factors, including chemicals, drugs, hormones, and nutritional factors, induce cytochrome P-450 in expression patterns that are highly specific for a particular inducer (see Table 44–1). Induction of a particular P-450 enzyme substantially increases the oxidative metabolism of drugs that are substrates of that specific enzyme. As a consequence, there is an increased rate of elimination of the drug and, in certain instances, an increased rate of formation of reactive and potentially toxic intermediate metabolites.

C. COMPETITIVE INHIBITION

Drugs that share the same P-450 specificity for their biotransformation (see Table 44–1) may competitively inhibit this biotransformation. This important type of drug interaction can lead to substantial blood and tissue accumulation of drugs metabolized by P-450. For ex-

Table 44–1. Examples of hepatic cytochrome P-450.

P-450[1]	Substrates	Reaction Type	Inducers
1A2	Caffeine	N-Demethylation	Hydrocarbons in cigarette smoke
	Theophylline	N-Demethylation	
2B1	Testosterone	Hydroxylation	Phenobarbital
2C9	Tolbutamide	Hydroxylation	None identified
	Ticrynafen[2]	Hydroxylation	
2D6	Debrisoquin	Hydroxylation	None identified
	Perhexiline		
2E1	Acetaminophen		Ethanol
	Ethanol		Isoniazid
3A	Erythromycin	N-Demethylation	Rifampin
	Cyclosporine		Anticonvulsants
	Ketoconazole		Glucocorticoids

[1]The number/letter/number P-450 nomenclature designates family/subfamily/individual gene product.
[2]This uricosuric diuretic was withdrawn because of its severe hepatotoxicity.

ample, patients undergoing organ transplantation who receive both the immunosuppressive drug cyclosporine and the antifungal agent ketoconazole markedly accumulate cyclosporine as a result of ketoconazole inhibition of P-450-3A. Drug interactions at the level of P-450 biotransformation may also reduce the rate of formation of toxic intermediates generated by specific P-450 enzymes and thus offer a potential therapeutic strategy. For example, in mice, 8-methoxypsoralen prevents acetaminophen-induced hepatotoxicity via the inhibition of P-450, with a marked reduction in the formation of reactive acetaminophen intermediates generated by P-450.

Predictable & Unpredictable Hepatotoxicity

Conventionally, drugs with the potential for producing liver injury are divided into predictable, or direct, hepatotoxins and unpredictable, or idiosyncratic, hepatotoxins. Typically, direct hepatotoxins produce liver damage in a predictable, dosage-dependent fashion, whereas idiosyncratic hepatotoxins produce damage in an unpredictable manner, usually while being administered within an accepted therapeutic range. Although there are several excellent examples of drug-induced liver injury that support this categorization, the division is often somewhat arbitrary. For example, although direct hepatotoxins, such as acetaminophen and carbon tetrachloride, will produce liver injury in all individuals who ingest a sufficient quantity, there is substantial variation among individuals in susceptibility to injury in the subtoxic dosage range. Also, there are numerous examples of drugs commonly viewed as idiosyncratic hepatotoxins that will produce milder levels of liver damage in a larger proportion of patients and often in a dosage-related manner. Table 44–2 compares some of the essential features of direct and indirect drug-induced liver disease.

Molecular Mechanisms of Drug-Induced Hepatocellular Injury

Most direct hepatotoxins that produce serious liver disease require activation to reactive electrophiles or free radicals via the cytochrome P-450 system (Table 44–3 and Figure 44–2). Others undergo repeated cycles of enzymatic bioreduction, followed by oxidation by molecular oxygen (redox cycling), a process that results in the generation of large amounts of reactive oxygen species, including superoxide anion radicals and hydrogen peroxide. Both electrophiles and free radicals can form covalent adducts with cellular macromolecules, including proteins, lipids, and nucleic acids, and this leads to disruption of their function. In the case of proteins, binding to thiol groups by electrophilic com-

Table 44–2. Predictable and unpredictable hepatotoxins.

Characteristic	Predictable	Unpredictable
Dosage dependence	Invariable	Unusual
Latent period[1]	Hours to days	Weeks to months
Dependence on host factors	Low	High
Histologic findings	Zonal necrosis Steatosis	Necrosis Cholestasis Granulomas Duct lesions
Systemic features	Multiorgan toxicity	Drug allergy
Examples	Acetaminophen Aspirin Carbon tetrachloride	Approximately 900 therapeutic agents

[1]The interval between starting the drug and the onset of the hepatotoxic reaction.

pounds inactivates enzymes and disrupts membrane cation transporters. One of the more devastating effects of the latter is the collapse of calcium compartmentation in the mitochondria and endoplasmic reticulum. This results in an influx of calcium into the cytoplasmic and nuclear compartments, with activation of phospholipases and nucleases and, eventually, cell death. Factors that contribute to the final pathway of cell injury and death in drug-induced liver injury include inflammatory mediators such as Fas ligand and tumor necrosis factor-α.

Table 44–3. Mechanisms of drug-induced hepatotoxicity.

Mechanism	Example
Conversion to reactive intermediates	
Electrophiles producing covalent adducts with tissue macromolecules	Acetaminophen
Electrophiles acting as oxidants	Acetaminophen
Free radicals producing lipid peroxidation	Carbon tetrachloride
Redox cycling with production of reactive oxygen species	Nitrofurantoin
Alteration of membrane physical properties	Estrogens
Inhibition of membrane enzymes	Chlorpromazine
Interference with hepatic uptake processes	Rifampin
Impairment of cytoskeletal function	Chlorpromazine
Formation of insoluble complexes in bile	Chlorpromazine

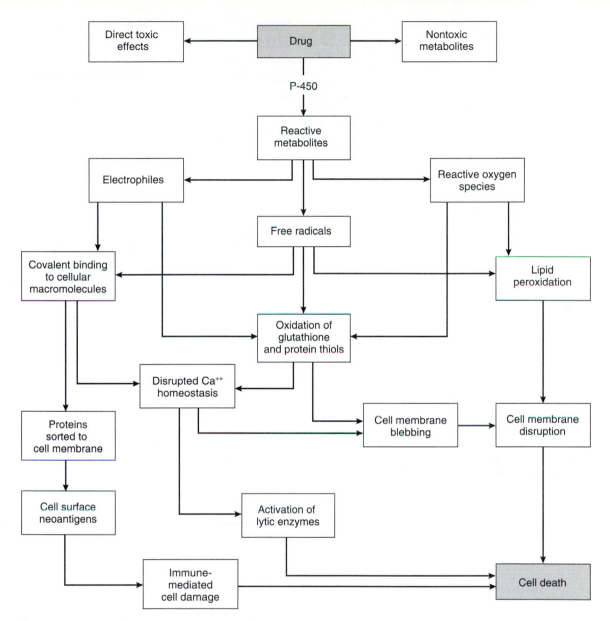

Figure 44–2. Mechanisms of drug-induced hepatotoxicity.

The so-called covalent-binding hypothesis of cellular injury by drugs has stressed the importance of the covalent modification of cellular macromolecules by reactive drug intermediates in the production of cellular damage. In some experimental models, however, the extent of covalent binding of drug intermediates to cellular proteins does not correlate with the severity of cellular necrosis, and this brings into question the importance of this mechanism. The specificity of the proteins attacked by a particular reactive intermediate may be more significant than the amount of covalent modification per se. In addition, oxidative processes are of fundamental importance in the pathogenesis of cell damage. For example, the reactive electrophile produced by the P-450 metabolism of acetaminophen, in addition to forming covalent adducts with key cellular proteins, may also act as a cellular oxidant, producing oxidation of protein thiol groups. Free radicals are, in general, more reactive than electrophiles and attack lipids, proteins, or nucleic acids closer to the vicinity of their formation. Lipid peroxidation initiated by free radical attack on polyunsaturated fatty acids leads to the formation of free lipid radicals, which are subsequently oxidized by molecular oxygen to form lipid peroxy radicals. These can initiate a further cycle of lipid peroxidation. In this manner, lipid peroxidation may proceed in a chain reaction, amplifying the injurious effects of the original free radicals. Certain solvents, such as carbon tetrachloride, in addition to producing liver damage via free radical formation, may in native form cause an early, direct disruption of cellular membranes. Alteration of the physical properties of cell membranes and inhibition of membrane enzymes are also important mechanisms in the hepatotoxicity produced by drugs such as estrogens and chlorpromazine.

Drugs that cause unpredictable hepatotoxicity often form covalent adducts with cellular proteins in experimental models; this raises the question of why these drugs produce liver disease in only a minority of patients. There clearly exist other, often poorly understood, host factors in the production of liver disease by these agents (Table 44–4). In some instances (eg, the idiosyncratic acute hepatitis caused by isoniazid), the reactive metabolite responsible for the liver injury is overproduced in only some individuals. Troglitazone, a drug used for the treatment of diabetes mellitus, provides a recent example of apparently infrequent idiosyncratic severe hepatotoxicity that, on closer analysis, overshadows a more frequent incidence of milder, probably direct toxicity. This drug was withdrawn from the market because of the association of its use with several cases of severe, often fatal hepatotoxicity. Estimates based on postmarketing surveillance suggest that 2% of patients receiving troglitazone developed serum alanine transaminase values greater than three times normal, approximately 1:1,250 developed jaundice and 1:40,000 to 50,000 had irreversible liver failure leading to death or liver transplantation. The drug is predominantly metabolized by conjugation to sulfate or glucuronic acid, but metabolism to a quinone intermediate by cytochromes P-450-2C8, -3A4, and -2C19 also occurs; polymorphisms in these enzymes may account for variations in individual susceptibilty to hepatotoxicity. Other types of idiosyncratic hepatic drug reactions are accompanied by marked immunologic or hypersensitivity phenomena, including fever, rash, eosinophilia, serum sickness syndrome, and even the emergence of classic autoimmune serologic markers. In these instances, immunologic processes play a major pathogenic role. Thus, in liver disease produced by halothane, diclofenac, and ticrynafen (tienilic acid, a uricosuric diuretic withdrawn from use because of its hepatotoxicity), there is strong evidence for a mechanism in which reactive intermediates of these drugs form cova-

Table 44–4. Host factors as determinants of individual susceptibility to hepatotoxicity.

Host Factor	Increased Susceptibility
Age	
Older adults	Isoniazid, NSAIDs[1]
Infancy	Valproic acid
Gender	
Female	Isoniazid, halothane, zidovudine
Male	Amoxicillin-clavulanic acid
Race	
African	Isoniazid
Asian	Isoniazid
Renal insufficiency	NSAIDs, methotrexate
Hypoalbuminemia	Aspirin, methotrexate
Preexisting liver disease	Isoniazid, acetaminophen, methotrexate
Obesity	Halothane, methotrexate
HIV positive or AIDS	Oxacillin, trimethoprimsulfamethoxazole
Other drugs	
Alcohol	Acetaminophen, NSAIDs, methotrexate
Isoniazid	Acetaminophen
Anticonvulsants	Acetaminophen, valproic acid
Rifampin	Isoniazid
Genetic polymorphism or defect	
N-Acetyltransferase 2	Isoniazid
P-450-2D6	Perhexiline maleate
Urea cycle	Valproic acid
Mitochondrial β-oxidation	Valproic acid, aspirin
Uridine diphosphate glucuronosyl transferase	Acetaminophen
Glutathione synthase	Acetaminophen

[1]NSAIDs, nonsteroidal antiinflammatory drugs.

lent adducts with specific microsomal proteins, including the cytochrome P-450 enzymes involved in their biotransformation. The adduct-modified microsomal proteins are next transported to the plasma membrane, where they are expressed as neoantigens that are recognized as foreign by the immune system, and this elicits an immune-mediated attack upon the liver. For example, patients who developed hepatitis after taking the diuretic ticrynafen demonstrated a high incidence of circulating anti-liver–kidney microsome (anti-LKM$_2$) autoantibodies that recognize epitopes specific to cytochrome P-450-2C9, the major P-450 enzyme involved in the metabolism of ticrynafen. Anti-LKM$_2$ autoantibodies are highly specific for drug-induced autoimmune-like chronic hepatitis, and differ from the anti-LKM$_1$ antibody characteristic of idiopathic type 2 autoimmune hepatitis, which, by contrast, reacts specifically with P-450-2D6 (see Chapter 36).

Cellular Defenses against Toxic Injury

Liver cells possess several important defenses against drug-induced injury. Most important is the tripeptide glutathione, which is present in millimolar concentration intracellularly. Glutathione provides a reactive thiol group that forms conjugates with electrophilic compounds, either spontaneously or catalyzed by the glutathione S-transferases, which are abundantly present in the cytosol of liver cells. The resulting conjugates are excreted in the bile. Glutathione also performs a major antioxidant function by maintaining the reduced state of protein thiols in the cell. Glutathione, as a substrate for glutathione peroxidases, reduces both hydrogen peroxide and organic hydroperoxides such as polyunsaturated fatty hydroperoxides, which arise during lipid peroxidation. Finally, along with vitamin E, carotenoids, and ascorbic acid, glutathione scavenges free radicals within the cell. Superoxide dismutase disposes of the superoxide radical, while catalase, along with the glutathione peroxidases, also prevents accumulation of hydrogen peroxide in the cell. Impairment of the above defenses may constitute an important factor in determining individual susceptibility to toxic liver injury. Thus, impairment of glutathione synthesis and its depletion in the hepatocyte is implicated in the marked susceptibility to the toxicity of acetaminophen, and possibly other medications, in chronic alcoholics, patients with acquired immunodeficiency syndrome (AIDS), and malnourished individuals (see Table 44–4). Also, the liver's ability to produce antiinflammatory cytokines (eg, interleukins 10, 6, 4, and 3) and prostaglandins may function to prevent allergic hepatitis as well as acute hepatotoxicity through inhibition of γδ T cells.

Determinants of Individual Susceptibility to Toxic Liver Damage

A variety of host factors—some more definite than others—determine individual susceptibility to both direct and indirect hepatotoxins (see Table 44–4). The variation in individual susceptibility to drug-induced liver injury depends both on the production of a toxic derivative of a drug and on the effectiveness of the defenses responsible for its elimination. Thus, for a drug to cause liver injury, a given set of conditions affecting toxic species production or removal, or both, must exist. For drugs regarded as predictable hepatotoxins, the necessary conditions exist in most persons, whereas

for idiosyncratic hepatotoxins, the necessary conditions rarely coexist. Induction of cytochrome P-450 enzymes, as discussed above, may markedly increase the rate of toxic species production and the risk of liver damage. Well-recognized examples include induction of P-450-2E1 by chronic exposure to alcohol and anticonvulsant medication, which leads to enhanced acetaminophen toxicity, and increased isoniazid toxicity due to coadministration of rifampin. Depletion of glutathione in patients with AIDS may explain their increased susceptibility to drug toxicity from agents including oxacillin and sulfa drugs. Decreased plasma protein binding that leads to increased tissue levels of a drug may be the underlying reason for the association of hypoalbuminemia with an increased risk of toxicity from aspirin and methotrexate. The increased susceptibility of the elderly to hepatotoxicity from a number of drugs, especially the nonsteroidal antiinflammatory drugs (NSAIDs), may depend on several age-related changes in hepatic enzyme activities and pharmacokinetics, including reduced hepatic blood flow and mass and prolonged drug half-lives.

Specific inborn errors of metabolism that are phenotypically subtle or quiescent may reveal themselves as a marked susceptibility to particular types of liver dysfunction with certain drugs. For example, congenital abnormalities of the mitochondrial β-oxidation and urea cycles may cause increased susceptibility to hepatic dysfunction, with microvesicular fat infiltration in children exposed to aspirin (Reye's syndrome) or valproic acid. In many other varieties of idiosyncratic drug-induced liver injury, abnormal production or elimination of toxic drug metabolites resulting from genetic polymorphisms in drug-metabolizing enzymes is likely to play a key role. Examples include the greater apparent susceptibility to isoniazid and possibly sulfonamide hepatotoxicity in individuals with a slow acetylator phenotype (polymorphic N-acetyltransferase 2), and an association between the poor metabolizer phenotype for debrisoquin hydroxylation (which is a result of a defect in P-450-2D6 gene expression) and hepatotoxicity from perhexilene maleate. Also, deficient glucuronidation in individuals with Gilbert's syndrome or deficiency of the enzyme glutathione synthase may impose an increased susceptibility to acetaminophen hepatotoxicity. Similarly, the lymphocytes of individuals (and their first-degree relatives) who have sustained hepatic damage with phenytoin or amineptine are abnormally susceptible to in vitro damage from P-450-generated metabolites of these drugs; this points to a defect in defenses against these reactive metabolites.

The concept of "metabolic idiosyncrasy" in hepatic drug toxicity emphasizes the accumulation in susceptible individuals of a particular reactive intermediate, with production of cellular damage via either the covalent or oxidative disruption of protein structure and function. However, as discussed above, both metabolic and immunologic processes play a prominent role in some types of idiosyncratic hepatotoxicity. In such instances, the generation of drug hapten neoantigens by reactive metabolites appears to be of significance. Neoantigen formation on the hepatocyte surface by certain drugs occurs far more commonly than liver injury produced by these drugs. This suggests that immunologic rather than metabolic idiosyncrasy is the main determinant of liver damage developing after exposure to these drugs. For example, probably all individuals exposed to halothane produce adducts of trifluoroacetic acid (a highly reactive intermediate produced by the oxidative hepatic biotransformation of halothane) with hepatic microsomal proteins, which can be expressed on the hepatocyte surface membrane. Only the sera of patients afflicted with halothane hepatitis contain antibodies directed against these hepatic trifluoroacetylated proteins, however; this suggests the existence of a defect in immunologic tolerance to these drug-induced neoantigens. "Molecular mimicry" may also be an important component of halothane hepatitis. Recent studies have demonstrated that the unmodified E2 subunit of pyruvate dehydrogenase reacts strongly with the sera of patients who had developed halothane hepatitis. This subunit, which is the major autoantigen recognized by the M2 antimitochondrial antibodies characteristic of primary biliary cirrhosis, contains lipoic acid as a prosthetic group. Lipoic acid mimics the epitopic structure of the N-ε-trifluoroacetyl-L-lysine moiety common to the trifluoroacetylated proteins arising after halothane exposure. Thus, the recognition of the pyruvate dehydrogenase E2 subunit by halothane hepatitis sera results from a form of molecular mimicry, in which a normal hepatic protein is rendered autoantigenic after sensitization by drug-induced neoantigens. The molecular basis for such immunologic idiosyncrasy is poorly understood. An association of particular "autoimmune" HLA alleles (eg, HLA-B8) with a susceptibility to drug-induced autoimmunelike hepatitis is an attractive possibility but currently lacks experimental support.

CLINICAL & MORPHOLOGIC PATTERNS OF DRUG-INDUCED LIVER INJURY

Drugs produce a wide variety of clinical and histologic patterns of liver injury. The two most common types of injury are termed hepatocellular, or cytotoxic, and cholestatic. Some drugs produce more than one pattern of damage (eg, oral contraceptives may cause cholestasis, adenoma, sinusoidal dilatation, or peliosis hepatis) (Table 44–5).

Drug-induced liver injury is designated **hepatocellular injury** if the alanine aminotransferase (ALT) level

Table 44–5. Patterns of drug-induced liver disease.

Category	Examples
Zonal necrosis	Acetaminophen, bromfenac, carbon tetrachloride
Hepatitis	
Viral hepatitis-like reaction	Halothane, isoniazid, phenytoin, diclofenac
Focal hepatitis	Aspirin, oxacillin
Chronic hepatitis	
Autoimmune hepatitis-like reaction	Methyldopa, dantrolene, diclofenac
Viral hepatitis-like reaction	Isoniazid, halothane, troglitazone
Cholestasis	
Noninflammatory cholestasis	Estrogens, androgenic and anabolic steroids
Inflammatory cholestasis	Amoxicillin-clavulanic acid, piroxicam
Ductal cholestasis	Flucloxacillin, thiabendazole
Sclerosing cholangitis	Floxuridine
Steatosis	
Macrovesicular fatty liver	Ethanol, corticosteroids
Microvesicular fatty liver	Tetracycline, valproic acid, didanosine
Phospholipidosis	Amiodarone, perhexiline maleate
Steatohepatitis	Amiodarone, perhexiline maleate, nifedipine, tamoxifen
Granulomas	Phenylbutazone, allopurinol, quinidine
Firbrosis	Methotrexate, hypervitaminosis A
Vascular lesions	
Hepatic vein thrombosis	Estrogens
Venoocclusive disease	Anticancer agents, azathioprine
Peliosis hepatis	Androgenic and anabolic steroids, estrogens
Hepatic arteritis	Allopurinol, floxuridine
Nodular regenerative hyperplasia	Azathioprine, anticancer agents
Tumors	
Adenoma	Estrogens
Hepatocellular carcinoma	Estrogens, androgenic and anabolic steroids
Angiosarcoma	Vinyl chloride, thorium dioxide

is increased to more than twice the upper limit of normal, or if the ratio of ALT to alkaline phosphatase is equal to or greater than 5, where both enzymes are expressed as multiples of the upper limit of normal. Liver injury is designated **cholestatic injury** if the alkaline phosphatase level is increased to twice the upper limit of normal, or if the ratio of ALT to alkaline phosphatase is less than or equal to 2. Mixed patterns of injury are common, and are characterized by elevations in both ALT and alkaline phosphatase levels to greater than twice the upper limit of normal for these enzymes, with the ratio of ALT to alkaline phosphatase greater than 2 but less than 5. The specific morphologic patterns of liver injury that are recognized in drug-induced hepatotoxicity are summarized in Table 44–5 and are discussed briefly below.

Zonal Necrosis

The typical injury caused by most direct hepatotoxins is liver cell necrosis largely confined to a particular zone of the liver lobule. Centrilobular or perivenous necrosis is typical of carbon tetrachloride, acetaminophen, and *Amanita* mushroom toxins. This pattern is explained by the greater abundance of P-450 drug-metabolizing enzymes in the centrizonal region and possibly also the relative hypoxemia of this region. Periportal zonal necrosis is much rarer and is produced by allyl alcohol and yellow phosphorus. In severe cases of liver injury by zonal toxins, the necrosis may extend further throughout the liver lobule and may progress to submassive or massive necrosis. Extremely high levels of serum aminotransferase are typical with this type of injury, which may also result in severe disturbance of liver cell function or even fulminant hepatic failure.

Hepatitis

The term hepatitis connotes a morphologic pattern of drug-induced liver damage in which hepatocellular necrosis with accompanying inflammatory cell infiltrates is prominent. Three patterns of drug-induced hepatitis are commonly encountered.

A. VIRAL HEPATITIS-LIKE REACTIONS

This is a common pattern of hepatotoxicity produced by idiosyncratic hepatotoxins. The pathologic features resemble those of acute viral hepatitis, with diffuse hepatocellular necrosis, acidophil bodies, and variable inflammatory infiltration. In severe cases, the lesion may progress to bridging, submassive or massive liver necrosis, and fulminant liver failure. Drugs producing this type of injury pattern include halothane, isoniazid, ketoconazole, and phenytoin.

B. FOCAL HEPATITIS (NONSPECIFIC HEPATITIS)

Scattered foci of liver cell necrosis with mononuclear cell infiltrates may result from many forms of drug injury, including those due to aspirin and oxacillin. This is usually a mild type of injury that resolves completely upon discontinuation of the drug.

C. CHRONIC HEPATITIS

Ongoing hepatocellular injury with features of chronic hepatitis both temporally and histologically has been associated with many drugs, including amiodarone, dantrolene, diclofenac, isoniazid, methyldopa, nitrofurantoin, hydralazine, phenytoin, propylthiouracil, troglitazone, sulfonylureas, and sulfonamides. This type of lesion is characterized by a chronic, progressive process leading to cirrhosis in some instances. The clinical, serologic, and histologic features resemble those of autoimmune hepatitis most closely when oxyphenisatin, nitrofurantoin, or ticrynafen is the offending drug. With other drugs such as isoniazid, the manifestations are more like those of chronic viral hepatitis.

Cholestasis

In drug-induced cholestatic liver injury, the symptoms of pruritus and jaundice may be prominent; an elevated serum alkaline phosphatase level is the dominant biochemical finding (see beginning of this section). There are at least four distinct forms of cholestatic drug-induced liver injury.

A. NONINFLAMMATORY (BLAND) CHOLESTASIS

This is caused principally by estrogens and 17α-substituted androgenic and anabolic steroids. There is impairment of bile secretion by the hepatocytes, with little or no evidence of hepatocellular necrosis or parenchymal inflammation.

B. INFLAMMATORY CHOLESTASIS

This pattern of injury, sometimes referred to as cholestatic hepatitis, is characterized by significant hepatocellular necrosis and portal lobular inflammation, and prominent cholestasis. Systemic symptoms include rash, fever, and athralgias. Agents that typically cause inflammatory cholestasis include phenothiazines, amoxicillin-clavulanic acid (co-amoxiclav), sulfonylureas, propylthiouracil, and erythromycin estolate. The prognosis is usually favorable.

C. DUCTAL CHOLESTASIS

This lesion is characterized by progressive destruction of the small bile ducts, producing a clinical syndrome similar to that of primary biliary cirrhosis. Profound cholestasis may persist for months to years before resolving, or progress to secondary biliary cirrhosis. This "vanishing bile duct syndrome" is a variant of the cholestatic injury produced by chlorpromazine, carbamazepine, sulfonylureas, and flucloxacillin.

D. SCLEROSING CHOLANGITIS

This is a unique type of drug-induced liver injury that has followed intrahepatic arterial infusion chemotherapy with floxuridine. The lesion, in many respects, resembles the diffuse ductal strictures of primary sclerosing cholangitis and results from ischemic duct injury secondary to a drug-induced chemical arteritis.

Steatosis (Fatty Liver)

Triglyceride accumulation in hepatocytes may occur as a major or associated manifestation of hepatotoxicity. Two main patterns of fat accumulation in the liver are recognized.

A. MACROVESICULAR STEATOSIS (LARGE-DROPLET FATTY LIVER)

Fat droplets coalesce to form large vacuoles, which may occupy most of the hepatocyte volume. In spite of the dramatic appearance of this type of fat infiltration, it is usually associated with little disturbance in liver cell function. This pattern of injury is typically produced by corticosteroids, alcohol, and other direct hepatotoxins. It resembles the fatty liver seen in systemic conditions such as obesity and poorly controlled diabetes mellitus.

B. MICROVESICULAR STEATOSIS (SMALL-DROPLET FATTY LIVER)

This pattern is less commonly encountered and is seen in association with tetracycline, valproic acid, nucleoside analogues (didanosine, fialuridine), and hypoglycin poisoning (Jamaican vomiting sickness). Although distinct in some features, this type of hepatotoxicity is similar to the rare systemic disorders of Reye's syndrome (which in many cases appears to be related to aspirin usage) and acute fatty liver of pregnancy. Mitochondrial dysfunction appears to be an important factor common to the different causes of microvesicular steatosis. The fat is deposited in small droplets throughout the liver cell, producing a foamy appearance under conventional light microscopy. It is usually associated with a profound disturbance of hepatocellular function and may produce a picture of fulminant hepatic failure. The distinction between the clincopathologic entities of macro- and microvesicular steatotic liver injury may not always be that clear. For example, alcoholic liver damage may produce a mixed pattern of macro- and microvesicular steatosis, often with profound hepatic dysfunction. Also, the nucleoside analog zidovudine has been implicated in several cases of liver disease charac-

terized by hepatomegaly and macrovesicular steatosis, in which profound hepatic dysfunction occurred, with fatal lactic acidosis.

C. PHOSPHOLIPIDOSIS

A distinctive type of hepatic phospholipid accumulation resembling the inherited disorders of phospholipid metabolism, Niemann-Pick disease and Tay-Sachs disease, occurs following the use of certain drugs, including amiodarone, perhexiline maleate, and 4,4′-diethylaminoethoxyhexestrol. The lesion results from lysosomal phospholipid storage secondary to inactivation of lysosomal phospholipases by these drugs.

Nonalcoholic Steatohepatitis (NASH)

A liver lesion resembling the typical histologic finding of alcoholic hepatitis, with hepatocellular necrosis, neutrophil inflammatory infiltrates, fatty change, fibrosis, and Mallory bodies, can be seen in some patients treated with amiodarone, perhexilene maleate, tamoxifen, methotrexate, diltiazem, nifedipine, or the industrial toxin, dimethylformamide. Progression to cirrhosis occurs in some instances.

Granulomas

Medications may account for up to a third of cases of granulomatous hepatitis (see Chapter 36). Drug-induced granulomas are typically noncaseating and are often associated with granulomas in other tissues and prominent systemic features of hypersensitivity and systemic vasculitis. Commonly responsible agents include quinidine, allopurinol, phenytoin, phenylbutazone, hydralazine, and sulfonamides.

Fibrosis

Some agents will produce an increase in collagen deposition, with minimal or absent features of necrosis or inflammation. This type of fibrosis may progress to cirrhosis and portal hypertension, although the latter may also occur as a result of portal fibrosis, even in the absence of cirrhosis. This type of injury has been observed following chronic administration of methotrexate and also with prolonged ingestion of high dosages of vitamin A, inorganic arsenicals, thioguanine, and azathioprine.

Vascular Lesions

Direct damage to the hepatic vascular endothelium may be the basis for the wide variety of vascular lesions caused by toxins and medications. Hepatic venoocclusive disease, first recognized as a result of the ingestion of bush teas containing hepatotoxic pyrrolizidine alkaloids, is now seen most commonly in patients treated with azathioprine as an immunosuppressive agent and in patients receiving combination chemotherapy for bone marrow transplantation. Oral contraceptives may cause focal sinusoidal dilatation. Both contraceptives and anabolic steroids may lead to peliosis hepatis, a more striking lesion characterized by extrasinusoidal blood-filled spaces. Nodular regenerative hyperplasia, a lesion associated with hyperviscosity syndromes and vasculitic diseases, has also been linked to azathioprine and antineoplastic drugs.

Tumors

Neoplastic lesions have in some cases been ascribed to prolonged exposure to certain drugs or toxins. These tumors include hepatic adenoma and hepatocellular carcinoma associated with either oral contraceptives or androgenic-anabolic steroids, and angiosarcoma caused by exposure to vinyl chloride monomer, thorium dioxide, or arsenic.

SPECIFIC DRUGS CAUSING LIVER INJURY

Acetaminophen

Hepatotoxicity from this widely used analgesic is most commonly seen as a result of intentional or accidental overdosage, but toxicity even in the therapeutic range is increasingly encountered in chronic alcoholics. The mechanism of acetaminophen-induced liver necrosis has been extensively studied (Figure 44–3). When taken in therapeutic dosages, acetaminophen is eliminated mainly via hepatic conjugation with sulfate and glucuronic acids. A small proportion of the drug undergoes biotransformation via cytochrome P-450-2E1 to a reactive metabolite, N-acetyl-p-benzoquinone imine (NAPQI), which subsequently undergoes phase 2 conjugation with glutathione. When a large dose of acetaminophen is ingested, usually more than 10–15 g in an adult, the capacities of the glucuronidation and sulfation pathways of elimination become saturated, and a greater proportion of the drug is directed toward the P-450-mediated formation of NAPQI. As more NAPQI is formed, glutathione is rapidly consumed at a rate faster than the ability of the glutathione synthetic pathway to replenish hepatic stores. When the glutathione pool available for NAPQI conjugation is critically depleted, the reactive metabolite arylates hepatic macromolecules, leading to the formation of protein thiol adducts, with subsequent alteration in protein function. Among the most important of these are membrane-associated calcium pumps, damage to which results in disruption of intracellular calcium homeostasis. In particular, mitochondrial calcium homeostasis is believed to play an important role in the subsequent events that occur leading to liver cell necrosis following acetaminophen overdosage.

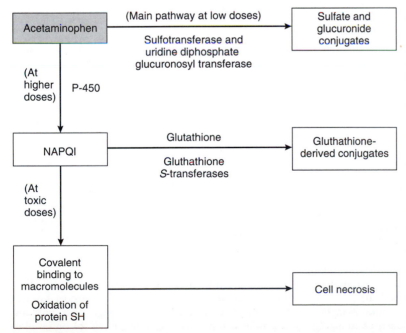

Figure 44–3. Mechanism of acetaminophen-induced hepatotoxicity. At usual therapeutic dosages, acetaminophen is metabolized predominantly by conjugation reactions. The capacity of these pathways becomes saturated at higher dosages of acetaminophen, leading to greater diversion of the drug to the P-450-mediated pathway that generates the reactive electrophile N-acetyl-p-benzoquinone imine (NAPQI), which subsequently undergoes phase 2 conjugation with glutathione. After ingestion of acetaminophen at toxic dosages, NAPQI formation leads to glutathione depletion, allowing the electrophile to exert damaging effects within the cell via covalent binding to cellular macromolecules and via the oxidation of protein thiol groups.

In chronic alcoholics, severe hepatocellular necrosis has been observed with acetaminophen taken at doses of 2–6 g/d for several days. The markedly increased susceptibility of alcoholics to acetaminophen hepatotoxicity is the result of two major processes. The first is induction of cytochrome P-450-2E1 by alcohol, which increases the flux of acetaminophen through this pathway and hence the rate of formation of NAPQI. The second is the depletion of hepatic glutathione stores as a result of both consumption of glutathione and inhibition of its synthesis. Other factors that may increase susceptibility to acetaminophen toxicity include starvation (depletion of glutathione) and concurrent treatment with drugs that induce cytochrome P-450 (eg, phenobarbital). Acetaminophen is a classic zonal toxin, producing necrosis in the perivenular (zone 3) region of the liver lobule, corresponding to the predominant region of cytochrome P-450-2E1 expression.

In the first few hours following acetaminophen overdosage, patients may develop nausea and vomiting. These symptoms are followed by a relatively asymptomatic phase lasting approximately 24 hours, following which clinical and laboratory signs of liver damage become evident. Serum aminotransferase levels often rise to more than 5000–10,000 U/L. Severe liver injury may lead to progressive liver failure, with encephalopathy, coagulopathy, hypoglycemia, and acidosis. Acute renal failure may also develop as a sequela of direct acetaminophen toxicity.

The plasma level of acetaminophen is the most reliable means for assessing prognosis following an overdosage (Figure 44–4). Levels in excess of 200 mg/L at 4 hours, 100 mg/L at 8 hours, or 50 mg/L at 12 hours after ingestion are predictive of severe liver damage and indicate that treatment with acetylcysteine is needed. Although often useful, plasma levels of acetaminophen should not be relied upon exclusively in deciding whether to administer this antidote. When uncertainty exists regarding the quantity of acetaminophen ingested or the time interval between ingestion and presentation, it is prudent to treat with N-acetylcysteine. In patients presenting very early after an overdosage, oral administration of activated charcoal may help to reduce further absorption of the drug. N-Acetylcysteine, which is a highly effective antidote, should be administered without delay. Its efficacy is based upon stimulation of endogenous glutathione synthesis. In patients who receive N-acetylcysteine within 16 hours of acetaminophen overdosage, severe liver injury is rarely observed. The initial dose is 140 mg/kg orally, followed by a maintenance dose of 70 mg/kg every 4 hours for 48–72 hours. In the United Kingdom, an intravenous formulation of N-acetylcysteine is available that is given in an initial dose of 150 mg/kg over 15 minutes in 200 mL of 5% dextrose, with subsequent doses of 50 mg/kg

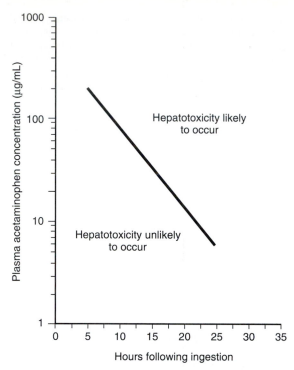

Figure 44–4. The Rumack-Matthew nomogram showing the relationship between the plasma acetaminophen concentration at various times after ingestion and the likelihood of liver damage. (Adapted, with permission, from Rumack BH, Matthew H: Acetaminophen poisoning and toxicity. Pediatrics 1975;55:871.)

administered at 4-hour intervals thereafter, to a total dose of 300 mg/kg. Although it is clear that the hepatoprotective effect of N-acetylcysteine is greatest if it is given within the first 16 hours following an overdosage, there is evidence to suggest that later administration, even up to 36 hours following ingestion, may afford some benefit. Patients who survive acute acetaminophen toxicity recover fully, without evidence of progressive or residual liver damage. Among those who develop fulminant hepatic failure, recovery is still the rule, although advanced encephalopathy, severe coagulopathy, and acidosis are associated with a poor outcome. In this circumstance, expedited referral for liver transplantation is indicated.

Amiodarone

This iodinated benzofuran used in the treatment of refractory arrhythmias can produce an unusual form of liver injury. Subclinical liver damage with mild increases in serum aminotransferase levels is seen in up to

20% of patients who receive this drug. However, 1–3% of patients develop a more severe liver injury that histologically resembles acute alcoholic hepatitis, with steatosis, focal necrosis, fibrosis, polymorphonuclear leukocyte infiltrates, and Mallory bodies. This lesion may progress to a micronodular cirrhosis, portal hypertension, and liver failure. Hepatomegaly is common, but jaundice is rare. Evidence of liver damage may persist for several months after the drug is discontinued. On electron microscopy, most patients receiving amiodarone demonstrate unusual lysosomal morphologic characteristics, with concentric, electron-dense myeloid bodies resulting from phospholipid accumulation. This acquired phospholipidosis results from the fact that amiodarone concentrates in lysosomes and inhibits lysosomal phospholipases. This effect of the drug is seen in most patients who receive it, and appears to bear little relationship to the risk of development of pseudoalcoholic hepatitis with amiodarone.

Chlorpromazine

This drug, as well as other phenothiazines, may produce a cholestatic reaction in up to 1% of patients after 3–5 weeks of treatment. Symptoms of fever, anorexia, nausea, upper abdominal pain, rash, and arthralgias may be present at the onset. Pruritus and jaundice soon follow, and eosinophilia is commonly present. Liver biopsy reveals cholestasis with canalicular bile plugs and prominent portal inflammation with a cellular infiltrate consisting of mononuclear, polymorphonuclear, and eosinophilic leukocytes, with variable focal liver cell necrosis. Symptoms usually subside over a period of weeks following discontinuation of the drug, but, rarely, a syndrome of prolonged cholestasis resembling primary biliary cirrhosis may occur.

Erythromycin

A cholestatic reaction with components of inflammation and necrosis of liver cells may result from the use of the lauryl sulfate salt of propionyl erythromycin (erythromycin estolate). It is also occasionally associated with the ethylsuccinate, lactobionate, and propionate salts of this antibiotic. Hepatotoxicity typically presents as an acute syndrome of right upper quadrant pain, fever, and variable cholestatic symptoms. The clinical picture may closely mimic that of acute cholecystitis or cholangitis and has resulted in surgical exploration in some instances. The prognosis is usually excellent, but the reaction typically recurs if the drug is readministered. The prognosis is uniformly excellent for the cholestatic reaction observed with oral erythromycin preparations, but fulminant hepatitis has resulted from the intravenous administration of this antibiotic.

Halothane

This halogenated alkane anesthetic rarely causes a viral hepatitis-like reaction, which in severe cases has progressed to fatal massive hepatic necrosis. Cross-sensitization may occur among halothane, methoxyflurane, and enflurane, although hepatic injury appears to be less common with the latter two anesthetic agents. Isoflurane appears to have the least hepatotoxic potential of all halogenated alkane anesthetic agents in current use. Susceptibility to halothane hepatitis is increased in older persons, women, and obese individuals, and severe reactions are more likely after previous or multiple exposures to this anesthetic. Symptoms typical of viral hepatitis occur 7–10 days after anesthesia, but this interval may shorten considerably after repeated exposure. Symptoms at the onset include severe fever, chills, and sweats, followed by jaundice. Features of hypersensitivity such as rash and eosinophilia are less frequent. The course may progress to fulminant hepatic failure within days, with a high mortality rate. Some patients develop a more protracted course, with either slow recovery or evolution into progressive liver failure. Halothane is metabolized along two pathways, which result in different mechanisms of liver damage. In the presence of high oxygen tension, oxidative biotransformation yields trifluoroacetic acid, which, as previously described (see section, "Mechanisms of Drug-Induced Liver Disease"), forms adducts with microsomal proteins that are sorted to the hepatocyte membrane. These trifluoroacetic acid–protein adducts act as neoantigens that trigger humoral and cell-mediated immune responses leading to hepatocellular necrosis. At low oxygen tension, biotransformation occurs along a reductive pathway that yields a free radical metabolite capable of producing necrosis directly.

Isoniazid

A mild increase in aminotransferase levels is observed in up to 20% of individuals taking isoniazid for single-drug chemoprophylaxis within the first few weeks of therapy. These abnormalities subside in most patients, despite continued administration of the drug. About 0.6% of patients receiving isoniazid develop significant liver injury, which follows a viral hepatitis-like pattern. The onset is usually within 2–3 months after commencing the drug, and initial symptoms are often nonspecific, with malaise and anorexia preceding signs of liver disease. Clinical features of hypersensitivity are distinctly unusual. The liver disease may present as an initially mild acute process but may progress to a subacute or chronic hepatitis or fatal massive liver necrosis. Older individuals are far more susceptible to severe isoniazid liver injury, the incidence of which increases significantly after age 35 years and probably exceeds 2% among individuals over age 50 years.

Isoniazid appears to injure the liver through a toxic metabolite, the formation of which may be increased in individuals with a slow-acetylator phenotype. Both hydrazine and toxic derivatives of monoacetylhydrazine formed during the metabolism of isoniazid have been implicated in the mechanism of hepatotoxicity. The formation of the nontoxic derivative diacetylhydrazine from monoacetylhydrazine may be impaired in slow acetylators, thus favoring the formation of more toxic derivatives of monoacetylhydrazine via cytochrome P-450-mediated metabolism. Induction of P-450 by rifampin may account for a severe form of isoniazid hepatitis in patients receiving both drugs.

Patients receiving isoniazid should be followed at regular intervals and advised to report intercurrent symptoms. If these are associated with evidence of disturbed liver function, the drug should be discontinued pending further evaluation. Because minor liver abnormalities are a common and transient finding, particularly in the early course of isoniazid treatment, routine monitoring of liver tests in patients taking the drug is not usually recommended, except in those over age 35 years. In these individuals, given the increased risk-to-benefit ratio of isoniazid chemoprophylaxis, a conservative approach to chemoprophylaxis is warranted, along with appropriate monitoring of liver function tests. A four-fold or increasing elevation in serum aminotransferases in this older age group should be regarded as potentially serious and may justify discontinuation of the drug, particularly as the prognosis is closely related to the severity of hepatic dysfunction at the time of presentation.

Methotrexate

Chronic treatment of patients with psoriasis and rheumatoid arthritis with methotrexate may rarely lead to significant fibrosis and cirrhosis. Concomitant alcohol consumption, diabetes, obesity, and impaired renal function may all increase the risk of methotrexate-induced hepatic fibrosis. In most patients, the disease is subclinical and nonprogressive. The insidious development of fibrosis due to methotrexate means that routine tests of liver function are often normal and therefore unsuitable for patient monitoring. Instead, liver biopsy must be considered once the total dose exceeds 1.5 g. For patients receiving chronic treatment with methotrexate, both the need for and the timing of a liver biopsy is debated, however. The presence of significant disease on liver biopsy is considered a relative contraindication to continued use of the drug.

Methyldopa

As with isoniazid, patients taking methyldopa have minor, apparently inconsequential abnormalities in

liver function in up to 6% of cases. Clinically overt hepatotoxicity is much less common and usually presents as acute viral hepatitis or chronic hepatitis within 20 weeks after the drug is started. The Coombs' test is often positive but does not correlate with the occurrence of hepatic injury. Furthermore, clinical manifestations of drug hypersensitivity are unusual. Injury usually abates when the drug is discontinued, but full recovery may be delayed by months; progression to a fatal outcome despite discontinuation of the drug has been reported.

Penicillins

Penicillin G and ampicillin have little hepatotoxic potential. Amoxicillin is also considered safe, but when it is in combination with the β-lactamase inhibitor clavulanic acid (co-amoxyclav), its use has resulted in delayed cholestatic liver injury presenting up to several weeks after treatment has ended. Elderly males are most frequently affected. Jaundice is a consistent feature, and histologic studies of the liver show cholestasis with minimal necrosis or inflammation. Hypersensitivity manifestations are unusual. The clinical course has been benign in most cases, with complete recovery within 4–6 months. A less benign course has accompanied flucloxacillin treatment in some individuals. This drug appears to target the biliary epithelium selectively to produce a form of idiosyncratic cholestatic liver injury that has affected several hundred individuals to date. Older patients treated for longer than 2 weeks seem to be at particular risk, with the onset of jaundice and pruritus usually 1–3 weeks after cessation of therapy. Although resolution of clinical symptoms usually occurs within 2 months, abnormalities in serum liver enzymes may persist for months to years. In a minority of patients, the injury has pursued a progressive course characterized by bile duct damage and depletion of intralobular bile ducts (vanishing bile duct syndrome), with the ultimate development of secondary biliary cirrhosis over several years.

Phenytoin

This anticonvulsant has rarely been associated with a severe, viral hepatitis-like liver injury with pronounced hypersensitivity features. The onset is usual within 6 weeks of starting the drug and is characterized by malaise, fever, lymphadenopathy, and a striking rash. Leukocytosis, atypical lymphocytosis, and eosinophilia may be present. Histologic studies of the liver resemble acute viral hepatitis but with greater abundance of eosinophils. Progression to liver failure and death has ensued. In spite of the marked hypersensitivity features that characterize phenytoin hepatotoxicity, a toxic metabolite may participate in its pathogenesis. Phenytoin is partly converted in the liver to highly reactive arene oxides, and a genetically determined impairment in detoxifying these reactive intermediates may underlie individual susceptibility to hepatotoxicity.

Valproic Acid

This medium branched-chain fatty acid used principally in the treatment of petit mal epilepsy may produce hepatotoxicity that is fatal in about 1 in 800 children under the age of 2 years. Infants and young children are at appreciably higher risk. There is an incidence of 10–40% of transient, slight increases in serum aminotransferase levels after several weeks of therapy. Severe liver injury occurs more rarely, with clinical and histologic features reminiscent of Reye's syndrome, although with a greater frequency of jaundice. Histologically, the lesion is characterized by centrilobular necrosis, small-droplet fat infiltration, and bile duct injury. The mechanism of valproate-induced liver injury is uncertain, but available evidence suggests that a valproate metabolite impairs the mitochondrial oxidation of long-chain fatty acids possibly through the induction of L-carnitine deficiency. Underlying inherited abnormalities in mitochondrial β-oxidation or urea synthesis may predispose to this form of hepatotoxicity. Oral supplementation with L-carnitine of children at high risk for valproate hepatotoxicity and intravenous L-carnitine administration to patients with established valproate hepatotoxicity have been recommended.

ENVIRONMENTAL & INDUSTRIAL HEPATOTOXINS

Botanical Hepatotoxins

A diverse range of naturally occurring substances derived from plants or fungi may cause liver damage, usually in a dosage-dependent manner. These substances may be ingested in increasingly popular medicinal herbal teas or remedies (Table 44–6) or, as in the case of *Amanita* mushroom poisoning, accidentally ingested. *Amanita* species contain a variety of hepatotoxic cyclopeptides, including α-amanitine and phalloidin. The onset of symptoms is delayed for up to 24 hours after ingestion of the mushrooms, with abdominal pain and profuse watery diarrhea that may lead to profound dehydration being prominent initially. Over the subsequent 48 hours, gastrointestinal symptoms subside but liver test abnormalities become marked, with progression to fulminant hepatic failure. Liver transplantation has been life-saving in severe cases. Liver damage from *Amanita* mushroom poisoning is characterized by fatty change and zone 3 necrosis.

Table 44–6. Herbal and alternative remedies associated with liver injury.

Pyrrolizidine alkaloids
  Crotolaria
  Gordolobo herbal tea
  Heliotropium
  Mate (Paraquay) tea
  Senecio aureus
  Symphytum officinale (comfrey)
Chaparral leaf
Germander
Chelidonium majus (greater celandine)
Pennyroyal (squawmit oil)
Traditional Chinese herbs
  Jin Bu Huan
  Sho-saiko-to
Kava (rhizome of pepper plant)
Kombucha mushroom (tea)
Valerian root and skullcap
Mistletoe
Margosa oil
Senna fruit extracts
Asafetida
Cascara sagrada
Megavitamin A therapy
Shark cartilage
Hydrazine sulfate

Among hepatotoxic principals derived from plants, the pyrrolizidine alkaloids present in *Senecio*, *Heliotropium*, *Crotalaria*, and *Symphytum* (comfrey) species are the best known and have been responsible for outbreaks of venoocclusive disease, largely in developing countries. Poisoning with pyrrolizidine alkaloids may present acutely or more chronically, with features of hepatic venous outflow obstruction (ie, portal hypertension and ascites) and variable features of hepatocellular failure.

Herbal remedies are increasingly being recognized as potential hepatotoxins. In France, a number of cases of toxic hepatitis recurring on rechallenge have been attributed to drinking tea brewed from the wall germander *(Teucrium chamaedrys)*. The onset of symptoms has occurred 3–18 weeks after initial ingestion of this remedy, which has been taken for weight reduction. Jaundice has been common, with histologic features of hepatocellular necrosis, particularly in zone 3.

Industrial Hepatotoxins

Industrial solvents and other compounds used in the manufacturing industries have given rise to liver disease ranging from asymptomatic elevation of serum aminotransferase levels to fulminant hepatic failure and hepatic cancer. The best known and most extensively characterized of these compounds is carbon tetrachloride; its use has been abandoned because of its extreme hepatotoxic potential. Carbon tetrachloride is a classic, direct hepatotoxin, which produces a dosage-dependent hepatocellular necrosis most severe in zone 3. Other solvents that have been more recently implicated in cases of hepatotoxicity include 2-nitropropane, 1,1,1-trichloroethane, and dimethylformamide.

DIAGNOSIS & MANAGEMENT OF DRUG- & TOXIN-INDUCED LIVER INJURY

It is often difficult to establish a causal relationship between the use of a drug and a liver injury, because drugs may produce abnormalities similar to those of other common hepatic disorders. Also, hepatotoxicity often occurs in patients who are receiving multiple therapeutic agents. Because of the severity of hepatic damage and dysfunction that may accompany many types of drug-induced liver disease, early diagnosis is essential and will rely on a thorough drug history, including details of recent and past exposure to therapeutic agents. Exposure to hepatotoxic drugs in the form of combination over-the-counter and prescription formulations should not be overlooked. For example, severe hepatic necrosis can occur from acetaminophen contained in over-the-counter preparations such as Nyquil, or in combination with other analgesics such as hydrocodone, propoxyphene, and oxycodone. Details of the patient's occupation and work environment should be routinely obtained, and information about the use of herbal preparations and "traditional" medications should be sought. From a practical point of view, no histologic or clinical features specific for drug-induced liver disease exist, although zonal necrosis on liver biopsy is highly suggestive of a toxic cause. Accordingly, the diagnosis of drug-induced liver disease will ultimately depend upon a history of exposure, consistent clinical, laboratory, and, in select cases, liver biopsy findings, and resolution of the liver injury after the presumed toxin is discontinued. In instances where a single agent is involved, the diagnosis may be relatively straightforward. Conditions are far more complex when several drugs are being used. The role of a particular drug in the causation of idiosyncratic liver injury can often be established through rechallenge with the drug, but this is rarely justified because of the risk of severe or even fatal liver injury. Usually, it is not necessary to incriminate the responsible drug unambiguously by rechallenge, because alternative agents are often available. To facilitate the diagnosis of drug-induced hepatic injury, several groups have developed clinical scales for causality assessment. However, these potentially useful tools are yet to be prospectively validated.

The most important initial step in managing drug-induced liver disease is to discontinue the implicated drug, with supportive care of acute hepatitis and hepatic failure as required. In the case of severe drug-induced liver failure, urgent liver transplantation may be life-saving. Specific drug treatment is limited to the administration of acetylcysteine for acetaminophen overdosage. L-Carnitine is considered potentially valuable in the prevention and treatment of valproate toxicity. In general, corticosteroids have no established value in the treatment of drug-induced liver disease, although they may suppress the marked systemic hypersensitivity features associated with certain idiosyncratic reactions (eg, allopurinol, diclofenac, and azulfidine-induced liver disease). Management of protracted drug-induced cholestasis is similar to that for idiopathic chronic cholestatic liver diseases such as primary biliary cirrhosis. Basic principles of management include the alleviation of pruritus with cholestyramine, supplementation with fat-soluble vitamins, administration of ursodeoxycholic acid, and, ultimately, liver transplantation for cases that progress to secondary biliary cirrhosis.

REFERENCES

Aithal PG, Day CP: The natural history of histologically proved drug induced liver disease. Gut 1999;44:731.

Aithal GP, Rawlins MD, Day CP: Clinical diagnostic scale: a useful tool in the evaluation of suspected hepatotoxic adverse drug reactions. J Hepatol 2000;33:949.

Bass NM, Ockner RK: Drug-induced liver disease. In: *Hepatology: A Textbook of Liver Disease,* 3rd ed. Zakim D, Boyer TD (editors). Saunders, 1995.

Bessems JG, Vermeulen NP. Paracetamol (acetaminophen)-induced toxicity: molecular and biochemical mechanisms, analogues and protective approaches. Crit Rev Toxicol 2001; 31:55.

Bissell DM et al: Drug-induced liver injury: mechanisms and test systems. Hepatology 2001;33:1009.

Bissuel F et al: Fulminant hepatitis with severe lactic acidosis in HIV-infected patients on didanosine therapy. J Intern Med 1994;235:367.

Bjorkman D: Nonsteroidal antiinflammatory drug-associated toxicity of the liver, lower gastrointestinal tract, and esophagus. Am J Med 1998;105:17S.

Brackett CC, Bloch JD: Phenytoin as a possible cause of acetaminophen hepatotoxicity: case report and review of the literature. Pharmacotherapy 2000;20:229.

Buckley NA at el: Oral or intravenous N-acetylcysteine: which is the treatment of choice for acetaminophen (paracetamol) poisoning? J Toxicol Clin Toxicol 1999;37:759.

Caravati EM: Unintentional acetaminophen ingestion in children and the potential for hepatotoxicity. J Toxicol Clin Toxicol 2000;38:291.

Chitturi S, Farrell GC: Etiopathogenesis of nonalcoholic steatohepatitis. Semin Liv Dis 2001;21:27.

Clarke S et al: Late onset hepatitis and prolonged deterioration in hepatic function associated with nevirapine therapy. Int J Std AIDS 2000;11:336.

Davies MH et al: Antibiotic-associated acute vanishing bile duct syndrome: a pattern associated with severe, prolonged, intrahepatic cholestasis. J Hepatol 1994;20:112.

De Vivo DC et al: L-Carnitine supplementation in childhood epilepsy: current perspectives. Epilepsia 1998;39:1216.

Desmet VJ: Vanishing bile duct syndrome in drug-induced liver disease. J Hepatol 1997;26(Suppl 1):31.

Draganov P et al: Alcohol-acetaminophen syndrome. Even moderate social drinkers are at risk. Postgrad Med 2000;107:189.

Erlinger S: Drug-induced cholestasis. J Hepatol 1997;26(Suppl 1):1.

Farrell GC: *Drug-Induced Liver Disease.* Churchill-Livingstone, 1994.

Fontana RJ et al: Acute liver failure associated with prolonged use of bromfenac leading to liver transplantation. The Acute Liver Failure Study Group. Liver Transplant Surg 1999;5:480.

Forman LM, Simmons DA, Diamond RH: Hepatic failure in a patient taking rosiglitazone. Ann Intern Med 2000;132:118.

Kaplowitz N: Causality assessment versus guilt-by-association in drug hepatotoxicity.[Editorial]. Hepatology 2001;33:308.

Kim BK et al: Liver disease during the first post-transplant year in bone marrow transplantation recipients: retrospective study. BMT 2000;26:193.

Konig SA et al: Fatal liver failure associated with valproate therapy in a patient with Friedreich's disease: review of valproate hepatotoxicity in adults. Epilepsia 1999;40:1036.

Larrey D: Drug-induced liver diseases. J Hepatol 2000;32 (Suppl 1):77.

Larrey D, Pageaux GP: Genetic predisposition to drug-induced hepatotoxicity. J Hepatol 1997;26(Suppl 2):12.

Lee WM: Assessing causality in drug-induced liver injury. (Editorial) J Hepatol 2000;33:1003.

Lewis JH: Drug-induced liver disease. Med Clin North Am 2000; 84:1275.

Makin A, Williams R: Paracetamol hepatotoxicity and alcohol consumption in deliberate and accidental overdose. Q J Med 2000;93:341.

McClain CJ et al: Acetaminophen hepatotoxicity: an update. Curr Gastroenterol Rep 1999;1:42.

Murphy EJ et al: Troglitazone-induced fulminant hepatic failure. Acute Liver Failure Study Group. Dig Dis Sci 2000;45:549.

O'Donohue J et al: Co-amoxiclav jaundice: clinical and histological features and HLA class II association. Gut 2000;47:717.

Ohno M et al: Slow N-acetyltransferase 2 genotype affects the incidence of isoniazid and rifampicin-induced hepatotoxicity. Int J Tuberculosis Lung Dis 2000;4:256.

Perry MC: Chemotherapeutic agents and hepatotoxicity. Semin Oncol 1992;19:551.

Pessayre D et al: Hepatotoxicity due to mitochondrial dysfunction. Cell Biol Toxicol 1999;15:367.

Raskind JY, El-Chaar GM: The role of carnitine supplementation during valproic acid therapy. Ann Pharmacother 2000;34: 630.

Schiodt FV et al: Acetaminophen toxicity in an urban county hospital. N Engl J Med 1997;337:1112.

Seeff LB et al: Complementary and alternative medicine in chronic liver disease. Hepatology 2001;34:595.

Selim K, Kaplowitz N: Hepatotoxicity of psychotropic drugs. Hepatology 1999;29:1347.

Shah RR: Drug-induced hepatotoxicity: pharmacokinetic perspectives and strategies for risk reduction. Adverse Drug React Toxicol Rev 1999;18:181.

Tolman KG: Defining patient risks from expanded preventive therapies. Am J Cardiol 2000;85:15E.

Wong WM et al: Antituberculosis drug-related liver dysfunction in chronic hepatitis B infection. Hepatology 2000;31:201.

Zimmerman HJ: Drug-induced liver disease. Clin Liver Dis 2000; 4:73.

The Liver in Systemic Disease

45

Adil Habib, MD & Brent A. Neuschwander-Tetri, MD

The liver is commonly involved in systemic diseases or diseases that primarily affect other organ systems because of its central role in the body's metabolic and immunologic functions. This involvement can vary from trivial to substantial, and the spectrum of the clinical sequelae can range from minor pathologic findings to life-threatening liver dysfunction. An awareness of the hepatic manifestions of systemic disease is essential for recognizing and appropriately evaluating liver abnormalities that develop in patients with systemic disease.

The liver handles a wide variety of metabolic stresses. It is exposed to the mesenteric blood flow, which is not only enriched with physiologic fuels and metabolic precursors but is also laden with potentially antigenic food components, ingested toxins, and potentially toxic metabolites generated by the colonic flora. To handle some of these products, active scavenging by resident hepatic macrophages, the Kupffer cells, is an essential component of the immune system. Like many macrophages, Kupffer cells may release potent cytotoxic agents, and these factors have the capacity to injure neighboring hepatocytes and the vascular endothelium of the liver.

The unique circulatory anatomy of the liver accounts, in part, for its response to systemic disease. The low sinusoidal hydrostatic pressure within the liver prevents the loss of massive quantities of fluid through the fenestrated hepatic endothelium into the perisinusoidal space of Disse. The endothelial fenestrations allow intimate contact between hepatocytes and circulating plasma proteins such as albumin, the protein that transports fatty acids from peripheral adipose tissue to the liver. Although the fenestrated vascular endothelium is essential for the normal function of the liver, this high-capacitance, low-pressure vascular tree makes the liver particularly sensitive to conditions that obstruct blood flow anywhere between the hepatic central vein and the left ventricle.

Although the liver is complex in its functions, this organ is limited in its phenotypic response to injury or metabolic abnormalities (Table 45–1). Whereas most liver abnormalities are potentially reversible if effective therapy for the underlying disorder is applied, the extreme consequence of sustained liver injury, cirrhosis (severe fibrosis with regenerative nodules), is usually irreversible (see Chapter 43). Therefore, the management of patients with liver abnormalities as a consequence of extrahepatic diseases should focus on preventing irreversible liver injury while treating the underlying disease.

CHOLESTASIS OF SEPSIS

ESSENTIALS OF DIAGNOSIS

- *Elevations of serum bilirubin (usually 5–15 mg/dL) and alkaline phosphatase (up to three times the upper limit of normal) occur in the setting of many bacterial infections.*
- *The diagnosis is confirmed by negative imaging of the biliary tract and improvement following treatment of the underlying infection.*
- *Liver biopsy is generally not needed to establish the diagnosis.*

General Considerations

Systemic bacterial infections, especially those caused by gram-negative bacteria and pneumococcus, cause intrahepatic cholestasis. The mechanism of cholestasis is impaired hepatocellular transport at the sinusoidal and canalicular membranes mediated by the cytokine tumor necrosis factor-α (TNF-α), endotoxin, or other factors. The onset of cholestasis can sometimes precede the diagnosis of bacterial infection.

Clinical Findings

A. SYMPTOMS AND SIGNS

The cholestasis is generally asymptomatic other than the development of jaundice. Pruritus, a feature of other cholestatic syndromes, has not been described as a major feature of the cholestasis of sepsis.

B. LABORATORY FINDINGS

The serum bilirubin is typically 5–15 mg/dL but can be elevated as high as 30 mg/dL. Fractionation demonstrates that it is primarily conjugated hyperbilirubine-

Table 45–1. Limited major phenotypic expressions of liver injury.

Extracellular matrix alterations	Fibrosis, cirrhosis
Hepatocellular changes	Steatosis, ballooning
	Atrophy
	Necrosis
Bile duct changes	Atrophy
	Proliferation
Inflammatory changes	Granulomas
	Lymphocytic infiltration
	Neutrophilic infiltration
Vascular changes	Sinusoidal dilatation
	Endophlebitis

mia. Serum alkaline phosphatase levels can be elevated up to three times the upper limit of normal. Aminotransferases typically remain normal or are only mildly elevated, up to two times the upper limit of normal. The bilirubin and alkaline phosphatase levels gradually normalize following effective treatment of the underlying infection.

C. LIVER BIOPSY

The diagnosis is usually established on clinical grounds and a biopsy is generally not needed. When a biopsy is obtained, it most often demonstrates relatively bland cholestasis with minimal inflammation or cellular injury.

Differential Diagnosis

Bacterial cholangitis must be considered in the patient with jaundice and bacteremia or sepsis. Biliary tract obstruction should be excluded by appropriate imaging [ultrasonography, computed tomography (CT), or magnetic resonance (MR) cholangiography as is clinically indicated]. The diagnosis is further confirmed by observing gradual improvement following appropriate antibiotic therapy. In the critically ill hospitalized patient, drug-induced cholestasis is often a consideration. When possible, drugs commonly associated with cholestasis should be withdrawn.

Complications

The cholestasis of sepsis is generally a relatively benign process without specific complications.

Treatment & Prognosis

Treatment is directed to the underlying infectious process. In the case of undrained abscesses, surgical drainage in addition to appropriate antibiotics is neces-

sary. The prognosis is guarded if the underlying infectious process is not recognized and treated in a timely manner.

Franson TR, Hierholzer WJ, LaBrecque DR: Frequency and characteristics of hyperbilirubinemia associated with bacteremia. Rev Infect Dis 1985;7:1.

Moseley RH: Sepsis-associated cholestasis. Gastroenterology 1997: 112:302.

CARDIAC DISEASE

1. Low-Flow States & Shock Liver

 ESSENTIALS OF DIAGNOSIS

- A sudden rise in serum aminotransferases after a period of systemic hypotension, followed by rapid normalization after restoration of normal perfusion.

- Recurrent transient increases of serum aminotransferases that correlate with episodes of poor systemic perfusion in the patient with marginal left ventricular function.

- Concomitant ischemic injury of the kidneys and central nervous system after a prolonged period of hypotension.

General Considerations

Although the liver is relatively protected from ischemic injury by virtue of its dual blood supply, acute low-flow states caused by hemorrhagic or cardiogenic shock can cause ischemic liver injury. After an isolated episode of hypoperfusion severe enough to cause liver injury, evidence of renal and central nervous system ischemic injury are usually seen as well. In the patient with marginal left ventricular output and evidence of ischemic liver injury, altered mental status and evidence of renal insufficiency are usually evident. Acute left heart failure in a patient with long-standing right heart failure is also a classic setting for the development of ischemic liver injury.

Clinical Findings

A. SYMPTOMS AND SIGNS

The symptoms and signs are usually dominated by sequelae outside of the liver such as altered mentation and hypotension. The presence of stigmata of chronic liver disease suggests preexisting liver disease.

B. LABORATORY FINDINGS

Serum aminotransferase levels may rise to more than 100 times the upper limit of normal with severe ischemic liver injury. With injury of this severity, the prothrombin time will be elevated and the bilirubin levels will rise 1–5 days after the insult. With less severe injury, the aminotransferase elevations will be less pronounced yet characteristic in the rapidity with which they rise after the initial insult (over 1–2 days). Typical of ischemic injury is the rapid normalization of aminotransferases that follows the restoration of adequate perfusion. Only after toxin-induced liver injury (eg, acetaminophen) or passage of a gallstone is such prompt normalization of aminotransferase levels also seen. This prompt improvement in the elevations of the aspartate aminotransferase (AST) and alanine aminotransferase (ALT) corresponds to the rapid elimination rate of circulating aminotransferases ($t_{1/2}$ of serum AST, 12–24 hours; $t_{1/2}$ of serum ALT, 36–48 hours). Because ALT has a longer circulating half-life, the ALT level is typically greater than the AST level during the recovery phase.

C. LIVER BIOPSY

The rapid improvement in serum aminotransferases after resolution of the precipitating event allows the diagnosis of ischemic injury to be made on a clinical basis, and biopsy is rarely, if ever, needed. Persistent aminotransferase elevations should raise the possibility of ongoing injury due to other causes such as viral hepatitis, drug toxicity, or autoimmune hepatitis.

Differential Diagnosis

Dramatic, acute elevations of aminotransferases greater than 2000 U/L are caused by a limited number of insults to the liver. The five major causes are viral hepatitis (hepatitis A, B, D, and E), autoimmune hepatitis, drugs/toxins, ischemia, and transient biliary obstruction caused by passage of a gallstone. Prompt resolution of aminotransferase elevations does not occur during the resolution of acute infectious hepatitis. Therefore, the diagnosis of ischemic hepatitis is confidently based on the clinical setting and the rate at which the enzyme elevations improve.

Complications

The remarkable regenerative capacity of the liver promotes the return to normal liver function after a substantial acute ischemic insult. Irreversible hepatic necrosis is unusual, and death in the setting of ischemic liver usually occurs from multiorgan failure. Because the injury is typically transient, significant coagulopathy caused by impaired synthetic function of the liver rarely develops.

Treatment & Prognosis

Optimization of cardiac output and removal of precipitants to hypoperfusion, where possible, are the required treatments for ischemic liver injury. When recurrent hepatic ischemia is caused by severe left ventricular failure, efforts to reduce cardiac afterload pharmacologically can further compromise organ perfusion and thus perpetuate ongoing liver injury, as evidenced by persistently fluctuating aminotransferase elevations. When this happens, the outlook is poor, unless definitive therapy for the failing heart can be provided. On the other hand, potentially avoidable liver injury caused by other factors such as drugs should be considered when the aminotransferase elevations persist despite well-preserved cardiac function.

2. Congestive Hepatopathy

 ESSENTIALS OF DIAGNOSIS

- *Jugular venous distention is a key examination finding.*
- *Hepatomegaly and ascites can develop.*
- *Jaundice can develop with a normal or near normal alkaline phosphatase measurement.*

General Considerations

Congestive hepatopathy can present in any patient with impeded blood flow across the heart. The specific predisposing conditions include constrictive pericarditis, tricuspid insufficiency, severe right ventricular failure, cor pulmonale, mitral stenosis, and severe left ventricular failure. In patients with left ventricular failure, a mixed picture of hepatic congestion and a low-flow state leading to ischemic liver injury can be present (see preceding section). Unrecognized chronic congestion of the liver may in some circumstances lead to cirrhosis ("cardiac cirrhosis"), although this sequela is rarely observed in current clinical practice.

Clinical Findings

A. SYMPTOMS AND SIGNS

Patients will occasionally complain of aching right upper quadrant pain, likely due to stretching of the liver capsule (Table 45–2). Those with severe left ventricular failure often have prominent symptoms of pulmonary vascular congestion (eg, orthopnea). Hepatomegaly is a frequent but not essential finding. Jugular venous distention is an important physical finding that suggests congestive hepatopathy as an explanation of bilirubin and liver enzyme elevations. This physical finding is especially important in the patient without recognized heart disease who presents with jaundice or ascites and may have constrictive pericarditis. Manual pressure on the distended liver during physical examination can measurably increase the jugular venous pressure (hepatojugular reflex), although this finding does not imply that the liver is pathologically congested. Ascites may be present and reflects the elevated sinusoidal pressure within the liver.

B. Laboratory Findings

Bilirubin levels and prothrombin time are typically elevated out of proportion to the true degree of liver dysfunction. Additionally, a normal or only minimally elevated alkaline phosphatase measurement helps to differentiate hyperbilirubinemia caused by hepatic congestion from biliary obstruction (see Chapter 33). Fluctuating aminotransferase elevations suggest intermittent underperfusion causing episodic ischemic injury. Evaluation of ascitic fluid demonstrates a high serum to ascites albumin gradient (serum albumin minus ascites albumin >1.1 g/dL), a finding characteristic of portal hypertension. Yet, the total protein concentration is high (>2.5 g/dL), a finding that is unusual in chronic liver disease (see Chapter 43). A low protein concentration of both serum and ascites suggests the progression of congestive hepatopathy to cirrhosis with concomitant impaired liver synthetic function. Other causes of liver disease must be excluded routinely during the evaluation of ascites; in patients with congestive heart failure, diagnostic considerations include genetic hemochromatosis as well as viral hepatitis and other less common causes of chronic liver disease.

C. Liver Biopsy

The diagnosis of congestive hepatopathy is usually established on clinical grounds without the need for liver biopsy. The patient undergoing evaluation for heart transplantation may require liver biopsy, however, to rule out otherwise silent cirrhosis, which would adversely affect the likelihood of a successful transplant outcome. Grossly, the liver has a "nutmeg" appearance because of the pericentral congestion. Histologically, sinusoidal dilatation and congestion are evident, accompanied by atrophy of the hepatocyte cords.

Treatment

Treatment of the underlying cause of the hepatic congestion is indicated when possible. For the patient with heart failure, this usually includes afterload reduction and use of inotropes and diuretics. Recognizing constrictive pericarditis as a cause of congestive hepatopathy can lead to definitive treatment, which may save the liver from permanent damage. Similarly, correcting severe valvular dysfunction can alleviate hepatic congestion and avoid further liver injury.

Prognosis

The prognosis is determined by the severity of the underlying cardiac disease. Because an elevated prothrombin time and the presence of jaundice do not necessarily imply end-stage liver disease, these findings should not preclude definitive surgical correction of the responsible cardiac abnormality.

Table 45–2. Clinical features of congestive hepatopathy and ischemic liver injury.

	Congestive Hepatopathy	Ischemia
Clinical setting	Blood flow obstruction between right atrium and aorta	Systolic hypotension
Symptoms	Right upper quadrant pain	
Signs	Jugular venous distention; hepatomegaly; ascites; lower extremity edema	Altered mentation due to CNS hypoperfusion
Laboratory findings	Elevated bilirubin, elevated prothrombin time alkaline phosphatase and aminotransferase < four times upper limit of normal	Rapid rise and fall of aminotransferases

Arcidi JM, Gorre GW, Hutchins GM: Hepatic morphology in cardiac dysfunction: a clinicopathologic study of 1000 subjects at autopsy. Am J Pathol 1981;104:159.

Dunn GD et al: The liver in congestive heart failure: a review. Am J Med Sci 1973;265:174.

Runyon BA: Cardiac ascites: a characterization. J Clin Gastroenterol 1988;10:410.

BUDD–CHIARI SYNDROME

 ESSENTIALS OF DIAGNOSIS

- *Disease can develop acutely or chronically.*
- *Acute progression is characterized by right upper quadrant pain, hepatomegaly, and ascites.*
- *Indolent progression is characterized by the development of ascites, varices, jaundice, and liver failure.*
- *Imaging of hepatic blood flow is needed to confirm the diagnosis.*
- *Liver biopsy is helpful to establish the severity of liver injury and guide therapy.*

General Considerations

Hepatic congestion can occur with obstruction of blood flow at any level from the centrilobular vein to the aortic valve. Budd–Chiari syndrome should be thought of as obstructed venous blood flow between the hepatic venules and the right atrium; congestive hepatopathy (arbitrarily) connotes obstruction from the right atrium to the aortic valve with transmission of elevated pressure back to the liver. By comparison, the term hepatic venoocclusive disease is used to describe the nonthrombotic occlusion of central veins and their immediate tributaries within the liver. Venoocclusive disease will cause many of the hepatic manifestations also seen with congestive hepatopathy and Budd–Chiari syndrome, but because it has its own set of predisposing conditions, it differs clinically in its course and response to therapy (see Chapter 49).

Pathophysiology

Budd–Chiari syndrome is a disease with many similarities to congestive hepatopathy in its hepatic manifestations but a different pathogenesis and spectrum of predisposing diseases. Whereas congestive hepatopathy classically describes venous congestion transmitted from the cava and right atrium, Budd–Chiari syndrome is a disease of intrahepatic venous congestion caused by obstruction of blood flow within the liver. Truly a syndrome rather than a specific disease, this disorder can result from obstruction of either large- or small-caliber veins. Recognized predisposing factors are numerous but can be categorized as thrombophilic, mechanical, infectious, or related to a variety of other diseases that lead to obstruction of hepatic venous outflow (Table 45–3). Myeloproliferative disorders and their treat-

Table 45–3. Predisposing factors to venous outflow obstruction (Budd-Chiari syndrome).

Hypercoagulable states
  Myeloproliferative disorders
  Polycythemia vera
  Oral contraceptives
  Postpartum status
  Paroxysmal nocturnal hemoglobinuria
  Lupus anticoagulant
  Antithrombin III deficiency
  Protein C deficiency
  Essential thrombocytosis
Mechanical disorders
  Membranous septae
  Congenital abnormalities of hepatic venous system
  Tumors: renal cell carcinoma, hepatocellular carcinoma, Wilms' tumor, adrenal carcinoma, leiomyosarcoma
  Infections: amebic abscess, hydatid cysts, aspergillosis
  Adult polycystic disease
Collagen vascular diseases
  Systemic lupus erythematosus
  Mixed connective tissue disease
  Sjögren's syndrome
  Behçet's disease
Miscellaneous
  Ulcerative colitis
  Syphilis
  α_1-Antitrypsin deficiency
  Sarcoidosis
  Trauma

ments account for about a third of cases. Recently, a polymorphism of the coagulation factor V (factor V Leiden mutation) has been associated with hypercoagulability and the development of Budd–Chiari syndrome. One of the mechanical causes of hepatic vein thrombosis is the presence of hepatic vein webs. These may be acquired in origin following abdominal trauma with subclinical injury to the attachment of the liver to the inferior vena cava at the cava–hepatic vein junction.

Clinical Findings

A. SYMPTOMS AND SIGNS

The presentation of hepatic vein thrombosis is highly variable. Whereas some patients may present with asymptomatic hepatomegaly and slowly accumulating ascites, others present with fulminant liver failure. The difference is thought to depend on the time course of venous obstruction, the development of compensatory collateral blood flow, and the degree of acute hepatocyte injury. Right upper quadrant abdominal pain and hepatomegaly are characteristic of Budd–Chiari syndrome and should prompt further investigation. The absence of jugular venous distention is a key finding that differentiates it from congestive hepatopathy (see the preceding section). Ascites is frequently present and may contribute to abdominal pain and a sensation of fullness. The presence of severe lower extremity edema and distended abdominal veins suggests concomitant obstruction of the inferior vena cava. Hepatic encephalopathy is a terminal manifestation.

B. LABORATORY FINDINGS

The alkaline phosphatase and aminotransferase levels may be elevated (more than 10 times the upper limit). The bilirubin levels and prothrombin time are elevated with progression of disease to severe liver injury. Analysis of the ascites would be expected to reveal a difference between serum and ascites albumin of more than 1.1 g/dL, although this has not been directly demonstrated in clinical studies.

C. IMAGING STUDIES

Establishing the patency of the hepatic venous outflow is the cornerstone of diagnosing Budd–Chiari syndrome. Absence of blood flow in the hepatic veins is usually evident by ultrasonography. Some patients exhibit reversal of flow through the portal vein because of retrograde egress of hepatic arterial blood out of the liver through the portal vein into collaterals. Pulsed doppler ultrasound is currently the best diagnostic imaging modality because of its 85% sensitivity in identifying hepatic vein thrombosis. Magnetic resonance imaging (MRI) can also be used to assess hepatic blood flow. Dynamic abdominal CT scanning with intravenous contrast material will show delayed drainage of contrast material from involved sections of the liver and can reveal rapid drainage from the caudate lobe, which has direct venous connections to the inferior vena cava. The uninvolved venous drainage of the caudate lobe may lead to caudate lobe hypertrophy. When these indirect measures of hepatic blood flow are equivocal, retrograde hepatic angiography can be performed to directly assess the localization and extent of venous outflow obstruction.

D. LIVER BIOPSY

Liver biopsy can help establish the severity of liver injury and guide the therapeutic approach. Centrilobular sinusoidal dilatation occurs early in the disease and may not be uniform throughout the liver. Similar to congestive hepatopathy, hepatocyte atrophy is present and can progress to the point of complete dropout of cell plates surrounding the central vein. Congestion of sinusoids with blood and accumulation of red cells within the subendothelial space confirm the presence of congestion and differentiate the lesion from other causes of sinusoidal dilatation. Organized thrombus within central

veins and sublobular veins can also be seen in about one-half of the cases and distinguishes Budd–Chiari syndrome from congestive hepatopathy. Late in the disease, progression to cirrhosis is evident, with extensive fibrosis involving the centrilobular regions.

Differential Diagnosis

There is nothing in the clinical presentation and no changes in serum biochemical findings that are specific for Budd–Chiari syndrome. The approach to the patient with right upper quadrant pain, hepatomegaly, and modestly elevated liver enzymes should include evaluation of the common infectious and metabolic causes of liver disease (see Chapter 33). A high index of suspicion for this disease is required to guide the diagnostic evaluation to the correct conclusion. The diagnosis is typically established by imaging studies to assess blood flow and a liver biopsy when the absence of significant coagulopathy or ascites permits.

Complications

Patients with acutely developing Budd–Chiari syndrome can succumb rapidly to liver failure. Those with a more indolent form of the disease can develop esophageal varices, hepatic encephalopathy, and the hepatorenal syndrome. None of these complications is an impediment to liver transplantation.

Treatment

Treatment of Budd–Chiari syndrome is tailored to the specific cause, if one can be identified, and reestablishment of hepatic venous outflow. This can be accomplished in some patients by radiologic or surgical techniques. The best treatment approach depends on the severity of liver disease and the patency of the inferior vena cava and portal vein. Anticoagulation may prevent the progression of disease when it is detected early in its course. When the patient's symptoms are related to portal hypertension rather than liver insufficiency, decompression of the liver vasculature can be accomplished surgically and, in selected patients, by transjugular intrahepatic portosystemic shunting (TIPS). When liver insufficiency dominates the clinical picture, liver transplantation should be considered as an option. Anticoagulation therapy following transplantation may be required in these patients to prevent recurrence of the disease.

Prognosis

Without definitive therapy, most symptomatic patients with Budd–Chiari syndrome will die of liver failure or its complications within months to several years after diagnosis. Asymptomatic patients diagnosed during evaluation of liver enzyme abnormalities develop significant functional vascular collaterals and have a much better outlook.

Asherson RA, Khamashta MA, Hughes GRV: The hepatic complications of the antiphospholipid antibodies. Clin Exp Rheum 1991;9:341.

Dilawari JB et al: Hepatic outflow obstruction (Budd-Chiari syndrome): experience with 177 patients and a review of the literature. Medicine 1994;73:21.

Hadengue A et al: The changing scene of hepatic vein thrombosis: recognition of asymptomatic cases. Gastroenterology 1994; 106:1042.

Knoop M et al: Treatment of the Budd-Chiari syndrome with orthotopic liver transplantation and long-term anticoagulation. Clin Transplant 1994;8:67.

Kohli V et al: Management of hepatic venous outflow obstruction. Lancet 1993;342:718.

SARCOIDOSIS

ESSENTIALS OF DIAGNOSIS

- *Noncaseating granulomas on liver biopsy.*
- *Elevated serum angiotensin-converting enzyme activity is usually present.*
- *Negative antimitochondrial antibody.*
- *Exclusion of drugs and other causes of granulomatous disease.*

General Considerations

Pulmonary disease typically predominates in the patient with sarcoidosis. Liver involvement is found in most patients (60–95%) and is characterized by noncaseating epithelioid granulomas primarily in portal tracts and sometimes in the liver parenchyma. These are rarely significant in terms of liver function or impedance to blood flow. Chronic intrahepatic cholestasis, portal hypertension, and cirrhosis are uncommon complications, each being found in less than 1% of patients with sarcoidosis. The syndrome of chronic cholestasis that occurs in some patients shares numerous features with primary biliary cirrhosis, including progression to biliary cirrhosis over several decades. Because of this similarity, primary biliary cirrhosis should be excluded by measuring the antimitochondrial antibody titer. This titer is normal in patients having sarcoidosis but is elevated in 95% of patients with primary biliary cirrhosis (see Chapter 51).

Pathophysiology

Sarcoidosis is a systemic disease of unknown etiology manifested by noncaseating granulomas involving lymph nodes, lungs, liver, heart, and many other organs.

Clinical Findings

A. SYMPTOMS AND SIGNS

Active sarcoidosis manifested by fever and arthralgias is predictive of liver involvement, although the involvement is usually asymptomatic. In rare cases, portal hypertension manifested as ascites and esophageal varices has been documented. Similarly, significant cholestasis with jaundice and pruritus is an unusual complication that can develop. None of the signs and symptoms is specific for sarcoidosis, and the diagnosis is based on laboratory and histologic findings.

B. LABORATORY FINDINGS

Hyperglobulinemia and elevations in serum alkaline phosphatase levels (up to 25 times normal) are commonly present in hepatic sarcoidosis. The aminotransferases can be moderately elevated (up to five times the upper limit) in sarcoidosis, but synthetic function is preserved, as indicated by a normal prothrombin time. Serum angiotensin-converting enzyme levels are often elevated in other granulomatous and nongranulomatous conditions. During the treatment of sarcoidosis, serial measurements can help assess the response to therapy and predict disease relapse.

C. IMAGING STUDIES

The liver on CT scanning is typically unremarkable. In 10% of patients, intrahepatic nodules and hepatomegaly may be seen. Intrahepatic hypodense nodules on CT imaging must be distinguished from malignant lesions and abscesses based on the clinical setting and sometimes invasive testing.

D. LIVER BIOPSY

The granulomas of sarcoidosis are typically found in the portal tracts, although they can also be found throughout the parenchyma. Bile duct injury should suggest primary biliary cirrhosis (PBC), although an unusual variant of hepatic sarcoidosis can cause progressive bile duct loss. Sarcoidosis may coexist with PBC and, less often, with primary sclerosing cholangitis.

Differential Diagnosis

Although sarcoidosis is one of the most common causes of hepatic granulomas, a large number of other diseases can also be responsible for granulomas observed on liver biopsy (see Chapter 36). Thus, the diagnosis of hepatic sarcoidosis is based on establishing sarcoid involvement of other organs and excluding other causes of hepatic granulomas. Symptomatic sarcoidosis rarely involves the liver without extrahepatic disease and, when it does, firmly establishing the diagnosis can be problematic.

Treatment

Because liver complications of sarcoidosis are unusual, therapy with corticosteroids is generally reserved for active sarcoidosis involving other organs (eg, pulmonary sarcoidosis) but is not indicated for asymptomatic hepatic involvement. Despite resolution of systemic symptoms, hepatic granulomas remain after corticosteroid therapy.

Prognosis

Because functionally significant liver disease attributable to sarcoidosis is rare, the prognosis of patients is usually determined by the extent of other organ involvement and the response to corticosteroid therapy. Patients with portal hypertension due to cirrhosis have irreversible structural changes within the liver and are unlikely to have improved liver function following treatment with corticosteroids. In such patients, liver transplantation should be considered as a treatment option. The outcome of liver transplantation is not adversely affected by sarcoidosis.

Hercules DM, Bethlem NM: Value of liver biopsy in sarcoidosis. Arch Pathol Lab Med 1984;108:831.

James DG, Sherlock S: Sarcoidosis of the liver. Sarcoidosis 1994; 11:2.

Murphy JR et al: Small bile duct abnormalities in sarcoidosis. J Clin Gastroenterol 1990;12:555.

Pereira-Lima J, Schaffner F: Chronic cholestasis in hepatic sarcoidosis with clinical features resembling primary biliary cirrhosis: report of two cases. Am J Med 1987;83:144.

Valla D et al: Hepatic sarcoidosis with portal hypertension: a report of seven cases with a review of the literature. Q J Med 1987; 63:531.

Warshauer DM et al: Abdominal CT findings in sarcoidosis: radiologic and clinical correlation. Radiology 1994;192:93.

ULCERATIVE COLITIS & CROHN'S DISEASE

ESSENTIALS OF DIAGNOSIS

- *Aminotransferase elevations in patients with inflammatory bowel disease are not specific and deserve evaluation looking for other causes of liver injury.*

- *An elevated alkaline phosphatase level should prompt the evaluation for primary sclerosing cholangitis or cholangiocarcinoma.*

- *Jaundice and symptomatic liver dysfunction suggest cirrhosis, primary sclerosing cholangitis, choledocholithiasis, or liver diseases that are unrelated to inflammatory bowel disease.*

General Considerations

Hepatic manifestations of varying severity can be found in nearly all patients with ulcerative colitis and Crohn's disease at the time of autopsy. Clinically evident biochemical abnormalities are much less common and warrant further evaluation when detected. The presence of hepatic abnormalities in patients with ulcerative colitis and Crohn's disease is unrelated to the severity or duration of inflammatory bowel disease. Nonetheless, in those patients who do have liver involvement, biochemical evidence of liver injury can fluctuate in parallel with disease activity.

Pathophysiology

The major hepatobiliary complications of inflammatory bowel disease are listed in Table 45–4. The pathophysiology of these liver abnormalities remains unclear. A postulated role for abnormal permeability of the inflamed gut mucosa and exposure of the liver to toxic bacterial products has been proposed. However, the development of the most important complication, primary sclerosing cholangitis, despite disease remission or surgical colectomy, suggests that other etiologic factors play a role (see Chapter 51). A primary defect in cellular immunity may predispose the epithelia of the gut, biliary tract, and liver to damage by unregulated inflammation and thus explain the independent development of disease in these tissues.

Clinical Findings

A. SYMPTOMS AND SIGNS

Most patients with inflammatory bowel disease are asymptomatic from the standpoint of liver disease. The presence of jaundice or pruritus suggests primary sclerosing cholangitis, although biliary obstruction from gallstones or the development of cholangiocarcinoma must also be considered. Hepatomegaly and splenomegaly can be found but are unusual. Progression of sclerosing cholangitis to cirrhosis is characterized by worsening jaundice and the development of portal hypertension with ascites and esophageal varices. Fever, rigors, and right upper quadrant pain may signal bacte-

Table 45–4. Prevalence of hepatobiliary complications of inflammatory bowel disease.

	Ulcerative Colitis	Crohn's Disease
Primary sclerosing cholangitis	5–10%[1]	< 1%[2]
Cholangiocarcinoma[3]	< 1%[4]	< 1%[4]
Hepatic steatosis	6%	4%
Chronic hepatitis[5]	?	?
Cirrhosis[5]	< 1%	< 1%
Gallstones	—	< 1%[6]
Hepatic granulomas	—	< 1%[7]
Amyloidosis	—	< 1%[7]
Liver abscess	Rare	Rare

[1]In patients with primary sclerosing cholangitis, ulcerative cholitis can be found in 90%, although it may be clinically quiescent.
[2]Ten percent of patients with primary sclerosing cholangitis have Crohn's disease.
[3]Cholangiocarcinoma occurs only in the presence of primary sclerosing cholangitis.
[4]Cholangiocarcinoma develops in 10% of patients with primary sclerosing cholangitis.
[5]The prevalence of chronic hepatitis and cirrhosis in inflammatory bowel disease is unknown when hepatitis C is excluded as a cause.
[6]Significant ileal disease or ileal resection is a risk factor for developing gallstones.
[7]Complication can regress with resection of involved bowel.

rial cholangitis in the patient with sclerosing cholangitis or the development of a liver abscess in the patient with Crohn's disease. Cholangitis is particularly common if there has been previous surgical revision of the biliary tract or recent ductal manipulation during cholangiography.

B. LABORATORY FINDINGS

Mild elevations of the serum aminotransferases and alkaline phosphatase commonly occur in both ulcerative colitis and Crohn's disease. These are often sequelae of malnutrition, sepsis, fatty liver, or administration of total parenteral nutrition. Rigorous evaluation of other causes of chronic hepatitis should always be undertaken with the first presentation of biochemical evidence of liver disease in the patient with inflammatory bowel disease to exclude drug reactions, viral hepatitis, and metabolic causes as contributing factors. An elevated alkaline phosphatase level suggests sclerosing cholangitis, although this biochemical marker can be normal in the early stages of primary sclerosing cholangitis. Hyperbilirubinemia should also raise the possibility of sclerosing cholangitis, although end-stage liver disease or other

types of liver disease such as drug toxicity from sulfasalazine or viral hepatitis must be excluded.

C. IMAGING STUDIES

Primary sclerosing cholangitis is diagnosed by visualization of the intrahepatic and extrahepatic bile ducts, generally by endoscopic retrograde cholangiopancreatography (ERCP), revealing bile duct strictures and beaded dilatations. Distinguishing between the benign strictures of primary sclerosing cholangitis and early cholangiocarcinoma can prove difficult radiologically. Brush cytologic studies of the biliary tract obtained at the time of ERCP are helpful.

D. LIVER BIOPSY

Over one-half of all patients with inflammatory bowel disease have abnormal liver biopsies. **Macrovesicular fatty liver (steatosis)** is a common finding when bowel disease is active and there is biochemical evidence of liver disease (ie, elevated aminotransferase, alkaline phosphatase, or bilirubin levels). **Varying degrees of inflammation** characterized by portal and lobular infiltrates with mononuclear inflammatory cells have been described in patients with inflammatory bowel disease, although concomitant hepatitis C was not excluded in older studies. The diagnosis of primary sclerosing cholangitis is confirmed by imaging of the bile ducts (see preceding section) because there are no pathognomonic findings of this disorder on liver biopsy. **Pericholangitis** is an outmoded term once commonly used to describe the inflammatory cells within the portal triad in patients in Crohn's disease and ulcerative colitis as well as other intraabdominal inflammatory processes. **Bile duct proliferation** is common, as it is in any chronic portal-based inflammatory process. Intrahepatic bile duct cell injury is not a feature of inflammatory bowel disease, and its presence suggests primary biliary cirrhosis. Varying degrees of fibrosis, including cirrhosis, can be found in a small percentage of patients with ulcerative colitis or Crohn's disease.

Hepatic amyloidosis is an infrequent but well-documented complication of active Crohn's disease and is due to the deposition of a poorly soluble fragment of serum amyloid A protein (see the following section).

Differential Diagnosis

Because of the potential for severe liver disease to develop as a consequence of inflammatory bowel disease, patients should be evaluated at least annually with liver enzyme testing. Those found to have elevated liver enzymes should be further evaluated in the same manner as any other patient, ruling out viral hepatitis, drug toxicity, and other causes. Diagnostic considerations in the patient with an elevated alkaline phosphatase or bilirubin levels include primary sclerosing cholangitis, cholangiocarcinoma, or common bile duct stones. Gallstone disease, which is relatively common in the general population, is more common in patients who have had ileal resection because of alterations in the bile salt pool.

Complications

Primary sclerosing cholangitis is the major hepatobiliary complication of inflammatory bowel disease. Although it can slowly progress in a benign fashion for a decade or more, cholangiocarcinoma eventually develops in about 10% of patients, and biliary cirrhosis with liver failure eventually develops in most, if not all, patients over time.

Treatment

Although biochemical evidence of liver disease can fluctuate with disease activity, treatment of the bowel disease with corticosteroids and salicylates does not clearly improve the outcome from associated liver disease. Similarly, surgical resection of the involved bowel does not improve sclerosing cholangitis or fatty liver. For the patient with severe deterioration of liver function, liver transplantation is an effective option. The presence of cholangiocarcinoma as a complication of primary sclerosing cholangitis precludes transplantation because of the high likelihood of tumor recurrence posttransplant.

Prognosis

How the presence of liver disease in patients with ulcerative colitis and Crohn's disease affects the overall outcome depends on the nature of the liver disease. Steatosis is a benign lesion. Primary sclerosing cholangitis is an indolent disease, but death from liver failure or cholangiocarcinoma is inevitable over time. When the diagnosis is established early (as is often the case with the evaluation of asymptomatic elevations of alkaline phosphatase by ERCP), 10–20 years may elapse before impaired liver function becomes clinically significant.

Broome U et al: Liver disease in ulcerative colitis: an epidemiological and follow-up study in the county of Stockholm. Gut 1994;35:84.

Rankin GB: Extraintestinal and systemic manifestations of inflammatory bowel disease. Med Clin North Am 1990;74:39.

Schrumpf E et al: Hepatobiliary complications of inflammatory bowel disease. Semin Liver Dis 1988;8:201.

Vakil N et al: Liver abscess in Crohn's disease. Am J Gastroenterol 1994;89:1090.

Wewer V et al: Prevalence of hepatobiliary dysfunction in a regional group of patients with chronic inflammatory bowel disease. Scand J Gastroenterol 1991;26:97.

DIABETES MELLITUS

 ESSENTIALS OF DIAGNOSIS

- *Hepatomegaly is an occasional finding and is due to hepatic steatosis in patients with type 1 and type 2 diabetes.*
- *Serum aminotransferases and alkaline phosphatase range from normal to four times the upper limit of normal.*
- *Nonalcoholic steatohepatitis (NASH) can develop in some patients with diabetes and is diagnosed by liver biopsy.*

Pathophysiology

The liver is adversely affected by several of the metabolic derangements of both type 1 and type 2 diabetes mellitus. Episodic hyperglycemia, increased fatty acid delivery from peripheral stores in times of hypoglycemia, hyperinsulinism in patients with type 2 diabetes, and insufficient insulin in patients with type 1 diabetes all participate in the hepatic complications. The accumulation of fat in the liver of the patient with type 1 diabetes reflects poor glucose control. During periods of insulin deficiency, peripheral fat stores are mobilized, and the free fatty acids released into the circulation are taken up by the liver for conversion to alternative energy forms (eg, ketone bodies). Fatty acids that do not undergo mitochondrial β-oxidation in the liver are recycled back into triglycerides and transported to the peripheral stores by very low density lipoproteins. Any interference in the complex process of synthesizing and secreting triglycerides from hepatocytes is manifested histologically as steatosis. In patients with type 2 diabetes, obesity is the primary cause of fatty liver due to ongoing oversupply of the liver with fatty acids from peripheral stores because of peripheral insulin resistance. Although the accumulation of fat in the liver can cause biochemical evidence of liver injury, diabetes itself rarely, if ever, is a cause of cirrhosis. Impaired liver function caused by other factors (eg, chronic viral or alcoholic cirrhosis) can unmask latent diabetes by increasing peripheral insulin resistance. Thus, an overrepresentation of diabetes in patients with cirrhosis cannot be interpreted as the former causing the latter.

Clinical Findings

A. SYMPTOMS AND SIGNS

Hepatomegaly is occasionally detectable on physical examination and can be a source of vague right upper quadrant pain. Patients with stigmata of chronic liver disease must be further evaluated for causes apart from diabetes (eg, chronic viral hepatitis, hemochromatosis).

B. LABORATORY FINDINGS

The serum alkaline phosphatase and aminotransferase levels may be mildly elevated but cannot be used to distinguish steatosis alone from coexisting inflammation or fibrosis that characterize nonalcoholic steatohepatitis.

C. LIVER BIOPSY

Macrovesicular steatosis (large cytoplasmic droplets that displace nuclei to the periphery) is found in about one-half of patients with type 2 diabetes and a minority of patients with type 1 diabetes. In the presence of steatosis, the finding of inflammatory cells (neutrophils and mononuclear leukocytes) within the parenchyma and evidence of cell injury (Mallory bodies, necrosis, and fibrosis) establish the diagnosis of nonalcoholic steatohepatitis. Hepatocyte glycogen stores are nearly always increased, and glycogen nuclei (clear vacuoles within hepatocyte nuclei) are frequently present.

Differential Diagnosis

There are no specific tests that establish the cause of liver abnormalities in diabetes. Aminotransferase elevations in a patient with diabetes should be evaluated as in any other individual, ruling out viral and metabolic causes as well as alcohol abuse. An elevated alkaline phosphatase level should be further evaluated with ultrasonographic study of the biliary tree. Iron studies (serum iron, transferrin, ferritin) are indicated in any adult with new-onset diabetes to rule out hemochromatosis, because of its association with both liver disease and diabetes.

Complications

Hepatic steatosis without the additional findings of NASH does not confer a risk of progressive fibrosis and cirrhosis. On the other hand, about 15–40% of patients with NASH develop fibrosis and must be considered at risk for developing cirrhosis over time.

Treatment

Maintenance of euglycemia in patients with type 1 diabetes will improve hepatic steatosis. Gradual weight reduction in the overweight patient with type 2 diabetes may be helpful; whereas improved glycemic control through the use of insulin and sulfonylureas has not been found to improve liver abnormalities.

Prognosis

Hepatic steatosis in the absence of inflammation or fibrosis in the patient with diabetes is not associated with any adverse outcomes. The degree to which it predisposes to nonalcoholic steatohepatitis, liver fibrosis, and cirrhosis is unknown, and specific therapies for these latter sequelae have not been established.

Falchuk KR, Conlin D: The intestinal and liver complications of diabetes mellitus. Adv Intern Med 1993;38:269.

Neuschwander-Tetri BA: Nonalcoholic steatohepatitis. Clin Liver Dis 1998;2:149.

Petrides AS et al: Pathogenesis of glucose intolerance and diabetes mellitus in cirrhosis. Hepatology 1994;19:616.

Powell EE et al: The natural history of nonalcoholic steatohepatitis: a follow-up study of forty-two patients for up to 21 years. Hepatology 1990;11:74.

Wanless IR, Lentz JS: Fatty liver hepatitis (steatohepatitis) and obesity: an autopsy study with analysis of risk factors. Hepatology 1990;12:1106.

OBESITY

 ESSENTIALS OF DIAGNOSIS

- *Hepatomegaly is often present due to hepatic steatosis (fatty infiltration).*
- *Stigmata of chronic liver disease should raise the suspicion of cirrhosis caused by NASH or other types of chronic liver disease.*
- *Serum aminotransferase levels typically range from normal to four times the upper limit of normal.*
- *Liver biopsy usually demonstrates steatosis.*
- *NASH is present in 20–70% of obese patients.*
- *Alcohol abuse must be excluded as a cause of liver disease.*

Pathophysiology

Fatty infiltration of the liver is a nearly invariable finding in morbidly obese patients (>20% above ideal body weight) and can be associated with inflammatory changes and varying degrees of parenchymal fibrosis (NASH). Insulin resistance is common in obesity and predisposes to the development of type 2 diabetes and possibly NASH.

Clinical Findings

A. SYMPTOMS AND SIGNS

Fatty infiltration is generally asymptomatic, although some patients may complain of vague right upper quadrant abdominal pain, possibly due to capsular stretching. Chronic liver disease, if present, rarely exhibits clinical manifestations other than nonspecific fatigue until quite advanced. Physical examination can reveal hepatomegaly, which is commonly present but difficult to detect.

B. LABORATORY FINDINGS

Serum aminotransferase and alkaline phosphatase levels can be mildly elevated (up to four times the upper limit) and normalize with weight loss. Unlike alcoholic liver disease, where AST is characteristically higher than ALT, in obese patients with elevated aminotransferases due to fatty infiltration or NASH, the ALT is usually higher than the AST. Triglyceride levels are often elevated in adults with NASH and almost always elevated in obese children with NASH.

C. IMAGING STUDIES

Fatty infiltration of the liver can be revealed as a diffusely echogenic liver on ultrasonography. A homogeneously low-density liver when compared with the spleen on CT scanning is a more sensitive indication of fatty liver. Imaging studies cannot distinguish between steatosis alone, which has a benign course, and NASH.

D. LIVER BIOPSY

Hepatic steatosis is commonly found in obese patients. The morphologic changes of NASH are found in 20–70% of patients with morbid obesity with the prevalence correlating directly with the magnitude of obesity. Lipogranulomas are a common finding in fatty livers.

Differential Diagnosis

The obese patient with an enlarged fatty liver cannot be assumed to have benign steatosis of obesity until other causes have been ruled out. Alcohol abuse and drug toxicity must be considered as contributing factors. Persistently elevated aminotransferases with a negative evaluation for viral, autoimmune, or metabolic causes of liver disease (see Chapter 33) should be further evaluated by liver biopsy, especially if no response to weight loss occurs. The liver biopsy in these patients excludes other unsuspected causes of liver disease and helps to establish prognosis based on the presence or absence of fibrosis.

Complications

Fatty infiltration of the liver is generally a benign condition although in can cause abdominal pain. About 15–40% of patients with NASH develop fibrosis and are at risk of developing cirrhosis.

Treatment

Gradual weight loss attained with a well-balanced diet can improve aminotransferase elevations and the extent of hepatic steatosis. The impact of weight loss on inflammation and fibrosis is less certain.

Prognosis

The prognosis of fatty liver alone is benign. When inflammation and fibrosis are evident on liver biopsy, the progression to cirrhosis may be possible over time.

Nanji AA, French SW, Freeman JB: Serum alanine aminotransferase to aspartate aminotransferase ratio and degree of fatty liver in morbidly obese patients. Enzyme 1986;36:266.

Neuschwander-Tetri BA: Nonalcoholic steatohepatitis. Clin Liver Dis 1998;2:149.

Palmer M, Schaffner F: Effect of weight reduction on hepatic abnormalities in overweight patients. Gastroenterology 1990; 99:1408.

Ranlov I, Hardt F: Regression of liver steatosis following gastroplasty or gastric bypass for morbid obesity. Digestion 1990; 47:208.

Silverman JF et al: Liver pathology in morbidly obese patients with and without diabetes. Am J Gastroenterol 1990;85:1349.

SICKLE CELL DISEASE

 ESSENTIALS OF DIAGNOSIS

- *Severe right upper quadrant pain with nausea, often in the setting of a typical crisis.*
- *Tender hepatomegaly.*
- *Markedly elevated aminotransferases and profound hyperbilirubinemia in severe hepatic crises.*
- *Differentiating hepatic crisis from ascending cholangitis and acute cholecystitis requires rapid clinical assessment and diagnostic imaging.*

Pathophysiology

The obstruction of sinusoidal blood flow by sickled erythrocytes can cause acute episodes of severe ischemic injury or recurrent subclinical episodes of injury. Concomitant hemolysis further contributes to hyperbilirubinemia during episodes of severe hepatic crisis. About 7–10% of hospitalizations for sickle cell anemia are complicated by hepatic crisis.

Clinical Findings

A. SYMPTOMS AND SIGNS

Severe right upper quadrant abdominal pain characterizes hepatic crisis and can be associated with other symptoms of sickle crisis such as back and joint pain and fever. Tender hepatomegaly is usually detectable.

B. LABORATORY FINDINGS

The biochemical evidence of liver injury in sickle crisis reflects a combination of ischemic injury and hemolysis, with markedly elevated aminotransferases (more than 10 times the upper limit of normal), elevated prothrombin time, and profound hyperbilirubinemia (can exceed 50 mg/dL). Leukocytosis is also frequently seen and does not necessarily signify cholangitis or cholecystitis.

C. IMAGING STUDIES

Cholelithiasis with radiopaque calcium bilirubinate gallstones is common in sickle cell disease. Thus, sonography should be performed to rule out acute biliary obstruction as a cause of right upper quadrant pain and jaundice. If doubt persists about the patency of the common bile duct, ERCP should be performed. Ultrasonography is also useful for detecting acute cholecystitis as a cause of right upper quadrant pain. Radionuclide scanning can effectively exclude cholecystitis if it shows normal filling of the gallbladder. This imaging modality is ineffective in the presence of severe hepatocellular dysfunction, however.

D. LIVER BIOPSY

Hepatic sickle crisis is characterized by focal hepatocellular necrosis due to ischemic injury. Sinusoidal congestion and engulfed red blood cells within sinusoidal macrophages can also be seen during a crisis, as well as in baseline states in sickle cell disease. Cirrhosis occurs in 15–20% of patients with sickle cell anemia and may reflect the repeated ischemic insults from sickling, transfusion-acquired viral hepatitis, or massive hemosiderosis.

Differential Diagnosis

The constellation of symptoms and laboratory findings in hepatic crisis is distinctive and readily suggests the diagnosis. Fever and leukocytosis may suggest infection but can also be attributed to hepatic crisis after appropriate exclusion of other causes. Acute drug toxicity and viral hepatitis must be excluded by reviewing the patient's history and obtaining viral serologic studies (see Chapter 33). Hepatitis A in the patient with sickle cell disease can lead to fulminant hepatitis, which is an otherwise unusual complication of acute hepatitis A. Other important diagnostic considerations include choledocholithiasis and acute cholecystitis. These are difficult to distinguish from hepatic crisis on clinical grounds alone, and the biliary tree must be imaged sonographically in patients with hepatic crisis. The patient without right upper quadrant pain but abnormal aminotransferases should be evaluated for other causes of liver disease, especially hepatitis C acquired from repeated blood transfusions.

Complications

Fulminant liver failure as a consequence of hepatic crisis can occur but is rare. Previous cocaine use predisposes to more severe liver injury during hepatic crisis and should be sought in the patient's history. Progressive chronic liver injury due to either repeated acute injury or coexisting transfusion-related viral hepatitis is probably the cause of the 20% incidence of cirrhosis in these patients. Transfusion-associated hemosiderosis is found on biopsy, but the role of iron accumulation in chronic liver injury has not been established.

Treatment

Treatment of hepatic crisis is no different from the treatment of sickle crisis in general, with transfusion, hydration, analgesia, and optimization of hemoglobin oxygenation. Acetaminophen-containing analgesics should be avoided because of their hepatotoxic potential. Vaccination for hepatitis A would prevent the complications of this infection in this susceptible population.

Hassell KL, Eckman JR, Lane PA: Acute multiorgan failure syndrome: a potentially catastrophic complication of severe sickle cell pain episodes. Am J Med 1994;96:155.

Pearson HA: The kidney, hepatobiliary system, and spleen in sickle cell anemia. Ann NY Acad Sci 1989;565:120.

COLLAGEN VASCULAR DISEASES

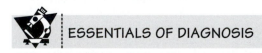 ESSENTIALS OF DIAGNOSIS

- *Hepatomegaly is an occasional finding in many forms of collagen vascular diseases.*

- Liver enzymes are usually normal or mildly elevated (up to four times the upper limit).
- Hepatic artery vasculitis in a patient with systemic lupus erythematosus or polyarteritis nodosa can cause fatal hepatic infarction or aneurysm rupture, presenting as severe right upper quadrant abdominal pain.

General Considerations

Liver involvement is common but usually mild in patients with systemic lupus erythematosus, polyarteritis nodosa, rheumatoid arthritis, Felty's syndrome, Sjögren's disease, polymyalgia rheumatica, or adult Still's disease. Although there can be serologic overlapping of these diseases with primary liver diseases such as primary biliary cirrhosis and chronic autoimmune hepatitis, the appropriate diagnosis can usually be made on clinical grounds. The historic use of the term "lupoid hepatitis" to refer to autoimmune liver disease has sometimes led to confusion. This entity is now called autoimmune hepatitis and is completely distinct from systemic lupus erythematosus (see Chapter 36).

Clinical Findings

A. SYMPTOMS AND SIGNS

Hepatomegaly can be found on examination, but symptoms referable to liver involvement are unusual. A notable exception is the rupture of an intrahepatic arterial aneurysm in patients with polyarteritis nodosa or systemic lupus erythematosus. This catastrophic complication can lead to severe right upper quadrant pain, shock, and death.

B. LABORATORY FINDINGS

Mild elevations (up to four times the upper limit of normal) of the serum aminotransferases and alkaline phosphatase of liver origin are frequent. Substantial elevations of bilirubin and aminotransferases are rare and should guide the investigation toward other causes such as drug toxicity, autoimmune liver disease, and viral hepatitis.

C. IMAGING STUDIES

Abdominal CT scanning is indicated in patients with systemic lupus or polyarteritis nodosa who have severe right upper quadrant pain to identify hepatic infarction or rupture of an arterial aneurysm. Active vasculitis of the hepatic artery can be further pursued by angiography in the patient with right upper quadrant pain, fever, and an elevated sedimentation rate.

D. LIVER BIOPSY

Liver biopsy should be performed when there is clinical suspicion of significant liver dysfunction (physical findings, elevated bilirubin, elevated prothrombin time). Hepatic steatosis is not typically present and when evident may be the result of corticosteroid therapy. Periportal inflammation and liver fibrosis occur in a small fraction of patients with collagen vascular diseases. Nodular regenerative hyperplasia is an unusual histologic finding that is sometimes seen in patients with Felty's syndrome. Secondary hepatic amyloidosis (see following section) may develop in patients with uncontrolled rheumatoid arthritis.

Differential Diagnosis

Drug-induced hepatotoxicity must be excluded in the patient with significant liver enzyme elevations. Nonsteroidal antiinflammatory drugs can cause liver injury, and fulminant hepatitis has been described in patients treated with aspirin and nonsteroidal antiinflammatory agents for collagen vascular diseases.

Treatment

Active vasculitis of the hepatic artery should be treated with corticosteroids. The patient with severe right upper quadrant pain should be evaluated for surgical or radiologic intervention to prevent exsanguinating hemorrhage from a ruptured aneurysm. Otherwise, specific treatment for the hepatic manifestations of collagen vascular diseases has not been identified.

Ilan Y, Ben-Chetrit E: Liver involvement in giant cell arteritis. Clin Rheumatol 1993;12:219.

Leggett B: The liver in systemic lupus erythematosus. J Gastroenterol Hepatol 1993;8:84.

Matsumoto T et al: The liver in systemic lupus erythematosus: pathologic analysis of 52 cases and review of the Japanese Autopsy Registry Data. Hum Pathol 1992;23:1151.

Zimmerman H: Hepatotoxicity. Disease-a-Month 1993;39:747.

AMYLOIDOSIS

 ESSENTIALS OF DIAGNOSIS

- Fatigue, weight loss, and peripheral edema can be long-standing before the diagnosis is considered.
- Hepatic involvement is frequent, but liver-specific symptoms are rare.

- *Hepatomegaly, peripheral edema, macroglossia, peripheral neuropathy, skin capillary fragility, and congestive heart failure are found with varying frequency.*

- *Fat, skin, or rectal biopsies are preferable to liver biopsy to establish the diagnosis.*

General Considerations

The shared feature of all forms of amyloidosis is the perivascular deposition of protein fragments folded in the highly stable and insoluble β-pleated sheet configuration. This configuration is responsible for the birefringent microscopic appearance observed under polarized light and is a common internal structural arrangement of many proteins. Molecular techniques have identified many of the protein fragments responsible for amyloidosis, as well as the function of the intact proteins from which the fragments are derived. With this new information, a rational approach to treatment is now possible for many forms of amyloidosis.

There are two common types of amyloidosis, and their prevalence varies depending on the population studied. One type, caused by the deposition of excessively produced immunoglobulin light chain fragments, has been termed primary, or AL, amyloidosis. This light chain excess can result from monoclonal expansion of a plasma cell or B cell line, either as multiple myeloma or a subclinical myeloid cell dyscrasia. The disease may respond to cytotoxic therapy. The other common type of amyloidosis has been termed secondary, or AA, amyloidosis and is caused by the perivascular deposition of fragments of a protein called serum amyloid A. This protein is an apolipoprotein synthesized by the liver that circulates in the plasma bound to high-density lipoprotein. Like C-reactive protein, it is one of the acute phase reactants that responds most robustly to inflammation (100- to 1000-fold increase). This type of amyloidosis is associated with lymphomas and chronic inflammatory states, including untreated inflammatory bowel disease, rheumatoid arthritis, osteomyelitis, tuberculosis, leprosy, and familial Mediterranean fever.

Mutations of genes encoding several other proteins have also been recognized to cause deposition of specific protein fragments, which appear microscopically as perivascular amyloid. These include transthyretin, β-amyloid protein P, apolipoprotein A1, procalcitonin, and $β_2$-microglobulin. Establishing the molecular identities of the proteins causing these types of amyloidosis is important. For examinationple, the thyroxin-binding protein transthyretin is susceptible to point mutations, which lead to its deposition as amyloid. Clinically, this particular form of amyloidosis causes fatal neurologic and cardiac complications. Because transthyretin is synthesized by the liver, identification of this disease early in its course and treatment with liver transplantation have proved effective in preventing an otherwise fatal outcome.

Pathogenesis

The term amyloidosis connotes an etiologically diverse group of diseases sharing the common feature of perivascular accumulation of protein folded in the stable β-pleated sheet configuration.

Clinical Findings

A. Symptoms and Signs

Liver deposition of amyloid protein has been associated primarily with light chain disease (primary amyloidosis) and serum amyloid A disease (secondary amyloidosis). The clinical presentation of amyloidosis was defined before the identification of specific types of amyloidosis by molecular techniques. Thus, our understanding of each type of amyloidosis may evolve with further elucidation of the diverse pathogenetic mechanisms.

In general, nonspecific complaints of fatigue, unintentional weight loss, edema, and dyspnea are longstanding by the time the diagnosis is considered. Symptoms due to liver dysfunction are generally not present, even in advanced disease. Occasionally, ascites occurs, but congestive heart failure and nephrotic protein loss may be contributory factors. Rarely, hepatic involvement can cause cholestasis with associated pruritus.

Hepatomegaly is a common finding on examinationination. Dependent edema is also frequent and may reflect associated congestive heart failure or nephrotic syndrome. Macroglossia, although an infrequent finding, can be helpful in suggesting the diagnosis. Skin fragility (sloughing, purpura, easy bruisability), carpal tunnel syndrome, and peripheral neuropathy may be seen.

B. Laboratory Findings

Serum alkaline phosphatase levels are usually mildly elevated (up to four times normal), and the aminotransferases are normal or mildly elevated (up to four times normal). Coagulation abnormalities may be present, associated with reduced levels of factors IX and X, due to their binding to the amyloid proteins.

C. Imaging Studies

Imaging of the liver by CT scanning or sonography can identify hepatomegaly. A radionuclide liver-spleen scan is generally not required but may show patchy uptake of tracer material consistent with inhomogeneous liver involvement.

D. LIVER BIOPSY

The diagnosis of hepatic amyloidosis is confirmed by the finding of eosinophilic protein within the subendothelial space of Disse, which exhibits green birefringence when stained with Congo red. The site of amyloid protein within the liver does not establish the type of amyloidosis. Hepatocyte atrophy is commonly found, possibly caused by compromised transfer of oxygen and nutrients from the vascular space to the cell. Cirrhosis is not a feature. Performing a liver biopsy may be associated with an increased risk of bleeding due to deficient clotting factors and capillary abnormalities. Therefore, biopsies must be undertaken cautiously, especially in the patient with a history of purpura, which suggests capillary fragility.

Complications

The liver generally tolerates the accumulation of perivascular protein well compared to the heart and central nervous system, and patients typically present with dysfunction of organs other than the liver. Occlusion of the sinusoidal space can lead to clinically evident portal hypertension in a minority of cases.

Treatment

Specific therapies for each type of amyloidosis are evolving as individual pathogenetic mechanisms are elucidated. Cytotoxic therapy has been successful for the paraproteinemia of primary immunoglobulin light chain amyloidosis, even in the absence of multiple myeloma. For secondary amyloidosis, treatment of the underlying inflammatory disorder is the mainstay of therapy. Colchicine is beneficial in preventing amyloidosis in patients with familial Mediterranean fever and in some patients with other chronic inflammatory diseases. Familial amyloidosis caused by dominant mutations of the transthyretin gene has now been successfully treated with liver transplantation. These new therapeutic options emphasize the need to make an early and accurate diagnosis of amyloidosis.

Benson M, Wallace M: Amyloidosis. In: *The Metabolic Basis of Inherited Disease,* 6th ed. Scriver C et al (editors). McGraw-Hill, 1989.

Buck F, Koss M: Hepatic amyloidosis: morphological differences between systemic AL and AA types. Hum Pathol 1991;22:904.

Gertz M, Kyle R: Primary systemic amyloidosis: a diagnostic primer. Mayo Clin Proc 1989;64:1505.

Rienhoff H et al: Molecular and cellular biology of serum amyloid A. Mol Biol Med 1990;7:287.

Mass Lesions & Neoplasia of the Liver

46

Douglas R. LaBrecque, MD

The rapid advances in medical technology over the past two decades have greatly increased the ease and accuracy of diagnosing hepatic tumors. However, the wide availability of ultrasonography and computed axial tomography has also spawned additional frustration and expense in pursuing incidental findings that eventually prove insignificant. Ignoring the lesion is rarely an option, however, due to the difficulty in treating primary and metastatic neoplasms of the liver and the frequency with which they occur. The liver is the major site of blood-borne metastases from within the abdomen and a very common site of metastases from tumors above the diaphragm. It is the most common site of metastatic disease in patients who die from neoplasia; 36–42% of patients dying from primary extrahepatic tumors have liver metastases. Metastatic liver tumors are about 20–40 times more common than primary hepatic tumors. The most frequently identified hepatic mass is a benign hemangioma, which occurs in 7% or more of patients.

HEPATOCELLULAR CARCINOMA

ESSENTIALS OF DIAGNOSIS

- *Frequently asymptomatic with normal or minimally abnormal liver tests.*
- *Elevated α-fetoprotein in 50% or more of hepatocellular carcinomas.*
- *Physical examination may reveal rock hard hepatomegaly, tender hepatomegaly, or signs of chronic liver disease, or may be completely normal.*
- *Presence of a bruit or friction rub over the liver strongly suggests liver tumor.*
- *Imaging studies are the key to diagnostic evaluation.*
- *Biopsy is usually necessary to confirm and differentiate malignancies.*

General Considerations

The liver is comprised of a variety of cell types, including hepatocytes, biliary epithelium, vascular endothelium, Kupffer cells, stellate (Ito) cells, lymphoid cells, and neuroendocrine cells. Any of these cells may give rise to malignant or benign tumors (Table 46–1). However, 90–95% of all primary liver tumors are hepatocellular carcinomas (HCC) that arise from the parenchymal cell. This chapter will focus primarily on HCC, but will touch briefly on the other noninfectious causes of liver mass lesions.

Although HCC is an uncommon tumor in the Western world, where it represents only 0.5–2.0% of all cancers, and has an incidence of only three to five cases per 100,000 population per year in the United States, it has an attack rate as high as 150 per 100,000 population in areas of Sub-Saharan Africa and Southeast Asia. Worldwide, it is the most common visceral cancer and may be the single most common cancer.

Pathophysiology

A number of factors have been associated with the pathogenesis of HCC, including physical, chemical, infectious, and metabolic/hereditary etiologies (Table 46–2). The rodent liver is one of the most successful models of chemical carcinogenesis and has contributed a great deal to our current understanding of the common steps in the pathogenesis of malignant transformation. This multistep model of hepatocarcinogenesis (Figure 46–1) includes four steps. **Initiation** occurs when an infection or chemical exposure produces a fixed genetic change that makes the initiated cell responsive to promotion. During **promotion,** hepatocyte necrosis, inflammation with production of cytokines and growth factors, or exposure to specific chemicals (anabolic steroids, alcohol, iron) leads to liver regeneration and active or inactive cirrhosis. This "fixes" the genetic defect, preventing the liver from eliminating the cell with its altered genome. **Progression** occurs when these "growth-advantaged" malignant cells are stimulated to produce microscopic foci of HCC by clonal expansion. Phenobarbital and other chemicals are particu-

Table 46–1. Simple classification of major liver tumors.

Malignant	Benign
Epithelial	**Epithelial**
Hepatocellular carcinoma	Hepatocellular adenoma
Fibrolamellar carcinoma[1]	Focal nodular hyperplasia
Hepatoblastoma[2]	Nodular regenerative hyperplasia
Cholangiocarcinoma	Bile duct adenoma
Biliary cystadenocarcinoma	Biliary cystadenoma
Carcinoid tumor	Intrahepatic biliary papillomatosis
Mesodermal	**Mesodermal**
Hemangiosarcoma	Hemangioma (cavernous hemangioma)
Epithelial hemangioendothelioma	Infantile hemangioendothelioma[2]
Undifferentiated (embryonal) sarcoma[2]	
Embryonal rhabdomyosarcoma[2]	
Lymphoma	
Other sarcomas, rare tumors,	
and mixed tumors	
	Tumor-like
	Peliosis hepatis
	Simple cyst
	Mesenchymal hamartoma[2]
	Hepatic abscess

[1]An important histologic variant of hepatocellular carcinoma with a significantly better prognosis.
[2]Occurs in infants and children.

larly effective in producing progression. Ultimately, continued growth stimulation and clonal expansion of the malignant cells lead to one or more macroscopic foci of HCC and clinically apparent cancer. Most explanations of hepatocellular carcinogenesis attempt to recapitulate these steps and generally no single agent is felt to be sufficient by itself to induce HCC.

A. PHYSICAL AND CHEMICAL AGENTS

1. Radiation—Ionizing radiation causes liver tumors in mice, but does not appear to be a significant factor in the development of human HCC. Long-term follow-

Table 46–2. Risk factors for develoment of hepatocellular carcinoma.

Definite	Possible
Chronic hepatic B virus infection	Oral contraceptives
Chronic hepatitis C virus infection	Androgenic/anabolic
Aflatoxin	steroids
Cirrhosis	α_1-Antitrypsin deficiency
Hereditary tyrosinemia	Ataxia telangiectasia
Vinyl chloride monomer[1]	Alcohol
Thorotrast[1]	

[1]Primarily hemangiosarcomas.

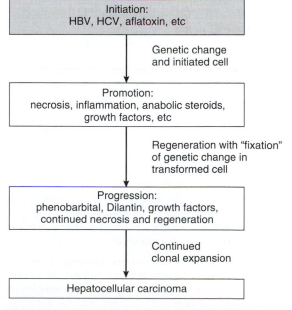

Figure 46–1. Multistep pathogenesis of hepatocellular carcinoma.

up of those who survived the atomic bombing of Nagasaki and Hiroshima has not demonstrated an increase in HCC, although venoocclusive disease and the Budd-Chiari syndrome are increased following radiation exposure. The low rate of cell turnover in the adult liver with the limited opportunity for fixation of genetic alterations may account for resistance to radiation-induced tumors. Long-term continuous exposure to radiation, however, can produce tumors in the human liver. The unfortunate use of **thorotrast,** one of the original radiologic contrast agents and the radionuclide of choice from the late 1920s to the mid-1950s, has produced hemangiosarcomas and even HCCs. This α-radiation emitter has a biological half-life of approximately 400 years, and well over 50,000 adults remain at risk for the development of HCC.

2. Chemical carcinogenesis—Because of the liver's unique anatomic position in the body, and its dual blood flow, everything taken by mouth traverses the liver via the portal drainage of the abdominal viscera before reaching the systemic circulation. Compounds that enter the body via other routes also find their way to the liver, which receives 25% of the cardiac output. Over 12,350,000 unique chemical compounds have been identified and this total grows by more than 11,500 each week as new compounds are synthesized or found in the environment. Over 90,000 are in regular use, including some 800 as food additives. In animal models, more than 3,000 chemicals are known to be carcinogenic and, as noted above, the rodent liver has been the standard model used to delineate the multistep model of hepatic carcinogenesis. Despite the overwhelming evidence of carcinogenicity of chemicals, and the massive daily exposure of the human liver to chemicals, only two chemicals are clearly documented human hepatic carcinogens: **aflatoxin** and **vinyl chloride monomer.** The former, a contaminant of foodstuffs (eg, nuts and grains), is produced by the mold *Aspergillus flavus.* It contaminates food stored for long periods in a hot or humid environment and is clearly associated with HCC, particularly as a cofactor with the hepatitis B virus in many sections of Africa and Southeast Asia. It is the most powerful human hepatocarcinogen known and promotes tumors, in part, by leading to inactivation of p53 through specific G-T mutations at codon 249. Vinyl chloride monomer induces angiosarcomas in animal models as well as in industrial workers manufacturing polyvinyl chlorides.

3. Viral and other infectious agents—There are many examples of virus-induced tumors in animal models. In most cases, the viral genome becomes incorporated into the host cells' genetic material either directly, if it is a DNA virus, or following reverse transcriptase production of a DNA copy, if it is an RNA virus. Insertion of the viral material into the host cell genome may then act as a mutagen or as a promoter to alter gene expression to produce new proteins, particularly oncogenes, or may cause overexpression of normal genes, which leads to malignant transformation. The hepatitis B virus has the strongest association with the development of HCC and hepatitis B viral DNA has been found integrated into the genome of the host DNA in up to 80% of patients with HCC who are hepatitis B carriers. However, there is no consistent site of integration. In contrast, hepatitis C, which is also strongly associated with HCC, is an RNA virus with no reverse transcriptase activity; thus, it is unlikely that it exerts its effect by insertion into the host cell genome. In Japan, where 70% of patients with HCC are hepatitis C positive, patients with chronic hepatitis C are three times more likely to develop HCC than those with chronic hepatitis B. Unlike in hepatitis B, however, HCC occurs only after the development of cirrhosis and the continuous necroinflammatory reaction with subsequent regeneration may account for its tumorigenic behavior.

4. Trematodes (liver flukes)—Oriental cholangiohepatitis, caused primarily by the liver fluke, *Clonorchis sinensis,* has a strong association with the development of cholangiocarcinoma. Unfortunately, the blood flukes that cause chronic schistosomiasis often occur in patients who also have chronic active hepatitis B with cirrhosis, and HCC is common in these patients. In pure hepatosplenic schistosomiasis, however, portal fibrosis is the primary lesion, and the parenchyma is relatively undamaged.

5. Cirrhosis—Cirrhosis is a common feature in almost all cases of HCC. In some cases, such as hepatitis C, it may be the necroinflammatory reaction and continuous regeneration that ultimately "fix" the mutation that leads to malignant transformation and allows it to flourish. In other cases, such as hereditary hemachromatosis in which 3–27% of patients develop HCC, tumor develops only in patients with cirrhosis. If timely phlebotomy is performed in hemachromatosis prior to the development of cirrhosis, the lifelong risk of developing HCC is reduced to that of the normal population.

However, cirrhosis is clearly only another cofactor in the development of HCC. In Western industrialized countries where HCC is uncommon, 80–90% of patients who develop HCC will have underlying cirrhosis and it occurs primarily in older individuals. In contrast, in Africa, where chronic hepatitis B and aflatoxin exposure are common cofactors, HCC occurs at an earlier age, and only 60–70% of patients have underlying cirrhosis. A combination of hepatitis B with cirrhosis increases the risk of developing HCC by at least four-fold over those who are hepatitis B negative. Virtually any form of cirrhosis appears to increase the risk of developing HCC, but the overall rates may vary from 40 to 50% in those with hepatitis B to 5 to 15% in those whose cirrhosis is caused by alcohol. The highest rate is found in hereditary tyrosinemia.

6. Drugs and alcohol—In the Western industrialized world, HCC is most commonly associated with alcohol. The lifetime risk of developing HCC appears to be about 15% in alcoholic cirrhosis, and this continues even after cessation of alcohol ingestion. In one study, 55% of patients who had stopped drinking had HCC at autopsy. As noted in the section on chemicals, many drugs act as initiators, promotors, or progression factors in the development of HCC in animals. Surprisingly few have been proven to produce HCC in humans. Possible exceptions are anabolic steroids and estrogens, which may play a role in the development of HCC, hepatic adenomas, and hemangiomas as discussed below. Phenobarbitol and diphenylhydantoin (Dilantin) are among the most potent promotors and inducers in animals, but have shown no association with HCC in humans. Similarly, tolazamide, oxytetracycline, and aminopyrine have not been recognized as hepatic carcinogens in humans, despite their ability to be metabolized to carcinogenic nitrosamines.

7. Genetic—Hereditary tyrosinemia has the clearest association with the development of HCC. Close to 40% of patients in one study developed HCC despite good dietary control. Tumors have also been reported in association with ataxia telangiectasia. Most other associations have not been borne out by more careful study, and convincing evidence of a genetic predisposition to the development of HCC is lacking. Familial clustering of HCC is seen in patients with chronic hepatitis B, but this is probably related to vertical and horizontal transmission of the hepatitis B. Differences between ethnic and geographic groups have been discussed above, and are probably more environmental than genetic. The association with Fanconi's anemia is probably related to the androgens used to treat the anemia rather than the underlying disease. Probably the best recognized and most striking association of an hereditary disease with the development of HCC is that with hereditary hemachromatosis.

B. Epidemiology

The incidence of HCC varies dramatically around the globe, ranging from 150 cases per 100,000 population per year in areas such as Taiwan, Mozambique, and Southeast China to a low of three to seven cases per 100,000 population in North and South America, North and Central Europe, and Australia. Intermediate rates from 5 to 20 cases per 100,000 population per year are found in Japan, the Middle East, and European

countries bordering on the Mediterranean. The attack rate in Western developed countries is rising, however, with the incidence in the United States increasing by 71% between 1976–1980 and 1991–1995. Similar changes have been noted in France, Italy, the United Kingdom, Canada, Australia, and Japan. This increasing incidence is particularly linked to the rising numbers of patients with chronic hepatitis C.

Although these generalities hold true, marked differences can be seen within the same geographic area. Native black South Africans and native Maori males in New Zealand have attack rates 28- and 7-fold greater than whites in their respective countries. Blacks in Southern California have an attack rate four times greater than that of whites. Although the above findings suggest racial and/or genetic factors, environmental differences may play an even bigger role. It is commonly found that when natives move from areas with a high attack rate to one with a low attack rate, the incidence falls as they adapt the Western life-style. In contrast, individuals who move from highly developed countries to third-world countries tend to retain their low attack rate, possibly because they maintain their original life-style rather than that of their adopted country. HCC is considerably more common in males (8:1 in areas of high incidence and 2:1 to 3:1 in areas of low incidence).

C. Summary

The precise pathogenesis of HCC is most likely multifactorial, representing the end result of a multistep process in which more than one factor must interact.

Clinical Findings

A. History

The various risk factors described in the section on Pathogenesis should be sought in the history. Thus, high-risk activities that would expose the patient to hepatitis B or C; travel in countries in which ingestion of raw fish could lead to liver fluke infection; a family history of metabolic diseases, prior liver disease, or liver cancer; known inflammatory bowel disease; primary sclerosing cholangitis or congenital biliary anomaly; ingestion of certain medications, such as oral contraceptives or anabolic androgenic steroids; or exposure to environmental carcinogens such as vinyl chloride can point in certain directions in the evaluation of the patient.

B. Symptoms and Signs

Often, the patient has no symptoms or signs of liver disease. Rapid, unexplained weight loss, or the finding of an hepatic bruit or friction rub on physical examination, strongly suggests underlying tumor. Stigmata of chronic liver disease point to the liver as the possible site of such a tumor. Presentation with severe right upper quadrant pain, shoulder pain, or an acute abdomen should lead to the consideration of hemoperitoneum due to the rupture of HCC or hepatocellular adenoma. Jaundice is uncommon unless the patient has extremely advanced liver disease, a tumor compressing the biliary tree, or a primary tumor of the biliary tree. Hypertension with diarrhea, flushing, or vasomotor abnormalities suggests carcinoid syndrome, which frequently metastasizes to the liver.

Findings on physical examination of the liver may vary from an entirely normal liver to one that is large and rock-hard. The latter strongly suggests tumor. The presence of a distended, very tender liver suggests possible hemorrhage into HCC or hepatic adenoma or hemangioma, or could be due to tension on the liver capsule due to a large, rapidly expanding tumor. If clinical signs of liver disease, particularly cirrhosis with ascites, splenomegaly, abdominal collateral vessels, spider angiomata, and jaundice, are present, HCC is more likely, as it most often occurs in patients with cirrhosis. Invasion of the portal and hepatic veins, which occurs frequently with HCC, may also produce portal hypertension.

C. CLINICAL PRESENTATION

The clinical presentation varies dramatically throughout the world. In developing countries with a high incidence of HCC, the disease occurs most often in younger individuals between the ages of 20 and 50 years, and almost always presents as a massive tumor that is easily diagnosed. Right upper quadrant or epigastric pain, sometimes radiating to the right shoulder, is a common presentation. A dramatic increase in the pain usually indicates hemorrhage into the tumor or hemoperitoneum. Marked weakness and rapid weight loss often accompany these complaints, and patients are frequently aware of the recent development of a right upper quadrant mass or swelling. Cirrhosis is present in only 40–50% of patients, so signs of chronic liver disease may not be present.

In contrast, in Western countries the development of HCC is usually insidious. Patients are older, usually 50–70 years of age. Fatigue, weight loss, right upper quadrant pain, abdominal swelling (from ascites), or a change in a previously stable cirrhosis usually herald the development of HCC. Despite the frequently mild complaints, it is discouraging how often large and multiple tumors are found at the time of presentation. Diagnosis and death frequently follow within a few months. In these patients, signs of liver disease are common due to the advanced stage of the underlying cirrhosis. Common signs and symptoms include spider angiomata, palmar erythema, prominent muscle wast-

ing, which may have become much more noticeable shortly before diagnosis, and marked fatigue.

HCC must always be suspected in a patient with rapid and dramatic change in a previously stable cirrhosis. On routine visits, liver size (both and right and left lobes), the presence or absence of ascites, numbers of spider angiomata, and degree of palmar erythema, as well as status of nutrition, muscle mass, and presence or absence of jaundice, should be recorded. Significant or rapid changes in any of these parameters, as well as the development of new symptoms or signs, should prompt the immediate search for possible development of HCC.

A number of **paraneoplastic syndromes** may also develop in the patient with HCC. The most common problems are hypoglycemia, erythrocytosis, and hypercholesterolemia, which may be the only presenting signs or symptoms of HCC in 4–5% of patients.

D. LABORATORY FINDINGS

Often the most striking laboratory finding in HCC is the lack of abnormal tests. Transaminases [aspartate aminotransferase (AST) and alanine aminotransferase (ALT)] are most often normal or only minimally elevated. Alkaline phosphatase (AP) and γ-glutamyltransferase are the most frequently abnormal tests, but are rarely more than two- to three-fold elevated. Lactate dehydrogenase (LDH) can be strikingly and disproportionately elevated in patients with metastatic liver disease, particularly if of hematogenous origin.

The most useful and specific liver test commonly available is the α-fetoprotein, which will be elevated in 70–90% of patients with HCC. However, it is also frequently elevated in patients with very active hepatocellular necrosis and some tumors metastatic to the liver. Thus, it is most useful when it is either extremely high (greater than 300–500 ng/mL), presents as a new elevation, or is steadily rising. Other tests are either not readily available or not particularly helpful.

E. IMAGING

The greatest advance in the diagnosis of HCC has come with the dramatic technological improvements in real time ultrasonography (US) (Figure 46–2A), computed axial tomography (CT) (Figure 46–2B), and magnetic resonance imaging (MRI) (Figure 46–2D and 46–2E). Hepatic angiography (Figure 46–2F) is probably still the single most accurate technique, but it is invasive, requires exposure to contrast media and high doses of radiation, and is quite expensive. At the other extreme, ultrasound is readily available and significantly less expensive but is unable to clearly distinguish malignant masses from other hyper- and hypoechoic masses. The combination of liver ultrasound and triphasic CT, in which rapid images of the lesion in question are

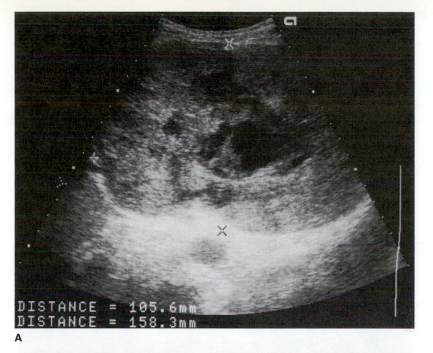

A

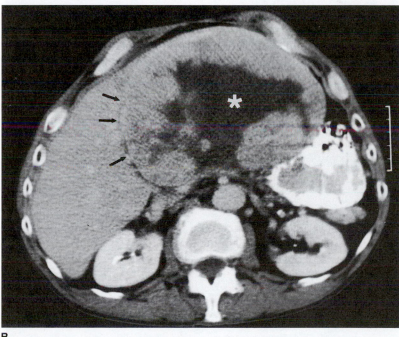

B

Figure 46–2. Imaging of hepatocellular carcinoma by multiple modalities. **A:** A 66-year-old male former alcoholic complained of a painless mid-abdominal mass. α-Fetoprotein was negative. Ultrasound showed a 10.5 × 15.8 cm hyperechoic mass in the left lobe of the liver with central hypodense areas due to fluid or necrosis (edges marked by Xs). **B:** CT with contrast of the same patient shows a large hepatocellular carcinoma occupying virtually the entire left lobe of the liver and penetrating the right lobe. Note that the tumor is almost isodense with the normal liver **(small arrows along border)** and, were it not for the hypodense center (*) caused by tumor necrosis, the tumor could have been easily overlooked.

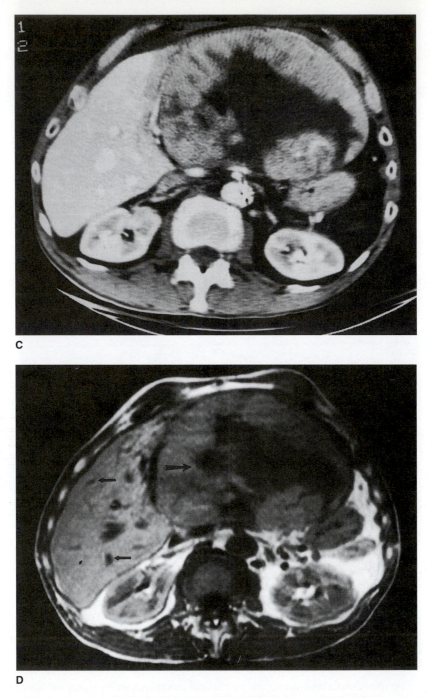

Figure 46–2. **C:** CTAP (CT arterioportography) of the same patient shows dramatic difference in density between normal liver and tumor, highlighting the low-density tumor around the necrotic center and readily delineating the border between normal and neoplastic tissue. **D:** Axial MRI of same patient. The decreased intensity on the T1-weighted images *(large arrow)* indicates fluid in the center of the mass. Note the similar low intensity of vessels in the right lobe *(small arrows).*

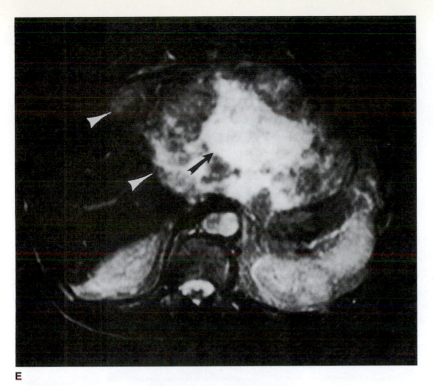

E

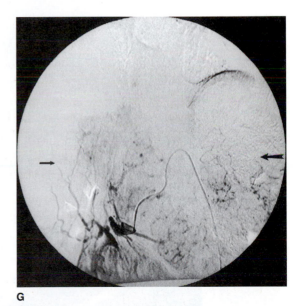

F   G

Figure 46–2. **E:** T2-weighted axial MRI shows a marked increase in signal intensity in the center of the mass *(arrow),* indicative of central tumor necrosis. The signal intensity of the tumor itself is also greater than that of the normal right lobe due to its increased vascularity *(white arrowheads at edge of the tumor).* **F:** An angiogram catheter can be seen selectively placed in the left hepatic artery (*) of the same patient where it supplies the tumor. The hepatocellular carcinoma demonstrates a typical bizarre vascular pattern resulting from tumor neovascularity *(large arrow)* and a tumor blush *(small arrow).* **G:** An angiogram with the same projection as in **F** following embolization with Gelfoam. Note the almost complete absence of blood flow in the tumor *(large arrow)* with good flow to the right lobe *(small arrow).*

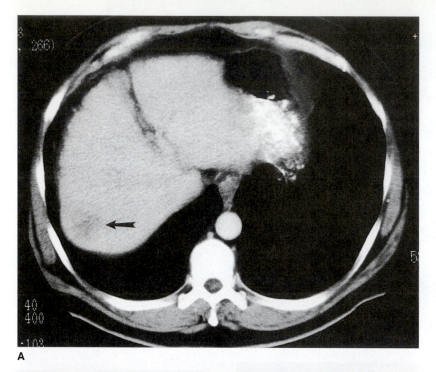

A

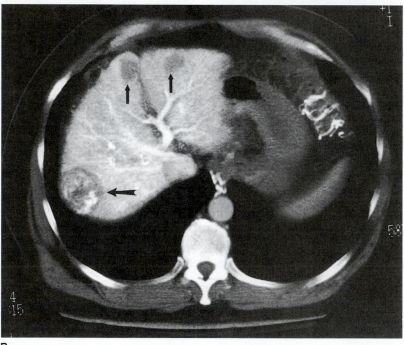

B

Figure 46–3. Sensitivity of CTAP versus CT. **A:** Regular CT with contrast shows area of slightly decreased density in the lower right lobe of the liver *(arrow).* **B:** CTAP in the same plane as **A** makes the lesion in the right posterior lobe obvious and identifies two additional anterior lesions *(arrows).*

taken before contrast injection and during the arterial and venous phases following a bolus injection of contrast material, is usually sufficient to produce a reliable diagnosis. However, CT arterioportagraphy (CTAP), in which a CT is performed during arterial portography, is considerably more sensitive in identifying lesions that may be missed by regular US or CT, and is quite helpful in mapping out the lesion or lesions for the surgeon prior to attempted resection (Figure 46–3). The limitation of this technique is the frequency of false positives in the patient with severe underlying cirrhosis, in whom most of the bolus is shunted around the liver due to portal hypertension. In that situation, high-resolution fast-spin echo magnetic resonance imaging, with or without contrast, is superior, although much more expensive. By far, the most sensitive and accurate technique is intraoperative ultrasonography, which provides the surgeon with the best road map for resection, when resection is possible. Imaging studies along with biochemical tests will usually allow the malignant mass to be distinguished from the nonmalignant one. However, in the majority of cases, tissue diagnosis is required. Tissue can be obtained by ultrasound or CT-guided fine-needle aspiration cytology, if an experienced hepatocytologist is available, or by standard core biopsy via one of the same techniques. Because the histology of well-differentiated HCC and hepatic adenomas can so closely mimic normal hepatic histology, it may be necessary to request outside consultation from an experienced hepatopathologist to rule out malignancy.

F. Hepatocellular Carcinoma Surveillance

Because HCC has such a dismal prognosis and surgical resection remains the only curative option, it is of vital importance to discover the tumor when it is as small as possible. As discussed above, most patients do not present with clinical disease until they already have massive or multiple tumor nodules. Thus, attempts have been made to identify patients at high risk for the development of HCC, and follow them closely via periodic ultrasound and α-fetoprotein studies. The growth rate of HCC is remarkably varied. The time required for tumor nodules to double in size ranges from 30 to 400 days, making selection of an ideal interval for screening difficult. This area is controversial and recommendations vary, but studies in Japan, China, and among American Eskimos have clearly shown that close surveillance every 6 months significantly increases the identification rate of resectable lesions. This appears to be a reasonable interval based on a median doubling time in one study of 117 days. The fastest growing tumor in this study took 5 months to grow from 1 cm to 3 cm. Similar data have not yet been produced to document the utility of such a program, particularly its cost effectiveness, in whites.

Differential Diagnosis

HCC must be distinguished from all of the other malignant and benign masses noted in Table 46–1. Usually the use of appropriate imaging studies, plus testing for α-fetoprotein, is sufficient. In fact, in a patient with cirrhosis with another risk factor such as hepatitis C, hepatitis B, hemochromatosis, or alcohol, the presence of a typical lesion on ultrasound and CT imaging, plus a high or rapidly rising α-fetoprotein, is sufficient to make the diagnosis without histologic verification.

Major Complications

Deaths from HCC occur for a variety of reasons, but most often from liver failure due to underlying cirrhosis. Severe hemorrhage from tumor rupture or variceal bleeding, severe hypoglycemia, sepsis, and bacterial peritonitis are also frequent terminal events. Many patients with HCC suffer from debilitating ascites, and marked palliation can be provided by repeated large volume paracentesis. Standard diuretic therapy is of limited benefit in these patients. The ascites is usually transudative in nature and lacks direct evidence of HCC, which rarely metastasizes to the peritoneum; thus, malignant cells are not often found in the ascites. Direct extension of the tumor to the diaphragm or surrounding areas is uncommon, but two-thirds or more will expand directly into the hepatic vascular system or the vena cava. At autopsy, almost half of the cases will show metastases, most often in the portal, pancreatic, and paraaortic lymph nodes. The lung is the next most common site of metastasis, with occasional metastases to the adrenal, bone, and myocardium.

Treatment

Clinicians have been remarkably creative in devising innovative and complex approaches to the treatment of HCC (Table 46–3). **However, HCC remains remarkably resistant to cure.** Of chemotherapeutic agents, only doxorubicin (Adriamycin) has shown a better than 20% response rate. There have been essentially no cures with chemotherapy given systemically, either as a single agent or in combination. Site-directed chemotherapy via intraarterial perfusion has shown only a modest increase in response rate by allowing delivery of larger doses of chemotherapeutic agents directly to the tumor site. More promising, but primarily for short- or long-term palliation, is the recent approach of embolizing the vessels feeding the tumor with Gelfoam (see Figure 46–2F and 46–2G) or Lipiodol, an oily substance that becomes trapped in the tumor (Figure 46–4). An extension of these two approaches combines embolization of the tumor vessels with chemotherapy, thus producing a combination of anoxic necrosis with high local concen-

Table 46–3. Therapeutic options for HCC.

Generally accepted modalities
    One to three nodules, < 5 cm in diameter
        1. Surgical resection
        2. Percutaneous ethanol injection[1]
        3. Cryosurgery[1] or radiofrequency ablation[1]
        4. Chemoembolization with or without liver transplantation[2]
    More than three nodules or > 5 cm in diameter
        1. Percutaneous ethanol injection[1]
        2. Chemoembolization[1]
        3. Cryosurgery[1] or radiofrequency ablation[1]
Experimental modalities
    1. Surgical resection with adjuvant chemotherapy
    2. Liver transplantation with or without chemoembolization before transplant with or without adjuvant chemotherapy[2]
    3. Immunotargeting with monoclonal or polyclonal antibodies[1] to α-fetoprotein, ferritin, or "tumor-associated antigens," as palliative treatment or cytoreduction therapy to allow resection of large tumors
        a. Monoclonal antibodies alone
        b. Antibodies conjugated to chemotherapeutic agents
        c. Antibodies conjugated to ^{131}I, ^{125}I, ^{90}Y, ^{99m}Tc (radioimmunodetection and therapy)
    4. Proton irridation[1]

---

[1]Do not require open surgery. Performed percutaneously via laparoscopy or under ultrasound guidance.
[2]Liver transplantation with its many multimodal approaches is clearly still experimental but is listed in both categories because of its widespread use and availability.

trations of trapped chemotherapeutic agents. This approach with **chemoembolization** has shown some promise. For small tumors, less than 5 cm and preferably less than 3 cm in size, percutaneous ethanol, acetic acid, and even hot saline injections have proved quite beneficial in improving 3- to 5-year survival. Encapsulation of Adriamycin in liposomes, and a variety of attempts to target the tumor with monoclonal antibodies, or antibodies to molecules produced in high concentration by the tumor (α-fetoprotein, ferritin), have also been used experimentally, but to date have either been used only in animals, or have shown no significant improvement over other modalities when used in humans. Recently, cryosurgery and radiofrequency ablation by laparoscopic or percutaneous techniques have been applied to patients with small tumors and poor hepatic reserve or other comorbid conditions that eliminate the option of surgical resection or liver transplantation. Data are limited at present and these techniques should still be considered experimental.

The only technique currently available with a reasonable chance of cure is **surgical resection.** However, this is true only for single nodules less than 3 cm in size. Larger nodules or the presence of multiple nodules make recurrence almost inevitable. **Liver transplantation** removes the entire liver, and with it all intrahepatic micrometastases and dysplastic, preneoplastic cells.

It is beneficial in the treatment of small (<5 cm) single lesions, often in combination with chemoembolization and posttransplant adjuvant chemotherapy. Such approaches have been reported to produce 5-year survival rates of 60–70% in highly selected patients.

The use of historic, untreated controls, or controls treated with only systemic chemotherapy, makes it very difficult to evaluate the variety of treatment modalities currently available. Controlled trials will be necessary to determine whether any of the more aggressive treatments offer an advantage over a simple resection or chemoembolization. Meanwhile, the limitations of treatment remain the lack of highly effective chemotherapeutic agents and the poor surgical candidacy of the majority of patients with HCC due to the large size of the tumor at presentation or the severity of the underlying cirrhosis. Estimates have been made that <5% of patients with HCC are acceptable risks for resection. The major complication following liver resection in such patients is liver failure. The likelihood of new tumors developing remains high when the native liver and the risk factors for HCC due to cirrhosis and continued necroinflammatory change remain in place. Currently, in most cases it is best to identify patients at high risk for developing HCC, follow them with careful surveillance in hopes of identifying very early lesions, and have an experienced surgeon perform resec-

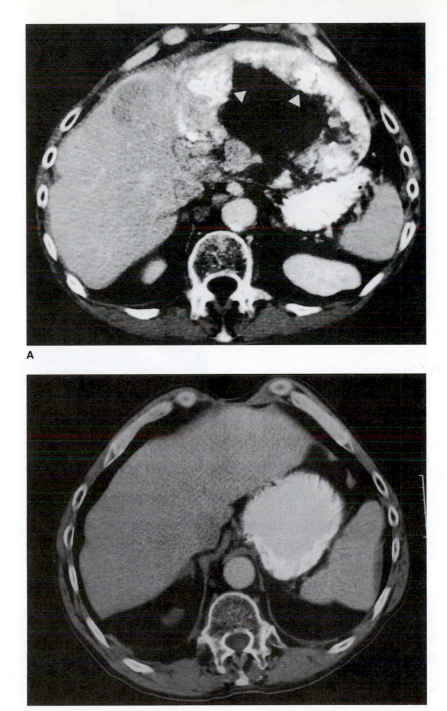

A

B

Figure 46–4. **A:** CT shows Lipiodal trapped in the tumor of the patient in Figure 46–2 following chemoemboliza-tion of the tumor *(arrowheads).* **B:** CT shows a normal liver 1 year following chemoembolization and transplanta-tion of the patient in Figure 46–2.

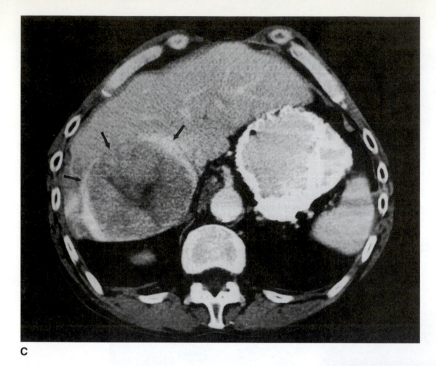

C

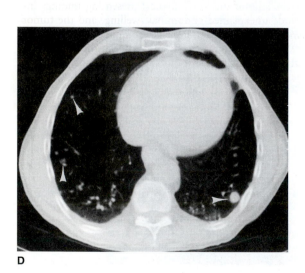

D

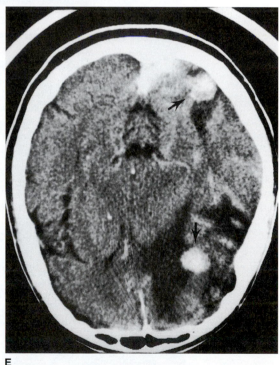

E

Figure 46–4. **C–E:** CT 6 months later (18 months posttransplantation) shows tumor recurrence in the right lobe of the transplanted liver. Note rim enhancement of this hypervascular lesion *(arrows)* and hypodense necrotic center. Boney metastases (not shown) and lung metastases were also apparent *(**arrowheads,** D)*. Two months later the patient developed slurring speech and an ataxic gait. Brain metastases were found in the right frontal and right parietooccipital lobes *(**arrows,** E)*.

tion. Referral to a liver transplant center for those with one to three small lesions should also be considered. All other approaches should remain in the hands of those conducting clinical trials so that useful data will be developed to improve future therapy. Aggressive universal immunization against hepatitis B on a worldwide basis, elimination of food contaminated by aflatoxin and other hepatocarcinogenic toxins, reduction of alcoholism, and careful screening of blood products will ultimately have the greatest impact on HCC incidence by eliminating the major factors contributing to its pathogenesis. Also of great interest are recent studies showing that treatment with interferon-α may delay and possibly even prevent the development of HCC in patients with hepatitis C. Additional long-term studies of this finding are currently underway.

Prognosis

The overall prognosis for HCC remains very poor. Mean survival after diagnosis of large tumors, if not treated, is less than 6 months. Small tumors have a considerably better prognosis, with one study reporting 90% survival at 3 years in patients with tumors smaller than 3 cm; another found 63% survival at 3 years in patients with tumors less than 5 cm in size, and Child–Pugh class A cirrhosis (undecompensated cirrhosis). Surgical resection of small tumors or possibly percutaneous ethanol injection or radiofrequency ablation provides the only reasonable chance for cure. Liver transplantation is probably most successful in this group of patients as well, but limited data and a lack of controls make it difficult to interpret the transplant literature. Long delays prior to transplantation due to a shortage of donor organs also limit the practicality of this approach. The same is true for most other approaches to HCC. There is currently no adequate staging system that takes into account all prognostic factors identified in individual studies, and virtually all studies use historic controls or no controls at all. Until there is better information on the natural history of HCC and more carefully controlled comparative trials, it is difficult to recommend the more aggressive approaches to HCC outside of experimental trials. For small tumors (<3 cm), simple resection is probably the best approach; for large tumors, chemoembolization may offer significant palliation.

OTHER MALIGNANT TUMORS

1. Fibrolamellar Carcinoma

This important variant of HCC is characterized by its occurrence primarily in younger patients between the ages of 20 and 40 years and by the absence of cirrhosis.

It has no gender preference or known risk factors, and α-fetoprotein is usually normal. Over 50% of the tumors occur in the left lobe, making it particularly amenable to surgical resection. Histologically, it is characterized by monotonous benign-looking cells with extremely rare mitoses and the presence of fibrous bands that traverse the tumor in a lamellar fashion dividing it into cords and nodules. The prognosis is considerably better than that for HCC, and long-term survival is frequent with either resection or liver transplantation.

2. Minute or Encapsulated HCC

This unusual variant accounts for 10% of the HCC cases in Japan, and is found almost exclusively in Southeast Asia. It is a slow growing tumor, usually only 3–5 cm in diameter, with a thick fibrous capsule. It is well differentiated histologically, and vascular invasion is quite rare. No risk factors are known, and only 50% are α-fetoprotein positive. Because of its small encapsulated nature and lack of vascular invasion, it has a very high surgical cure rate.

3. Hepatoblastoma

This rare liver tumor of infancy presents almost exclusively before 3 years of age, and most often before 2 years of age. It is the most common liver tumor of infants, but is the cause of only 0.2–5.8% of malignancies of childhood. Two-thirds are solitary, most often in the right lobe of the liver. Typical presenting findings include unexplained abdominal swelling, and the tumor may already be quite large at the time of birth. Associated findings may include anorexia, diarrhea, vomiting, abdominal pain, irritability, weight loss, and failure to thrive. Tumor rupture may produce hemoperitoneum. A variety of associated congenital anomalies have been noted, including hemihypertrophy, talipes, macroglossia, right diaphragmatic defect, Meckel's diverticulum, cardiac and renal malformations, and polyposis coli. Approximately twice as many males are affected as females. α-Fetoprotein levels are increased in 80–90% of patients, but routine liver tests are usually normal or show only minor abnormalities. Ectopic production of human chorionic gonadotropin may produce precocious puberty, in addition to osteopenia with fractures, hypoglycemia, and isosexual precocity. Cystathioninuria has been reported. Metastases to the lung may be identified. The lesion is avascular on angiography and frequently shows calcification. Because of its large size and aggressive growth (mean 10–12 cm, range 3–20 cm), hepatoblastoma is rapidly fatal in most cases. Surgical resection should be performed immediately if possible. If not, aggressive chemotherapy may debulk the tumor sufficiently to allow curative surgery. A combination of chemotherapy and radiotherapy following surgery may improve prognosis.

4. Angiosarcoma

Although it is the most common mesenchymal tumor of the liver, fewer than 25 cases occur in North America each year, and the attack rate is 0.14–0.25 cases per million. Four out of five cases occur in males, generally in their sixth or seventh decades. Thorotrast and vinyl chloride monomer have been the most carefully documented causes of this tumor, but it has also been associated with arsenic and potassium arsenite ("Fowler's solution"), which was previously used to treat psoriasis. Also implicated have been radium, inorganic copper, and phenylethylhydrazine. Workers exposed to polyvinyl chloride have a 400-fold greater risk of developing angiosarcoma, but the incidence of this tumor has been decreasing with better manufacturing controls and the declining number of patients alive who received thorotrast.

Abdominal pain or discomfort, abdominal swelling, rapidly progressive liver failure, malaise, weakness, weight loss, anorexia, and vomiting can all be presentations of the disease. Fifty percent of the patients will have splenomegaly, and 25% will have jaundice and ascites, which may be blood tinged. Low platelet counts are found in 50% of patients, and 15% present with hemoperitoneum. There is no association with hepatitis B or other viruses, and α-fetoprotein and carcinoembryonic antigen (CEA) are normal. Hepatic arteriography demonstrates displacement of hepatic arteries by tumor, with a tumor blush and "puddling" during the mid-phase of arteriography. Central enhancement may not occur due to tumor necrosis. Liver biopsy is generally avoided because of the high risk of hemorrhage. Life expectancy from the time of diagnosis is 6 months, with 50% or more of the patients dying of liver failure. To date, no successful therapy has been found.

5. Cholangiocarcinoma

Cholangiocarcinoma is an uncommon disease in the Western world, with an incidence of 2–2.8 per 100,000 population per year. However, the incidence is much higher in the Far East due to the frequency of biliary parasites. It is associated with a variety of liver and biliary tract diseases, including (1) inflammatory bowel disease, even in the absence of sclerosing cholangitis; (2) congenital biliary anomalies including choledochal cysts, polycystic liver disease, and Caroli's disease; (3) Oriental cholangiohepatitis (*Clonorchis sinensis*); and (4) chemical exposure including thorotrast, benzidine, 3'3-dichlorobenzidine, and *m*-toluenediamide. The best recognized of these associations is with primary

sclerosing cholangitis (see Chapter 51). Of patients coming to liver transplant for sclerosing cholangitis, 7–15% are found to have cholangiocarcinoma, often first identified in the explant.

Pathophysiology

At least 50% of the tumors occur at the confluence of the right and left hepatic ducts (Klatskin tumor). Another ~20% are in the mid and ~20% in the distal common bile duct; 5% are diffuse. Most are adenocarcinomas that arise from the biliary epithelium, and there is a heavy, fibrous reaction to the tumor. This strong desmoplastic reaction, along with the presence of inflammation, may make it difficult to diagnose from brushings, or even full thickness biopsies, as the tumor cells may be sparse and well separated.

 ESSENTIALS OF DIAGNOSIS

- *A 3:1 male-to-female ratio.*
- *Most frequent in the sixth and seventh decades.*
- *Presentation with jaundice occurs most often when the tumor is located at the bifurcation of the right and left hepatic ducts (Klatskin tumor).*
- *Weight loss, diarrhea, and acholic stool in 60–75% of cases.*
- *Epigastric distress with weight loss is common.*
- *Elevated alkaline phosphatase and γ-glutamyltransferase are uniformly present; bilirubin is elevated only if there is total or near total obstruction at the bifurcation of the common duct.*
- *Anorexia and fat malabsorption are common if jaundice is present.*
- *Bacterial cholangitis occurs usually only in late-stage disease or if a stent is in place.*

Clinical Findings

A. SYMPTOMS AND SIGNS

The symptoms and signs depend on the location of the tumor (at the bifurcation of the right and left hepatic duct, or more distal) and the degree of obstruction. Patients with unilateral bile duct obstruction may have a normal bilirubin. If there is significant obstruction, jaundice, acholic stools, dark urine, and pruritus may be present. Anorexia, epigastric distress, weight loss, and diarrhea are also present in up to 60–70% of cases. Bacterial cholangitis is uncommon, except late in the disease when total or near total obstruction has occurred or if the duct has been instrumented.

B. LABORATORY FINDINGS

Mild to marked elevations in alkaline phosphatase and γ-glutamyltransferase are uniformly found. Bilirubin may be normal, unless significant obstruction is present. Transaminases (AST and ALT) are generally minimally abnormal. α-Fetoprotein is negative but CA 19-9 and CEA are frequently positive, although not pathognomonic.

C. IMAGING

Ultrasound demonstrates dilated intrahepatic ducts if a Klatskin lesion is present and extrahepatic duct dilation will occur to the level of obstruction if there is a distal obstruction. CT scan will not reveal a mass lesion until late in the disease, but can confirm the dilated ducts. Angiography is indicated only if surgical resection is contemplated as vascular invasion is a contraindication to surgical resection. Magnetic resonance cholangiopancreatography (MRCP) will identify the site of obstruction, but endoscopic retrograde cholangiopancreatography (ERCP) or percutaneous transhepatic cholangiography (PTC) will demonstrate the biliary obstruction at the site of the tumor and allow brushings for cytologic examination as well. A good cytologic specimen will be positive in approximately 75% of cases.

Differential Diagnosis

Cholangiocarcinoma must be differentiated from all other biliary obstructive lesions. Particularly problematic is the differentiation from primary sclerosing cholangitis, which frequently serves as a substratum for the development of cholangiocarcinoma. ERCP and PTC are the most useful in ruling out other causes of cholestasis and attempting to document the presence of malignancy. However, even good cytologic brushings will be negative in the presence of tumor at least 25% of the time.

Complications

Patients most often die of liver failure due to the development of biliary cirrhosis, although sepsis, cholangitis, and metastatic destruction of the liver can also occur.

Treatment

Curative resection is rarely possible because of the advanced stage of disease at which patients present. Liver transplantation has been equally disappointing due to the 100% recurrence rate of cholangiocarcinoma following transplantation. There is no effective chemotherapy. Very aggressive approaches to unresectable

tumor are being pursued in a few centers currently, utilizing external beam radiotherapy, brachyradiotherapy with iridium-192 implants placed by ERCP, and combinations of the above with liver transplantation. Sufficient data have not been published at present to form a definite opinion as to the long-term efficacy of such approaches but early reports appear promising. Significant palliation can be produced by dilation and stenting of strictures when resection is not possible. Endoscopic stent placement provides an advantage over externally drained stents because it maintains biliary enteric continuity, and should be possible in 85% of cases when a well-trained endoscopist is available. The stent tends to become obstructed over time, and many centers routinely exchange the stents at least every 4 to 6 months on an outpatient basis.

Prognosis

Five-year survival is only 4–10%. Patients die from liver failure or infectious complications due to problems with biliary drainage. Anorexia, malaise, and inanition are frequent accompaniments of end-stage disease. Local invasion of the portal vein and hepatic artery may also produce the standard complications of portal hypertension, ascites, and variceal bleeding.

NONMALIGNANT EPITHELIAL TUMORS

Nonmalignant hepatic masses can range from simple cysts and hemangiomas to hepatocellular adenomas and focal nodular hyperplasia. Although all are benign, some can produce significant morbidity and even mortality if inaccurately diagnosed and treated. Others can lead to unnecessary, costly, and sometimes mischievous interventions when they would be better left alone.

1. Hepatocellular Adenoma

Hepatocellular adenomas are benign epithelial cell tumors that were extremely rare in the United States prior to 1954. Only two were found in 50,000 autopsies at the Los Angeles County General Hospital prior to that time and none during surgery at the Mayo Clinic over the same period. However, since 1960 there has been a dramatic rise, which has been attributed to the common use of estrogens in oral contraceptives. The estimated incidence is 3–4 per 100,000 users per year. This ranges from a low of 1–1.3 per 100,000 individuals who never used oral contraceptives to 34 per 100,000 individuals with long-term use of oral contraceptives. The individuals at greatest risk were over 30 years of age and had used high-dose estrogens for more than 5 years. Over the past decade, the incidence has dropped dramatically as oral contraceptives have been produced with progressively lower concentrations of estrogen.

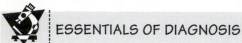

ESSENTIALS OF DIAGNOSIS

- Sixty percent have a history of oral contraceptive use.
- Ninety percent are solitary lesions.
- Liver tests are normal or minimally abnormal.
- Regression after discontinuing hormonal therapy.
- Anabolic androgenic steroids and certain metabolic diseases are also risk factors.
- Complications of intratumor hemorrhage and hemoperitoneum from tumor rupture.
- Resection is required in most cases.

Pathophysiology

Estrogen exposure is the major risk factor for the development of hepatocellular adenoma, and the risk correlates with the dose and duration of estrogen ingestion. Hepatocellular adenomas have been identified in men taking anabolic androgenic steroids, which can be aromatized to estrogens, indicating a possible common pathway. This benign tumor has also been reported in patients with glycogen storage disease type 1, tyrosinemia, and galactosemia. When it occurs in association with a metabolic disease, it is primarily a male disease with a high risk of malignant transformation.

An unrelated condition, **multiple hepatocellular adenomatosis,** presents with multiple adenomas, usually more than four, scattered among the hepatic lobes. It is not associated with other liver diseases or estrogen intake.

Clinical Findings

A. SYMPTOMS AND SIGNS

Patients may present in crisis with intraabdominal hemorrhage due to rupture of an adenoma, with complaints of right upper quadrant pain due to intratumor hemorrhage, after noting a palpable mass, or, most frequently, following the incidental finding of a liver mass during an ultrasound or CT examination performed for another purpose.

B. PHYSICAL EXAMINATION

There are usually no findings on physical examination. A palpable and sometimes tender mass may be noted in the right upper quadrant. When hemoperitoneum is present, findings typical of an acute abdomen and possibly shock, depending on the severity of the hemorrhage, will predominate.

C. LABORATORY FINDINGS

Laboratory findings are not helpful and most often are normal. Minor elevations of alkaline phosphatase, γ-glutamyltransferase, or transaminases may be noted. α-Fetoprotein is normal.

D. IMAGING

Ultrasound and CT examinations will usually identify the lesion without difficulty (Table 46–4). Because of its lack of Kupffer cells, it will present as a defect on radioactive sulfur colloid scan. There are no diagnostic findings on ultrasound or CT. The lesion is hypervascular, which can be noted on MRI. Angiography may demonstrate large peripheral vessels with centrifugal flow; central avascular scars may be present due to internal hemorrhage. However, some adenomas will be hypovascular.

Differential Diagnosis

The hepatocellular adenoma must be differentiated from malignant lesions and focal nodular hyperplasia (Table 46–5). It is most often solitary, and frequently quite large, often being greater than 10 cm in size. Histologically, it may also be difficult to differentiate from normal liver and highly differentiated HCC. Adjacent normal hepatocytes should be distinguishable from the "neohepatocytes" of the tumor. Kupffer cells are absent. The failure to find portal tracts or bile ducts, producing "free floating" intralobular arterioles without their usual accompanying bile ducts and portal veins, is a particularly useful histologic difference. Giant cell formation, cholestasis, alcoholic hyaline, and α_1-antitrypsin inclusions may also be found.

Complications

Up to one-third of patients may present with acute hemoperitoneum, requiring emergent resection or hepatic artery ligation. This is the major risk, although occasional progression to HCC has been noted, primarily in those related to underlying metabolic disorders.

Treatment

The majority of hepatocellular adenomas should be resected whenever possible; this may be possible laparascopically in some cases. For readily accessible adenomas some centers are now utilizing US-guided radiofrequency ablation, thus avoiding a major incision and shortening recovery time. Experience with this technique is limited, however. Controversy exists concern-

Table 46–4. Imaging techniques and hepatic masses.[1]

Technique	Discussion
US	Noninvasive, low cost, readily available; with Doppler imaging, also provides information on vascular patency and volume and direction of flow; sensitivity to 1 cm; ideal screening technique; diagnostic for simple cysts; unable to convincingly determine etiology of solid or mixed masses; excellent technique for guided biopsy; marked obesity or bowel gas interferes with the examination; generally the screening test of first choice
CT	Radiation and contrast exposure; readily available and provides "normal anatomy" for nonradiologist; sensitivity to 1 cm; nearly isodense lesions may be missed due to volume averaging or timing of imaging to contrast injection; will screen for extrahepatic lesions simultaneously, thus identifying metastatic disease beyond the liver
Triphasic helical CT	Increased radiation exposure (must first localize lesion and then take multiple timed images); correctly identifies two-thirds of hemangiomas
CTAP	Invasive, requiring placement of angiography catheter for bolus injection; superior delineation of anatomic location of lesions to help with surgical planning; more sensitive than standard CT and will often save unnecessary surgery by identifying additional tumor nodules not noted on standard CT or US; may produce increase in false-positive findings in presence of severe cirrhosis
MRI	Totally noninvasive but very expensive; excellent biplanar images with sensitivity to 1.0 cm; more accurate than CTAP in the presence of severe cirrhosis; problems identifying lesions near the diaphragm due to cardiac motion-induced artifacts; provides additional information on vascular supply and patency
Angiography	Most invasive with high contrast dose and high radiation exposure; most expensive (along with MRI); provides most accurate information on vascular supply, patency, and flow, including pressures if needed
Nuclear medicine	Minimally invasive, less costly (except for US), and readily available; less sensitive (2 cm minimum); primarily useful to distinguish hepatic adenomas from focal nodular hyperplasia (due to the lack of Kupffer cells for colloid uptake in the adenomas) and identifying hemangiomas (with the ^{99m}Tc-tagged RBC-SPECT study)

[1]US, ultrasound; CT, computed axial tomography; CTAP, computed axial tomography arterioportogram; MRI, fast-spin echo magnetic resonance imaging; RBC-SPECT, ^{99m}Tc-tagged red blood cell study utilizing single photon emission computed tomography.

ing the smaller lesions in patients on oral contraceptives, as they will usually regress with discontinuation of the oral contraceptives. If the adenoma is not surgically removed, patients should be closely followed in case there is an increase in size or malignant transformation. Estrogens and pregnancy should be avoided. Pregnancy is safe following successful resection of a hepatic adenoma, if no recurrence is noted.

Table 46–5. Focal nodular hyperplasia and hepatic adenoma.[1]

	FNH	HA
Healthy young women	+	+
Induced by OC	±	+
Hemorrhage	–	+
Malignant transformation	–	+
Treatment	Observation	Resection

[1]FNH, focal nodular hyperplasia; HA, hepatocellular adenoma; OC, oral contraceptive.

Prognosis

Prognosis is excellent with discontinuation of estrogens and resection.

2. Focal Nodular Hyperplasia

Focal nodular hyperplasia (FNH) is the most common benign hepatic tumor, other than vascular tumors. In one large series from the University of Southern California, approximately 8% of all primary hepatic tumors were FNH, which represented 66% of all benign, non-hemangiomatous lesions in the autopsy study of 96,625 patients. A more recent study of 549 patients undergoing MRI examination found that 23% of 805 benign lesions were FNH, which represented 86% of all non-hemangiomatous lesions.

Pathogenesis

FNH has been described as a benign tumor, a hamartoma, or a manifestation of liver regeneration. Most likely it develops because of a congenital vascular malformation with subsequent cellular hyperplasia and possibly hepatocellular metaplasia in response to hyperperfusion by the anomalous arteries characteristically found in the center of these lesions. Its association with oral contraceptive agents is unclear, and it occurs in men, in children, and in women not on oral contraceptive agents, thus making the association considerably weaker than with hepatic adenomas. However, it is most common in females (8 or 9:1) between the ages of 20 and 50 years.

ESSENTIALS OF DIAGNOSIS

- *Two-thirds to three-fourths are discovered incidentally.*
- *Ninety percent are solitary lesions.*
- *Normal laboratory studies.*
- *Occasionally there is pain due to rupture or hemorrhage.*
- *"Spoked-wheel" appearance on hepatic angiography.*
- *Gadolinium-enhanced MRI is 98% specific and 70% sensitive.*
- *Not premalignant, and generally no therapy is required.*
- *Avoid oral contraceptives and pregnancy.*

General Considerations

This is not felt to be a premalignant lesion, and is most often discovered incidentally and best left alone.

Clinical Findings

A. SYMPTOMS AND SIGNS

The vast majority of these benign tumor-like lesions are found incidentally. If symptoms or signs are present, most commonly a mass is noted in the upper abdomen. Pain is occasionally present, usually in association with hemorrhage into the nodule or rupture. Hemorrhage most often occurs in women taking oral contraceptives.

B. LABORATORY FINDINGS

The laboratory findings are almost always normal. α-Fetoprotein is normal.

C. IMAGING

The imaging findings are better understood when correlated with the histology. FNH usually occurs as a sin-gle subcapsular lesion less than 5 cm in size. The characteristic finding is a central fibrous scar with fibrous septae radiating to the periphery of the lesion. Early reports described this as "focal cirrhosis," and large arterial vessels with fibromuscular hyperplasia as well as multiple bile ductules travel along the septae. Kupffer cells are present, providing another means to differentiate it from hepatocellular adenomas. Ultrasound and CT readily identify the lesion, but have no characteristic findings, although the central scar is often noted on CT. The same scar will be hyperdense on gadolinium-enhanced MRI T2-weighted images, and an enhanced MRI study is 98% specific and 70% sensitive. Angiography may demonstrate the hypervascular lesion with a hypovascular central scar and vessels radiating toward the center in a "spoked-wheel" fashion.

Differential Diagnosis

This lesion must be differentiated from all other benign and malignant mass lesions of the liver (Table 46–6). Usually, the characteristic imaging findings are sufficient to make the diagnosis. In up to two-thirds of cases, when the lesion is found incidentally at surgery, it is biopsied and the histology is characteristic.

Treatment

Because the lesion is rarely symptomatic and there is no convincing evidence of malignant predisposition, no treatment is necessary. On the rare occasion when pain or hemorrhage occurs, a definitive diagnosis is elusive, or an unusually large lesion is present (>8 cm), surgical resection is appropriate.

Prognosis

The prognosis is excellent and, other than the rare case of abdominal crisis from rupture and hemorrhage, FNH is unlikely to produce morbidity or mortality. There is no clear predisposition to malignancy. However, it is probably best to avoid the use of oral contraceptives, and most authorities do not recommend pregnancy, although a recent study of 216 women found no effect of oral contraceptives on size, number, or change in size of FNH lesions. The same study documented successful completion of 12 of 12 pregnancies with no FNH complications. Still, this is one study with small numbers and it would seem prudent to avoid oral contraceptives or pregnancy if a large FNH nodule is present.

3. Nodular Regenerative Hyperplasia

This unusual and uncommon condition is characterized by nodules of hyperplastic hepatocytes surrounded

Table 46–6. Differential diagnosis of hepatic mass lesions.[1]

	Hepatocellular Carcinoma	Metastatic Carcinoma	Hepatocellular Adenoma	Focal Nodular Hyperplasia	Cavernous Hemangioma	Simple Cyst
Incidence/100,000[3]	1–4800[3]	8–20	3–4	3–4	400–7500	170
Solitary	20–40%	5–10%	90%	90%	90%	?
Coexisting liver disease	HBV, HCV, cirrhosis hemochromatosis	Uncommon in cirrhotic liver	None	None	None	None
Pathogenesis	HBV, HCV, alcohol, aflatoxin, cirrhosis	Hematogenous, lymphatic or direct spread	Estrogens, anabolic steroids	Congenital, ?estrogens	Congenital, estrogens	Congenital
Imaging[4]	US, CT	US, CT, CTAP	US, CT, ^{99m}Tc	US, CT, MRI, ^{99m}Tc	Triphasic spiral CT, ^{99m}Tc–RBC–SPECT scan MRI	US, CT
α-Fetoprotein	> 300–500 ng/mL	Normal	Normal	Normal	Normal	Normal
Characteristic gross features	Hemorrhage, necrosis, vascular invasion/obstruction	Hemorrhage, Necrosis; umbilicated	Hemorrhage, necrosis	Central scar	Blood-filled "cyst"	Thin-walled cyst with clear fluid
Characteristic microscopic features	"Thick" (> 3–4 cells) trabeculae	Replacement of hepatocytes by malignant cells	"Neohepatocytes," normal cord structure, no portal structures	"Focal cirrhosis" with pseudoductules	Blood-filled spaces lined by single layer of flat endothelium	Simple cuboidal endothelium
Diagnosis[5]	FNAB or core biopsy	FNAB or core biopsy	Imaging, biopsy	Imaging, biopsy	Imaging	Imaging
Treatment	"Curative resection" or ethanol injection if solitary, < 5.0 cm; ? transplantation with or without chemoembolization	"Curative resection" if < 3.0 cm and three or fewer nodules	Discontinue estrogens/androgens; resect if possible, especially if large; otherwise periodic imaging; malignant potential	Discontinue estrogens; periodic imaging	Surgical resection only if symptomatic or > 10.0 cm; discontinue estrogens; periodic imaging	Usually no treatment; percutaneous aspiration or surgical enucleation if symptomatic

[1] US, ultrasound; CT, computed axial tomography; triphasic spiral CT, rapid sequential CT images taken at plane of the mass before contrast injection, with delayed images up to 20 minutes after contrast to capture arterial and venous phases; CTAP, computed axial tomography arterioportogram; MRI, fast-spin echo magnetic resonance imaging; ^{99m}Tc, ^{99m}Tc-labeled sulfur colloid scan; RBC-SPECT, ^{99m}Tc-tagged red blood cell study utilizing single photon emission computerized tomography; FNAB, fine-needle aspiration biopsy for cytology.

[2] From autopsy series.

[3] Varies with geographic origin.

[4] Most useful imaging technique with which to obtain a diagnosis.

[5] Definitive test required for confident diagnosis.

by compressed and distorted adjacent hepatocytes, giving a superficial appearance of cirrhosis, although no fibrosis is present. The hyperplastic hepatocytes are arranged in plates more than one cell thick and the lesion is best demonstrated on reticulin stain.

Pathogenesis

The etiology of this lesion is unclear, but may involve occlusion of multiple intrahepatic portal vein branches, producing local ischemia and atrophy with subsequent compensatory regeneration of surrounding hepatocytes leading to compression of adjacent lobules. A possible association with arterial and/or portal venous inflammation has been suggested, and pathology has always been required for diagnosis. Although usually idiopathic, it has often been reported in association with rheumatoid arthritis, Felty's syndrome, subacute bacterial endocarditis, CRST syndrome, and the long-term use of certain drugs (corticosteroids and oral contraceptives). It has also been noted in association with hematologic diseases such as myeloma, polycythemia vera, and myelofibrosis. Hereditary hemorrhagic telangiectasia, polyarteritis nodosa, diabetes mellitus, and the toxic oil syndrome have also been reported associations.

Clinical Findings

A. SYMPTOMS AND SIGNS

Nodular regenerative hyperplasia is rarely recognized other than as an incidental finding. Occasionally, development of portal hypertension or its complications will lead to the diagnosis.

B. LABORATORY FINDINGS

Laboratory tests are normal, unless the patient develops portal hypertension. Laboratory abnormalities related to associated diseases are frequently present and may lead to the suggestion of nodular regenerative hyperplasia, when the primary disease has been diagnosed. α-Fetoprotein is normal.

C. IMAGING

Ill-defined nodules may be noted on US or CT, but they have no defining characteristics, and histology is required for diagnosis.

Differential Diagnosis

Nodular regenerative hyperplasia must be distinguished from focal nodular hyperplasia, hepatocellular adenoma, and HCC, as well as cirrhosis. Histology is required to make this distinction.

Complications

Portal hypertension, if present, may require the usual therapy for ascites, bleeding varices, or hepatic encephalopathy, although all of these are uncommon. Most often the treatment is directed at the underlying associated disease. On rare occasion, nodular regenerative hyperplasia can lead to liver failure, and patients have required liver transplantation. Rupture of the liver has also been a rare event. As with the other benign conditions discussed above, female patients are advised not to use contraceptive steroids.

4. Other Uncommon Conditions

Anabolic Steroid-Associated Hepatocellular Adenoma

C-17 alkylated forms of anabolic steroids have been reported as potential inducers of a variety of liver problems, including peliosis hepatis, hepatocellular adenoma, and possibly cholangiocarcinoma and HCC. **Peliosis hepatis** is a condition in which multiple small, dilated, blood-filled cavities, with no supporting stroma, develop. These cavities usually do not have any lining endothelium. They are less than 5–10 mm in diameter and are associated with the use of anabolic steroids as well as estrogenic compounds. They have also been associated with *Bartonella quintana* infection in human immunodeficiency virus (HIV) disease (see Chapter 38). They may also be seen as a precursor to the development of hemangiosarcoma in patients exposed to vinyl chloride monomer. For the past 20–30 years, increasing numbers of hepatocellular adenomas have been reported in patients taking anabolic steroids, but this still remains an infrequent occurrence.

Seventy-five percent of cases occur in males of virtually all ages, but particularly adolescence. Hepatomegaly and pain are the usual presenting symptoms, although hemoperitoneum may occur. It is rare for tumors to be noted unless patients have been taking steroids for more than 40–80 months. Laboratory studies are not helpful, and α-fetoprotein is normal. If α-fetoprotein is elevated, underlying cholangiocarcinoma or HCC should be suspected.

Multiple small tumors or numerous small nodules are the usual finding, although they can range up to 11 cm in size. Tumor nodules usually resolve with discontinuation of steroid therapy, but may persist. Clearly documented progression to HCC has not been demonstrated, although long-term follow-up without development of tumor after 10–15 years of use has been reported. Overall prognosis is generally excellent and is more dependent on the underlying condition than the benign tumors associated with it.

Microregenerative Nodules

Microregenerative nodules related to prior submassive hepatic necrosis or cirrhosis are occasionally noted. They contain normal portal areas, as well as hyperplastic hepatocytes, and lack neoplastic characteristics or potential.

Partial Nodular Transformation

This condition is extremely rare, and may be related to nodular regenerative hyperplasia. Nodules of hyperplastic hepatocytes up to 4 cm in size are found in the perihilar area in association with portal hypertension. A marked reduction in the number and size of portal vein branches is found, and is most likely the cause of the portal hypertension rather than compression by the nodules. Cavernous transformation of the portal vein may also be found.

OTHER LIVER MASSES & TUMOR-LIKE CONDITIONS

1. Hepatic Cysts

Up to 0.17% of livers at autopsy will have incidental small cysts and a similar prevalence has been noted on US examination. Classic hepatic cysts have a thin, poorly cellular, fibrous wall, lined by a single cuboidal epithelium, and contain clear fluid. Ultrasound examination will demonstrate no internal echoes and through transmission of the sound waves (Figure 46–5A). With such findings, there is essentially no differential diagnosis. Abscesses, HCC, metastases, hematomas, and echinococcal cysts should not be confused with a simple cyst because the later will ordinarily have a variety of irregular internal echos and well-defined borders, making their distinction quite simple. Cysts also display a sharply demarcated, smooth wall and water density interior on CT; however, in cysts that are smaller than 2 cm in size, volume averaging may make them difficult to identify on CT. MRI is rarely necessary to distinguish simple cysts, and generally no treatment is required. On occasion, hemorrhage into the cyst or superinfection of the cyst will require percutaneous drainage or surgical excision or enucleation.

2. Biliary Cystadenoma

This benign epithelial cystic tumor is multilocular and has a dense fibrous capsule that clearly separates it from the surrounding liver parenchyma. It is relatively rare and found most frequently in young women. Presenting symptoms and signs include abdominal pain and/or a large palpable mass. Differentiation is primarily from a simple cyst and is usually not difficult because of the unilocular nature of simple cysts and the very thin, diaphanous wall of simple cysts, both of which are readily appreciated on imaging studies. The distinction is an important one because up to 25% of biliary cystadenomas are, or may become, malignant. Thus, in contrast to simple hepatic cysts, biliary cystadenomas should be resected.

3. Cavernous Hemangioma

Among hepatic masses, hemangiomas probably present the greatest diagnostic challenge and create the most problems for the physician and radiologist. Occurring in up to 7% of the population, they are generally benign, and require no therapy but may prove quite difficult to distinguish from malignancies.

 ESSENTIALS OF DIAGNOSIS

- *Eighty-five percent are asymptomatic.*
- *Triphasic helical CT scan is the diagnostic study of choice.*
- *Confirmation is usually possible with MRI or red cell (SPECT) study.*
- *Follow-up imaging study should be done at 3–6 months.*
- *Large (>10 cm) cavernous hemangiomas should be resected if possible.*

General Considerations

These benign blood-filled mesenchymal tumors have a normal endothelial cell lining, with a thin fibrous stroma producing multiple cavernous spaces. Usually solitary, they range in size from 2 mm to greater than 20 cm. More than 85% are asymptomatic, and are picked up incidentally by US or CT performed for other reasons.

Clinical Findings

A. SYMPTOMS AND SIGNS

Fewer than 15% have any symptoms. The most common symptom is pain, often quite sharp, and usually related to hemorrhage into the hemangioma. An abdominal crisis may occur if there is rupture of the hemangioma. Asymptomatic detection may cause concern for the patient, particularly when the possibility of a

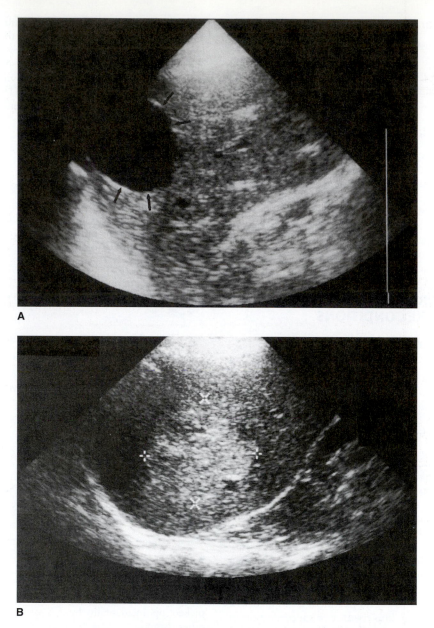

A

B

Figure 46–5. Imaging of an hepatic cyst and an hemangioma. **A:** A benign hepatic cyst *(arrows)* is clearly seen on this ultrasound image. The cyst is completely anechoic with a sharply defined, thin wall. Compare with the mixed hyper- and hypochoic areas in Figure 46–2A (hepatocellular carcinoma) and the hyperchoic mass in **B** (cavernous hemangioma). **B:** A 5-cm × 5-cm hyperechoic mass is readily seen on this ultrasound image. The edges of the mass are marked with crosses. Color Doppler ultrasound (not shown) revealed virtually no flow, strongly suggesting a diagnosis of cavernous hemangioma.

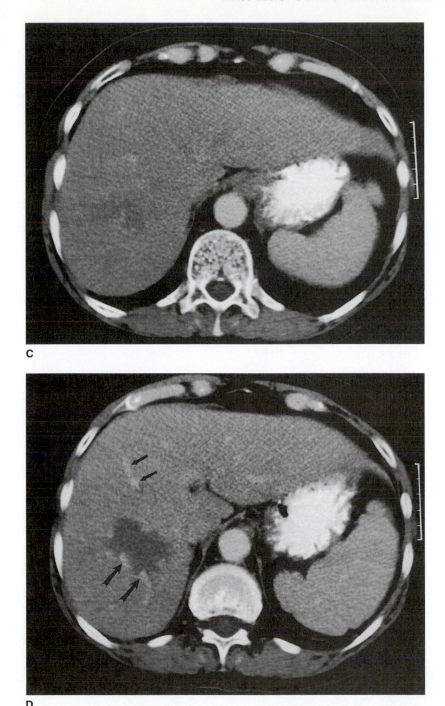

Figure 46–5. **C–D:** Diagnosis was confirmed by a dynamic bolus CT. Just before injection of the contrast bolus **(C)**, the hemangioma is virtually indiscernible from the normal liver. Within 20 seconds of injecting the bolus **(D)**, the hypodense hemangioma is readily apparent with some puddling of contrast at the periphery of the lesion ***(large arrows)***; blood vessels are easily identified ***(small arrows).***

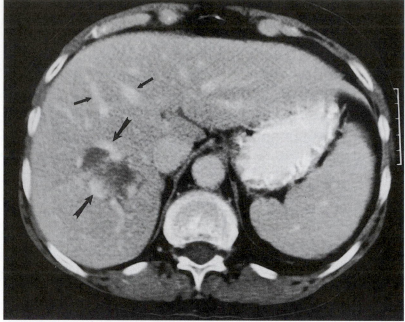

E

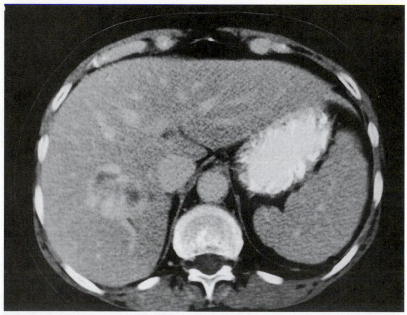

F

Figure 46–5. **E–F:** The puddling of contrast at the periphery is more apparent by 1 minute and blood vessels are more apparent **(E)**; at 5 minutes **(F)**, the lesion has begun filling in from the periphery but a hypodense core is still apparent.

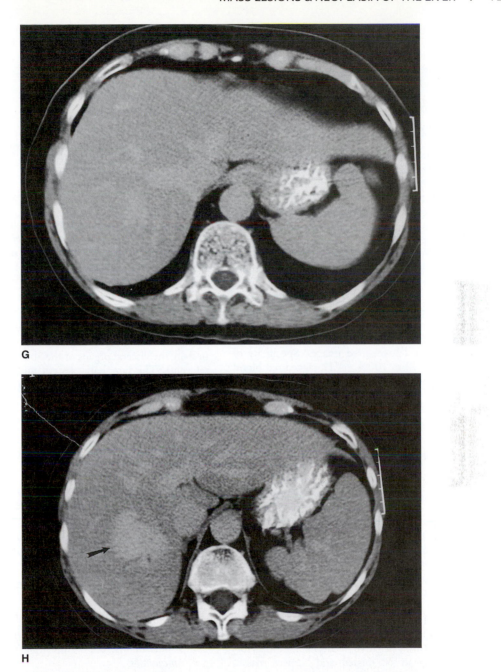

Figure 46–5. **G–H:** By 18 minutes **(G)**, the entire lesion is isodense with the liver parenchyma and cannot be discerned; 1 minute later **(H)**, the lesion is hyperdense compared with the rest of the liver as the contrast agent drains more slowly from the hemangioma ***(large arrow).***

malignancy is raised (see Figure 46–5B). The laboratory findings are not helpful, other than ruling out other possible diagnoses. Thus, negative α-fetoprotein and CEA tests are useful indirect evidence that the patient does not have an HCC.

B. IMAGING STUDIES

The most readily available and generally reliable test is the triphasic helical CT scan. In this study, the lesion is first identified on CT scan. Sequential cuts are later taken of the same area over at least a 20-minute interval, before and following bolus contrast injection, in order to evaluate the lesion without contrast and during the arterial and venous phases with contrast. With a cavernous hemangioma the lesion, which is usually hypodense at the outset, fills in from the periphery and gradually becomes isodense with the surrounding liver, and then hyperdense as the contrast puddles within the hemangioma on delayed scans (see Figure 46–5C–H). Approximately one-third of cases will not meet all of these criteria. In those cases, a fast-spin echo MRI is quite sensitive and specific, demonstrating a low signal intensity on T1-weighted images and a very high signal intensity on T2-weighted images. Specificity of MRI ranges from 92 to 100%. ^{99m}Tc-tagged red blood cell studies utilizing single-photon emission computerized tomography (SPECT) are equally sensitive and specific. If the radionuclide study is available, it is often less expensive than an MRI.

Differential Diagnosis

In most cases diagnosis can be confidently made by the finding of a hyperechoic, well-defined lesion on ultrasound (see Figure 46–5A), and confirmed by a triphasic helical CT scan, enhanced MRI, or tagged red cell SPECT study. On occasion, however, the diagnosis is still unclear because of problems in distinguishing it from an abscess, focal fatty infiltration, or malignancy. This problem is particularly difficult if the patient has a known or prior malignancy. In such cases, fine-needle aspiration biopsy is generally safe, as long as there is sufficient hepatic parenchyma between the lesion and the liver surface to tamponade any potential hemorrhage. However, even with a negative needle aspiration cytology, malignancy can be missed and suspect masses should be followed up at 3- to 6-month intervals to be certain that the lesion is not changing.

Complications

Most hemangiomas are benign and asymptomatic and require no treatment. Large (>10 cm) cavernous hemangiomas should be resected if possible because of the high risk of rupture with hemorrhagic crisis. Symptomatic hemangiomas, usually due to hemorrhage into the hemangioma, should also be resected as they will usually hemorrhage again.

Prognosis

Prognosis is excellent. Estrogenic compounds should be avoided and pregnancy should be discouraged if the hemangioma cannot be resected.

METASTATIC TUMORS

The most common neoplasms in the liver are metastatic ones. Approximately 40% of patients with primary or extrahepatic tumors have evidence of hepatic metastases at the time of death (Table 46–7).

Pathophysiology

The liver's unique dual blood supply provides bloodborne access to the liver from all organs of the body, especially the visceral organs of the abdomen (via the portal vein). The lymphatic system and direct extension from other organs also serve as sources of metastatic liver disease.

 ESSENTIALS OF DIAGNOSIS

- *Jaundice is rare and laboratory studies are frequently normal, despite extensive liver involvement.*
- *Symptoms include malaise, fatigue, weight loss, hepatic pain, and right upper quadrant distension or mass.*
- *Rock-hard hepatomegaly occurs in approximately one-third of cases.*
- *Hepatic friction rub or bruit suggests tumor.*
- *Alkaline phosphatase, γ-glutamyltransferase, and 5'-nucleotidase are the most likely liver test abnormalities.*
- *AST and ALT are rarely elevated.*
- *Disproportionately increased lactate dehydrogenase (LDH) is a red flag for malignancy, particularly hematogenous.*
- *Underlying cirrhosis is rare; the tumor in a cirrhotic liver is HCC until proven otherwise.*

Table 46–7. Frequency of tumor metastasis to liver.[1]

Primary Tumor	Percent with Liver Metastasis
Gallbladder	77.6
Pancreas	70.4
Unknown primary	57.0
Colon	56.0
Breast	53.2
Melanoma	50.0
Ovary	48.0
Stomach	44.0
Bronchogenic	41.8

[1]Data derived from Craig JR, Peters RL, Edmondson HA: *Tumors of the Liver and the Intrahepatic Bile Ducts.* Armed Forces Institutes of Pathology, 1989:257.

General Considerations

Metastatic liver disease is frequently the first sign of tumor elsewhere and in many cases the primary tumor cannot be identified. Unexplained malaise, fatigue, and weight loss should always prompt a consideration of occult malignancy and any biochemical liver abnormalities should prompt the use of imaging studies. Typical sites of primary tumors include colon, bile duct, pancreas, ovary, and breast.

Clinical Findings

A. SYMPTOMS AND SIGNS

Most patients have no signs of underlying liver disease and jaundice is rare until late in the disease unless the biliary tree is obstructed. Symptoms are nonspecific, although severe malaise and weight loss should suggest underlying tumor. The presence of an hepatic friction rub or bruit strongly suggests underlying tumor.

B. LABORATORY FINDINGS

Laboratory studies are often remarkably normal despite massive infiltration of the liver by tumor. Alkaline phosphatase, γ-glutamyltransferase, and 5′-nucleotidase are most often elevated and the transaminases (ALT, AST) are rarely elevated. A disproportionate rise in the LDH should strongly suggest the possibility of underlying malignancy when other causes for LDH elevation (hemolysis, muscle necrosis) have been eliminated. This is a particularly common finding in patients with infiltration of the liver by tumors of hematogenous origin (lymphomas and leukemias).

C. IMAGING

Any of the imaging techniques currently available will demonstrate metastatic lesions in most cases. Ultrasound (see Figures 46–2A and 46–5A) and CT (see Figure 46–6A–C) are generally the most useful as they will distinguish cystic from solid lesions. CT may also show areas of low attenuation within the tumor, suggesting hemorrhage and necrosis (see Figures 46–2B and 46–6A). Unenhanced CT, without contrast, is particularly helpful, especially with vascular neoplasms such as carcinoid and islet cell tumors, which may be isodense with the normal liver and missed entirely if scans are not taken immediately after peak enhancement.

Differential Diagnosis

Metastatic liver tumors must be distinguished from primary liver tumors and benign conditions. A tissue diagnosis is almost always required, which is best performed under US or CT guidance. A single pass blind liver biopsy in a patient with multiple metastatic lesions will be positive in 40–50% of cases. A second pass at a slightly different angle along with cytology and a touch preparation of the specimen will improve the yield to 60–70%. However, use of CT or US-guided biopsy will increase the yield to 90–95%. Fine-needle aspiration cytology is frequently sufficient to diagnose the general class of metastatic tumor and dictate further evaluation to identify the primary tumor, but this is not always successful.

Treatment & Prognosis

The finding of multiple metastatic lesions is generally a very poor prognostic sign, although it varies depending on the type of tumor. Making a tissue diagnosis is always worthwhile as certain tumors are remarkably responsive to therapy and thus significant palliation, and occasionally cure, can be obtained. Surgical resection of isolated metastases, if they are fewer than three in number, can provide significant long-term palliation in certain tumors, particularly adenocarcinoma of the colon, if all other disease has been resected. Often a single metastasis is the first evidence of tumor recurrence and surgical removal will provide another prolonged period of disease-free survival. Resection has also shown some success with carcinoid tumors and long remissions have been noted with breast cancer, malignant melanoma, and occasionally sarcoma. However, such an approach is applicable to only 5–10% of patients and in most cases, until more successful chemotherapeutic regimens become available, the prognosis is dismal. Liver transplantation is not an option except in very limited research protocols utilizing aggressive chemoembolization

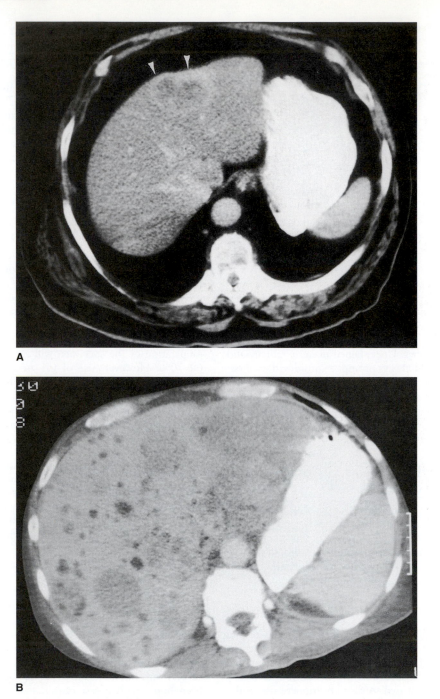

Figure 46–6. Metastatic and hematologic malignancies in liver. **A:** Rim enhancement of hypodense liver metastasis from lung cancer is present on this CT following contrast injection ***(arrowheads).*** **B:** A 54-year-old white male with hepatomegaly. Numerous hypodense areas of varying size could represent tumor, candidiasis, or microabscesses. In this case, liver tissue was replaced by infiltrating chronic lymphatic leukemia.

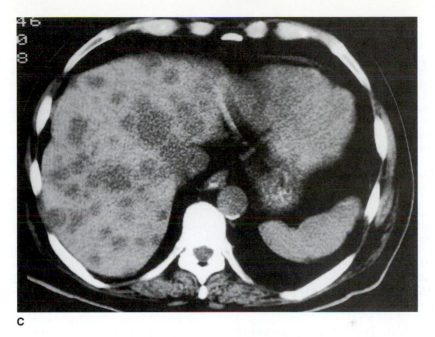

C

Figure 46–6. C: A 67-year-old male renal transplant patient with similar CT performed without contrast. His lesions were due to lymphoma.

followed by transplantation in selected cases of carcinoid tumor and sarcomas.

REFERENCES

Arnoletti JP, Brodsky J: Surgical treatment of benign hepatic mass lesions. Am Surg 1999;65(5):431.

Baffis V et al: Use of interferon for prevention of hepatocellular carcinoma in cirrhotic patients with hepatitis B or hepatitis C virus infection. Ann Intern Med 1999;131(9):696.

Bennett WF, Bova JG: Review of hepatic imaging and a problem-oriented approach to liver masses. Hepatology 1990;12(4 Pt 1):761.

Bismuth H, Chiche L: Surgery of hepatic tumors. Prog Liver Dis 1993;11:269.

Bottles K, Cohen MB: An approach to fine-needle aspiration biopsy diagnosis of hepatic masses. Diagn Cytopathol 1991; 7(2):204.

Bruix J et al: Phase II study of transarterial embolization in European patients with hepatocellular carcinoma: need for controlled trials. Hepatology 1994;20(3):643.

Bruix J et al: Transarterial embolization versus symptomatic treatment in patients with advanced hepatocellular carcinoma: results of a randomized, controlled trial in a single institution. Hepatology 1998;27(6):1578.

Camma C et al: Interferon and prevention of hepatocellular carcinoma in viral cirrhosis: an evidence-based approach. J Hepatol 2001;34:593.

Castells A et al: Treatment of small hepatocellular carcinoma in cirrhotic patients: a cohort study comparing surgical resection and percutaneous ethanol injection. Hepatology 1993;18(5): 1121.

Chang MH et al: Universal hepatitis B vaccination in Taiwan and the incidence of hepatocellular carcinoma in children. Taiwan Childhood Hepatoma Study Group. N Engl J Med 1997;336(26):1855.

Chen MF et al: Postoperative recurrence of hepatocellular carcinoma. Two hundred five consecutive patients who underwent hepatic resection in 15 years. Arch Surg 1994;129(7): 738.

Craig J, Peters R, Edmondson H: *Tumors of the Liver and Intrahepatic Bile Ducts. Atlas of Tumor Pathology.* Armed Forces Institute of Pathology, 1989.

Di Bisceglie AM: Hepatitis C and hepatocellular carcinoma. Hepatology 1997;26(3 Suppl 1):34S.

Di Bisceglie AM: *Clinics in Liver Disease-Liver Tumors,* Vol. 5, 1st ed. W.B Saunders, 2001.

El Serag HB, Mason AC: Rising incidence of hepatocellular carcinoma in the United States. N Engl J Med 1999;340(10):745.

Harnois DM et al: Preoperative hepatic artery chemoembolization followed by orthotopic liver transplantation for hepatocellular carcinoma. Liver Transpl Surg 1999;5(3):192.

Heinemann LA et al: Modern oral contraceptive use and benign liver tumors: the German Benign Liver Tumor Case-Control Study. Eur J Contracept Reprod Health Care 1998;3(4):194.

Hepatocellular Carcinoma Study Group: Effect of interferon-alpha on progression of cirrhosis to hepatocellular carcinoma: a retrospective cohort study. International Interferon-alpha. Lancet 1998;(351):1535.

Hytiroglou P, Theise ND: Differential diagnosis of hepatocellular nodular lesions. Semin Diagn Pathol 1998;15(4):285.

Ikeda K et al: Effect of interferon therapy on hepatocellular carcinogenesis in patients with chronic hepatitis type C: a long-term observation study of 1,643 patients using statistical bias correction with proportional hazard analysis. Hepatology 1999;(29):1124.

Imai Y et al: Relation of interferon therapy and hepatocellular carcinoma in patients with chronic hepatitis C. Ann Intern Med 1998;(129):94.

Irie H et al: MR imaging of focal nodular hyperplasia of the liver: value of contrast-enhanced dynamic study. Radiat Med 1997; 15(1):29.

Kubo S et al: Risk factors for recurrence after resection of hepatitis C virus-related hepatocellular carcinoma. World J Surg 2000; (24):1559.

Kubo S et al: Effects of long-term postoperative interferon alpha therapy on intrahepatic recurrence after resection of hepatitis C virus-related hepatocellular carcinoma. Ann Intern Med 2001;134(10):963.

LaBrecque D: Neoplasia of the liver. In: *Liver and Biliary Diseases*. Kaplowitz N (editor). Williams & Wilkins, 1992.

Lau WY et al: Adjuvant intra-arterial iodine-131-labelled lipiodol for resectable hepatocellular carcinoma: a prospective randomised trial. Lancet 1999;353(9155):797.

Leconte I et al: Focal nodular hyperplasia: natural course observed with CT and MRI. J Comput Assist Tomogr 2000;24(1):61.

Llovet JM, Fuster J, Bruix J: Intention-to-treat analysis of surgical treatment for early hepatocellular carcinoma: resection versus transplantation. Hepatology 1999;30(6):1434.

Llovet JM et al: Natural history of untreated nonsurgical hepatocellular carcinoma: rationale for the design and evaluation of therapeutic trials. Hepatology 1999;29(1):62.

Llovet JM et al: Increased risk of tumor seeding after percutaneous radiofrequency ablation for single hepatocellular carcinoma. Hepatology 2001;33(5):1124.

Marsh JW et al: The prediction of risk of recurrence and time to recurrence of hepatocellular carcinoma after orthotopic liver transplantation: a pilot study. Hepatology 1997;26(2):444.

Mathieu D et al: Oral contraceptive use and focal nodular hyperplasia of the liver. Gastroenterology 2000;118(3):560.

Mazzaferro V et al: Liver transplantation for the treatment of small hepatocellular carcinomas in patients with cirrhosis. N Engl J Med 1996;334(11):693.

McMahon BJ et al: Hepatocellular carcinoma in Alaska Eskimos: epidemiology, clinical features, and early detection. Prog Liver Dis 1990;9:643.

Mergo PJ, Ros PR: Benign lesions of the liver. Radiol Clin North Am 1998;36(2):319.

Miller WJ et al: Malignancies in patients with cirrhosis: CT sensitivity and specificity in 200 consecutive transplant patients. Radiology 1994;193(3):645.

Oka H et al: Prospective study of alpha-fetoprotein in cirrhotic patients monitored for development of hepatocellular carcinoma. Hepatology 1994;19(1):61.

Prospective validation of the CLIP score: a new prognostic system for patients with cirrhosis and hepatocellular carcinoma. The Cancer of the Liver Italian Program (CLIP) Investigators. Hepatology 2000;31(4):840.

Ravikumar TS et al: Intraoperative ultrasonography of liver: detection of occult liver tumors and treatment by cryosurgery. Cancer Detect Prev 1994;18(2):131.

Ringe B et al: Surgical treatment of hepatocellular carcinoma: experience with liver resection and transplantation in 198 patients. World J Surg 1991;15(2):270.

Rizzi PM et al: Accuracy of radiology in detection of hepatocellular carcinoma before liver transplantation. Gastroenterology 1994;107(5):1425.

Rodes J, Sherlock S: Focal nodular hyperplasia in a young female. J Hepatol 1998;29(6):1005.

Rubin RA, Mitchell DG: Evaluation of the solid hepatic mass. Med Clin North Am 1996;80(5):907.

Sato M et al: Well-differentiated hepatocellular carcinoma: clinicopathological features and results of hepatic resection. Am J Gastroenterol 1995;90(1):112.

Schwartz ME: Primary hepatocellular carcinoma: transplant versus resection. Semin Liver Dis 1994;14(2):135.

Sheiner PA, Brower ST: Treatment of metastatic cancer to the liver. Semin Liver Dis 1994;14(2):169.

Sheu JC et al: Growth rate of asymptomatic hepatocellular carcinoma and its clinical implications. Gastroenterology 1985;89(2):259.

Shouval D, Adler R: Tumor site-directed therapy for hepatocellular carcinoma using monoclonal antibodies against hepatoma-associated antigens. Prog Liver Dis 1993;11:251.

Tang ZY et al: Surgery of small hepatocellular carcinoma. Analysis of 144 cases. Cancer 1989;64(2):536.

Tsai JF et al: Hepatitis B and C virus infection as risk factors for liver cirrhosis and cirrhotic hepatocellular carcinoma: a case-control study. Liver 1994;14(2):98.

Wahlstrom HE: Liver transplantation for hepatocellular carcinoma—is it worth it? Mayo Clin Proc 1994;69(6):599.

Weimann A et al: Benign liver tumors: differential diagnosis and indications for surgery. World J Surg 1997;21(9):983.

Weimann A et al: Pregnancy in women with observed focal nodular hyperplasia of the liver. Lancet 1998;351(9111):1251.

Yoshida H et al: Interferon therapy reduces the risk for hepatocellular carcinoma: national surveillance program of cirrhotic and noncirrhotic patients with chronic hepatitis C in Japan. IHIT Study Group. Inhibition of Hepatocarcinogenesis by Interferon Therapy. Ann Intern Med 1999;131(3):174.

Liver Disease in Pregnancy

47

Rebecca W. Van Dyke, MD

Interactions between the pregnant state and liver disease will be reviewed in this chapter. The discussion will be divided into three areas: (1) the effects of pregnancy on the liver and liver function, (2) the effects of common liver diseases when they occur during pregnancy, and (3) a review of liver diseases unique to the pregnant state.

■ EFFECTS OF PREGNANCY ON THE LIVER

CHANGES IN LIVER BIOCHEMICAL TESTS

Most liver functions, including production of clotting factors, are not affected by a normal pregnancy. However, due to a 50% increase in blood volume in late pregnancy, serum albumin is diluted and levels fall by up to 60%. In contrast, plasma concentrations of acute phase reactant proteins and ceruloplasmin are increased during pregnancy. Because of an increase in triglyceride flux and fatty acid metabolism, hepatic production of lipoproteins is increased during pregnancy, as are levels of plasma triglycerides, cholesterol, and phospholipids. Metabolism of individual drugs may be increased, decreased, or not altered during pregnancy.

Biochemical tests of liver injury, including aspartate aminotransferase (AST) and alanine aminotransferase (ALT), remain normal throughout pregnancy; however, serum alkaline phosphatase and leucine aminopeptidase activities rise progressively, owing to placental synthesis and release of these enzymes. At term, over one-half of women have elevated alkaline phosphatase levels, however these levels are rarely greater than two-fold normal. Therefore, serum alkaline phosphatase levels that are increased to more than three to five times the upper limit of normal or increases in serum aminotransferase measurements are reliable indicators of hepatobiliary disease during pregnancy and should prompt further investigation. In contrast, palmar erythema and cutaneous vascular spiders frequently appear during pregnancy and do not reliably indicate liver disease.

CHOLESTASIS

Normal pregnancy is associated with a progressive, albeit mild, decline in hepatic transport of bile salts and other organic anions (eg, bilirubin) and in the formation of hepatic bile. Because of reduced hepatic secretion of bile salts, serum levels of bile salts rise throughout pregnancy. Although in most women values do not exceed the upper limit of normal, a subset of women, probably those susceptible to development of intrahepatic cholestasis of pregnancy (see discussion later in this chapter), exhibits serum bile acid levels late in pregnancy that are two-fold or three-fold the upper limit of normal. This mild pregnancy-related cholestasis is of no clinical significance; however, changes in bile formation during pregnancy potentiate formation of gallstones.

GALLSTONE FORMATION

Pregnancy predisposes women both to the formation of gallstones and to their becoming clinically symptomatic. The risk of developing cholesterol gallstones is related epidemiologically to the female gender, the use of exogenous female steroid hormones, and the number and frequency of pregnancies; these factors reflect, in part, the effects of estrogens. Exposure to estrogens increases hepatic secretion of cholesterol, decreases hepatic secretion of bile salts, and increases cholesterol saturation in gallbladder bile. Development of gallstones also is potentiated by estrogen/progesterone-induced decreases in gallbladder emptying. Impaired gallbladder motility, combined with increased biliary cholesterol saturation, leads to formation, during pregnancy, of biliary sludge in about one-third of women and to development of cholesterol gallstones in about 10% of women. Most biliary sludge disappears during the postpartum period, but only one-third of small stones resolve. Finally, studies of both men and women exposed to high levels of estrogens suggest that estrogen use also accelerates development of symptoms in patients with preexisting gallstones.

During pregnancy, biliary colic occurs in up to one-third of women with existing stones and other complications of gallstones, such as acute cholecystitis, obstructive jaundice, or gallstone pancreatitis, may also occur. Because many pregnant women will respond to medical therapy, cholecystectomy often may be deferred until after delivery. However, women with recurring or worsening symptoms or obstructive jaundice need urgent treatment. Endoscopic therapy may be employed for gallstone pancreatitis and obstructive jaundice. Open or laparoscopic cholecystectomy can be undertaken for biliary colic or acute cholecystitis with excellent maternal outcome and low (<5–10%) rates of fetal loss. Indeed, acute cholecystitis is a common cause of nonobstetric surgery during pregnancy, occurring in one to eight cases per 10,000 pregnancies.

HEPATIC ADENOMA

Hepatic adenomas are estrogen-sensitive neoplasms. Enlargement with development of symptoms (abdominal pain, nausea, and vomiting) and rupture has been reported during pregnancy, presumably related to increased estrogen levels. Screening for adenomas in all pregnant women is not indicated; however, for patients previously known to have small adenomas, the size of the tumors can be monitored during pregnancy by ultrasonography. If adenomas grow rapidly and become large, thereby increasing the risk of rupture, termination of pregnancy or early delivery should be considered. Elective surgical resection of large adenomas to prevent their growth and rupture during a future pregnancy should be considered in women with known adenomas who wish to bear children.

HYPEREMESIS GRAVIDARUM

Hyperemesis gravidarum is not a liver disease per se, but the liver may be involved in women with severe hyperemesis who require hospitalization for dehydration. Ten to thirty percent of women who require hospitalization for vomiting and dehydration develop mild liver injury. Clinical signs include mild hyperbilirubinemia, occasionally pruritus, and moderate increases in serum transaminases (up to two to three times normal levels). On rare occasions, values of aminotransferase activity up to 10–20 times the upper limit of normal have been noted. Alkaline phosphatase activities are elevated above the level expected for pregnancy in only a few patients. These modest changes in liver biochemical tests are of little clinical significance and resolve rapidly as vomiting is controlled and dehydration and malnutrition are reversed.

■ LIVER DISEASES OCCURRING DURING PREGNANCY

ACUTE VIRAL HEPATITIS

Any of the acute viral hepatitides may occur during pregnancy; moreover, viral hepatitis is the most common cause of jaundice during pregnancy in the United States. For most of the hepatitis viruses (A, B, C, and D), viral hepatitis in well-nourished women with normal liver function has little effect on the mother or the fetus, although some epidemiologic studies suggest a minor increase in fetal and perinatal mortality rates.

In Asia and India, where the waterborne hepatitis E virus (HEV) is endemic and women are often poorly nourished, acute hepatitis E is associated with a high frequency (15–20%) of fulminant hepatic failure and maternal and fetal death. This may reflect a unique and as yet unknown interaction between HEV and pregnancy.

HERPES SIMPLEX HEPATITIS

Herpes simplex hepatitis is rare in healthy adults, but over one-half the reported cases have been pregnant women. The mortality rate in this group is at least 50%. Typical clinical features include a 4- to 14-day history of fever, systemic symptoms typical of viral infection, and abdominal pain. Laboratory findings include high aminotransferase levels (>1000 IU/L), liver synthetic failure as documented by an increased prothrombin time, and a modest degree of hyperbilirubinemia (serum levels typically <3 mg/dL). Liver biopsy may be diagnostic, revealing typical intranuclear inclusions. Liver, vaginal, cervical, or throat cultures for herpes simplex virus (HSV) are often positive.

Immediate therapy with acyclovir can successfully treat both mother and infant. Thus, pregnant women who have symptoms and signs of severe viral hepatitis should be evaluated aggressively for HSV, with immediate institution of acyclovir, based on the clinical presentation, biopsy, or positive culture results. Vertical transmission of HSV to the fetus *in utero* or the infant after delivery can occur, and infants should be monitored closely and treated appropriately.

CHRONIC HEPATITIS & CIRRHOSIS

The effect of chronic hepatitis or cirrhosis on the mother and fetus is related primarily to the degree of liver dysfunction and portal hypertension. Women with mild chronic hepatitis, including most women with hepatitis C, and normal liver synthetic function have normal fertility rates and tolerate pregnancy well. Indeed, serum aminotransferase values in women with hepatitis C often normalize during pregnancy and return to prepregnant values after delivery.

Women with severe chronic hepatitis or cirrhosis have reduced fertility rates and rarely become pregnant. If pregnancy does occur, liver biochemical tests, including serum bilirubin, alkaline phosphatase, and serum transaminase measurements, may worsen, although these tests often return to baseline values after delivery. For women with known cirrhosis who do become pregnant, mortality rates as high as 10% have been reported, primarily because of liver failure or variceal hemorrhage, or both. It is unknown whether these rates are higher than would be expected if the women were not pregnant.

Bleeding from esophageal varices is common during pregnancy in women with cirrhosis or extrahepatic portal vein thrombosis. Bleeding occurs in 18–30% of women with cirrhosis and in up to 50% of women known to have established portal hypertension, reflecting, in part, the expansion of intravascular volume during the second and third trimesters. Bleeding from esophageal varices is not precipitated by vaginal delivery. Mortality rates from episodes of variceal hemorrhage are high in women with cirrhosis but lower in women with extrahepatic portal vein thrombosis, in whom liver function usually is normal.

Mothers and babies have survived pregnancies complicated by one or more episodes of variceal bleeding, although the numbers of such cases are small. Bleeding episodes can be managed using variceal banding, sclerotherapy, or transjugular intrahepatic portal-systemic shunts (TIPS). Prophylactic shunts or sclerotherapy are justified although prophylactic banding, a procedure thought to be associated with fewer complications than sclerotherapy, can be considered.

Fetal outcome is compromised in the face of severe maternal liver disease with or without variceal hemorrhage. Pregnancies in such women are associated with a high rate of spontaneous abortion, stillbirth, and perinatal death. Surviving fetuses are phenotypically and developmentally normal.

Fertility often returns after successful liver transplantation. Although pregnancies in women after liver transplantation are considered high risk, 70% of reported pregnancies in such women have resulted in live, healthy babies.

VERTICAL TRANSMISSION OF HEPATITIS VIRUSES

An important aspect of viral hepatitis and pregnancy is vertical transmission of the virus to the fetus or newborn infant, particularly when maternal infection, acute or chronic, is present during the third trimester. Vertical transmission of hepatitis B virus (HBV) has been studied extensively and is common, in 50–90%, when a chronically infected mother with high levels of viral replication [as indicated by detectable HBV DNA and hepatitis B e antigen (HBeAg) in the serum] gives birth. Vertical transmission from a mother with acute or chronic hepatitis B and low viral replication is less frequent. Most children infected at birth fail to clear the virus and become lifelong HBV carriers. Vertical transmission of HBV may be prevented if the newborn infant of a woman with serum hepatitis B surface antigen (HBsAg) is treated immediately after delivery with one intramuscular dose of hepatitis B immune serum globulin and the first of three injections of hepatitis B vaccine (Table 47–1). Thus, current recommendations are to screen all pregnant women during the third trimester for HBsAg and prepare to treat their offspring at birth, if necessary.

Vertical transmission of hepatitis C virus (HCV) is uncommon but does occur in about 5% of infants of infected mothers. It is more frequent when mothers are coinfected with the human immunodeficiency virus (HIV). No immunoprophylaxis is currently available. Vertical transmission of hepatitis A virus (HAV), hepatitis D virus (HDV), HEV, and other non-A, non-B viruses occurs rarely, and only if the mother is viremic at the time of delivery.

■ LIVER DISEASES UNIQUE TO PREGNANCY

INTRAHEPATIC CHOLESTASIS OF PREGNANCY

Intrahepatic cholestasis of pregnancy (pruritus gravidarum; cholestasis of pregnancy) is an uncommon and usually benign cholestatic disorder that appears late in

Table 47–1. Prevention of vertical transmission of hepatitis B.

Test all women in the third trimester of pregnancy for HBsAg	
Administer prophylaxis within hours of delivery to all infants of HBsAg-positive women	
Hepatitis B immume globulin	0.5 mL intramuscularly[1]
Hepatitis B vaccine	0.5 mL intramuscularly,[1] with follow-up doses at 1 and 6 months
Test and vaccinate other family members of HBsAg-positive women	

[1]Dosage recommendations should be checked using current manufacturer's specifications.

pregnancy. The syndrome disappears rapidly after delivery but often recurs either during subsequent pregnancies or with the use of oral contraceptives.

Pathophysiology

Intrahepatic cholestasis of pregnancy is thought to reflect a genetic predisposition to the known cholestatic effects of estrogens, possibly due to polymorphisms of hepatic bile salt transporters. It frequently affects female relatives of index cases and has been identified in up to three generations in some families. Patients and female relatives often develop cholestasis when taking oral contraceptives. Even male family members of women with intrahepatic cholestasis of pregnancy demonstrate exaggerated impairment of biliary secretion of organic anions if exposed to estrogens. In Scandinavia and Chile, the disorder is seen in up to 5% of pregnancies, but it is much less common in the United States.

Clinical Findings

A. Symptoms and Signs

Intrahepatic cholestasis of pregnancy can present at any age and any degree of parity (Table 47–2). Seventy percent of cases present during the third trimester. The major clinical feature is intense pruritus, which often prevents sleep and leads to skin excoriations, minor skin infections, and depression. The onset of pruritus is usually at 28–30 weeks. In approximately 10–25% of patients with more severe cholestasis, jaundice is also seen. Nausea, vomiting, abdominal pain, and hepatomegaly are observed in a few patients.

Table 47–2. Clinical findings in intrahepatic cholestasis of pregnancy.

Incidence	~ 0.5 to –3% of pregnant women
Onset	Third trimester (median onset, 29 weeks)
Symptoms and signs	
Pruritus	100%
Jaundice	10–25%
Nausea and vomiting	5–75%
Abdominal pain	10–25%
Usual laboratory findings	
Alkaline phosphatase	2- to 5-fold increase
Bilirubin	1–4 mg/dL
Aminotransferases	3- to 4-fold increase
Serum bile salts	5- to 10-fold increase
Prothrombin time	Modest increase in 15% of patients

B. Laboratory Findings

Laboratory features are those of cholestasis, with alkaline phosphatase levels usually two- to five-fold the upper limit of normal, a mild hyperbilirubinemia averaging 3 mg/dL, and modest elevations of transaminases (usually, 100–200 IU/L; rarely, as high as 1000 IU/L). Serum bile acid levels are markedly elevated but rarely measured. In women with severe, long-lasting cholestasis, vitamin K deficiency and steatorrhea may occur, with modest elevation of the prothrombin time.

Differential Diagnosis

The history, physical examination, and laboratory tests should reliably differentiate intrahepatic cholestasis of pregnancy from acute viral hepatitis, acute fatty liver of pregnancy, or preeclamptic liver disease. The histologic appearance of the liver on a biopsy specimen is usually diagnostic, showing intense intrahepatic cholestasis with little inflammation or hepatocellular necrosis; however, biopsy is rarely necessary, because the diagnosis can usually be made on the basis of the clinical findings.

Treatment & Prognosis

Intrahepatic cholestasis of pregnancy is a self-limited entity that rapidly resolves after delivery. In rare instances, cholestasis may persist for several weeks into the postpartum period; however, the pruritus usually disappears within 24–48 hours. Patients with severe pruritus may respond to ursodeoxycholic acid, a hydrophilic bile salt that promotes hepatic secretion of other, potentially toxic, bile salts. In several clinical studies ursodeoxycholic acid appears to be safe in pregnancy and, when given at doses of either 10–15 mg/kg per day or 1 g/d, rapidly improves pruritus and abnormal liver tests in most patients. Pruritus may, in some patients, also respond to treatment with oral cholestyramine or phenobarbital. Hypnotics may be helpful, as nocturnal pruritus may be severe. Vitamin K administration near the time of delivery is indicated in patients with steatorrhea or an elevated prothrombin time.

The prognosis of intrahepatic cholestasis of pregnancy for mothers is excellent except for an increased lifetime incidence of gallstones. The prognosis for the fetus may not be as benign; several studies from Chile and Scandinavia suggest an increase in fetal distress during late pregnancy, premature labor, and unexpected neonatal death. Experts have recommended close monitoring of women and fetuses during the third trimester with plans for early delivery. However, even frequent fetal monitoring does not prevent all fetal deaths. Delivery at 34 weeks is recommended for babies with mature lungs if mothers develop jaundice, if the onset of intrahepatic cholestasis of pregnancy occurred before 32 weeks, if the pregnancy is multiple, or if there was a previous stillbirth. For other mothers with less severe cholestasis, delivery at 38 weeks is recommended unless fetal distress is observed. Delivery should be undertaken promptly for fetal distress.

ACUTE FATTY LIVER OF PREGNANCY

Acute fatty liver of pregnancy is a rare, sporadic disease that occurs in late pregnancy and is associated with acute liver failure and considerable risk of maternal and fetal morbidity and death.

Pathophysiology

Acute fatty liver of pregnancy is characterized by infiltration of hepatocytes with microvesicular droplets of fat, a histologic picture strikingly similar to that seen in Reye's syndrome, Jamaican vomiting sickness, valproic acid hepatotoxicity, and acyl-CoA dehydrogenase deficiency, a group of diseases known as the hepatic microvesicular steatoses. Although most cases of acute fatty liver of pregnancy are sporadic and nonrecurrent, genetic abnormalities in fatty acid oxidation, especially long chain 3-hydroxyacyl-CoA dehydrogenase deficiency in the mother and the fetus, predispose to its development. In pregnancy, hepatic metabolism of triglycerides and fatty acids increases greatly. Impairment of mitochondrial β-oxidation of fatty acids (resulting from the combined effects of estrogens, genetic abnormalities in acyl-CoA dehydrogenases, inflammatory cytokines, and/or drugs such as salicylates) may, in rare instances, cause sufficient impairment of β-oxidation to lead to elevated hepatic levels of potentially toxic fatty acids and liver injury.

Clinical Findings

A. SYMPTOMS AND SIGNS

The onset of acute fatty liver of pregnancy is usually in the third trimester (at approximately 35 weeks), although onset as early as 26 weeks and as late as the immediate postpartum period has been reported (Table 47–3). The early clinical signs are nonspecific and include nausea, fatigue, malaise, vomiting, and right upper quadrant or epigastric pain. Fever, headache, diarrhea, and myalgias are seen in some patients. Clinical signs of liver disease may ensue within days. Physical findings may be minimal but may include right upper quadrant tenderness. The appearance of jaundice, edema, ascites, and hepatic encephalopathy signal impending liver failure. Signs and symptoms of preeclampsia, such as hypertension and proteinuria, are seen in at least 30% of cases. This high degree of overlap between acute fatty liver of pregnancy and preeclampsia suggests

Table 47–3. Clinical findings in acute fatty liver of pregnancy.

Incidence	1 in 7,000–16,000 pregnancies
Onset	Third trimester (median onset, 35 weeks)
Symptoms and signs	
Nausea and vomiting	80%
Abdominal pain	50%
Hypertension, proteinuria, and edema	20–25%
Jaundice	90%
Encephalopathy	55%
Hypoglycemia	40%
Ascites (modest)	30%
Usual laboratory findings	
Alkaline phosphatase	2- to 5-fold increase
Bilirubin	2–30 mg/dL
Aminotransferases	5- to 20-fold increase
Prothrombin time	Marked increase in severe disease to > 20 seconds
Platelet count	Decrease late in severe disease with evidence of disseminated intravascular coagulation
Serum uric acid	Modest elevation in most patients

an underlying common pathophysiologic process, as yet not identified.

Although patients may have only mild degrees of liver damage, the feared clinical course of acute fatty liver of pregnancy is rapid progression to liver failure. Severely affected women exhibit all of the complications of fulminant hepatic failure, including hypoglycemia, coagulopathy, hepatic encephalopathy, and cerebral edema.

B. LABORATORY FINDINGS

Laboratory abnormalities include evidence of liver damage but with only modest elevations of alkaline phosphatase and serum transaminases. Transaminase levels average 200–400 IU/L, but values exceeding 1000 IU/L have been reported. Serum bilirubin levels are characteristically elevated; however, the range of values reported is broad, from normal to 36 mg/dL. Evidence of liver failure is frequent, as exemplified by hypoglycemia and a rising prothrombin time. Hematologic studies suggest the presence of disseminated intravascular coagulation in severely affected patients. Nucleated red blood cells, red blood cell fragments, and thrombocytopenia may be present. The white blood cell count is usually elevated, in the range of 12,000–46,000/μL.

Serum uric acid levels are always mildly elevated, and renal function is usually impaired, with serum creatinine averaging 3 mg/dL. Although a computed tomography (CT) scan may suggest a fatty liver, it is insensitive in identifying acute fatty liver of pregnancy.

Differential Diagnosis

Disorders most commonly confused with acute fatty liver of pregnancy include acute viral hepatitis and preeclamptic liver disease, such as the HELLP syndrome (see following discussion). Both of the latter disorders are characterized by intense hepatocellular necrosis and are most readily distinguished from acute fatty liver of pregnancy by high levels of serum aminotransferase activity. Other distinguishing features include early evidence of thrombocytopenia and disseminated intravascular coagulation in preeclamptic liver disease, and serologic evidence of viral infection in acute viral hepatitis. Liver biopsy is usually diagnostic of acute fatty liver of pregnancy, especially if fat staining is performed on frozen sections of tissue to identify microvesicular steatosis; however, in severe cases, coagulopathy may be a contraindication to liver biopsy.

Treatment & Prognosis

Acute fatty liver of pregnancy resolves spontaneously and rapidly after delivery. Therefore, treatment is based on prompt delivery as well as supportive care for the complications of liver failure. Women with mild disease (no evidence of impaired liver function as monitored by the serum prothrombin time, hypoglycemia, hepatic encephalopathy), no evidence of fetal distress, or carrying a fetus with immature lungs can be monitored closely. In these patients, there should be contingency plans for rapid delivery by induction of labor or cesarean section in the event that maternal hepatic function deteriorates or fetal distress is observed. For patients who present with severe liver involvement and liver synthetic failure (as exemplified by an increased prothrombin time), labor should be rapidly induced followed by cesarean section if indicated.

Although treatment by rapid delivery has never been studied in a controlled clinical trial, maternal and fetal outcomes in acute fatty liver of pregnancy have improved since this approach has been used. Patients should be followed by both the appropriate obstetric and neonatal services and a physician experienced in the care of patients with fulminant hepatic failure. Because acute fatty liver of pregnancy usually resolves spontaneously after delivery, evaluation for liver transplantation for severely affected women is usually not necessary.

Maternal and fetal mortality rates of approximately 50% were previously reported. In more recent studies, maternal mortality rates of 5–15% and infant mortality rates of 8–20% have been reported in which mild cases were identified and rapid delivery undertaken. The high rate of fetal mortality in this disorder probably reflects not only maternal decompensation and premature delivery, but also maternal disseminated intravascular coagulation with fibrin deposition in the placenta, leading to placental infarcts and fetal asphyxia.

PREECLAMPTIC LIVER INJURY

Preeclampsia, characterized by hypertension, proteinuria, and edema in the third trimester of pregnancy, is not primarily a liver disease, but the liver may be involved in severe cases. The two best characterized hepatic syndromes observed in women with preeclampsia or eclampsia include HELLP syndrome (an acronym for the characteristic laboratory features of *h*emolysis, *e*levated *l*iver enzymes, and *l*ow *p*latelet count) and acute hepatic rupture.

Pathophysiology

Preeclampsia is thought to arise from abnormalities in placental development and perfusion, leading to maternal endothelial activation, sensitivity to endogenous pressor agents, hypertension, intense vasoconstriction, and progressive endothelial damage resulting in fibrin and platelet deposition and a picture resembling that of disseminated intravascular coagulation. Renal involvement occurs in virtually all affected women, but hepatic involvement is seen in at least 10% of patients. Hepatic disease is marked by deposition of fibrin along hepatic sinusoids, ischemic necrosis (either focal or confluent), and periportal and portal tract hemorrhage, with little or no inflammation. In cases with severe confluent liver necrosis, large intrahepatic hematomas may form and rupture. As discussed above (see section, "Acute Fatty Liver of Pregnancy") preeclampsia occurs more often than expected in women with acute fatty liver of pregnancy. Further, liver biopsies in women with preeclampsia may show mild microvesicular steatosis in addition to the characteristic changes of preeclamptic liver damage.

1. HELLP Syndrome

HELLP syndrome, first defined in 1982, probably represents the middle of the spectrum of liver involvement in preeclampsia (ie, the point at which clinically significant liver necrosis and disseminated intravascular coagulation occur, but not confluent necrosis).

Clinical Findings

A. SYMPTOMS AND SIGNS

Patients with HELLP syndrome exhibit the signs or symptoms of preeclampsia, including hypertension, proteinuria, and edema (Table 47–4). Patients are usually in their first pregnancy, and the onset commonly occurs at around 33 weeks. Nonspecific signs or symptoms such as nausea, vomiting, epigastric and right upper quadrant pain, headache, and hepatic tenderness are often, although not invariably, present.

B. LABORATORY FINDINGS

The diagnosis is suggested by the characteristic laboratory features, primarily thrombocytopenia. A platelet count of less than 100,000/μL is required to make the diagnosis. Fibrinogen levels are modestly decreased. Evidence of disseminated intravascular coagulation and intravascular hemolysis may be found in many patients, if sensitive tests are employed such as those for fibrin degradation products, D-dimer levels, and morphologic studies of red blood cells. Abnormal clotting times, measured by both the prothrombin time and partial thromboplastin time, are common. Liver involvement

Table 47–4. Clinical findings in HELLP syndrome.

Incidence	~ 1% of all pregnancies, especially first pregnancies
	~ 10% of women with preeclampsia
Onset	Third trimester (median-on set, 33 weeks)
Symptoms and signs	
Hypertension, proteinuria and edema	90%+
Headache	50%
Nausea and vomiting	30%
Abdominal pain	50%
Usual laboratory findings	
Thrombocytopenia	95%, early onset
Abnormal morphologic studies of RBCs	Frequent (fragments, schistocytes)
Prothrombin time	Modest increase in 15%
Fibrin degradation products	Increased early
Aminotransferases	5- to 20-fold increase
Alkaline phosphatase	Normal or modest increase (2-fold)
Bilirubin	Low, unless extensive hemolysis and hepatic necrosis occur
Serum creatinine	Mild increase

is typified by moderate elevations of serum transaminases, typically in the range of 200–500 IU/L, although values up to several thousand international units per liter are seen in more severe cases. Serum bilirubin levels are commonly, but modestly, elevated, in part reflecting the degree of intravascular hemolysis. Impaired renal function is virtually universal, as indicated by increases in serum blood urea nitrogen and creatinine. Complications include bleeding due to the underlying coagulopathy, progressive hepatic hemorrhage, and development of hepatic rupture (see following discussion), and, rarely, fulminant hepatic failure.

Differential Diagnosis

HELLP syndrome can be differentiated from acute viral hepatitis and acute fatty liver of pregnancy (Table 47–5) by the early appearance and more severe degree of thrombocytopenia and evidence of disseminated intravascular coagulation. The transaminase values may be modest or as high as those seen in acute viral hepatitis and may be similar to or higher than those typically seen in acute fatty liver of pregnancy. Liver biopsy can be diagnostic but is higher risk because of the patient's underlying coagulopathy. Differentiation of HELLP syndrome from acute fatty liver of pregnancy may be difficult, because some cases appear to reflect an overlap syndrome, with features of both acute fatty liver of pregnancy and preeclamptic liver disease. In such cases, laboratory values may represent a combination of those typical for each disease, and liver biopsy may show both microvesicular fatty infiltration and evidence of fibrin deposition and hepatocyte necrosis. Because the treatment for both entities is virtually identical (ie, prompt delivery), differentiation of acute fatty liver of pregnancy from HELLP syndrome may not be essential.

Treatment & Prognosis

Preeclampsia resolves spontaneously and rapidly after delivery, and the clinical signs or symptoms of HELLP syndrome usually resolve within 24–48 hours. Thus, the principal treatment for this disorder is rapid identification of HELLP syndrome and urgent vaginal or abdominal delivery. In patients with mild liver involvement and mild coagulopathy, the maturity of the fetus should be assessed and its well-being closely monitored. Delivery may be cautiously postponed if the lungs are not mature, although fetuses are at risk due to poor placental function. In all other cases, it is preferable to move toward rapid delivery. The peak of thrombocytopenia and liver abnormalities may not occur until 1–2 days following delivery, but laboratory abnormalities should return to normal within 72 hours. In rare

Table 47–5. Differential diagnosis of acute liver disease in pregnancy.

	Viral Hepatitis	Biliary Tract Disease	Intrahepatic Cholestasis of Pregnancy	Acute Fatty Liver of Pregnancy	HELLP Syndrome
Time of onset	Variable	Variable	Third trimester	Third trimester	Third trimester
Nausea and vomiting	Yes	Variable	Rare	Yes	Occasionally
Abdominal pain	Variable	Variable	Rare	Yes	Yes
Associated with preeclampsia	No	No	No	Often	Yes
Cholestasis	Mild to marked	Marked	Marked	Modest and late	Mild or absent
Transaminase elevation	High	Low	Low	Modest	Modest to high
Coagulopathy	Rare and late	No	No	Common but late	Early, thrombo-cytopenia; late, disseminated intravascular coagulation
Hepatic failure	Variable	No	No	Yes	Rare
Hepatic ultrasound or CT scan	Nonspecific	Dilated bile ducts	Normal	No change or low density	Areas of infaction and necrosis
Liver biopsy	Inflammatory infiltrate, spotty hepatocyte necrosis	Cholestasis, variable inflammation	Cholestasis	Microvesicular fatty infiltration	Patchy hemorrhagic necrosis, fibrin deposition, mild microvesicular fatty infiltration

cases in which thrombocytopenia persists for more than 72 hours after delivery, treatment with prednisone or exchange transfusions have been suggested as a potential therapy.

Because the clinical outcome for both mother and fetus is worse in those women with preeclampsia who also develop HELLP syndrome, some investigators advocate screening all women with preeclampsia, especially those with abdominal pain, for this syndrome, using laboratory tests for liver injury and coagulation. Those with HELLP syndrome should undergo close monitoring and rapid delivery, as previously outlined.

Maternal prognosis is related to the severity of liver involvement and coagulopathy. In those with no bleeding complications, the outcome is excellent. Fetal outcome is not as good; retardation of intrauterine growth is common and sudden death can occur because of rapid changes in placental blood flow. The chances of fetal survival are clearly better when delivery is prompt. The maternal mortality rate is 2.5% or less, although the fetal mortality rate is 6–37%. The recurrence rate of HELLP syndrome in subsequent pregnancies is about 3%.

2. Hepatic Rupture

Clinical Findings

Hepatic rupture in pregnancy was first described in 1844, and is due to confluent hepatic necrosis from preeclamptic liver disease. It is reported in 1–77 of every 100,000 deliveries, and in 1–2% of women with preeclampsia.

A. SYMPTOMS AND SIGNS

Hemorrhage may occur up to 48 hours after delivery in women with severe liver necrosis. Virtually all patients have clinical and histologic features of preeclampsia, and most would satisfy the criteria for HELLP syndrome. Contained intrahepatic hemorrhage is more common than free rupture into the peritoneal cavity. Both types of rupture are heralded by the sudden onset of abdominal pain, usually in the right upper quadrant. Clinical findings include hepatic tenderness, diffuse abdominal pain, peritoneal findings, chest and shoulder pain, and shock. These signs and symptoms are seen in a variety of intraabdominal catastrophes, including rupture of hepatic adenoma, abruptio placentae, perforated viscus, and intestinal infarction.

B. DIAGNOSTIC STUDIES

Diagnosis is based on clinical suspicion, laboratory or clinical evidence of preeclampsia, and imaging of the liver. Abdominal CT is the most sensitive test for either contained or free hepatic rupture. Magnetic resonance imaging (MRI) can identify intrahepatic hematomas but is more sensitive for chronic, rather than acute, hematomas.

Treatment & Prognosis

Women with contained hepatic hematomas, diagnosed by abdominal CT or another radiologic procedure, often do well without surgery if they receive adequate hemodynamic support and are followed closely. Patients with free hepatic rupture require immediate treatment to survive. Approaches include angiographic embolization of bleeding arterioles and/or laparotomy with drainage and packing of the ruptured areas.

Overall, the maternal and fetal mortality rates for acute hepatic rupture are high (>50%). The mortality rate is lower in women with contained hematomas; in such individuals, the hematomas gradually resolve over several weeks. Recurrence of acute hepatic rupture is possible, as preeclampsia and liver involvement may recur in subsequent pregnancies, and, indeed, recurrence has been reported.

REFERENCES

Liver Disease in Pregnancy. Sem Perinatol 1998;22:entire April issue (issue 2).

Riely CA: Liver disease in the pregnant patient. Am J Gastroenterol 1999;94:1728.

Su G, Van Dyke RW: Liver disease in pregnancy. In: *Diseases of the Liver.* Bacon BR, Di Bisceglie AM (editors). Churchill Livingstone, 2000.

Van Dyke RW: The liver in pregnancy. In: *Hepatology: A Textbook of Liver Disease,* 3rd ed. Zakim D, Boyer TD (editors). WB Saunders, 1996 (4th edition in press, 2002).

Pediatric Liver Disease

48

Joel E. Lavine, MD, PhD

■ NORMAL LIVER ANATOMY & FUNCTION

Pediatrics is unique in the diversity of its patient population, with the passage from birth to adolescence marked by profound growth and development. Many liver diseases present primarily in the pediatric age group, when rapid diagnosis and treatment can prevent death or significant morbidity. Chronic liver disease in children presents an additional challenge to the practitioner: enabling the affected child to achieve optimal growth and to lead as normal a life as possible.

ANATOMY & DEVELOPMENT

The liver originates as a diverticulum of endodermal cells arising from the primitive foregut within the first weeks following conception. By the third week of gestation, the diverticulum divides into the solid cranial pars hepatica, destined to become the liver, and the hollow, caudal pars cystica, which will become the gallbladder and extrahepatic biliary ducts. The lumen of these ducts becomes occluded with endodermal cells, but is normally recanalized by the seventh week. By the sixth week, bile canaliculi form between the hepatoblasts, with duct formation occurring by the ninth week. After 3 months, the intra- and extrahepatic biliary structures have joined, with initiation of bile formation and bile excretion into the duodenum, giving meconium its characteristic color. Failure of either recanalization of the nascent extrahepatic biliary ducts at week 7, or joining of the intra- and extrahepatic biliary drainage systems at week 12, results in malformation or atresia of the biliary tree, with consequent derangement of normal bile metabolism. The cause of these anatomic malformations is unknown.

Pediatric hepatic anatomy is identical to adult hepatic anatomy. The liver is composed of right, left, quadrate, and caudate lobes. The left and right hepatic ducts join outside the porta hepatis to form the common hepatic duct. The gallbladder is united with this system via the cystic duct, which becomes the common bile duct after joining with the common hepatic duct. The common bile duct ends in the papilla of Vater, where it is also united with the pancreatic duct to form the ampulla of Vater, circumscribed by the sphincter of Oddi. The latter regulates secretion of bile into the duodenum.

At the cellular level, hepatocytes are specialized in their concentration of drug- and toxin-metabolizing enzymes located in the smooth endoplasmic reticulum. In the newborn period, these enzymes, including the glucuronyl transferases involved in bilirubin metabolism, have reduced activity. This leads to inefficient and sometimes insufficient metabolism of drugs and endogenous toxins such as bilirubin, especially when the newborn is stressed (eg, sepsis, hemolysis). This decreased enzymatic activity predisposes the neonate to a common sign of illness, hyperbilirubinemia.

FUNCTION

The fetal liver is relatively inactive, relying on the maternal liver to perform its chores via the placenta. As gestation nears completion, the fetus prepares for birth and cessation of this dependency by stockpiling glycogen and lipids, substances critical for survival in the immediate postnatal period. The primary functions of the postnatal liver include (1) conversion of nutrients to storage forms that are readily accessible; (2) synthesis of proteins (including albumin and clotting factors); (3) synthesis of bile acids, key in intestinal fat absorption; and (4) toxin disposal, including excretable derivatives of bilirubin and ammonia. These functions develop rapidly after birth, with closure of the ductus venosus, maturation of microsomal enzymes, and use of the gastrointestinal tract (stimulation of bile secretion).

Storage of Nutrients

The liver plays a primary role in glucose homeostasis. After a meal, it replenishes depleted glycogen stores with surplus glucose; in the fasting state, the liver must break down the glycogen to supply energy to the body. With depletion of the glycogen stores in a prolonged fast (longer than 8–12 hours), the liver must synthesize glucose from amino acids supplied through muscle breakdown (gluconeogenesis). This capacity is utilized from birth, as the newborn infant compensates for the loss of maternal support by mobilizing greater than 90% of stored glycogen in the first 2 hours of life.

Synthetic Function

The fetal liver possesses full synthetic function by 3 months gestation. Albumin is quantitatively the most important plasma protein synthesized by the liver. Others include coagulation factors (fibrinogen, II, V, VII, IX, and X). Of these, factors II, VII, IX, and X depend on vitamin K as a cofactor. Vitamin K is synthesized in the gut by colonic flora.

Newborns initially have sterile gastrointestinal tracts, and thus require exogenous vitamin K supplementation at birth to prevent hemorrhagic disease. The prothrombin time, often used as a gauge of hepatic synthetic function in fulminant hepatic failure, depends on the presence of factors II, V, VII, and fibrinogen.

Bile Acids & Fat Absorption

The newborn absorbs dietary fat inefficiently because of immaturity in production and intestinal reabsorption of bile acids. The neonatal bile acid pool is not only smaller than the adult, but differs in composition as well. The fetal liver contains more chenodeoxycholic acid than cholic acid, whereas in the term infant and adult, these ratios are reversed. Fetal livers also contain bile acids not found in the adult liver. There are few endogenous secondary bile acids in the neonatal liver, because the intestine is sterile at birth and secondary bile acids are formed by the action of colonic bacteria on primary bile acids. A small amount can be transplacentally acquired from the maternal supply. Newborns are also prone to excessive fecal bile acid losses that result from poor reabsorption. In the adult, enterohepatic circulation of bile acids occurs via three mechanisms: (1) passive jejunal absorption, (2) active absorption in the distal ileum, and (3) passive colonic transport. In the neonate, all reabsorption is passive. There is also impaired hepatic uptake of bile acids from the circulation. This leads to increased serum bile acid levels in the neonate, a useful indicator of hepatic dysfunction. This immaturity of the newborn bile acid system not only results in inefficient fat absorption, but also in inefficient absorption of fat-soluble vitamins (A, D, E, and K) and a tendency toward cholestasis.

Toxin Clearance

Postnatally, the liver must assume many of the detoxification functions previously handled by the placenta. Monooxygenase and conjugative microsomal enzymes are central to the conversion of hydrophobic metabolites to hydrophilic derivatives more readily excreted in bile and poorly reabsorbed from the intestine. Although these microsomal enzymes are minimally active antenatally, their maturation is triggered at birth. The importance of the liver in detoxification, and the impact that the immaturity of these systems may have on the individual, is illustrated best by the following examination of bilirubin metabolism in the neonate.

Once the placental clearance of bilirubin is abolished, there is an immediate need for an alternative clearance mechanism. Bilirubin is predominantly a breakdown product of heme; neonates are burdened with an increased load (greater than twice that accommodated by adults) because of a reduced erythrocyte life span (80–90 days) and greater contributions from nonheme sources of bilirubin. Substrate load is further augmented by prematurity, hypoxia, acidosis, sepsis, hypoglycemia, inherited defects of conjugation, and hemolysis from conditions such as ABO-fetal-maternal blood group incompatibility or red cell enzymopathies.

Bilirubin must be conjugated for excretion, because it is insoluble in water at pH less than 7.8. The liver conjugates bilirubin by transfer of one or two glucuronic acid residues from uridine diphosphoglucuronic acid (UDPGA); this reaction is catalyzed by a specific microsomal glucuronyltransferase. In neonates, conjugation is hindered by lack of UDPGA (which may be conserved by forming monoglucuronides rather than diconjugates), and by an incompletely developed bilirubin uridine diphosphate (UDP) glucuronyltransferase activity. Conjugated bilirubin is excreted in the adult feces as a nonabsorbable urobilinogen derivative formed by intestinal microorganisms. In neonates, bacterial conversion is inhibited by lack of the appropriate colonic flora. Also, newborn stool and colonic mucosa contain active β-glucuronidase that hydrolyzes bilirubin glucuronide to absorbable free pigment. Thus in the neonate, enterohepatic shunting of bile may further contribute to substrate load for an already taxed system. Bilirubin travels in plasma attached to proteins with a high affinity for hydrophobic compounds, such as albumin. Drugs, such as sulfonamides, salicylates, or organic anions, such as fatty acids, may reduce the affinity of albumin for bilirubin, leading to segregation in hydrophobic environments such as plasma membranes, meninges, adipose tissue, and the brain. **Kernicterus** is the term applied to bilirubin staining of the basal ganglia. This causes a toxic encephalopathy that can result in death or permanent sequelae ranging from cerebral palsy and mental retardation to mild cognitive impairment.

A final mechanism contributing to inefficient bilirubin clearance involves neonatal vascular anatomy. At birth, the blood supply to the left lobe of the liver changes from the highly oxygenated umbilical venous blood to portal venous blood. Flow via the hepatic arteries is minimal. The ductus venosus remains patent for several days, creating a potential shunt away from the liver that would contribute to delayed plasma bilirubin clearance.

With all of these mechanisms contributing to delayed and inefficient bilirubin clearance by the neonatal liver, it is not surprising that jaundice is a frequent presenting sign in the neonatal period. Jaundice refers to the yellow staining of the skin, sclerae, and deeper tissues from excess serum bile pigments. It can be cholestatic, resulting from an excess of conjugated bile due to the impedance of normal flow in the biliary system, or noncholestatic, reflecting an increase in the absolute amount of serum bile without an associated decrease in bile flow. The majority of cases of noncholestatic jaundice result from an abundance of unconjugated bilirubin, effectively trapping the excess bilirubin within the circulation. Two presentations of neonatal hyperbilirubinemia reflect the temporary inefficiency of neonatal hepatic excretion of bilirubin as outlined above. **"Physiologic" jaundice,** common between the second and sixth days of life, is noncholestatic and predominantly results from nonconjugated bilirubin, which accumulates before adequate maturation of the UDP glucuronyl transferase conjugation system is achieved. **Breast milk jaundice** is another type of unconjugated hyperbilirubinemia sometimes confused with physiologic jaundice. Breast milk jaundice is often characterized by more pronounced hyperbilirubinemia (15–20 mg/dL) that persists longer (up to 2–3 weeks). The breast milk component causing the problem is undefined. Theories have included agents such as 3α,20β-pregnanediol or free fatty acids. Often many of the siblings within a family are affected. Cessation of breastfeeding leads to immediate diminution of the bilirubin level.

Although most neonatal jaundice is benign, jaundice can be the first clue to significant underlying hepatic pathology. The key is to pursue a logical, stepwise evaluation guided by clinical presentation and persistence of symptoms. An algorithm for a sample approach to this problem is presented in Figure 48–1.

■ LIVER DISEASES PRESENTING IN CHILDHOOD: AN ETIOLOGIC CLASSIFICATION

Common presenting signs and symptoms of pediatric liver disease include jaundice, hepatomegaly, coagulopathy, encephalopathy, or elevation of liver enzymes or waste products such as ammonia; this represents a relatively limited repertoire to herald a wide array of diseases. To most efficiently review the spectrum of pediatric liver disease, I will categorize by cause rather than by symptom into the following groups: anatomic abnormalities, infections, metabolic defects, toxin exposure, vascular anomalies, and oncologic problems.

ANATOMIC ABNORMALITIES

Pathophysiology

Most anatomic anomalies occur in the biliary tract. There are several points in gestation at which malformations are believed to arise, including failure of recanalization of the occluded ducts at 7 weeks, and failure of the intra- and extrahepatic drainage systems to join, occurring at the close of the first trimester.

General Considerations

Biliary tract malformations are divided into disorders of **intrahepatic** and **extrahepatic** ducts. Diagnosis must include determination of the exact location and type of malformation and an estimation of surgical correctability. Rapid diagnosis is essential to prevent irreversible hepatic damage.

Differential Diagnosis

1. Disorders of intrahepatic bile ducts
   a. congenital hepatic fibrosis
   b. intrahepatic paucity of bile ducts
      (1) syndromic (Alagille's)
      (2) nonsyndromic
   c. Caroli's disease
2. Disorders of extrahepatic bile ducts
   a. extrahepatic biliary atresia
   b. choledochal cyst
   c. extraluminal compression resulting from extrinsic compression (cyst, tumor)
   d. spontaneous perforation of extrahepatic bile ducts
   e. intraluminal obstruction (gallstones)

Clinical Findings

A. SYMPTOMS AND SIGNS

It is difficult to establish the primary cause from clinical presentation alone, although there are some diagnostic clues. Intrahepatic lesions can be silent until fibrosis leads to cirrhosis and portal hypertension, heralded by the development of splenomegaly or variceal bleeding. This is often the case with **congenital hepatic fibrosis,** an autosomal recessive disorder, unless associated renal anomalies facilitate earlier detection of the occult disease, or the less common presentation with abdominal pain and cholangitis spurs investigation. Intrahepatic paucity of ducts can be associated with jaundice and pruritus. With

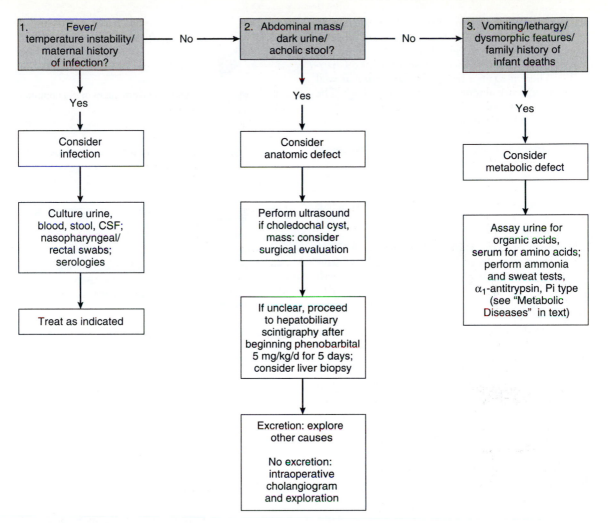

Figure 48–1. Evaluation of hyperbilirubinemia in the neonate. In a neonate older than 7 days with a direct bilirubin of greater than 4 mg/dL, consideration of possible pathologic causes should be initiated. In the sample approach outlined *below,* the physician *AIM*s toward the diagnosis, in recognition of the three major etiologic groups: *A*natomic, *I*nfectious, and *M*etabolic. Also consider potential contributory toxic effects of medications and parenteral nutrition.

Alagille's syndrome, diagnosis is facilitated by recognition of the characteristic constellation of signs, including a typical facial appearance with deeply set, widely spaced eyes, a small, pointed chin, and a flat nasal bridge. Other associations include a cardiac murmur, often caused by peripheral pulmonic stenosis, atrial septal defect, or tetralogy of Fallot; butterfly anomalies of the vertebrae; and ocular anomalies (posterior embryotoxon). **Nonsyndromic paucity of interlobular bile ducts** also exists. Another intrahepatic defect is **Caroli's disease,** a congenital cystic malformation of the biliary tract often associated with autosomal recessive polycystic kidney disease. There is a female predominance. A common presentation is recurrent abdominal pain, icterus, emesis, and hepatomegaly.

Anomalies of the extrahepatic biliary tree are less subtle in presentation. Impedance of bile flow, whether the result of stasis from a cystic dilatation, absence or diminution of ducts, or the occlusion of ducts by extrinsic masses or intrinsic stones, results in progressive jaundice and cholestasis. **Choledochal cysts** usually present as abdominal masses (exclusion of other causes, specifically tumors, can often be performed with imaging studies—see below). Choledochal cysts are congenital cystic dilatations of the biliary tree, and as such form a continuum with Caroli's disease (see also Chapter 53). There is again a female predominance, as well as a high incidence among those of Asian heritage. The five types of cysts are presented schematically in Figure 48–2. Choledochal cysts account for 2–5% of cases of extrahepatic neonatal cholestasis.

Spontaneous perforation of the extrahepatic ducts, although rare, presents as sudden jaundice, abdominal distention from ascites, and acholic (white) stools in the absence of hepatomegaly in a previously healthy newborn. The ascitic fluid is bilious if sampled; extravasation of fluid often stains the umbilicus and scrotum green, an important diagnostic clue.

Diagnosis of **extrahepatic biliary atresia (EHBA)** remains the greatest challenge. Presenting as progressive jaundice, pruritus, and hepatomegaly in a neonate with acholic stools and dark urine, it cannot readily be distinguished from other entities with similar presentations, including idiopathic neonatal (giant cell) hepatitis. **Giant cell hepatitis** is a nonspecific reaction of the neonatal liver to a variety of insults, including infections or metabolic anomalies, although in the vast majority of cases a cause cannot be identified (see Figure 48–3A for histology). EHBA occurs with a frequency of 1 in 10,000 live births. Its cause remains obscure, with both environmental and genetic factors implicated in pathogenesis. There are several cases in the literature of

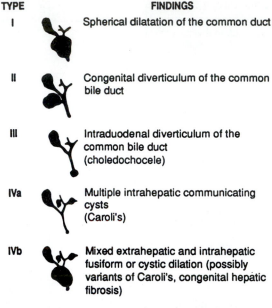

Figure 48–2. Schematic representation of types of cystic dilatations of the biliary tract. Types I–III are extrahepatic. [Reproduced, with permission, from Hathaway WE et al (editors): *Current Pediatric Diagnosis & Treatment,* 11th ed. Appleton & Lange, 1993.]

Figure 48–3. Characteristic histology in six examples of pediatric liver disease. **A:** Neonatal giant cell hepatitis. Note the central cluster of multinucleated hepatocytes with ballooning degeneration. Autopsy specimen from a 2-month-old infant with fulminant hepatic failure of unknown etiology. Magnification: ×100. Hematoxylin and eosin stain. **B:** Congenital hepatic fibrosis. There is a broad fibrous septum that occupies a significant percentage of the biopsy. Multiple cystically dilated tortuous bile ducts can be seen within the septum. Hepatocytes appear normal. From a 2-year-old child presenting with portal hypertension and hematemesis. Magnification: ×400. Hematoxylin and eosin stain. **C:** Biliary atresia. Extension of portal tract by fibrosis, with proliferation of bile ducts characteristic of biliary atresia. Macro/micronodular cirrhosis is evident. Wedge biopsy from liver excised prior to transplant in an 8-month-old child following Kasai portoenterostomy, with recurrent episodes of cholangitis, growth failure, and progressive jaundice. Magnification: ×100. Hematoxylin and eosin stain. **D:** α_1-Antitrypsin deficiency. Note diffuse hepatocellular disarray with ballooning, steatosis, and fibrosis. Intracytoplasmic inclusions resistant to diastase confirm the diagnosis (*arrowhead*). Magnification: ×400. Diastase-treated periodic acid–Schiff stain. **E:** Neonatal hemochromatosis. Hematoxolin and eosin-stained sections show marked architectural disarray, hepatocellular damage, and micro/macronodular cirrhosis. Diffuse intracellular iron deposition, evident here, was mirrored in salivary gland biopsies. From a neonate presenting with fulminant hepatic failure. Magnification: ×400. Iron stain. **F:** OTC deficiency/Reye's-like syndrome. Note moderate fibrosis of the portal tract in the center with bridging, prominent microvesicular steatosis, hepatocyte disarray, and glycogenated nuclei. This biopsy is from a previously healthy 14-year-old boy presenting with encephalopathy and hyperammonemia after taking aspirin during a viral illness. Although initially diagnosed as Reye's syndrome, urinary orotic acid levels were elevated, and the hepatic fibrosis was suggestive of a chronic phenomenon. Enzymatic analysis of liver tissue revealed a deficiency in ornithine transcarbamylase. Magnification: ×400. Hematoxylin and eosin stain.

concordance in twins, although there is a greater number of discordant twins. A "2-hit" phenomenon has been hypothesized, where manifestation of EHBA is dependent on a genetic vulnerability with subsequent exposure to unknown precipitants (eg, toxins, ischemia, infection). Ten percent of neonates with EHBA have an associated vascular or situs anomaly.

B. LABORATORY FINDINGS

Laboratory findings are not specific in disorders of the biliary system. Bilirubin is usually elevated if jaundice is present. The predisposition of the newborn to cholestasis is exacerbated if there is mechanical impedance to flow as described above; this can result in higher elevations in

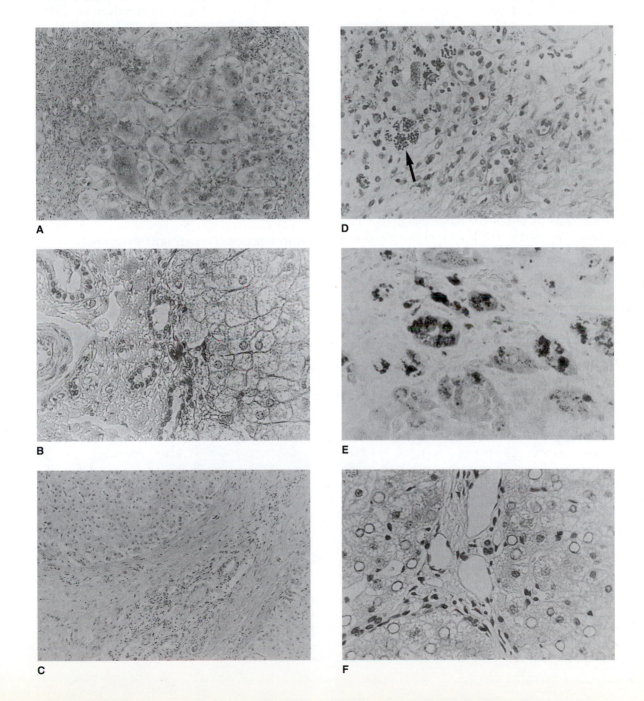

serum bile acids. Markers of biliary tract irritation, including alkaline phosphatase and γ-glutamyltransferase (GGT), may be elevated but are rarely helpful diagnostically. Transaminases may be slightly elevated as well, but synthetic function is usually preserved at presentation.

C. IMAGING

Radiologic studies are key to the diagnosis of anatomic malformations. Sonographic imaging can identify the presence or absence of a gallbladder (often absent in EHBA) as well as the presence of cysts or dilatations, stones, or inhomogeneity in the surrounding hepatic parenchyma. Figure 48–4 illustrates a sonogram of a choledochal cyst. Estimations of the caliber of the biliary tract are readily made; this can be helpful when a proximal dilatation has occurred, but the offending obstruction has passed. Doppler flow studies can detect the early development of portal hypertension with reversal of flow in key vessels such as the portal vein.

Direct imaging of the biliary tree with contrast agents can be performed via intraoperative or percutaneous cholangiogram, or by endoscopic retrograde cholangiography (ERC) with cannulation of the ampullae and injection of radiopaque dye. Figure 48–5 illustrates a fluoroscopic view of a percutaneous cholangiogram revealing a choledochal cyst.

Hepatobiliary scintigraphy is also a useful technique, especially in the diagnosis of EHBA. Utilizing intravenous injection of one of several common radiolabeled tracers, including 99mTc-labeled diethyliminodiacetic acid (DIDA) and 99mTc-labeled p-isopropylacetanilidoiminodiacetic acid (PIPIDA), the scan estimates both integrity of the hepatic parenchyma via visualization of its ability to concentrate tracer, and patency of the biliary drainage system, as the tracer is accumulated in the gallbladder and excreted into the small intestine in normal controls within 4 hours of administration. EHBA is likely if after hepatic uptake the gallbladder is not visualized and if no intestinal excretion occurs on delayed images. Hepatobiliary scans can also be helpful in the diagnosis of choledochal cysts. Figure 48–6 illustrates examples of several hepatobiliary scans.

The **liver biopsy** is diagnostic in congenital hepatic fibrosis, with characteristic dense bands of fibrous tissue containing distorted bile ducts (see Figure 48–3B). In Caroli's disease, biopsy reveals normal hepatic parenchyma with an abundance of dilated channels lined by biliary epithelium. In EHBA, biopsy reveals cholestasis, giant cell transformation of the hepatocytes, and proliferation of bile ductules with a paucity of interlobular ducts (see Figure 48–3C).

Complications/Treatment/Prognosis

The options for treatment of anatomic abnormalities depend on the diagnosis. For congenital hepatic fibro-

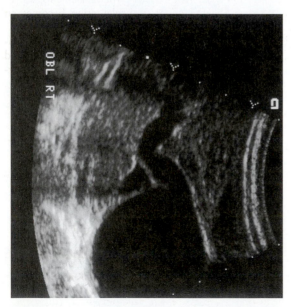

Figure 48–4. Ultrasonographic view of a choledochal cyst, with cystic dilatation of the common duct discernible as a lucent area at the bottom. (Courtesy of Carlo Buonomo, MD, Children's Hospital, Boston, MA.)

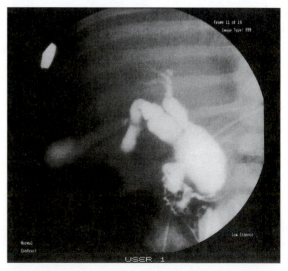

Figure 48–5. Fluoroscopic view of a percutaneous cholangiogram demonstrating large spherical dilatation of the common duct typical of a choledochal cyst. (Courtesy of Carlo Buonomo, MD, Children's Hospital, Boston, MA.)

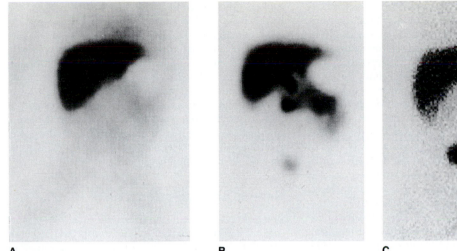
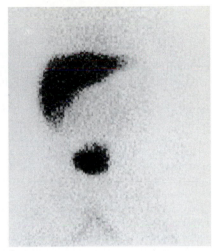

A   B   C

Figure 48–6. Hepatobiliary scintigraphy. **A, B:** Normal study. **A:** Initial view confirming uniform, facile uptake and concentration of the tracer by healthy hepatic parenchyma. **B:** Excretion of tracer into the duodenum *(arrow)* at 15 minutes. A small amount of tracer is visible in the bladder, an alternative route of excretion. **C:** View at 60 minutes from a patient with EHBA; although the hepatic parenchyma concentrated the tracer well, there is no visible excretion. (Courtesy of Carlo Buonomo, MD, Children's Hospital, Boston, MA.)

sis, Alagille's syndrome, and Caroli's disease, treatment is supportive. Supportive measures include treatment of the consequences of cholestasis, including pruritus, jaundice, malabsorption, steatorrhea, and fat-soluble vitamin deficiency (Table 48–1). There is an increased risk of cholangitis with Caroli's disease, presenting as fever without other source, and progressive jaundice. Treatment requires several weeks of broad-spectrum intravenous antibiotics. Progression of fibrosis to cirrhosis can lead to the complication of portal hypertension, with consequent development of varices and an associated risk of spontaneous hemorrhage. Bleeding varices can be treated with sclerotherapy or banding. If cirrhosis or complications of portal hypertension progress to end-stage hepatic failure, transplantation becomes an option.

Extrahepatic biliary abnormalities are treated surgically. Cystic dilatations of the biliary tract are excised with subsequent portojejunal anastomosis. Spontaneous perforation of the bile ducts requires surgical repair. Obstruction or ductal dilatation due to intraluminal causes (ie, retained stone, constriction) can often be

Table 48–1. Sequelae of chronic cholestasis, with suggested management.

Symptom	Pathophysiologic Findings	Treatment
Jaundice	Obstructed biliary tract, decreased bile flow	Ursodiol
Pruritus	Increased serum bile acids or their metabolites	Cholestyramine, diphenlydramine
Malabsorption steatorrhea	Reduced enteric bile acids, with diminished micelle formation and consequent fat malabsorption	Medium-chain triglyceride oil, vitamins A, D, E, K
Malnutrition	Steatorrhea, anorexia, early satiety	Increase calories
Ascites	Portal hypertension, fluid overload, low serum oncotic pressure	Fluid and salt restriction, diuretics, propranolol paracentesis
Bleeding	Varices, coagulopathy from factor deficiency and thrombocytopenia	Vitamin K, fresh-frozen plasma, cryoprecipitate
Encephalopathy	Decreased clearance of neurotoxins	Lactulose, dietary protein restriction, plasmapheresis

remedied via ERC with sphincterotomy or stent placement. Without operative intervention, the natural history of EHBA is progressive cirrhosis resulting in death by 12–18 months. Treatment was revolutionized in 1959 by the development of the Kasai portoenterostomy procedure, in which an intestinal conduit is anastomosed to the transected ductal remnants at the liver hilum, with drainage of bile established via the remaining intrahepatic bile ductules. The procedure has the best chance of reestablishing bile flow if performed by an experienced surgeon on a patient younger than 2 months of age, and before the patient develops significant fibrosis. Although a successful procedure relieves the immediate biliary obstruction, its effect on long-term outcome is variable, as the mechanism of the underlying disease remains unknown. The majority of patients go on to develop chronic liver disease requiring transplantation despite the portoenterostomy. The Kasai procedure usually allows time for patient growth and development. Transplantation is technically easier in a larger child, and whole donor organs are more readily available for recipients who weigh more than 15 kg. Portoenterostomy and liver transplantation are thus complementary approaches to treating EHBA.

INFECTIOUS DISEASES

Pathophysiology

Infections involving the liver can be caused by bacterial, viral, fungal, or protozoal organisms. Primary hepatic infections are caused by hepatotropic viruses (for example, the hepatitis viruses A through E) or by parasites with an affinity for the liver (including *Entamoeba* and *Echinicoccus*). **Liver abscesses** are rare in children. The liver may also be secondarily affected by agents causing disseminated infection. Examples include cytomegalovirus, adenovirus, brucellosis (unpasteurized dairy products), leptospirosis (animal urine), and perihepatitis associated with pelvic inflammatory disease (Fitz-Hugh-Curtis syndrome). The route of infection varies, especially in the neonatal period, and can be congenital (transplacental), perinatally acquired (ascending infection with ruptured membranes, swallowed blood, or other fluid at delivery), or postnatally acquired (breast milk, hospital personnel). Older children and adolescents are prone to fecal–oral, parenteral (blood products, injecting drug abuse), or sexual modes of transmission. Liver abscesses, often polymicrobial, result from ascending infection via the portal system (pancreatitis, omphalitis); spread from contiguous structures (cholangitis); systemic bacteremia (via the hepatic artery—cystitis, endocarditis, osteomyelitis); or direct inoculation (trauma, surgery, transplantation).

Infections generally cause hepatic damage in two ways: either via direct toxic/cytopathic effect, as in the case of herpes simplex virus (HSV) infection or endotoxin release, or via immune-mediated damage, as with cirrhosis from chronic hepatitis B infection. Immunocompromised individuals have a heightened susceptibility to hepatic infection; examples include fungal infection of the liver in a neutropenic oncology patient, or *Mycobacterium avium-intracellulaire* hepatic infection in a pediatric patient with acquired immunodeficiency syndrome (AIDS). Neonates are also functionally more susceptible to infection because of immune immaturity.

General Considerations

Presenting signs and symptoms of infection can be myriad yet subtle, and include nonspecific systemic manifestations such as persistent fever, malaise, or lethargy in addition to more localizing signs of hepatic involvement, including right upper quadrant pain, jaundice, or elevated transaminases. Important history to assist in diagnosis includes maternal exposures and medications in the case of a neonate, or in an older child, age of onset, recent diet, travel history, pets, or pica. Once an infection has been identified, specific treatment can be prescribed.

Differential Diagnosis

1. Viral
   a. hepatitis A–E
   b. rubella
   c. cytomegalovirus (CMV)
   d. herpes simplex virus (HSV)
   e. human immunodeficiency virus (HIV)
   f. adenovirus
   g. Epstein–Barr virus (EBV)
   h. enterovirus (Coxsackie, echovirus)
2. Bacterial
   a. *Escherichia coli*
   b. *Listeria monocytogenes*
   c. *Treponema pallidum* (syphilis)
3. Protozoal/Parasitic
   a. *Toxoplasma gondii* (toxoplasmosis)
   b. *Entamoeba histolytica* (amebiasis)
   c. *Toxocara cani* (toxocariasis)
   d. *Echinococcus granulosis* (hytatid disease)
   e. *Schistosoma mansoni* and *S japonicum* (schistosomiasis)
4. Fungal

Clinical Findings

A. SYMPTOMS AND SIGNS

Presentation varies depending on the age of the child and the particular infection in question. **Congenital infections** often present with vomiting, lethargy, temperature instability, anorexia, jaundice, and hepatomegaly. Associated malformations can provide important additional diagnostic clues to congenital infections; these include microcephaly, intracranial calcifications (toxoplasmosis, CMV), hydrocephalus (toxoplasmosis), cataracts, congenital heart disease, sensorineural hearing deficit (rubella), and growth failure, whether intrauterine (CMV, rubella) or postnatal (HIV). **Bacterial infections in the neonate** often have a more abrupt onset (48–72 hours postdelivery) with shock and disseminated intravascular coagulopathy. Bacterial infections can also be secondary to an underlying metabolic disorder such as galactosemia, known to predispose to *E coli* infections. **Liver abscesses** can present in a variety of ways, with fever, nausea, vomiting, malaise, weight loss, abdominal pain, right upper quadrant tenderness, and jaundice. These symptoms can be part of fulminant sepsis or a smoldering nonspecific illness, or can follow abdominal trauma, surgery, or immunocompromise. Liver abscesses, more common in children with sickle cell disease as liver or intestinal infarcts resulting from sickling, can serve either as a nidus for abscess formation or allow ascent of organisms such as *Salmonella.* Immunocompromised patients, including those with malignancy, AIDS, or X-linked chronic granulomatous disease, are also more prone to liver abscesses, with common agents including *Candida, Mycobacterium avium-intracellulaire,* or gram-negative enteric bacteria.

TORCH infections result from a group of organisms causing similar, sometimes devastating congenital infections, affecting 0.5–2.5% of all births. They include *t*oxoplasmosis, *r*ubella, *c*ytomegalovirus, *h*erpes virus, and usually syphilis and HIV ("*o*ther"). Toxoplasmosis, caused by the obligate intracellular organism *Toxoplasma gondii,* can be transmitted transplacentally if an acute infection occurs during gestation. The earlier in the pregnancy infection occurs, the more devastating the outcome. The fetus is protected, however, by pregestational maternal antibodies to toxoplasma. Rubella and syphilis are rare in the era of screening, vaccination, and antibiotics, which makes them more difficult to diagnose when they do occur. Cytomegalovirus affects 2% of all live births, and unlike toxoplasmosis, maternal immunity does not prevent virus reactivation or control spread, although infants infected *in utero* by maternal CMV reactivation are less likely to demonstrate significant sequelae.

The **hepatitis viruses (A–E)** share similarities in clinical presentation despite their diverse genetic origins. Hepatitis A (HAV) is endemic in many developing countries. In the United States, populations at risk include day care workers, international travelers to known endemic areas, and those with known contact with a hepatitis A-positive individual or with contaminated food or water. Transmission is fecal–oral. Anicteric infection in children is more common, and 90% of infected children younger than 5 years of age are asymptomatic. These children are highly infectious, nevertheless, with virus particles shed in feces concurrent with transaminase elevation and peak of anti-HAV immunoglobulin M (IgM). These asymptomatic children serve as a reservoir for adult infection. There is life-long immunity established after infection, with no chronic phase. Active immunization is protective.

Hepatitis B virus (HBV) infection is endemic in the Far East, Africa, and Southeast Asia. In the United States, it affects approximately 300,000 people yearly. Unlike hepatitis A, some of those infected with HBV go on to develop chronic infection with complications of cirrhosis and hepatic failure, and increased risk of primary hepatocellular carcinoma. Similar to hepatitis A, childhood infection with HBV can be asymptomatic, leading to underestimation of prevalence. Transmission can be perinatal, parenteral, or sexual. *In utero* transmission is rare. Risk of perinatal transmission is highest if maternal infection occurs in the third trimester; if the mother is hepatitis B e antigen (HBeAg) positive, there is a 70–90% chance of transmission. Although occasionally the neonate develops fulminant hepatic failure, the more typical clinical scenario is chronic infection, defined as failure to clear hepatitis B surface antigen (HBsAg) and persistent presence of viral particles for at least 6 months.

Hepatitis C (HCV) Transmission is often parenteral, although there is evidence for occasional vertical transmission. One percent of adult blood donors in the United States possess antibodies to HCV. Presentation may be asymptomatic, or characterized by mild jaundice and malaise in the setting of elevated transaminases. Diagnosis is based on detection of antibodies to HCV. High-risk children include those with a significant blood product requirement: hemophiliacs, cancer survivors, transplant recipients, and patients with thalassemia or undergoing dialysis.

Parasitic infections affecting the liver have been infrequent in the United States, but this is changing with increased immigration from endemic countries and the prevalence of international travel. Amebiasis results from ingestion of cysts in feces or contaminated meat or water. Liver involvement occurs when activated trophozoites invade the gut mucosa and are directed by the portal blood to form a solitary abscess in the right lobe. Ingestion of infected cat or dog feces leads to toxocariasis, typical in toddlers with sandboxes and a tendency toward pica. Symptoms are variable in toxocariasis and infections are often asymptomatic, unless the inoculum is large or a significant allergic response is generated.

B. LABORATORY FINDINGS

Clues to hepatic involvement include elevation of transaminases, bilirubin, alkaline phosphatase, and γ-glutamyltransferase. More problematic is identifying the specific etiologic agent. In the neonatal period, infections are the prime suspect for any unusual symptom. Maternal history; bacterial cultures from blood, urine, and cerebrospinal fluid (CSF); and viral cultures from urine, CSF, and rectal and nasopharyngeal swabs are often diagnostic. Serologic testing is also important, including maternal and infant TORCH titers, IgM anti-HAV, anti-HCV IgG, and detection of HBsAg. In older children, stool ova and parasite testing may be informative. Liver biopsies can often be supportive if not diagnostic, as with identification of acidophilic intranuclear inclusions in HSV infection. Biopsy cultures may also be informative.

C. IMAGING

Imaging studies, specifically ultrasonography and computed tomography, are useful for characterizing the location and size of hepatic abscesses. These can be solitary right lobe lesions (amebiasis, hytatid disease) or multiple disseminated lesions more common with fungal or mycobacterial infection.

Complications/Treatment/Prognosis

Bacterial infections are effectively treated with broad-spectrum antibiotics that are narrowed once specific etiologic agents are identified. Abscesses need surgical drainage if antibiotic therapy is incompletely effective. Effective antiviral therapies are more limited and lack the specificity of antibiotics. Ganciclovir and foscarnet for CMV infection can be supplemented by globulin preparations containing high titers against the virus. Acyclovir is used with varicella as well as herpes simplex infections.

Prevention of hepatitis A infection is accomplished by avoidance of infected persons and tainted food or water, and by delivery of γ-globulin for passive transient protection from pooled antibodies. A safe, formalin-inactivated vaccine is available. Greater than 95% of children are protected after two doses. Current recommendations call for immunization of travelers to endemic countries, military recruits, food handlers, and day care workers or sewage workers. Mandatory vaccination of children entering kindergarten is being considered.

The risk of developing chronicity after HBV infection is up to 90% for those infected at younger than 1 year of age, with a 25% lifetime risk of end-stage complications such as cirrhosis or primary hepatocellular carcinoma. Some children who are HBeAg positive as well as HBV DNA positive clear their infection before reaching adulthood. Few progress to cirrhosis by the time of initial liver biopsy. The best treatment is prevention, with education about the risks of intravenous drug abuse and unprotected sexual activity. The widely available recombinant vaccine containing surface antigen elicits formation of protective antibodies in greater than 95% of those vaccinated. Initial attempts to target at-risk populations failed to significantly reduce the number of HBV infections.

Guidelines established by the American Academy of Pediatrics and the Advisory Committee on Immunization Practices call for **universal immunization at birth** regardless of the HBV status of the mother, with booster doses at 2 and 6 months. If the mother is HBsAg positive, hepatitis B immune globulin (HBIG) should be given in addition to the vaccine; this combination generally prevents infection in the newborn.

Treatment of chronic HBV infections with lamivudine or interferon-α appears efficacious in children (although interpretation of success is complicated by the rate of spontaneous improvement). Children adopted from other countries in which HBV infection is endemic and horizontal transmission is known to occur pose a risk to adoptive families, whose members should be serologically screened and vaccinated. The risk is associated only with repetitive, intimate contact, however; classmates at school or day care are not at risk unless the infected child exhibits aggressive behavior such as biting, or has a bleeding disorder.

The natural history of hepatitis C infection in children is largely unknown, although recent reports suggest a higher rate of clearance than in adults. The only available treatment is interferon-α, shown to be beneficial in aminotransferase reduction and viral clearance in a minority of patients.

METABOLIC DEFECTS

Pathophysiology

As might be expected from its diverse yet essential roles in glucose homeostasis, protein and lipid synthesis, and detoxification, the liver is the primary organ affected by a wide range of metabolic derangements, many of which initially manifest in infancy and childhood. These abnormalities include defects in carbohydrate, protein, and amino acid metabolism; fatty acid oxidation; bilirubin conjugation and bile acid synthesis; and copper transport. In most cases the exact biochemical defect has been characterized; in some, the actual genetic defect has been identified as well. Careful study of these experiments of nature has contributed substantially to the understanding and appreciation of the complexities of normal liver function.

Glycogen storage disorders represent a series of enzymatic defects in the pathways devoted to glycogenolysis or gluconeogenesis in the liver. Galactosemia and hereditary fructose intolerance are characterized by defects in the ability to metabolize galactose and fructose, respectively. **Abnormalities of protein metabolism** include enzymatic defects in the urea cycle, the principal mechanism for disposal of waste nitrogen. Enzymatic defects in fatty acid oxidation are exposed during periods of prolonged fasting or increased energy demands, when glycogen is no longer available and metabolism of fats provides the major energy source. **Defects in lipid metabolism** also lead to a variety of lysosomal storage defects, including Wolman's disease, cholesterol ester storage disease, Gaucher's disease, and Niemann-Pick disease. α_1-Antitrypsin deficiency is another storage defect, in which a defective protease inhibitor accumulates as diastase-resistant glycoprotein in hepatocytes, interfering with normal function (see Figure 48–3D). **Disorders of bilirubin metabolism** include the Crigler-Najjar syndromes, in which a deficiency of UDP glucuronyl transferase results in a profound unconjugated hyperbilirubinemia. **Defects in bile acid synthesis** are rare and extremely difficult to accurately diagnose, given the protean number of enzymatic steps involved. At least one bile acid synthesis defect is attributable to absence of functioning peroxisomes (Zellweger's syndrome). Both cystic fibrosis and Wilson's disease result from **defects in ion transport;** in cystic fibrosis, there is a defective chloride channel, the cystic fibrosis transmembrane regulator (CFTR), whereas in Wilson's disease, copper accumulation occurs because of a defective copper transporter, a P-type ATPase. The pathophysiology of **neonatal hemochromatosis** remains obscure, but this disorder results in progressive and almost invariable fatal hepatic insufficiency, with significant hepatic (as well as extrahepatic) iron deposition (see Figure 48–3E). The defect responsible for the decreasingly prevalent **Reye's syndrome** has never been identified, although possible candidates have included toxic exposures (aspirin, insecticides) or unusual presentations of fatty acid or urea cycle defects, manifest under conditions of starvation and stress from illness (see Figure 48–3F, and page 750).

General Considerations

Although individually rare, these conditions collectively comprise a significant proportion of chronic liver disease in children. Initial clinical manifestations are often nonspecific. It is important to suspect possible metabolic disease when repeated episodes of vomiting, lethargy, hyperammonemia, or hypoglycemia occur. This is espe-cially true during the neonatal period, when prompt diagnosis and treatment can prevent death or crippling sequelae. Although many metabolic diseases present nonspecifically, some present in ways that provide unique clues to the appropriate diagnosis. For example, persistent jaundice and unconjugated hyperbilirubinemia suggest Crigler-Najjar syndrome; the temporal association of symptom onset and introduction of fructose to the diet suggests hereditary fructose intolerance. Diagnosis is usually confirmed by the lack of demonstrable enzymatic activity in liver or other tissue; by demonstration of the accumulation of a toxic metabolite in blood, urine, or liver; or by identification of the abnormal genotype (cystic fibrosis) or phenotype (α_1-antitrypsin deficiency).

Differential Diagnosis

1. Disorders of carbohydrate metabolism
   a. glycogen storage disorders
   b. galactosemia
   c. hereditary fructose intolerance
2. Disorders of protein or amino acid metabolism
   a. tyrosinemia
   b. urea cycle defects
3. Disorders of fatty acid oxidation
   a. medium-chain acyl-CoA dehydrogenase deficiency
   b. long-chain acyl-CoA dehydrogenase deficiency
   c. primary carnitine deficiency (systemic)
4. Disorders of bilirubin and bile acid metabolism
   a. Crigler-Najjar types I and II
   b. bile acid synthesis defects
5. Disorders of storage
   a. α_1-antitrypsin deficiency
   b. lysosomal storage
      (1) Wolman's disease
      (2) cholesterol ester storage disease
6. Disorders of ion transport
   a. cystic fibrosis
   b. Wilson's disease
7. Idiopathic metabolic disorders
   a. neonatal hemochromatosis
   b. Reye's syndrome

Clinical Findings

A. SYMPTOMS AND SIGNS

The diagnosis of a metabolic defect involves pattern recognition based on clinical presentation and history, as well as a high index of suspicion. Metabolic disease must be considered as part of the differential diagnosis in any situation involving unexplained lethargy, poor feeding, recurrent vomiting, hypoglycemia, hyperbilirubinemia, or hyperammonemia, especially in a neonate. Suspicion must remain high even into adolescence, as teenagers can present with mental status changes (Wilson's disease), hyperammonemia in the setting of a viral illness (Reye's-like syndrome, urea cycle defects), or cryptogenic cirrhosis (α_1-antitrypsin deficiency). Other important clues include parental consanguinity, unexplained sibling deaths, or deaths ascribed to sudden infant death syndrome or Reye's syndrome.

The **glycogen storage diseases (GSD)** are a heterogeneous group of disorders involving derangements in glucose or glycogen metabolism. Although there are more than 10 forms, not all have liver disease as a primary component. Type I, or Von Gierke's disease, is the most common as well as the most severe GSD, involving a deficient enzyme important in gluconeogenesis. Type Ib differs from Ia in that the enzyme in question, glucose-6-phosphatase, cannot be detected in fresh tissue but is detectable when tissue microsomes are disrupted. Long-term complications besides growth failure include the formation of hepatic nodules potentially associated with adenoma or hepatocellular carcinoma, as well as the development of renal failure. Type III GSD (Cori's disease, limit dextrinosis) results from an autosomal recessive defect in a debrancher enzyme important in glycogenolysis. It presents with hepatomegaly, hypoglycemia, and growth failure, with later complications of hepatic fibrosis, cardiomyopathy, and muscle weakness related to undegradable glycogen in these tissues. In GSD type IV, a deficiency in a brancher enzyme results in formation of a glycogen similar to a plant starch. Hepatomegaly, growth failure, and splenomegaly develop soon after birth, with fibrosis quickly progressing to cirrhosis as a result of the foreign glycogen. Type VI GSD results from a defect in phosphorylase, and presents with marked hepatomegaly and growth failure.

Other disorders of carbohydrate metabolism include **galactosemia,** a deficiency of galactose-1-phosphate uridyltransferase resulting in an inability to tolerate dietary galactose. This defect is perhaps best known for its association in the neonatal period with frequent infections, notably *E coli* urinary tract infections. **Fructose intolerance** can take three forms: fructokinase deficiency, causing benign essential fructosuria, and the more serious fructose-1,6-diphosphatase and fructose-1-phosphate aldolase deficiencies. The latter results in hereditary fructose intolerance characterized by vomiting, hypoglycemia, jaundice, hepatomegaly, reducing substances in the urine, and a metabolic acidosis upon exposure to fructose. The toxic effects on liver, intestine, and kidney are related to sequestration of phos-

phate as fructose-1-phosphate, with a consequent decrease in intracellular stores of phosphate and adenosine triphosphate (ATP). Fructose-1,6-diphosphatase deficiency has a similar presentation without jaundice.

Disorders of protein or amino acid metabolism present in the neonatal period after initiation of feeding. These defects include the urea cycle defects as well as hereditary tyrosinemia. The latter is a defect in fumaryl acetoacetic acid hydrolase (FAH), leading to increased serum and tissue concentrations of tyrosine. There are two phenotypes; in the acute form, vomiting, jaundice, hepatomegaly, anemia, hypoglycemia, and metabolic acidosis develop within the first few months of life. A renal Fanconi syndrome is also often part of the clinical picture, with glycosuria, phosphaturia, hypercalcuria, and renal bicarbonate wasting leading to hypophosphatemia and a hypochloremic metabolic acidosis. The chronic form has a much more indolent course, with slowly progressive cirrhosis complicated by a 37% incidence of hepatocellular carcinoma.

The **urea cycle defects** as a group impair the functioning of the primary pathway for waste nitrogen excretion via ammonia detoxification. Whereas many liver diseases result in secondary hyperammonemia because of generalized impairment of liver metabolism, the urea cycle defects represent a primary derangement in this specific pathway. Clinical hallmarks include hyperammonemia leading to vomiting, lethargy, and other central nervous system (CNS) effects including coma, seizures, and apnea. Ornithine transcarbamylase (OTC) deficiency is the most common urea cycle defect, affecting 1 out of every 50,000 newborns. It is the only X-linked defect, with classic presentation being a catastrophically ill male neonate with hyperammonemic coma and respiratory failure. Female carriers have variable penetrance due to lyonization of the affected X chromosome; their symptoms can include episodic vomiting, aversion to high protein foods, headaches, intermittent lethargy, seizures, and hepatomegaly. They are prone to hyperammonemia during acute illnesses or following other precipitants such as excessive protein ingestion, surgery, or vaccine administration (myolysis). There is also a small subgroup of males with milder late-onset OTC deficiency due to a less severe gene defect or mosaicism; it is easy to misdiagnose these late-onset atypical presentations as Reye's syndrome if careful diagnostic evaluations are not conducted. The second most common urea cycle defect is argininosuccinic aciduria, an autosomal recessive deficiency of argininosuccinic acid lyase leading to accumulation of argininosuccinic acid (ASA) in blood, urine, and tissues. Carbamyl-phosphate synthetase (CPS) deficiency has a presentation almost identical to OTC deficiency, with a severe, usually fatal neonatal onset as well as a milder form apparent in the first year (with 10–25% residual enzyme activity).

Fats supply energy to the body during prolonged fasts when glycogen stores have been depleted. **Fatty acid oxidation defects** present with persistent vomiting, cardiomegaly, hepatomegaly, hypotonia, developmental delay, and sometimes seizures in the setting of decreased food intake (gastroenteritis) or increased energy demands (fever). Medium-chain acyl-CoA dehydrogenase deficiency (MCAD) specifically presents as recurrent episodes of illness in the first 2 years of life, with prolonged fasting leading to vomiting, lethargy, hypoglycemia, and often coma and death. The risk of mortality exceeds 50% for affected individuals from 15 to 26 months of age. Long-chain acyl-CoA dehydrogenase deficiency (LCAD) presents similarly, but with a more severe involvement manifest at a younger age, with more pronounced cardiac and skeletal muscle involvement. Carnitine is responsible for ferrying long-chain fatty acids into mitochondria for oxidation. Synthesized in the liver, carnitine is transported via the serum into muscle, where it is present in high concentrations. Primary carnitine deficiency is an autosomal recessive defect affecting the carnitine uptake mechanism. Systemic manifestations include weakness, cardiomyopathy, and episodic hepatic encephalopathy with hypoglycemia and hypoketosis.

Some presentations of metabolic diseases are unique, as with the persistently elevated total bilirubin levels without any detectable conjugates in serum or bile seen in an otherwise healthy infant with **Crigler-Najjar syndrome.** Crigler-Najjar types I and II are distinguished by responsiveness to phenobarbital. As type I involves a total absence of the conjugating enzyme UDP glucuronyltransferase, phenobarbital is of little efficacy in reducing the unconjugated pool. Type II, by contrast, is defined by clinical responsive to phenobarbital, supporting the existence of a small pool of functioning enzyme.

Bile acids serve vital roles in the elimination of cholesterol, promotion of bile flow, and facilitation of fat and fat-soluble vitamin absorption. **Derangements in bile acid synthesis** result in significant illness, as seen in four of the known syndromes involving such defects. Cerebrotendinous xanthomatosis is a lipid storage disease presenting with progressive neurologic compromise, ataxia, and xanthomatous lesions in the brain and tendons. Its biochemical abnormalities include reduced synthesis of primary bile acids and markedly elevated cholestanol levels. **Cerebrohepatorenal or Zellweger's syndrome** is a disorder of reduced or absent peroxisomes. The resulting interference with β-oxidation of fatty acids causes abnormal bile acid synthesis (among many other defects). Two of the other known disorders of bile acid synthesis are associated with neonatal cholestasis and familial giant cell hepatitis. 3β-Hydroxysteroid dehydrogenase/isomerase deficiency is charac-

terized by jaundice, acholic (white) stools, dark urine, cholestasis, hepatocellular damage, and fat-soluble vitamin malabsorption. No chenodeoxycholic or cholic acids are detectable in the plasma. Hepatoxicity is thought to result from impaired bile flow or direct toxic effect of the mutant bile acid species synthesized. δ^4-3-Oxosteroid 5β-reductase deficiency presents in a similar fashion with cholestasis and increased urinary bile acid secretion. Interestingly, in addition to giant cell transformation on liver biopsy, the bile canaliculi are noted to be small with few microvilli, suggesting a possible role for adequate bile acid concentration in normal morphologic development.

α_1-Antitrypsin deficiency has a broad range of clinical manifestations, including primary lung disease (emphysema) in addition to isolated liver involvement. A missense mutation leads to retention of this protease inhibitor in the endoplasmic reticulum, resulting in accumulation of diastase-resistant glycoprotein deposits in periportal hepatocytes (see Figure 48–3D) and consequent interference with normal hepatocyte function. Cirrhosis frequently develops. This secretory defect results in diminished serum α_1-antitrypsin levels. The natural history and prevalence of this defect have been well documented in the Swedish cohort studies of Sveger; 20% of those carrying the PiZZ phenotype develop liver disease in childhood. Newborns can present with cholestasis, failure to thrive, and hepatosplenomegaly; alternatively, silent progression to cirrhosis or portal hypertension also occurs. There is evidence for increased intracellular aggregate formation of defective protein in settings of stress or fever, as with intercurrent illnesses. Some of those afflicted with the defective gene remain asymptomatic until lung disease, exacerbated by smoking, develops in middle age.

Two other storage diseases involve defects in the same enzyme, acid lipase, which is important in degradation of lipoproteins. **Wolman's disease** is an autosomal recessive defect presenting in the newborn period with abdominal distension, hepatosplenomegaly, ascites, anemia, widespread lipid storage, and bilateral adrenal calcification, an essentially pathognomonic finding. Liver biopsy reveals marked accumulation of lipid within lysosomes. Stored lysosomal fat is also found in intestinal mucosa, vascular endothelium, spleen, lymph nodes, bone marrow, and circulating leukocytes. Death occurs before 6 months of age in 90% of patients. **Cholesterol ester storage disease** results from a deficiency of the same enzyme, and is thought to represent a milder allelic variant. Often the only presenting symptoms are hepatomegaly and hyperlipidemia. Birefringent crystals of cholesterol esters can be demonstrated within lysosomes on liver biopsy.

Cystic fibrosis (CF) can present as cholestasis in infancy related to inspissated bile, with hepatomegaly related to protein malabsorption and fatty infiltration, or with biliary cirrhosis in the adolescent (20% of adolescents with CF have cirrhosis). Gallbladder anomalies are also frequently found in these patients. The cirrhosis may be asymptomatic (apart from hepatosplenomegaly) or present as ascites or variceal bleeding. The underlying defect involves mutations in the chloride channel protein, CFTR. **Wilson's disease** also results from an ion (copper) transport defect (see Chapter 41). A defective P-type ATPase is responsible for the toxic accumulation of copper in brain (neuropsychiatric symptoms), eyes (Kayser-Fleischer rings), kidneys, and liver. The absorption of copper is normal. Wilson's disease is among the most difficult of the metabolic defects to diagnose accurately given its range of presentation, from mild lethargy and malaise, abdominal pain, jaundice, and decreased school performance, to outright psychosis or fulminant hepatic failure.

Neonatal hemochromatosis is an uncommon idiopathic liver disease characterized by early fulminant hepatic failure in the setting of extensive intra- and extrahepatic iron deposition. The iron is readily detectable in both hepatocytes and in additional sites such as salivary glands by staining of tissue sections (see Figure 48–3E). No specific defect has been identified.

Rarely diagnosed today, **Reye's syndrome** was first described in 1963 in Australia, and was characterized by a severe encephalopathy, marked cerebral edema, and diffuse fatty infiltration of the viscera, especially the liver. Onset was innocuous, 2–5 days after the start of a viral illness, with a resurgence of malaise and emesis that would progress quickly. In addition to the characteristic viral prodrome, there was frequent association with recent consumption of aspirin. This association fueled today's practice of using acetaminophen as an antipyretic in the pediatric age group, especially in children with varicella. The cause of Reye's syndrome has never been elucidated, and the frequency has decreased to almost zero. It is conjectured that many cases represented previously undiagnosed metabolic derangements existing as *forme frustes* or partial defects uncovered by conditions of stress, fasting, fever, etc. Candidate categories include urea cycle defects, especially late-onset male or carrier female OTC deficiencies, or fatty acid oxidation defects.

B. Laboratory Findings

Demonstration of deficient enzyme activity in a liver biopsy sample or cultured skin fibroblasts is a frequent key to diagnosis in many metabolic diseases. Histologic examination of the liver biopsy itself can also yield important diagnostic clues, such as the abnormal glycogen deposition seen in many of the GSD, or the birefringent lysosomal cholesterol ester crystals in the cholesterol ester storage diseases.

A few unique approaches deserve special mention. One of the earliest diagnostic clues to the presence of a fatty acid oxidation defect is the presence of a low serum glucose (<50) in the absence of urinary ketones. Although easily and rapidly performed using commercially available "on the spot" blood sugar estimator sticks and urine dipsticks, these results reveal the central problem in this disorder, the inability to break down fats for energy during prolonged fasts with exhausted glycogen storage.

Two urea cycle defects, OTC deficiency and CPS deficiency, have extremely similar presentations. Prior to enzyme assay of affected tissue to identify the precise defect, a diagnostic clue can be provided by measurement of urinary orotic acid. This substance is elevated in OTC deficiency but not in CPS deficiency.

Unique technology is utilized to diagnose suspected bile acid synthesis defects: fast atom bombardment-mass spectrometry (FAB-MS). In concert with gas chromatography (GC-MS), FAB-MS facilitates identification of abnormal bile acid metabolites in urine samples. In healthy individuals, there is negligible urinary bile acid excretion, but this changes in conditions of cholestasis, as in bile acid synthesis defects.

C. Liver Biopsy

For many metabolic diseases, it is the enzymatic assay rather than characteristic histology that makes liver biopsy diagnostic. Percutaneous needle biopsies often provide insufficient material for enzymatic assay, necessitating open wedge biopsy.

Complications/Treatment/Prognosis

In addition to the dietary restrictions traditionally used to treat many metabolic diseases, including galactosemia, fructose intolerance, and tyrosinemia, there are increasing numbers of innovative pharmacologic therapies with a design based on a comprehensive understanding of the affected biochemical pathways. These therapies usually facilitate alternative enzymatic pathways, or block the synthesis of precursors that become toxic in excess. Examples include therapies for urea cycle defects and tyrosinemia. For urea cycle defects, treatment involves not only a restriction of protein intake (decreasing nitrogen load), but also the use of sodium benzoate and phenyl acetate to divert nitrogen from urea synthesis to other waste products (hippurate and phenylacetyl glutamine). Long-term prognosis in these disorders still depends on the severity of hyperammonemic crises, and the rapidity with which the metabolic derangement is normalized. Hereditary tyrosinemia has traditionally been treated with dietary restriction of tyrosine, phenylalanine, and methionine. Recently, 2-(2-nitro-4-trifluromethyl-benzoyl)-1,3-cyclohexanedione (NTBC) has been successfully utilized in this disorder. This compound acts to block tyrosine metabolism proximal to the enzymatic defect by inhibition of 4-hydroxyphenylpyruvate dioxygenase. Use of this substance in conjunction with dietary restriction lessens the high incidence of hepatocellular carcinoma in individuals with the chronic form of this disease.

Other metabolic diseases treated pharmacologically include Wilson's disease (use of penicillamine as a copper chelator) and cystic fibrosis and the bile acid synthesis defects (oral bile acids, which stimulate bile flow and inhibit synthesis of potentially toxic novel bile acids). Although the first line therapy for Crigler-Najjar type I disease remains phototherapy, there has been investigation into use of metalloporphyrin injections as a means of inhibiting *de novo* bilirubin production. As with urea cycle defects and the risks of long-term sequelae from repeated episodes of hyperammonemia, the risk of kernicterus with permanent neurologic deficit or even death remains high in Crigler-Najjar type I disease, even after the patients have reached adulthood.

Liver transplantation is almost always an option, if the disease condition is confined to the liver, or if the key systemic proteins are hepatically synthesized. Correctable examples include the urea cycle defects, Crigler-Najjar type I, hereditary tyrosinemia, and some of the bile acid synthesis deficiencies. Difficulties arise in choosing the optimal timing for the transplant. The procedure must be performed prior to accrual of irreversible effects of the underlying disease, yet the child must be old enough so that the risks of the transplant are minimized. Liver transplantation is not necessarily curative if other areas of primary disease exist in the body, such as with cystic fibrosis (depending on the extent of lung involvement) or lysosomal defects such as Gaucher's disease. Although a patient with Gaucher's disease was reported to experience temporary resolution of symptoms after an orthotopic liver transplant, symptoms returned within 2 years as Gaucher cells infiltrated the allograft.

Antenatal diagnosis is possible for many of these diseases. This may be beneficial from a therapeutic point of view, for example, by permitting initiation of appropriate dietary restrictions during pregnancy to prevent accrual of damage *in utero*. Antenatal diagnosis also allows the option of abortion if, after counseling, this choice is selected by the mother.

TOXINS

(See Chapter 44.)

Pathophysiology

The liver plays a primary role in detoxification of a variety of endogenous and exogenous substances, including bilirubin and various drugs. The role can be viewed as a balance between two processes:

- Activation: A compound is altered to an unstable or reactive intermediate by one of the cytochrome P-450 enzymes or an inducible monooxygenase.
- Detoxification: The usually hydrophobic intermediate is transformed to a hydrophilic compound suitable for excretion in urine or bile.

These processes place the liver at considerable risk should there be an imbalance of activation and detoxification, with an excess of reactive intermediates. The activated metabolites can be directly hepatotoxic, or can act as neoantigens, eliciting an autoimmune response with the potential for significant toxicity of its own. Damage is primarily hepatocellular, often concentrated in zone 3, the location of many of the drug-metabolizing enzymes.

Toxicity related to total parenteral nutrition (PN) represents a special, more complex situation. Most reports of PN-associated cholestasis have been in the pediatric age group, where 65% of cases are in neonates with a birth weight of less than 2000 g. By contrast, adults receiving parenteral nutrition are more likely to present with a reversible steatosis sometimes accompanied by cholestasis; only 15% have histologically significant lesions related to PN usage. Risk factors associated with the development of PN cholestasis in a neonate include prematurity, sepsis, lack of enteral stimulation, a history of hypoxia or abdominal surgery, and duration of PN use greater than 2 weeks. The pathophysiology remains obscure but is likely multifactorial, related to the immaturity of neonatal bile secretion resulting in an overall decrease in bile flow, to the frequent simultaneous use of multiple potentially hepatotoxic drugs in sick premature neonates, and to the frequent coexistence of sepsis or urinary tract infection, with associated endotoxin release also acting as a hepatotoxin. Additional factors include an increase in the proportion of potentially toxic secondary bile acids (lithocholate) in the bile acid pool. The solutions used in parenteral nutrition have also been implicated, with hepatic damage attributed to lack of tyrosine, cysteine, or taurine (found in high levels in breast milk), toxicity of photodegraded tryptophan, and excessive caloric contributions of dextrose or amino acids.

General Considerations

The possibility of toxin-induced damage should be included in the differential diagnosis of any pediatric liver disease. Such instances are probably less common than in the adult population, due to use of fewer simultaneous medications and absence of many hormonal and noxious influences contributing to the development of hepatotoxicity (obesity, ethanol abuse). In addition to being a less frequent occurrence, manifestations of toxin-mediated hepatic damage differ in children, because of developmental changes and maturation occurring in the detoxification systems; this further complicates facile diagnosis. Important information to gather when considering toxin-mediated liver damage includes a complete list of medications including over-the-counter preparations, the dosage of medications given, and the timing of initiation and discontinuation of the medications in relation to onset of hepatic pathology.

Differential Diagnosis (partial list)

1. Antipyretics
   a. acetaminophen
   b. acetylsalicylic acid
2. Anticonvulsants
   a. phenytoin
   b. carbamazepine
   c. phenobarbital
   d. valproate
3. Antibiotics
   a. sulfonamides
   b. erythromycin
   c. isoniazid
4. Immunomodulators
   a. cyclosporine
   b. methotrexate
5. Miscellaneous
   a. halothane
   b. parenteral nutrition

Clinical Findings

A. SYMPTOMS AND SIGNS

The range of presentation of toxin-induced liver damage is broad, from mild transaminase elevation to fulminant hepatic failure. The extent of hepatocellular damage determines the degree of transaminase elevation or cholestasis. Hypersensitivity or autoimmune reactions lead to more systemic manifestations, including fever, rash, and eosinophilia.

For cholestasis associated with parenteral nutrition, diagnosis is suggested by the presence of a rising conjugated hyperbilirubinemia in a neonate on parenteral nutrition for greater than 2 weeks.

B. LABORATORY FINDINGS

In general, laboratory findings reflect underlying hepatocellular damage, with increased transaminases, hyper-

bilirubinemia, cholestasis, and coagulopathy, depending on the extent and duration of damage. Eosinophilia suggests a hypersensitivity reaction. With PN-associated cholestasis, the serum bile salt concentrations will be increased, as will the proportion of lithocholate in the pool. Rising conjugated bilirubin and elevated GGT are also important diagnostic clues.

C. IMAGING

Diagnostic imaging is generally not helpful with diagnosis, although steatosis can be demonstrated on ultrasound or computed tomography.

D. LIVER BIOPSY

Most biopsies with toxin-associated pathology demonstrate focal necrosis, with concentration of hepatocellular damage in zone 3. Microvesicular steatosis is a frequent finding in valproate toxicity, as is eosinophilic infiltration in erythromycin-associated toxicity. Biopsy characteristics supportive of PN-associated cholestasis include early steatosis and periportal inflammation, progressing to cholestasis, fibrosis, and widening of the portal tracts with bile duct proliferation, giant cell transformation, and eventual cirrhosis. PN-associated cholestasis is a diagnosis of exclusion; other potential causes of cholestasis, especially infection, metabolic defects, or biliary tract obstruction, must be considered.

Complications/Treatment/Prognosis

In most cases, discontinuation of the offending medication is sufficient and will result in cessation of symptoms and reversal of damages except for fibrosis. Treatment of PN-associated cholestasis is more complex, not only because the cause is unknown but because most patients receiving PN are extremely ill with limited nutritional options. Compromises include concurrent initiation of small amounts of enteral feeding, limitation of calories delivered as dextrose or amino acids (not to exceed 3.5 g/kg/d), and allowing several hours per day free from nutrient infusion ("cycling"). Phenobarbital and ursochenodeoxycholic acid may minimize cholestasis by facilitating bile flow. Steroids may benefit in hypersensitivity reactions.

VASCULAR DISORDERS

(See Chapters 43 and 45.)

Pathophysiology

The liver receives a dual vascular supply, with both hepatic and portal veins supplying blood to the extensive network of sinusoids bathing the hepatic parenchyma. Unimpeded blood flow is needed to sustain the liver and to allow successful performance of its myriad functions, including detoxification of waste products and metabolism of drugs, dissemination of synthesized proteins, and maintenance of glucose homeostasis. Because its function is so closely dependent on its vascular supply, the liver is susceptible to a variety of vascular insults. These can be arbitrarily divided on an anatomical basis into pre-, intra-, and posthepatic problems.

Portal hypertension can be of pre-, intra-, or posthepatic cause (see Chapter 43). Prehepatic causes are a result of portal vein occlusion, whether from a congenital malformation such as a web or a result of infection or instrumentation in the neonatal period. Intrahepatic portal hypertension is usually a result of cirrhosis impeding blood flow. As described in the previous sections, cirrhosis can be the end result of numerous hepatic derangements, including those of anatomic, infectious, metabolic, and toxic causes. Posthepatic portal hypertension results from hepatic vein or inferior vena cava thrombosis (Budd–Chiari syndrome), a rare condition in children.

The liver is subject to damage from sudden changes in cardiac output, even if transient. **Decreased cardiac output** with consequent ischemia can lead to hepatocellular damage indicated by elevated transaminases as well as cholestasis. The extent of damage is determined by the duration of the ischemic episode. Right-sided heart failure (cor pulmonale), often associated with end-stage lung disease in cystic fibrosis, can lead to hepatomegaly from passive congestion of the liver.

Other intrahepatic vascular disturbances include **venoocclusive disease** (VOD), characterized by the triad of an enlarged, tender liver, ascites or unexplained weight gain, and jaundice (with or without elevated transaminases) (see Chapter 49). Although the precise cause is unknown, this disorder frequently follows allogeneic bone marrow transplantation, with associated factors of high-dose chemotherapy, total body irradiation, or graft-versus-host disease. The clinical picture mimics the result of ingestion of pyrrolizidine alkaloids (Jamaican bush tea), which leads to occlusion of small hepatic veins and hepatocyte congestion and necrosis.

Differential Diagnosis

1. Prehepatic
   a. portal hypertension secondary to portal vein thrombosis
      (1) congenital anomalies
      (2) omphalitis
      (3) umbilical venous catheter placement
   b. ischemia
2. Intrahepatic
   a. portal hypertension secondary to cirrhosis
      (1) biliary atresia

   (2) infectious disease with chronic sequelae
   (3) metabolic diseases
   (4) toxins
   b. VOD
3. Posthepatic
   a. portal hypertension secondary to hepatic venous or inferior vena cava occlusion (Budd–Chiari)
      (1) congenital anomalies
      (2) trauma
      (3) tumor
      (4) clotting abnormality
   b. passive congestion

Clinical Findings

A. SYMPTOMS AND SIGNS

The presentation of portal hypertension can often be dramatic, heralded by gastrointestinal bleeding from esophageal or gastric varices. If due to post- or intrahepatic causes, there can be significant hepatomegaly with or without splenomegaly. The latter often results in sequestration of white blood cells and platelets within the enlarged spleen (hypersplenism), leading to neutropenia and thrombocytopenia. The liver is normal size in prehepatic portal hypertension. Passive congestion and venoocclusive disease often present with hepatomegaly.

B. LABORATORY FINDINGS

In cases of suspected vascular disease, especially portal hypertension, it is important to obtain a complete blood count with differential and platelets, coagulation studies, and liver function tests. If hemorrhage is present, a type and cross for a possible transfusion is indicated. Prehepatic causes of portal hypertension are often associated with normal laboratory values.

C. IMAGING

Ultrasonography with Doppler is the most facile way to confirm a suspected diagnosis of portal hypertension. In addition to detection of reversed or hepatofugal flow, the presence of clots and the caliber of vessels can be assessed. The hepatic parenchyma can be examined as well. Computed tomography with and without contrast can detect fixed vascular anomalies such as cavernous transformation of the portal vein. It is also useful in the evaluation of hemangiomas of the liver. The technique of magnetic resonance angiography is becoming popular as a substitute for traditional angiography in documenting hepatic vasculature. Invasive angiography may be necessary to document vascular anatomy prior to operative procedures, or to assess intravascular or intrasplenic pressure.

D. LIVER BIOPSY

Biopsy is not a useful diagnostic technique in portal hypertension except to assess the presence or extent of cirrhosis. Findings consistent with passive congestion or ischemia are supportive but not illuminating as to cause. Histopathologic lesions in VOD may be helpful in demonstrating central venous congestion, centrilobular hemorrhage, and necrosis with minimal inflammatory response.

Complications/Treatment/Prognosis

Treatment of portal hypertension depends on presentation. Gastrointestinal hemorrhage requires transfusion followed by endoscopy for diagnosis and possible treatment with sclerotherapy or banding. Agents to lower portal pressure (eg, vasopressin, somatostatin) may also be useful in decreasing variceal bleeding. Ascites requires a low-salt diet and use of diuretics such as spironolactone or furosemide. For intrahepatic causes of portal hypertension, it is important to treat the cause of the cirrhosis. Congenital webs or other anomalies require surgical repair. Persistent variceal bleeding with continued hepatic deterioration is an indication for liver transplantation. Treatment for the remainder of vascular defects discussed is supportive. Hepatic damage from transient ischemia is reversible if the episode was isolated.

NEOPLASTIC DISORDERS

(See Chapter 46.)

Pathophysiology

Primary liver tumors represent the third largest group of abdominal neoplasms in children. One-third are benign, with the most common being mesenchymal hamartomas and hemangioendotheliomas. Two-thirds are malignant, and include hepatoblastoma, hepatocellular carcinoma, and metastases. Common childhood tumors metastatic to the liver include Wilms', stage IV neuroblastoma, and leukemia. A literature survey of primary pediatric liver tumors revealed hepatoblastoma to be the most common (43%), followed by hepatocellular carcinoma (23%), hemangiomas/hemangioendotheliomas (13%), and mesenchymal hamartomas (6%).

Hemangiomas are the most common benign liver tumors. They usually present within the first 6 months of life, grow rapidly for the first year, then gradually involute over 5–8 years. Cavernous hemangiomas are often asymptomatic and small, but capillary hemangiomas, or hemangioendotheliomas, are large, frequently multiple, and often hemodynamically significant. Intrahepatic lesions are often accompanied by

cutaneous ones. Hemangiomas often result in congestive heart failure and consumptive coagulopathy (Kasabach-Merritt syndrome). Mesenchymal hamartomas arise from mesenchymal rest cells of the portal tract. A usual patient would be a male younger than 2 years old. The lesions usually consist of large septated cysts filled with mucoid material and lined by flattened biliary epithelium.

Hepatoblastomas are of mesodermal origin, and are formed from incompletely differentiated hepatocytes. They usually present before 3 years of age. They occur more frequently in males, in the right lobe, and are generally large and multinodular. The cellular components can be diverse; most recapitulate a stage of normal fetal hepatic development. This variety complicates evaluation, because treatment and prognosis are tightly linked to histology. The worst prognosis is associated with tumor composed of small undifferentiated cells. There is a broad spectrum of genetic alterations associated with hepatoblastomas. In the tumor itself, trisomy 2, trisomy 20, and various translocations and partial deletions have been documented. There is a clear association with familial adenomatous polyposis, with a 1000-fold increased incidence of hepatoblastoma in children from affected families compared with the general population.

Hepatocellular carcinoma (HCC) occurs more frequently in older children, with an increased frequency in males. The spectrum of cell types involved is similar to the adult presentation. Hepatocellular carcinoma has a much higher incidence in chronic carriers of HBV and in various metabolic disorders, including the glycogen storage diseases, type I tyrosinemia, and α_1-antitrypsin deficiency.

General Considerations

Once an abdominal mass has been identified, swift and accurate diagnosis is imperative, because many liver tumors will have already grown to considerable dimensions. The primary decisions center around the questions of benign or malignant and resectable or nonresectable. Imaging studies are vital to characterization of the mass, revealing diagnostic clues in addition to important information concerning vascularity and hence resectability.

Differential Diagnosis

1. Benign tumors
   a. hemangiomas, cavernous
   b. hemangioendotheliomas
   c. mesenchymal hamartomas
2. Malignant tumors

    a. hepatoblastoma
    b. hepatocellular carcinoma
3. Metastatic
    a. neuroblastoma
    b. Wilms'

Clinical Findings

A. SYMPTOMS AND SIGNS

The most frequent presentation is an asymptomatic abdominal mass. It is often discovered by the primary physician during a routine "well-child" check-up, or by a parent during bath time or play. Masses often grow to sizable proportions prior to discovery. Other common features include abdominal pain, anorexia, weight loss, vomiting, diarrhea, and jaundice with or without pruritus, if tumor growth causes impedance of bile flow. In cases of large hemangioendotheliomas or vascular or mesenchymal hamartomas, the presentation can involve congestive heart failure as well as hepatomegaly. With hemangioendotheliomas, there are also often cutaneous lesions or a bruit audible on auscultation of the liver.

B. LABORATORY FINDINGS

As with any disruption of normal hepatic architecture, transaminase elevation and hyperbilirubinemia may accompany tumor growth. Anemia can sometimes be found in association with hepatoblastoma, as can thrombocytopenia with hemangioendotheliomas (Kasabach-Merritt syndrome). Substances that can be used as tumor markers to aid in diagnosis and to follow efficacy of therapeutic regimens include α-fetoprotein, elevated in 80–90% of hepatoblastoma patients and 60–90% of those with hepatocellular carcinoma; serum ferritin, almost universally elevated in cases of HCC; and descarboxyprothrombin, also elevated in HCC.

C. IMAGING

As with primary vascular anomalies, radiologic imaging is essential for diagnosis of liver masses. Ultrasonography is especially useful for delineation of cystic lesions or for guidance of fine-needle aspirates. Computed tomography (CT) with and without contrast is best for lesions that are exceptionally small or difficult to assess by ultrasound, for documentation of metastases, and for preoperative assessment of vascular involvement. Figure 48–7 illustrates an hepatoblastoma on CT scan with contrast. Magnetic resonance angiography (MRA) is becoming the best noninvasive way of accurately imaging tumor vascularity and potential encroachment on hepatic vessels. Therapeutic angiography can be used to selectively embolize vessels supplying a hemangioendothelioma.

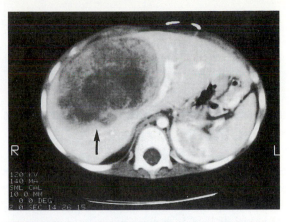

Figure 48–7. CT scan of the liver with contrast. Note the large, circumscribed hepatoblastoma ***(arrow)***. Necrotic areas are visible within the tumor. The portal vein is displaced. (Courtesy of Carlo Buonomo, MD, Children's Hospital, Boston, MA.)

Complications/Treatment/Prognosis

The major therapeutic goal for liver neoplasms is complete excision. The staging mechanism reflects this goal, with stage I consisting of complete resection; stage II, microscopic residual tumor; stage III, gross residual tumor; and stage IV, metastatic disease. The primary barriers to excision include size, location, and vascularity of the tumor. If the tumor is too large for resection at presentation, an attempt at tumor reduction with chemotherapy or radiotherapy is made. Hepatoblastoma has proven responsive to doxorubicin as well as to regimens including vincristine, cyclophosphamide, 5-fluorouracil, and cisplatinum. HCC responds poorly to chemotherapy, however; only 10–25% are resectable, and postresection adjuvant chemotherapy cures less than one-third of patients. Liver transplantation for HCC is generally unsuccessful because of rapid reinfiltration of the allograft with tumor. The best tool to combat HCC is prevention of chronic HBV infection using aggressive vaccination, and careful surveillance in clinical situations known to predispose to HCC (ie, tyrosinemia).

The treatment of hemangiomas also depends on presentation. As described earlier, the natural history of these benign tumors involves rapid growth over the first year of life with subsequent gradual involution. Treatment in an attempt to reduce the size of lesions becomes important in the case of large or multiple lesions compromising vital structures or their function. For lesions localized to the liver, resection or selective embolization is possible. For disseminated lesions, treatment in the past has involved radiation, cyclophosphamide, or more recently, steroids to accelerate the rate of involution. Interferon-α2a may be effective in life-threatening cases in which steroid therapy fails. Benign mesenchymal hamartoma need be excised only if symptomatic.

■ PEDIATRIC LIVER TRANSPLANTATION

(See also Chapter 54.) Liver transplantation has become an important therapy for a number of previously fatal pediatric diseases including metabolic derangements such as tyrosinemia and ornithine transcarbamylase deficiency. Approximately 350 children annually receive liver transplants in the United States.

There are three major indications for transplantation in a pediatric patient:

- Primary progressive liver disease resulting in failure without intervention (acute idiopathic hepatic failure, biliary atresia, sclerosing cholangitis);
- Primary static liver disease with morbidity significant enough to overshadow the risks of transplantation (refractory pruritus, severe growth failure);
- Metabolic disease.

Lesser indications include liver disease secondary to systemic illness primarily affecting another organ system (cystic fibrosis) or primary hepatic malignancy (hepatocellular carcinoma). Indications for transplantation as listed in the SPLIT registry are shown in Table 48–2. As in most series, biliary atresia is the most frequent indication. The second most common indication is acute failure, and the third is the metabolic diseases as a group.

Timing of transplantation is obviously critical. Technically, liver transplantation is easier in an older child, and donor organs are easier to obtain. Older children are also less likely to have growth problems. Delaying transplantation can be hazardous, however. Chronic liver disease can itself lead to growth failure because of a variety of reasons including fat and fat-soluble vitamin malabsorption, early satiety, and anorexia (see Table 48–1 for treatment options). Some complications, such as variceal hemorrhage, spontaneous bacterial peritonitis, or recurrent cholangitis, can be life threatening. In the case of metabolic diseases, the passage of time increases the chances of accumulation of central nervous system damage from recurrent episodes of hyperammonemia or hyperbilirubinemia, or of development of hepatocellular carcinoma. Attempts to

Table 48–2. Frequency of liver transplantation for various disorders.[1]

Disorder	Number	Percentage of Total
Biliary atresia	304	43
Fulminant hepatic failure	96	14
Metabolic disease	55	8
Urea cycle	(13)	2
Tyrosinemia	(10)	1
Neonatal hemochromatosis	(8)	1
α_1-Antitrypsin deficiency	28	4
Neonatal hepatitis	10	1
Hepatoblastoma	23	3
Autoimmune hepatitis	25	4
Sclerosing cholangitis	19	3
Parenteral nutrition associated	13	2
Alagille syndrome	21	3
Other	112	16

[1]Data from 12 center compilation 1995–2000. Percentage totals are approximations.

develop methods to aid in prediction of optimal timing of transplantation have not been successful.

Once the difficult decision to proceed with transplantation has been made, timing ultimately is controlled through the ranking system of the United Network for Organ Sharing (UNOS). This system is necessary because of the severe shortage of cadaveric donor organs. Pediatric donors commonly arise from accident victims, with the most frequent susceptible age range being toddlers and school age children. Most children waiting for a liver are younger than 2 years of age and less than 30 kg. Innovative graft surgery has helped to lessen the impact of this critical shortage. Approaches include the use of reduced-size cadaveric organs, in which a large organ is trimmed to accommodate the recipient's size, and living-related donor transplants, in which a portion of the donor's left lobe (or left lateral lobe) is resected. This latter procedure ensures graft quality and has enabled transplants to be performed electively before the deterioration of the child's health. Donors are usually parents who are screened and evaluated for suitability. Additionally, auxiliary transplants are being developed for the treatment of transient insults or metabolic diseases, where temporary support or minimal auxiliary function is sufficient to augment native liver function.

The central goal of the pediatrician caring for a child with liver disease is to optimize the child's growth and development. Although liver transplantation often represents the cure for underlying disease, it brings new problems as well. For example, immunosuppression is required for successful graft maintenance, but predisposes to infection as well as to secondary malignancy (posttransplant lymphoproliferative disease associated with EBV infection). Additionally, these medications contribute to transplant-associated growth failure, especially during the first 6 months, when regimens are most stringent. Transplantation in children younger than 2 years of age results in poor growth. There are also a variety of factors leading to poor oral intake, including nausea from medications or infections, gastric dysmotility, and persistent malabsorption. With children, behavioral factors are important as well, with frequent noxious stimuli such as suctioning or intubation leading to residual oral aversion and refusal to feed.

Despite these potential complications, it is important to emphasize that the vast majority of pediatric transplant recipients grow and develop normally in a fashion that would not have been possible without the transplant. In many centers, survival rates as high as 80–90% are reported. Many children lead fully normal lives with regular school attendance and normal maturation into adulthood.

REFERENCES

Alonso MH, Ryckman FC: Current concepts in pediatric liver transplant. Semin Liver Dis 1998;18:295.

Becht MB et al: Growth and nutritional management of pediatric patients after orthotopic liver transplantation. Gastroenterol Clin North Am 1993;22:367.

Burton BK: Inborn errors of metabolism: the clinical diagnosis in early infancy. Pediatrics 1987;79:359.

Codona-Franch P, Bernardo O, Alvarez F: Long-term follow-up of growth in height after successful liver transplantation. J Pediatr 1994;124:368.

Finegold MJ: Tumors of the liver. Semin Liver Dis 1994;14:270.

Knisely AS: Iron and pediatric liver disease. Semin Liver Dis 1994;14:229.

Peter G et al (editors): *2000 Red Book: Report of the Committee on Infections and Diseases,* 23rd ed. American Academy of Pediatrics, 2000.

Romero R, Lavine JE: Viral hepatitis in children. Semin Liver Dis 1994;14:289.

Treem WR, Sokol RJ: Disorders of the mitochondria. Semin Liver Dis 1998;18:237.

Wolf AD, Lavine JE: Hepatomegaly in neonates and children. Pediatr Rev 2000;21:303.

Hepatic Complications of Marrow & Stem Cell Transplantation

49

George B. McDonald, MD

Hepatic diseases are common in marrow and peripheral blood stem cell transplantation recipients. Diagnoses are often difficult, as the transplantation milieu is complex and patients are susceptible to toxic, infectious, and immunologic liver diseases, sometimes concurrently.

■ HEPATOBILIARY DISEASES IN CANDIDATES FOR TRANSPLANTATION

FUNGAL INFECTION IN THE LIVER

Patients who are candidates for transplantation and have a history of granulocytopenia, fever, and fungal sepsis may have fungal abscesses in the liver. These should be identified and treated before transplantation, if possible. Antifungal therapy (usually liposomal amphotericin) should be given throughout the transplantation procedure until the fungal lesions have resolved completely before transplant.

HEPATIC METASTASES

Liver involvement with tumor is common in patients who are undergoing transplantation for a malignant disorder, and this is not a contraindication to transplantation. It is important to be sure that filling defects seen on liver imaging tests do not represent abscesses rather than metastases.

HEPATITIS

Elevated serum transaminase levels are common before transplantation because of viral hepatitis B and C infections (from prior blood products), steatohepatitis, or drug toxicity. Liver inflammation predisposes patients to fatal venoocclusive disease of the liver following high-dose cytoreductive therapy. Cirrhosis is a contraindication to high-dose myeloablative conditioning therapy. Viral hepatitis B may cause fulminant hepatitis

after transplantation, but the usual course is asymptomatic viral replication after conditioning therapy, followed by mild hepatitis after Day 60, followed by chronic hepatitis. Patients with chronic hepatitis B should receive lamivudine throughout their transplant course, until full immunologic recovery. There is little morbidity associated with hepatitis C after transplant.

GALLSTONES

Asymptomatic gallstones can be watched throughout the transplantation process, but symptomatic biliary disease (biliary colic, cholecystitis, or common duct stones) is an indication for surgical correction before the start of conditioning therapy.

■ LIVER DISEASES IN THE FIRST 100 DAYS AFTER TRANSPLANTATION

The approach to hepatic diseases after transplantation starts with a review of the individual patient's risk factors for these diseases (Table 49–1). The differential diagnosis becomes more manageable if certain diseases can be dismissed on the basis of a low probability that they are present. The timing of liver dysfunction in relation to conditioning therapy, marrow or stem cell infusion, and immune system reconstitution is also useful in constructing a list of likely diagnoses. The height of serum bilirubin is correlated with survival from the transplant process (Table 49–2).

VENOOCCLUSIVE DISEASE OF THE LIVER

Venoocclusive disease (also called sinusoidal obstruction syndrome) is the most common cause of jaundice in the first few weeks following marrow or stem cell infusion. Cytoreductive therapy ("conditioning therapy") given before marrow or stem cell infusion may cause widespread damage to zone 3 of the liver acinus (the area surrounding the central veins). This damage includes injury

Table 49–1. Overview of liver diseases commonly seen in marrow transplantation patients.

Hepatic Disease after Transplantation	Risk Factors[1]	Timing
Venoocclusive disease (sinusoidal obstruction syndrome)	High-dosage conditioning regimens: total body irradiation dose > 13 Gy; cyclophosphamide-based regimens; multiple alkylating agents; Mylotarg Elevated serum transaminase levels before cytoreductive therapy Persistent fever before and during cytoreductive therapy Mismatched or unrelated donor allogeneic marrow Second conditioning regimen and transplantation	Onset from before marrow infusion to Day +20 posttransplantation Onset differs with various regimens of cytoreductive therapy
Fungal liver disease	Pretransplantation filling defects in liver Fungal colonization or infection Venoocclusive disease or graft-versus-host disease of liver Granulocytopenia Absence of prophylaxis	During granulocytopenia, usually before day 50
Cholangitis lenta	Persistent fever Sepsis syndrome	During sepsis, usually before Day 50.
Acute graft-versus-host disease	Allogeneic marrow donor, especially HLA-mismatched or unrelated donor Lack of prophylactic immunosuppressive drugs (cyclosporine, tacrolimus, methotrexate) Donor, lymphocyte infusion	Onset day +15–60 Note "hyperacute graft-versus-host disease" in patients who do not receive prophylactic drugs
Biliary sludge disease	Minimal oral intake Prolonged parenteral nutrition Conditioning therapy Use of medications that precipitate in bile (cyclosporine, ceftriaxone)	Found on ultrasound by Day +10 Symptoms by Day +20–35
Drug- or TPN-induced liver injury	Known hepatotoxic drug Prolonged, noncyclic TPN ± sepsis	At any time
Bacterial infection of the liver	Prior infection with M tuberculosis Prior BCG vaccination	Early, during granulocytopenia Later, during immunosuppression
Epstein–Barr virus lymphoproliferative disease	T lymphocyte-depleted marrow Acute graft-versus-host disease High-dosage, prolonged immunosuppression therapy Anti-T lymphocyte antibody therapy	Later, usually Day +50–100
Malignant cells in the liver	Pretransplantation malignant disease Transplantation in leukemic relapse	Day +50–100
Nodular regenerative hyperplasia	High burden of chemotherapy before transplantation High-dosage cytoreductive therapy for marrow transplantation Signs of venoocclusive disease before Day 20	Day +50–100
Acute viral hepatitis	Evidence of active or latent viral infection before transplantation (herpes simplex virus, varicella-zoster virus, hepatitis B or C virus, cytomegalovirus) Restitution of cell-mediated immunity after transplantation (hepatitis B or C virus) Exposure to adenovirus	For herpesviruses and adenovirus, Day +30–150 For hepatitis viruses, after immune reconstitution, Day +60–120

[1]TPN, total parenteral nutrition; BCG, bacille Calmette–Guérin.

Table 49–2. Frequency of mortality after allogeneic hematopoietic cell transplantation as a function of total serum bilirubin at various times after transplant.

Total Serum Bilirubin (mg/dL)	At Day 10 (%)	At Day 30 (%)	At Day 60 (%)
1–4	25	19	15
4–7	51	51	55
7–10	55	75	70
>10	73	83	88
>19	80	87	100

to endothelial cells lining the sinusoids and venules, hepatocyte necrosis, deposition of thrombotic material in venular walls, and, in severe cases, fibrosis of hepatic venules and sinusoids. Risk factors for the development of severe venoocclusive disease are the intensity of the conditioning regimen (higher-dosage regimens, especially those containing cyclophosphamide, are more likely to cause severe disease) and factors individual to each patient, such as the presence of hepatitis before transplantation, persistent fever during conditioning therapy, and the degree of mismatching between patient and marrow donor. Patients who receive a second course of high-dose conditioning therapy, particularly adults, are also predisposed to severe venoocclusive disease. Treatment of relapsed acute myeloid leukemia after transplant with gemtuzumab ozogamicin (Mylotarg) may also lead to severe sinusoidal injury.

Clinical Findings

A. SYMPTOMS AND SIGNS

The triad of painful hepatomegaly, weight gain caused by fluid retention, and jaundice is present in most patients with venoocclusive disease. The clinical onset is usually within 7–14 days of the start of regimens that include busulfan plus cyclophosphamide, cyclophosphamide plus total body irradiation, or carmustine (BCNU) plus cyclophosphamide plus etoposide. In some cases, the onset is before Day 0, the day of marrow infusion. The clinical onset develops later with regimens that include multiple alkylating agents (eg, busulfan plus melphalan plus thiotepa).

Hepatomegaly and weight gain are the initial manifestations, followed by jaundice 4–7 days later, on average. The onset can be abrupt, with severe abdominal pain from rapid hepatic enlargement. In some cases, the onset is insidious and the diagnosis is not apparent until Day 15–30, when ascites and jaundice are noted.

B. DIAGNOSTIC STUDIES

In patients with a classic presentation, biopsy may not be necessary. If the clinical presentation is atypical or other liver diseases are present simultaneously with venoocclusive disease, accurate diagnoses can be achieved with transvenous liver biopsy and measurement of the hepatic venous pressure gradient (>10 mm Hg is highly predictive of venoocclusive disease in this setting).

Serum transaminase and alkaline phosphatase levels are usually normal or minimally elevated; in some patients, however, transaminase levels can exceed 1000 IU/L, probably as a result of ischemic hepatocyte necrosis. Platelet counts are lower than expected in patients with severe venoocclusive disease, probably because of rapid consumption.

Differential Diagnosis

Hepatomegaly can be seen with tumor or fungal infiltration of the liver, hepatic vein obstruction (Budd–Chiari syndrome), right heart failure, or constrictive pericarditis. Jaundice in the early posttransplantation period can be caused by persistent septicemia (cholangitis lenta), liver injury due to drug toxicity or total parenteral nutrition, or acute graft-versus-host disease. Ascites can also result from the spreading of intraperitoneal tumor or pancreatitis.

Complications

Venoocclusive disease is a major risk factor for renal failure, cardiac enlargement, respiratory insufficiency, septicemia, neurologic symptoms, and intestinal bleeding. The cause of death in patients with severe venoocclusive disease is usually not fulminant hepatic failure but rather multiorgan failure.

Treatment & Prognosis

Several approaches have been used to prevent venoocclusive disease. Using lower dosages of conditioning therapy will result in less liver toxicity, but the risk of recurrence of the underlying cancer is then increased. When busulfan is part of the conditioning regimen, individualized dosages based on pharmacokinetic measurements from the first doses may result in less venoocclusive disease. Current research is examining individualized dosing of cyclophosphamide, substitution of fludarabine for cyclophosphamide, and use of nonmyeloablative conditioning regimens as methods of preventing venoocclusive disease. Prophylactic heparin infusions are ineffective.

Treatment of established venoocclusive disease is largely supportive. Minimizing the amount of retained fluid will lessen cardiac and pulmonary congestion and the volume of ascites. Limiting sodium intake and increasing urinary sodium excretion with diuretics will accomplish this goal, but in patients with severe venoocclusive disease, it is often difficult to maintain a negative sodium balance without resorting to hemodialysis or hemofiltration. Uncontrolled experience with thrombolytic therapy and with an investigational drug, defibrotide, suggests a limited role for these treatments in patients with severe venoocclusive disease. Fatal bleeding has been described in marrow transplantation patients who have received thrombolytic therapy. Liver transplantation has been undertaken in some patients with severe venoocclusive disease, but there are no reports of long-term survivors. Use of transhepatic shunts does not appear to be effective.

Of patients who develop venoocclusive disease, 85% recover spontaneously, usually by Day 30–40 following transplantation, and 15% have a more severe illness associated with multiorgan failure and death. Patients whose course will be severe can be identified soon after the clinical onset, because they gain weight more rapidly and become more deeply jaundiced than those who recover.

FUNGAL LIVER INFECTION

Fungal liver abscess is a complications of fungal infection in the bloodstream. *Candida* species are the usual cause, but unusual fungi and molds can also be seen. Major risk factors include granulocytopenia, colonization or superficial infection with fungi, deep fungal infection (particularly bloodstream infections), and the presence of severe liver disease caused by venoocclusive disease and graft-versus-host disease. The most common portal of entry for fungi is the intestine, which allows yeast forms to pass directly into the portal circulation.

Fungal infection isolated to the liver occurs in less than 3% of marrow transplantation patients who receive prophylactic fluconazole; most infected patients have fungal lesions in other organs (spleen, kidneys, lungs) as well.

Clinical Findings

A. SYMPTOMS AND SIGNS

Persistent fever may be the only sign. Hepatomegaly and pain in the liver are signs of extensive fungal infiltration.

B. DIAGNOSTIC STUDIES

In marrow transplantation patients, the diagnosis of fungal infection is difficult because of a high frequency of liver dysfunction and fever that is unrelated to infection, and the unreliability of imaging studies [computed tomography (CT), and ultrasound studies are

only 20–30% sensitive]. If imaging studies are positive, however, fungal abscesses will be found more than 90% of the time. Diagnosis is often based on evidence of persistent colonization with fungi or prior fungal sepsis and a compatible clinical picture. Definitive diagnosis requires study of liver tissue via fine-needle aspiration or open biopsy.

Differential Diagnosis

The differential diagnosis of painful hepatomegaly includes venoocclusive disease, right heart failure, and tumor infiltration. A common problem is deciding whether a defect on CT scanning, or ultrasound studies represents fungal infection, tumor in the liver, or a preexisting lesion such as a liver cyst, hemangioma, or focal fibrosis, and whether the defect is related to signs and symptoms.

Complications

If the diagnosis is not made and the patient is not treated, *Candida* lesions may coalesce and grow into the biliary ducts and gallbladder. *Aspergillus* and *Mucor* species may invade the hepatic veins to cause Budd–Chiari syndrome and may extend beyond the liver capsule. These are rare events.

Treatment & Prognosis

Prevention of fungal liver infection is based on four strategies: prevention of colonization with fungi, prompt treatment of superficial fungal infections (especially those involving the oropharynx and esophagus), treatment of fungal bloodstream infections with intravenous amphotericin, and early restoration of granulocyte function. Fluconazole and itraconazole have proved to be very effective in preventing visceral infections caused by *Candida albicans* in marrow transplantation patients, but there may be emergence of *Candida* species resistant to these agents. Candidal liver abscesses are treated with intravenous amphotericin. The end point of therapy may be ill defined, because filling defects seen on imaging studies may persist despite eradication of fungal elements from the liver.

Treatment is usually successful if granulocyte counts return to normal and immunosuppressive drug dosages can be minimized. Patients with fungal liver infection almost never die because of liver infection; rather, they die because of the persistence of the underlying diseases that led to the infection. In rare patients, the liver fungi become encapsulated by fibrous material and cause no clinical signs or symptoms, despite the presence of viable fungi within these lesions. Immunosuppressive drugs may activate such lesions.

CHOLANGITIS LENTA (CHOLESTASIS CAUSED BY SEPSIS)

Jaundice may develop after prolonged fever or infection distant from the liver. Although earlier reports implicated bacterial cell wall components and endotoxin, recent evidence points to the inflammatory response, particularly the cytokine interleukin-6, as leading to cholestatic liver injury.

Clinical Findings

A. SYMPTOMS AND SIGNS

Cholangitis lenta is probably a common cause of mild jaundice in febrile marrow transplantation patients but an unusual cause of severe jaundice. It occurs after fungal or bacterial infections.

The presentation is usually that of hyperbilirubinemia that follows persistent fever or sepsis syndrome by days or weeks. Liver synthetic function is preserved, and there is no evidence of liver failure.

B. DIAGNOSTIC STUDIES

There may be elevation of serum alkaline phosphatase levels and a rise in total serum bilirubin levels to 15 mg/dL when cholangitis lenta occurs in isolation. When it occurs in patients who already have liver dysfunction, serum bilirubin levels may rise to more than 50 mg/dL. Liver biopsy shows either pericentral canalicular cholestasis or periportal ductular cholestasis, but the portal inflammation often seen with this condition in septic patients may be absent in marrow transplantation patients. In many cases, this diagnosis is made in retrospect.

Differential Diagnosis

The diseases that lead to isolated hyperbilirubinemia in this setting include hemolytic anemia, venoocclusive disease of the liver, graft-versus-host disease, drug-induced cholestasis (especially with cyclosporine), and liver injury related to total parenteral nutrition.

Complications

There are no complications from this form of cholestasis per se. If graft-versus-host disease is mistaken for sepsis-related cholestasis and high-dosage immunosuppressive therapy is begun in error, the patient may have an adverse course.

Treatment & Prognosis

There is no specific treatment other than treatment of the underlying infection. Patient outcomes are related to immune competence and control of the underlying infection.

ACUTE GRAFT-VERSUS-HOST DISEASE

Graft-versus-host disease results from infusion of alloimmune lymphoid cells into a host that is unable to reject them. Epithelial cells of small bile ducts, hepatocytes in zone 1 of the liver acinus, and periductular glandular epithelial cells are the target cells of graft-versus-host disease. Necrosis of target bile duct cells in the liver occurs by apoptosis, or programmed cell death, a result of cell-to-cell interaction between lymphoid cells and target cells. The molecular events leading to apoptosis in graft-versus-host disease are not well understood. Release of cytokines, both locally and systemically, is also a cause of tissue damage and symptoms.

Clinical Findings

A. SYMPTOMS AND SIGNS

Hepatic graft-versus-host disease occurs almost exclusively in recipients of allogeneic marrow or stem cell infusions, often in conjunction with the development of a skin rash and intestinal symptoms (nausea, vomiting, anorexia, diarrhea, and pain) caused by acute graft-versus-host disease. A similar presentation can be seen in <5% of autologous graft recipients. Diagnosis of acute hepatic graft-versus-host disease is frequently made on clinical grounds, that is, the onset or worsening of jaundice in proximity to skin and gut symptoms, plus the exclusion of infectious causes of this clinical picture. Hepatic graft-versus-host disease can develop without apparent skin and gut disease, but this is unusual. The average time of onset of acute graft-versus-host disease is Day 14–19; graft-versus-host disease may occur earlier if the patient received stem cells rather than marrow or if prophylactic medications were not given.

B. DIAGNOSTIC STUDIES

Progressive elevations of serum bilirubin, transaminases (usually 10 or more times the upper limit of normal), and alkaline phosphatase (2–10 times normal) are characteristic. Liver biopsy may be needed to determine whether graft-versus-host disease is present. Histologic findings of acute disease include necrosis and dropout of epithelial cells of small bile ducts, mild hepatocyte necrosis, and cholestasis. In severe cases, portal areas devoid of recognizable small bile ducts are seen.

In recipients of allogeneic marrow, particularly when there is an HLA-mismatched or unrelated donor, liver graft-versus-host disease is always under consideration in the jaundiced patient. The diagnosis of graft-versus-host disease is not difficult when it develops in skin, gut, and liver by Day 20 following transplantation. Recognition of graft-versus-host disease in the liver can be difficult when a patient already has significant liver disease (eg, venoocclusive disease and cholangitis lenta) at the time graft-versus-host disease starts, or when the onset of graft-versus-host disease is concurrent with the onset of sepsis and multiorgan failure.

Total serum bilirubin and alkaline phosphatase levels usually rise in parallel, but in some cases, early elevations of transaminase enzymes are seen. Skin lesions, gut symptoms, and fever are present in typical cases. The liver may be slightly enlarged and tender. The disease is primarily cholestatic; in the early phases of graft-versus-host disease, liver failure and ascites are absent. Bilirubin elevations occur rapidly when graft-versus-host disease develops in the presence of venoocclusive disease. When hemolysis or renal failure develops in patients with graft-versus-host disease, the level of serum bilirubin may exceed 50–60 mg/dL.

Differential Diagnosis

From Day 7 to 20, the differential diagnosis includes venoocclusive disease, cholangitis lenta, and liver injury caused by drugs. After Day 20, venoocclusive disease becomes less of a consideration but can obscure the onset of graft-versus-host disease of the liver if present previously. From Day 20 to 60, cholangitis lenta, fungal liver infection, liver injury caused by drugs, extrahepatic obstruction caused by biliary sludge, and viral infections with herpes viruses or adenovirus are considerations. After Day 60, engraftment is usually more advanced and infections less common, but viral hepatitis B and C may appear after restoration of cell-mediated immunity. At all times, the major difficulty is determining which combination of liver disorders is present, not which single disease.

Complications

Hepatic graft-versus-host disease, although prognostically important, is not a common cause of liver failure. The complications of graft-versus-host disease relate to damage to target organs, severe immunosuppression that results from the disease itself, and the medications used to treat it. The most common cause of death is infection. Prolonged, unremitting hepatic graft-versus-host disease may lead to portal hypertension and ascites.

Treatment & Prognosis

Prevention of graft-versus-host disease is important because treatment of severe multisystem graft-versus-host disease is usually futile. Prevention strategies include better donor–host genetic matches, depletion of donor T lymphocytes, and pharmacologic modulation of the grafted marrow with drugs (usually combinations of cyclosporine, methotrexate, tacrolimus, and mycophenolate mofetil). Treatment of acute graft-versus-host disease is usually with prednisone, 2 mg/kg/d, in addition to the prophylactic medications being given. The approach to treatment failures varies among centers; some increase the prednisone dosage to 4–8 mg/kg/d and others give antithymocyte globulin. Experimental therapies under current study include modulation of cytokine effects and targeting of putative lymphoid effector cells with specific antibodies. Because hepatic graft-versus-host disease is primarily a cholestatic process, ursodiol should be given at 15–30 mg/kg/d.

Treatment of acute graft-versus-host disease is successful 50–75% of the time, depending on the degree of donor–host genetic disparity and the success of delivery of prophylactic drugs. Persistent hepatic involvement with graft-versus-host disease is an independent predictor of a fatal outcome, usually from sepsis. Acute disease is a risk factor for chronic graft-versus-host disease of the liver.

BILIARY SLUDGE DISEASE

The combination of cytoreductive therapy, prolonged gallbladder stasis resulting from the patient's inability to eat, and increased biliary excretion of precipitable material (calcium bilirubinate, cyclosporine, antibiotics) leads to a 60–70% prevalence of sonolucent gallbladder sludge by Day 14. The exfoliation of mucus-containing cells from the gallbladder mucosa caused by cytoreductive therapy may provide nucleating material. Symptoms may result when gallbladder sludge is lodged in the cystic duct, common bile duct, or ampulla of Vater.

Clinical Findings

A. SYMPTOMS AND SIGNS

Postprandial epigastric pain, nausea, and vomiting are typical symptoms of the passage of common bile duct sludge; these symptoms may last for 7–10 days before resolution. Jaundice is unusual, but transient increases in liver enzymes may occur. Acute pancreatitis is heralded by the onset of steady abdominal pain.

B. DIAGNOSTIC STUDIES

Ultrasound studies of the gallbladder in asymptomatic patients will often reveal sludge and thickening of the gallbladder wall. A careful history is therefore more useful than ultrasound in deciding when symptoms are caused by biliary sludge. The diagnosis of cholecystitis in the marrow transplantation setting may also depend on the history and physical findings, unless gallbladder imaging gives unequivocal evidence of mucosal necrosis, perforation, or gas in the gallbladder wall. The diagnosis of common bile duct obstruction and pancreatitis depends on demonstrating common bile duct dilatation and elevations of pancreatic amylase and lipase enzymes.

Because so many patients have gallbladder sludge after transplantation, the usefulness of gallbladder imaging as a diagnostic tool in patients with vague symptoms is questionable. The eventual elimination of sludge from the gallbladder, brought on by eating, sometimes leads to biliary symptoms and pancreatitis. In most patients, these are transient problems that are not life threatening.

Differential Diagnosis

The abrupt onset of abdominal pain during the period from Day 20 to 35 can be due to acute graft-versus-host disease, infectious enteritis, liver abscess, intestinal perforation, or acute pancreatitis. Cholecystitis may also be caused by infections (cytomegalovirus, fungal invasion) and pancreatitis by viral infections and drug toxicity.

Complications

Although severe symptoms can occur, most patients have a self-limited illness. Acute cholecystitis is a relatively unusual event, despite the presence of sludge. Acute pancreatitis occurs sporadically; some cases are severe, especially if extensive retroperitoneal bleeding occurs because of thrombocytopenia.

Treatment & Prognosis

Supportive care and analgesia usually suffice, because the gallbladder empties itself of most of its sludge with continued eating. The duration of symptoms is 1–10 days.

The prognosis is usually good, although cholecystitis and pancreatitis can present problems.

LIVER INJURY INDUCED BY DRUG TOXICITY OR TOTAL PARENTERAL NUTRITION

The major drug toxicity is caused by cytoreductive therapy (see section, "Venoocclusive Disease"). Other drugs may cause hepatotoxicity in a dose-dependent manner (eg, methotrexate), but the dosages used in the transplantation setting seldom cause clinically evident liver damage. Cyclosporine interferes with canalicular excretion of bile at the cellular level at therapeutic doses. The reactions to other drugs are idiosyncratic (see Chapter 44).

Clinical Findings

The usual guilt-by-association diagnosis of drug-induced liver injury is difficult to prove in a setting where there are so many other causes of hepatic disease. Transient elevations of aspartate aminotransferase (AST) may follow use of methotrexate. Drugs that are known to cause idiosyncratic injury (eg, trimethoprim-sulfamethoxazole, fluconazole, itraconazole) can be discontinued in problematic cases. Liver histologic studies are seldom helpful in this setting.

Evidence of hepatocyte necrosis and cholestatic liver disease can be seen in serum liver enzymes. With some medications such as trimethoprim-sulfamethoxazole, anorexia and nausea may accompany liver toxicity.

Differential Diagnosis

All of the liver disorders discussed in the preceding sections must be considered.

Complications

In general, drugs are an uncommon cause of severe liver disease in the transplantation setting. An exception is liver damage caused by gemtuzumab ozogamicin (Mylotarg) for treatment of relapsed acute myeloid leukemia after transplant (see page 760). Continued use of any toxic drug may cause progressive liver damage.

Treatment & Prognosis

The treatment is discontinuation of the offending drug. Unless a toxic drug is continued despite ongoing liver injury, the outcome is usually good.

LIVER INFECTION WITH BACTERIA

Bacterial liver infections are rare after transplant. Bacteria reach the liver via the bloodstream or the bile ducts but seldom lead to abscesses. Mycobacteria may exist in the liver in a latent form before transplantation and become active while immunosuppressive therapy is being given.

Clinical Findings

A. SYMPTOMS AND SIGNS

Pyogenic bacterial abscesses present with fever and painful hepatomegaly. There is usually a history of septicemia or biliary infection. Mycobacterial infections are activated from latency and present in a more subtle manner, with fever, anorexia, and hepatomegaly.

B. DIAGNOSTIC STUDIES

Liver abscesses are identified by imaging tests showing characteristic lesions in the liver parenchyma; directed needle aspiration may be necessary to identify the organism. Mycobacterial infections cause granulomas in the liver but seldom gross abscesses; skin tests before transplantation may or may not identify patients at risk, depending on the level of immunity. Liver biopsy is needed for diagnosis of mycobacterial infection, unless the organisms are found elsewhere (marrow, lungs).

Pyogenic bacterial liver abscesses are rare in the transplantation setting, probably because of empiric use of antibiotics for fever. Mycobacterial infections (*Mycobacterium tuberculosis, M avium* complex, bacille Calmette–Guérin) are likewise rare, because screening before transplantation identifies most patients at risk.

Differential Diagnosis

Bacterial liver abscesses are greatly outnumbered by fungal lesions, which usually involve the kidneys and spleen as well as the liver. Lesions seen on liver imaging studies that could be confused with abscesses include cysts, hemangiomas, and tumor nodules. Mycobacterial infections have a broader differential diagnosis that encompasses cholestatic liver diseases such as graft-versus-host disease, cytomegalovirus hepatitis, and liver injury caused by drugs.

Complications

Pyogenic infections are usually a manifestation of granulocytopenia and uncontrolled sepsis, which is the usual cause of death. Unrecognized mycobacterial infections cause inanition and marrow failure.

Treatment & Prognosis

Broad-spectrum antibiotics are used to treat bacterial infection. Antimycobacterial therapy depends on the organism identified by biopsy.

Uncontrolled bacterial infections are fatal. Mycobacterial infections can be effectively treated if host immunity recovers.

EPSTEIN–BARR VIRUS LYMPHOPROLIFERATIVE DISEASE

This is a disease seen in patients who have received prolonged immunosuppressive therapy, usually to treat acute graft-versus-host disease, or in recipients of T lymphocyte-depleted donor marrow, or in patients treated with potent anti-T cell antibodies. Epstein–Barr virus infection of B lymphoid cells transforms them into immunoblasts that infiltrate tissues.

Clinical Findings

A. SYMPTOMS AND SIGNS

Liver involvement is characterized by rapidly progressive hepatomegaly and abdominal pain. Infiltration of other organs occurs in parallel. Fever is common.

B. DIAGNOSTIC STUDIES

The diagnosis is suggested by the clinical situation and clinical findings. Imaging tests may show a diffuse infiltrative process in the liver, in addition to nodal enlargement and infiltration of other viscera. Tissue biopsy of affected organs (eg, liver, intestine, lymph nodes, lungs) is required for diagnosis. The morphologic characteristics of the infiltrative process are usually diagnostic, although there can be difficulty in differentiating an intense inflammatory response from this lymphoma-like process.

Differential Diagnosis

Rapidly progressive infiltrative liver lesions are unusual; the only common cause is recurrent malignant tumors. Unrecognized fungal infection and fatty liver could be mistaken for lymphoproliferative disease.

Complications

This is usually a progressive, lymphoma-like illness that leads to death.

Treatment & Prognosis

Until recently, discontinuation of immunosuppressive drugs was the only treatment that could be offered, and that was usually unsuccessful. Most patients who presented with visceral infiltration have died rapidly. Successful treatment with infusion of donor T cells has been reported. Current research employs early detection of circulating Epstein–Barr virus using polymerase chain reaction and anti-B lymphocyte therapy for patients found to be viremic.

MALIGNANT CELLS IN THE LIVER

When conditioning therapy given to eradicate malignant cells is not successful, recurrent tumor may involve the liver, whether or not there was liver involvement at the start of therapy. In rare instances, there may be contamination of autologous marrow or peripheral blood stem cells with tumor cells; infusion of these cells following conditioning therapy may lead to liver seeding.

Recurrent tumor in the liver should be considered when the original malignant tumor involved the liver or when the indication for transplantation was a leukemia with a propensity to recur.

Clinical Findings

Progressive hepatomegaly, elevation of serum alkaline phosphatase measurements, and signs of portal hypertension may be early indications of recurrent tumor in the liver. There may also be evidence of recurrent tumor in the marrow and other organ systems.

Clinical signs and symptoms lead to imaging studies (CT or MR) that show filling defects if the tumor burden is large. Directed needle aspiration cytology or biopsy is useful if positive; however, recurrent tumor in the liver may be microscopic and focal. Detection of tumor cells in other sites (particularly marrow) makes the identification of liver tumor of little additional value.

Differential Diagnosis

Most recurrences of tumor occur beyond Day 50. The differential diagnosis includes fungal liver infection, graft-versus-host disease, constrictive pericarditis, Epstein–Barr virus lymphoproliferative disease, nodular regenerative hyperplasia, and persistent venoocclusive disease.

Complications

Rapid growth of tumor may result in portal hypertension and ascites, but liver metastases are not the usual cause of illness in patients with recurrent malignant tumors.

Treatment & Prognosis

No treatment is available in most cases. The outcome is poor.

NODULAR REGENERATIVE HYPERPLASIA

The pathogenesis of nodule formation in the liver is unknown, but most authors speculate that vascular injury precedes the formation of hyperplastic nodules. This lesion has been described following conventional chemotherapy as well as after marrow transplantation.

Nodular hyperplasia is probably not a major cause of clinical liver disease in marrow transplantation patients but can be found at autopsy. It could be responsi-ble for signs of portal hypertension that are seen months after transplantation.

Clinical Findings

Portal hypertension, hepatorenal syndrome, and ascites, occurring months after transplantation, can be due to nodular regenerative hyperplasia. Esophageal varices are rare.

Inspection of the surface of the liver is useful, as there are multiple small nodules (usually <5 mm in diameter) diffusely present in the liver. Imaging studies may fail to detect nodularity. Definitive diagnosis requires a large liver biopsy; the nodules are encircled by bands of collapsed reticulin. Reticulin and antitrypsin staining may be useful.

Differential Diagnosis

Venoocclusive disease is the major cause of portal hypertension after transplantation. Cirrhosis of the liver has an appearance similar to that of nodular regenerative hyperplasia on gross inspection, but histologic studies show fibrosis rather than collapsed reticulin.

Complications

It is difficult to define a symptom complex or complications that result from nodular regenerative hyperplasia alone in these patients.

Treatment & Prognosis

Portacaval shunts are often curative in non-marrow transplantation patients whose portal hypertension is problematic. The overall prognosis is good, because liver function is preserved.

ACUTE VIRAL HEPATITIS

Hepatitis viruses B and C can be transmitted from marrow or stem cell donors but more commonly have been acquired from previous blood products. These viruses replicate after conditioning therapy and circulate in high titers immediately following transplantation, but do not appear to cause liver injury until after the immune system has been reconstituted. Some of the viruses that infect the liver in the transplantation setting cause hepatocyte necrosis in the absence of cellular immunity (eg, adenovirus, varicella-zoster virus, herpes simplex virus). Cytomegalovirus causes microabscesses in the liver and can infect the biliary epithelium. Epstein–Barr virus may cause a lymphoma-like illness (see above).

The viruses that cause fulminant hepatitis usually occur soon after conditioning therapy has ablated the immune system, or during immunosuppressive treatment of acute graft-versus-host disease. Fortunately, effective prophylaxis with acyclovir and ganciclovir has almost eliminated infection with herpes group viruses in this setting, leaving adenovirus as the most common (but still rare) cause of fulminant viral hepatitis. Despite high viral titers, hepatitis B virus is not a cause of hepatitis in the first 30–60 days following transplantation, but may lead to fulminant hepatic failure after immune reconstitution.

Clinical Findings

Table 49–3 shows the major diagnostic features of infection with the most frequent viral causes of liver injury. Because most of these infections are caused by reactivation of latent viruses, it is important to review pre-marrow-transplant serologic studies (herpes simplex virus, cytomegalovirus, varicella-zoster virus, hepatitis B or C virus) to identify these latent viruses; however, false-negative serologic findings can be seen in immune-deficient transplantation candidates. Diagnosis of pretransplant infection with hepatitis B or C virus may require detection of hepatitis B virus DNA or hepatitis C virus RNA. Posttransplantation infection with adenovirus, herpes simplex virus, or varicella-zoster virus is heralded by rapid rises in serum transaminases to over 1000 IU/L, with clinical deterioration and death in 2–10 days in severe cases. Although these viruses commonly cause hepatic necrosis as part of a disseminated disease, liver involvement can be the initial presentation. Liver biopsy and immunohistologic searching for viral antigens in liver tissue comprise the ultimate diagnostic test. However, polymerase chain reaction of serum or a skin lesion for varicella zoster virus or herpes simplex virus may confirm these diagnoses without liver biopsy. Almost all cases of posttransplantation hepatitis B and C can be predicted by examining the pretransplant hepatitis virus status of both patient and donor. Posttransplant determination of hepatitis B virus antigens and DNA and hepatitis C virus RNA is reliable, but antibodies may not be present because of inadequate B cell function.

Differential Diagnosis

Other diseases that present with transaminase elevation before Day 60 are venoocclusive disease (where the serum AST may rarely rise to 2000–10,000 IU/L), acute graft-versus-host disease (where the serum AST may range to 1200 IU/L in severe cases), liver injury caused by drugs, and liver ischemia related to septic shock or low cardiac output states. Severe venoocclusive disease and graft-versus-host disease are usually clinically obvious, but their presence does not preclude a viral infection. The differential diagnosis of hepatitis after Day 60 is narrower; it includes flare-ups of acute graft-versus-host disease during attempts at tapering immunosuppressive therapy, *de novo* onset of chronic graft-versus-host disease (see below), and liver injury caused by drugs. Discerning the cause of rising liver enzymes following the tapering of doses of immunosuppressive drugs can be difficult when both graft-versus-host disease and hepatitis B or C are present, because all of these diseases respond similarly. Higher alkaline phosphatase levels and more extensive bile duct destruction on liver biopsy favor graft-versus-host disease.

Complications

Fulminant hepatitis and death are major but rare complications of viral liver infection. Viral hepatitis in a liver already affected by venoocclusive disease or graft-versus-host disease may also lead to a fatal outcome. Reactivation or acquisition of hepatitis B or C leads to chronic hepatitis in high frequency among transplant patients, but a number of fulminant hepatitis B cases have also been described.

Treatment & Prognosis

Prevention of viral infection is outlined in Table 49–3. Effective prophylaxis is limited to herpes group viruses (valacyclovir) and hepatitis B virus (lamivudine). There is evidence that transplantation of marrow or stem cells from a donor who is naturally immune to hepatitis B virus will allow a hepatitis B virus-infected patient to clear the virus. A clinical suspicion of fulminant viral hepatitis caused by varicella-zoster virus or herpes simplex virus should lead to prompt empiric acyclovir therapy before the final diagnosis is available. Adenovirus hepatitis may be treated with cidofovir, but experience with this nephrotoxic agent is limited. Hepatitis C that appears following tapering of immunosuppressive drugs does not usually require treatment, and interferon-α and ribavirin therapy are seldom effective until the immune system recovers fully. Hepatitis B virus DNA, when detected posttransplant, should prompt treatment with lamivudine until the immune system has recovered.

Adenovirus, herpes simplex virus, and varicella-zoster virus hepatitis may be fatal unless diagnosed and treated early. Cytomegalovirus hepatitis is usually seen only with disseminated cytomegalovirus disease, and the liver disease is almost never severe. There is a high frequency of chronic hepatitis and cirrhosis among long-term survivors of transplantation who are infected with hepatitis C virus.

Table 49–3. Viruses that infect the liver in marrow transplantation patients.[1]

Virus	Presentation in Transplantation Patients	Diagnosis	Prevention	Treatment
Adenovirus	Fulminant hepatitis	Rapidly rising trans- aminases Gut, lung, urinary infection Viral cultures, PCR Liver histologic studies and culture	None for latent infection Hand washing, avoidance of infected visitors, for primary infection	Cidofovir Immune globulin, donor T lymphocyte infusions may be effective
Varicella- zoster virus	Fulminant hepatitis	Rapidly rising trans- aminases Skin lesions Abdominal pain common Viral cultures, PCR Liver histologic studies and culture	Acyclovir	Acyclovir
Herpes simplex virus	Fulminant hepatitis	Rapidly rising trans- aminase levels Skin lesions Viral cultures, PCR Liver histologic studies and culture	Acyclovir	Acyclovir
Cytomegalovirus	Mild abnormalities of liver enzymes	Cytomegalovirus disease usually obvious in lungs, gut Viral cultures, PCR Liver histologic studies (microabscesses)	Ganciclovir, for latent infection Cytomegalovirus seronegative blood products ± ganciclovir, for primary infection	Ganciclovir Foscarnet
Hepatitis B virus	Acute hepatitis, rarely fulminant	Pre-BMT presence of hepatitis B virus or anti-HBc or hepatitis B-positive donor Transaminase eleva- tions after Day 60 HBsAg, hepatitis B virus DNA Liver histologic studies	Infusion of marrow from donor/naturally immune to hepatitis B virus	Lamivudine prophylaxis
Hepatitis C virus	Acute hepatitis	Pre-BMT presence of hepatitis C virus RNA or hepatitis C-posi- tive donor Transaminase elevations after Day 60 Hepatitis C virus RNA Liver histologic studies	Treatment of donor with IFN-α pre-BMT	IFN-α, ribavirin after recovery

[1]PCR, polymerase chain reaction; BMT, bone marrow transplant; HBc, hepatitis B core antigen; HBsAg, hepatitis B surface antigen; IFN, interferon.

■ LIVER DISEASES IN LONG-TERM TRANSPLANTATION SURVIVORS

With increasing intervals from the day of transplantation, the prevalence of liver dysfunction is reduced and the differential diagnosis of liver disease narrows (Table 49–4).

CHRONIC GRAFT-VERSUS-HOST DISEASE

Chronic graft-versus-host disease of the liver can be an insidious process leading to prolonged cholestasis, or an abrupt process that rapidly destroys small bile ducts. Chronic disease affects many organs in the body and is associated with profound immunodeficiency; unless recognized and treated aggressively, it can lead to death.

Chronic graft-versus-host disease may follow acute graft-versus-host disease, or may appear after acute disease has resolved, or may appear *de novo*. Chronic graft-versus-host disease has many autoimmune features and is caused by abnormalities of both cellular and humoral immunity. It is almost exclusively a result of allogeneic hematopoietic cell transplantation.

Table 49–4. Overview of liver diseases in long-term survivors of marrow transplantation.

Hepatic Disease	Risk Factors
Chronic graft-versus-host disease	Allogeneic marrow graft recipient
	Prior acute graft-versus-host disease
	Unrelated or mismatched marrow donor
Chronic viral hepatitis	Serologic or virologic evidence of hepatitis B or C virus before or after transplantation
	Hepatitis C virus RNA-positive marrow donor
	Hepatitis B virus DNA marrow donor
Iron overload	Multiple transfusions
	Prolonged ineffective erythropoiesis
	Thalassemia
Malignant cells in the liver	Pretransplantation malignant disease
	Transplantation in leukemic relapse
	Secondary cancer

Clinical Findings

A. SYMPTOMS AND SIGNS

Although liver involvement can be seen as an isolated finding, it is more common to find dry eyes, oral mucositis, and skin involvement, along with liver disease. In the early phases, elevated serum alkaline phosphatase levels may be the only abnormality, but most patients become jaundiced unless treated. Patients who have a rapid, *de novo* onset may have elevated serum transaminase levels initially.

B. DIAGNOSTIC STUDIES

Elevations of serum alkaline phosphatase and bilirubin are characteristic of liver involvement with chronic graft-versus-host disease. When these are seen in a patient with clinically obvious lacrimal gland, oral, and skin involvement, a clinical diagnosis can be made. Definitive diagnosis requires liver biopsy. Histologic features include abnormal small bile ducts (leading to ductopenia), lymphoid infiltration of the epithelium, and cholestasis.

Differential Diagnosis

Viral hepatitis C may mimic mild chronic graft-versus-host disease, because both diseases cause mild elevations of serum transaminase measurements and histologic abnormalities of small bile ducts; both may also respond to immunosuppressive therapy with decreased levels of serum liver enzymes. Serum alkaline phosphatase elevations are likely to be higher in chronic graft-versus-host disease, especially if the disease is severe. Cholestatic liver injury caused by drugs, biliary tract disease, and, rarely, granulomatous hepatitis should also be considered. When *de novo* chronic graft-versus-host disease develops rapidly, acute viral hepatitis is also included in the differential diagnosis (varicella-zoster virus, herpes simplex virus, hepatitis B and C viruses).

Complications

If left untreated, chronic graft-versus-host disease of the liver may progress to severe cholestatic liver injury and eventually cirrhosis. Immunodeficiency associated with chronic graft-versus-host disease and its treatment predispose patients to fatal bacterial infections.

Treatment & Prognosis

Immunosuppressive therapy, usually with prednisone and cyclosporine or tacrolimus, is standard. Other drugs that are in current trials include sirilimus, mycophenolate mofetil, and thalidomide. Ursodiol at a dose of 15–30 mg/kg/d may play a role in modulating the severity of cholestatic injury.

Immunosuppressive therapy is usually successful in reducing the activity of this chronic inflammatory disease. Some patients, however, require therapy indefinitely; in others, dosages of immunosuppressive drugs can be tapered without flare-ups of chronic graft-versus-host disease.

CHRONIC VIRAL HEPATITIS

The pathophysiology of hepatitis is discussed in Chapter 35. In hematopoietic cell transplantation patients, viremia from hepatitis B and C are common when chronic graft-versus-host disease is present or immunosuppressive drugs are being given. Some patients who were chronically infected with hepatitis B virus before transplantation have cleared virus after receiving stem cells from a donor who was naturally immune to hepatitis B virus.

The prevalence of chronic viral hepatitis in patients who underwent transplantation before 1991 is high but has been reduced considerably since the advent of effective hepatitis C screening of blood products.

Clinical Findings

The presentation and laboratory findings of chronic hepatitis are discussed in Chapters 35 and 36. There may be progression of chronic hepatitis C to cirrhosis in marrow transplantation patients over a period of 10–20 years.

Measurement of hepatitis B surface and core viral antigens (HBs, HBc) and nucleic acids (hepatitis B virus DNA, hepatitis C virus RNA) is reliable, even when patients are immunodeficient or receiving immune globulin. Liver biopsy is needed when both viral hepatitis and chronic graft-versus-host disease are under consideration. The histologic distinction between hepatitis C and chronic graft-versus-host disease is difficult, because both diseases cause lymphoid infiltration and abnormalities of small bile ducts. Immunosuppressive therapy may alter the histologic appearance of hepatitis C virus infection. In some patients, chronic viral hepatitis and chronic graft-versus-host disease coexist.

Differential Diagnosis

Chronic graft-versus-host disease and drug-induced liver injury are usually the only other considerations.

Complications

Chronic viral hepatitis C may lead to cirrhosis. Some of the extrahepatic manifestations of hepatitis C could be confused with the autoimmune manifestations of chronic graft-versus-host disease. Patients who came to transplant with latent hepatitis B (anti-HBc positive)

may have reactivated virus after transplant and then present with rapidly progressive hepatitis. Such patients should be tested for HBV DNA serially posttransplant so that viremia is detected and treatment with lamivudine begun before clinical hepatitis develops.

Treatment & Prognosis

Chronic hepatitis C may lead to cirrhosis in long-term survivors of marrow transplantation, with a rising prevalence of cirrhosis after 15 years. Iron overload may be a contributory factor (see below). Patients with chronic hepatitis C should avoid alcohol and should be immunized against hepatitis A and B. Little has been published concerning the safety and efficacy of antiviral agents in hematopoietic cell transplantation patients with chronic hepatitis C. Antiviral therapy appears to be ineffective in patients who have chronic graft-versus-host disease or who are receiving immunosuppressive therapy. Some transplant survivors have very labile platelet and neutrophil counts while receiving therapy with interferon-α and ribavirin. The presence of residual liver iron (from prior transfusions) may affect a patient's response to interferon (see below). Liver transplantation should be considered if incipient liver failure develops.

IRON OVERLOAD

Significant accumulation of iron can be seen after transplant as a result of multiple transfusions, intestinal hyperabsorption of iron because of ineffective erythropoiesis, and/or unrecognized genetic iron overload disorders. Patients transplanted for thalassemia are especially at risk as their iron stores may be very high by the time they come to transplant.

Clinical Findings

A. SYMPTOMS AND SIGNS

Hepatic and splenic enlargement can be seen, but the most common clinical manifestations of extreme iron overload result from skin, joint, pancreas, heart, and pituitary iron deposition (see Chapter 41). Fortunately, the degree of iron overload after transplant is seldom extreme, and iron stores decline with time after the underlying disease is cured.

B. DIAGNOSTIC STUDIES

Minor elevations of AST and alanine aminotransferase (ALT) can be seen. All survivors of transplantation should be screened for their degree of iron overload with serum ferritin and transferrin saturation, but ferritin levels may be falsely high in patients with chronic graft-versus-host disease because it is an acute phase reactant. The iron content of marrow biopsies correlates well with liver iron concentration in these patients. As most patients have a marrow biopsy done for staging purposes after recovery from the transplant process, assessment of marrow iron can be used to identify patients at risk for dangerous levels of tissue iron. In these patients, liver biopsy is needed to quantify iron, and patients with liver iron >7000 μg/g dry weight should undergo iron mobilization. Heavily iron overloaded patients should also be screened for the HFE gene mutation.

Differential Diagnosis

Iron overload may coexist with any liver process that occurs in transplant survivors, but the greatest concern is in patients who have hepatitis C, in whom progression to cirrhosis may be accelerated in the presence of iron overload. By chance, some transplant survivors will carry an HFE gene mutation. These patients will need lifelong followup, whereas iron mobilized from other transplant survivors should not reaccumulate.

Complications

Iron overload may lead to skin, joint, pancreas, heart, and pituitary dysfunction and to a more rapid progression to cirrhosis, particularly when hepatitis C is present. Rarely, patients with iron overload are susceptible to unusual infections (*Listeria,* molds, *Vibrio, Yersinia*).

Treatment & Prognosis

Prognosis is dependent on the amount of iron overload. Patients with liver iron >15,000 μg/g dry weight have a high frequency of diabetes and cardiac death and should undergo aggressive iron mobilization with deferoxamine and phlebotomy. Follow-up studies of heavily iron-overloaded transplant survivors suggest marked improvement in both cardiac and hepatic parameters following iron mobilization. Patients with liver iron from 7000 to 15,000 μg/g dry weight can be managed with phlebotomy alone. Patients with lower amounts of liver iron can be followed, as they will slowly mobilize iron stores.

MALIGNANT CELLS IN THE LIVER

The liver may be a site of recurrence of the original malignant tumor or the appearance of a secondary malignant tumor. The latter is usually lymphoid in origin. The clinical findings and differential diagnosis are the same as during the first 100 days following transplantation (see preceding section).

Some patients with recurrent or secondary cancers have undergone second transplantations; most of the successes with this approach have been in children. The prognosis is poor.

REFERENCES

Angelucci E et al: Phlebotomy to reduce iron overload in patients cured of thalassemia by bone marrow transplantation. Blood 1997;90:994.

Murakami CS et al: Biliary obstruction in hematopoietic cell transplant recipients: an uncommon diagnosis with specific causes. Bone Marrow Transplant 1999;23:921.

Shulman HM et al: Utility of transvenous liver biopsies and wedged hepatic venous pressure measurements in sixty marrow transplant recipients. Transplantation 1995;59:1015.

Strasser SI, McDonald GB: Hepatitis viruses and hematopoietic cell transplantation: a guide to patient and donor management. Blood 1999;93:1127.

Strasser SI, McDonald GB: Hepatobiliary complications of hematopoietic cell transplantation. In: *Schiff's Diseases of the Liver,* 9th ed. Schiff ER, Sorrell MF, Maddrey WC (editors). J.B. Lippincott, in press.

Strasser SI et al: Iron overload in bone marrow transplant recipients. Bone Marrow Transplant 1998;22:167.

Strasser SI, Shulman HM, McDonald GB: Cholestasis after hematopoietic cell transplantation. Clin Liver Dis 1999;3:651.

Strasser SI et al: Cirrhosis of the liver in long-term marrow transplant survivors. Blood 1999;93:3259.

Strasser SI et al: Hepatitis C virus infection after bone marrow transplantation: a cohort study with 10 year follow-up. Hepatology 1999;29:1893.

Strasser SI et al: Chronic graft-vs-host disease of the liver: presentation as an acute hepatitis. Hepatology 2000;32:1265.

van Burik JH et al: The effect of prophylactic fluconazole on the clinical spectrum of fungal diseases in bone marrow transplant recipients with special attention to hepatic candidiasis. An autopsy study of 355 patients. Medicine (Baltimore) 1998;77:246.

Gallstones

Ira M. Jacobson, MD

Cholelithiasis is one of the most common gastrointestinal diseases seen in clinical practice. Most patients with gallstones are asymptomatic. The clinical manifestations of gallstones can include episodic pain, acute cholecystitis, or obstructive jaundice, cholangitis, and pancreatitis, the latter three complications resulting from gallstone migration into the common bile duct.

The clinical approach to gallstones has undergone major revision because of the development of laparoscopic cholecystectomy. As a result, pharmacologic and other nonoperative approaches have been relegated to a secondary role. Moreover, the widespread availability of endoscopic retrograde cholangiopancreatography (ERCP) has dramatically decreased the need for surgical removal of common bile duct stones.

Classification

Gallstones are usually classified as cholesterol or pigment stones, but this is an oversimplification for two reasons. First, stones containing only one component or the other are uncommon. Second, pigment stones can themselves be divided into two major groups with different pathogeneses: Black pigment stones consist of polymers of bilirubin with large amounts of mucin glycoproteins, whereas calcium salts of unconjugated bilirubin (calcium bilirubinate) make up the chief component of brown pigment stones.

Most gallstones in patients in the United States and Europe are cholesterol rich, often containing mucin glycoproteins in layers alternating with cholesterol crystals. Even cholesterol-rich stones usually contain some degree of bilirubin-derived material, however. A large proportion of gallstones in Asian patients are pigment stones, especially brown pigment stones rich in calcium bilirubinate. These may originate in the gallbladder but may also form as primary bile duct stones. As outlined below, the composition of gallstones in a particular patient can often be linked to specific epidemiologic risk factors.

Pathogenesis

A. CHOLESTEROL STONES

The three main constituents of normal bile are cholesterol, bile salts, and phospholipids, over 90% of which is lecithin. Most biliary cholesterol is derived from *de novo* hepatic synthesis rather than secretion of dietary cholesterol. The primary bile acids, chenodeoxycholic acid and cholic acid, are secreted into the bile after conjugation in the liver with taurine or glycine. The conjugated primary bile acids are reabsorbed in the terminal ileum via the enterohepatic circulation, and a small proportion is deconjugated by bacteria in the distal bowel. The deconjugated bile acids may themselves be reabsorbed, or they may be dehydroxylated by colonic bacteria, forming the secondary bile acids deoxycholic acid and lithocholic acid. These, in turn, also undergo partial absorption. Bile acids within the enterohepatic circulation down-regulate hepatic bile acid synthesis.

Normally insoluble in aqueous solution, cholesterol depends for its solubility in bile on the formation of mixed micelles containing aggregates of cholesterol, bile acids, and lecithin. Micelle formation is based on the ability of lipid molecules to align themselves so that their hydrophilic regions form the external environment and their hydrophobic regions form the internal environment. In addition to micelles, phospholipids and cholesterol in bile form spherical bilayers, or vesicles, in which hydrophobic portions are aligned inward and hydrophilic groups outward. With increasing concentrations of cholesterol in vesicles, the vesicles fuse into multilamellar forms. Cholesterol crystals form on the surface of these multilamellar vesicles, and subsequently nucleate into the solid form.

Essential to cholesterol gallstone formation is the hepatic synthesis of bile with supersaturated cholesterol concentrations. In patients with equivalent degrees of supersaturation, bile will form cholesterol crystals at variable rates; this indicates the existence of other factors that contribute to stone formation. Biliary proteins, including mucous glycoproteins, appear to play a role as promoters of the nucleation of cholesterol crystals. An additional role has been ascribed to impaired gallbladder motility in patients with supersaturated bile, leading to stasis and the promotion of gallstone formation. Other postulated contributing factors for cholesterol gallstone formation include altered gallbladder synthesis of prostaglandins and excessive biliary calcium concentrations.

A precursor to the formation of stones in some patients is biliary sludge, consisting of viscous mucoproteins containing cholesterol crystals. Such sludge may be visible sonographically and may be the only abnormality in patients presenting with biliary pain, pancreatitis, or cholangitis. Because sludge may be a transient finding, particularly in fasting patients, its specificity is somewhat limited. Recent publications have emphasized, however, that sludge is pathogenic in some patients with biliary-related illnesses, particularly pancreatitis, that would otherwise be classified as "idiopathic." When sludge is not visible on sonographic studies in such patients, some clinicians collect gallbladder bile by duodenal intubation after stimulating the gallbladder contractility with cholecystokinin. The bile is then analyzed under polarizing microscopy for cholesterol crystals, which, if found, purportedly establish a causal relationship sufficient to warrant cholecystectomy. The value of this approach is not universally accepted, however.

B. PIGMENT STONES

Black pigment stones form primarily in the gallbladder in patients with cirrhosis or chronic hemolytic diseases such as sickle cell anemia. Brown pigment stones, on the other hand, may form either in the gallbladder or the bile duct; primary bile duct stones are usually of this type. Bacterial infection, the usual cause for the formation of primary bile duct stones, leads to deconjugation of bilirubin by bacterial β-glucuronidases. The deconjugated bilirubin then binds with calcium to form insoluble calcium bilirubinate, which in turn becomes the nidus for primary duct stone formation. Primary bile duct stones are particularly common in Asia, where bacterial contamination of the bile may be attributable to biliary parasites such as *Clonorchis* or other factors not well understood. Brown pigment stones may also form primarily in the gallbladder; this may occur in patients receiving total parenteral nutrition, who commonly have gallbladder stasis.

Epidemiologic Findings

The prevalence of gallstones increases with age (Table 50–1). Gallstones are more prevalent in females than males in all adult age groups, with ratios exceeding 3:1 in women in their reproductive years and falling to under 2:1 in persons over 70. The gender difference is at least partly due to endogenous estrogens, which inhibit the enzymatic conversion of cholesterol to bile acids, thereby increasing the cholesterol saturation of bile. Pregnancy increases the risk of gallstones, and it is common for women to present with symptomatic gallstones for the first time during pregnancy or shortly thereafter (see Chapter 47). Impaired gallbladder emptying, promoted by progesterone, combines with the

Table 50–1. Risk factors for gallstones.

Increasing age
Female gender
Pregnancy
Estrogens
Obesity
Ethnicity (eg, native Americans)
Cirrhosis
Hemolytic anemia (eg, sickle-cell disease, hereditary spherocytosis)
Total parenteral nutrition

influence of estrogens to increase the lithogenesis of bile in pregnancy. Pharmacologically administered estrogens also increase the risk of gallstone formation. Patients with extensive ileitis or a history of ileal resection, in whom the enterohepatic circulation is impaired, have a high risk of cholesterol gallstones because of excess loss of bile acids.

Obese persons have an increased risk of cholesterol gallstones associated with excess biliary cholesterol secretion. Certain ethnic groups are also particularly susceptible, most strikingly the Pima Indians of the western United States, in whom the prevalence is over 75%. The prevalence is also relatively high in other Native Americans. Whites in the United States and Europe have a higher prevalence than Asians and Africans, in whom pigment stones have historically been more common. More recently, however, cholesterol stones are increasing in prevalence in Asian and African populations, particularly in Japan, where dietary and life-style patterns have become more westernized.

Clinical Findings

Most people with gallstones (approximately 80%) are asymptomatic. The clinical features in symptomatic patients include episodic pain of variable severity and frequency, acute cholecystitis, and complications related to passage of gallstones into the bile duct, including pain, jaundice, cholangitis, and pancreatitis.

A. SYMPTOMS AND SIGNS

1. Cystic duct obstruction—Most episodes of gallstone-induced pain occur when a stone transiently obstructs the cystic duct. Pain arising from gallstones is usually felt in the right upper quadrant or epigastrium. With right upper quadrant pain particularly, the pain may radiate around to the right side of the back or the right shoulder. Alternatively, pain perceived by the patient as arising in the midline within the epigastrium may radiate to the right side secondarily. Occasionally, pain may be felt in the substernal area, where it may be mistaken for myocardial ischemia. Pain primarily in the left upper quadrant of the abdomen may occasionally be seen.

Gallstone pain is steady rather than wavelike, cramping, or colicky, and therefore the classic description "biliary colic" is somewhat of a misnomer. Many patients develop pain between 15 minutes and 2 hours after eating, with fatty foods being the most notorious (but far from universal) offender. Indeed, fatty food intolerance is actually no more common in patients with gallstones than in those with other disorders such as nonulcer dyspepsia. Nevertheless, clinicians regularly see patients with gallstones and classic biliary colic whose episodes are brought on by fatty foods and diminished in frequency by avoiding fatty foods, and whose pain is ultimately alleviated by cholecystectomy. Some patients have pain unrelated to eating.

The duration of an episode of biliary colic pain may range from a few minutes to 1–4 hours or even longer. There may be concomitant nausea with or without vomiting. Nocturnal pain awakening the patient is a common presentation.

Gastrointestinal symptoms in the absence of pain conforming to one of the variants described above should not be attributed to gallstones without considering other diagnoses. For example, belching, heartburn, and bloating might indicate reflux or peptic disease. The discovery of gallstones on imaging studies concomitant with these symptoms does not, therefore, mean that cholecystectomy is indicated.

The physical examination in patients with episodic biliary pain is typically normal between episodes. Right upper quadrant tenderness usually is present only in patients with very frequent episodes and usually indicates significant chronic inflammation of the gallbladder.

2. Acute cholecystitis—In acute cholecystitis, unlike biliary colic, there is sustained obstruction of the cystic duct, producing gallbladder distention and a self-perpetuating inflammatory process involving prostaglandins and other inflammatory mediators. Bacterial infection is probably a secondary event occurring later in the course in some patients. Corresponding to its pathogenesis, the pain of acute cholecystitis is distinguished from that of "biliary colic" by its intensity and persistence for more than several hours. Nausea and vomiting are frequent, and there is localization of the pain in the right upper quadrant. The presence of fever in a patient with protracted biliary pain signifies that the process has transcended "biliary colic" and that cholecystitis or another complication, such as cholangitis or pancreatitis, has supervened.

Physical examination in patients with acute cholecystitis reveals right upper quadrant tenderness often extending into the epigastrium. The classic **Murphy's sign** refers to the presence of marked tenderness and inhibition of inspiration on deep palpation under the right subcostal margin.

Mild to moderate leukocytosis is common in acute cholecystitis. Serum liver tests may be mildly abnormal, but substantial elevations should raise the possibility of bile duct obstruction concomitant with, or instead of, acute cholecystitis. Serum amylase levels usually are normal; again, more than minimal elevations raise the possibility of pancreatitis.

3. Bile duct obstruction—Pain arising from obstruction of the bile duct by a gallstone is similar to the pain of cystic duct obstruction. Patients who have had their gallbladders removed and present for the first time with symptomatic common bile duct stones frequently say the pain reminds them of what they felt before surgery. If obstruction of the bile duct by a stone is of sufficient duration and severity, jaundice may develop. Painless jaundice is less common with stones than with tumors that obstruct the bile duct, but it may occur.

If obstruction of the bile duct is accompanied by infection resulting in cholangitis, fever will develop. The temperature often is higher than in patients with cholecystitis, sometimes exceeding 40°C. In addition, rigors are far more common with cholangitis than with cholecystitis or pancreatitis. Septic patients with cholangitis are commonly hypotensive. The manifestations of pancreatitis are discussed in detail elsewhere (see Chapter 30).

Physical examination in patients with bile duct obstruction by stones is characterized by less abdominal tenderness than in patients with gallbladder inflammation. Fever or jaundice may be pronounced. Murphy's sign is not present.

Most patients with biliary obstruction from stones have elevated liver enzymes, even if the symptoms are transient. The degree of enzyme elevation far exceeds the levels seen in patients with cystic duct obstruction. In acute bile duct obstruction, alanine aminotransferase (ALT) and aspartate aminotransferase (AST) rise quickly, and may reach or exceed levels 10 times the upper limit of normal. Even if obstruction persists, these enzymes fall rapidly toward normal, whereas the alkaline phosphatase level progressively rises. Hyperbilirubinemia may not occur if obstruction is transient.

B. DIAGNOSTIC STUDIES

1. Ultrasonography—Ultrasonography is the critical diagnostic procedure in patients with suspected cholelithiasis; its sensitivity in detecting gallstones is greater than 96%. The characteristic finding is an echogenic focus that casts a shadow (Figure 50–1). The mobility of an echogenic focus may help to distinguish

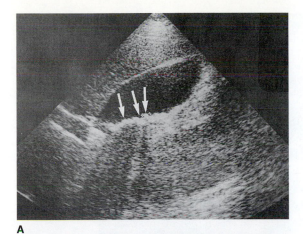

A

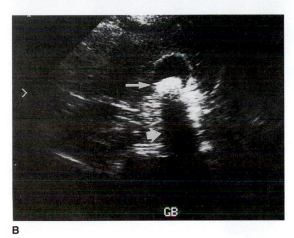

B

Figure 50–1. Sonogram demonstrating multiple small echogenic foci *(arrows)* with shadowing diagnostic of gallstones **(A)**, and single large stone *(thin arrow)* with shadowing *(thick arrow)* in another patient **(B)**.

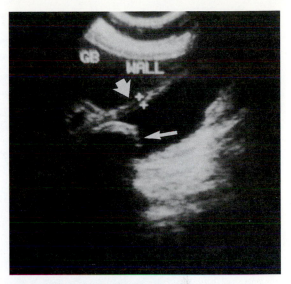

Figure 50–2. Ultrasound demonstrating gallstone in the neck of the gallbladder *(thin arrow)* with thickened gallbladder wall *(thick arrow)*, consistent with acute cholecystitis.

gallstones from other filling defects such as polyps. Ultrasonography also demonstrates gallbladder wall thickness, conformation, and size, which all reflect the presence and degree of acute or chronic inflammation (Figure 50–2). Pericholecystic fluid is a highly specific sign of acute rather than chronic cholecystitis. Ultrasonography can also accurately identify common bile duct dilatation, as well as hepatic or pancreatic parenchymal lesions. Common bile duct stones may be identified by ultrasonography, although the sensitivity is no greater than 50% (Figure 50–3).

2. Oral cholecystography—Ultrasonography has almost completely replaced oral cholecystography as the initial diagnostic procedure of choice for investigating patients with suspected gallstones, although oral chole-

cystography may still be valuable in specific situations. Uncommonly, it may detect stones when sonographic studies have been negative, and thus may be appropriate when the clinical suspicion for gallbladder disease is high but sonographic studies have not revealed disease. Oral cholecystography is also useful in assessing patients for nonsurgical therapy of gallstones, because it provides information about gallbladder function, the size and number of gallstones, and gallbladder composition. For example, calcified stones are generally not amenable to dissolution therapy, whereas small stones that float are likely to be rich in cholesterol and more likely to dissolve.

3. Computed tomography (CT)—CT is infrequently used for primary screening for gallstones. It is less sensitive and more expensive than other screening approaches and requires exposure to radiation. CT may, however, reveal gallstones and visualize the biliary system in patients being evaluated for acute abdominal disease or suspected biliary obstruction.

4. Magnetic resonance imaging (MRI)—Although not routinely useful for the detection of gallbladder stones, MRI has in recent years been increasingly used as a noninvasive means to detect bile duct stones with the use of T2-weighted images. This adaptation of MRI, called magnetic resonance cholangiopancreatography (MRCP), has a sensitivity of approximately 85% for bile duct stones, even more so if the bile duct is di-

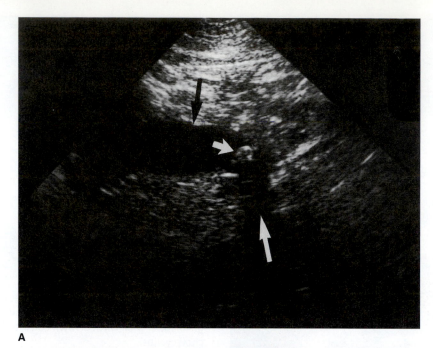

A

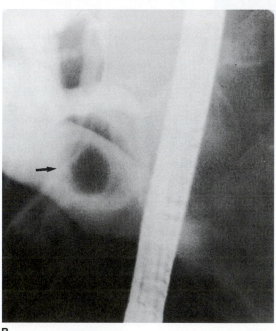

B

Figure 50–3. **A:** Ultrasound demonstrating a dilated bile duct with stone *(short arrow)* and shadowing *(long arrow).* **B:** ERCP revealed the same findings *(arrow).*

lated. MRCP is an excellent option when there is a low to intermediate level of suspicion for bile duct stones before laparoscopic cholecystectomy, because a negative MRCP can obviate the need for ERCP. The technique does detect gallbladder stones accurately, but its role in patients with negative ultrasound has yet to be defined.

5. Endoscopic retrograde cholangiopancreatography (ERCP)—ERCP reportedly can be used to diagnose gallstones within the gallbladder when noninvasive imaging studies have been negative, but it should rarely if ever be used for this purpose alone if bile duct stones are unlikely.

6. Hepatobiliary scintigraphy—Hepatobiliary scintigraphy is not useful in detecting gallstones, but it is an important procedure in patients with suspected acute cholecystitis. Scintigraphy relies on uptake by the gallbladder of an intravenously administered ^{99m}Tc-labeled iminodiacetic acid (IDA) derivative. The isotope is excreted by the liver into the bile ducts, where it is visualized by gamma counting. Several IDA compounds have been used, including diisopropyliminodiacetic acid (DISIDA), which has the advantage of hepatic uptake even in the presence of hyperbilirubinemia.

Acute cholecystitis is almost always accompanied by cystic duct obstruction. Therefore, a normal DISIDA scan, in which the isotope is seen in the gallbladder within 30–45 minutes, rules out the diagnosis of acute cholecystitis (Figure 50–4). Conversely, failure of the

isotope to appear within 4 hours is highly specific for acute cholecystitis (Figure 50–5). The isotope can be seen in intermediate degrees in the gallbladder of patients with chronic cholecystitis who have partial cystic duct obstruction, a contracted gallbladder, or stasis due to prolonged fasting.

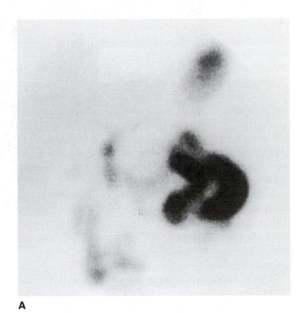

A

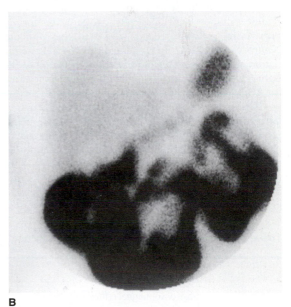

B

Figure 50–4. DISIDA scan showing normal gallbladder uptake within 30 minutes, ruling out acute cholecystitis.

Figure 50–5. DISIDA scan with nonvisualization of gallbladder after 2 hours (**A**) and 4 hours (**B**), consistent with acute cholecystitis

Some clinicians additionally rely upon DISIDA scanning to evaluate patients with suspected bile duct obstruction, but the author's experience does not support the use of this procedure routinely.

Differential Diagnosis

The differential diagnosis of gallstone-related pain includes peptic ulcer disease, gastroesophageal reflux, esophageal dysmotility, nonulcer dyspepsia, irritable bowel syndrome, renal colic, and cardiac disease (Tables 50–2 and 50–3).

The pain of peptic ulcer disease is usually more frequent, even occurring daily, and may be relieved by eating, a characteristic almost never shared by gallstone-related pain. Conversely, ulcer pain rarely conforms to the episodic pattern of distinct attacks caused by gallstones. Occasionally, patients with gallbladder disease have a steady ache in the right upper quadrant, but this presentation is less common.

Reflux symptoms are readily distinguished from biliary pain by their burning quality, substernal location, and occasional positional dependence (with symptoms worsening when the patient is supine). Regurgitation is common, and symptoms are usually relieved with antacids or acid-suppressive therapy.

The term **nonulcer dyspepsia** encompasses a variety of symptoms and underlying causes, not all well defined (see Chapter 21). Gastroduodenal dysmotility and gastritis or duodenitis may each contribute. When nonulcer dyspepsia includes epigastric pain, the distinction from gallstone-related pain can be difficult. Nonetheless, biliary pain is distinguished by its sporadic nature, greater intensity, and pattern of radiation to the right upper quadrant or right shoulder. Nocturnal awakenings are uncharacteristic of nonulcer dyspepsia or irritable bowel syndrome, and alterations or irregularities in bowel habits are features of irritable bowel syndrome but not biliary pain. Renal colic may produce pain that predominates in the anterior abdomen rather than the more characteristic location in the back or flank. When renal colic is suspected, urinalysis and imaging studies of the kidneys are indicated. Because

Table 50–2. Differential diagnosis of biliary colic.

Peptic ulcer disease
Esophageal spasm
Gastroesophageal reflux
Nonulcer dyspepsia
Irritable bowel syndrome
Renal colic
Coronary artery disease

Table 50–3. Differential diagnosis of acute cholecystitis.

Acute appendicitis
Acute pancreatitis
Acute bile duct obstruction (with or without cholangitis)
Perforated or penetrating ulcer
Intestinal obstruction
Nephrolithiasis
Acute myocardial infarction

biliary pain may appear in the substernal area, it may potentially be confused with angina, although biliary pain is not related to exertion. Any suspicion that chest pain may be cardiac in origin, even when gallstones have been documented, warrants rigorous cardiac evaluation.

A dilemma in evaluating patients with suspected biliary pain and documented gallstones is the absence of a test that conclusively establishes gallstones as the source of the pain. Any uncertainty regarding the likelihood of relief from surgery should be shared with the patient. More extensive evaluation may be necessary in patients with less specific symptoms. Therefore, barium studies, endoscopic studies, imaging of the kidneys, cardiac evaluation, and other tests all have a potential role but not an invariable one. In typical patients with documented gallstones, it may be appropriate to proceed directly to cholecystectomy without further testing.

The differential diagnosis of acute cholecystitis includes an acute event related to peptic ulcer disease, such as penetration or perforation, acute pancreatitis, acute hepatitis, Fitz-Hugh-Curtis syndrome, appendicitis, diverticulitis, or acute intestinal diseases. The physical findings in patients with perforated ulcers are usually more diffuse, and the presence of free air on plain films of the abdomen confirms a perforated viscus. The pain and physical findings in acute pancreatitis are less focal than in acute cholecystitis and are associated less often with peritoneal signs. A pattern of pain "boring through" to the back and partially relieved by sitting up is typical of pancreatitis. Fever and leukocytosis may be similar in both diseases, but the serum amylase level is far higher in acute pancreatitis than in cholecystitis. In severe pancreatitis, signs of systemic toxicity are more pronounced. A small percentage of patients with gallstone pancreatitis have concomitant acute cholecystitis. In this circumstance, the sonographic appearance of the gallbladder is critical, as a thickened wall or related findings may indicate cholecystitis (see following discussion).

Distinguishing hepatitis from cholecystitis should not be difficult. On those occasions when severe pain is present in hepatitis, the pain has a serosal character, as it arises from Glisson's capsule rather than the liver parenchyma itself. A careful physical examination can generally distinguish the tender, enlarged liver from the right subcostal tenderness of cholecystitis, even when the gallbladder is palpably enlarged. Serum chemistry measurements feature much more striking liver enzyme abnormalities in acute hepatitis (eg, ALT and AST). Acute hepatitis A, unlike the other forms of acute hepatitis, has been reported to cause acute cholecystitis by infecting the gallbladder epithelium. **Fitz-Hugh-Curtis syndrome** should be distinguishable from acute cholecystitis by the presence of adnexal tenderness on pelvic examination and positive findings on cervical gram-stained smears and culture for *Gonococcus* or *Chlamydia*.

Although the pain of appendicitis characteristically evolves in the right lower quadrant, its tendency to begin with pain in the periumbilical area, and the diversity of locations in which the appendix may lie, may occasionally lead erroneously to a diagnosis of acute cholecystitis. Imaging studies, including sonography or CT scanning, or both, should enable the distinction to be made.

Occasionally, pulmonary disease involving the right lower lobe may mimic gallbladder disease, and the pain of cholecystitis may have a pleuritic component when there is peritoneal irritation. The differential diagnosis in such cases depends on the presence of other pulmonary signs and symptoms and the findings on chest x-ray.

Treatment & Prognosis

A. CONSIDERATIONS IN PLANNING TREATMENT

Because most persons with gallstones are asymptomatic, a clear understanding of the natural history of this disorder is essential in formulating management.

1. Asymptomatic gallstones—Prospective cohort studies in the past 15 years have uniformly shown that only a minority of patients with asymptomatic gallstones develop symptoms or biliary complications over many years. In one study of 123 persons with asymptomatic gallstones followed for 11–24 years, biliary pain developed in 2% during each of the first 5 years, followed by a decreasing incidence thereafter. Complications were seen in only three persons and were preceded by pain in all cases. There are occasional patients who present with a complication, especially gallstone pancreatitis, in the absence of prior symptoms, but even in this setting, death is rare.

Based on these data, asymptomatic gallstones should be left alone in otherwise healthy people. Diabetics with gallstones have traditionally been considered high-risk patients, and prophylactic cholecystectomy has been recommended. It appears, however, that the com-

plications of surgery in such patients are related more closely to the systemic complications of the diabetes itself.

Prophylactic cholecystectomy has also been advocated in patients with sickle cell disease, as they are at increased risk of pigment stones. This recommendation is based on the difficulty in distinguishing pain crises from cholecystitis, the likelihood that true cholecystitis will precipitate a pain crisis, and the increased risk of emergent surgery in this population.

One caveat to the expectant management of asymptomatic gallstones is concern about gallbladder carcinoma (see Chapter 52). Indeed, when carcinoma of the gallbladder develops, it is almost always in persons with gallstones, but most persons with gallstones do not develop carcinoma. In asymptomatic persons, the risk of cancer is not considered sufficient to justify surgical treatment. The main exceptions are patients with calcified or "porcelain" gallbladder and Native Americans with gallstones, as both groups have a higher incidence of gallbladder carcinoma. Prophylactic cholecystectomy should therefore be considered in such persons, even when they are asymptomatic. Gallbladder cancer is more common in persons with symptomatic gallstones.

2. Symptomatic gallstones—In contrast to those with asymptomatic gallstones, patients with symptomatic stones have a higher risk of future problems, so that cholecystectomy is generally warranted. Up to two-thirds of patients with biliary pain will have recurrent episodes within 1–2 years. Moreover, about 3% will develop biliary complications annually. Decision analysis has indicated that elective cholecystectomy in symptomatic patients produces a small but real increase in life expectancy of 3–4 months.

B. SURGICAL TREATMENT

Until the past decade, cholecystectomy by laparotomy was the only treatment for gallstones, with a mortality rate of less than 1%. The need for prolonged hospitalization with this technique and the lengthy period of convalescence have fueled interest in less invasive alternatives.

1. Laparoscopic cholecystectomy—Laparoscopic cholecystectomy, introduced in 1987, rapidly became the standard method of cholecystectomy in patients with symptomatic gallstones. Despite the absence of controlled trials, its advantages are obvious. Patients are usually discharged within 1–2 days postoperatively, there is decreased scar tissue, and the return to normal activities is rapid. The number of cholecystectomies in the United States has increased recently, and this has been attributed in part to less hesitation by physicians to recommend surgery for "high-risk," reluctant, or mildly symptomatic patients.

Approximately 10% of laparoscopic cholecystectomies must be converted to open procedures in the operating room because of excessive inflammation, adhesions, or complications such as bile duct injuries requiring repair. Laparoscopy was initially considered to be contraindicated in patients with acute cholecystitis but may be performed safely in the hands of experienced surgeons.

Although the incidence of wound infections and cardiopulmonary complications appears to be reduced by laparoscopic cholecystectomy, the incidence of bile duct injuries initially appeared to increase, reportedly to 0.1–0.5%. The risk of bile duct injury is greatest with less experienced surgeons. With the maturation of laparoscopy, the incidence of this complication appears to have declined.

Surgical bile duct injuries are either recognized at the time of surgery or become apparent days to months later. The most common short-term postoperative problem is leakage of bile from the cystic duct remnant; this is not a true duct "injury," however. Patients complain of pain and may have low-grade fever or leukocytosis. The diagnosis may be apparent from a fluid collection on ultrasound or CT scanning, and can be confirmed by DISIDA scanning. Large fluid collections may require percutaneous drainage. The preferred treatment is stent placement, with or without sphincterotomy (preferences among endoscopists vary), to diminish the outflow resistance intrinsic to the intact ampulla and divert bile from the leak. This approach usually permits the leak to heal spontaneously.

Late complications of cholecystectomy are more difficult to manage because they usually result from bile duct stricturing. Patients may develop jaundice or cholangitis and are at high risk for secondary biliary cirrhosis if untreated. Endoscopic treatment with balloon dilation and stent placement may be effective, but surgery is often required, especially for proximal lesions involving the hepatic duct bifurcation.

2. Laparotomy (open cholecystectomy)—Acute cholecystitis or the finding of dense adhesions involving the gallbladder may lead the surgeon to perform open cholecystectomy at the outset of the operation or, more commonly, to convert laparoscopy to an open operation. In addition, patients with common bile duct stones that cannot be removed by endoscopic means may undergo open cholecystectomy and bile duct exploration. Finally, if there is suspicion of gallbladder cancer, many surgeons advocate open cholecystectomy.

C. Nonsurgical Treatment

1. Ursodeoxycholic acid—Ursodeoxycholic acid is a bile acid currently approved for gallstone dissolution in appropriate patients. The drug reduces cholesterol saturation by inhibiting hydroxymethylglutaryl-coenzyme A (HMG-CoA) reductase, a critical enzyme in cholesterol biosynthesis. Ursodeoxycholic acid also forms highly soluble multilamellar vesicles and prolongs the nucleation time of bile. The only significant adverse effects are diarrhea and hair thinning, which are uncommon and generally mild when they do occur. The overall efficacy of this agent in dissolving stones (at a dosage of 10–13 mg/kg/d) is about 50%, with dissolution complete within 6–12 months. The ideal candidate for dissolution therapy has small floating (ie, cholesterol-rich) noncalcified stones in a gallbladder demonstrated to be functional on oral cholecystography. Nonfloating stones are not an absolute contraindication to treatment. Stones over 1.5 cm in size will rarely dissolve. Pigment stones are not responsive to ursodeoxycholic acid.

Despite the initial enthusiasm for ursodeoxycholic acid, the expense, need for serial imaging studies, and high recurrence rates (at least 50%) after completion of therapy have diminished interest in this treatment. Interest in dissolution therapy waned further with the advent of laparoscopic cholecystectomy. For these reasons, dissolution therapy with bile acids is limited to patients who are at unusually high risk or who simply refuse surgery.

2. Contact dissolution therapy—Solvents that dissolve cholesterol stones can be instilled directly into the gallbladder via a percutaneously or endoscopically placed catheter. The prototype agent, methyl-*tert*-butyl ether, dissolves cholesterol gallstones within 1–3 days. Adverse effects include complications of catheter placement, hemorrhagic duodenitis, and sedation related to systemic absorption of the agent. As with oral bile acid dissolution therapy, gallstones may recur. This treatment is of largely historical interest.

3. Extracorporeal shock wave lithotripsy (ESWL)—ESWL for gallbladder stone fragmentation was developed because of its initial success in renal stone dissolution. Results in gallstone fragmentation have been less impressive, however. In ESWL, high-amplitude shock waves generated by external electrohydraulic or piezoelectric devices are focused on gallbladder stones by ultrasonographic guidance. The goal of ESWL is the production of tiny fragments, which are then amenable to oral bile acid dissolution therapy. The selection criteria are similar to those for primary bile acid dissolution therapy; preferred patients are those with a small number of stones, ideally a solitary stone. The lower rate of efficacy in patients with multiple stones excludes many patients with gallstones from this therapy. Moreover, gallstones commonly recur even after successful treatment, although less often than with dissolution therapy alone. Adverse effects of ESWL include postprocedure biliary colic, pancreatitis (rarely), and transient injury to the right lung or kidney.

Despite the clear benefit of ESWL in some patients, the expense of the lithotripsy units, limited spectrum of eligible patients, potential for recurrence, need for subsequent medical therapy, and evolution of laparoscopy have limited enthusiasm for this option.

D. TREATMENT OF COMPLICATIONS

1. Acute cholecystitis—Patients admitted with suspected acute cholecystitis should initially be made NPO (nothing by mouth) and intravenously hydrated. Administration of broad-spectrum antibiotics early in the course is recommended, because secondary infection often supervenes in what is initially a noninfectious process. If the diagnosis of acute cholecystitis is made within 24–48 hours of onset of symptoms, early surgery leads to reduced morbidity and mortality rates. If the diagnosis has been delayed, surgery may be technically more difficult. Therefore, some surgeons prefer to postpone surgery for several weeks, in the hope that the acute inflammation will subside with medical therapy. Surgery without delay is sometimes necessary in patients who fail to respond to medical therapy. In severely ill or elderly patients at high surgical risk, percutaneously placed cholecystostomy catheters may temporize the situation.

Although complications of cholecystitis almost always require surgery, definitive cholecystectomy may not be feasible in all cases at the time of the initial operation. Such complications can include free or localized perforation, with pericholecystic abscess; fistulization to bowel, most commonly the duodenum or hepatic flexure of colon; gallbladder empyema; emphysematous cholecystitis with gas-producing organisms; or **Mirizzi's syndrome,** in which a stone impacted in the gallbladder neck or cystic duct obstructs the adjacent common bile duct. Mirizzi's syndrome frequently is diagnosed by ERCP because of the prominence of biliary obstruction in the patient's presenting illness. Endoscopic stent placement may provide temporary benefit if cholangitis or jaundice is dominating the clinical picture. Endoscopic techniques, such as electrohydraulic lithotripsy, have been used successfully to clear the obstructing stone in patients with Mirizzi's syndrome. In such situations, subsequent cholecystectomy is still usually advised.

Gallstone passage from the gallbladder into the bowel via a fistula may cause intestinal obstruction if the stone is sufficiently large ("gallstone ileus"). Obstruction usually occurs in the ileum, but duodenal and even colonic obstruction have been encountered. The clinical presentation is similar to that of obstruction from other causes, although the presence of gallstones and air in the biliary tree may provide clues. At surgery,

the obstructing stone must be removed by enterotomy; cholecystectomy can be performed simultaneously if deemed feasible by the surgeon.

2. Common bile duct stones—There are several modes of presentation in patients with common bile duct stones. Most common is the patient presenting with biliary pain accompanied by abnormal liver tests, with or without jaundice. Jaundice from common bile duct stones may be painless, although the possibility of malignant bile duct obstruction must also be considered.

Most patients with symptoms suggestive of bile duct stones have stones in the gallbladder. Thus, treatment plans must consider adjunctive cholecystectomy. Recommendations for cholecystectomy in patients with primarily common bile duct complications have evolved rapidly since the advent of laparoscopic cholecystectomy. There is a low threshold of hesitation to remove the gallbladder given the minimal discomfort and rapid recovery in patients who undergo this procedure. Therefore, endoscopic stone removal is now often followed by laparoscopic surgery. The combination of the two techniques is the usual approach for patients with common duct and gallbladder stones.

Because some patients may have a self-limited episode with spontaneous stone passage, it may be difficult to determine when ERCP is necessary. Factors favoring persistent choledocholithiasis include imaging of duct stones or dilatation of the bile duct on sonography, or persistent abnormalities in liver tests after presentation, or both. Patients with transient pain, rapidly resolving liver enzyme abnormalities, and negative sonographic studies of the gallbladder usually have normal cholangiograms; therefore, ERCP is not usually performed in such patients. Depending on the level of suspicion, the surgeon may elect to obtain an intraoperative cholangiogram, which, in centers with the necessary expertise, may be followed by laparoscopic removal of bile duct stones via the transcystic route or by laparoscopic choledochotomy. Many surgeons, confident of their endoscopic colleague's expertise, defer removal of bile duct stones in favor of postoperative ERCP.

The treatment of choice in patients with bile duct stones who have had prior cholecystectomy is endoscopic sphincterotomy and stone extraction. The success rate exceeds 95% at experienced centers. Complications can be anticipated in 5–10%, however, with mortality rates of 0.5–1%. The major complications include iatrogenic pancreatitis, bleeding, perforation, and infection. Infection is a major concern when the bile duct is not drained adequately, either by complete clearing of stones or placement of a biliary stent. Pancreatitis usually resolves with conservative therapy, but in exceptional circumstances, a protracted course with pseudocyst or abscess formation may occur. Perforation is retroperitoneal and usually responds to antibiotics, preferably with nasobiliary drainage if the complication is recognized during ERCP. Surgery may be required, however, and should be considered early if there is any evidence of sepsis or fluid collections.

3. Biliary pancreatitis—This subject is covered in more detail elsewhere (see Chapter 30). A key decision in managing gallstone pancreatitis is whether to intervene early or treat conservatively. Most cases of gallstone pancreatitis are mild, resolve spontaneously, and can be managed expectantly. Once the acute episode has subsided, it is generally preferable to perform cholecystectomy prior to discharge to prevent recurrent attacks. Routine preoperative ERCP in patients with resolved biliary pancreatitis is not recommended unless there are signs of persistent bile duct obstruction.

In contrast, early ERCP may be warranted in severe gallstone pancreatitis. A British study of patients with severe pancreatitis demonstrated that urgent ERCP and sphincterotomy reduced the duration of hospitalization and overall complication rate, and showed a trend toward reduced mortality rates. Another study from Asia documented that early ERCP reduced the incidence of cholangitis in biliary pancreatitis, although the nature of stone disease (ie, more primary bile duct stones and bacterial contamination) may differ from that of Western patients. Complications in patients with severe pancreatitis were also reduced in the British study. However, a third study from Gremany failed to reveal an advantage for early ERCP, even in patients with severe pancreatitis, in the absence of jaundice or cholangitis. Thus this area remains controversial, but many clinicians do perform early ERCP in patients with severe gallstone pancreatitis. Fortunately, ERCP in patients with already established acute pancreatitis does not appear to exacerbate the disease.

4. Cholangitis—ERCP has assumed an important role in the management of acute cholangitis because it provides a prompt, nonsurgical method of bile duct drainage, with or without stone extraction. For septic, acutely ill patients, this offers a distinct advantage over surgery. In particularly unstable patients with cholangitis, placement of a stent or nasobiliary tube may be the most expeditious way to rapidly drain the bile duct without prolonging the procedure.

Some patients with cholangitis are not overtly toxic at presentation, and their acute illnesses resolve with antibiotics. During this time, vigilant observation is required, with endoscopic intervention if the patient fails to defervesce promptly. The likelihood of persistent common bile duct stones in these patients is high even after clinical improvement has occurred, indicating that ERCP is still warranted to clear the ducts.

5. Acalculous cholecystitis—Cholecystitis in the absence of gallstones is seen most often in critically ill patients in intensive care units. Its pathogenesis involves ischemia, with distention of the wall of the gallbladder and bile stasis. Immunocompromised patients, especially those with human immunodeficiency virus (HIV) infection, are also at risk for cytomegalovirus-related acalculous cholecystitis (see Chapter 38).

The presentation of acalculous cholecystitis may be similar to that of gallstone-associated cholecystitis, or it may be more subtle, with fever or leukocytosis but no focal abdominal symptoms or signs. Acalculous cholecystitis is associated with a high mortality rate, in part because patients often have severe underlying multisystem disease. Thus, a high index of suspicion is essential in making a diagnosis early enough to prevent death.

Hepatobiliary scintigraphy with hepatic IDA (HIDA) scanning frequently is abnormal in patients with acalculous cholecystitis. The utility of this test is reduced in severely ill patients, however, because of prolonged fasting. In contrast, sonographic studies and CT scanning may reveal thickening of the gallbladder wall and the presence of pericholecystic fluid even in the absence of stones and should be considered early.

The optimal treatment for acalculous cholecystitis is cholecystectomy, but underlying critical illness may preclude laparotomy. Surgical or percutaneous cholecystostomy is an established alternative, the latter requiring radiologic guidance. Most recently, transpapillary endoscopic drainage of the gallbladder has been reported; this technique may be most appropriate in patients with ascites and coagulopathies. The choice of treatment will depend on local expertise within the institution.

6. Sphincter of Oddi dysfunction—Also called biliary dyskinesia and papillary stenosis, this disorder is recognized most frequently in postcholecystectomy patients with recurrent biliary pain. Its incidence has been much debated, as have diagnostic criteria and appropriate therapy. Sphincter of Oddi dysfunction encompasses both actual stenosis due to fibrosis of the sphincter and spasm of the smooth muscle within the sphincter.

Criteria used by clinicians to diagnose this dysfunction include abnormal liver enzymes not attributable to parenchymal liver disease, dilatation of the bile duct beyond 12 mm in a postcholecystectomy patient, and delayed drainage of contrast material from the biliary tree more than 45 minutes after ERCP (Table 50–4). Sphincter of Oddi manometry has become the "gold standard" in diagnosing this disorder, although the technique remains confined to relatively few centers and poses a risk of postprocedure pancreatitis higher than that following routine diagnostic ERCP. This risk

Table 50–4. Proposed criteria for sphincter of Oddi dysfunction.

Biliary pain
Dilated common bile duct over 12 mm (postcholecystectomy)
Delayed drainage of contrast beyond 45 minutes (postcholecystectomy)
Abnormal liver enzymes beyond twice normal
Delayed drainage from bile duct to duodenum on DISIDA scan
Abnormal sphincter of Oddi manometry:
    Basal sphincter of Oddi pressure beyond 40 mm
    Tachyoddia (over 8 sphincter contractions per minute)
    Paradoxical response to cholecystokinin
    Excessive number of retrograde contractions

---

may be reduced with the use of an aspirating catheter. In an attempt to reduce the invasiveness of diagnostic testing for this entity, some clinicians use DISIDA scanning to assess the rapidity of flow from the bile duct into the intestine. The level of confidence in this modality varies widely, however, and at best, it furnishes supplementary rather than definitive data on which to base management decisions.

Sphincter of Oddi manometry can help to predict which patients will respond to endoscopic sphincterotomy, usually considered the treatment of choice for this condition. An accurate diagnosis is essential, because the risk of sphincterotomy for sphincter of Oddi dysfunction is greater than when performed for bile duct stones. Investigators in specialized centers have shown that patients who meet the laboratory and radiologic criteria for sphincter of Oddi dysfunction almost always have abnormal sphincter pressures, so that manometry prior to sphincterotomy may not always be necessary. More commonly, however, patients with postcholecystectomy biliary pain have only one or two of these criteria, and the results of manometry cannot be predicted. Manometry findings in patients with an uncertain diagnosis of sphincter of Oddi dysfunction correlate most clearly with the results of sphincterotomy. The approach to patients with biliary pain alone but no other criteria for sphincter of Oddi dysfunction is less well defined. Even in patients with laboratory or imaging abnormalities, some endoscopists prefer to rely on clinical judgment rather than manometry in deciding whether to perform sphincterotomy.

REFERENCES

Abei M et al: Identification of human biliary acid glycoprotein as a cholesterol crystallization promoter. Gastroenterology 1994; 106:231.

Berdah SV et al: Follow up of selective endoscopic ultrasonography and/or endoscopic retrograde cholangiography prior to laparoscopic cholecystectomy: a prospective study of 300 patients. Endoscopy 2001;33:216.

Everhart JE: Contributions of obesity and weight loss to gallstone disease. Ann Intern Med 1993;119:1029.

Folsch UR et al: Early ERCP and papillotomy compared with conservative treatment with acute biliary pancreatitis. N Engl J Med 1997;336:237.

Gracie WA, Ransohoff DF: The natural history of silent gallstones: the innocent gallstone is not a myth. N Engl J Med 1982; 798.

Habib FA et al: Role of laparoscopic cholecystectomy in the management of gangrenous cholecystitis. Am J Surg 2001;181:71.

Jacobson IM: ERCP in patients undergoing cholecystectomy. In: *ERCP and Its Applications.* Jacobson IM (editor). Lippincott-Raven, 1998; 95.

Johnston DE, Kaplan MM: Pathogenesis and treatment of gallstones. N Engl J Med 1993;328:412.

Kohut M et al: The frequency of bile duct crystals in patients with presumed biliary pancreatitis. Gastrointest Endosc 2001;54: 37.

Lezoche E et al: Technical considerations and laparoscopic bile duct exploration: transcystic and choledochotomy. Semin Laparosc Surg 2000;7:262.

Neoptolemos JP et al: Controlled trial of urgent endoscopic retrograde cholangiopancreatography and endoscopic sphincterotomy versus conservative treatment for acute pancreatitis due to gallstones. Lancet 1988;2:979.

Sackmann M et al: The Munich gallbladder lithotripsy study: results of the first 5 years with 711 patients. Ann Intern Med 1991;114:290.

Sackmann M et al: Gallstone recurrence after shock-wave therapy. Gastroenterology 1994;106:225.

Southern Surgeons Club: A prospective analysis of 1518 laparoscopic cholecystectomies. N Engl J Med 1991;324:1073.

Strasberg S, Clavien P-A: Cholecystolithiasis: lithotherapy for the 1990s. Hepatology 1992;16:820.

Primary Disease of the Bile Ducts

51

Keith D. Lindor, MD

PRIMARY BILIARY CIRRHOSIS

Primary biliary cirrhosis is a chronic cholestatic liver disease characterized by inflammatory destruction of interlobular and septal bile ducts. The disease affects middle-aged women in 9 out of 10 cases, and is typically marked by the presence of antimitochondrial antibodies. It is usually slowly progressive, with eventual development of cirrhosis and portal hypertension and its complications.

Primary biliary cirrhosis is uncommon, with an estimated incidence of 10–12 cases per year per million persons, and a prevalence of 100–150 cases per million, although higher prevalence is being reported. Many of these patients are identified because of increased serum alkaline phosphatase levels found during routine health evaluations or during evaluation of unrelated complaints. Most patients at this stage are asymptomatic; some may manifest symptoms specific for primary biliary cirrhosis (see following discussion) or symptoms from diseases known to be associated with primary biliary cirrhosis, such as Hashimoto's thyroiditis or keratoconjunctivitis sicca.

Primary biliary cirrhosis is being recognized with increasing frequency. Ursodeoxycholic acid has emerged as the recognized therapy for these patients, but liver transplantation still plays an important role in the management of end-stage disease.

Pathophysiology

Although the cause of primary biliary cirrhosis is not established, immunologic mechanisms may play a primary role. As immunologic destruction of bile ducts progresses, chronic cholestasis ensues. Many of the complications of primary biliary cirrhosis are related to chronic cholestasis and the resultant hepatic dysfunction. Treatment has been used to alter immunologic function and improve the chronic cholestasis.

A. IMMUNOLOGIC MECHANISMS

Immunologic mechanisms are most strongly suggested by the presence of T cells, sometimes activated, in the inflammatory infiltrates surrounding the damaged bile ducts. A widespread defect in immune function is suggested by the association of primary biliary cirrhosis with other autoimmune diseases characterized by lymphocytic destruction of glandular epithelial tissues, including thyroid, salivary, and lacrimal glands.

Several immunologic abnormalities have been demonstrated, but it is not known whether these are etiologic or a secondary phenomenon. Precipitating agents, such as toxins or viruses, have been unsuccessfully sought. Genetic factors do not appear to play a major role in the development of this disease, although there is a clearly increased risk of developing primary biliary cirrhosis in relatives of affected patients. Abnormalities of cellular immunity include defective suppressor cell function, increased autoreactivity to autoantigens, and aberrant expression of autoantigens on biliary epithelium. As noted previously, however, it is uncertain whether these are primary or secondary phenomena. Similarly, the presence of antimitochondrial antibodies has been recognized as a characteristic and diagnostic feature of this disease. In recent years, characterization of the antigens recognized by this antibody has been greatly advanced, but their role in the pathogenesis of primary biliary cirrhosis is uncertain.

B. CHOLESTASIS

Progressive immunologically mediated destruction of bile ducts leads to impaired intrahepatic bile flow and chronic cholestasis. Animal models indicate that it is likely that cholestasis causes accumulation of hydrophobic and potentially toxic bile acids within the liver, creating a self-perpetuating liver injury. Although copper was once considered to be pathogenically important, it is now recognized that accumulation of copper is a passive consequence of cholestasis and is without pathogenic significance.

Clinical Findings

A. SYMPTOMS AND SIGNS

The most common symptom in patients with primary biliary cirrhosis is fatigue (Table 51–1), but this is nonspecific. Of the specific symptoms, pruritus is the most important; it can occur at any stage of the disease, and its intensity does not correlate with the severity of the underlying liver disease. Symptoms of more advanced disease, such as jaundice, variceal bleeding, ascites, or encephalopathy, are rare at presentation but can occur late in the course of the disease. As noted above, an in-

Table 51–1. Symptoms and signs of primary biliary cirrhosis.

Symptoms and Signs	Incidence (%)
Fatigue	60–70
Pruritus	50–60
Asymptomatic	30–40
Associated with advanced disease	
Jaundice	16
Variceal bleeding	2
Ascites	3

creasing number of patients (in some series, up to 40%) are now being recognized without symptoms. A number of diseases that share a presumed autoimmune basis have been associated with primary biliary cirrhosis (Table 51–2). There also appears to be an associated increased risk of breast cancer in women with primary biliary cirrhosis.

B. DIAGNOSTIC STUDIES

The diagnosis of primary biliary cirrhosis should be considered, in particular, in middle-aged women with chronic cholestasis. The most characteristic biochemical abnormality is an increase in the serum alkaline phosphatase level to at least three or four times normal or higher. Occasional patients may have nearly normal alkaline phosphatase levels but positive antimitochondrial antibody and liver biopsies consistent with the diagnosis of primary biliary cirrhosis. Antimitochondrial antibodies (AMA) are usually present in high titers; 90–95% of patients will have an antimitochondrial antibody titer greater than 1:40. Every patient should undergo ultrasound study or computed tomography (CT) scanning to exclude biliary obstruction, although the presence of an antimitochondrial antibody is unusual (<2%) in biliary obstruction from other causes. Liver biopsy has been used to confirm the diagnosis histologi-

Table 51–2. Diseases associated with primary biliary cirrhosis.

Disease	Incidence (%)
Keratoconjunctivitis sicca	50
Thyroid disease	15
Arthritis	10
Less commonly associated diseases	
Raynaud's phenomenon	9
Scleroderma	2
Renal stones	3
Breast cancer	2

cally as well as to provide information regarding histologic staging. The need for liver biopsy in middle-aged women with chronic cholestasis and a strongly positive AMA is now being questioned. Ordinarily, cholangiography is not necessary, unless atypical features are present, such as the absence of an antimitochondrial antibody, occurrence in a male, or the suggestion of biliary obstruction on imaging studies.

1. Laboratory findings—Elevated alkaline phosphatase is the most commonly found abnormality in patients with primary biliary cirrhosis; usually, this is elevated to four to five times normal or higher. The transaminases are typically only mildly elevated, and most patients have serum bilirubin levels ranging from normal to less than 2 mg/dL at presentation. Serum immunoglobulin M (IgM) levels are elevated in approximately 95% of patients. Hypercholesterolemia is common and found in nearly 80% of patients. Serum albumin levels and prothrombin times are usually normal until late in the course of the disease. Antimitochondrial antibodies are present in approximately 95% of patients. The M2 component of this antibody, which recognizes the pyruvate dehydrogenase complex, is the most specific for primary biliary cirrhosis.

Some patients may have features of primary biliary cirrhosis but lack antimitochondrial antibodies. These patients are classified as "antimitochondrial antibody-negative primary biliary cirrhosis," or "autoimmune cholangitis" (see Chapter 36). Ninety-five percent of antimitochondrial antibody-negative patients will have either antinuclear antibody or anti-smooth muscle antibodies. These patients with AMA-negative primary biliary cirrhosis autoimmune cholangitis follow a course that is identical to that of primary biliary cirrhosis.

2. Histologic findings—Histologic changes have been divided into four stages, as shown in Figure 51–1.

- The portal stage (stage 1) is characterized by inflammation of the portal tracts surrounding the bile ducts.
- Stage 2 is characterized by more bile duct destruction, proliferation of bile ductules, and piecemeal necrosis, with inflammation spilling from the portal areas into the hepatic parenchyma.
- Stage 3 is characterized by fibrosis extending from the portal tracts.
- The so-called septal stage (stage 4) is defined as the presence of regenerative nodules surrounded by fibrosis.

Histologic progression occurs over many years. At present, most patients have advanced histologic changes at the time of diagnosis, although they may follow a benign asymptomatic course for many years after the diagnosis is established.

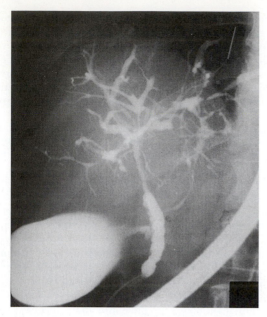

Figure 51–1. The typical cholangiographic features of primary sclerosing cholangitis as seen here include diffuse multifocal stricturing of the intra- and extrahepatic bile ducts.

3. Imaging studies—The most important imaging studies are those used to exclude biliary obstruction. Ordinarily, ultrasound studies and CT scans are adequate for this purpose in middle-aged women with chronic cholestasis and a positive antimitochondrial antibody test. In a patient who is antimitochondrial antibody-negative or male, the author has usually recommended endoscopic retrograde cholangiopancreatography to exclude other diagnoses. Magnetic resonance cholangiography is a new technique that is noninvasive yet allows exclusion of biliary tract disease quite effectively. In the great majority of patients, however, routine cholangiography is not indicated.

Differential Diagnosis

The differential diagnosis of patients with chronic cholestasis includes extrahepatic biliary obstruction due to biliary stones, strictures, or tumors; ultrasonography or CT scanning will help exclude these possibilities. Several other conditions may not be excluded by these imaging studies, however, including primary sclerosing cholangitis (see Table 51–7), drug-induced cholestasis, overlap with autoimmune hepatitis, hepatitis C, and, occasionally, sarcoidosis or idiopathic adulthood ductopenia (Table 51–3).

Table 51–3. Differential diagnosis of primary biliary cirrhosis.

Extrahepatic biliary obstruction due to stones, strictures, tumors
Primary sclerosing cholangitis
Drug-induced cholestasis
Overlap with autoimmune hepatitis
Sarcoidosis
Idiopathic adulthood ductopenia
Autoimmune cholangitis

Primary sclerosing cholangitis (see following discussion) should be considered, especially in patients with inflammatory bowel disease. In primary sclerosing cholangitis, cholangiography is the critical diagnostic study. Liver biopsy can suggest primary sclerosing cholangitis but may not adequately distinguish between primary biliary cirrhosis and primary sclerosing cholangitis, because both conditions may be associated with periductular inflammation, bile duct injury, and cholestasis.

The use of drugs, such as phenothiazines, estrogens, androgens, and those associated with granulomatous involvement of the liver, should be considered. In some patients autoimmune hepatitis may be confused with primary biliary cirrhosis, particularly because up to 25% of these patients may also have antimitochondrial antibodies. In contrast to primary biliary cirrhosis, however, patients with autoimmune hepatitis usually have antimitochondrial antibody titers of 1:40 or less. Liver biopsy will also help distinguish the condition because patients with autoimmune hepatitis rarely have bile duct destruction.

Hepatitis C must also be considered in the differential diagnosis of patients with primary biliary cirrhosis because the infection is sometimes associated with granulomatous inflammation around bile ducts. Increasingly, cases of hepatitis C associated with a cholestatic profile are being described.

Sarcoidosis may present with cholestasis and hepatic granulomas; however, its histologic features are otherwise different from those of primary biliary cirrhosis. Florid duct lesions are not a part of sarcoidosis. Antimitochondrial antibody tests are negative, and characteristic chest x-ray abnormalities are present in the great majority of patients with sarcoidosis.

Idiopathic adulthood ductopenia is a recently described entity. It typically occurs in men who have normal cholangiography and do not have autoantibodies or a history of colitis. The cholestasis is usually more rapidly progressive than in primary biliary cirrhosis and often results in referral for liver transplantation. Idiopathic biliary ductopenia is similar to idiopathic adulthood ductopenia but follows a benign course and usually responds to ursodeoxycholic acid therapy. As the name implies, the cause of these conditions is unknown.

Complications

Complications of primary biliary cirrhosis include those of chronic liver disease, such as portal hypertension with variceal bleeding, ascites, and hepatic encephalopathy, as well as consequences of cholestasis, including osteopenia, fat-soluble vitamin deficiency, and hypercholesterolemia (Table 51–4).

A. Osteopenia

The osteopenia found in patients in North America with primary biliary cirrhosis is nearly always osteoporosis. Osteomalacia has been described primarily in the United Kingdom and has been related to decreased exposure to sunlight. Nevertheless, osteomalacia should be considered in these patients because of the increased risk of vitamin D deficiency in the setting of malabsorption of fat-soluble vitamins (see following discussion). Approximately 35% of patients with primary biliary cirrhosis have bone mineral densities of the lumbar spine below the fracture threshold. The exact incidence of spontaneous compression fractures, however, is not known but appears to be about 5% per year. No specific measures have yet been identified for management of these patients with osteoporosis of cholestasis. Vitamin D deficiency should be identified and corrected (see following discussion). General measures to treat postmenopausal osteoporosis are recommended, including supplemental calcium and adequate exercise. The utility of estrogens in these patients is less well defined; our experience has shown that estrogens are safe, well tolerated, and lead to stabilization or actual improvement in the bone density. Because of concerns about worsening cholestasis, however, estrogens should be used with caution and at low dosages (ie, transdermal estrogen, 0.05 mg twice weekly), with liver tests carefully monitored after initiating therapy. Supplemental vitamin D in the absence of deficiency does not appear to have a role. Agents such as calcitonin, fluoride, and bisphosphonates have not been adequately evaluated in patients with cholestatic osteopenia.

B. Fat-Soluble Vitamin Deficiency

Fat-soluble vitamin deficiency, especially of vitamin A, is common. Although no clinical trials have optimized the approach to vitamin A deficiency, the author's policy has been to measure serum levels in patients with advanced disease and to replace deficiencies as needed with 50,000–150,000 units per week when levels are below normal. Others have followed a less aggressive approach, instead replacing vitamin A only after the onset of changes in dark adaptation. If vitamin A therapy is used, levels should be monitored to ensure adequacy without overreplacement, because of concerns regarding vitamin A hepatic toxicity, with therapy continued as needed to maintain normal serum levels.

Vitamin D deficiency occurs in particular in patients with advanced disease. Approximately 12% of the author's patients have had vitamin D deficiency. Vitamin D can be replaced with a dosage of 50,000–150,000 units per week of vitamin D_2 (ergocalciferol). These patients usually do not have difficulty in hydroxylation of 25-hydroxycholecalciferol, and, therefore, do not require the more expensive 1,25-dihydroxycholecalciferol or 25-hydroxyergocalciferol replacement.

Vitamin K deficiency can be inferred from a prolonged prothrombin time. If an elevated prothrombin time responds to vitamin K replacement, chronic therapy with water-soluble vitamin K, 5 mg/d, is indicated.

Vitamin E deficiency is rare. When symptomatic, it causes usually irreversible neurologic abnormalities characterized by areflexia, loss of proprioception, and ataxia. Patients with symptomatic vitamin E deficiency may not respond to replacement therapy, and it has been the author's policy to measure levels, particularly in patients with advanced disease, and institute replacement therapy with 100 mg orally twice daily in those who are deficient.

Treatment

Treatment for primary biliary cirrhosis has been based on measures to reverse abnormalities observed clinically and histologically.

A. Drug Treatment

Drugs that have been tested are those designed to modify cholestasis, suppress the immune response, and alter fibrogenesis.

Table 51–4. Complications of cholestatic liver disease.

Associated with chronic liver disease
    Portal hypertension
    Variceal bleeding
    Ascites
    Hepatic encephalopathy
Specific for cholestasis
    Osteopenia
    Fat-soluble vitamin deficiency
    Hypercholesterolemia

1. Ursodeoxycholic acid—The most important advance in recent years has been the use of ursodeoxycholic acid. The drug may be effective by displacing hepatotoxic endogenous bile acids. Ursodeoxycholic acid may also have immunomodulatory effects that modify the underlying immunologic abnormalities of primary biliary cirrhosis. Controlled trials have now indicated that ursodeoxycholic acid leads to clear-cut biochemical improvement. In some series, symptomatic and histologic improvement has been reported, and a controlled trial cites improvement in survival rates and a decreased need for liver transplantation for the treatment of primary biliary cirrhosis. This drug is approved by the Food and Drug Administration and is endorsed by the American Association for the Study of Liver Disease.

Several other agents described below have undergone clinical testing with limited success.

2. Corticosteroids—Corticosteroids led to some improvement in symptoms, biochemical measurements, and histologic findings in patients with primary biliary cirrhosis in the only small randomized trial that has been reported. Improvement in the liver disease was offset by worsening of the osteopenia from the corticosteroids. Although, with further follow-up, this osteopenia was less of a problem, the small study size and the large number of dropouts prevent any conclusions to be drawn regarding efficacy. Thus, corticosteroids should be considered experimental and potentially hazardous therapy. Budesonide, a steroid with extensive hepatic metabolism when combined with ursodeoxycholic acid in untreated patients, led to improved biochemical response but when added to ursodeoxycholic acid in patients already receiving the drug but with persistently abnormal liver tests was ineffective and worsened osteoporosis.

3. Other drugs—Azathioprine has been studied in controlled trials, the largest of which showed no benefit with respect to clinical symptoms, biochemical measurements, histologic findings, or survival rates. At present, this treatment is seldom used for patients with primary biliary cirrhosis. Cyclosporine has been tested because of its immunomodulatory activity, but trials to date have shown little benefit and a high risk of drug-induced renal dysfunction. Methotrexate was initially reported in a small series to be effective in slowing the progression of primary biliary cirrhosis, but recent trials show little benefit. A large-scale randomized trial is underway comparing methotrexate plus ursodeoxycholic acid to ursdoeoxycholic acid alone. Penicillamine has been tested but found to be of no value. Colchicine has been studied in three large trials and appears to be of limited, if any, benefit in patients with primary biliary cirrhosis.

B. LIVER TRANSPLANTATION

Liver transplantation clearly benefits patients with end-stage primary biliary cirrhosis and is also considered on rare occasions for patients with intractable pruritus or fatigue (see Chapter 54). The osteoporosis associated with primary biliary cirrhosis may be worsened initially following liver transplantation. Thus, patients with severe osteoporosis should probably be referred early to a liver transplantation program.

Prognosis

There has been an increased appreciation of the natural history of primary biliary cirrhosis in recent years. The disease is slowly progressive, with an initial asymptomatic presentation followed by the gradual development of symptoms in most patients. Earlier studies suggested that asymptomatic patients with primary biliary cirrhosis had a normal life expectancy; however, continued follow-up studies suggest that such interpretations were based on a lead time bias, so that, ultimately, almost all patients develop progressive, symptomatic disease. The author believes that both asymptomatic and symptomatic patients should be considered for treatment.

In general, the course of primary biliary cirrhosis may exceed 10–15 years, but the prognosis varies among patients. Survival models have been developed that allow for better prediction of the course of the disease and that are particularly useful for timing of liver transplantation. The best validated model relies on simple clinical features such as age of the patient, serum bilirubin and albumin levels, prothrombin time, and the presence or absence of edema or ascites.

Liver transplantation can now be performed with a 1-year survival rate of 90–95% in most centers and a 5-year survival rate in the 70–80% range. Patients with primary biliary cirrhosis should be considered for liver transplantation when the serum bilirubin level approaches or exceeds 4–6 mg/dL, when hepatic synthetic function deteriorates, or, as noted above, for relief of symptoms such as disabling fatigue or pruritus. Other indications include uncontrolled ascites, hepatic encephalopathy, and variceal bleeding not controlled by endoscopic or pharmacologic means. Recurrence of primary biliary cirrhosis after transplantation has been described in approximately 10% of patients, but the disease in this setting follows a relatively benign course thus far.

PRIMARY SCLEROSING CHOLANGITIS

Primary sclerosing cholangitis is a chronic cholestatic liver disease that, like primary biliary cirrhosis, often progresses to cirrhosis, with complications of portal hypertension. The characteristic pathologic feature of this disease is inflammation, with obliterative fibrosis of intra- and extrahepatic bile ducts. Primary sclerosing cholangitis frequently occurs in association with chronic ulcerative colitis and, less commonly, with Crohn's colitis. The prevalence of primary sclerosing cholangitis is approximately 10–40 persons per million, making it much less common than primary biliary cirrhosis.

The cause of primary sclerosing cholangitis is unknown, and adequate therapy has not yet been defined. Like primary biliary cirrhosis, a variety of complications of cholestasis can occur in patients with primary sclerosing cholangitis. A major problem unique to primary sclerosing cholangitis is the occurrence of cholangiocarcinoma in approximately 1% of patients per year.

The presentation of primary sclerosing cholangitis can vary greatly, from asymptomatic disease to advanced liver disease. Nearly 70% of patients with primary sclerosing cholangitis have chronic colitis, which usually precedes the development of primary sclerosing cholangitis but may occur years after the onset of liver disease. Moreover, the liver disease can occur even after proctocolectomy. It is estimated that 5% of patients with ulcerative colitis will develop primary sclerosing cholangitis.

Pathogenesis

The cause of primary sclerosing cholangitis is unknown. A variety of mechanisms have been investigated, including toxins, viral agents, and immunologic abnormalities. Environmental toxins have not been found. An attractive hypothesis based on animal studies is that toxins absorbed from an inflamed colon, including bacterial peptides such as *N*-formylated chemotactic peptides and endotoxins, lead to the release of inflammatory cytokines, which cause bile duct injury.

Several viral infections have been considered as precipitating agents in primary sclerosing cholangitis because of the role of cytomegalovirus in the cholangiography associated with human immunodeficiency virus (HIV). Typical hepatitis viruses such as hepatitis A, B, and C do not appear to play a role; reovirus type 3 has also been excluded. Although hepatic artery damage due to chemotherapeutic agents such as floxuridine has been associated with biliary features of sclerosing cholangitis, no such arteriopathy has been identified in the primary disease.

Immunologic mechanisms may be important. Haplotypes HLA-B2 and HLA-DR3 are often present in both primary sclerosing cholangitis and other autoimmune diseases. Autoantibodies and defects in cellular immune function have been described in primary sclerosing cholangitis, but, as in primary biliary cirrhosis, a pathogenic role for such immunologic abnormalities has not been established.

Clinical Findings

A. SYMPTOMS AND SIGNS

Sixty to seventy percent of patients with primary sclerosing cholangitis are male, with a mean age at diagnosis of 43 years. Symptoms include progressive fatigue, pruritus, and jaundice. One (or more) of these symptoms is present in 75% of patients, whereas 25% may be asymptomatic, with abnormal liver tests noted incidentally (Table 51–5). Other symptoms such as fever, abdominal pain, and cholangitis are less common. Cholangitis is more common after surgical or endoscopic biliary tract manipulation.

B. DIAGNOSTIC STUDIES

Primary sclerosing cholangitis should be considered in patients with chronic cholestasis, particularly in the setting of inflammatory bowel disease. Cholangiography is the most important diagnostic study. Endoscopic retrograde cholangiopancreatography is the preferred method to visualize the biliary system (see the following section on "Imaging Studies"). Transhepatic cholangiography is technically difficult because the intrahepatic bile ducts are often sclerotic. Liver biopsy suggesting primary sclerosing cholangitis is often obtained prior to cholangiography; biopsy obtained even after the diagnosis is established can provide prognostic information, but sampling variability limits the usefulness of liver biopsies in patients with primary sclerosing cholangitis. Although autoantibodies are found in primary sclerosing cholangitis, their role in diagnosis is less certain than in primary biliary cirrhosis. Antimitochondrial antibodies are seldom found, and antinuclear antibodies can be found on occasion. Pericytoplasmic

Table 51–5. Symptoms and signs at presentation of primary sclerosing cholangitis.

	Incidence (%)
Symptoms	
Fatigue	75
Pruritus	60
Fever	20
Cholangitis	10
Asymptomatic	25
Signs	
Hepatomegaly	50
Splenomegaly	30
Hyperpigmentation	25
Xanthomas	5

antineutrophil cytoplasmic antibodies (p-ANCA) have been described in patients with inflammatory bowel disease as well as primary sclerosing cholangitis, suggesting that these autoantibodies may prove useful diagnostically in the future.

1. Laboratory findings—An elevated serum alkaline phosphatase level is the most important laboratory finding and is seen in nearly all patients at some point in the disease. The alkaline phosphatase levels may fluctuate considerably and, at times, may be normal. Transaminases are almost always elevated to less than three to five times normal. Serum bilirubin levels may rise as the disease progresses. Antinuclear antibody and p-ANCA are being identified more commonly. The antimitochondrial antibody is uncommon. Unlike primary biliary cirrhosis, primary sclerosing cholangitis is not commonly associated with autoimmune diseases.

2. Histologic findings—Surgical biopsies from the extrahepatic bile duct are not specific for primary sclerosing cholangitis, as stricturing conditions may give an identical histologic appearance. Findings from liver biopsy may strongly support the diagnosis of primary sclerosing cholangitis by demonstrating the absence of intralobular bile ducts in some portal tracts (ductopenia), with duct proliferation in other tracts. Fibrous cholangitis with duct obliteration is nearly diagnostic for primary sclerosing cholangitis but is an uncommon finding. In some patients, the histologic findings of primary sclerosing cholangitis cannot be distinguished from those of primary biliary cirrhosis; as was noted previously, cholangiographic abnormalities on endoscopic retrograde cholangiopancreatography would establish the diagnosis of primary sclerosing cholangitis in this setting.

Recently, the entity of **small duct primary sclerosing cholangitis** has been described. This condition, which occurs in the setting of chronic colitis, is characterized by a histologic appearance identical to primary sclerosing cholangitis but with cholangiographically normal ducts. Small duct primary sclerosing cholangitis may represent the initial phase of primary sclerosing cholangitis.

As in primary biliary cirrhosis, the histologic abnormalities in primary sclerosing cholangitis are divided into four stages:

1. The portal stage, which involves inflammation in the portal triad;
2. The periportal stage, in which there is inflammation spilling into the periportal area;
3. The septal stage, characterized by septal formation;
4. The cirrhotic stage, characterized by the development of regenerative nodules.

3. Imaging studies—Cholangiography is the most important diagnostic study. Endoscopic retrograde cholangiopancreatography, as noted above, is the procedure of choice. Typical findings include multifocal stricturing and irregularity usually involving both the intra- and extrahepatic biliary system. These strictures are usually diffuse, short, and annular, with intervening segments of normal to dilated bile ducts giving a beaded appearance. Marked dilation, a polypoid mass, or progressive stricture formation suggest a complicating bile duct carcinoma (see section on "Complications"). Magnetic resonance cholangiography can help establish the diagnosis but does not allow dilatation, stone extraction, or histologic sampling.

Differential Diagnosis

The differential diagnosis includes primary biliary cirrhosis, drug-induced cholestasis, idiopathic adulthood ductopenia, cholestatic alcoholic hepatitis, or chronic viral hepatitis.

Abnormalities of the bile ducts that may give a similar cholangiographic appearance include the following:

- The cholangiopathy associated with HIV infection, which is due to *Cryptosporidium, Microsporidia,* or cytomegalovirus (see Chapter 38);
- The cholangiopathy arising after manipulation of the hepatic artery, such as following infusions of the chemotherapeutic agent floxuridine; and
- Extrahepatic bile duct obstruction caused by stones, surgical strictures, choledochal cysts, or the presence of cholangiocarcinoma or other malignant tumors involving the bile ducts such as lymphoma or metastatic adenocarcinomas (Table 51–6).

A comparison of the features of primary biliary cirrhosis and primary sclerosing cholangitis is shown in Table 51–7.

Complications

Complications of primary sclerosing cholangitis include those resulting from advancing liver failure, such as variceal bleeding, ascites, and encephalopathy, and sequelae of cholestasis, such as osteopenia and fat-soluble vitamin deficiency (see section on "Complications of primary biliary cirrhosis"). Complications relatively unique to primary sclerosing cholangitis include cholangitis, dominant strictures, biliary stone disease, cholangiocarcinoma, and peristomal varices.

A. CHOLANGITIS

Cholangitis can occur spontaneously but is much more likely following surgical or radiologic manipulation of the biliary tree. Cholangiography should be considered

Table 51–6. Differential diagnosis of primary sclerosing cholangitis.

Primary biliary cirrhosis
Drug-induced cholestasis
Idiopathic adulthood ductopenia
Cholestatic alcoholic hepatitis or chronic viral hepatitis
Abnormalities of bile ducts
   AIDS
      Cryptosporidium
      Microsporidium
      Cytomegalovirus
Damage to hepatic artery (floxuridine infusions)
Extrahepatic bile duct obstruction from stones
Surgical strictures
Choledochal cysts
Cholangiocarcinoma
Lymphoma
Metastatic adenocarcinoma

---

in a patient with an otherwise stable course who develops cholangitis. Clinical features of cholangitis may range from mild fevers, chills, and pain, to life-threatening sepsis with shock. Empiric antibiotic therapy is indicated if cholangitis is suspected. The aggressiveness of the therapy should be matched to the severity of the cholangitis. Some episodes of cholangitis will respond to oral antibiotics that are effective for the most commonly found organisms, such as *Enterobacteriaceae, Enterococcus,* and *Clostridia* species; others require intravenous drugs such as the aminoglycosides. Oral agents, including ampicillin (500 mg four times a day), trimethoprim-sulfamethoxasole (one double-strength tablet twice a day), ciprofloxacin (500 mg twice a day), and metronidazole (250 mg three times a day), have been used. For patients with a more severe clinical presentation, ampicillin or mezlocillin in conjunction with an aminoglycoside is usually used. Cefotaxime or other third-generation cephalosporins can also be used, but these do not cover *Enterococcus,* and metronidazole should probably be added for increased anaerobic coverage if these drugs are chosen.

B. BILIARY TREE STRICTURES

Dominant strictures of the biliary tree in primary sclerosing cholangitis can lead to a rapid but reversible deterioration in liver function. Cholangiography is indicated in this setting, with possible balloon dilatation. Cytologic brushings should be obtained to exclude the presence of complicating cholangiocarcinoma as a cause of the stricture. Dominant strictures may also require stenting for 3–6 months after dilatation to maintain patency of the bile duct, but this may lead to complications.

C. BILIARY STONE DISEASE

Biliary stone disease is also a potential explanation for worsening liver tests, the onset of pruritus, or cholangitis. Endoscopic cholangiography is usually diagnostic and can be combined with sphincterotomy and stone removal. Biliary stone disease is a common complication in patients with primary sclerosing cholangitis, occurring in approximately 25% of these patients, but the stones are usually confined to the gallbladder. Patients with recurrent cholangitis may also develop intraductal pigment stones due to recurrent infection.

D. CHOLANGIOCARCINOMA

As noted above, cholangiocarcinoma may develop in up to 10–15% of patients with primary sclerosing cholangitis, usually in those with advanced disease. Differentiation of cholangiocarcinoma from preexisting primary sclerosing cholangitis is difficult, and detection early

Table 51–7. Comparison of the features of primary biliary cirrhosis and primary sclerosing cholangitis.

	Primary Biliary Cirrhosis	Primary Sclerosing Cholangitis
Mean age	53 years	41 years
Gender (M:F)	1:9	2:1
Inflammatory bowel disease	< 1%	70%
Sicca	50%	2%
Biochemical findings	Cholestatic	Cholestatic
Antimitochondrial antibodies	90–95%	< 5%
Cholangiography	Normal (or changes of cirrhosis)	Characteristic multifocal strictures
Liver histologic findings	Paucity of bile ducts, granulomatous cholangitis	Paucity of bile ducts, fibrous obliterative cholangitis

enough to allow surgical cure is unusual. Liver transplantation is seldom successful for patients with cholangiocarcinoma but may be useful in highly selected patients with localized disease.

E. PERISTOMAL VARICES

Another complication in patients with primary sclerosing cholangitis and portal hypertension is the development of peristomal varices around an ileostomy site in patients with colitis who have had a colectomy. These varices may bleed severely, and local measures are usually unable to control the bleeding. Portacaval shunts have been used but may make subsequent liver transplantation more difficult. The role of angiographic portal decompression by transjugular intrahepatic portasystemic shunting (TIPS) is uncertain.

Treatment

A. SURGICAL TREATMENT

Aggressive surgical approaches have been attempted to relieve strictures in primary sclerosing cholangitis; however, there is considerably less enthusiasm now for this approach. Because of the widespread intrahepatic disease, it is unlikely that surgical correction of isolated abnormalities of the extrahepatic biliary system will be sufficient in most cases. Aggressive endoscopic dilatation and stenting are advocated by some but has not been evaluated in controlled studies.

B. DRUG TREATMENT

Ursodeoxycholic acid has been intensively investigated. Biochemical improvement has been reported in several series, and isolated reports have suggested improvement in symptoms, histologic findings, and cholangiographic findings. A regimen of 10–15 mg/kg/d in three or four divided doses has been used in most studies. In the largest ones, only biochemical benefit was seen. Higher doses of ursodeoxycholic acid (20–30 mg/kg/d) appear promising. The results of ongoing, randomized trials should help clarify the role of this agent.

Aggressive control of concurrent inflammatory bowel disease by measures such as colectomy or use of antibiotics has not been successful, as the severity of the biliary and bowel disease does not correlate in most patients. Copper depletion therapy with penicillamine is ineffective. Immunosuppressive therapy with corticosteroids, whether administered topically or systemically, is not beneficial for primary sclerosing cholangitis and may worsen the associated osteopenia. Similarly, methotrexate has no proved effect. Oral nicotine, colchicine, pentoxifylline, and pirfenidone have not been shown to be useful.

C. LIVER TRANSPLANTATION

Liver transplantation has been reserved for patients with end-stage primary sclerosing cholangitis and is successful in most of these patients (see Chapter 54). Previous colectomy or biliary surgery may make transplantation technically more difficult. In theory, the choledochojejunostomy used in transplantation increases the risks of biliary complications. However, the 5-year survival rate of patients transplanted for primary sclerosing cholangitis is similar to that of patients with primary biliary cirrhosis. Retransplantation is more common in patients with primary sclerosing cholangitis than primary biliary cirrhosis, however. Recurrence of the primary sclerosing cholangitis occurs in up to 20% of patients and accelerated risks of developing colon cancer in patients with underlying inflammatory bowel disease are noted. Monitoring for colon cancer is appropriate, but the increased risk should not influence the decision to perform transplantation in patients with primary sclerosing cholangitis.

Prognosis

The prognosis of primary sclerosing cholangitis varies considerably. The average survival is approximately 10 years, with progression of liver disease over this interval. In a study from the author's institution, one-third of patients followed for 6 years developed liver failure. Progression of disease may be asymptomatic or symptomatic. Models for predicting survival rates and aiding in the timing of transplantation have been developed based on age of the patient, bilirubin levels, aspartate aminotransferase (AST) levels, and history of variceal bleeding.

OTHER DISEASES OF THE BILE DUCTS

Other diseases of the bile ducts include extrahepatic biliary obstruction and papillary stenosis. Incomplete mechanical obstruction of the bile duct may be difficult to differentiate from primary biliary cirrhosis and primary sclerosing cholangitis. Frequently, however, dilated bile ducts will be present on abdominal imaging and provide an important diagnostic clue to mechanical obstruction. This diagnosis should not be overlooked, because liver disease is reversible before secondary biliary cirrhosis arises. Secondary biliary cirrhosis can occur within 6 months of the onset of mechanical obstruction, but more typically develops over several years. Cholangiography is usually diagnostic. Liver biopsy may suggest features of mechanical obstruction such as bile infarcts, edema in the portal area, bile duct proliferation, and neutrophilic infiltrates. Mechanical obstruction should be considered when a biopsy shows edema and neutrophilic infiltrates. In contrast, in primary sclerosing cholangitis there is primarily fibrosis rather than edema, and the inflammatory cells are frequently mononuclear rather than neutrophilic.

Papillary stenosis or sphincter of Oddi dysfunction may occasionally be confused with primary problems of the bile duct in a patient complaining of upper abdominal pain who has abnormal liver tests (see Chapter 50). The existence of this process is controversial, and optimum management has not yet been established. A sphincterotomy has been used most often, but this has not been well studied in controlled trials.

REFERENCES

Angulo P et al: Magnetic resonance cholangiography in the evaluation of the biliary tree: its role in patients with primary sclerosing cholangitis. J Hepatol 2000;33(4):520.

Brentnall TA et al: Risk and natural history of colonic neoplasia in patients with primary sclerosing cholangitis and ulcerative colitis. Gastroenterology 1996;110:331.

Combes B et al: A randomized, double-blind, placebo-controlled trial of ursodeoxycholic acid in primary biliary cirrhosis. Hepatology 1995;22:759.

Goulis J, Leandro G, Burroughs AK: Radomised controlled trials of ursodeoxycholic acid therapy for primary biliary cirrhosis: a meta-analysis. Lancet 1999;354:1053.

Harnois DM et al: High-dose ursodeoxycholic acid as a therapy for patients with primary sclerosing cholangitis. Am J Gastroenterol 2001;96(5):1558.

Kaplan MM: Primary biliary cirrhosis. N Engl J Med 1996;335:1570.

Lindor KD and the Mayo PSC/UDCA Study Group: Ursodiol for primary sclerosing cholangitis. N Engl J Med 1997;336:691.

Metcalf JV et al: Natural history of primary biliary cirrhosis. Lancet 1996;348:1399.

Metcalf JV et al: Incidence and prevalence of primary bilary cirrhosis in the city of Newcastle upon Tyne, England. Int J Epidemiol 1997;26(4):830.

Poupon RE et al: Combined analysis of French, American, and Candian randomized controlled trials of ursodeoxycholic acid in primary biliary cirrhosis. Gastroenterology 1997;113: 884.

Tumors of the Ampulla & Bile Ducts   52

Sarah A. Little, MB, ChB & William R. Jarnagin, MD

Tumors of the ampulla and bile ducts comprise a heterogeneous group of diseases with a generally unfavorable prognosis. Their leading symptom is jaundice secondary to biliary tract obstruction and investigations are targeted toward determining the cause and level of bilary obstruction and delineating disease extent to determine whether resection is possible. Management paradigms for these malignancies continue to evolve as diagnostic imaging modalities, surgical techniques, and perioperative care improve. Indeed, despite the historically dismal reputation of these tumors, recent advances have meant that potentially curative resection can be safely accomplished and may lead to long-term survival in selected patients. Therefore, every patient who presents with malignant obstruction of the bile ducts deserves careful investigation before being consigned to palliative therapy.

CHOLANGIOCARCINOMA

Cholangiocarcinoma is an uncommon malignancy with a poor prognosis. Most patients present with jaundice, pruritus, fever, or weight loss. Median life expectancy is around 6–12 months from diagnosis, with death resulting from liver failure or infectious complications secondary to biliary obstruction. Surgery is the treatment of choice for cure, with chemoradiation having shown poor results. However, the majority of patients present at an advanced disease stage, when palliation is the only option.

This section will briefly review the epidemiology, etiology, and pathology of these lesions and then discuss the appropriate management of patients with suspected primary malignancy of the bile ducts.

Epidemiology & Etiology

Cholangiocarcinoma has an annual incidence of 1–2 per 100,000 population in the United States. It is more common in Native Americans, with an incidence of 6.5 per 100,000 population, and Japanese Americans, with an incidence of 5.5 per 100,000 population. It generally occurs in patients older than 65 years of age, with peak incidence in the eighth decade of life. The exact etiology of cholangiocarcinoma is not known, however,

there are several well-defined conditions that confer an excess risk. More recently, mutations in the *p53* tumor suppressor gene have been associated with peripheral cholangiocarcinoma and K-*ras* mutations with extrahepatic cholangiocarcinoma.

Primary sclerosing cholangitis (PSC) is an autoimmune condition that causes a diffuse inflammation of the periductal tissues and results in multifocal strictures throughout the biliary tree. The incidence of cholangiocarcinoma is variable in patients with this condition, however, in autopsy series, tumors have been found in up to 40% of patients and in 36% of liver explants. These patients may have multifocal tumors and the tumor develops earlier than in other patients, around the fifth decade of life. Around 70–80% of patients with PSC will have associated ulcerative colitis; in contrast, only a minority of patients with ulcerative colitis will develop PSC. Medical or surgical treatment for ulcerative colitis does not remove the subsequent risk of developing cholangiocarcinoma.

Biliary infestation is prevalent throughout Asia. *Chlonorchis senensis* and *Opisthorchis viverrini,* parasites common in Asia, migrate into the intrahepatic biliary tree via the portal circulation and cause biliary obstruction, inflammation, and periductal fibrosis, which is probably a premalignant lesion.

Hepatolithiasis (also known as recurrent pyogenic cholangiohepatitis or Oriental cholangiohepatitis) is again prevalent in Japan and other Asian countries. It involves formation of intrahepatic pigment stones and is thought to arise from recurrent episodes of biliary infection and portal phlebitis that result in stricture development. These patients have a 10% lifetime risk of developing cholangiocarcinoma.

Congenital biliary cystic disease (choledochal cysts, Caroli's disease) is well known to confer an increased risk of cholangiocarcinoma, especially in those patients who do not have diagnosis and cyst excision until later in life (older than 20 years of age). The cause for malignant transformation of the biliary tree in these patients may be an abnormal junction between the pancreatic duct and the common bile duct, which predisposes to reflux of pancreatic juice into the biliary tree, with resulting chronic inflammation.

Chemical carcinogens, although less well characterized, are other causative agents. They include thorium dioxide, asbestos, and nitrosamines.

Pathologic Findings

Although cholangiocarcinomas may arise in any part of the biliary tree, they are most often found at the biliary confluence (so-called Klatskin tumors). Tumors in this area comprise around 40–60% of cases, with around 10% in the intrahepatic biliary tree (peripheral cholangiocarcinoma) and the remainder in the extrahepatic ducts, either at the mid-duct or distally. Distal cholangiocarcinomas comprise around 10% of all periampullary tumors. Tumor location within the biliary tree probably has little influence on survival, provided full resection can be achieved. A small number of patients will have multifocal disease; this is almost never amenable to surgery and the prognosis is poor.

Macroscopically, tumors of the extrahepatic bile ducts fall in to three distinct subtypes: sclerosing, nodular, and papillary. Sclerosing is the most common type of tumor and is usually found at the hilus, where it forms a firm ring-like thickening of the bile duct. There is often extensive subepithelial or longitudinal spread of tumor, emphasizing the role of frozen section intraoperative analysis of bile duct margins during resection. Nodular tumors are also firm tumors but project into the lumen of the bile duct. Features of both subtypes are often seen in the one tumor (nodular–sclerosing type). The papillary variant, which is the least common, forms a soft pedunculated mass and may grow to sizable proportion, thereby expanding the bile duct. It occurs in around 10% of cases, but is often resectable and carries a better prognosis than the other subtypes. The majority of cholangiocarcinomas are adenocarcinomas; they are often well differentiated and may be mucin producing. They may express carcinoembryonic antigen (CEA) or the serum carbohydrate antigen CA 19-9, although these are not usually helpful diagnostically.

Historically considered a slow growing, locally invasive cancer, recent evidence suggests that metastatic disease is common with cholangiocarcinoma. Up to one-third of patients will have metastases to the peritoneal cavity, liver parenchyma, or regional lymph nodes at presentation and these may not be identified on preoperative radiologic studies.

Clinical Findings

The clinical presentation of cholangiocarcinoma is in part dependent on its location within the biliary tree. Unfortunately, most patients present when the tumor has advanced locally or metastatic disease has occurred, both features that preclude resection and, therefore, cure.

A. SYMPTOMS AND SIGNS

Early symptoms are nonspecific and may include malaise, anorexia, weight loss, jaundice, or upper abdominal pain. Although bacterial contamination of bile (bacterbilia) is fairly common, cholangitis is unusual at the outset and fever is not usually a presenting symptom. The majority of patients will be asymptomatic initially and cholangiocarcinoma is discovered during investigation for abnormal serum liver function values or jaundice. Most patients will become jaundiced at some point in the course of their disease, however, this may not be seen at first, particularly if there is obstruction of only the right or left hepatic duct or peripheral segmental obstruction. A distal cholangiocarcinoma will result in biliary obstruction early in the course of disease and a progressive jaundice is seen in 75–90% of these patients. Papillary lesions may cause intermittent jaundice.

On examination, there may be few specific signs, however, a thorough clinical evaluation is essential as part of the presurgical assessment. The patient may appear cachectic, and jaundice is usually clinically obvious at serum bilirubin levels greater than 40 mmol/L; pruritus may result in extensive skin excoriations. Biliary obstruction may cause firm hepatomegaly, although the gallbladder is usually not palpable. However, a distal obstruction may result in a distended, palpable, gallbladder (Courvoisier's sign). Occasionally there may be features of portal hypertension, if biliary or portal vein obstruction has been prolonged or cirrhosis is present. Ascites is uncommon, unless there is portal vein occlusion or carcinomatosis.

B. LABORATORY FINDINGS

Initial laboratory tests will show an obstructive pattern, including elevated serum bilirubin, alkaline phosphatase, and γ-glutamyltransferase. There may be a mild hypoalbuminemia and anemia. CEA and α-fetoprotein (AFP) are not generally elevated and hepatitis serologies are usually negative. Serum CA 19-9 is not diagnostically helpful, although very high levels may be associated with advanced disease.

C. IMAGING STUDIES

The diagnosis of cholangiocarcinoma is usually made during the investigation for obstructive jaundice. It is important to bear in mind that cholangiocarcinoma may coexist with a variety of biliary lesions such as gallstones, primary biliary sclerosis, or choledochal cystic disease. Therefore, a thorough investigation of the level and nature of biliary obstruction must be carried out so that a carcinoma is not missed. High-quality imaging studies are vital, both to elucidate the cause of obstruction and to delineate the lesion and its associated features, so that it may be determined whether resection is possible. If the tumor is amenable to resection, then a definitive tissue diagnosis prior to surgery is not mandatory. Patients who have an appropriate clinical history and are found on imaging to have a focal stenotic lesion can be given the presumptive diagnosis of cholangiocarcinoma, which will prove to be correct in most cases. However, if only palliative treatment is planned, then a percutaneous or endoscopic biopsy is usually performed. Patients for whom surgical intervention is proposed should also receive a full cardiorespiratory assessment to ensure that they are fit to undergo a major surgical procedure, which will often include a partial hepatectomy for proximal lesions, or a pancreatic resection for distal lesions.

Nearly all patients can be fully investigated with noninvasive studies, specifically duplex ultrasonography and magnetic resonance cholangiopancreatography (MRCP). These noninvasive studies are preferred since they avoid biliary instrumentation and the subsequent increase in perioperative morbidity. An ultrasound examination is usually the first imaging modality. Although operator dependant, it is extremely useful to de-

termine the level of biliary obstruction, the presence of dilated ducts, and whether there is involvement of vascular structures, particularly the portal vein, for which it has at least 95% specificity and sensitivity (Figure 52–1). It can also delineate the extent of tumor invasion within the bile duct and periductal tissues. MRCP is a cross-sectional noninvasive imaging study that can show the extent of tumor involvement in the hepatic parenchyma, patency of vascular structures at the liver hilus, and the presence of nodal or distant metastatic disease. A computed tomography (CT) scan, which is more widely available than MRCP, is an alternative investigation and high-quality CT scan can also adequately show the level of biliary obstruction, vascular involvement, or liver atrophy (Figure 52–2).

Percutaneous transhepatic cholangiography has been used in the past to delineate tumor location and extent of involvement of the biliary tree. It is an invasive study and can substantially increase the risk of cholangitis prior to surgery, which is undesirable. It has largely been replaced by MRCP for the investigation of cholangiocarcinoma, although surgical centers in Japan continue to use it extensively, often combined with direct cholangioscopy. Patients with evidence of cholan-

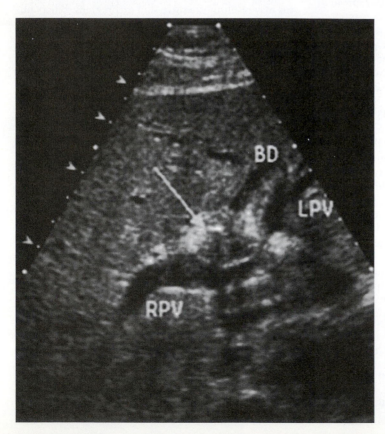

Figure 52–1. Duplex ultrasonography illustrating a hilar cholangiocarcinoma **(arrow)** invading the bifurcation of the right (RPV) and left (LPV) portal vein. This demonstrates the utility of ultrasound, by an experienced operator, in delineating vascular invasion by cholangiocarcinoma. BD, bile duct.

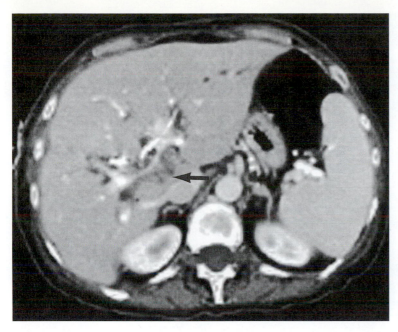

Figure 52–2. CT scan demonstrating a hilar cholangiocarcinoma **(arrow)** encasing the main portal vein—a contraindication to resection.

gitis clearly require adequate biliary decompression if resection is considered.

Differential Diagnosis

Most patients who present with a stricture of the biliary hilus and jaundice will have cholangiocarcinoma, although an alternative diagnosis may occur in around 10% of patients and should be considered. The most common differential diagnosis is gallbladder cancer and distinguishing between the two can be difficult. Patients with gallbladder cancer may have a thickened, irregular gallbladder on cross-sectional imaging, often with invasion into segments IV and V of the liver, with concomitant obstruction of the common hepatic duct or cystic duct.

There are also benign conditions that may mimic cholangiocarcinoma. The first of these is Mirizzi syndrome, which results from the impaction of a large gallstone in the neck of the gallbladder (Figure 52–3). This may cause secondary periductal and pericystic inflammation and proximal bile duct obstruction. More rarely, idiopathic benign focal strictures may occur at the hilus (so called "malignant masquerade"). Whenever there is diagnostic uncertainty, it is unwise to exclude cholangiocarcinoma based on the results of biliary brush cytology or percutaneous biopsy, as the false negative rate is high. Surgical exploration is required in these patients, or the opportunity to resect an early malignant lesion may be missed. Furthermore, many of the alternative diagnoses are best treated by operative intervention in any case.

Distal cholangiocarcinoma is one of many tumors that may be classified as periampullary carcinoma. These include carcinoma of the head of the pancreas and papillary tumors (vide infra); often the precise pathologic diagnosis is not known until after resection. A dilated common bile duct, with a distal stricture and a normal appearing pancreatic duct, is suggestive of bile duct or ampullary cancer, rather than pancreatic cancer.

Treatment

Complete resection remains the only treatment modality with the potential for cure of cholangiocarcinoma. It is therefore prudent that all patients are fully and carefully evaluated for a proposed resection by an experienced team before any palliative treatments, such as biliary decompression, are performed. The placement of biliary stents may cause local infection and inflammation that can make subsequent resection challenging and so should be avoided before a full assessment of the extent of disease has taken place. If surgery is clearly not appropriate, as will be the case in the majority of patients, there are several palliative options available. It should always be remembered that these patients have a relatively short life expectancy; therefore the potential benefits of any palliative interventions must be balanced against procedure-related morbidity, increased hospital stay, and the subsequent affect on quality of life.

Several centers have attempted to use orthotopic liver transplant for the treatment of cholangiocarcinoma. However, the results are disappointing, with few

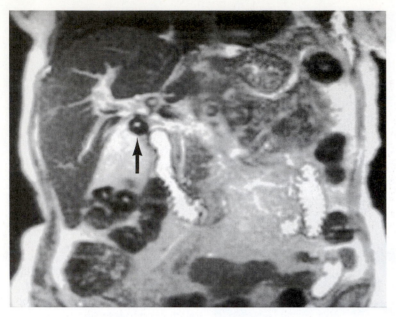

Figure 52–3. Magnetic resonance cholangiopancreatography (MRCP) (sagittal image) demonstrating Mirrizi syndrome—a large gallstone *(arrow)* is impacted at the neck of the gallbladder and compressing the common bile duct.

survivors beyond 2 years. Particularly in the current climate of national shortage of donor organs, liver transplantation is not currently recommended for cholangiocarcinoma except in experimental protocols.

A. RESECTION

A potentially curative resection for cholangiocarcinoma will involve complete resection of all gross disease with negative histologic margins and restoration of biliary-enteric continuity. The preoperative evaluation must first confirm the patient's fitness for a major surgical procedure, which will frequently include a liver resection. Patients who have chronic liver disease or portal hypertension are generally not candidates for surgery. In addition, if biliary tract sepsis is present, this must be treated and the patient resuscitated prior to resection. In patients with hilar cholangiocarcinoma, high-quality radiologic studies prior to operative intervention are extremely important and are required to investigate the four main determinants of resectability: (1) the extent of tumor within the biliary tree, (2) vascular invasion, (3) hepatic lobar atrophy, and (4) metastatic disease. The importance of lobar atrophy in patients with hilar cholangiocarcinoma cannot be overemphasized. Atrophy may result from longstanding ipsilateral biliary obstruction, but more commonly implies tumor involvement of the ipsilateral portal vein. The finding of an atrophic lobe, which appears small and is often hypoperfused with crowded and dilated intrahepatic bile ducts, has several clinical implications (Figure 52–4). First, if the tumor is resectable, then partial hepatec-

tomy will be required. Second, the presence of lobar atrophy with tumor extension to second-order biliary radicles on the contralateral lobe or tumor involvement of the contralateral portal vein is a contraindication to resection. Also, if the tumor is not resectable, biliary drainage must be performed using the contralateral, hypertrophic lobe, since drainage of the atrophic liver will not relieve jaundice. The criteria that render a patient unresectable are detailed in Table 52–1. For distal bile duct tumors, extension into adjacent organs and blood vessels must be delineated.

The critical determinant of outcome for cholangiocarcinoma is a complete resection with a negative margin. To achieve this, patients with proximal tumors generally will require a partial hepatectomy via a bilateral subcostal incision. Indeed, several recent studies have documented the positive relationship between the use of hepatectomy and a complete resection (Table 52–2). The resection may be preceded by laparoscopy, which can identify small peritoneal or liver nodules not seen on preoperative imaging studies and thus prevent some patients from being subjected to a major procedure that would not improve outcome. Small tumors may be managed with a limited resection, but this still necessitates removal of the entire supraduodenal bile duct, gallbladder, extrahepatic bile ducts, and related lymph nodes. Distal bile duct tumors are usually resected with a pancreaticoduodenectomy (Whipple procedure). A hepaticojejunostomy via a Roux-en-Y loop of jejunum is created to restore biliary-enteric continuity.

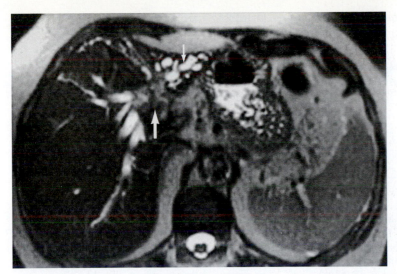

Figure 52–4. Magnetic resonance cholangiopancreatography (MRCP) (axial image) demonstrating atrophy of the left lobe of the liver, secondary to a mass at the biliary confluence ***(large arrow).*** The bile ducts ***(small arrow)*** appear dilated and crowded, with little normal hepatic parenchyma interposed

B. Chemotherapy and Radiation

No studies have yet shown that chemotherapy or radiation can improve survival significantly when given as an adjuvant therapy (after surgery) for cholangiocarcinoma. Similarly, chemotherapy alone has not improved survival when given palliatively and should not be used outside a clinical trial. Patients with advanced local disease, but no metastatic disease, may be candidates for palliative radiation either intraluminally or externally. This may provide symptomatic relief, but again does not appear to alter long-term outcome.

C. Palliation

The majority of patients with cholangiocarcinoma, especially those with proximal lesions, are not suitable for surgical resection and so will be managed in a palliative setting. This will include supportive care and usually some form of biliary decompression, either percutaneously or endoscopically. However, this can often cause substantial procedure-related morbidity and so jaundice alone does not necessarily mandate drainage. Indications usually include intractable pruritus or cholangitis or the need to restore hepatic parenchymal function prior to chemotherapy administration. Hilar tumors are best managed with percutaneous transhepatic biliary drainage and placement of one or more metallic endoprostheses (Wallstents). These may remain patent for around 6 months, although around 25% will occlude, requiring reintervention. Patients who are found to be unresectable at operation may have a surgical bypass performed using the segment III bile duct. Distal bile duct tumors may be managed with an endoscopically placed prosthesis.

Prognosis

Over the past decade, there has been increasing acceptance of the requirement for liver resection in order to

Table 52–1. Criteria for unresectability in patients with hilar cholangiocarcinoma.

Factor	Description
Patient factors	Medically unfit for operation
	Cirrhosis/portal hypertension
Local factors	Encasement or occlusion of the main portal vein proximal to its bifurcation
	Hepatic duct involvement up to secondary radicles bilaterally
	Atrophy of one lobe with encasement of contralateral portal vein branch
	Atrophy of one lobe with contralateral involvement of secondary biliary radicles
Distant disease	Liver, lung, or peritoneal metastases
	Histologically proven metastases to N2 lymph nodes

Adapted, with permission, from Burke EC et al: Hilar cholangiocarcinoma: patterns of spread, the importance of hepatic resection for curative operation, and a presurgical clinical staging system. Ann Surg 1998;228:385.

Table 52–2. Influence of partial hepatectomy on histologic margins in patients who underwent a potentially curative resection for hilar cholangiocarcinoma: summary of recent studies.

Author	Potential Curative Resection (n)	Hepatectomy (%)	Negative Margins (%)
Burke et al (1998)	30	73	83
Klempnauer et al (1997)	147	79	79
Cameron et al (1990)	39	20	15
Hadjis et al (1990)	27	60	56
Nimura et al (1990)	55	98	83

achieve a margin-negative excision for hilar cholangiocarcinoma. This has been responsible for the gradual increase in survival rates for these patients, such that the median survival is now around 40 months after a potentially curative surgery (5-year survival is 45–56%). For resection of distal bile duct tumors, the 5-year survival is around 30%, which is probably better than the survival rate for pancreatic adenocarcinoma. Unfortunately, the presentation of cholangiocarcinoma usually late in its natural history means that the majority of patients are candidates only for palliative care, and as such, have a median survival of 6–12 months.

GALLBLADDER CARCINOMA

The late presentation and paucity of effective treatments for gallbladder cancer have meant that its diagnosis is often met with a sense of therapeutic nihilism. The 5-year survival is around 5% and few patients are alive more than 6 months after diagnosis. In recent years, however, advances in anesthesia and perioperative care have made radical liver resection increasingly safe and may allow a select group of patients the opportunity for longer survival.

Epidemiology & Etiology

Gallbladder cancer is the most common biliary tract neoplasm and is the fifth most common gastrointestinal malignancy in the United States, with an estimated annual incidence of around 1.2 cases per 100,000 population. However, it has a heterogeneous geographic and racial distrubution worldwide. Highest incidences are found in Chile, Israel, and northeastern Europe, and in American Indian populations and in Americans of Mexican descent. Within the Western world, the incidence is inversely related to socioeconomic status—this possibly may be due to delayed access to cholecystectomy. It most commonly occurs in the seventh decade of life, and women are two to six times more commonly affected than men. In the United States, the incidence of gallbladder cancer is currently stable or in decline, which coincides with the increase in the number of cholecystectomies performed in recent years.

The main etiologic factor for gallbladder cancer seems to be chronic epithelial irritation and inflammation, arising usually as the result of gallstones. The geographic and racial variances of gallbladder cancer are directly related to the incidence of gallstones. However, the incidence of gallbladder cancer in population groups with high prevalences of gallstones ranges from only 0.3 to 3% in epidemiologic studies, which suggests that some other factors are involved. It may be that chronic inflammation is a promoter, which can incite damage by environmental carcinogenic agents, although this has been difficult to replicate in animal models. Bacterial contamination of the biliary tree is common in conjunction with gallstones and chronic cholecystitis and may be a factor. Other chemical carcinogens implicated include isoniazid, methyldopa, and the oral contraceptive pill, although all are, as yet, unproven.

One well-known association is with calcification of the gallbladder wall (porcelain gallbladder), which is thought to arise as a result of longstanding inflammation and scarring. These patients have a 25% risk of developing gallbladder cancer, and should undergo prophylactic open cholecystectomy. In the general population, however, the low incidence of gallbladder cancer relative to the fairly high incidence of gallstones means that cholecystectomy should still be performed only in symptomatic patients.

Pathologic Findings & Staging

As with many gastrointestinal malignancies, gallbladder cancer is thought to occur from a progression along a pathway from dyplasia to carcinoma *in situ* to invasive carcinoma. The time to progression from early dysplastic lesions to carcinoma is thought to be around 15 years. Grossly, these tumors may be classified as infiltrative, nodular, combined infiltrative–nodular, papillary, and combined papillary–infiltrative forms. Infiltrative is the most common type and spreads along the subserosal tissue plane (the same plane used for cholecystectomy) and, as such, can easily be disseminated at surgery. Prognostically, the papillary subtype has a significantly better outcome. Around 60% of tumors arise in the fundus, 30% in the body, and 10% in the neck of the gallbladder.

Most gallbladder tumors are adenocarcinomas, although squamous, adenosquamous, or oat cell carcinomas may occur more rarely. Histologically, they may be graded from G1 (well differentiated) to G4 (undifferentiated), although this has little influence on outcome and most are graded G3 (poorly differentiated). Again, *p53* and K-*ras* mutations are the most common genetic changes identified, being found in 92% and 39% of invasive carcinomas, respectively. Other mutations thus far identified include decreased expression of the nm23 gene product and over expression of the c-*erb*B-2 gene product.

Gallbladder cancer is an exceptionally aggressive malignancy and has an unrivaled capacity to seed in the peritoneal cavity, needle biopsy tract, and laparoscopic port sites. It tends to metastasize early and the thin lamina propria and single muscle layer of the viscus allows early tumor invasion into the lymphatic system, liver, and other adjacent organs. At initial presentation, only 10% of patients will have disease confined to the gallbladder. Of the remainder, around 60% of patients will have hepatic invasion, 45% regional lymph node metastasis, and 20% extrahepatic blood-borne metastases. It is important to accurately stage patients, since this has been shown to be the most consistent predictor of outcome. Several staging systems have been developed for gallbladder cancer, however, the AJCC/UICC tumor/node/metastasis (TNM) system is most commonly used in the United States (Table 52–3).

Table 52–3. Summary of the AJCC/UICC tumor/node/metastasis (TNM) staging system for gallbladder cancer.

Stage	Description
1	Mucosal or muscular invasion (T1N0M0)
2	Perimuscular invasion (T2N0M0)
3	Transmural invasion, liver invasion <2 cm; lymph node metastasis to hepatoduodenal ligament (T2N0M0, T1–3M1M0)
4A	Liver invasion >2 cm (T4N0M0, T4N1M0)
4B	Distant nodule (outside porta hepatitis) or hematogenous metastasis (TxN2M0, TxNxM1)

Clinical Findings

A. Symptoms and Signs

The presenting symptoms of gallbladder cancer are very similar to those of biliary colic and chronic cholecystitis and so the tumor is often unsuspected prior to cholecystectomy. However, a thorough history may reveal a change to longstanding and constant upper abdominal pain from the more typical cramping right upper quadrant pain associated with biliary colic. The diagnosis should be considered in elderly patients, particularly if other symptoms consistent with malignancy are present, such as anorexia and weight loss. The presence of such symptoms, or jaundice, often indicates advanced, irresectable disease.

B. Laboratory Findings

Serum tumor markers are occasionally helpful when radiologic investigations are ambiguous. A CEA level greater than 4 ng/mL is 93% specific and 50% sensitive for gallbladder cancer in patients in whom the disease is suspected. CA 19-9 is more useful, with 79.4% sensitivity and 79.5% specificity at levels greater then 20 U/mL. An elevated CA 19-9 is less specific in jaundiced patients, presumably because the antigen metabolism is altered by decreased liver function. Elevations of serum bilirubin and alkaline phosphatase generally indicate advanced disease. Solitary elevations of alkaline phosphatase may occur at an early stage secondary to isolated obstruction of the right hepatic duct.

C. Imaging Studies

The initial radiologic investigations for gallbladder cancer usually involve an ultrasound examination and CT scan. Over the past decades, the increase in the use of these two imaging modalities has meant that at least 75% of gallbladder cancers are now diagnosed prior to cholecystectomy. The ultrasound features of gallbladder cancer include discontiguous or echogenic mucosa or echolucency of the submucosa, in addition to a discrete mass. Ultrasound may also demonstrate the presence of gallstones, gallbladder polyps, biliary tree dilatation, and the level of biliary obstruction and provide information on the relationship of the tumor to major vascular structures. A CT scan may identify regional lymph node or intraperitoneal metastases. Endoscopic ultrasound can also demonstrate peripancreatic and periportal lymphadenopathy and can be used to direct a needle biopsy and thus prevent a laparotomy.

For advanced tumors causing obstructive jaundice, a percutaneous transhepatic cholangiogram (PTC) or endoscopic retrograde cholangiopancreatography (ERCP) may be useful to differentiate gallbladder cancer from other benign or malignant causes of obstructive jaundice, or for palliative intervention. If a malignant stricture of the mid-bile duct is present, gallbladder cancer should be assumed until proven otherwise. Since gallbladder cancer has a great ability to seed the tract of a percutaneous biopsy, such a procedure is not recommended if a curative resection is planned; it should, however, be done for all patients who are to be managed palliatively. An alternative method for obtaining a definitive tissue diagnosis is the use of bile cytology, which should be performed in all patients undergoing ERCP or PTC. The sensitivity of this test has been reported as between 50% and 73% for gallbladder cancer, with a false positive rate of less than 1%.

Treatment

A. RESECTION

As with cholangiocarcinmoma, surgery is the only potentially curative treatment for gallbladder cancer. The precise surgical intervention required is largely determined by the extent of invasion through the gallbladder wall. Stage I tumors may be safely treated with simple cholecystectomy and in fact are often noted incidentally on pathologic examination after such a procedure, for presumed benign disease. However, controversy still exists about the correct management for stage II and III tumors and recommendations vary between centers and countries. For those patients diagnosed preoperatively, en bloc resection of the gallbladder, segments IVb and V of the liver, and a regional lymphadenectomy should be performed. Patients with stage II and stage III disease discovered after laparoscopic cholecystectomy should undergo a reresection. This should include a partial hepatectomy and lymph node dissection, since it is likely that the subserosal plane used for the initial cholecystectomy will have left microscopic tumor *in situ* (vide supra) and these patients will frequently have nodal metastases. In a recent series from Memorial Sloan-Kettering Cancer Center, patients with T2 cancers submitted to reresection had a 5-year survival of 61% compared with just 19% in those who had cholecystectomy alone. Additionally, patients with apparently resectable T3 and T4 tumors who did not undergo reresection all died of disease within 1 year. Laparoscopic port sites should also be excised since the risk of recurrence there is high. More radical procedures, such as hepatic trisegmentectomy, may occasionally be justified for a large tumor without lymph node metastases or a small tumor at the infundibulum of the gallbladder that involves the right bile duct and portal vein. Stage IV disease usually indicates an advanced, unresectable malignancy, although rarely an extended resection may be curative for patients without lymph node metastases. Again the potential procedure-related

mortality and morbidity should be considered carefully before embarking on radical surgery for stage III and IV disease, which are aggressive malignancies with relatively low rates of long-term survival.

Centers in Japan advocate radical resection for all patients, including hepatectomy, pancreaticoduodenectomy, and lymph node dissection. Thus far, the survival after such radical resections is insufficient (and the morbidity too high) to routinely recommend this.

B. PALLIATION

Palliation of gallbladder cancer is directed at relief of pain, jaundice, and bowel obstruction, in the context of progressive malignancy where life expectancy is short. For patients found to be unresectable at operation, surgical bypass of biliary obstruction may be appropriate, using a hepaticojejunostomy to a dilated segment III duct. However, the potential prophylactic benefit of such a procedure must always be balanced against the risk of developing a postoperative anastomotic leak, which may result in patients spending much of the rest of their life hospitalized. Alternatively, percutaneous drainage may be performed once symptoms of advanced disease, such as pruritus, occur.

Gallbladder cancer had thus far proven to be relatively resistant to chemotherapy agents. For unresectable patients, systemic agents such as 5-fluorouracil, adriamycin, gemcitabine, and nitroureases have shown some response, but not high enough to be recommended routinely. The mode of spread of gallbladder cancer through the peritoneal cavity means that palliative radiotherapy is difficult to target and has proven to be of little benefit.

Prognosis

Overall, gallbladder cancer is an aggressive disease with a poor prognosis; disease stage is the most significant predictor of outcome. However, definitive resection at the initial procedure may provide a cure. Therefore, careful preoperative scrutiny of radiologic studies in patients with suspicious clinical features is mandatory. The overall 5-year survival rate is consistently less than 5%, with a median survival of 5–8 months and only 25% of all patients being suitable for surgical resection. On the other hand, for patients submitted to a complete resection, the 5-year survival is 100% for stage I disease, although this falls to around 67% and 33% for stage III and stage IV disease, respectively.

AMPULLARY CARCINOMA

Carcinoma of the ampulla is one of a heterogeneous group of neoplasms that may arise at the choledochoduodenal junction and comprise periampullary cancer. It accounts for 6–12% of these tumors, with carcinoma of the head of the pancreas comprising around 30% and the remainder a variety of other neoplasms such as duodenal tumors, distal bile duct tumors, and islet cell tumors. The management of these malignancies is broadly similar, with surgery again the only curative treatment modality. Their prognoses may vary widely and is largely dependent on the underlying pathology—carcinoma of the ampulla is thought to confer the most favorable prognosis following a complete resection.

Epidemiology & Etiology

Carcinoma of the ampulla is a relatively rare neoplasm, with an annual incidence of 0.57 per 100,000 population. These tumors represent around 2% of all gastrointestinal malignancies and account for approximately 20% of all tumors of the extrahepatic biliary tree. They usually occur from the seventh decade of life onward and are slightly more common in males.

The main population thus far identified at risk for ampullary cancer is composed of people with the hereditary condition familial adenomatous polyposis (FAP). These people develop multiple colon and small intestine polyps. Even for those who undergo a prophylactic colectomy, the most common cause of death is from ampullary cancer later in life. FAP confers a 100–200 times greater risk of developing ampullary cancer than the general population; 90% of these patients will develop ampullary and periampullary adenomas

Pathologic Findings

The majority of ampullary masses are carcinomas, although adenomas are common and neuroendocrine tumors have been reported; the exact diagnosis may be difficult to determine from a biopsy alone and the presence of malignancy is often not known until definitive pathologic examination after excision. The tumor may arise on the duodenal surface of the ampulla or its inner epithelial lining. Distant metastases are uncommon, although a recent series reported a 40% mean incidence of lymph node metastases at presentation, most commonly to the pancreaticoduodenal nodes. This is significant since several series have shown that the presence of positive nodal metastases is the most important predictor of survival (Table 52–4). The improved prognosis of these tumors compared with other biliary or pancreatic neoplasms is probably a reflection of their earlier presentation in combination with more favorable tumor biology. This may be because these tumors often have a morphology that is more similar to intestinal tumors than biliary or pancreatic tumors. In addition, the frequency with which these tumors occur in patients with FAP suggests they have some common genetic alteration with colonic neoplasms. Likewise, K-*ras* mutations also occur in these tumors in a pattern similar to colon cancers.

Clinical Findings

These tumors generally present as biliary obstruction and the history and physical examination will reflect that. Initial investigations are directed at determining the cause of obstruction and therefore the appropriate management.

A. SYMPTOMS AND SIGNS

Patients may give a history of fluctuating jaundice, in contrast to the progressive jaundice caused by other malignant biliary obstructions. This may be due to intermittent sloughing of tumor. Despite this, persistent jaundice is often a feature. Other nonspecific symptoms include anorexia, weight loss, or pruritus. Tumors that ulcerate can result in a moderate anemia and its symp-

Table 52–4. Clinicopathologic factors associated with survival in ampullary carcinoma.

Factor	Number of Patients	Median Survival (months)	P Value: Univariate Multivariate[1]
Resected	101	58.8	<.01
Unresected	22	9.7	—
Margins negative	89	59.5	<.01
Margins positive	4	11.3	.02
Negative nodes	55	69.7	<.01
Positive nodes	46	23.6	.04
Well/moderately differentiated	77	69.8	<.01
Poorly differentiated	22	20.8	.18

[1]Multivariate analysis performed for resected tumors only. Reproduced, with permission, from How JR et al: Factors predictive of survival in ampullary carcinoma. Ann Surg 1998;228:87.

toms thereof. On examination, hepatomegaly and a palpable distended gallbladder may be felt.

B. LABORATORY FINDINGS

As with other causes of malignant biliary obstruction, the most striking biochemical abnormalities will be an elevated serum bilirubin and alkaline phosphatase, although the transaminases may also be modestly elevated.

C. IMAGING STUDIES

An ultrasound examination is usually the first imaging investigation and can demonstrate the level of obstruction and resulting biliary dilatation. If an ampullary tumor is suspected, then a CT scan is preferred for further evaluation. This can delineate the tumor's relationship to the pancreas and other surrounding structures better than ultrasound, which is often limited in assessing distal structures due to the presence of overlying bowel. A CT scan can differentiate between alternative causes of distal biliary obstruction, such as carcinoma of the head of the pancreas, and demonstrate lymph node metastases. An MRCP is an alternative study, which is reportedly 85–100% accurate for predicting site and level of obstruction.

An ERCP and/or endoscopic ultrasound with biopsy may be useful for small lesions when the diagnosis is unclear or ultrasound and CT have failed to demonstrate the ampulla, as frequently occurs. However, ERCP with stent placement should not be routine practice in patients with minimal jaundice, since it often serves only to introduce infection into the biliary tree and complicate any subsequent resection. PTC is rarely indicated for distal bile duct lesions, except where palliative biliary decompression is required and endoscopic stenting has failed.

Treatment

A greater proportion of ampullary tumors is suitable for surgical resection than other biliary tumors, possibly due to their earlier presentation. Halstead performed the first transduodenal ampullary excision in 1898. However, it was not until 1935 that A.O. Whipple first reported a two-stage en bloc resection of the duodenum and the head of the pancreas for ampullary cancer; this was later refined to a one-stage procedure and so effective surgery for ampullary cancer was initiated. Unfortunately, even in the modern surgical era and when performed by experienced operators, pancreaticoduodenectomy still may result in considerable postoperative morbidity and mortality.

The alternative procedure, an ampullectomy, has been reported by some centers to provide comparable long-term survival with less operative risk. This operation may be associated with a high rate of local tumor recurrence and so long-term endoscopic surveillance is mandatory. In addition, an intraoperative frozen section to distinguish a carcinoma from a benign lesion is often unreliable, with patients subsequently having to undergo interval pancreaticoduodenectomy. Therefore, a Whipple procedure remains the operation of choice, even in patients thought preoperatively to have a benign pathology. Ampullectomy is appropriate only when a benign lesion is certain.

The factors associated with increased survival after resection for ampullary cancer are detailed in Table 52–4. As with other biliary tumors, the presence of a negative resection margin correlates most strongly with long-term survival. For patients who are unsuitable surgical candidates, endoscopic sphincterotomy and endoscopic or percutaneous placement of biliary stents may achieve palliation of jaundice and pruritus.

Prognosis

Because ampullary cancer tends to present early in the course of disease, the majority of patients may undergo a potentially curative surgical resection. This is reflected in substantially better long-term survival rates compared with tumors discussed previously. Median survival is 30–50 months for all patients, with 5-year survival rates of 30–50% for surgically resected patients.

MISCELLANEOUS TUMORS OF THE BILE DUCTS

A variety of tumors may metastasize to the biliary tree and clinically and radiologically mimic primary biliary tumors. The most common of these are melanoma and carcinoma of the breast, stomach, and colon. When the primary malignancy is documented, bile cytology or endoscopic biliary brushings may provide a diagnosis and treatment is largely palliative. However, highly selected patients, with absence of disease elsewhere, may occasionally be suitable for surgical resection.

Several biliary abnormalities have been described in patients with acquired immunodeficiency syndrome (AIDS). These include bile duct lymphomas, papillary stenosis and a type of sclerosing cholangitis probably secondary to cytomegalovirus infection (Chapter 38).

REFERENCES

Bartlett DL: Gallbladder cancer. Sem Surg Oncol 2000;19(2):145.

Bartlett DH et al: Long-term results after resection for gallbladder cancer, implications for staging and management. Ann Surg 1996;224:639.

Blumgart LH, Fong Y (editors): *Surgery of the Liver and Biliary Tract,* 3rd ed. Churchill Livingstone, 2000.

Burke EC et al: Hilar cholangiocarcinoma: patterns of spread, the importance of hepatic resection for curative operation, and a presurgical clinical staging system. Ann Surg 1998;228:385.

Cameron JL et al: Management of proximal cholangiocarcinomas by surgical resection and radiotherapy. Am J Surg 1990; 159:91.

Chamberlain RS, Blumgart LH: Hilar cholangiocarcinoma: a review and commentary. Ann Surg Oncol. 2000;7(1):55.

Fong Y, Jarnagin WR, Blumgart LH: Gallbladder cancer: comparison of patients presenting initially for definitive operation with those presenting after prior noncurative intervention. Ann Surg 2000;232(4):557.

Hadjis NS et al: Outcome of radical surgery in hilar cholangiocarcinoma. Surgery 1990;107:597.

Howe JR et al: Factors predictive of survival in ampullary carcinoma. Ann Surg 1998;228:87.

Jarnagin WR et al: Staging, analysis of resectability and outcome in 225 patients with hilar cholangiocarcinoma. Ann Surg 2001; 234:507.

Klempnauer J et al: Resectional surgery of hilar cholangiocarcinoma: a multivariate analysis of prognostic factors. J Clin Oncol 1997;15:947.

Nakeeb A et al: Cholangiocarcinoma: a spectrum of intrahepatic, perihilar and distal tumors. Ann Surg 1996;224:463.

Nimura Y et al: Hepatic segmentectomy with caudate lobe resection for bile duct carcinoma of the hepatic hilus. World J Surg 1990;14:535.

Tsao J et al: Management of hilar cholangiocarcinoma: comparison of an American and Japanese experience. Ann Surg 2000; 232:166.

Cystic Diseases of the Bile Duct & Liver

53

Rowen K. Zetterman, MD

The fibrocystic diseases of the liver include congenital hepatic fibrosis, biliary microhamartomas (von Meyenburg's complexes), polycystic liver disease, Caroli's disease, and choledochal cysts. These congenital diseases, some of which are inherited, occur in varying combinations, with congenital hepatic fibrosis the most frequently recurring disorder. Cysts can be macroscopic or microscopic and arise from embryonic biliary components. Depending on the disorder, these cysts may or may not communicate with or be an integral part of the biliary tree. There is an increased risk of cholangiocarcinoma in those with choledochal cysts, Caroli's disease, congenital hepatic fibrosis, polycystic liver disease, and microhamartomas.

Biliary microhamartomas, or von Meyenburg's complexes, are common and often found when a liver biopsy is obtained for other reasons. On gross examination of the biopsy specimen, microhamartomas may appear as small white deposits in the parenchyma, and on histology be seen as enlarged fibrotic portal areas with increased numbers of bile duct-like structures and nerve fibers (Figure 53–1). Associated cholangiocarcinoma has been observed in patients with von Meyenburg's complexes.

Congenital hepatic fibrosis is characterized by enlarged portal areas with extensive fibrosis and numerous bile ductules creating broad bands of fibrosis that can result in portal hypertension. When portal hypertension is present in patients with cystic liver diseases, congenital hepatic fibrosis should be considered, although portal hypertension may also occur in these disorders for other reasons (see Chapter 48).

SOLITARY CYSTS

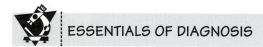

ESSENTIALS OF DIAGNOSIS

- *Typically unilocular and single in number.*
- *More common in women.*

General Considerations

Solitary liver cysts are common, occurring in 1–2.5% of the adult population. They are more often found in the right hepatic lobe than the left, are more frequent in women than men, and are usually identified in persons 20–50 years of age. Although most are small, cysts as large as 20 cm in diameter have been described. Larger cysts are more likely to be identified in older adults. Multiple simple cysts may be present. If aspirated, cystic fluid is usually clear but may be bile stained.

Pathophysiology

Solitary cysts of the liver are thought to be congenital, arising from aberrant bile duct remnants. Most are true cysts lined by biliary-type epithelium, although "pseudocysts" lined by fibrous tissue also occur.

Clinical Findings

A. SYMPTOMS AND SIGNS

Isolated liver cysts are usually asymptomatic, although vague right upper quadrant discomfort may develop from the mass effect if cysts are large. Compression of adjacent viscera or bile ducts can cause nausea and vomiting or jaundice. If cysts are pedunculated, torsion can result in severe pain, hemorrhage, or rupture. A palpable mass may be rarely noted on physical examination. Large cysts may be mistaken for ascites.

B. LABORATORY FINDINGS

There are no abnormalities in biochemical liver tests in the absence of major bile duct compression.

C. IMAGING STUDIES

Cysts are typically round or ovoid, well circumscribed, and more common in the right lobe. The location and size of the cyst can affect radiographic findings, sometimes producing elevation of the right diaphragm, displacement of adjacent organs, or compression of major bile ducts. The cyst wall may calcify and be confused with an echinococcal cyst. The absence of daughter cysts in a simple liver cyst should assist in the differentiation.

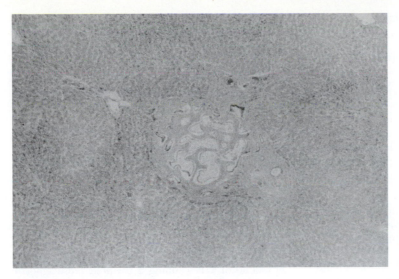

Figure 53–1. Microhamartoma with increased portal area size, multiple enlarged bile ducts, and fibrosis.

Ultrasound is the most cost-effective imaging study. Technetium liver–spleen scans will demonstrate only a cold filling defect, whether the cyst is benign or infectious. Ultrasound will identify the simple cyst as a well-defined, thin-walled, noncomplex cyst lacking internal echoes. Ultrasound can also note cysts that might arise in other organs such as the kidney or pancreas.

Computed tomography (CT) scanning offers little additional information and need not be obtained when ultrasound has identified a simple liver cyst. CT scanning will define a smooth-walled filling defect that lacks internal structures and has attenuation similar to that of water. If magnetic resonance imaging (MRI) is utilized, solitary cysts may be confused with hemangiomas, as both are hyperdense on a T2-weighted image and hypodense with T1 weighting. If gadolinium enhancement is added, there is no increase in signal intensity in a simple cyst.

Differential Diagnosis

Other diseases may produce solitary cysts with an appearance similar to that of the solitary liver cyst. These include infectious cysts (both bacterial and echinococcal), cystic tumors such as biliary cystadenoma, endometriosis involving the liver, old intrahepatic hematomas, ciliated hepatic foregut cysts, and pseudocysts that arise from the pancreas and erode into the liver. Certain features may assist in differentiation (eg, bacterial and echinococcal cysts are thick walled with internal echoes, and cystic tumors are often multiloculated). Old hematomas from either endometriosis or trauma may be difficult to differentiate radiographically, although a history of endometriosis or trauma is helpful.

Complications

Complications of solitary cysts are rare. Cystic rupture into the biliary tree or peritoneal cavity, intracystic hemorrhage, cyst infection, and enlargement causing bile duct obstruction, visceral compression, or pain may occur.

Treatment

Treatment of a solitary cyst is usually not required. If symptomatic, smaller cysts of less than 8 cm in diameter may be aspirated and injected with a sclerosant such as absolute ethanol or minocycline. Large cysts may require operation. The cyst wall, however, may contain large blood vessels, with risk of hemorrhage. Biliary fistulas may also follow resection. Simply unroofing the cyst to permit continuing drainage of contents into the peritoneal cavity may be preferable. Infected cysts should be drained externally with a percutaneously placed catheter.

Prognosis

As solitary cysts are usually asymptomatic, the prognosis is excellent. Aspirated cysts may recur. Recurrence is unusual following resection.

CHOLEDOCHAL CYST

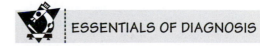

ESSENTIALS OF DIAGNOSIS

- *Single or multiple dilatations of the extrahepatic biliary tree.*

• *Occurs as concentric bile duct dilatation or a diverticulum of the common bile duct.*

General Considerations

Choledochal cysts may be identified at any age. Two percent present in infancy, 60% before age 10 years, and 75% by age 20 years. Females are four times more likely to be affected, except with choledochoceles, where the incidence is similar in males and females. Choledochal cysts may be more prevalent in Asia.

There are multiple types of choledochal cysts:

Type I: Fusiform or saccular dilatation of the common bile duct with distal duct narrowing (85%).
Type II: Diverticulum of the common bile duct (1–2%).
Type III: Choledochocele (dilatation of the intraduodenal segment of the common bile duct) (1–5%).
Type IV: Generalized involvement of both the extrahepatic and intrahepatic ducts (>10%).
Some classification schemes include Caroli's disease as Type V.

Choledochal cysts may be associated with other anomalies of the biliary tree, including common duct or gallbladder duplication and accessory hepatic ducts or congenital hepatic fibrosis. There may also be coexisting hypoplastic or polycystic kidneys.

Pathophysiology

An anomalous junction of the pancreatic duct and common bile duct proximal to the sphincter of Oddi is frequently observed in patients with choledochal cysts, creating a common channel of up to 2 cm in length. This is thought to permit reflux of pancreatic secretions into the common bile duct, weakening the duct wall and resulting in duct enlargement. Choledochal cysts also appear to be part of the spectrum of fibrocystic disorders, as congenital hepatic fibrosis is frequently associated. Biliary atresia may occur in 2% of cases, raising the possibility of distal bile duct obstruction and duct wall weakness as a cause of choledochal cysts.

Clinical Findings

A. SYMPTOMS AND SIGNS

The classic triad of pain, abdominal mass, and jaundice develops in approximately one-third of patients, most commonly in children. Overall, two-thirds will present with jaundice, 60% with a mass, and 55% with pain. The clinical presentation in infants with cholestasis is similar to the clinical presentation in infants with bil-iary atresia. A palpable mass may extend from the liver to the umbilicus. Cholangitis, typically with enteric organisms, may result in fever and chills. At diagnosis, portal hypertension may be evident due to coexisting biliary cirrhosis or congenital hepatic fibrosis. Recurrent abdominal pain from pancreatitis is described.

B. LABORATORY FINDINGS

Cholestasis with elevation of alkaline phosphatase and γ-glutamyltransferase (GGT), hyperamylasemia from associated pancreatitis, and conjugated hyperbilirubinemia are observed. Histologic findings in the liver may be normal or demonstrate cholestasis or biliary cirrhosis. Biliary atresia or congenital hepatic fibrosis may coexist.

C. IMAGING STUDIES

Ultrasound or CT scanning is the preferred diagnostic study and will identify a dilated segment of the common bile duct with an abrupt change between the dilated portion and the normal duct. Biliary scans may show accumulation of isotopes in a dilated common bile duct or a choledochocele. Cholangiography may be used (Figure 53–2). Magnetic resonance cholangiography can also identify the dilated segment. Debris or stones may accumulate within the cyst and result in pancreatitis or cholangitis.

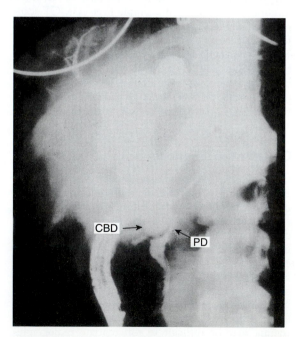

Figure 53–2. Retrograde cholangiography of a choledochal cyst. CBD, common bile duct; PD, pancreatic duct.

Differential Diagnosis

Other causes of common bile duct obstruction must be excluded. In infants, biliary atresia and choledochal cysts may have similar presentations. A pseudocyst of the pancreatic head that causes jaundice from biliary obstruction may be confused with a choledochal cyst on ultrasound or CT scan.

Complications

Choledochal cysts may develop spontaneous or traumatic rupture, rupture during pregnancy, produce obstructive jaundice, accumulate sludge and develop stones within the cyst, cause liver abscesses, or result in secondary biliary cirrhosis. Choledochoceles cause obstructive jaundice in one-fourth and pancreatitis in approximately one-third of cases. Portal hypertension may result from secondary biliary cirrhosis, associated congenital hepatic fibrosis, or local compression of the portal vein by the cyst.

Denudation and ulceration of the cystic mucosa occur and are associated with development of bile duct neoplasm (usually adenocarcinomas). Up to 15% of patients over age 20 years with choledochal cysts will develop carcinomas, especially those with type I and IV cysts. The presence of a solid mass on ultrasound or CT scanning associated with a choledochal cyst should alert the clinician to a possible adenocarcinoma.

Treatment

Treatment is operative in all but type III cysts (choledochoceles), where the risk of carcinoma is low and adequate drainage may be achieved by sphincterotomy. Internal drainage that does not remove the entire cyst is associated with a continuing risk of carcinoma. When portal hypertension precludes resection, internal drainage may be the best treatment. If resection is attempted, as much duct as possible should be resected and the remaining biliary epithelium excluded from contact with pancreatic secretions. Complete excision of the cyst with a Roux-en-Y hepaticojejunostomy is preferred.

Prognosis

The prognosis is excellent for those with complete cyst excision.

POLYCYSTIC LIVER DISEASE

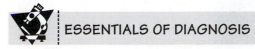
ESSENTIALS OF DIAGNOSIS

- Multiple, uncomplicated nonbiliary liver cysts of varying size.

- Disease may be localized to one area such as the left lobe.

General Considerations

Polycystic liver disease is more prevalent in women and is commonly identified with increasing age, typically in the fourth or fifth decade of life. Liver cysts may be identified during evaluation of worsening renal function from polycystic kidney disease. Infantile polycystic liver disease results in small cysts at the periphery of portal areas and portal fibrosis. Associated congenital hepatic fibrosis and portal hypertension may also occur in polycystic disease.

Pathophysiology

Polycystic liver diseases are inherited disorders. A possible locus for adult polycystic liver disease has been identified on chromosome 19p13.2–13.1. Adult disease is inherited as an autosomal dominant disorder, and infantile disease as an autosomal recessive disorder. Both result in embryonic hepatic maldevelopment with failed involution of interlobular bile ducts, and associated cysts in other organs such as the kidney, pancreas, lung, and spleen in up to 50% of patients. Cerebrovascular aneurysms may also be present. Cysts are lined with biliary-type epithelium and filled with fluid similar to the bile-salt independent fraction of bile.

Clinical Findings

A. SYMPTOMS AND SIGNS

Patients are frequently asymptomatic, although large or multiple cysts may result in continuous pain due to stretching, mass effect, or compression of other structures. Nausea from stomach compression and jaundice from bile duct obstruction may develop. Palpation may suggest normal liver size or massive enlargement. The texture may be nodular and firm due to large cysts (adult polycystic disease) or enlarged, smooth, and firm (infantile polycystic disease).

B. LABORATORY FINDINGS

Liver tests are usually normal in the absence of bile duct obstruction from cyst compression. Histologic examination of the liver will reveal a preserved architecture with cysts. Biliary microhamartomas may be present.

C. IMAGING STUDIES

Ultrasound or CT scanning will identify multiple uncomplicated liver cysts of varying sizes (up to 10 cm in diameter). Cysts may also be seen in other organs (eg, in kidneys in 50% of patients). Radionuclide scans, MRI, and arteriography are of little additional assistance in diagnosis.

Differential Diagnosis

The large nodular liver on physical examination can be confused with metastatic disease or cirrhosis. Hepatic imaging will also identify the multiple cystic structures in Caroli's disease and rarely with biliary cystadenomas. If only a few cysts are present, simple cysts may be a more likely cause.

Complications

Cystic rupture, intracystic hemorrhage, and infection (especially with *Klebsiella* or *Enterobacter* species) may develop. Cysts rarely obstruct bile ducts, cause pain, or result in portal hypertension. Bile duct obstruction and portal hypertension can develop from cyst compression of adjacent structures. Cholangiocarcinoma may rarely occur.

Treatment

When cystic disease is asymptomatic, no therapy is required. If there are only a few cysts near the liver surface, symptoms may be controlled by aspiration, cyst sclerosis by ethanol injection, surgically unroofing the cysts laparoscopically or by open laparotomy, or surgical cystojejunostomy. Localized collections of cysts can be resected, while severe diffuse symptomatic disease has been treated with orthotopic liver transplantation.

Prognosis

The prognosis is excellent in those asymptomatic or when operation or aspiration can easily control cysts. The prognosis also depends in part on the severity of cystic disease in other organs such as the kidney, where renal failure may be a larger risk.

CAROLI'S DISEASE

 ESSENTIALS OF DIAGNOSIS

- *Documentation of saccular intrahepatic bile ducts of varying size that communicate with normal or dilated bile ducts.*
- *Caroli's disease may be diffuse or localized.*

General Considerations

Most patients with Caroli's disease have coexisting congenital hepatic fibrosis. A choledochal cyst or Laurence-Moon-Biedl syndrome may coexist. Symptoms usually begin in adulthood, although Caroli's disease should be considered at any age, especially in children who present with bacterial cholangitis.

Pathophysiology

Caroli's disease is a congenital malformation of the bile ducts that is associated with other fibrocystic diseases,

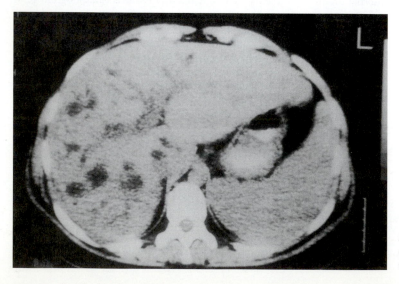

Figure 53–3. CT scan of Caroli's disease, with multiple cystic structures within the liver.

including choledochal cysts and congenital hepatic fibrosis.

Clinical Findings

A. SYMPTOMS AND SIGNS

Presentation is typically as fever and recurrent sepsis, which sometimes coexist with right upper quadrant pain or jaundice. For those with biliary stones, obstruction of the common bile duct may be the cause of jaundice. If congenital hepatic fibrosis coexists, complications of portal hypertension, including splenomegaly, variceal hemorrhage, ascites, and edema, may lead to the diagnosis. Right upper quadrant tenderness occurs. The liver is usually enlarged.

B. LABORATORY FINDINGS

Biochemical liver tests are typically normal, although there may be mild elevation of alkaline phosphatase or γ-glutamyltransferase. With sepsis, leukocytosis is also present. Histologic examination of the liver may identify coexisting congenital hepatic fibrosis.

C. IMAGING STUDIES

Hepatobiliary scans may define initially cold areas that become isotope dense with time. Ultrasound and CT scanning will identify low-density saccular structures within the liver, which may be diffuse or localized (Figure 53–3). When localized, the left lobe is more typically involved. Radiographic "dots" within cysts correspond to portal vein branches, which protrude into the cyst lumen. Intracystic stones also occur. Endoscopic retrograde cholangiography identifies the integral nature of the cystic structures within the biliary tree (Figure 53–4). This procedure may lead to infection of the cysts by organisms introduced during contrast injection.

Differential Diagnosis

Polycystic liver disease, dilated ducts due to biliary obstruction, and ectatic ducts associated with primary sclerosing cholangitis may present with similar findings on ultrasound or CT scanning.

Complications

Recurrent bacterial cholangitis with septicemia or formation of intrahepatic or subdiaphragmatic abscesses may develop. With recurrent infection, secondary amyloidosis may occur. Intracystic calculi of calcium bilirubinate may serve as a nidus for persisting infection. Pancreatitis and biliary tract cholangiocarcinoma are associated findings in some patients.

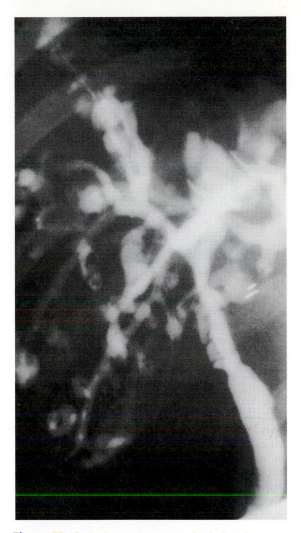

Figure 53–4. Endoscopic retrograde cholangiogram of Caroli's disease, with multiple cystic areas communicating with the bile ducts.

Treatment

Sepsis should be controlled with antibiotics as needed. The ability to intervene surgically is limited, unless there is localized disease and the involved lobe can be resected. Orthotopic liver transplantation following control of sepsis has been successful in management of recurrent cholangitis.

Prognosis

For those with recurrent sepsis, the prognosis is poor, as many die of complications. Stones that form within cysts may migrate to the common bile duct and cause obstruction, cholangitis, or pancreatitis.

REFERENCES

Desmet VJ: What is congenital hepatic fibrosis? Histopathology 1992;20:465.

Dotey JE, Tompkins RK: Management of cystic disease of the liver. Surg Clin North Am 1989;69:285.

Forbes A, Murray-Lyon IM: Cystic disease of the liver and biliary tract. Gut 1991(Suppl):S116.

Fulcher AS, Turner MA: Benign diseases of the biliary tract: evaluation with MR cholangiography. Semin Ultrasound CT MR 1999;20:294.

Harris KM et al: Clinical and radiographic features of simple and hydatid cysts of the liver. Br J Surg 1986;73:835.

Lee SS et al: Choledochal cyst: a report of nine cases and a review of the literature. Arch Surg 1969;99:19.

Mercadier M et al: Caroli's disease. World J Surg 1984;8:22.

O'Neill JA Jr: Choledochal cyst. Curr Probl Surg 1992;29:365.

Pirenne J et al: Liver transplantation for polycystic liver disease. Liver Transpl 2001;7:238.

Rocken C et al: Cholangiocarcinoma occurring in a liver with multiple bile duct hamartomas (von Meyenburg complexes). Arch Pathol Lab Med 2000;124:1704.

Sarris GE, Tsang D: Choledochocele: case report, literature review, and proposed classification. Surgery 1989;105:408.

Shimonishi T, Sasaki M, Nakamuma Y: Precancerous lesions of intrahepatic cholangiocarcinoma. J Hepatobiliary Pancreat Surg 2000;7:542.

Taylor AC, Palmer KR: Caroli's disease. Eur J Gastroenterol Hepatol 1998;10:105.

Vauthey J-N, Maddern GJ, Blumert LH: Adult polycystic disease of the liver. Br J Surg 1991;78:524.

Watanatittan S, Niramis R: Choledochal cyst: review of 74 pediatric cases. J Med Assoc Thai 1998;81:586

Liver Transplantation

54

John R. Lake, MD

Orthotopic liver transplantation is now the therapy of choice for liver failure resulting from acute or chronic liver disease. It also has a role in the treatment of several inborn errors of metabolism that do not ultimately affect the liver itself. Initially described by Starzl and colleagues in 1963, the procedure did not gain widespread acceptance until improved methods of immunosuppression and refinements in surgical technique led to enhanced patient and graft survival rates. In 2000, nearly 10,000 liver transplants were performed worldwide, with about half performed in the United States. Current 1-year patient survival rates in this country are 85–90%, and 5-year survival rates are 70–75%.

The success of transplantation in treating end-stage liver disease has led to a dramatic increase in the number of patients referred for evaluation and then placed on waiting lists for the procedure (Figure 54–1). Because the number of cadaveric donors appears to be relatively constant, the shortage of donor organs has become acute, and more patients are dying while awaiting transplantation (Figure 54–2). This has led to a renewed interest in innovative surgical approaches to address the organ shortage. These include splitting livers to serve two recipients and adult-to-adult live donor transplants using full right lobes for the graft.

The clinical profile of patients transplanted will probably continue to change over the next several years. The number of patients transplanted for liver disease caused by chronic hepatitis C will continue to rise. Likewise, patients with hepatocellular carcinoma related to hepatitis C will be referred in increasing numbers for orthotopic liver transplantation. As more and more patients are referred for transplantation and then return to the community, it will become increasingly important for physicians in all fields, including primary care, to understand the basic principles involved in patient selection, transplantation surgery, and postoperative complications and management.

INDICATIONS & CONTRAINDICATIONS FOR LIVER TRANSPLANTATION

Indications

A. TREATMENT OF CERTAIN DISEASES

Diseases for which liver transplantation might be a therapeutic option are shown in Table 54–1.

1. Hepatocellular diseases—Postnecrotic cirrhosis is the most common cause of end-stage liver disease necessitating liver transplantation. Previously, patients with hepatitis B virus-induced cirrhosis suffered a high incidence of recurrent infection and aggressive posttransplant liver disease, with disappointing postoperative survival rates. However, now through the use of antiviral agents (lamivudine) and passive immunoprophylaxis, hepatitis B virus reinfection can be prevented in most cases. Patients with hepatitis C virus-induced cirrhosis have survival rates at 5 years that are not significantly different for other diagnoses, in spite of a high rate of recurrent infection. This reflects a relatively more benign course than for recurrent hepatitis B. Alcoholic liver disease is a common cause of cirrhosis in the Western world and a not uncommon reason for transplant referral. Autoimmune hepatitis with resulting cirrhosis is a relatively uncommon indication for transplantation. Even though this disease can also recur, outcomes have been excellent.

Up to 30% of patients undergoing orthotopic liver transplantation have no discernible cause of cirrhosis and are thus described as having cryptogenic cirrhosis. Recent studies show that many of such patients have risk factors associated with nonalcoholic steatohepatitis. A yet-to-be-identified viral agent or toxin may also be responsible for some cases (see Chapter 36).

Other less common causes of hepatocellular disease that may be effectively treated by transplantation include acute liver failure and Budd–Chiari syndrome, and neonatal hepatitis in the pediatric population (see Chapters 34, 45, and 48).

2. Cholestatic liver diseases—Primary biliary cirrhosis, primary and secondary sclerosing cholangitis, and extrahepatic biliary atresia may all lead to liver failure and require liver transplantation. Although primary biliary cirrhosis and primary sclerosing cholangitis can recur, this does not seem to be a significant short-term clinical problem following transplantation.

3. Inborn errors of metabolism—Liver transplantation may correct an inborn error of metabolism, even when its effect does not primarily involve the liver, eg, familial amyloidosis or hereditary oxalosis, as the liver allograft retains its native metabolic potential. In adults, this is a relatively uncommon indication for liver transplantation. However, in children, up to one-third of such procedures are performed for this reason. Exam-

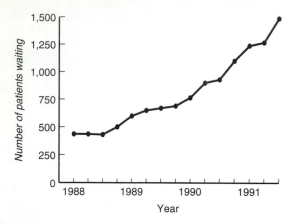

Figure 54–1. Number of patients on the UNOS liver transplantation waiting list, 1988–1991.

ples of metabolic diseases necessitating transplantation are shown in Table 54–2.

In the case of α_1-antitrypsin deficiency, the serum phenotype of the recipient will become that of the donor. Patients with concomitant pulmonary disease may achieve stabilization of the lung disease following transplantation. Copper metabolism becomes normal in patients with Wilson's disease, and liver transplantation may improve neurologic deficits. In contrast, diseases such as genetic hemochromatosis, in which the liver is damaged by enhanced iron uptake by the intestine, are not "cured" by transplantation. The liver disease is corrected, but ongoing enhanced iron uptake could eventually damage the allograft, although this would take decades.

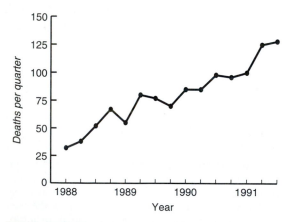

Figure 54–2. Number of patients on the UNOS liver transplantation waiting list who died before transplantation, 1988–1991.

Table 54–1. Hepatic disorders successfully treated by liver transplantation.

Hepatocellular disease
Postnecrotic cirrhosis
Alcoholic cirrhosis
Budd–Chiari syndrome
Fulminant liver failure
α_1-Antitrypsin deficiency
Autoimmune hepatitis
Wilson's disease
Trauma
Hemochromatosis
Neonatal hepatitis[1]
Congenital hepatic fibrosis[1]
Cholestatic liver disease
Biliary cirrhosis (primary and secondary)
Primary sclerosing cholangitis
Biliary atresia[1]
Inborn errors of metabolism[1]

[1]More common in pediatric patients.

B. PREVENTION OF DEATH IN SEVERE DISEASE

In general, patients on the waiting list who have the greatest risk of death are given the highest priority (Table 54 –3). To get on the waiting list in the United States, a Child–Pugh score of 7 is needed. The criteria for listing at a higher status are shown in Table 54–3. The natural history of many hepatic diseases is poorly defined, and prediction of survival time may be difficult. Recently, the multifactorial end-stage liver disease score (MELD) has been shown to be an excellent predictor of mortality on the waiting list. This score, which uses only three laboratory measures, prothrombin time, bilirubin, and creatinine, will be used beginning in 2002 in the United States to prioritize patients on the waiting list.

Table 54–2. Inborn errors of metabolism treated by liver transplantation.

α_1-Antitrypsin deficiency
Wilson's disease
Tyrosinemia
Type I and IV glycogen storage disease
Niemann–Pick disease
Crigler–Najjar syndrome
Type I hyperoxaluria
Urea cycle enzyme deficiency
C protein deficiency
Hemophilia A, B

Table 54–3. Disease severity indications for liver transplantation.

Cholestatic liver disease
Serum bilirubin > 10 mg/dL
Hepatocellular disease
Hepatorenal syndrome
Spontaneous bacterial peritonitis
Serum albumin concentration < 2.5 mg/dL
Prothrombin time > 5 seconds prolonged
Serum bilirubin concentration > 5 mg/dL

C. Improvement of Quality of Life

Symptoms resulting from hepatic dysfunction that markedly impair the quality of life but do not pose an immediate threat to survival may also be considered an indication for liver transplantation (Table 54–4). Some of these symptoms are more common in early cholestatic liver disease and others in hepatocellular disease or advanced cholestatic liver disease. Determining whether fatigue is a result of hepatic insufficiency may be difficult, and this symptom is seldom the sole indication for transplantation.

Contraindications

A. Absolute Contraindications

Commonly accepted absolute contraindications are listed in Table 54–5. The presence of these conditions sufficiently reduces the potential success of transplantation so that long-term benefits are unlikely. In cases of concomitant renal, heart, or pulmonary disease, consideration may be given to multiple-organ transplantation. Contraindications to orthotopic liver transplantation vary widely among different programs and may depend on the experience of the transplantation team (hepatologists, transplantation surgeons, and nursing staff). Contraindications may change not only within centers

Table 54–4. Quality-of-life indications for liver transplantation.

Cholestatic liver disease
Intractable pruritus
Metabolic bone disease with fracture
Recurrent episodes of biliary sepsis
Xanthomatous neuropathy
Hepatocellular liver disease
Intractable ascites
Hepatic encephalopathy
Variceal hemorrhage
Fatigue

Table 54–5. Absolute contraindications to liver transplantation.

Human immunodeficiency virus seropositivity
Extrahepatic cancer
Advanced cardiac or pulmonary disease
Chronic hepatitis B with viremia
Medical noncompliance
Active substance abuse
Anatomic abnormalities precluding transplantation surgery

as experience increases, but also among the transplantation community at large, as surgical techniques and management of these disorders evolve.

B. Relative Contraindications

Relative contraindications (Table 54–6) may also reduce the success of orthotopic liver transplantation or increase its cost, but not to the same extent as absolute contraindications. The presence of extrahepatic infection does not preclude transplantation, but therapy should be initiated prior to the procedure. In patients with spontaneous bacterial peritonitis, a 48-hour course of antibiotics is probably sufficient, whereas other infections should be treated more aggressively for longer periods. Transplantation may be performed successfully in some patients with partially treated infections if antibiotics are continued postoperatively.

The use of thrombectomy and jump grafts has allowed successful transplantation in many patients with portal vein thrombosis, although operative blood loss and overall financial costs may be greater than with conventional therapy. Surgical (ie, portacaval) shunts do not preclude successful transplantation; however, angiography should be performed preoperatively to help plan vascular anastomoses.

Table 54–6. Relative contraindications to liver transplantation.

Advanced malnutrition
Renal insufficiency
Extrahepatic or hepatobiliary infection
Portal vein thrombosis
Surgical portacaval shunt
Mild impairment of cardiac function
Chronic, unremitting encephalopathy

Controversial Indications

A. ALCOHOLIC LIVER DISEASE

Initially, centers were reluctant to perform orthotopic liver transplantation in patients with alcoholic liver disease for several reasons:

- concern that the patient would return to drinking;
- concern that the presence of alcohol-mediated damage to other organs would lead to unacceptable complications; and
- concern about societal disapproval of treating a disease that was perceived to be self-inflicted.

Initial data from several centers suggested that recurrent alcoholic liver disease following transplantation is uncommon and death from recurrent drinking is rare. Success rates were similar to those of transplantation performed for other causes of liver disease, although some studies suggested that transplantation for alcoholic liver disease might be more costly. More recent data with longer term follow-up have shown that return to alcohol use is more common than previously thought, and that complications of alcohol use is the most common cause of death long term. However, patients with a history of alcohol abuse appear no more likely to be noncompliant with medical therapy than a control group of patients without prior alcohol use.

B. HEPATITIS B VIRUS (HBV) INFECTION

The initial enthusiasm for performing liver transplantation in patients with chronic HBV infection was tempered by the high rate of severe, recurrent infection of the allograft. Recurrent infection, defined as the appearance following transplantation of detectable hepatitis B surface antigen (HBsAg) in serum, occurred in 80–90% of patients who are HBsAg positive preoperatively. Histologic findings of hepatitis were seen in most patients including the lesion "fibrosing cholestatic hepatitis." This lesion is marked by overexpression of HBV proteins in hepatocytes, with cellular swelling and cholestasis but only minimal inflammation. These observations have suggested that HBV may be directly cytopathic in the posttransplant setting. Fortunately, most patients who remained HBsAg negative following transplantation have a normal liver on histologic studies and a benign clinical course.

Patients at risk of developing recurrent HBV infection were those with chronic hepatitis and, in particular, those with detectable HBV DNA or hepatitis B "e" antigen (HBeAg) in the serum before transplantation. Patients at lower risk of reinfection include those with fulminant HBV infection and those who are coinfected with hepatitis D, which appears to suppress HBV replication.

A major breakthrough came when several studies demonstrated that hepatitis B immune globulin given in high doses during and following transplantation can substantially reduce the risk of recurrence, leading to improved survival rates. This approach is more effective in those at lower risk for recurrent infection. However, administration of hepatitis B immune globulin, which is quite costly, may be required for life. The nucleoside analogue lamivudine has also been shown to markedly decrease the rate of HBV reinfection following liver transplantation. Lamivudine is very well tolerated and much less expensive than hepatitis B immune globulin. The limitation to its use is the development of resistance through viral mutation. Recently many programs have combined the use of lamivudine with hepatitis B immune globulin. The optimal dosage and treatment interval have not been established, nor has the utility of measuring HBsAg titers to monitor therapy in this setting. It appears, however, that much lower doses of hepatitis B immune globulin are required when combined with lamivudine, and that the rate of acquired viral resistance is much lower. With such regimens, the rate of HBV infection is now less than or equal to 5%.

Lamivudine is also the most effective therapy for posttransplant hepatitis B. It can rescue patients who develop fibrosing cholestatic hepatitis. Other antiviral agents such as famciclovir or ganciclovir transiently reduce viral replication but do not eliminate detectable HBsAg from the serum.

C. HEPATITIS C VIRUS (HCV) INFECTION

Chronic HCV infection with cirrhosis is now the most common indication for orthotopic liver transplantation in the United States. HCV reinfection, determined by detection of HCV RNA in serum, is nearly universal following transplantation. Reinfection of the allograft may occur either from extrahepatic sites of HCV replication or from circulating virus perioperatively. Recurrent infection commonly leads to hepatitis, however, the hepatitis that develops is less aggressive than the hepatitis B that develops posttransplant, and, in most cases, the natural history is much more benign than with recurrent hepatitis B. As with hepatitis B, the lesion fibrosing cholestatic hepatitis B has been seen with HCV reinfection but this occurs relatively infrequently. Similar to hepatitis B, the prognosis once this lesion develops is poor. Short-term graft loss secondary to recurrent disease is uncommon and, in general, 5-year graft survival rates are not significantly different from those seen with other pretransplant diagnoses.

Several studies have identified pretransplant factors associated with an increased risk of graft loss from recurrent hepatitis C. These factors include pretransplant viral load, nonwhite race, older age, and more advanced pretransplant liver disease. Some studies have also suggested that patients infected with the genotype 1b virus do less well. In contrast to patients transplanted for other diseases, patients with HCV infection who develop rejection have a significantly greater risk of graft loss.

In considering treatment, recurrent hepatitis C usually does not respond to interferon-α, although circulating virus levels may be transiently reduced. It is unclear how effective interferon combined with ribavirin is and, similarly, there are very few data on the effect of pegylated interferons. It is clear that toxicity of all of these agents is significant and often dose reductions are required, particularly with ribavirin.

D. Carcinoma of the Liver and Biliary System

1. Hepatocellular carcinoma—In principle, orthotopic liver transplantation is an attractive treatment for hepatocellular carcinoma, as tumors are often not amenable to partial hepatectomy, either because the uninvolved liver is cirrhotic or the tumor is too extensive. Unfortunately, the early results of transplantation for hepatocellular carcinoma were poor, with 3-year survival rates of only 20–30%, because of high recurrence rates. Most of these patients had extensive tumor bulk pretransplant. However, smaller tumors (<5 cm in diameter) have lower rates of recurrence. In fact, tumors discovered incidentally at the time of transplantation have a good prognosis and do not often recur. To qualify for listing at a higher priority status in the United States, patients with hepatocellular carcinoma must have no evidence of major vascular invasion and either a single lesion <5 cm in diameter or three or fewer lesions, the largest of which is <3 cm in diameter.

Posttransplant recurrence of hepatocellular carcinoma may be reduced through the use of adjuvant therapy given prior to and possibly following transplantation. Given the ever-lengthening waiting times for cadaveric organs, adjuvant therapy is probably indicated in most patients at present. Current adjuvant therapies include intraarterial chemoembolization, percutaneous alcohol injection, cryoablation, and radio frequency wave ablation, although their relative efficacy has not been established.

Hepatocellular carcinoma has also emerged as one of the more common indications for live donor transplants.

2. Cholangiocarcinoma—Three-year survival rates for patients with cholangiocarcinoma who have undergone transplantation are less than 20%. Unlike hepatocellular carcinoma, cholangiocarcinoma discovered incidentally recurs in most cases, with poor survival rates. One recent study has suggested that patients treated with a very aggressive regimen of intraductal and external beam radiation combined with chemotherapy can experience satisfactory outcomes. However, most pa-

tients in the study failed to respond to this therapy and were not offered transplantation. In general, cholangiocarcinoma should not be treated by orthotopic liver transplantation.

3. Epithelioid hemangioendothelioma—This low-grade, uncommon hepatic neoplasm is sometimes curable by orthotopic liver transplantation.

E. Fulminant Hepatic Failure (Acute Liver Failure)

Because medical therapy for fulminant hepatic failure is associated with a 40–80% mortality rate, transplantation has emerged as the treatment of choice for fulminant liver failure (see Chapter 34). These patients are listed as the highest priority for transplantation on the waiting list. In carefully selected patients, survival rates following transplantation are comparable to those for other indications. Recognition of several indications that predict a poor prognosis has recently optimized patient selection (Table 54–7). These indicators differ significantly, depending on whether liver failure results from acetaminophen toxicity or other causes. Intracranial pressure monitoring, which allows for earlier diagnosis and treatment of elevated pressure, is also a useful adjunct in the preoperative management of potential transplantation candidates. Increased pressure resulting in cerebral perfusion pressures of less than 40 mm Hg

Table 54–7. Indications for liver transplantation in fulminant (acute) hepatic failure.[1,2]

Patients with acetaminophen-induced FHF
  pH < 7.3 (irrespective of stage of encephalopathy)
  or
  PT > 100 seconds (INR >6.5) and serum creatinine
    > 3.4 mg/dL in patients with stage 3 or 4
    encephalopathy
Other causes of FHF
  PT > 100 seconds (INR > 6.5) (irrespective of stage of en-
    cephalopathy)
or
Any three of the following:
  Age < 10 or > 40 years
  Any cause other than acetaminophen-induced disease
    or hepatitis A or B
  Duration of jaundice prior to onset of encephalopathy
    > 7 days
  PT > 50 seconds (INR > 3.5)
  Serum bilirubin >17.5 mg/dL

[1]Adapted, with permission, from O'Grady JG et al: Early indicators of prognosis in fulminant hepatic failure. Gastroenterology 1989;97:439.
[2]PT, prothrombin time: INR, international normalized ratio.

for at least an hour results in irreversible neurologic damage; in this situation, transplantation should be withheld. In the future, it is hoped that liver support devices will lead to even better outcomes in these patients, but none has been approved for clinical use yet.

PRETRANSPLANTATION MEDICAL EVALUATION

The preoperative medical evaluation of potential candidates for liver transplantation includes the following steps.

Evaluation of Cause of Liver Disease

One approach to determining the cause of liver disease in potential transplantation candidates is outlined in Table 54 –8, and should include several tests.

A. SEROLOGIC TESTING

Serologic testing should include tests for hepatitis A, B, C, and D virus, antinuclear antibody, antimitochondrial antibody, and anti-smooth muscle antibody. Antibody testing should be performed for Epstein–Barr virus, cytomegalovirus, human immunodeficiency virus (HIV), and syphilis.

B. OTHER TESTS

α_1-Antitrypsin levels, ceruloplasmin levels, and serum iron studies might be obtained depending on the situation. Skin testing for tuberculosis (PPD) with appropriate controls is necessary. Patients without immunity to hepatitis A virus or hepatitis B virus should be vaccinated. A liver biopsy may be helpful in determining the cause of hepatic disease but is generally nonspecific if cirrhosis is advanced. Endoscopic retrograde cholangiopancreatography (ERCP) is indicated if there is a suspicion of sclerosing cholangitis or cholangiocarcinoma.

Table 54–8. Preoperative evaluation of liver transplantation candidates: evaluation of cause of disease.

Serologic testing
  Hepatitis A, B, C, and D
  Antinuclear, antimitochondrial, anti-smooth muscle
    antibodies
Other testing
  α_1-Antitrypsin phenotype
  Ceruloplasmin
  Iron studies
When indicated
  Liver biopsy
  Endoscopic retrograde cholangiopancreatography

Evaluation of Severity of Liver Disease

The severity of hepatic dysfunction is determined by a clinical evaluation for the presence and severity of encephalopathy, ascites, and evidence of muscle wasting. Other helpful studies are shown in Table 54–9. Prothrombin time and measurements of serum albumin, alanine aminotransferase (ALT) and aspartate aminotransferase (AST), alkaline phosphatase, and bilirubin may be helpful in assessing hepatic reserve.

There is no ideal "liver function" test that reliably identifies patients in need of transplantation. As previously mentioned, a Child–Pugh score of 7 is needed to be listed in the United States for liver transplantation, to be replaced by the MELD score in 2002 (Table 54–10).

Evaluation of Hepatic Reserve & General Health

Determining whether the patient is an appropriate candidate for liver transplantation requires evaluation of both liver reserve and general health. The protocol includes the following evaluations.

A. HEPATIC EVALUATION

Esophagogastroduodenoscopy may reveal varices or peptic ulcer disease. In the patient with asymptomatic small varices, prophylactic sclerotherapy or ligation is not indicated. Patients with primary sclerosing cholangitis should undergo ERCP in most cases for biliary cytologic examination to exclude cholangiocarcinoma as a cause of sudden clinical deterioration. Doppler ultrasonography can exclude mass lesions and ensure patency of the portal vein and other vessels. Any sus-

Table 54–9. Preoperative evaluation of liver transplantation candidates: assessment of disease severity.

Laboratory evaluation
  Complete blood count
  Electrolytes, blood urea nitrogen, creatinine
  Serum aminotransferase activities
  Alkaline phosphatase activity, total serum
    bilirubin concentrations
  Total protein, albumin serum concentrations
  Prothrombin time, partial thromboplastin time
Other testing
  Abdominal ultrasound with Doppler studies of
    hepatic vessels
  Endoscopic evaluation where indicated
  Liver biopsy where indicated

Table 54–10. Child–Pugh and MELD classifications.

Variable	Child–Pugh Classification[1]		
	1 Point	2 Points	3 Points
Bilirubin (mg/dL)	< 2	2–3	> 3
Albumin (g/dL)	> 3.5	2.8–3.5	< 2.8
Prothrombin time (seconds prolonged)	1–3	4–6	> 6
Ascites	None	Slight	Moderate
Encephalopathy	None	Stages 1–2	Stages 3–4
MELD Classification[2]			

The formula for the MELD score is $3.8 \times \log_e$ [bilirubin (mg/dL)] $+ 11.2 \times \log_e$ (INR) $+ 9.6 \times \log_e$ [creatinine (mg/dL)] $+ 6.4 \times$ (etiology: 0 if cholestatic or alcoholic, 1 otherwise)

[1]Class A: 1–6 total points; B: 7–9 points; C: 10–15 points.
[2]An on-line worksheet is available over the Internet at *www.mayo.edu/int-med/gi/model/mayomodl.htm.*

pected vascular abnormalities should be further evaluated with angiography. Patients with elevated serum α-fetoprotein concentrations (ie, >100 μg/mL) require computed tomography (CT) or magnetic resonance imaging (MRI) scanning to exclude hepatocellular carcinoma.

B. Cardiopulmonary Evaluation

A chest radiograph is necessary, with thorough evaluation of any abnormalities. Pulmonary function testing is indicated, especially in patients with a history of lung disease or tobacco use. Patients with hypoxemia or increased alveolar–arterial oxygen gradients suggesting hepatopulmonary syndrome should have the diagnosis confirmed by contrast echocardiography or injection of radiolabeled albumin microaggregates to document intrapulmonary shunting. Echocardiography is helpful in evaluating general cardiac function and in screening for the presence of pulmonary hypertension. Patients with right heart dysfunction or elevated pulmonary vascular resistance are not candidates for liver transplantation. Patients with abnormal echocardiographic examinations or significant risk factors for coronary artery disease should undergo additional testing to exclude coronary artery insufficiency.

C. Psychosocial Evaluation

The potential candidate's social situation should be evaluated to ensure that adequate support mechanisms exist for posttransplant care and rehabilitation. The patient must be judged likely to comply with medical therapy, postoperative instructions, and evaluations. In patients with a history of substance abuse, the likeli-

hood of recidivism should be estimated, with arrangements made for further rehabilitation prior to transplantation if necessary.

Special Considerations

A. Renal Failure

In patients with pretransplant renal dysfunction, the cause should be determined using urine electrolyte measurements, glomerular filtration rates, ultrasonography, and renal biopsy where indicated. Patients with hepatorenal syndrome usually regain some renal function following transplantation, but commonly have some renal insufficiency posttransplant. Patients with chronic renal disease may require combined liver and kidney transplantation.

B. Pulmonary Disorders

Patients with pulmonary infiltrates should be carefully investigated prior to orthotopic liver transplantation. Those with infectious disease should be treated with appropriate antibiotics. Patients with adult respiratory distress syndrome usually have poor survival rates following transplantation. It now appears that the hepatopulmonary syndrome is reversible with transplantation, but these patients may require oxygen supplementation for several months postoperatively.

Preoperative Management of Complications of Hepatic Failure

A. Variceal Hemorrhage

Esophageal variceal hemorrhage may be managed acutely by variceal sclerotherapy or variceal band ligation. In patients who continue to hemorrhage despite these therapies, transjugular intrahepatic portasystemic shunt (TIPS) placement is usually effective in controlling bleeding, and provides an effective "bridge" to transplantation. Optimal therapy for gastric variceal hemorrhage is not defined, but anecdotal experience supports the use of TIPS. Surgical portacaval shunts are also an option in the candidate refractory to other measures, but surgical complications and transfusion requirements during the transplantation procedure are increased compared with healthier patients.

B. Ascites

In patients who do not respond adequately to diuretic therapy, large-volume paracenteses may be necessary to control ascites. Peritoneovenous shunts are another option but can be associated with complications, including shunt occlusion and disseminated intravascular coagulation. TIPS has now emerged as the treatment of choice for diuretic refractory ascites. TIPS, however, is restricted to patients with relatively good liver function. Patients with low-protein ascites (<1 g/dL) may benefit from antibiotic prophylaxis against spontaneous bacterial peritonitis with norfloxacin, ciprofloxacin, or trimethoprim-sulfamethoxazole. Patients with a prior history of spontaneous bacterial peritonitis should certainly receive prophylaxis while awaiting transplantation.

C. RENAL FAILURE

In patients who develop renal insufficiency, it is important to discontinue agents that adversely affect renal function in cirrhosis, particularly nonsteroidal antiinflammatory drugs (NSAIDs). The development of hepatorenal syndrome portends a poor prognosis and patients with this complication achieve a high priority for transplantation. Prostaglandins, peritonovenous shunts, and TIPS have had limited success in treating this complication.

TIMING OF LIVER TRANSPLANTATION

Patients who meet minimal listing criteria for liver transplantation should be referred for evaluation. Appropriate candidates must be placed on the waiting list as soon as possible. Allocation of available donor organs is currently based on a priority system developed by the Unified Network of Organ Sharing (UNOS), in which the sickest patients are given the highest priority, according to the MELD score.

Ideally, the timing should be based on detailed information about the natural history of the underlying disease process, with the goal of avoiding transplantation too early (ie, when extended survival time is possible without it) or too late (ie, when posttransplant survival time is impaired or the course prolonged) in the course of the illness.

Table 54–11 illustrates variables for predicting survival rates in patients with primary biliary cirrhosis or primary sclerosing cholangitis based on the various clinical factors. A formula is used to calculate a risk score, which predicts survival times and thus allows decisions about the timing of transplantation to be made with more precision. Higher risk scores correlate with both increased costs and reduced survival rates following transplantation. The implication is that patients should be considered for the procedure before the risk becomes unacceptably high. MELD appears to fulfill a similar role for other chronic liver diseases.

SURGICAL CONSIDERATIONS

Donor Operation

A. DONOR SUITABILITY

Livers from older patients are more prone to preservation injury and primary graft nonfunction. Most studies suggest, however, that when carefully selected, these organs are almost as effective as livers from younger donors.

The donor should be hemodynamically stable prior to organ donation. Long-term, high-dosage vasopressor support may lead to ischemic liver damage and increase the risk of posttransplant graft dysfunction. Serologic testing for HIV and HBV and HCV should be performed. Elevated liver tests do not necessarily preclude donation of the organ, but histologic evidence of significant macrovesicular steatosis or viral hepatitis should exclude it.

The use of organs from donors testing positive for HCV is no longer controversial. Although there is a clear risk of transmission to the recipient, when transplanted into HCV-positive recipients the outcome is no worse than when organs from donors testing negative for HCV are transplanted. In some cases, the decision to use the organ will depend on the extent of histologic damage.

B. ORGAN RETRIEVAL AND PRESERVATION

The donor liver is inspected at time of harvest, with biopsy performed to evaluate the parenchyma. Cold preservation solution is flushed through the arterial supply and portal vein prior to removal. The liver, together with its vascular and biliary structures, is then removed *en bloc*. Immediately prior to transplanting the organ into the recipient, all extraneous tissues are removed and vascular structures are prepared for anastomosis.

The preservation solution most commonly used is the University of Wisconsin solution, which allows storage times of up to 24 hours. The risk of preservation injury, primary graft nonfunction, and biliary complications increases with time, however, so the cold-ischemia time should be minimized, ideally <12 hours.

Table 54–11. Independent clinical variables predictive of survival in primary biliary cirrhosis and primary sclerosing cholangitis.[1]

Primary Biliary Cirrhosis	Primary Sclerosing Cholangitis
Age	Age
Bilirubin	Bilirubin
Albumin	Histologic stage
Prothrombin time	Hemoglobin
Edema	Inflammatory bowel disease

[1]Reproduced, with permission, from Weisner RH et al: Selection and timing of liver transplantation in primary biliary cirrhosis and primary sclerosing cholangitis. Hepatology 1992;16:1291.

Recipient Operation

The goal is to replace the diseased liver with a donor graft matched as closely as possible for size and blood group. The liver is devascularized, the biliary tree is ligated, and the portal vein is dissected. The inferior vena cava is clamped. The resulting reduction in cardiac output may not be well tolerated. Underlying portal hypertension makes the surgery more difficult; to circumvent this problem, many programs use venovenous bypass (Figure 54–3), which decompresses the venous system below the diaphragm, shunting the blood to the superior vena cava via the axillary vein. This procedure allows for more stable hemodynamic status and blood volume and less bowel edema. Venovenous bypass may reduce intraoperative bleeding, according to some, but not all, studies.

Following removal of the diseased liver, the donor liver is placed into the abdominal cavity and the anastomoses are performed in the following order:

1. Suprahepatic vena cava
2. Intrahepatic vena cava
3. Portal vein
4. Hepatic artery
5. Bile duct.

Adequate hepatic arterial flow is usually assessed intraoperatively by Doppler ultrasound or flowmeters. A portal vein thrombosis can be managed by thrombectomy or iliac vein grafts. The biliary anastomosis is most commonly a choledochocholedochostomy, with choledochojejunostomy being used more commonly in patients with known disease of the biliary tree (Figure 54–4). Fewer centers now use a T-tube to stent the anastomosis. One advantage of a T-tube is it allows assessment of bile production and duct patency during the immediate postoperative course. The transplantation operation usually lasts 4–8 hours.

Newer Surgical Techniques

The large number of patients awaiting orthotopic liver transplantation has prompted innovative approaches to expand the donor pool. Using livers from older donors is one option (see the preceding discussion). More promising is the use of reduced-size liver grafts.

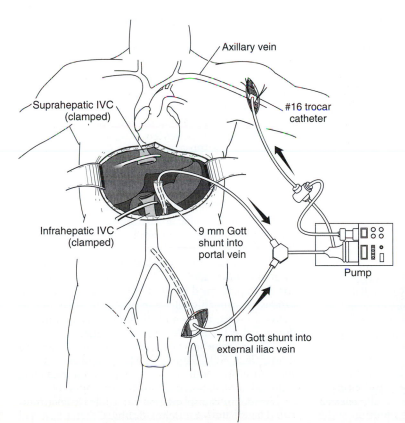

Figure 54–3. Venovenous bypass. Bypass may be initiated at any time during the procedure and is usually most helpful in situations in which very high portal pressures create bleeding problems. [Reproduced, with permission, from Miller CM et al: Operative techniques and strategies in liver transplantation. In: *Guide to Liver Transplantation.* Fabry TL, Klion FM (editors). Igaku-Shoin, 1992.]

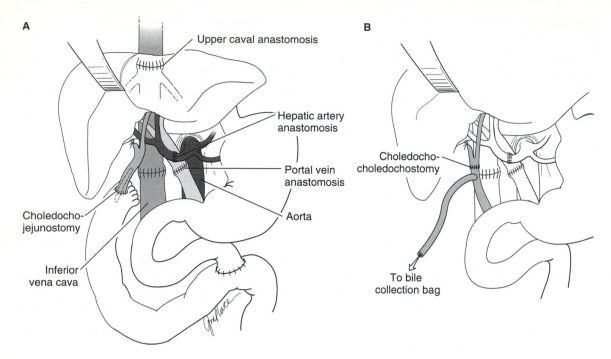

Figure 54–4. Types of biliary anastomoses performed. **A:** Choledochojejunostomy, most commonly performed in patients with prior biliary tract abnormalities. **B:** Choledochocholedochostomy with T-tube drainage. [Reproduced, with permission, from Miller CM et al: Operative techniques and strategies in liver transplantation. In: *Guide to Liver Transplantation.* Fabry TL, Klion FM (editors). Igaku-Shoin, 1992.]

A. SPLIT-LIVER TRANSPLANTATION

In this operation, a single donor liver is used to provide grafts to two patients with end-stage liver disease. The smaller recipient receives the left lobe or, if the recipient is a child, the left lateral segment of the donor organ may be sufficient. Thus far, biliary complications have been a major postoperative complication, and survival rates have been less than those of conventional orthotopic liver transplantation.

B. AUXILIARY LIVER TRANSPLANTATION

A portion of the diseased liver is removed, usually the left lobe lateral segment, and the reduced-size graft is implanted alongside the remaining native organ. This operation can correct metabolic defects in pediatric patients with otherwise normally functioning livers. Another indication is fulminant liver disease in adults, where the graft provides metabolic support until the native liver has recovered function.

C. LIVE DONOR TRANSPLANTATION

This technique has been used primarily in pediatric patients but is being increasingly used in carefully selected adults. In the case of pediatric patients, a portion of the left lobe from the donor is resected and placed into the recipient following removal of the diseased liver. The resected lobe must be of adequate size to support the smaller patient. Experienced programs report donor survival rates of 100%, and recipient survival rates of 80–90% after 1 year. Hepatic artery thrombosis was once the major postoperative complication, but in a series reported by Emond, the incidence was about 10%, similar to that seen in adults. The incidence of rejection and graft loss is similar to that in patients undergoing cadaveric liver transplantation. However, primary nonfunction is virtually never seen.

Although left lobe transplants have been performed in adults, most adult-to-adult live donor transplants have been performed using full right lobes. The complications are primarily biliary in origin, most commonly leaks. However, this is a much larger operation for the donor. It has become clear that the operation is not indicated for recipients with severely decompensated liver disease (ie, UNOS status 2A). This procedure will continue to evolve both in terms of the indications and technical factors associated with success.

Live donor transplantation for adults is controversial. There have been donor deaths. Criteria have not been defined to determine whether a program has the appropriate skills and facilities to perform this procedure, but not every center performing orthotopic liver transplantation can necessarily perform live donor transplantation.

POSTOPERATIVE COMPLICATIONS & MANAGEMENT

Complications following orthotopic liver transplantation may be divided into those occurring early (within the first 10 days) and those occurring later, although there is significant overlap in the timing. A basic approach to evaluating liver dysfunction following transplantation is outlined in Figure 54–5.

Early Complications

A. PRIMARY GRAFT NONFUNCTION

Primary graft nonfunction occurs in 2–10% of transplants and often results in death if retransplantation is not performed immediately. The wide range of reported incidence likely reflects differences in definition. Technical problems are the cause in less than 10% of adults but are more common in children. Primary nonfunction is usually the result of ischemic damage of the allograft sustained during harvest and transport, but the exact mechanisms are not well characterized. Less common causes are hepatic artery thrombosis, portal vein thrombosis, and hyperacute rejection. Risk factors for primary nonfunction identified by Ploeg, et al are shown in Table 54–12. Primary nonfunction should be suspected if coagulopathy is severe and does not resolve following transplantation, if encephalopathy occurs or does not clear, if serum transaminase activities remain persistently elevated, or if lactic acidosis develops. Reduced bile production in the first 24–48 hours following transplantation may also suggest poor graft function. Primary nonfunction may be seen immediately postoperatively or may develop within 2–3 days. There is no recognized medical therapy for this condition.

B. INITIAL POOR FUNCTION OR EARLY ALLOGRAFT DYSFUNCTION

These terms have been used by some investigators to describe a marginally functioning graft that recovers adequate function only after days to weeks. Sometimes these organs fail, and retransplantation is required. There is an increased risk of death, often from bacterial or fungal infections. The risk factors for initial poor function are similar to those for primary nonfunction.

C. PRESERVATION INJURY

This refers to hepatocyte injury that results from cold preservation or reperfusion of the allograft. Some degree of preservation injury is common following cadaveric liver transplantation, but severe injury may result in initial poor function or primary nonfunction. Typical laboratory abnormalities include a marked increase in serum transaminase activities during the first 24–48 hours following surgery, with a subsequent slow decrease. Later, serum alkaline phosphatase and bilirubin levels are elevated. These changes occur in the absence of other recognized causes of graft failure. The diagnosis may be made by liver biopsy, but vascular thrombosis can cause a similar histologic appearance and must be excluded by Doppler studies.

D. HYPERACUTE REJECTION

Preformed antidonor antibodies may cause arterial endothelial damage resulting in hepatic necrosis and liver failure within days of transplantation. This type of rejection is seen more commonly following kidney transplantation and can be distinguished histologically from other causes of early graft loss by the presence of portal inflammatory infiltrates, which are not typically seen in primary nonfunction or preservation injury. Fortunately, hyperacute rejection is uncommon following liver transplantation.

Later Complications

A. ALLOGRAFT REJECTION

This is a common problem in the posttransplant setting. The incidence appears to be decreasing, perhaps related to improved immunosuppressive regimens. Because of overlap in the timing of different types of rejection following transplantation, terms such as acute and chronic rejection are being replaced by more descriptive ones such as cellular and ductopenic rejection. Characteristics of cellular and ductopenic rejection are summarized in Table 54–13.

1. Mechanisms of rejection—Both cellular and ductopenic rejection appear to be T cell mediated. Host CD4-positive T cells recognize donor class II major histocompatibility antigens on biliary epithelial and vascular endothelial cells. Activated CD4-positive cells produce cytokines such as interleukins 1 and 6, tumor necrosis factor-α, and interferon-γ, which stimulate maturation and proliferation of CD8-positive cytotoxic T cells. These effector cells damage the biliary epithelium and vasculature. Expression of adhesion molecules also plays a role in the final pathologic response. Because of the relative paucity of major histocompatibility antigens on hepatocytes, these cells are often left undamaged during rejection. Despite the apparent importance of the major histocompatibility antigens in this process, there has been no consistent benefit demonstrated of HLA matching of donor with recipient.

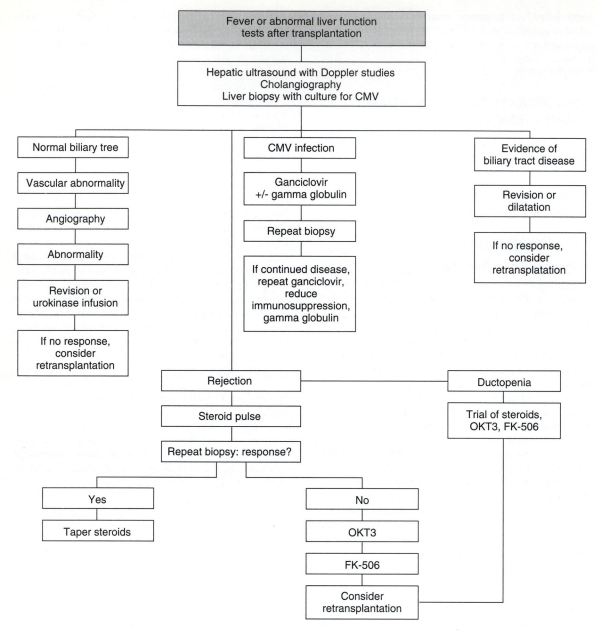

Figure 54–5. Suggested algorithm for evaluation of abnormal liver function tests or fevers following liver transplantation. See text for details.

2. Cellular rejection—Cellular rejection is usually seen in the first 3 weeks (average 10 days) following orthotopic liver transplantation, but may occur at any time. Acute cellular rejection is seen in about two-thirds of patients; risk factors include dual immunosuppressive therapy (versus triple therapy using cyclosporine,

azathioprine, and prednisone), young age, and complete HLA-DR donor–recipient mismatching.

Episodes of rejection may be asymptomatic or associated with fevers, malaise, abdominal pain, or, occasionally, manifestations of elevated portal pressure such as ascites. Protocol liver biopsies may be useful in diag-

Table 54–12. Risk factors for the development of primary graft nonfunction following liver transplantation.

Reduced-size livers
Donor liver steatosis
Older donor age
Retransplantation
Renal insufficiency
Prolonged cold ischemia time

nosing rejection in the early postoperative period, as biochemical changes are relatively nonspecific during this time. Histologically, cellular rejection is characterized by a mixed infiltrate containing neutrophils, eosinophils, and lymphocytes in the portal tracts. Destructive nonsuppurative cholangitis or centrilobular necrosis also may be seen. Inflammatory changes around the endothelial cells of the portal or hepatic vein branches (endotheliitis) are seen less commonly but are relatively specific for the diagnosis of rejection. Therapy is additional immunosuppression with steroids or OKT3 (see the following discussion).

3. Ductopenic rejection—This type of rejection occurs in 5–10% of patients undergoing orthotopic liver transplantation and is usually diagnosed between 6 weeks and 6 months postoperatively. Risk factors include recurrent bouts of acute rejection, primary sclerosing cholangitis as the indication for transplantation, dual immunosuppression, and, possibly, a positive cytotoxic lymphocyte cross-match. The process tends to be progressive and responds poorly to additional immunosuppression. Retransplantation may be required, but ductopenic rejection tends to recur in subsequent allografts. Histologically, this type of rejection is characterized by little inflammation, with the loss of interlobular and septal bile ducts in at least 50% of examined portal tracts. A so-called foam cell arteriopathy also suggests ductopenic rejection but is seen in only a minority of cases.

4. Prevention of rejection—Prophylaxis against rejection necessitates starting immunosuppression imme-

diately after transplantation of the donor organ (primary or induction immunosuppression). Various combinations of immunosuppressive agents, including prednisone, cyclosporine, tacrolimus, azathioprine, and mycophenylate-mofetil in a triple-drug or dual-drug regimen, are currently used for immunosuppression. Most centers have designed their regimens to maximize immunosuppression during the early posttransplant period when the risk of rejection is highest. The doses of the various agents are subsequently tapered with most programs withdrawing prednisone because of the increased cardiovascular risk associated with long-term use of the drug. Exceptions are patients with autoimmune hepatitis and inflammatory bowel disease where the disease may flare with steroid withdrawal. Ideally, patients can be maintained on a single immunosuppressive agent, generally either tacrolimus or cyclosporine. The exact maintenance regimen is generally determined by what toxicity the patient experiences with the various agents. One major difference between liver transplants and other solid organ transplants is that with the exception of patients with hepatitis C, episodes of mild rejection seem to have no negative impact on outcome. Thus the focus of designing regimens is primarily on limiting toxicity. Common side effects of cyclosporine and tacrolimus are listed in Table 54–14. Cyclosporine-induced hypertension is usually managed with calcium channel blockers, as angiotensin-converting enzyme inhibitors may exacerbate cyclosporine-induced hyperkalemia or fluid retention. Some patients may also require magnesium supplementation. Drug interactions are important to consider because many commonly used medications alter blood levels through their effect on the metabolism of cyclosporine or tacrolimus by the cytochrome P-450 system, leading to either rejection or toxicity. Common drug interactions are shown in Table 54–15.

5. Treatment of rejection episodes—Because of the risks involved with additional immunosuppressive therapy, liver biopsy should be performed to confirm rejection. A biopsy may be commonly performed following the completion of treatment to document an adequate response. Cellular rejection often responds to additional

Table 54–13. Hepatic allograft rejection: terminology and characteristics.

	Acute Cellular Rejection	Chronic Ductopenic Rejection
Histology	Mixed, but predominantly mononuclear portal-based infiltrate, with bile duct damage with or without endotheliitis	Duct loss, arteriopathy
Timing	Earlier, but may occur any time	Later, but may occur any time
Reversibility	Usually reversible	Rarely reversible

Table 54–14. Adverse effects of cyclosporine therapy.

Nephrotoxicity
Hypertension
Hypertrichosis
Gastrointestinal symptoms: anorexia, nausea, vomiting, gingival hyperplasia
Neurotoxicity: headache, tremors, seizures, cortical blindness, quadriplegia, coma
Opportunistic infections
Cancer: B cell lymphoma

---

immunosuppression with corticosteroids, usually in two or three daily boluses, followed by tapering of the prednisone dosage. Episodes of cellular rejection that are refractory to steroid pulse therapy (about 15% of patients) usually respond to a 7- to 14-day course of OKT3, a mouse-derived antihuman antibody directed at the CD3 determinant on human T cells. Use of OKT3 usually causes fever, diarrhea, and headache and additionally may cause rigors, hypotension, pulmonary edema, aseptic meningitis, or seizures.

B. INFECTIOUS COMPLICATIONS

Infections are still the most common cause of death following orthotopic liver transplantation. Most patients develop a bacterial infection, 10–25% develop a clinically recognized viral infection, and fungal infections may also occur. In particular, *Aspergillus* infections can be quite difficult to manage. Virtually any pathogen can cause infection following transplantation; this emphasizes the need to thoroughly investigate fevers in these patients.

Table 54–15. Common cyclosporine drug interactions.

Drugs that may decrease cyclosporine concentrations
   Carbamazepine
   Phenobarbital
   Phenytoin
   Rifampin
Drugs that may increase cyclosporine concentrations
   Bromocriptine
   Diltiazem
   Erythromycin
   Fluconazole
   Itraconazole
   Ketoconazole
   Metoclopramide
   Verapamil

---

1. Cytomegalovirus infection—Infection with cytomegalovirus is the most frequent viral infection following transplantation, with an overall incidence of 15–25%. This infection may be fatal and may also increase the risk of superinfection with other organisms and, perhaps, chronic rejection. Patients at highest risk include seronegative patients who receive an organ from a cytomegalovirus-positive donor, those who receive antilymphocyte therapy for rejection, and those undergoing retransplantation.

Because of the potential for illness and death associated with cytomegalovirus infection, most patients receive prophylactic antiviral therapy. Ganciclovir, administered early in the postoperative course and followed by high-dosage acyclovir or oral ganciclovir when the patient is taking oral medications, may reduce the incidence and severity of cytomegalovirus disease. The administration of intravenous immunoglobulin directed at cytomegalovirus may also be helpful in high-risk patients such as cytomegalovirus-negative recipients of cytomegalovirus-positive donor organs, but this therapy is expensive and the overall impact on patient and graft survival rates is unclear. Nevertheless, most programs use some form of prophylaxis against cytomegalovirus infection during the first 6 months following transplantation.

Cytomegalovirus infection occurs an average of 30–50 days following transplantation and is currently diagnosed by either a surrogate culture assay (shell vial assay), the rapid antigen assay, or by assaying CMV DNA in serum. Recovery of virus in blood cultures represents infection, but cytomegalovirus "disease" is a term used to describe end-organ damage, such as cytomegalovirus pneumonitis, hepatitis, esophagitis, or gastroenteritis. Patients may present with fever, malaise, shortness of breath, problems in swallowing, diarrhea, or abdominal pain. Laboratory abnormalities may include elevated liver tests and leukopenia. Diagnosis is made by biopsy of the involved organ.

Treatment of cytomegalovirus requires intravenous ganciclovir, which eradicates disease in approximately 85% of patients. The usual dose is 5 mg/kg intravenously every 12 hours, with adjustment for renal dysfunction. Resistance to this agent has been reported. In patients not responding to ganciclovir, another antiviral agent, foscarnet, may be used. An attempt should be made to reduce immunosuppression in conjunction with antiviral therapy if possible. Newer agents such as valganciclovir are undergoing testing.

2. Posttransplant viral hepatitis—Hepatitis B virus infection either can recur following orthotopic liver transplantation or can result from inapparent infection of blood products or the donor liver, in particular, livers from donors who are HBcAb positive. HBV infections have been difficult to manage, however, treatment with antiviral medications such as lamivudine are often now successful in rescuing patients with this unfortunate complication. However, such recipients may require life-long therapy and the development of drug resistance is common. As stated earlier, HCV reinfection is essentially universal, but this infection is less likely to lead to graft loss. Other viruses that may cause hepatitis following transplantation include Epstein–Barr virus, herpes simplex virus, and adenovirus. Diagnosis of these infections is usually made on the basis of histologic appearance and increases in antibody titers from pretransplantation levels. Herpes simplex virus hepatitis and Epstein–Barr virus hepatitis may respond to treatment with acyclovir or ganciclovir, but treatment for adenovirus is largely supportive.

3. Bacterial infections—These usually occur within 2 months following orthotopic liver transplantation and are most often due to gram-positive aerobic bacteria. The risk of bacterial infection increases with the length of the operation and the need for retransplantation. The source of infection is often related to use of an intravenous catheter or to pneumonia; abdominal abscess and peritonitis are less common. Early use of empiric broad-spectrum antibiotics, such as a third-generation cephalosporin, is usually indicated in patients with fever, pending the results of further studies and cultures. Following discharge, transplanted patients most commonly develop infections with community-acquired bacteria (eg, pneumococcus).

A few published studies suggest that selective bowel decontamination using a drug combination against gram-negative and fungal organisms may reduce the incidence of these infections. Regimens used include oral quinolones alone or gentamycin, nystatin, and polymyxins in combination. The impact of this approach on graft and patient survival rates is unclear.

4. Fungal infections—Patients receiving immunosuppression or prolonged antibiotic therapy are susceptible to fungal infections. The incidence declines with time following discharge from the hospital. Superficial infections involving the skin or mouth may be treated with topical antifungals such as mycostatin or chlortrimazole. Candidal urinary tract infections are responsive to oral fluconazole or amphotericin B bladder irrigation. Invasive infections, however, must be treated with systemic amphotericin B, often for prolonged periods. *Aspergillus* infection may involve the lung, skin, or central nervous system. In contrast to persons with intact immune systems, immunosuppressed patients develop a diffuse, patchy infiltrate on chest radiography, rather than a fungus ball. Hematogenous spread is possible, and central nervous system infection is difficult to treat and usually fatal. Prolonged courses of ampho-

tericin are usually required, and combination therapy with itraconazole may be helpful.

Infections with *Cryptococcus, Mucor,* or *Rhizopus* may also be seen, but are less common. Treatment involves the combination of systemic amphotericin, surgical debridement of infected tissue where possible, and reduced immunosuppression.

5. Other infections—*Pneumocystis carinii* infections usually occur 2–3 months following transplantation and are eliminated by prophylactic trimethoprim-sulfamethoxazole, inhaled pentamidine, or dapsone. *Mycobacterium tuberculosis* infection may develop or reactivate following transplantation and often presents atypically.

C. BILIARY COMPLICATIONS

Once a major cause of illness following orthotopic liver transplantation, biliary problems are becoming less frequent because of improved surgical techniques and liver preservation. They are currently seen in 10–25% of patients.

1. Anastomotic leak—These usually occur either early in the postoperative course or much later following removal of the T-tube. Corticosteroids may mask symptoms and signs, but patients often present with right upper quadrant pain, fever, or other signs of peritonitis. The diagnosis is typically suggested by the presence of a biloma on ultrasonography or CT scanning. Any new fluid collection seen in the porta hepatis, even if the imaging studies were performed for other reasons, should prompt an investigation for a biliary leak. A cholangiogram should be obtained to rule out biliary obstruction or identify the site of leakage. A Doppler study is indicated to rule out hepatic artery thrombosis, which may lead to biliary ischemia and anastomotic leaks.

Management of an anastomotic leak includes antibiotics and opening the T-tube if it is still in place. For leakage at the exit site of the T-tube, successful therapy can include insertion of a biliary stent to allow bile diversion, or placement of a nasobiliary drain. Endoscopic sphincterotomy also can be effective. Associated fluid collections require percutaneous drainage if technically feasible.

2. Anastomotic stricture—Strictures at the site of anastomosis occur in 4–10% of patients following orthotopic liver transplantation. Patients may present with right upper quadrant pain or fevers following removal of the T-tube, or, more commonly, with asymptomatic elevations of liver tests. Ultrasonography may demonstrate dilated intrahepatic ducts. Liver biopsy, which is commonly abnormal, reveals a portal infiltrate composed of periductular neutrophils, suggesting cholangitis and proliferation of intralobular bile ductules. Percutaneous cholangiography or ERCP is usually diagnostic. Hepatic artery thrombosis can also explain these abnormalities. These strictures may be treated with balloon dilatation or stent placement, but surgical revision to a choledochojejunostomy may be required.

3. Nonanastomotic biliary strictures—These strictures occur predominantly at the bifurcation of the right and left hepatic ducts and in intrahepatic bile ducts. In one series, nonanastomotic strictures were seen following 19% of liver transplants. Important associations include hepatic artery thrombosis, transplantation across ABO blood barriers, ductopenic vascular rejection, extended cold preservation times (>10–14h), and pretransplant primary sclerosing cholangitis. They typically occur 1–4 months after transplantation; those occurring earlier usually have a worse prognosis. Patients with these types of strictures have lower 1-year graft survival rates and a higher rate of retransplantation, but their overall survival rate appears to be similar to that of other patients. The Mayo Clinic has described successful nonoperative management of these ischemic-type biliary strictures using percutaneously placed stents and serial dilatations, but approximately 25% of these patients eventually required retransplantation.

D. Pulmonary Complications

Pulmonary effusions are extremely common following orthotopic liver transplantation but are usually not clinically significant. They typically occur on the right side and usually resolve within 1–2 weeks after surgery. Rarely, pleurodesis may be required for persistent symptomatic effusions. Atelectasis is common and also is usually right-sided.

Pulmonary infiltrates occur in 12–50% of patients, with about half of these being infectious. Early pulmonary infections more commonly result from bacteria, with gram-negative organisms predominating. Opportunistic infections tend to occur later in the postoperative course; causes include *Pneumocystis carinii, Cryptococcus, Aspergillus,* and *Candida.* Cytomegaloirus is the most common viral pathogen. Bronchoscopy with bronchoalveolar lavage and, rarely, open-lung biopsy may be required to make a diagnosis. Noncardiogenic pulmonary edema has been reported with the use of OKT3. *Pneumocystis* and cytomegalovirus pneumonitis can be prevented using trimethoprim-sulfamethoxazole and ganciclovir prophylaxis, respectively.

In one retrospective study, preoperative pulmonary testing did not accurately predict postoperative pulmonary infections or pulmonary-related deaths. As noted previously, the hypoxemia associated with the hepatopulmonary syndrome may take weeks to months to resolve after successful liver transplantation.

E. Neurologic Complications

Neurologic complications occur in up to one-third of patients undergoing orthotopic liver transplantation and are more common following retransplantation. Alterations in mental status may be related to electrolyte abnormalities, metabolic encephalopathy suggesting graft dysfunction, situational psychoses, or medications. In patients receiving immunosuppression prior to transplantation, the possibility of central nervous system infection must be considered in the early postoperative period. Cyclosporine and tacrolimus have been incriminated in the development of extrapontine myelinolysis, which can present variably with tremor, confusion, cortical blindness, and seizures; this may be more common in patients with reduced serum cholesterol levels and more pretransplant encephalopathy. Less common causes of neurologic dysfunction include cerebral infarction, central pontine myelinolysis, and nonspecific psychoses. Management includes treatment of the underlying condition where possible; drug withdrawal or dose reduction, particularly in the case of corticosteroid-induced neurologic complications; and use of antiepileptics and antipsychotics when necessary. Treatment for seizures is generally needed for only a limited period (ie, 3 months).

F. Renal Complications

Pretransplant renal dysfunction is a risk factor for the development of posttransplant renal complications. Acute renal failure requiring hemodialysis occurs in 10–20% of patients. Most commonly, intraoperative hypotension or drug toxicity results in renal ischemia and acute tubular necrosis. Management includes withdrawal of the offending drug or dose reduction and, occasionally, dialysis. Survival rates in patients requiring dialysis are reduced, particularly in the presence of concomitant multiorgan failure or if hemodialysis is required for prolonged periods. Despite the prevailing notion that renal function in patients with hepatorenal syndrome is normal after successful transplantation, many patients with pretransplant functional renal failure are at increased risk for developing posttransplant renal failure and commonly develop long-standing renal insufficiency.

G. Other Complications

1. Bone disease—Bone loss is maximal during the first 3–6 months following orthotopic liver transplantation due to the effects of high-dosage corticosteroid therapy, bed rest, and, possibly, increased cytokine levels. In the absence of significant pretransplant bone disease, this loss is generally not clinically significant. Osteonecrosis can also occur, particularly of the hip. In patients with preexisting osteopenia, posttransplant calcium and vitamin D supplementation may be used but is of uncertain benefit. The role of pre- or posttransplant bisphosphonate administration appears much more effective in preventing significant bone disease posttransplant.

2. Graft-versus-host disease—Although common following bone marrow transplantation (see Chapter 49), graft-versus-host disease occurs only rarely following orthotopic liver transplantation. The clinical syndrome typically includes skin rash, diarrhea, severe neutropenia, and fever occurring 1–2 months following transplantation. The pathophysiology involves the migration of donor lymphocytes from the transplanted organ into the recipient, with a subsequent immune response against the host. Diagnosis of graft-versus-host disease requires biopsy of the involved organ, usually the skin or colon, and, if possible, HLA typing of peripheral mononuclear blood cells. Therapy usually includes increased immunosuppression with corticosteroids and antilymphocyte preparations, but very few patients respond.

3. Posttransplantation lymphoproliferative disorder—This disorder occurs in 1–3% of liver transplantation recipients, as early as 1 month or as late as 10 years following operation. The clinical presentation is variable, from an infectious mononucleosis-like illness with fevers and lymphadenopathy to weight loss and symptoms suggestive of bowel obstruction or perforation. Extrahepatic manifestations are common. The development of posttransplant lymphoproliferative disorder is thought to reflect the unrestricted proliferation of B cells stimulated by Epstein–Barr virus infection. Both polyclonal and monoclonal B cell proliferation have been described. The major risk factors are exposure to greater amounts of immunosuppression and lack of previous Epstein–Barr virus exposure. Posttransplantation lymphoproliferative disorder may respond to reduced immunosuppression and initiation of anti-Epstein–Barr virus therapy in some patients. Chemotherapy may be effective in some cases that fail to respond to decreased immunosuppression.

4. Ascites—Ascites may be a persistent problem for several weeks or months following transplantation, but resolves in the absence of complications. Worsening ascites usually indicates allograft rejection, hepatic venous outflow obstruction, or portal vein thrombosis.

5. Gastrointestinal complications—Gastrointestinal complications include gastrointestinal bleeding following a Roux-en-Y choledochojejunostomy biliary reconstruction, peptic ulceration, or hemorrhage related to varices that may persist for a few days following transplantation. Less common causes include intestinal obstruction secondary to adhesions or posttransplant lymphoma. Liver biopsy has a number of associated

complications, but these appear to be no more common in posttransplant patients than in other patients. Pancreatitis may occur secondary to operative trauma or medications.

Retransplantation

Approximately 10–20% of transplants performed in the United States are retransplants. The indications are listed in Table 54–16, with primary nonfunction the most common. Patients undergoing retransplantation have reduced survival rates compared with those of patients undergoing a first transplantation. Some recurrent disorders, such as hepatitis B and C infection and ductopenic rejection, have such a high risk of recurrence following retransplantation that the appropriateness of retransplantation is under debate. There is theoretically no limit on the number of transplants that may be performed in an individual patient, but, in reality, limits are imposed by concerns over worsening prognosis after retransplantation and the diversion of donor organs away from other deserving recipients.

Disease Recurrence

A. VIRAL HEPATITIS

As noted previously, patients undergoing liver transplantation for chronic hepatitis B or C infection frequently develop recurrent infection of the allograft. Herpes simplex virus infection is an uncommon indication for transplantation, and significant recurrent disease is uncommon. Hepatitis D virus infection may recur, even in the absence of detectable HBsAg, but is usually associated with only minor hepatitis on histologic studies and appears to be self-limited.

B. HEPATOCELLULAR CARCINOMA

Recurrence of hepatocellular carcinoma can be decreased following liver transplantation by appropriate patient selection.

C. ALCOHOLIC LIVER DISEASE

The recidivism rate following liver transplantation increases over time. Patients who return to alcohol abuse

Table 54–16. Indications for retransplantation.

Primary graft nonfunction
Chronic rejection
Nonresponsive acute rejection
Hepatic artery thrombosis
Portal vein thrombosis
Recurrent viral hepatitis
Biliary strictures

are also less likely to comply with medical therapy, and this may lead to graft loss.

D. OTHER RECURRENT DISEASES

Recurrence of Budd–Chiari syndrome has been reported but may be prevented by use of anticoagulants following transplantation. Controversy exists as to the importance of recurrent primary biliary cirrhosis. Although titers of antimitochondrial antibodies may become negative immediately following transplantation, they reappear in nearly 100% of patients. Defining histologic evidence of recurrent disease is difficult because there is overlap with the histologic changes associated with rejection. Nevertheless, characteristic histologic findings such as the florid duct lesion have been reported. Given the natural history of primary biliary cirrhosis, it may be years before clear-cut evidence of recurrent disease is seen. Similarly, recurrent primary sclerosing cholangitis is difficult to prove, since similar cholangiographic abnormalities may be caused by a number of events (eg, ischemia). Patients undergoing orthotopic liver transplantation for primary sclerosing cholangitis do have a higher incidence of biliary complications than those without the disorder. The timing of the development of strictures may help as patients with recurrent primary sclerosing cholangitis generally develop stricturing later than those with other etiologies. As with primary biliary cirrhosis, recurrent disease may become more evident with longer follow-up. It appears unlikely that recurrent primary biliary cirrhosis or primary sclerosing cholangitis will be a major problem in the early years following transplantation. Recurrent autoimmune hepatitis following transplantation also occurs but generally can be controlled by increasing the dose of corticosteroids.

Diseases Transmitted by Donor Organs

Diseases transmitted by donor organs include hepatitis B and C, HIV infection, factor XI deficiency, idiopathic thrombocytopenic purpura, Gilbert syndrome, and various malignant tumors. Donor organs are carefully screened for such diseases, but given the imperfect sensitivities of current assays, a small risk of transmission will likely persist. Donors with readily treatable infectious diseases such as syphilis are acceptable if antibiotics are administered following transplantation.

Multiple-Organ Transplantation

Liver transplantation may be performed in conjunction with renal transplantation in the presence of advanced renal dysfunction without adding significantly to rates of complications or death. The liver may also be transplanted in combination with the pancreas, heart, and lung. Visceral organ cluster transplantation involving the liver, pancreas, and entire gastrointestinal tract or a portion of intestine has also been performed.

COSTS & OUTCOME OF LIVER TRANSPLANTATION

Costs of Liver Transplantation

The total expense of performing a liver transplantation includes the costs of pretransplantation evaluation, hospital charges, costs associated with acquisition of the donor organ, and professional fees. The costs of medications and treatment of complications can be substantial but are difficult to analyze and therefore are not usually included in published cost estimates. The cost of hospitalization for transplantation itself appears to be declining, possibly as a result of better candidate selection and improved postoperative management.

In a review of expenses, Evans et al determined that the average cost of a liver transplantation in the United States was $145,795 of which $104,049 was hospital charges and the remainder included professional fees and donor acquisition costs. Private insurance pays for orthotopic liver transplantation in about 70% of cases, and government programs pay for most other cases. No reliable information is available on the long-term costs of caring for patients following transplantation.

Patient Outcomes

The rate of complications and death in patients surviving more than 1 year after liver transplantation is relatively low. Late deaths, occurring after more than 5 years, are most commonly related to disease recurrence, chronic rejection, or a malignant tumor.

In a study from the Mayo Clinic, 91% of patients surviving 1 year following transplantation reported subjective feelings of well-being and satisfaction with life. Of patients followed for 2 years, over 90% reported no health problems or only minor difficulties. More than 85% of patients working prior to transplantation were able to return to work and said they could perform their jobs well. Hence, despite debate regarding the costs of this procedure, it is clear that liver transplantation rehabilitates patients with advanced liver disease and contributes to an improved quality of life.

REFERENCES

Pimstone NR et al: Liver transplantation. In: *Hepatology: A Textbook of Liver Disease,* 2nd ed. Zakim D, Boyer TD (editors). Saunders, 1990.

UNOS Scientific Registry: Liver allocation data examined. UNOS Update 1991;7(issue 10):11.

INDICATIONS & CONTRAINDICATIONS FOR LIVER TRANSPLANTATION

Abu-Elmagd KM et al: Cholangiocarcinoma and sclerosing cholangitis: clinical characteristics and effect on survival after liver transplantation. Transplant Proc 1993;25:1124.

Ascher NL et al: Liver transplantation for fulminant hepatic failure. Arch Surg 1993;128:677.

Benner KG et al: Fibrosing cytolytic liver failure secondary to recurrent hepatitis B after liver transplantation. Gastroenterology 1992;103:1307.

Chazouilleres O et al: Quantitation of hepatitis C virus RNA in liver transplant recipients. Gastroenterology 1994;106:994.

Cohen C, Benjamin M: Alcoholics and liver transplantation. JAMA 1991;265:1299.

David E et al: Recurrence of hepatitis D (delta) in liver transplant patients: histopathologic aspects. Gastroenterology 1993;104:1122.

Delcore R et al: Risk of occult carcinomas in patients undergoing orthotopic liver transplantation for end-stage liver disease secondary to primary sclerosing cholangitis. Transplant Proc 1993;25:1883.

Ferrell LD et al: Hepatitis C viral infection in liver transplant recipients. Hepatology 1992;16:865.

Gordon RD, Van Thiel DH, Starzl TE: Liver transplantation. In: Diseases of the Liver, 7th ed. Schiff L, Schiff ER (editors). Lippincott, 1993.

Gores GJ: Liver transplantation for malignant disease. Gastroenterol Clin North Am 1993;22:285.

Gores GJ, Steers JL: Progress in orthotopic liver transplantation for hepatocellular carcinoma. (Editorial.) Gastroenterology 1993;104:317.

Gugenheim J et al: Long-term immunoprophylaxis of B virus recurrence after liver transplantation in HBs antigen-positive patients. Transplant Proc 1993;25:1349.

Konig V et al: Hepatitis C virus reinfection in allografts after orthotopic liver transplantation. Hepatology 1992;16:1137.

Kumar S et al: Orthotopic liver transplantation for alcoholic liver disease. Hepatology 1990;11:159.

Lake JR: Changing indications for liver transplantation. Gastroenterol Clin North Am 1993;22:213.

Lake JR, Wright TW: Liver transplantation for patients with hepatitis B: what have we learned from our results? Hepatology 1991;13:796.

Lake JR et al: Hepatitis B and C in liver transplantation. Transplant Proc 1993;25:2006.

Lidofsky SD: Liver transplantation for fulminant hepatic failure. Gastroenterol Clin North Am 1993;22:257.

Lidofsky SD et al: Intracranial pressure monitoring and liver transplantation for fulminant hepatic failure. Hepatology 1992;16:1.

Lucey MR: Liver transplantation for the alcoholic patient. Gastroenterol Clin North Am 1993;22:243.

Martin P, Munoz SJ, Friedman LS: Liver transplantation for viral hepatitis: current status. Am J Gastroenterol 1992;87:409.

Moss AH, Siegler M: Should alcoholics compete equally for liver transplantation? JAMA 1991;265:1295.

O'Grady JG et al: Early indicators of prognosis in fulminant hepatic failure. Gastroenterology 1989;97:439.

O'Grady JG et al: Hepatitis B virus reinfection after orthotopic liver transplantation. J Hepatol 1992;14:104.

Osario RW et al: Orthotopic liver transplantation for end-stage alcoholic liver disease. Transplant Proc 1993;25:1133.

Pageaux GP et al: Results and cost of orthotopic liver transplantation for alcoholic cirrhosis. Transplant Proc 1993;25:1135.

Rakela J: Hepatitis C viral infection in liver transplant patients: how bad is it really? (Editorial.) Gastroenterology 1992;103:38.

Samuel D, Bismuth H: Liver transplantation for hepatitis B. Gastroenterol Clin North Am 1993;22:271.

Samuel D et al: Liver transplantation in European patients with the hepatitis B surface antigen. N Engl J Med 1993;329:1842.

Shah G et al: Incidence, prevalence, and clinical course of hepatitis C following liver transplantation. Gastroenterology 1992;103:323.

Starzl TE, Demetris AJ, Van Thiel D: Liver transplantation. (Part 1 of 2 parts.) N Engl J Med 1989;321:1014.

Starzl TE et al: Orthotopic liver transplantation for alcoholic cirrhosis. JAMA 1988;260:2542.

Stone MJ et al: Neoadjuvant chemotherapy and liver transplantation for hepatocellular carcinoma: a pilot study in 20 patients. Gastroenterology 1993;104:196.

Tan CK et al: Orthotopic liver transplantation for preoperative early-stage hepatocellular carcinoma. Mayo Clin Proc 1994;69:509.

Wright H, Gavaler JS, Van Thiel DH: Preliminary experience with alpha 2b interferon therapy of viral hepatitis in liver allograft recipients. Transplantation 1992;53:121.

Wright TL: Liver transplantation for chronic hepatitis C viral infection. Gastroenterol Clin North Am 1993;22:231.

Wright TL et al: Recurrent and acquired hepatitis C viral infection in liver transplant recipients. Gastroenterology 1992;103:317.

PRETRANSPLANTATION MEDICAL EVALUATION

Conn HO: Transjugular intrahepatic portalsystemic shunts: the state of the art. Hepatology 1993;17:148.

Fabry TL, Klion FM (editors): Guide to Liver Transplantation. Igaku-Shoin, 1992.

Gines P et al: Paracentesis with intravenous infusion of albumin as compared with peritoneovenous shunting in cirrhosis with refractory ascites. N Engl J Med 1991;325:829.

Hoefs JC: Spontaneous bacterial peritonitis: prevention and therapy. (Editorial.) Hepatology 1990;12:776.

Ring EJ et al: Using transjugular intrahepatic portasystemic shunts to control variceal bleeding before liver transplantation. Ann Intern Med 1992;116:304.

Rossle M et al: The transjugular intrahepatic portasystemic stent-shunt procedure for variceal bleeding. N Engl J Med 1994;330:165.

Runyon B: Care of patients with ascites. N Engl J Med 1994;330:337.

Scott V et al: Reversibility of the hepatopulmonary syndrome by orthotopic liver transplantation. Transplant Proc 1993;25:1787.

TIMING OF LIVER TRANSPLANTATION

Starzl TE, Demetris AJ, Van Thiel D: Liver transplantation. (Part 1 of 2 parts.) N Engl J Med 1989;321:1014.

Wiesner RH et al: Selection and timing of liver transplantation in primary biliary cirrhosis and primary sclerosing cholangitis. Hepatology 1992;16:1290.

SURGICAL CONSIDERATIONS

Adam R et al: Liver transplantation from elderly donors. Transplant Proc 1993;25:1556.

Belzer FO et al: Update on preservation of liver grafts. Transplant Proc 1993;25:2010.

Broelsh CE et al: Application of reduced-size liver transplants as split grafts, auxiliary orthotopic grafts, and living related segmental transplants. Ann Surg 1990;212:368.

Emond JC: Clinical application of living-related liver transplantation. Gastroenterol Clin North Am 1993;22:301.

Gottesdiener KM: Transplanted infections: donor-to-host transmission with the allograft. Ann Intern Med 1989;110:1001.

Kalayoglu M et al: Surgical refinements in liver transplantation. Transplant Proc 1993;25(Suppl 3):48.

Langnas AN et al: The results of reduced-size liver transplantation, including split livers, in patients with end-stage liver disease. Transplantation 1992;53:387.

Masatoshi M et al: Donor hepatectomy for living related partial liver transplantation. Surgery 1993;113:395.

Miller CM et al: Operative techniques and strategies in liver transplantation. In: *Guide to Liver Transplantation.* Fabry TL, Klion FM (editors). Igaku-Shoin, 1992.

Moreno-Gonzalez E et al: Utilization of split liver grafts in orthotopic liver transplantation. Hepatogastroenterology 1993;40:17.

Pereira BJG et al: Transmission of hepatitis C virus by organ transplantation. N Engl J Med 1991;325:454.

Ringe B et al: An update of partial liver transplantation. Transplant Proc 1993;25:2198.

Zaballos JM et al: Venovenous bypass versus no bypass in orthotopic liver transplantation: metabolic values during reperfusion. Transplant Proc 1993;25:1865.

POSTOPERATIVE COMPLICATIONS & MANAGEMENT

Adams DH, Neuberger JM: Treatment of acute rejection. Semin Liver Dis 1992;12:80.

Ascher NL: Immunosuppression and rejection in liver transplantation. Transplant Proc 1993;25:1744.

Chazouilleres O et al: Preservation-induced liver injury: clinical aspects, mechanisms, and therapeutic approaches. J Hepatol 1993;18:123.

Clavien PA et al: Preservation and reperfusion injuries in liver allografts. Transplantation 1992;53:957.

de Groen P: Cyclosporin: a review and its specific use in liver transplantation. Mayo Clin Proc 1989;64:680.

Donaldson P et al: Influence of human leukocyte antigen matching on liver allograft survival and rejection: "the dualistic effect." Hepatology 1993;17:1008.

Greig PD et al: Treatment of primary liver graft nonfunction with prostaglandin E1. Transplantation 1989;48:447.

Krams SM, Ascher NL, Martinez OM: New immunologic insights into mechanisms of allograft rejection. Gastroenterol Clin North Am 1993;22:381.

Lake JR, Roberts JP, Ascher NL: Maintenance immunosuppression after liver transplantation. Semin Liver Dis 1992;12:73.

Mor E et al: Acute cellular rejection following liver transplantation: clinical pathologic features and effect on outcome. Semin Liver Dis 1992;12:28.

Peters DH et al: Tacrolimus: a review of its pharmacology, and therapeutic potential in hepatic and renal transplantation. Drugs 1993;46:746.

Ploeg, RJ et al: Risk factors for primary dysfunction after liver transplantation: a multivariate analysis. Transplantation 1993;55:807.

Schwartz ME et al: Immunosuppression and rejection. In: *Guide to Liver Transplantation.* Fabry TL, Klion FM (editors). Igaku-Shoin, 1992.

Vierling JM: Immunologic mechanisms of hepatic allograft rejection. Semin Liver Dis 1992;12:16.

Wiesner R et al: Hepatic allograft rejection: new developments in terminology, diagnosis, prevention, and treatment. Mayo Clin Proc 1993;68:69.

INFECTIOUS COMPLICATIONS

Chazouilleres O et al: Quantitation of hepatitis C virus RNA in liver transplant recipients. Gastroenterology 1994;106:994.

Cuevas-Mons V et al: Bacterial infections in liver transplant patients under selective decontamination with norfloxacin. Transplant Proc 1989;21:3558.

Dummer JS: Cytomegalovirus infection after liver transplantation: clinical manifestations and strategies for prevention. Rev Infect Dis 1990;12(Suppl 7):S767.

Dunn DL et al: A prospective randomized study of acyclovir versus ganciclovir plus human immune globulin prophylaxis of cytomegalovirus infection after solid organ transplantation. Transplantation 1994;57:876.

Gorensek MJ et al: Selective bowel decontamination with quinolones and nystatin reduces gram-negative and fungal infections in orthotopic liver transplant recipients. Cleve Clin J Med 1993;60:139.

Kizilisik TA, Preiksaitis JK, Kneteman NM: Cytomegalovirus disease in liver transplant recipients: impact of acyclovir prophylaxis. Transplant Proc 1993;25:2282.

Mollison L et al: High-dose oral acyclovir reduces the incidence of cytomegalovirus infection in liver transplant recipients. J Infect Dis 1993;168:721.

O'Grady JG et al: Hepatitis B virus reinfection after orthotopic liver transplantation: serological and clinical implications. J Hepatol 1992;14:104.

Paya CV et al: Incidence, distribution, and outcome of episodes of infection in 100 orthotopic liver transplantations. Mayo Clin Proc 1989;64:555.

Saliba F et al: Randomized controlled trial of acyclovir for the prevention of cytomegalovirus infection and disease in liver transplant recipients. Transplant Proc 1993;25:1444.

Snydman DR et al: Cytomegalovirus immune globulin prophylaxis in liver transplantation: a randomized, double-blind, placebo-controlled trial. Ann Intern Med 1993;119:984.

Stratta RJ et al: A randomized prospective trial of acyclovir and immune globulin prophylaxis in liver transplant recipients receiving OKT3 therapy. Arch Surg 1992;127:55.

Wright HI, Gavaler JS, Van Thiel DH: Preliminary experience with alpha-2b-interferon therapy of viral hepatitis in liver allograft recipients. Transplantation 1992;53:121.

Wright TL et al: Recurrent and acquired hepatitis C viral infection in liver transplant recipients. Gastroenterology 1992;103:317.

BILIARY COMPLICATIONS

Colonna JO et al: Biliary strictures complicating liver transplantation: incidence, pathogenesis, management, and outcome. Ann Surg 1992;216:344.

Donovan J: Nonsurgical management of biliary tract disease after liver transplantation. Gastroenterol Clin North Am 1993;22:317.

Li S et al: Diffuse biliary tract injury after orthotopic liver transplantation. Am J Surg 1992;164:536.

Sanchez-Urdazpal L et al: Ischemic-type biliary complications after orthotopic liver transplantation. Hepatology 1992;16:49.

Sanchez-Urdazpal L et al: Diagnostic features and clinical outcome of ischemic-type biliary complications after liver transplantation. Hepatology 1993;17:605.

Sanchez-Urdazpal L et al: Increased bile duct complications in liver transplantation across the ABO barrier. Ann Surg 1993;218:152.

Wolfsen HC et al: Role of endoscopic retrograde cholangiopancreatography after orthotopic liver transplantation. Am J Gastroenterol 1992;87:955.

OTHER COMPLICATIONS

Adams DH et al: Neurological complications following liver transplantation. Lancet 1987;ii:949.

Afessa B et al: Pulmonary complications of orthotopic liver transplantation. Mayo Clin Proc 1993;68:427.

de Groen PC et al: Central nervous system toxicity after liver transplantation: the role of cyclosporine and cholesterol. N Engl J Med 1987;317:861.

Gordon RD, Van Thiel DH, Starzl TE: Liver transplantation. In: *Diseases of the Liver.* Schiff L, Schiff ER (editors). Lippincott, 1993.

Hay JE: Bone disease in liver transplant patients. Gastroenterol Clin North Am 1993;22:337.

Ishitani M et al: Outcome of patients requiring hemodialysis after liver transplantation. Transplant Proc 1993;25:1762.

Krowka MJ, Cortese DA: Pulmonary aspects of liver disease and liver transplantation. Clin Chest Med 1989;10:593.

Lopez OL et al: Neurological complications after liver retransplantation. Hepatology 1992;16:162.

McCauley J et al: Dialysis in liver failure and liver transplantation. Transplant Proc 1993;25:1740.

Penn I: Cancers complicating organ transplantation. N Engl J Med 1990;323:1767.

Randhawa PS et al: Expression of Epstein–Barr virus-encoded small RNA (by the EBER-1 gene) in liver specimens from transplant recipients with posttransplantation lymphoproliferative disease. N Engl J Med 1992;327:1710.

Renard TH, Andrews WS, Foster ME: Relationship between OKT3 administration, EBV seroconversion, and the lymphoproliferative syndrome in pediatric liver transplant recipients. Transplant Proc 1991;23:1473.

Roberts JP et al: Graft versus host disease after liver transplantation. Hepatology 1991;14:274.

Wiesner RH et al: Long-term management of liver transplant recipients. Semin Gastrointest Dis 1993;4:151.

DISEASE RECURRENCE & RETRANSPLANTATION

Anthuber M et al: Liver retransplantation: indications, frequency, and results. Transplant Proc 1992;24:1965.

Crippen J et al: Retransplantation in hepatitis B: a multicenter experience. Transplantation 1994;57:823.

Ezio D et al: Recurrence of hepatitis D (delta) in liver transplants: histopathologic aspects. Gastroenterology 1993;104:1122.

Gores GJ: Liver transplantation for malignant disease. Gastroenterol Clin North Am 1993;22:285.

Halff G et al: Liver transplantation for Budd-Chiari syndrome. Ann Surg 1990;211:43.

Lucey MR: Liver transplantation for the alcoholic patient. Gastroenterol Clin North Am 1993;22:243.

Perrillo R, Mason AL: Hepatitis B and liver transplantation: problems and promises. (Editorial.) N Engl J Med 1993;329:1885.

Shah GA et al: Incidence, prevalence, and clinical course of hepatitis C following liver transplantation. Gastroenterology 1992;103:323.

Starzl TE, Demetris AJ, Van Thiel D: Liver transplantation. (Part 2 of 2 parts.) N Engl J Med 1989;321:1014.

Wright TL et al: Recurrent and acquired hepatitis C viral infection in liver transplant patients. Gastroenterology 1992;103:317.

DISEASES TRANSMITTED BY DONOR ORGANS & CELLULAR CHIMERISM

Aeder et al: Incidence and clinical impact of hepatitis C virus-positive donors in cadaveric transplantation. Transplant Proc 1993;25:1469.

Collins RH et al: Brief report: donor-derived long-term mutilineage hematopoiesis in a liver transplant recipient. N Engl J Med 1993;328:762.

Gottesdiener KM: Transplanted infections: donor-to-host transmission with the allograft. Ann Intern Med 1989;110:1001.

Pereira BJG et al: Transmission of hepatitis C virus by organ transplantation. N Engl J Med 1991;325:454.

Pereira BJG et al: Prevalence of hepatitis C virus RNA in organ donors positive for hepatitis C antibody and in recipients of their donor organs. N Engl J Med 1992;327:910.

Starzl TE et al: Systemic chimerism in human female recipients of male livers. Lancet 1992;340:876.

Starzl TE et al: Cell migration and chimerism after whole-organ transplantation: the basis of graft acceptance. Hepatology 1993;17:1127.

Starzl TE et al: Chimerism after liver transplantation for type IV glycogen storage disease and type I Gaucher's disease. N Engl J Med 1993;328:745.

Steinman RM, Inaba K, Austyn JM: Donor-derived chimerism in recipients of organ transplants. (Editorial.) Hepatology 1993;17:1153.

COSTS & OUTCOME OF LIVER TRANSPLANTATION

Eid A et al: Beyond 1 year after liver transplantation. Mayo Clin Proc 1989;64:446.

Evans RW, Manninen DL, Dong FB: An economic analysis of liver transplantation: costs, insurance coverage, and reimbursement. Gastroenterol Clin North Am 1993;22:451.

Krom RAF: Organ donation: are we moving in the right direction? (Editorial.) Mayo Clin Proc 1989;64:705.

Starzl TE, Demetris AJ, Van Thiel D: Liver transplantation. (Part 2 of 2 parts.) N Engl J Med 1989;321:101

Index

NOTE: A *t* following a page number indicates tabular material and an *f* following a page number indicates a figure.